DUCTAL CARCINOMA IN SITU OF THE BREAST
SECOND EDITION

DUCTAL CARCINOMA IN SITU
OF THE BREAST

SECOND EDITION

Editor

MELVIN J. SILVERSTEIN, M.D.

Professor of Surgery
Henrietta C. Lee Chair in Breast Cancer Research
Keck School of Medicine
University of Southern California
Director, Harold E. and Henrietta C. Lee Breast Center
USC/Norris Comprehensive Cancer Center
Los Angeles, California

Associate Editors

ABRAM RECHT, M.D.

Associate Professor
Department of Radiation Oncology
Harvard Medical School
Senior Radiation Oncologist and Deputy Chief
Department of Radiation Oncology
Beth Israel Deaconess Medical Center
Boston, Massachusetts

MICHAEL D. LAGIOS, M.D.

The Breast Cancer Consultation Service
Tiburon, California
Clinical Associate Professor of Pathology
Stanford University
Stanford, California

LIPPINCOTT WILLIAMS & WILKINS
A **Wolters Kluwer** Company

Philadelphia · Baltimore · New York · London
Buenos Aires · Hong Kong · Sydney · Tokyo

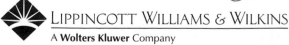

Acquisitions Editor: Jonathan Pine
Developmental Editor: Lisa Consoli
Production Manager: Toni Ann Scaramuzzo
Production Editor: Michael Mallard
Manufacturing Manager: Tim Reynolds
Compositor: Maryland Composition
Printer: Maple Press

© 2002 by LIPPINCOTT WILLIAMS & WILKINS
530 Walnut Street
Philadelphia, PA 19106 USA
LWW.com

Printed in the USA

Library of Congress Cataloging-in-Publication Data
Ductal carcinoma in situ of the breast / editor, Melvin J. Silverstein ; associate editors, Abram Recht, Michael D. Lagios.—2nd ed.
    p. ; cm.
  Includes bibliographical references and index.
  ISBN 0-7817-3223-9
    1. Breast—Cancer. I. Silverstein, Mel, 1940- II. Recht, Abram. III. Lagios, Michael D.
  [DNLM: 1. Breast Neoplasms. 2. Carcinoma, Intraductal, Noninfiltrating. 3. Carcinoma
  in Situ. 4. Carcinoma, Infiltrating Duct. WP 870 D843 2002]
  RC280.B8 D83 2002
  616.99′449—dc21
                                                                    2002016284

Care has been taken to confirm the accuracy of the information presented and to describe generally accepted practices. However, the authors, editors, and publisher are not responsible for errors or omissions or for any consequences from application of the information in this book and make no warranty, expressed or implied, with respect to the currency, completeness, or accuracy of the contents of the publication. Application of this information in a particular situation remains the professional responsibility of the practitioner.

The authors, editors, and publisher have exerted every effort to ensure that drug selection and dosage set forth in this text are in accordance with current recommendations and practice at the time of publication. However, in view of ongoing research, changes in government regulations, and the constant flow of information relating to drug therapy and drug reactions, the reader is urged to check the package insert for each drug for any change in indications and dosage and for added warnings and precautions. This is particularly important when the recommended agent is a new or infrequently employed drug.

Some drugs and medical devices presented in this publication have Food and Drug Administration (FDA) clearance for limited use in restricted research settings. It is the responsibility of the health care provider to ascertain the FDA status of each drug or device planned for use in their clinical practice.

10 9 8 7 6 5 4 3 2 1

To My Daughter
Sara Silverstein
1981-1999

Artist
Angel
Beautiful Child

Too much work
Patients first
Too little time
Nothing I can change
Much I would change
Sara, I love you and I miss you
Wait for me

CONTENTS

CONTRIBUTORS

D. Craig Allred, M.D. Professor of Pathology, Baylor College of Medicine, Houston, Texas

Benjamin O. Anderson, M.D. Associate Professor of Surgery, University of Washington, Seattle, Washington

Hugues Auvray, M.D. Department of Radiation Oncology, Centre Jean Perrin, Clermont-Ferrand, France

William Barrett, M.D. Department of Radiation Oncology, University of Cincinnati College of Medicine, Cincinnati, Ohio

Leslie Bernstein, Ph.D. Professor of Preventative Medicine and AFLAC Chair in Cancer Research, Keck School of Medicine, University of Southern California, Los Angeles, California

Simonetta Bianchi, M.D. Research Fellow in Pathology, Istituto di Anatomia, Università degli Studi di Firenze, Florence, Italy

Nina Bijker, M.D. Department of Radiotherapy, The Netherlands Cancer Institute, Amsterdam, The Netherlands

Roger W. Blamey, M.D., F.R.C.S., F.R.A.C.S. Professor Emeritus of Surgical Science, Department of Surgery, City Hospital NHS Trust, Nottingham, United Kingdom

Werner Böcker, M.D. Professor and Chief, Gerhard-Domagk-Institute of Pathology, Westfalische Wilhelmsuniversitat, Universitets Klinikum Münster, Münster, Germany

Patrick I. Borgen, M.D. Associate Professor of Surgery, Weill Medical College of Cornell University; Chief, Breast Service, Memorial Sloan-Kettering Cancer Center, New York, New York

Jacques Borger, M.D. Department of Radiotherapy, Netherlands Cancer Institute, Amsterdam Netherlands

Bruce A. Bornstein, M.D. Assistant Professor of Radiation Oncology, Harvard Medical School, Boston, Massachusetts

Erika M. Brinkmann, M.D. Assistant Professor of Surgery, Northwestern University; Director, Highland Park Hospital Breast Center, Evanston Northwestern Healthcare, Chicago, Illinois

Michael Buehner, M.D. Department of Gynecology and Obstetrics, Universitat Erlangen, Erlangen, Germany; Chief, Department of Obstetrics and Gynecology, Klinikum Bayreuth, Bayreuth, Germany

Horst Bürger, M.D. Gerhard-Domagk-Institute of Pathology, Westfalische Wilhelmsuniversitat, Universitets Klinikum Münster, Münster, Germany

Nigel J. Bundred, M.D. Professor of Surgical Oncology, South Manchester University Hospital, Manchester, United Kingdom

François Campana, M.D. Senior Radiation Oncologist, Department of Radiation Oncology, Institut Curie, Paris, France

Luigi Cataliotti, M.D. Professor of Surgery, Instituto di Clinica Chirurgica, Universita degli Studi di Firenze, Florence, Italy

Jean-Christophe Charpentier, M.D. MRC Statistics, Cernay les Reims, France

Claire Charra-Brunaud, M.D. Department of Radiation Oncology, Centre Alexis Vautrin, Vandoeuvre les Nancy, France

Stefano Ciatto, M.D. Department of Radiology, Instituto di Clinica Chirurgica, Universita degli Studi di Firenze, Florence, Italy

Krishna B. Clough, M.D. Chief, Breast and General Surgery, Institut Curie, Paris, France

Hiram S. Cody III, M.D. Memorial Sloan-Kettering Cancer Center, New York, New York

Christine Cohen-Solal-le Nir, M.D. Department of Radiation Oncology, Centre Rene Huguenin, St. Cloud, France

William J. Colburn, M.D. Director of Pathology, Encino-Tarzana Regional Medical Center, Tarzana, California

James L. Connolly, M.D. Professor of Pathology, Harvard Medical School; Beth Isreal Deaconess Medical Center, Boston, Massachusetts

Bruno Cutuli, M.D.   Chief, Department of Radiation Oncology, Polyclinique De Courlancy, Reims, France

James Dignam, Ph.D.   Assistant Professor, Department of Health Studies, University of Chicago, Chicago, Illinois

Suzanne M. Dintzis, M.D., Ph.D.   Department of Pathology, St. Luke's Hospital, Chesterfield, Missouri

Vito Distante, M.D.   Research Fellow in Surgical Pathology, Instituto di Clinica Chirurgica I, Università degli Studi di Firenze, Florence, Italy

J. Michael Dixon, M.D.   Senior Lecurer in Surgery, Department of Oncology, University of Edinburgh; Consultant Breast Surgeon, Edinburgh Breast Unit, Western General Hospital, Edinburgh, United Kingdom

William Dupont, Ph.D.   Professor and Director, Division of Biostatistics, Vanderbilt University School of Medicine, Nashville, Tennessee

Melinda S. Epstein, Ph.D.   Department of Microbiology and Immunology, University of California, Los Angeles, Los Angeles, California

Vincenzo Eusebi, M.D., F.R.C.Path.   Professor of Pathology, University of Bologna; Head, Department of Pathology, Bellaria Hospital, Bologna, Italy

Andrew J. Evans, M.R.C.P., F.R.C.P.   Breast Radiologist, Helen Garrod Breast Screening Unit and Trent Region Screening Quality Assurance Unit, Nottingham City Hospital, Nottingham, United Kingdom

Daniel R. G. Faverly, M.D.   Department of Pathology, National Expert and Training Centre for Breast Cancer Screening, Radboud University Hospital, Nijmegen, The Netherlands

Renaud Fay, Ph.D.   MRC Statistics, Cernay les Reims, Reims, France

Robert E. Fechner, M.D.   Professor of Pathology, University of Virginia Health Sciences Center, Charlottesville, Virginia

Ian S. Fentiman, M.D., F.R.C.S.   Professor of Surgical Oncology, Department of Oncology, Guy's Hospital, London, United Kingdom

Virginie Fichet, M.D.   Department of Radiation Oncology, Institut Paoli Calmettes, Marseille, France

Bernard Fisher, M.D.   Scientific Director, National Surgical Adjuvant Breast and Bowel Project, Allegheny General Hospital, Pittsburgh, Pennsylvania

Edwin R. Fisher, M.D.   Pathologist, Edwin R. Fisher Institute of Pathology, Shadyside Hospital; Chief Pathologist, National Surgical Adjuvant Breast and Bowel Project, Pittsburgh, Pennsylvania

Maria P. Foschini, M.D.   Anatomia Patologica, Ospedale Bellaria, Bologna, Italy

Alain Fourquet, M.D.   Chief of Service, Department of Radiation Oncology, Institut Curie, Paris, France

Barbara Fowble, M.D.   Senior Member Emeritus, Department of Radiation Oncology; Fox Chase Cancer Center, Philadelphia, Pennsylvania

Adel Gad, M.D.   Associate Professor of Pathology, Department of Pathology and Cytology, Huddinge University Hospital, Huddinge, Sweden

Csaba Gajdos, M.D.   Robert H. Lurie Comprehensive Cancer Center, Feinberg School of Medicine, Northwestern University Medical School, Chicago, Illinois

Parvis Gamagami, M.D.   Director of Radiology, The Breast Center, Van Nuys, California

W. David George, M.D.   Professor of Surgery, University of Glasgow, Western Infirmary, Glasgow, United Kingdom

Dianne Georgian-Smith, M.D.   Associate Professor of Radiology, Harvard Medical School, Boston, Massachusetts

Sylvia Giard, M.D.   Department of Surgery, Centre Oscar Lambret, Lille, France

Eugene D. Gierson, M.D.   Attending Surgeon, Northridge Medical Center, Van Nuys, California

Armando E. Giuliano, M.D.   Director, Joyce Eisenberg Keefer Breast Center and Chief of Surgical Oncology, John Wayne Cancer Institute, Saint John's Hospital and Health Center, Santa Monica, California

James C. Grotting, M.D., F.A.C.S.   Clinical Professor of Plastice Surgery, University of Alabama at Birmingham, Birmington, Alabama

Bruce Haffty, M.D.   Professor of Radiation Oncology, Yale University School of Medicine, New Haven, Connecticut

Nora M. Hansen, M.D.   Joyce Eisenberg Keefer Breast Center, John Wayne Cancer Institute, Saint John's Hospital and Health Center, Santa Monica, California

Steven E. Harms, M.D.   Professor of Radiology, University of Arkansas for Medical Services, Little Rock, Arkansas

James L. Henderson, M.D.,   Plastic Surgeon, Birmingham, Alabama

Roland Holland, M.D., Ph.D.   Professor of Pathology, University Medical Center Nijmegen; Director, National Expert and Training Center for Breast Cancer Screening, Nijmegen, The Netherlands

Joan Houghton, Ph.D. Senior Lecturer in Clinical Trials, CRC and UCL Cancer Trials Centre, London, United Kingdom

Wei-Chiang Hsiao, M.D. Clinical Instructor, Department of Surgery, National Cheng Kung University College of Medicine, Tainan, Taiwan

John Ingold, M.D. Department of Surgery, William Beaumont Hospital, Royal Oak, Michigan

Margaret J. Jeffrey, M.D. F.R.C.Path. Consultant Histopathology, Queen Alexandra Hospital, Cosham, Portsmouth, United Kingdom

Roy Jensen, M.D. Associate Professor of Pathology, Vanderbilt University School of Medicine, Nashville, Tennesee

V. Craig Jordan, Ph.D., D.Sc., M.D. Diana, Princess of Wales Professor of Cancer Research, Robert H. Lurie Comprehensive Cancer Center, Feinberg School of Medicine, Northwestern University, Chicago, Illinois

Patricia T. Kelly, Ph.D. Medical Geneticist, Saint Francis Memorial Hospital, San Francisco, California; Cancer Risk Assessment Services, Berkeley, California

Larry Kestin, M.D. Department of Radiation Oncology, William Beaumont Hospital, Royal Oak, Michigan

Jung-Soo Kim, M.D. University of Texas M.D. Anderson Cancer Center, Houston, Texas

John Kurtz, M.D. Chairman, Department of Radiation Oncology, University Hospital, Geneva, Switzerland

Robert R. Kuske, Jr., M.D. Professor, Department of Oncology, University of Wisconsin Hospitals and Clinics, Madison, Wisconsin

Brigitte de Lafontan, M.D. Department of Radiation Oncology, Institut Claudius Regaud, Toulouse, France

Michael D. Lagios, M.D. The Breast Cancer Consultation Service, Tiburon, California; Clinical Associate Professor of Pathology, Stanford University, Stanford, California.

Stephanie Land, Ph.D. Research Assistant Professor of Biostatistics, University of Pittsburgh, Associate Director, Biostatistics Facility of the Pittsburgh Cancer Institute

Christine Landmann, M.D. University Hospital, Geneva, Switzerland

Norbert Lang, M.D. Professor of Gynecology and Obstetrics, Department of Gynecology and Obstetrics, Universitat Erlangen, Erlangen, Germany; Chief, Department of Gynecology and Obstetrics, Klinikum Bayreuth, Bayreuth, Germany

Linda Larsen, M.D. Assistant Professor of Clinical Radiology, Keck School of Medicine, University of Southern California, USC/Norris Cancer Center, Los Angeles, California

Thomas Lawton, M.D. Assistant Professor of Pathology, University of Washington, Seattle, Washington

Claire Lemanski, M.D. Department of Radiation Oncology, Centre Val d'Aurelle, Montpellier, France

Bernard S. Lewinsky, M.D. Director, Western Tumor Medical Group, Sherman Oaks, California

Christopher I. Li, M.D., M.P.H. Post-Doctoral Fellow, University of Washington, Seattle, Washington

Marc E. Lippman, M.D. Professor of Medicine and Chairman, Department of Internal Medicine, University Michigan Health Systems, Taubman Health Center, Ann Arbor, Michigan

Jennifer I. MacGregor, M.D. Robert H. Lurie Cancer Center, Feinberg School of Medicine, Northwestern University, Chicago, Illinois

R Douglas Macmillan, M.D. Breast Surgeon and Senior Lecturer in Surgery, Breast Unit, Nottingham City Hospital, Nottingham, United Kingdom

Eleftherios Mamounas, M.D. Associate Professor of Surgery, Northeastern Ohio Universities College of Medicine, Rootstown, Ohio; Medical Director, Aultman Cancer Center, Canton, Ohio

Richard G. Margolese, M.D. Professor of Surgery, Jewish General Hospital, Montreal, Quebec, Canada

Alvaro A. Martinez, M.D. Chairman, Department of Radiation Oncology, William Beaumont Hospital, Royal Oak, Michigan

Beryl McCormick, M.D. Clinical Director and Attending Physician, Department of Radiation Oncology, Memorial Sloan Kettering Canter Center, New York, New York

Marsha McNeese, M.D. University of Texas M.D. Anderson Cancer Center, Houston, Texas

Hervé Mignotte, M.D. Department of Surgery, Centre Leon Berard, Lyon, France

Roger E. Moe, M.D. Professor Emeritus of Surgery, University of Washington, Seattle, Washington

Monica Morrow, M.D. Professor of Surgery, Feinberg School of Medicine, Northwestern University; Director, Lynn Sage Comprehensive Breast Center, Northwestern Memorial Hospital, Chicago, Illinois

Shelley Nakamura, M.D. Breast Fellow, USC/Norris Comprehensive Cancer Center, Keck School of Medicine, University of Southern California, Los Angeles, California

David B. Neeland, M.D. Co-Director, Baptist Breast Health Center, Baptist Medical Center, Montgomery, Alabama

Ivo Olivotto, M.D. British Columbia Center Agency, Victoria, British Columbia, Canada

Lorenza Orzalesi, M.D. Instituto di Clinica Chirurgica, Universita degli Studi di Firenze, Florence, Italy

David L. Page, M.D. Professor of Pathology and Epidemiology, Vanderbilt University School of Medicine, Nashville, Tennessee

Yuri Parisky, M.D. Associate Professor of Clinical Radiology, Keck School of Medicine, Los Angeles, California

Catherine C. Park, M.D. Assistant Professor, Department of Radiation Oncology, University of California School of Medicine, San Francisco, California

Steve H. Parker, M.D. Radiology Imaging Associates, Englewood, Colorado

Ward C. Parsons, M.D., R.T. Associate Professor of Radiology, University of Texas Southwestern Medical Center at Dallas, Dallas, Texas

Frédérique Penault-Llorca, M.D. Department of Pathology, Centre Jean Perrin, Clermont Ferrand, France

Lori Pierce, M.D. University of Michigan, Ann Arbor, Michigan

Sarah E. Pinder, M.R.C.Path. Breast Histopathologist, Breast Unit and Trent Region Screening Quality Assurance Unit, Nottingham City Hospital, Nottingham, United Kingdom

David N. Poller, M.D., F.R.C.Path. Honorary Reader, University of Portsmouth; Consultant Pathologist, Queen Alexandra Hospital Cosham, Cosham, Portsmouth, United Kingdom

Michael F. Press, M.D., Ph.D. Professor of Pathology and Harold E. Lee Chair in Cancer Research, Keck School of Medicine, University of Southern California, Los Angeles, California

Rajan S. Rampaul, M.D. Trainee Surgeon, Breast Unit, Nottingham City Hospital, Nottingham, United Kingdom

Peter M. Ravdin, M.D., Ph.D. Clinical Associate Professor of Medicine, University of Texas Health Science Center, San Antonio, Texas

Jackie Read Trent Performance Manager, Trent Region Screening Quality Assurance Unit, Nottingham City Hospital, Nottingham, United Kingdom

Abram Recht, M.D. Associate Professor of Radiation Oncology, Harvard Medical School; Senior Radiation Oncologist and Deputy Chief, Department of Radiation Oncology, Beth Israel Deaconess Medical Center, Boston, Massachusetts

Kristine Rinn, M.D. Medical Oncologist, Swedish Cancer Institute, Seattle, Washington

David S. Robinson, M.D. Professor of Surgery and Paul G. Koontz, Jr., M.D., Endowed Chair of Breast Disease, University of Missouri at Kansas City; Saint Lukes Hospital, Kansas City, Missouri

Anne de la Rochefordiere, M.D. Department of Radiation Oncology, Institut Curie, Paris, France

Lowell Rogers, M.D. Director of Anatomic Pathology, Long Beach Memorial Medical Center, Long Beach, California

Eva Rubin, M.D. Professor of Radiology, Chief, Mammography Section, University of Alabama at Birmingham, Birmingham, Alabama

Christy A. Russell, M.D. Associate Professor of Medicine, Keck School of Medicine, University of Southern California; Los Angeles, California

Emil J. T. Rutgers, M.D. Senior Surgeon, Department of Surgery, Netherlands Cancer Institute, Amsterdam, The Netherlands

Calogero Saieva, M.D. Instituto di Clinica Chirurgica, Università degli Studi di Firenze, Florence, Italy

Jennifer MacGregor Schafer, Ph.D. Robert H. Laurie Comprehensive Cancer Center Chicago, Illinois

Isabell A. Schmitt, M.D. Breast Cancer Research Program of the Lee Breast Center, Department of Pathology, Norris Comprehensive Cancer Center, University of Southern California, Los Angeles, California

Stuart J. Schnitt, M.D. Associate Professor, Department of Pathology, Harvard Medical School; Co-Director of Anatomic Pathology, Department of Pathology, Beth Israel Deaconess Medical Center, Boston, Massachusetts

Delray J. Schultz, Ph.D. Associate Professor of Mathematics, Millersville University, Millersville, Pennsylvania

Peggy A. Schuyler, R.N., B.A. Department of Preventive Medicine, Vanderbilt University, Nashville, Tennessee

Gordon Francis Schwartz, M.D., M.B.A. Professor of Surgery, Jefferson Medical College, Philadelphia, Pennsylvania

Véronique Servent, M.D. Department of Senology, Centre Oscar Lambret, Lille, France

Andy Sherrod, M.D. Professor of Pathology, Keck School of Medicine, University of Southern California, Los Angeles, California

Pulin A. Sheth, M.D. Assistant Professor of Clinical Radiology, Keck School of Medicine, University of Southern California, Los Angeles, California

D. Mark Sibbering, M.B.B.S., F.R.C.S. Breast Surgeon, Derby City Hospital, Derby, United Kingdom

Brigitte Sigal-Zafrani, M.D. Senior Pathologist, Department of Tumor Biology, Institut Curie, Paris, France

Melvin J. Silverstein, M.D. Professor of Surgery and Henrietta C. Lee Chair in Cancer Research, Keck School of Medicine, University of Southern California; Director, Harold E. and Henrietta C. Lee Breast Center, USC/Norris Comprehensive Cancer Center, Los Angeles, California

Roberta Simoncini, M.D. Instituto di Clinica Chirurgica I, Università degli Studi di Firenze, Florence, Italy

Sonja Eva Singletary, M.D. Professor of Surgery, Department of Surgical Oncology, The University of Texas M.D. Anderson Cancer Center, Houston, Texas

Lawrence J. Solin, M.D. Professor of Radiation Oncology, University of Pennsylvania; Hospital of the University of Pennsylvania, Philadelphia, Pennsylvania

Rashida Soni, M.D. Assistant Professor of Pathology, Keck School of Medicine, University of Southern California, Los Angeles, California

Richard Sposto, Ph.D. Associate Professor of Research, Department of Preventive Medicine, Keck School of Medicine, University of Southern California, Los Angeles, California

A. Thomas Stavros, M.D. Radiology Imaging Associates, PC, Englewood, Colorado

Oscar E. Streeter Jr, M.D., F.A.C.R. Associate Professor of Clinical Radiation Oncology, Keck School of Medicine, University of Southern California, Los Angeles, California

Lázló Tabár, M.D. Professor of Radiology, Director, Department of Mammography, Falun Central Hospital, Falun, Sweden

Marie Taylor, M.D. Mallinckrodt Institute of Radiology, Washington University School of Medicine, St. Louis, Missouri

Debra A. Tonetti, Ph.D. Assistant Professor of Pharmaceutics and Pharmacodynamics, University of Illinois at Chicago, Chicago, Illinois

Tibor Tot, M.D. Department of Pathology and Clinical Cytology, Falun Central Hospital, Falun, Sweden

Augustinus H. Tulusan, Prof. M.D. Professor, Department of Gynecology and Obstetrics, Universitat, Erlangen, Erlangen, Germany; Chief, Department of Gynecology and Obstetrics, Klinikum Bayreuth, Bayreuth, Germany

Poppy Valassiadou, M.D. Trainee Surgeon, Breast Unit, Nottingham City Hospital, Nottingham, United Kingdom

Kimberly J. Van Zee, M.D. Assistant Professor of Surgery, Weill Medical College of Cornell University; Associate Attending Surgeon, Memorial Sloan-Kettering Cancer Center, New York, New York

Frank A. Vicini, M.D., Ph.D. Department of Radiation Oncology, William Beaumont Hospital, Royal Oak, Michigan

Yasmin Wahedna, M.D. Breast Surgeon, Derby City Hospital, Derby, United Kingdom

James R. Waisman, M.D. Associate Clinical Professor of Medicine and Surgery, Keck School of Medicine, University of Southern California, Los Angeles, California

Mark R. Wick, M.D. Professor of Pathology, University of Virginia, University of Virginia Medical Center, Charlottesville, Virginia

Wendy A. Wells, M.D. Associate Professor of Pathology, Department of Pathology, Dartmouth Medical School; Dartmouth-Hitchcock Medical Center, Lebanon, New Hampshire

Norman Wolmark, M.D. Professor, Department of Human Oncology, MCP Habnemann; Chairman, Department of Human Oncology, Allegheny General Hospital, Pittsburgh, Pennsylvania

Carol Woo, M.D. Fellow in Breast Surgery, USC/Norris Comprehensive Cancer Center, Keck School of Medicine, University of Southern California, Los Angeles, California

I-Tien Yeh, M.D. Department of Pathology and Laboratory Medicine, University of Pennsylvania School of Medicine, Philadelphia, Pennsylvania

Constantinos Yiangou, B.Sc., M.B., B.S., F.R.C.S. Consultant Surgeon, Queen Alexandra Hospital, Cosham, Portsmouth, United Kingdom

PREFACE

In 1995, two years prior to the first edition of this textbook, the publishers asked me to defend the rationale for a volume on ductal carcinoma in situ (DCIS) of the breast when there were many excellent textbooks on breast cancer in general. The answer was simple: ductal carcinoma in situ was the most rapidly growing subset within the breast cancer spectrum and relatively little was known about it. The existing textbooks were focused almost entirely on invasive disease. Ductal carcinoma in situ represented and still represents a completely different class of lesions in which the complete malignant phenotype of unlimited growth, angiogenesis, genomic elasticity, invasion, and metastasis has not been fully expressed. It is the non-obligate precursor lesion of most invasive breast cancers. Some DCIS lesions, if untreated, may progress rapidly to invasive breast cancer; others, if untreated, change little over five to ten years. The challenge is knowing which ones to treat and how to treat them.

Until 1980, DCIS was rare a lesion, representing less than 1% of all breast cancers. Only an occasional physician treated more than a few cases and most had no special understanding or knowledge of the disease. Mastectomy was the accepted treatment at the time and most patients with DCIS were treated with mastectomy, their disease lumped into the spectrum of invasive breast cancer.

During the 1980s, this changed. With the acceptance and increased utilization of mammography, needle directed biopsies for nonpalpable mammographically detected abnormalities increased. DCIS began to be diagnosed routinely. Currently, DCIS represents more than 20% of all new breast cancer cases in the United States. In centers that rely on mammography, DCIS may represent as much as 30–40% of all new cases. The need for a textbook devoted entirely to this disease is clear.

During the 1980s, most physicians were not ready for the deluge of noninvasive lesions. Pathologists often disagreed on diagnostic criteria for DCIS. There was no widely accepted scheme for nuclear grading or classification. There was no uniform definition of microinvasion. Surgeons disagreed on the need for axillary dissection. There was no definition of what constituted a clear margin or how widely clear the margin should be. Routine inking of margins did not begin until 1985 and physicians were slow to accept the need for accurate margin assessment.

As surgeons began treating patients with small invasive breast cancers with breast conservation, most continued to treat less advanced noninvasive lesions with mastectomy. For many patients and even physicians, this was confusing.

DCIS is a heterogeneous group of lesions whose diagnosis, understanding, and treatment require special knowledge and expertise. This knowledge has only begun to be developed during the last decade. Until 1997 (the first edition of this textbook), no textbook had ever been devoted to DCIS. Breast cancer textbooks generally reserve only a chapter or two for the subject of DCIS. The only reference to DCIS in general oncologic treatises may be a few paragraphs within the chapter devoted to breast cancer.

There continues to be confusion and disagreement regarding what lesions constitute the DCIS spectrum. There is confusion and disagreement regarding the extent of treatment: which patients need radiation therapy in addition to complete excision, who can be treated with excision alone, when is mastectomy the procedure of choice, which patients, if any, require sentinel node biopsy? Which prognostic factors can be used to select patients who require treatment and can they be used to guide treatment?

Patients with DCIS commonly obtain numerous consultations, often getting multiple different opinions regarding treatment, in spite of the fact that four prospective randomized trials have been published (NSABP B-17, NSABP B-24, EORTC 10853, UK DCIS Trial). All of these trials have chapters devoted to them in this textbook. All have shown an overall relative reduction in local recurrence of approximately 50% with the addition of radiation therapy after excision. But none have shown in which subgroups of patients there will be little absolute benefit from the addition of radiation therapy. Two trials looked at the benefit from postoperative tamoxifen. One showed that tamoxifen decreased the local recurrence rate while the other did not.

Our current approaches to DCIS continue to be based on morphology rather than etiology, on phenotype rather than genotype. Significant genetic changes are known to precede morphologic evidence of malignant and invasive transformation and the second edition of this textbook looks carefully at that. We in medicine must learn how to recognize these genetic changes, how to exploit them, and in the future, how to prevent them. Breast cancer is a fertile field for study and DCIS is a prime candidate for preventive therapeutic strategies. As we begin the 21st century, we must expand our search for the biologic solutions.

This book provides, in a multidisciplinary fashion, the distinctive and detailed knowledge required to understand, diagnose, and treat patients with ductal carcinoma in situ of the breast. The basic sciences and clinical aspects of the disease are covered in depth by a wealth of outstanding international contributors. This edition has 30 completely new chapters and more than 35 completely revised and updated chapters with the latest data from many centers throughout the world. It includes a chapter by the NSABP with 12-year follow-up data from the B-17 Trial and 7-year data from the B-24 Trial. It includes an update of the EORTC DCIS Trial and the first published details of the UK/Australia New Zealand DCIS Trial.

This text does not answer all of the existing questions and it raises many more. The controversy between excision plus radiation therapy versus excision alone is covered in detail in many chapters and from many different perspectives. Some chapters are personal experiences, dealing with a personal series of patients. Other chapters are exhaustive reviews of the world's literature, others are updates of prospective randomized trials, while others present overviews in an attempt to tie together, in a usable fashion, the available knowledge.

My associate editors and I hope that this book will be a useful resource to scientists, clinicians, and patients. We have tried hard to bring you a balanced book where all sides of the controversial issues are covered fairly. We hope that this book will increase communication between basic researchers and clinicians and between clinicians and patients. And finally, we hope that it will stimulate even more rapid advances in our understanding and treatment of patients with breast cancer.

Melvin J. Silverstein, M.D.

ACKNOWLEDGEMENTS

I am deeply indebted to the more than 150 outstanding scientists and clinicians who contributed chapters to this book. Without their hard work, research, and clinical skills, there would be no book. I sincerely thank each and every one of them for their time, effort, expertise, and superb skill.

I thank my associate editors, Michael D. Lagios and Abram Recht. We shared many exciting hours over the phone, by fax, by e-mail, and in person as this book developed. Each editor contributed something different, something outstanding to this text.

I want to thank the more than 4,000 women with breast cancer who have allowed me to be their doctor during my 30 year tenure as a surgical oncologist. It has been a privilege and an honor to take care of them.

I pay tribute to the staff at Lippincott Williams & Wilkins without whom this book would not have been possible. I specifically want to thank Jonathan Pine, the senior executive editor who supported me from the beginning and took a chance on the first edition of this book, Lisa Consoli, the developmental editor who took me step by step though the textbook process once again, Paula Edelsack and Jill Roberts who oversaw the endless hours of copy-editing, Richard Diamanti who proof read the final product, Gerry Lynn Messner who indexed the volume, and Julie Sikora who oversaw marketing and promotion. I particularly want to thank Michael Mallard, my production editor, for his sage counsel, his wisdom, and his patience as he tirelessly coordinated the final product. I also want to thank the many Lippincott Williams & Wilkins people behind the scenes who I never met but who helped me. Finally, I want to thank the sales force, all of whom took a personal interest in this book.

Many of the chapters authored by me would not have been possible without the hard work and input of many of my previous colleagues at the Van Nuys Breast Center and my current colleagues here at the USC/Norris Comprehensive Cancer Center and the University of Southern California in Los Angeles. I am indebted to all the clinicians, scientists, and students who have worked with me during the last 30 years and who have contributed to various works that we have published.

I thank all of the Van Nuys Breast Center staff and all of the USC/Norris Comprehensive Cancer Center staff who put up with me during the years that it took to produce the first and second editions of this book. Special thanks to Lenore Aisoff, Constance St. Albin, and Linda Friedman for their never-ending administrative and editorial help.

I especially want to thank Mrs. Henrietta C. Lee for endowing the chair that I hold which enabled me to have sufficient time to work on this book and for her continued support of the Harold E. and Henrietta C. Lee Breast Center and the USC/Norris Comprehensive Cancer Center.

I am grateful to the staff at Snug Harbor in Santa Monica, California who served my colleagues and me great food and endless cups of coffee as we discussed DCIS, this textbook, world crises, male aging, and much more most Saturday mornings for the last 20 years.

I thank all of my colleagues throughout the United States and the world who have continuously encouraged me throughout this process.

I thank my children Max, Kate, Sara, Melinda, and Matthew for their never-ending love and support.

And finally, I want to thank my wife, Lynna who provided me with an intellectual and loving environment and constant support throughout the writing and editing of this book. Lynna was first my friend, then my love, and finally my partner.

Melvin J. Silverstein, M.D.

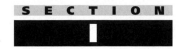

SECTION

I

HISTORY AND EPIDEMIOLOGY

HISTORY OF DUCTAL CARCINOMA IN SITU

ROBERT E. FECHNER

The history of ductal carcinoma in situ (DCIS) is temporally interwoven with the evolution of surgical pathology as a specific discipline. In a sense, the 1990s were the centennial of the diagnosis of DCIS as well as modern surgical pathology. In 1893, comedocarcinoma was first diagnosed by a surgeon on gross examination. (Comedocarcinoma is used in this chapter for DCIS having conspicuous necrosis regardless of cytologic grade. This criterion was used in the literature for more than the first half of the twentieth century.) DCIS, especially comedocarcinoma, continues to present as a clinically palpable and therefore visible mass. When the ducts are sufficiently dilated so that necrotic material can be expressed, the gross diagnosis can be made today with almost 100% certainty by a surgeon just as it was a century ago. Nevertheless, most cases of DCIS now lack a grossly recognizable mass and are found microscopically. Their diagnosis has become the sole domain of the pathologist.

In the nineteenth century and well into the twentieth century, surgeons usually served as their own pathologists. They operated only on a palpable breast abnormality, deciding whether it was benign or malignant on gross inspection at the operating table. The procedure was either terminated after biopsy or excision (for perceived benign disease), or a radical mastectomy was performed if their gross diagnosis was carcinoma. Until the early 1940s, nearly all the American literature on the gross and microscopic pathology of the breast was written by surgeons. Parenthetically, the few papers written by pathologists appeared in surgical journals.

Surgical pathology was the focus of very few pathologists in the first quarter of the twentieth century. Intraoperative consultation was uncommon, although a rapid frozen section technique developed by a gynecologist at Johns Hopkins Hospital was published in 1895 (1), and another was described in 1905 by Wilson, the first pathologist at the Mayo Clinic (2). Frozen section examination at Johns Hopkins Hospital had an inauspicious start in 1891 (3). The pathologist William H. Welch performed a frozen section on a breast lesion at the request of the surgeon William S.

Halsted. By the time a diagnosis was forthcoming, Halsted had not only made his own gross diagnosis but had completed the procedure.

Halsted's associate and successor was Joseph Colt Bloodgood. He was one of the most influential surgeons in the first third of the twentieth century and published voluminously on the gross and microscopic pathology of the breast, including a 97-page paper on fibrocystic changes in 1921 (4). Bloodgood was his own pathologist and ran the Surgical Pathology Laboratory at Johns Hopkins Hospital.

Bloodgood's writings on breast disease began early in the twentieth century. In a publication based on a "lantern-slide demonstration" before the American Association of Pathologists and Bacteriologists in 1906, he wrote: "The earlier the lesion of the breast is observed, the greater the difficulty in differentiating the benign from the malignant tumor. When it is impossible to make a clinical diagnosis of a malignant tumor, the diagnosis must be made from the appearance of the diseased area . . . or from the microscopic examination of a frozen section. For these requirements of the differential diagnosis, the *surgeon* [italics are mine] must have sufficient pathological training to recognize the gross and microscopic appearances of the different breast tumors and inflammations" (5). In 1908, Bloodgood discussed the role of frozen sections (6): "For the last three years I have made immediate frozen sections of fresh tissue received in the pathology laboratory, but up to the present time a stained frozen section has never been of aid in making the diagnosis when we have been unable to come to a conclusion from the fresh appearance of the tissue, nor, up to the present time, have I ever depended upon a frozen section to influence the operative procedure."

The widespread practice of the surgeon relying on the gross diagnosis of a breast lesion was sharply criticized by Mayo Clinic pathologists William C. MacCarty and Broders (7) in 1917 after a review of 1,800 breast lesions. They wrote: "Six months, a year or five years of training in gross pathology will not keep a surgeon from making a high percentage of error in gross diagnoses. . . . It must be fully realized by the medical profession that in many conditions a microscopic diagnosis is absolutely necessary." In 1919, MacCarty and Conner (8) stated that a combined "surgeon and pathologist would be an ideal individual and such a one was possible a few years ago when . . . pathological facts were limited. Today each represents specialism in the field of medical science the many branches of which have grown to such proportions that no one individual can comprehend all clinical facts, perform efficiently all operations or master the subject of pathology completely."

By the mid-1920s, Bloodgood (9) had changed his mind regarding frozen sections and began writing editorials in their support. He is quoted as saying, "Before 1915 it was rarely necessary for a surgeon well trained in gross pathology to need a frozen section to help him in diagnosis at the operating table. Since 1915, and especially since 1922, the public has become so enlightened that malignant disease formerly easily recognized either clinically or in the gross, now appears in our operating rooms devoid of its easily recognized clinical and gross appearance and can be properly discovered only by an immediate frozen section" (10). In 1935, near the end of his professional career, Bloodgood stated that "There is a greater demand today for pathologists and radiotherapeutists than for operators" (11).

During the early twentieth century, the practice of laboratory medicine and surgical pathology varied widely in different institutions. There were no formal training programs in pathology, and the scarcity of surgical pathologists can be appreciated by a statement made at the 1933 Annual Business Meeting of the American Society of Clinical Pathologists. It was "suggested that there should be in each state at least one tissue pathologist thoroughly competent to recognize malignancy" (12).

The diagnosis of mammary carcinoma in situ has existed de facto for a century. As previously noted, comedocarcinoma was recognized as an entity in 1893, albeit in an astoundingly arbitrary manner. Bloodgood wrote: "In 1893 . . . I assisted Dr. Halsted in exploring a clinically benign tumor of the breast. The moment we cut into and pressed on it, there exuded from its surface many grayish-white, granular cylinders, which I called at that time comedos. From the gross appearance the tumor was diagnosed as malignant, and the radical operation was performed. The nodes were not involved . . ." (13).

This statement is in Bloodgood's paper on comedocarcinoma published in 1934. A photomicrograph from the lesion in 1893 confirms the diagnosis (13). Although Bloodgood did not publish his series until 1934, his gross criteria for comedocarcinoma were disseminated and in use long before then. This is evidenced by the presence of the word comedocarcinoma accompanied by an accurate gross description in the book by Deaver (a surgeon) and McFarland (a pathologist) (14) published in 1917.

Two fundamental concerns at the turn of the twentieth century were the diagnosis of cancer and the cell of origin of

carcinoma. An English surgeon, A. Marmaduke Sheild (15), published a book on breast diseases in 1898. He wrote: "The earliest change usually observable by the microscope in carcinoma. . . . is a morbid proliferation of the acinous epithelium, which not only fills the acini, but also the ducts in immediate relation with them. The first certain sign of the dangerous nature of the affection, is furnished by a small-celled infiltration of the surrounding tissues. There seems every probability, that the infective cellular elements spread mainly along the lymphatic trunks, which commence by microscopical channels among the periacinous spaces."

Figure 1.1 illustrates the early stage of mammary carcinoma. For Sheild, the origin of invasive cancer is no different from our current concept. Nonetheless, it was not as clear to most investigators. There were devoted and often vocal adherents to cancer originating from embryonic rests, endothelial cells, or stromal cells. These concepts were rooted in the earliest thinking regarding neoplastic disease dating back to the 1830s. Numerous discussions focused on the origin of carcinoma. After considerable observations, a London surgeon, Sir G. Lenthal Cheatle (16), concluded in 1906 that invasive carcinoma arose from ducts.

Setting aside any consideration of origin, Rodman (17), a surgeon, used a classification of cancer in 1908 that he attributed to Halsted. The classification consisted of "adenocarcinoma, medullary and scirrhus carcinoma, carcinoma

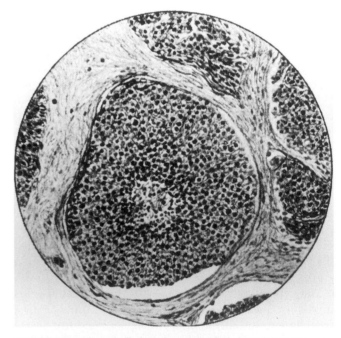

FIGURE 1.1. This small duct (or expanded ductule) appears to have a monomorphic population of cells with the solid pattern of ductal carcinoma in situ (DCIS). It is undoubtedly fortuitous that the duct seems to have a monomorphic cell population characteristic of DCIS. If the duct had been filled with cells of ordinary hyperplasia, it seems probable that the diagnosis would still have been the early stage of mammary carcinoma simply because of the hypercellularity. (From Sheild AM. *A clinical treatise on diseases of the breast.* London: MacMillan and Co. Ltd., 1898:313.)

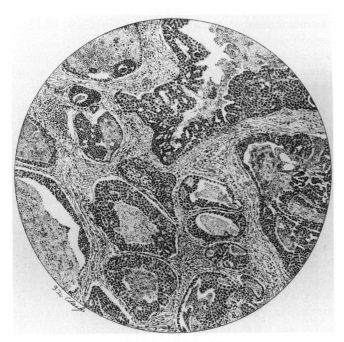

FIGURE 1.2. The original legend for this drawing reads: "Section showing areas of adenocarcinoma and medullary carcinoma." The proliferation appears to be micropapillary ductal carcinoma in situ (DCIS) with rare, small ducts having cribriform DCIS. The entire lesion, however, was viewed by the surgeon/author in 1908 as invasive carcinoma. (From Rodman WL. *Diseases of the breast with special reference to cancer.* Philadelphia: P. Blakiston's Son & Co., 1908:281.)

simplex, gelatinous carcinoma and carcinomatous cyst." Rodman made interesting observations on the category of adenocarcinoma. "Adenocarcinoma represents the first step in the deviation from epithelial proliferation . . . grows comparatively slowly . . . [and] the lymph nodes are rarely invaded until very late in the disease, when the tumor has been converted into one of the other forms of carcinoma." The histologic correlation for these clinical features is obvious when one looks at his illustrations for the category of adenocarcinoma. Comedocarcinoma, as well as low-grade cribriform and micropapillary carcinomas, are illustrated as adenocarcinoma without further modifiers. The fact that many or all the circumscribed nests of cells in a given tumor were actually confined to preexisting ducts was not appreciated (Fig. 1.2). It is understandable that DCIS was considered as invasive by looking at one paper that illustrates lymph node metastases with sharply circumscribed nests of cancer with a cribriform architecture (16). Each individual nest of cells in the lymph node is indistinguishable from a single duct of cribriform DCIS in the breast. Clearly, this particular case was an example of metastatic invasive cribriform carcinoma.

A well-illustrated and thoughtful paper published in 1911 by Mayo Clinic pathologist MacCarty (18) may be the first paper on the pathology of breast disease written by an American pathologist. It covers a variety of benign conditions and terminology, but, most important, he also copes

with the concept of preinvasive carcinoma by asking "Is it necessary to wait for the penetration of the basement membrane before making a diagnosis of carcinoma? . . . If the pathologist considers the penetration of the basement membrane the essential characteristic of carcinoma, then it must be admitted that the cells in adenoma are often just as irregular as in carcinoma." In 1913, he published a paper that demonstrated a spectrum of cytologic differences from normal cells to the cells of invasive carcinoma (19). It convincingly demonstrated that abnormal cells in the ducts of comedocarcinoma were cytologically identical to the cells of invasive carcinoma.

In every edition of the book *Neoplastic Diseases. A Treatise on Tumors* by James Ewing (20), first published in 1919, he illustrates the same two photomicrographs of DCIS. One is a cribriform/micropapillary carcinoma and the other is a comedocarcinoma with a cribriform pattern. In 1919, he apparently diagnosed these cases as DCIS based on "large cuboidal or cylindrical cells with hyperchromatic nuclei." In the final (fourth) edition in 1940, he added that such tumors "grow in distended ducts over considerable segments of the breast. Such tumors are slow to involve the lymph-nodes, but eventually they break through the basement membrane, and infiltrate the fat and connective tissue in the form of alveolar carcinoma [his term for infiltrating ductal carcinoma]" (21).

Cheatle (22) published a paper in 1921 with photographs of whole-mount sections and verified his earlier conclusion that carcinoma initially existed within ducts. The text and legends for his illustrations of micropapillary/cribriform DCIS stated that: "The cancer-containing cavities [ducts]" are not as numerous as they appear because the individual ducts are "tortuous and being cut repeatedly." In another publication in that same year, he has a photograph of cribriform DCIS that is associated with an invasive cribriform carcinoma (23). He refers to the "laciform and cart-wheel appearances . . . typical of this form of cancer." The phrase cribriform carcinoma was well established by 1933 when Schultz-Brauns (24) illustrated the sieve-like type of cribriform DCIS in a drawing and a photograph.

In 1931, Cheatle and Cutler (a radiotherapist) (25) published a book entitled *Tumors of the Breast.* Part of their text as well as several of their 18 color plates and 468 other illustrations embraced the existence of preinvasive carcinoma. There is a drawing of ducts "full of a malignant-looking epithelial neoplasia that is still confined within normal boundaries," and they illustrate microscopic stromal invasion from a duct in which there is a break in the "basement membrane." In 1981, this drawing was reprinted (26).

One of the most influential pioneers of surgical pathology, Arthur Purdy Stout (27), published a book on human cancer in 1932. He was aware of the concept of preinvasive carcinoma. Referring to mammary epithelial proliferations in women, Stout stated, "The decision as to whether a given lesion is still a simple hyperplasia or has passed the borderline and become a cancer is often a difficult one."

In 1934, Stout invited a young surgeon, Cushman D. Haagensen, to join his staff in the Surgical Pathology Laboratory at Columbia-Presbyterian Medical Center in New York. This collaboration of a surgeon turned pathologist (Stout) and a surgeon interested in breast pathology is reflected in Haagensen's (28) *Diseases of the Breast*, first published in 1956.

The concept of preinvasive carcinoma of the human breast seems to have been firmly established in the United Kingdom by the early 1930s. In 1933, the pathologist Dawson (29) concluded that carcinoma always arose in ducts and "in the majority of cases, in the terminal, intralobular ducts." Her observations on this particular point were confirmed and expanded with the meticulous study using the subgross method published by Wellings et al. (30) in 1975. Dawson also recognized what has come to be known (right or wrong) as cancerization of lobular ductules. She concluded that "Involvement of the ductules is not primary but secondary, and is evidence of extension of the cancerous process."

Muir, a Scottish pathologist, may have been the first to use the term intraduct carcinoma in 1935 (31). He noted that proliferating ductal epithelial cells "have acquired the essential characters of malignant neoplasia, and they acquire this character before they transgress the normal boundaries." In 1941, he wrote: "Although cells definitely recognizable as malignant can be seen in ducts or in acini before the ultimate break-through into tissue spaces occurs, it is not possible to state definitely at what stage cells acquire the malignant character" (32).

In 1932, Broders (33) coined the phrase "carcinoma in situ" and illustrated examples from five different organs, one of which was a lobule of the breast that he called "adenocarcinoma in situ." His photograph is an indubitable example of what was named by pathologists Frank W. Foote, Jr., and Fred W. Stewart (34) in 1941 as "lobular carcinoma in situ." Coincidentally, Muir (32), in his 1941 paper, illustrated an identical image that he called "intra-acinous carcinoma".

In 1945, Foote and Stewart (35,36), pathologists at Memorial Hospital for Cancer and Allied Diseases in New York, published very extensive papers covering benign and malignant conditions of the breast. In one paper, they illustrated a lesion diagnosed as "noninfiltrating papillary carcinoma of ducts" that is cytologically and architecturally identical to their illustration of an infiltrating papillary carcinoma (36). They observed that "The individual cells are usually of medium size and do not vary a great deal in configuration and stainability. Hyperchromatism is not impressive and the rate of cell division is low." Using today's terminology, their intraductal carcinoma is a low-grade cribriform carcinoma, and the infiltrating lesion is an infiltrating cribriform carcinoma. The difficulty of diagnosing intraductal lesions is evident in their statement "There is a zone of altered cell growth where the diagnosis of carcinoma versus atypical papillomatosis is a question of occult distinc-

tion and must be accepted or rejected on grounds of faith in the pathologist or lack of it" (Fig. 1.2).

Stewart (37), who wrote the first edition of the Armed Forces Institute of Pathology fascicle on tumors of the breast, published in 1950, used the same photograph of papillary intraductal carcinoma from the 1945 paper and added four other illustrations diagnosed as papillary cancer. In the legend of his Figure 2, the term "in situ duct carcinoma" appears. This may be the. first time, to paraphrase his words, that intraductal carcinoma was referred to as ductal carcinoma in situ. The aforementioned statement referring to "occult distinction" and "faith" was reiterated.

In the first edition (1953) of his classic textbook on surgical pathology, Lauren V. Ackerman (38) illustrated comedocarcinoma and a true papillary carcinoma with fibrovascular stalks. During the 1950s and 1960s, he was highly skeptical about the malignancy of intraductal lesions other than the ones that he illustrated (L. V. Ackerman, personal communication, 1991). The effect of his skepticism on this pathologist is mentioned at the end of the chapter.

Haagensen, whose writings influenced the surgical community, did nothing to illuminate the concept of DCIS, and, indeed, hampered the understanding of the concept. In the first edition of his book *Diseases of the Breast* (28), there was a subsection of his chapter on cancer entitled "Intraductal Carcinoma." In conjunction with Stout, he defined intraductal carcinoma as "the carcinomas that appear to grow predominantly within the mammary ducts. The so-called comedocarcinoma is a prototype of intraductal carcinoma. But there are a number of other cell patterns of intraductal growth. We know that all are infiltrating and fully malignant even though we do not happen to see actual infiltration." Under a section on incidence, he continues "intraductal carcinoma is the most frequent of the several special forms of carcinoma that have no special distinguishing clinical features. In his microscopical review, Dr. Stout classified 102 of a total of 668 carcinomas, or about 15 per cent, as intraductal." There are four photomicrographs that are fully acceptable as DCIS. One tumor is a typical comedocarcinoma and the others show solid, micropapillary, and cribriform patterns of DCIS. In his second edition (39) (1971), he dropped the illustration of the micropapillary pattern. He defined intraductal carcinoma more precisely than in the first edition (28) by acknowledging that Stout decided breast carcinomas were to be classified as intraductal when more than 50% of the lesion had an intraductal form. Obviously, this meant that an invasive carcinoma might be present. The category of intraductal carcinoma included pure DCIS and a mixture of DCIS and invasive cancer, but they were not separated.

Apparently working independently of Stout and Haagensen, Ozzello (40), a pathologist in the same Laboratory of Surgical Pathology, segregated 22 cases of pure intraductal carcinoma from the larger group defined by Stout and Haagensen. Ozzello's paper, published in 1959, was based on the incredibly limited sampling of two to nine blocks from mastectomy specimens. It is, therefore, not surprising that two patients had axillary metastases and another developed distant metastases in the absence of lymph node involvement.

In the third and final edition of his book in 1986 (41), Haagensen's lifetime experience with DCIS is summarized. Intraductal carcinoma was still viewed as a cancer with invasion as contrasted with lobular carcinoma in situ, which was viewed as a noninfiltrating breast carcinoma. He wrote that intraductal carcinoma tends to be confused "with noninfiltrating breast carcinoma, which is not a useful criterion in our opinion." Haagensen said "We know from experience . . . that although we may not see any infiltration of the mammary stroma, these lesions [intraductal carcinoma] must infiltrate because they metastasize. The pathologist who ventures to classify any one of them as noninfiltrating is misleading the surgeon, who may thereby be tempted to perform a less radical operation." Neither he nor Stout ever isolated a diagnostic category of pure DCIS.

As expected, all the lesions that Haagensen reported were palpable masses with an average diameter of 3.3 cm, which was comparable with the average diameter of 3.4 cm for all carcinomas of the breast. His and Stout's broad definition yielded many patients with DCIS who had metastases. The clinical follow-up of 223 patients diagnosed between 1931 and 1972 had 183 patients in clinical stage A (no clinically involved nodes or tumor fixed to chest wall); 21% of whom had axillary metastases. Forty patients were classified as stage B (clinically involved nodes) and 68% had metastases. Therefore, 29.2% of the 223 patients with radical mastectomy had axillary metastases that seemed to prove that intraductal carcinoma was a lesion capable of metastasizing. Haagensen noted that the survival rate in stage B intraductal carcinomas was higher than for carcinomas of all types and that this was "very convincing evidence that intraductal carcinoma is less malignant than most breast carcinomas." It is not surprising, given the breadth of what was included in the category of intraductal carcinoma, that he stated "it should not be an excuse for surgeons to treat intraductal carcinoma with anything less than a radical mastectomy; the disease is certainly malignant enough to justify it."

In each edition, Haagensen has the same gross photograph of an intraductal comedocarcinoma in which the lesion measures 8.0 cm in greatest dimension with many dozens of ducts grossly visible. The sampling of such a lesion to rule out invasion would be a nearly impossible task. The studies by Lagios et al. (42), published in 1982, indicated that a lesion of this size had a high risk of harboring invasive carcinoma if examined by the subgross method.

In 1960, Gillis et al. (43) published a paper from the Mayo Clinic on intraductal carcinoma. Their illustrations include noncomedo, low-grade DCIS, DCIS with low-grade cytology plus central necrosis, and the prototypical high-grade comedocarcinoma. This spectrum was thought to show that DCIS progressed from a low- to a high-grade tumor. They concluded that "preinvasive intraductal carcinoma of the breast, in its pure form, is an uncommon but distinctive manifestation of mammary carcinoma" and "the evidence from this study is that carcinoma of the breast does not involve the regional lymph nodes as long as it is still confined to the ducts."

After the publication of the paper by Gillis et al., there were no further publications on DCIS until the 1970s with two notable exceptions: the paper by Kraus and Neubecker (44) in 1962 and the study by Gallager and Martin (45) in 1969.

In 1962, Kraus, a former surgical pathology fellow of Ackerman, and Neubecker (44) attempted to provide several narrative criteria for distinguishing noncomedo DCIS from hyperplastic proliferations. They emphasized the cytologic monomorphism of some forms of DCIS, especially the cribriform type.

In 1969, Gallager and Martin (45) used huge, whole-organ tissue slides from mastectomy specimens. Two of eight cases of DCIS lacking recognizable invasion had positive lymph nodes. One other patient with DCIS had a distant metastasis but did not have a positive node. They stated that

> It is probable that the conventionally applied standards based on the work of Kraus and Neubecker, while clinically useful, actually define a point well beyond that at which cells are irreversibly committed to neoplastic proliferation. The diagnostic application of electron microscopy may eventually become commonplace as a means of recognizing noninvasive carcinoma in its earliest stages. Equally difficult to ascertain under the light microscope is the point of transition from noninvasive to invasive carcinoma. We have studied 2 patients, both of whom had axillary node metastases but in whose breasts subserial whole organ sections showed only intraductal carcinoma, lacking the classical criteria of invasion. It must be assumed that these apparently intraductal neoplastic cells were actually invasive, and that they formed cylindrical masses simply mimicking the configuration of ducts.

Ozzello (40), in 1959, had shown apparent discontinuity in the basement membrane by a modification of the periodic acid–Schiff stain. Ozzello and Santipak (46), in 1970, using electron microscopy, found gaps through which cytoplasmic protrusions of intraductal neoplastic cells extended. This observation proved that invasion could occur ultrastructurally when it was not demonstrable by light microscopy. They concluded that "the histologic diagnosis of intraductal carcinoma in situ is currently a hazardous one to make."

There were a few papers written about DCIS during the 1970s. As Brown et al. (47) said in 1976: "Because of its rarity, the diagnosis of non-invasive intraductal carcinoma of the breast has been of minimal clinical significance." We must keep in mind that up until this time, nearly 100% of the patients with DCIS were symptomatic; 52% had a mass and 46% had nipple discharge in one series published in 1975 (48).

Papers published in the 1970s continued to emphasize the especially confounding feature that hampered the concept of DCIS as noninvasive. Brown et al. (47) found one of 21 patients with DCIS had a positive node, and Carter and Smith (49) found positive nodes in one of 31 patients. Ashikari et al. (50) reported 112 patients with DCIS: one with a positive lymph node, one with negative nodes who died of metastases, and two with local recurrences after radical mastectomy.

The presence of invasive carcinoma in a mastectomy specimen after the initial biopsy showed only DCIS was also of considerable concern and seriously diluted the concept of pure DCIS from a patient management viewpoint. For example, Carter and Smith (49) found seven of 38 (18%) of breasts with DCIS in the biopsy had invasive cancer in the mastectomy specimen. Shah et al. (51) found eight of 45 (18%) patients with DCIS in the initial excision had infiltrating carcinoma in the mastectomy. Carter and Smith concluded that DCIS was synchronously associated with invasive cancer "with a sufficient frequency to indicate a modified radical mastectomy when that diagnosis [DCIS] is made."

Therefore, it was one thing to recognize and accept that infiltrating cancer originated in ducts. It was quite another idea to realize that carcinoma could be confined to ducts, might constitute a pathologic entity, be the only lesion, and have critical clinical ramifications. The patterns of noncomedo, low-grade types of DCIS were not well known in the pathology community until well into the 1970s or even early 1980s.

Interest in the clinical outcome of untreated patients with noncomedocarcinoma began in the late 1970s. There had been a 40-year hiatus since the report in 1938 by Lewis and Geschickter (52) on eight women with comedocarcinoma initially treated only with local excision. Six of their reported tumors locally recurred (four within 1 year), and in three cases, axillary lymph nodes were positive at the second operation.

In the late 1970s and early 1980s, four papers published within 5 years of each other provided follow-up for noncomedo types of DCIS. Most of the studies dealt with patients in whom the diagnosis had been overlooked in a breast biopsy at some time in the past. Betsill et al. (53), in 1978, reported on the outcome of patients with cribriform/micropapillary DCIS who were not further treated after the initial biopsy. Nine of their 25 patients had palpable disease; in the remaining 16 patients, there were incidental findings in a biopsy performed for another lesion. In a subsequent report in 1980, Rosen et al. (54) added five more patients to this group, giving a total of 15 with follow-up. Ten ultimately developed ipsilateral carcinoma, eight of which were invasive. Carter and associates (55), writing in 1983, provided follow-up data on women with intracystic

papillary carcinoma, a special form of DCIS. Patients treated with local excision did well except when there was DCIS in ducts beyond the confines of the cystic lesion. In 1982, Page et al. (56) reported the long-term follow-up of 25 women with cribriform/micropapillary DCIS that had been found as an incidental microscopic finding and not as a palpable mass. Seven of these women developed invasive carcinoma in the ipsilateral breast from 3 to 10 years later. The women who did not have a subsequent cancer were followed for 8 to 27 years (average, 16 years). This cohort has continued to be followed, and two additional women have developed invasive cancer in the ipsilateral breast 20 and 30 years after the initial biopsy (57). One other woman had extensive noncomedo DCIS identified 25 years later.

The prevalence of DCIS in the unscreened population has been assessed in a few autopsy studies beginning in 1973. Kramer and Rush (58) found that four of 70 (6%) of women beyond the age of 70 years had DCIS, and in half of the cases, it was bilateral. Alpers and Wellings (59) used the subgross method of examination on the breasts from 101 women and found nine (9%) with DCIS. The prevalence by decade was roughly the same from women in their 20s to women older than 60 years old. Nielsen et al. (60) also used the subgross method of examination in 110 forensic autopsies of women ranging from 20 to 54 years of age. Sixteen women (14%) had DCIS. Their study looked at one other interesting facet. Only seven of the 16 women with DCIS had specimen radiographs that would have been interpreted as suspicious if they had been clinical mammograms. Five were owing to microcalcification and two to a soft-tissue density. Thus, less than half of the cases of DCIS would have been mammographically detectable. Parenthetically, not all palpable lesions of DCIS have a positive mammogram. Howard et al. (61) found a 10% false-negative rate for palpable DCIS, which compares with the well-known false-negative rate of 15% for palpable invasive carcinomas.

The year 1982 marks the publication of a landmark paper by Lagios et al. (42), who studied mastectomy specimens from women with DCIS using the subgross method. They found that a small volume of DCIS (<2.5 cm) carried less risk of multicentricity and associated occult invasive carcinoma than did a larger volume of DCIS. Breasts with an area of DCIS less than 2.5 cm did not have invasion, whereas 11 (44%) of 25 cases with DCIS exceeding 2.5 cm had occult invasion, and one patient had a nodal metastasis. Their observations form the fundamental rationale justifying conservative therapy in patients with small-volume DCIS.

During the 1980s, DCIS came into progressively sharper focus as more and more lesions were discovered that were small and clearly had no invasive component. A flood of papers on DCIS began in the late 1980s and continues to the present. They form the basis of the more detailed information that appears in subsequent chapters of this volume.

PERSONAL NOTE

During the late 1960s, I became interested in lobular carcinoma in situ (LCIS) because of a few papers (in the surgical literature and in *Cancer*) regarding microscopic diagnosis and follow-up of untreated cases (62–65). The emphasis on detecting LCIS led me to search for lesions in ducts that might be a clue for LCIS located elsewhere in the unsampled breast. In 1972, I published a paper illustrating "epithelial proliferations" in the ducts of patients who had LCIS when additional blocks were submitted. I accurately noted that the ducts were populated by cells cytologically identical to the characteristic cells of LCIS (66). The proper categorization of these proliferations as either low-grade cribriform or micropapillary DCIS went unrecognized, and the diagnosis of DCIS was also missed by the reviewer or reviewers of the manuscript as well. I believe that the failure to recognize these lesions as DCIS stemmed from my time with Dr. Lauren V. Ackerman as a surgical pathology fellow and junior faculty member between 1962 and 1965. His skepticism of Dr. Stewart's cytologically low-grade micropapillary and cribriform types had made a major impact.

This skepticism was reinforced around 1966, when the manuscript of the second edition of the Armed Forces Institute of Pathology fascicle on tumors of the breast by McDivitt et al. (67) was being reviewed before acceptance for publication. I had the opportunity to see the illustrations, although I was not an official reviewer. They were shown to me by a highly respected former senior associate of Dr. Ackerman who was the formal reviewer. He thought that the lesions of micropapillary and cribriform carcinoma were only peculiar forms of hyperplasia. To the best of my recollection, this was based on the lack of necrosis and the nuclear uniformity. Nevertheless, the illustrations were published in 1968 with the legends and diagnoses of DCIS as submitted by the authors.

After this experience, I finally accepted DCIS of a small cell type without necrosis as illustrated by McDivitt et al. This was forcefully brought home by seeing a mastectomy specimen of infiltrating cribriform carcinoma with lymph node metastases. There was also an obviously noninvasive

component of cribriform DCIS in the breast. This case was presented at the Houston Society of Clinical Pathologists in 1972 or 1973 as some major breakthrough, i.e., intraductal carcinoma could have small uniform cells and lack necrosis. I then went back through 807 cases of fibrocystic disease that had been diagnosed by other pathologists between 1962 and 1966. This yielded 13 (1.5%) cases of LCIS or DCIS. There were six cases that were fully diagnostic micropapillary DCIS (68). This reflected an unawareness by pathologists of noncomedo DCIS. The photograph that I published in 1978 with the legend "micropapillary carcinoma" is interchangeable with one of the ducts published in 1972 that was merely called "papillary pattern of proliferation" and not further defined. A similar review by Page et al. (69) of 10,542 biopsy specimens between 1952 and 1968 yielded a frequency of 1.7% for undiagnosed LCIS or DCIS.

I have also been interested in the reproducibility of diagnosing DCIS. As discussed previously, Kraus and Neubecker (44) had addressed criteria for diagnosing DCIS in 1962. Another set of criteria for hyperplasia, atypical hyperplasia, and DCIS was illustrated and described in detail by Page et al. in 1982 (56) and 1985 (69). London et al. (70) subsequently validated the reproducibility and clinical relevance of these histologic criteria. The criteria of Page et al. have been widely accepted in the pathology community.

Two recent studies compare what happens when the criteria of Page et al. are followed and when they are not (Table 1.1). The first study was conducted by Rosai (71) and was presented at the Arthur Purdy Stout Scientific Meeting at the United States–Canadian Academy of Pathology in 1990. He selected five pathologists with special interest in mammary pathology and sent the same 17 tissue slides containing noninvasive epithelial proliferations to each of them. A small area was circled in ink, which ensured that each pathologist diagnosed precisely the same few ducts or lobules. The diagnostic choices were limited to usual hyperplasia, atypical hyperplasia, or carcinoma in situ. The pathologists used whatever criteria they employed in their daily practice. In none of the cases was there agreement by all pathologists. In only three cases (18%) did four of five

TABLE 1.1. INTEROBSERVER VARIABILITY ON DUCTAL LESIONS: AGREEMENT AS TO WHETHER HYPERPLASIA, ATYPICAL HYPERPLASIA, OR DUCTAL CARCINOMA IN SITU

Standardized Criteria (73) (24 Cases, 6 Pathologists)		No Standardized Criteria (72) (10 Cases, 5 Pathologists)	
No. of Pathologists in Exact Agreement	% of Cases	No. of Pathologists in Exact Agreement	% of Cases
6 of 6	58	5 of 5	0
5 of 6	71	4 of 5	20
4 of 6	92	3 of 5	50

pathologists agree, and in only nine cases (53%) did three of five pathologists agree. Moreover, six cases (35%) had diagnoses that spanned the spectrum of usual hyperplasia, atypical hyperplasia, and carcinoma in situ. To top it off, two of the pathologists were polarized. One pathologist called every lesion atypical hyperplasia or carcinoma in situ and another pathologist never diagnosed carcinoma in situ and diagnosed only four as atypical.

Schnitt et al. (72) organized a similar study using 24 tissue slides of ductal epithelial proliferations with a single small area visible on a slide that was otherwise covered with masking tape. There was one major difference, however. Before looking at the study slides, the six participating pathologists (three of whom had participated in the Rosai study) were given narrative and diagrammatic information regarding the criteria of Page et al. Additionally, Page et al. circulated 15 tissue slides that they had diagnosed as usual hyperplasia, atypical hyperplasia, or noncomedo DCIS for review. After this preparation, the study slides were circulated. All six pathologists agreed on the diagnosis in 14 (58%) of the 24 cases. Five of six pathologists agreed in 17 (71%) of cases, and four of six pathologists agreed in 22 (92%) of cases. Most of the discrepancies were between atypical hyperplasia and DCIS. Only two cases covered the diagnostic spectrum of usual hyperplasia, atypical hyperplasia, and DCIS. Furthermore, no pathologist was more malignant or benign as in their interpretations as measured by kappa analysis. The study demonstrates that a reasonable degree of reproducibility can be attained when standardized criteria are applied. It is important to realize that the cases of Schnitt et al. were intentionally selected for their morphologic complexity and unusual appearance cytologically and/or architecturally. They did not represent 24 consecutive breast biopsies accessioned as day-to-day specimens. In this latter real-life scenario, I would expect complete agreement between these pathologists in at least 95% of cases and perhaps 100%. I have discussed this point with Dr. Richard L. Kempson and Dr. Kevin O. Leslie, who agree with this admittedly undocumented statement (73).

Even when a classification system is developed for the express purpose of enhancing reproducibility, it is possible that lack of explicit criteria or ambiguity of criteria can result in diagnostic categories that are not mutually exclusive. Such classifications may have vague qualitative terms, imprecise quantitative terms, subjective variations in the interpretation of the relative importance for different criteria, and the fundamental problem of tumor heterogeneity with variable images that probably span an infinite spectrum in the breast.

The many issues involved in the diagnosis and treatment of DCIS have been a topic of interpretation for more than a century (74). It is inevitable that numerous facets of the pathologic diagnosis of DCIS and the subsequent clinical ramifications will continue to change for many years to come.

REFERENCES

1. Cullen TS. A rapid method of making permanent specimens from frozen sections by the use of formalin. *Johns Hopkins Hosp Bull* 1895;67.
2. Wilson LB. A method for the rapid preparation of fresh tissues for the microscope. *JAMA* 1905;45:1737.
3. Rosen G. Beginning of surgical biopsy. *Am J Surg Pathol* 1977;1:361–363.
4. Bloodgood JC. The pathology of chronic cystic mastitis of the female breast. With special consideration of the blue-domed cyst. *Arch Surg* 1921;3:445–542.
5. Bloodgood JC. Senile parenchymatous hypertrophy of female breast. Its relation to cyst formation and carcinoma. *Surg Gynecol Obstet* 1906;3:721–730.
6. Bloodgood JC. The clinical and pathological differential diagnosis of diseases of the female breast. *Am J Med Sci* 1908;135:157–168.
7. MacCarty WC, Broders AC. Studies in clinico-pathologic standardization and efficiency. I. Legitimate actual error in diagnosis of mammary conditions. *Surg Gynecol Obstet* 1917;25:666–673.
8. MacCarty WC, Conner HM. Clinicoefficiency and terminology in cancer of the breast. *Surg Gynecol Obstet* 1919;29:44–51.
9. Bloodgood JC. When cancer becomes a microscopic disease, there must be tissue diagnosis in the operating room. *JAMA* 1927;88:1022–1023.
10. Wright JR. The development of frozen section technique, the evolution of surgical biopsy, and the origins of surgical pathology. *Bull Hist Med* 1985;59:295–326.
11. Bloodgood JC. Biopsy in breast lesions. In relation to diagnosis, treatment and prognosis. *Ann Surg* 1935;102:239–247.
12. Stevenson GF. Ward Burdick award lecture: the history of the ASCP annual fall anatomic slide seminar. *Am J Clin Pathol* 1986;85:259–268.
13. Bloodgood JC. Comedo carcinoma (or comedo-adenoma) of the female breast. *Am J Cancer* 1934;22:842–853.
14. Deaver JB, McFarland J. *The breast: its anomalies, its diseases, and their treatment.* Philadelphia: P. Blakiston's Son & Co., 1917:485.
15. Sheild AM. *A clinical treatise on diseases of the breast.* London: MacMillan and Co. Ltd., 1898.
16. Cheatle GL. Clinical remarks on the early recognition of cancer of the breast. *BMJ* 1906;1:1205–1210.
17. Rodman WL. *Diseases of the breast with special reference to cancer.* Philadelphia: P. Blakiston's Son & Co., 1908:86.
18. MacCarty WC. Carcinoma of the breast. *Trans South Surg Gynecol Assoc* 1911;23:262–270.
19. MacCarty WC. The histogenesis of cancer (carcinoma) of the breast and its clinical significance. *Surg Gynecol Obstet* 1913;17:441–459.
20. Ewing J. *Neoplastic diseases. A treatise on tumors.* Philadelphia: WB Saunders, 1919:473, 494, 495.
21. Ewing J. *Neoplastic diseases. A treatise on tumors.* Philadelphia: WB Saunders, 1940:568.
22. Cheatle GL. Cysts, and primary cancer in cysts, of the breast. *Br J Surg* 1920–1921;8:149–166.
23. Cheatle GL. Benign and malignant changes in duct epithelium of the breast. *Br J Surg* 1920–1921;8:285–306.
24. Schultz-Brauns O. Die Geschwülste der Brustdrüse. In: Lubarsch O, Henke F, eds. *Handbuch der speziellen pathologischen Anatomie and Histologie.* Vol. 7, pt. 2. Berlin: Springer Verlag, 1933:291–292.
25. Cheatle GL, Cutler M. *Tumors of the breast.* Philadelphia: JB Lippincott, 1931:201–205.
26. Rosen PP. Clinical implications of preinvasive and small invasive breast carcinomas. *Pathol Annu* 1981;16(pt 2):337–356.

27. Stout AP. Human cancer. *Etiological factors; precancerous lesions; growth; spread; symptoms; diagnosis; prognosis; principles of treatment.* Philadelphia: Lea & Febiger, 1932:282.

28. Haagensen CD. *Diseases of the breast.* Philadelphia: WB Saunders, 1956:502–506.

29. Dawson EK. Carcinoma of the mammary lobule and its origin. *Edinburgh Med J* 1933;40:57–82.

30. Wellings SR, Jensen HM, Marcum RG. An atlas of subgross pathology of the human breast with special reference to possible precancerous lesion. *J Natl Cancer Inst* 1975;55:231–273.

31. Muir R. The pathogenesis of Paget's disease of the nipple and associated lesions. *Br J Surg* 1934–1935;22:728–737.

32. Muir R. The evolution of carcinoma of the mama. *J Pathol Bact* 1941;52:155–172.

33. Broders AC. Carcinoma in situ contrasted with benign penetrating epithelium. *JAMA* 1932;99:1670–1674.

34. Foote FW Jr, Stewart FW. Lobular carcinoma in situ. A rare form of mammary cancer. *Am J Pathol* 1941;17:491–495.

35. Foote FW Jr, Stewart FW. A histologic classification of carcinoma of the breast. *Surgery* 1945;17:74–99.

36. Foote FW Jr, Stewart FW. Comparative studies of cancerous versus noncancerous breasts. I. Basic morphologic characteristics. *Ann Surg* 1945;121:6–53.

37. Stewart FW. *Tumors of the breast. Atlas of tumor pathology.* Fascicle 34. Washington, DC: Armed Forces Institute of Pathology, 1950.

38. Ackerman LV. *Surgical pathology.* St. Louis: Mosby, 1953:598–599.

39. Haagensen CD. *Diseases of the breast,* 3rd ed. Philadelphia: WB Saunders, 1971.

40. Ozzello L. The behavior of basement membranes in intraductal carcinoma of the breast. *Am J Pathol* 1959;35:887–899.

41. Haagensen CD. *Diseases of the breast,* 3rd ed. Philadelphia: WB Saunders, 1986:782–789.

42. Lagios MD, Westdahl PR, Margolin FR, et al. Duct carcinoma in situ. Relationship of extent of noninvasive disease to the frequency of occult invasion, multicentricity, lymph node metastases, and short-term treatment failures. *Cancer* 1982;50:1309–14.

43. Gillis DA, Dockerty MB, Clagett OT. Preinvasive intraductal carcinoma of the breast. *Surg Gynecol Obstet* 1960;110:555–562.

44. Kraus FT, Neubecker RT. The differential diagnosis of papillary tumors of the breast. *Cancer* 1962;15:444–455.

45. Gallager HS, Martin JE. Early phases in the development of breast cancer. *Cancer* 1969;24:1170–1178.

46. Ozzello L, Santipak P. Epithelial-stromal junction of intraductal carcinoma of the breast. *Cancer* 1970;26:1186–1198.

47. Brown PW, Silverman J, Owens E, et al. Intraductal "non-infiltrating" carcinoma of the breast. *Arch Surg* 1976;111:1063–1067.

48. Westbrook KC, Gallager HS. Intraductal carcinoma of the breast. *Am J Surg* 1975;130:667–670.

49. Carter D, Smith RRL. Carcinoma in situ of the breast. *Cancer* 1977;40:1189–1193.

50. Ashikari R, Hajdu SI, Robbins GF. Intraductal carcinoma of the breast. *Cancer* 1971;28:1182–1187.

51. Shah JP, Rosen PP, Robbins GF. Pitfalls of local excision in the treatment of carcinoma of the breast. *Surg Gynecol Obstet* 1973;136:721–725.

52. Lewis D, Geschickter CF. Comedo carcinoma of the breast. *Arch Surg* 1938;36:225–244.

53. Betsill WL, Rosen PP, Lieberman PH, et al. Intraductal carcinoma. Long-term follow-up after treatment by biopsy alone. *JAMA* 1978;239:1863–1867.

54. Rosen PP, Braun DW Jr, Kinne DE. The clinical significance of pre-invasive breast carcinoma. *Cancer* 1980;46:919–925.

55. Carter D, Orr SL, Merino MJ. Intracystic papillary carcinoma of the breast. After mastectomy, radiotherapy or excisional biopsy alone. *Cancer* 1983;52:14–19.

56. Page DL, Dupont WD, Rogers LW, et al. Intraductal carcinoma of the breast. Follow-up after biopsy only. *Cancer* 1982;49:751–758.

57. Page DL, Dupont WD, Rogers LW, et al. Continued local recurrence of carcinoma 15–25 years after a diagnosis of low grade ductal carcinoma-in-situ of the breast treated only by biopsy. *Cancer* 1995;76:1197–2000.

58. Kramer WM, Rush BF Jr. Mammary duct proliferation in the elderly. *Cancer* 1973;31:130–137.

59. Alpers CE, Wellings SR. The prevalence of carcinoma in situ in normal and cancer-associated breasts. *Hum Pathol* 1985;16:796–807.

60. Nielsen M, Thomsen JL, Primdahl S, et al. Breast cancer and atypia among young and middle-aged women: a study of 110 medicolegal autopsies. *Br J Cancer* 1987;56:814–819.

61. Howard PW, Locker AP, Dowle CS, et al. In situ carcinoma of the breast. *Eur J Surg Oncol* 1989;15:328–332.

62. Godwin JT. Chronology of lobular carcinoma in the breast: report of a case. *Cancer* 1952;5:259–266.

63. Newman W. In situ lobular carcinoma of the breast: report of 26 women with 32 cancers. *Ann Surg* 1963;157:591–599.

64. Benfield JR, Jacobson M, Warner NE. In situ lobular carcinoma of the breast. *Arch Surg* 1965;91:130–135.

65. Newman W. Lobular carcinoma of the female breast. *Ann Surg* 1966;164:305–314.

66. Fechner RE. Epithelial alterations in the extralobular ducts of breasts with lobular carcinoma. *Arch Pathol* 1972;93:164–171.

67. McDivitt RW, Stewart FW, Berg JW. *Tumors of the breast. Atlas of tumor pathology,* 2nd series. Washington, DC: Armed Forces Institute of Pathology, 1968:42–49.

68. Harvey DG, Fechner RE. Atypical lobular and papillary lesions of the breast: a follow-up study of 30 cases. *South Med J* 1978;71:361–364.

69. Page DL, Dupont WD, Rogers LW, et al. Atypical hyperplastic lesions of the female breast. A long-term follow-up study. *Cancer* 1985;55:2698–2708.

70. London SJ, Connolly JL, Schnitt SJ, et al. A prospective study of benign breast disease and the risk of breast cancer. *JAMA* 1992;267:941–944.

71. Rosai J. Borderline epithelial lesions of the breast. *Am J Surg Pathol* 1991;15:209–221.

72. Schnitt SJ, Connolly JL, Tavassoli FA, et al. Interobserver reproducibility in the diagnosis of ductal proliferative breast lesions using standardized criteria. *Am J Surg Pathol* 1992;16:1133–1143.

73. Leslie KO, Fechner RE, Kempson RL. Second opinions in surgical pathology. *Am J Clin Pathol* 1996;106[Suppl 1]:558–S64.

74. Fechner RE. One century of mammary carcinoma in situ. What have we learned? *Am J Clin Pathol* 1993;100:654–658.

2

WHY STUDY DUCTAL CARCINOMA IN SITU?

MARC E. LIPPMAN

In some sense, the answer to the question "why study DCIS?" seems obvious. Ductal carcinoma in situ (DCIS) is a disease whose incidence is apparently increasing markedly (although the biases caused by improved means of mammographic detection are difficult to quantify). Unquestionably, some patients with DCIS can and will progress to invasive breast cancer if left untreated or treated inadequately. Current data suggest that approximately one-half of DCIS lesions that reappear in the same breast quadrant after local therapy show an invasive histology (1,2). We need far better understanding of the disease if we are to develop interventions that are based on mechanisms of disease pathogenesis rather than excision or irradiation. The usual goals in the management of any malignancy are stated easily enough. They are improved means of earlier detection (generally presuming that earlier detection lessens the extent and/or seriousness of treatment required), improved prognostication combined with a better understanding of natural history, improved therapy ranging from more precise allocation of patients to surgery of varying extents and/or radiation to the development of biologic treatments, and finally strategies for prevention. Interestingly, it is in the category of prevention that the greatest incremental change has been achieved since the previous edition. The results of the Breast Cancer Prevention Trial showed nearly 50% reduction in breast cancer including DCIS (3); the Multiple Outcomes of Raloxifene Evaluation (MORE) trial of raloxifene also demonstrated substantial efficacy in reducing both invasive and noninvasive breast cancer (4). Implicit in each of these separable goals involving improvements of detection, prognosis, therapy, and prevention is the premise that a clearer understanding of the etiologic factors of DCIS will have ramifications for disease management.

Unfortunately, at present, virtually none of our approaches to DCIS is based on specific etiologic considerations. Because we have no basis for considering any DCIS lesion to be nonprogressive, all cases are managed as though they share an approximately equivalent potential for malignant progression. We already know enough about cancer to be reasonably sure that this premise is false. Despite this, all

therapy currently involves surgical extirpation and/or sterilization with radiation (5,6). The same lack of mechanistic or etiologic approaches applies to detection. Virtually all efforts at earlier detection are based on radiographic changes visible on mammography rather than on any ability to analyze sera, urine, or nipple fluid aspirates for any products of sufficient specificity or sensitivity to diagnose noninvasive cancer. Recently, the ability to obtain large numbers of cells by duct lavage has become significantly more available (7). Whether analyses of cells or fluid obtained will enhance diagnostic techniques remains to be seen. Finally, essentially all prevention efforts to date are based on reasonable but oversimplified assumptions about hormonal promotion of cancer. More specific interventions based on genetic changes that accompany DCIS are hopes for the future at best.

ETIOLOGIC STUDIES

Possibly the most important reason to study DCIS is to obtain a fundamental understanding of its etiologic factors. DCIS presumably provides an early lesion in which the complete malignant phenotype of unlimited growth, invasiveness, metastatic potential, angiogenesis, and genomic elasticity has not been fully expressed. Because of the fact that at least some of these lesions will unequivocally progress to fully invasive and potentially lethal breast cancers, it is an additional reasonable presumption that interventions based on earlier changes responsible for noninvasive breast cancers could also have implications for invasive breast tumors.

Although most human breast cancers, invasive or otherwise, are made up of transformed epithelial cells of breast origin, their relatively similar morphology unquestionably masks a variety of diverse genetic changes that vary from one cancer to another. If we envision a series of phenotypic properties of malignancy such as growth or mitogenesis, immortalization, invasiveness, angiogenesis, metastasis, defeat of apoptosis, and normal senescence as steps along the pathway to full malignant potential, it is highly plausible that one or more members of groups of functionally nonover-

Metastasis	Angiogenesis	Invasion	Mitogenesis	Antiapoptosis	Immortalization
Met Gene 1	Ang Gene 1	Inv Gene 1	Mito Gene 1	Anti-ap Gene 1	Immort Gene 1
Met Gene 2	Ang Gene 2	Inv Gene 2	Mito Gene 2	Anti-ap Gene 2	Immort Gene 2
Met Gene 3	Ang Gene 3	Inv Gene 3	Mito Gene 3	Anti-ap Gene 3	Immort Gene 3
Met Gene 4	Ang Gene 4	Inv Gene 4	Mito Gene 4	Anti-ap Gene 4	Immort Gene 4

FIGURE 2.1. A theoretical explanation for the molecular diversity of breast cancer resulting in its highly variable clinical behavior.

lapping or partially overlapping genes may be responsible for each of these steps. Obviously, there are likely to be many other steps, each potentially dysregulated by more than one candidate gene (8). This is schematically shown in Figure 2.1.

Several different genes or groups of genes may each be able to render cells resistant to apoptosis, capable of inducing an angiogenic response, or unlimited growth, and so on. Each DCIS lesion, in theory, should be made up of most of whatever number of different steps or phenotypic effects must be expressed to derive a malignancy. Expression of all the phenotypic effects is the definition of invasive malignancy. Complexity and variability in natural history and response to therapy may be increased by having different genes or gene groups responsible for each of these phenotypic effects. Thus, as a simple model (Fig. 2.1), if there are four different genes that could induce angiogenesis, invasiveness, or growth, or defeat apoptosis and we hypothesize six different phenotypic effects required for a completed malignancy, there would be 4,096 combinations of genetic alterations that could lead to metastatic breast cancer. Thus, it is not difficult to explain the enormous diversity of behavior for both noninvasive and invasive breast cancers that share relatively common morphologies. It is likely that some combinations are substantially more common than others. In fact, perhaps a very limited number of genes may represent bottlenecks that are common targets for mutations in many cases. It is also likely that expression of one gene may specify other unique genes that will define a "pathway" to

malignancy. Thus, the overexpression of erbB2 (HER-2/neu) is never acquired after the development of DCIS.

In some cases, many more than four candidate genes have been identified that can drive some of these phenotypic effects. Figure 2.2 provides a few examples of candidate genes in each of the aforementioned phenotypic classes. Undoubtedly, there are many more. Mechanistically, it is important to distinguish between critical genes, which are epigenetically activated, e.g., as downstream targets of activated oncogenes, and genes actually targeted by genetic mechanisms such as gene amplification, mutation, and deletion because these are the true etiologic genes. Therapeutic strategies may be effective against either group.

Another remarkably interesting question raised by DCIS is whether there is any particular order in which the genes responsible for malignant transformation need to be either activated or inactivated. One could, for example, envision a DCIS lesion fully capable of invasiveness but limited in its growth because of the failure to express angiogenic molecules. In such a case, the expression of angiogenesis would potentially lead to an invasive breast cancer fully capable of metastasis. Conversely, a DCIS lesion lacking both angiogenic potential and invasiveness might grow to a large palpable mass if the genes controlling angiogenesis were activated while pathways for invasiveness remained dormant. It is also possible to hypothesize that there are hierarchical pathways for activation of these genes. For example, germline BRCA1 or 1 mutation, inactivation of p53 or overexpression of erbB2 occurring as relatively early events

Metastasis Genes (6,7)	Angiogenic Genes (8–10)	Invasion Genes (11, 12)	Mitogenic Genes (13–15)	Antiapoptosis Genes (16–18)	Immortalization Genes (19, 20)
nm23	VEGF's 1–3	UpA	EGFR	bcl-2	Telomerase
KA1	FGF's 1–9	MMP's	erbB-2	p53	
Multiple Candidate LOH's	PTN	Stromolysin 3	Heregulin	p16	
	Tie 1 & 2	Cathepsin D	EGFR ligands	Rb	
			IGF's		
			Cyclins		

FIGURE 2.2. LOH, loss of heterozygosity; VEGF, vascular endothelial cell growth factor; FGF, fibroblast growth factor; PTN, pleiotrophin; UPA, plasminogen activator; MMP, matrix metalloproteinase; EGFR, epidermal growth factor receptor; IGF, insulin-like growth factor; SAGE, serial analysis of gene expression.

may make other genetic changes more or less likely so that DCIS lesions may have preferred pathways for further malignant transformation.

Various other genes clearly are more difficult to categorize with respect to specific phenotypic effects but just as clearly can contribute to pathogenesis of DCIS. These include quantitative alterations in expression and/or mutations of estrogen receptor (24), myc (25), ras (26), BRCA1 (27), BRCA2 (28), and other genes critically involved in their signaling cascades. These signal transducing molecules may contribute to disease pathogenesis by either abrogating requirements for normal growth factors such as estrogens or altering the sensitivity to them or the pathways they control. Also critical in this category are genes that destabilize the genome and increase the rate of somatic mutation.

GENETIC CHANGES UNDERLYING DUCTAL CARCINOMA IN SITU

The current semidogmatic view of breast cancer suggests that the disease represents a clonal proliferation of malignantly transformed cells based on sequential acquisition of specific mutational changes. It is reasonable that genetic changes of profound significance may precede any morphologic evidence of transformation. The converse is not likely to be true. However, the genetic changes that underlie the disease, although beginning to be unearthed, clearly have a long way to go. There are remarkably sensitive and specific technologies evolving on an almost daily basis for identifying these genetic changes. These include measures of losses of heterozygosity such as single-strand conformation polymorphism, detection of amplicons involved in overexpression of specific genes, and chromosomal rearrangements leading to alterations in expression and point mutations. A series of technologies ranging from comparative genome hybridization, serial analysis of gene expression, subtraction hybridization, and other novel sequencing strategies are all yielding new information (29,30).

Three remarkable new technologies hold much promise for the molecular analysis of DCIS. First, laser capture microdissection provides a reliable, reasonably inexpensive means of sampling individual cells with a given lesion (31). Thus, DCIS cells can be obtained and compared with directly adjacent normal cells or regions of microinvasion. CDNA libraries can be constructed from these cells and used for gene array studies as described next.

Gene arrays have now made possible the semiquantitative analysis of thousands of expressed genes (32). Rather than focusing on individual genes, patterns of expression permit classification of tumors into known subsets and even, remarkably, the identification of new groupings unrecognizable on morphologic bases (33). Such analyses have been preliminarily applied to breast cancer with early indications suggesting that an eventual molecular classification

is likely to succeed (34). Parallel studies on DCIS are urgently needed.

Finally, once novel candidate genes of interest have been identified, they need to be analyzed for their biologic significance in the context of large data sets of DCIS material. The recent development of tumor array technology makes this possible (35). It is possible to serially array small core biopsies from preexistent pathology blocks such that 500 or more samples can be arrayed on a slide. Thus, entire retrospective data sets on clinical trials materials can be analyzed in a parsimonious way and the validity of potential markers associated with disease or outcome examined.

These various technologies will, it is hoped, allow the addressing of a series of critical questions that underlie disease pathogenesis.

First, what alterations of gene expression lead to DCIS? Obviously, as mentioned previously, it is virtually certain that genetic changes precede morphologic changes. Preliminary information from several groups has already suggested that cells that appear morphologically normal in the vicinity of DCIS can be shown to harbor some of the specific losses in heterozygosity (presumably reflecting inactivation of tumor suppressor genes) that are found in adjacent malignant cells. Once such candidate genes are identified, various strategies including knockout mice, transfection studies, and other approaches need to be employed to pathogenetically support a role for these genes in disease progression. Geographic mapping within the breast can be used to both molecularly stage disease extent and answer fundamental questions about the so-called field effects (discussed later) (36,37). If these criteria can be met, such genes (and their protein products) become obvious potential sites of attack in developing new therapies and/or products that may be useful in disease prognosis or detection. Expanding almost as rapidly as the field of genomics is that of proteomics (31,32). Analysis of nipple fluid as well as microdissected DCIS cells by these techniques may allow identification of critical proteins whose expression is either pathogenetically significant or a potential surrogate marker of malignancy.

Second, as previously alluded to, it is likely that multiple patterns of alteration in gene expression can lead to DCIS. Some of these patterns may either be more favored and therefore more common. These patterns of expression of multiple genes required for DCIS may also provide important evidence on pathways that are invoked in the malignant transformation process. Effective therapy need not be based on interference with a causative gene product but could involve interference with signaling through a specific pathway with therapy directed toward downstream effector molecules.

The third critical area that can be explored in such etiologic studies involves the natural history of DCIS. It is plausible (although largely unproven) that some DCIS lesions may eventually regress. Other lesions may be nearly certain to progress, whereas other lesions may, in fact, represent genetic dead ends with a very low likelihood of further progression. Morphologically, these three classes of lesions are likely to be nearly indistinguishable from each other, although histologic subtyping may provide some help. It is to be hoped that molecular dissection may permit specific therapies directed against these gene products to be employed eventually or to make decisions about their overall malignant potential.

Fourth, such etiologic studies may help to address one of the most vexing issues in DCIS. How much of DCIS represents a single cell that has undergone multiple genetic effects and how much represents field effects restricted to a region of the breast or to the entire breast or even the host in the form of genetic predisposition? An example of this could be altered host abilities to repair DNA damage. There are as yet no sufficiently powerful studies that actually allow a molecular understanding of either multifocality or multicentricity. How many of these lesions represent field effects, host effects, or true semisynchronous lesions is largely unknown and will remain so until their chromosomal and genetic lineage's can be traced to uncover common ancestors. These sorts of studies have the most profound importance for deciding how extensive therapy needs to be and, furthermore, at what point in time such therapy needs to begin. If multiple DCIS lesions scattered throughout either or both breasts (as in lobular neoplasia) can be traced to genetic defects that are preexistent to clinical disease by years or even decades, it is obvious that a variety of alternative strategies will need to be employed for optimal treatment of the disease.

CONCLUDING REMARKS

This introduction has tried to look at DCIS more from the viewpoint of the decades to follow than our current very restricted knowledge base. In many respects, we already have effective therapy for DCIS, it is simply too radical or noxious in many cases. Although it is always possible that empirically discovered agents or approaches will be able to successfully manage the patient with DCIS, it seems more likely that eventual biologic solutions to this disease will be based on the varying etiologic factors that underlie the disease.

ACKNOWLEDGMENT

Many colleagues including Vered Stearn, Craig Allred, Daniel Hayes, and the late Helene Smith improved this manuscript substantially by their helpful ideas or suggestions.

REFERENCES

1. Hetelekidis S, Schnitt SJ, Morrow M, et al. Management of ductal carcinoma in situ. *Cancer J Clin* 1995;45:244–253.
2. Page DL, Dupont WD, Rogers LW, et al. Continued local recurrence of carcinoma 15–25 years after a diagnosis of low grade ductal carcinoma in situ of the breast treated only by biopsy. *Cancer* 1995;76:1197–1200.
3. Fisher, B, Costantino JP, Wickerham DL, et al. Tamoxifen for prevention of breast Cancer: Report of the National Surgical Adjuvant Breast and Bowel Project P-1 Study. *J Natl Cancer Inst* 1998;90:1371–1388.
4. Cummings S, Eckert S, Krueger K, et al. The effect of raloxifene on risk of breast cancer in postmenopausal women under age 60. *Obstet Gynecol* 1999;95:104–110.
5. Silverstein MJ, Barth A, Poller DN, et al. Ten-year results comparing mastectomy to excision and radiation therapy for ductal carcinoma in situ of the breast. *Eur J Can* 1995;31A:1425–1427.
6. Solin LJ, Kurtz J, Fourquet A, et al. Fifteen-year results of breast-conserving surgery and definitive breast irradiation for the treatment of ductal carcinoma in situ of the breast. *J Clin Oncol* 1996;14:754–763.
7. Shen K-W, Shen Z-Z, Nguyen M, et al. Fiberoptic ductoscopy for patients with nipple discharge. 23rd Annual San Antonio Breast Cancer Symposium. *Breast Cancer Res Treat* 2000;64:30 (abst 18).
8. Murphy DS, Hoare SF, Going JJ, et al. Characterization of extensive genetic alterations in ductal carcinoma in situ by fluorescence in situ hybridization and molecular analysis. *J Natl Cancer Inst* 1995;87:1694–1704.
9. Howlett AR, Petersen OW, Steeg PS, et al. A novel function for the nm23-h1 gene: overexpression in human breast carcinoma cells leads to the formation of basement membrane and growth arrest. *J Natl Cancer Inst* 1994;86:1838–1844.
10. Hennessy C, Henry JA, May FE, et al. Expression of the antimetastatic gene nm23 in human breast cancer: an association with good prognosis. *J Natl Cancer Inst* 1991;83:281–285.
11. Fregene TA, Kellogg CM, Pienta KJ. Microvessel quantification as a measure of angiogenic activity in benign breast tissues lesions. A marker for precancerous disease? *Int J Oncol* 1994;4:1199–1202.
12. Mustonen T, Alitalo K. Endothelial receptor tyrosine kinases involved in angiogenesis. *J Cell Biol* 1995;129:895–898.
13. Lai S, Czubayko F, Riegel AT, et al. Structure of the human heparin-binding growth factor gene pleiotrophin. *Biochem Biophys Res Commun* 1992;187:1113–1122.
14. Ruoslahti E, Reed JC. Anchorage dependence, integrins, and apoptosis. *Cell* 1994;77:477–478.
15. Witty JP, Lempka T, Coffey RJ Jr, et al. Decreased tumor formation in 7,12-dimethylbenzanthracene-treated stromelysin-1 transgenic mice is associated with alterations in mammary epithelial cell apoptosis. *Cancer Res* 1995;55:1401–1406.
16. Goustin AS, Leof EB, Shipley GD, et al. Growth factors and cancer. *Cancer Res* 1986;46:1015–1029.
17. Mansour SJ, Matten WT, Hermann AS, et al. Transformation of mammalian cells by constitutively active MAP kinase kinase. *Science* 1994;265:966–970.
18. Quinn KA, Treston AM, Unsworth EJ, et al. Insulin-like growth factor expression in human cancer cell lines. *J Biol Chem* 1996;271:11477–11483.
19. Thompson CB. Apoptosis in the pathogenesis and treatment of disease. *Science* 1995;267:1456–1462.
20. Park JR, Hockenbery DM. BCL-2, a novel regulator of apoptosis. *J Cell Biochem* 1996;60:12–17.
21. Elledge RM, Lee WH. Life and death by p53. *Bioessays* 1995;17:923–930.
22. Hiyama E, Gollahon L, Kataoka T, et al. Telomerase activity in human breast tumors. *J Natl Cancer Inst* 1996;88:116–122.
23. Bacchetti S, Counter CM. Telomeres and telomerase in human cancer (review). *Int J Oncol* 7:423–432, 1995.
24. Leygue ER, Watson PH, Murphy LC. Estrogen receptor variants in normal human mammary tissue. *J Natl Cancer Inst* 1996;88:284–290.

25. Dubik D, Shiu RP. Mechanism of estrogen activation of *c-myc* oncogene expression. *Oncogene* 1992;7:1587–1594.

26. Clark GJ, Der CJ. Aberrant function of the ras signal transduction pathway in human breast cancer. *Breast Cancer Res Treat* 1995;35:133–144.

27. Shattuck-Eidens D, McClure M, Simard J, et al. A collaborative survey of 80 mutations in the brca1 breast and ovarian cancer susceptibility gene. implications for presymptomatic testing and screening. *JAMA* 1995;273:535–541.

28. Marcus JN, Watson P, Page DL, et al. Hereditary breast cancer. *Cancer* 1996;77:697–709.

29. Schrock E, du Manoir S, Veldman T, et al. Multicolor spectral karyotyping of human chromosomes. *Science* 1996;273:492–498.

30. Velculescu VE, Zhang L, Vogelstein B, et al. Serial analysis of gene expression. *Science* 1995;270:484–487.

31. Emmert-Buck MR, et al. Laser capture microdissection. *Science* 1996;274:998–1001.

32. Singh-Gasson S, Green RD, Yue Y, et al. Maskless fabrication of light-directed oligonucleotide microarrays using a digital micromirror array. *Nat Biotechnol* 1999;17:974–978.

33. Alizadeh AA, Eisen MB, Davis RE, et al. Distinct types of diffuse large B-cell lymphoma Identified by gene expression profiling. *Nature* 2000;403:503–511.

34. Perou CM, Jeffrey SS, van de Rijn M, et al. Distinctive gene expression patterns in Human mammary epithelial cells and breast cancers. *Proc Natl Acad Sci U S A* 1999;96:9212–9217.

35. Schraml P, Kononen J, Bubendorf L, et al. Tissue microarrays for gene amplification surveys in many different tumor types. *Clin Cancer Res* 1999;5:1966–1975.

36. Jensen RA, Page DL, Holt JT. Identification of genes expressed in premalignant breast disease by microscopy-directed cloning. *Proc Natl Acad Sci U S A* 1994;91:9257–9261.

37. Connolly JL, Harris JR, Schnitt SJ. Understanding the distribution of cancer within the breast is important for optimizing breast-conserving treatment. *Cancer* 1995;76:1–45.

3

THE NATURAL HISTORY OF DUCTAL CARCINOMA IN SITU OF THE BREAST

DAVID L. PAGE
LOWELL W. ROGERS
PEGGY A. SCHUYLER
WILLIAM D. DUPONT
ROY A. JENSEN

The original concept of carcinoma in situ (CIS) recognizes that cells in a normal location could have the appearance of invasive carcinoma. The biologic and clinical implications of CIS have been complicated by controversy at every body site. The variety of histologic and cytologic patterns of CIS and atypia found in the lobular units and ducts of the breast have further confounded the process of consensus. Recognition of the natural history of ductal carcinoma in situ (DCIS) of the breast and acceptance of these uncommon lesions as nonobligate but definite local precursors of invasive cancer is the topic of this chapter.

DCIS is a precursor of invasive carcinoma in the breast. The evidence comes from two remarkably similar studies from the premammographic era (1–3). This conclusion is forcefully supported by observations of recurrence patterns after local removal in the mammographic era; almost all recurrences after attempted excision are adjacent to the original lesion and represent reappearance of residual disease (4–6). Subsequent occurrence of invasive carcinoma in these local recurrences is of sufficient frequency to be of real clinical concern and necessitates therapeutic removal of DCIS lesions.

It is important to note that each piece of evidence is era-limited. We must also take into account that varied histologic definitions have applied to the diagnosis of DCIS. Recognition of atypical ducal hyperplasia (ADH) as a lesion limited in size (as well as completeness or purity of population of abnormal cells) has refined and confined the definition of DCIS (7–9). These ADH lesions are well proven to indicate increased risk anywhere in the breast as opposed to the local/regional indication of risk for DCIS (10–15): a fundamental and important difference.

HISTOLOGIC CASE DEFINITION

Precise case definition is importantly related to considerations of diagnostic and therapeutic patterns that change with time. Although small DCIS was not diagnosed in the 1950s and most of the 1960s (giving us the series of patients from Vanderbilt and Memorial discussed below) (1,2), ADH as we know it today was often diagnosed as DCIS in the 1970s. Thus, precise definition of lesions less than DCIS has diverse implications. In the cohorts studied by the major large series, the definitions seem quite close and consistent in incidence and natural histories (1–3).

The minimal lesions of DCIS recognized in the major follow-up studies are basically noncomedo, small, and low-grade (1–3). The classic patterns (usually cribriform) have uniform cytology and evenly placed cells. When measuring 5 to 8 mm in extent, the lesions are generally accepted as examples of DCIS (usually constituting minimal DCIS, because the even smaller lesions are usually ADH). Lesions of ADH are usually less then 3 mm in overall size and confined to an individual lobular unit (7,16,17). These size considerations provide guidelines rather than precise definitions in each case, because cytology and histologic pattern may vary. In most cases, pathologists agree if guidelines of histologic definition are given (9). The diversity of these lesions includes examples in which most spaces (bound by basement membrane) are not completely involved by the same population of cells; i.e., a polarized population remains related to the outer basement membrane while the atypical population is in the center of the space (7). Generally, even when two basement membrane–bound spaces (usually distended acini in a lobular unit) are involved, the overall size of the involved area is over 3 mm and the case is regarded as a minimal DCIS (2). Therefore, each diagnostic approach (extent and number of spaces completely involved) recognizes essentially the same cases. There are a small number of cases that may be most appropriately recognized as occupying the borderline between ADH and DCIS. Most of these cases are probably best understood as large examples of ADH. In our review of biopsies performed based on the indication of clinical palpation (thus the ADH and minimal DCIS lesions are clinically 'occult'), we used the guidelines that lesser lesions (ADH) had incomplete involvement of individual basement membrane–bound spaces because we did not have the whole lesion (by mammography or serial sectioning) (7,8). With complete removal of mammographically identified lesions, larger size became a more useful measure (18) when we had complete sampling of the cases and margins could be evaluated.

HETEROGENEITY OF HISTOLOGIC PATTERNS

With increased understanding of their differing natural histories, the importance of accepting high and low-grade variants, however recognized, is clear. Heterogeneity of DCIS is mentioned here to emphasize that the major underpinning of the natural history with long-term follow-up presented here is of the lower grade lesions only. Clear proof that DCIS that co-exists with an invasive carcinoma usually shares grade and known tumor markers has been found (19,20). We had some information about high-grade DCIS from the 1950s when excision of palpable, comedo DCIS was followed by recurrence within 3 to 4 years in over 50% of cases (21), of which many were invasive. Clearly, the time frame of the two follow-up cohort studies reported in 1978 and 1982 (1–3) is quite different from high-grade DCIS, because the later invasive carcinomas occurred much later (some occurring over 15 years later).

NATURAL HISTORY OF DUCTAL CARCINOMA IN SITU AFTER PARTIAL REMOVAL AT BIOPSY

When identified in biopsies from the premammographic era (1950s and 1960s) done for palpable lumps in which the ADH or minimal DCIS was not clinically apparent, a later incidence of invasive cancer in the same site of the same breast was found (approaching 50%). These recurrences in the premammographic era were prolonged over 15 to 20 years, although most cancers had been identified by 5 to 6 years (1–3).

In the series of patients followed after biopsy alone, a remarkable similarity was found: each researcher reviewing approximately 10,000 biopsies found an incidence of DCIS approaching 0.3% (1,3). The later event was not recurrence of DCIS [except for a single case (3)]; it was presentation of invasive carcinoma (in the premammographic era). More than a third of these patients died of breast cancer (3). The local/regional recurrence in all these cases is strong evidence for the largely committed nature of precursor status of these lesions (although prolonged in time). Since the last update of this series, another case of invasive carcinoma approximately 9 years after biopsy has been identified, with no further deaths (Fig. 3.1). One woman in the Vanderbilt series was diagnosed 25 years after original biopsy with a large DCIS (5 cm) detected by palpation (with minimal DCIS in the same area of the same breast at initial, entry biopsy).

A point of clarification with regard to the nature of the evidence from these two series of patients undergoing

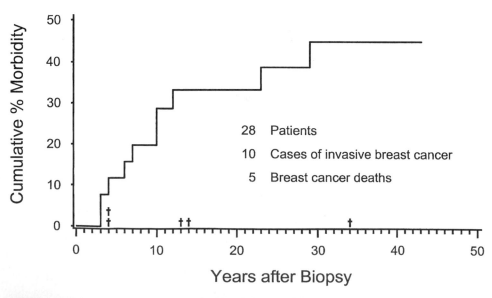

FIGURE 3.1. Morbidity and mortality graph of follow-up of the women with ductal carcinoma in situ diagnosed in biopsies performed in Nashville, Tennessee from 1950 to 1968 (2,3) updated as of 2001 by the authors. Deaths from breast cancer are noted by crosses at the bottom of the figure.

biopsy in the 1950s and 1970s: The natural history depends on the fact that some of the lesions sampled were probably removed entirely and some parts were left behind. These lesions were not recognized at the time of clinical biopsy and pathologic examination. Some evidence for this comes from two studies at about that time that recognized DCIS at biopsy and later sampled the mastectomies that were often negative for remaining DCIS (approximately 40% of the time) (22,23).

"MULTICENTRICITY" AS A MISCONCEPTION

It is now clear that the perceived multifocality of DCIS was partly the result of quite rare cases (usually with Paget's disease) that were extensive and in several or even in all quadrants of the breast. However, careful three-dimensional reconstruction of DCIS indicated that even extensive examples of DCIS are unifocal in three dimensions and usually confined to a single segment of the breast quadrant (24). The concept of multicentricity has been largely dispelled by the three-dimensional reconstruction studies of Lagios (25) and Holland and colleagues (24), but has been completely dispelled by the knowledge that recurrences of locally excised DCIS are almost overwhelmingly in the region of the original lesion and represent continued growth of inadequately excised lesions. One of the major reasons for believing in multicentricity was the inadequate sampling of mastectomy specimens (26,27) and the frequent apparent multicentricity of sampling in two (rather than three) dimensions, because the branching duct system often produces seemingly separated DCIS that is actually present in different branches of the same duct system (Fig. 3.2).

INCIDENCE OF DUCTAL CARCINOMA IN SITU AT AUTOPSY

Incidence at autopsy in women dying for other reasons is quite consistent in the literature, with the exception of one group from Denmark (28–33). If we delete the outlier, large incidence figures from Denmark, the evidence of the incidence of DCIS from autopsy series is clear, although widely misunderstood. The incidence of histologically, rigorously diagnosed DCIS is basically low (in the range of 1%), with variation for age and cancer incidence of the population studied. The most useful of these studies are those of Bartow et al. (34,35), which included mammographic detectability. Using the same criteria as Page and Rogers (7), the incidence of ADH and DCIS was similar to that found in a large premammographic biopsy series from the 1950s and 1960s (13). Further adding credibility to findings from this cohort was the lower incidence of these lesions in women from low-risk groups in New Mexico (34,35) and the clear restriction

to women dying suddenly from trauma although in apparent good health. This series is the most informative because it combines radiographic detection with a forensic series of women dying unexpectedly by trauma. The incidence is almost the same as that found in the Nashville cohort (8,13), and most lesions were ascertained by mammography (35).

The classic studies of Wellings and Jensen (36) also include breast evaluation at autopsy. The results are relevant and useful because the histology was rigorously and uniformly evaluated, focusing on the 'subgross' appearance of lesions that identified enlarged lobular units with subsequent classical histologic evaluation. Atypical hyperplastic lesions of level 3 to 4 (in a score of 1 to 5) were quite rare, with 5 (CIS) very uncommon, even in the 'cancer-associated' breasts.

Although often quoted as a foundation for a much higher incidence of "CIS" in breast at autopsy, the studies of Andersen, Nielsen, and colleagues (28–33) reported that "based on recent Danish autopsy studies, it has been estimated that about 25% of all women will develop in situ carcinoma, predominantly in the form of DCIS. Only a fraction of these lesions will evolve into a clinical manifest form." Of course, it is precisely this 'fraction' that makes us consider likelihood and degree of risk as a necessary part of our analysis. One of their studies was a medicolegal series of women averaging 39 years of age with a reported DCIS incidence of 18% (33). The flaw in these studies is that although the entire breast was sampled, the reports were made by several pathologists without rigorous, agreed on criteria. The record (as documented in photographs from this group) indicates a photo of ADH and other photos of common or usual forms of hyperplasia. For example, in 1989, they reviewed their experience with women dying with a clinical diagnosis of breast cancer (32). The frequency of "malignant" histologic changes in the opposite breast (metastases or invasive and in situ breast carcinomas) was unexpectedly high (80%): a result far beyond any meaningful verification.

The Nashville cohort reported since 1985 (3,13) also represents a useful reference here, because it presents biopsies done on the indication of palpability and concern of cancer prior to mammography (1950 to 1968). This system basically selects a group of women with areas of relative increased density from fibrocystic changes and lack of postmenopausal involution to the soft consistency of fat. The incidence of small DCIS was 0.28%. This was the same experience as the Memorial (New York) series published at approximately the same time (1).

SUMMARY

We now know that in the majority of cases DCIS is relatively uncommon and limited to a single focus. When partially removed, DCIS will often recur locally as in situ disease but also

The non-multifocality of DCIS
"overlapping" duct systems

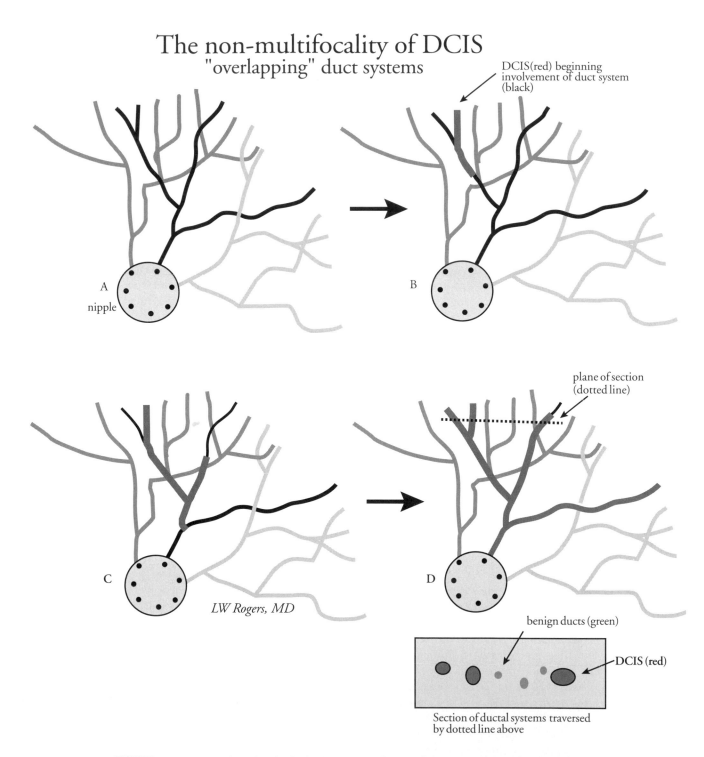

FIGURE 3.2. DCIS involves the single duct system in this case but may appear to be "multifocal" in two dimensional sampling. Intervening benign ducts in a tissue section seemingly suggest separate "foci" of DCIS, however three dimensional reconstructions (24) indicate that virtually all DCIS is continuous within ducts and thus unifocal.

frequently as invasive disease. When completely removed (a challenge for a disease traveling along the duct within a three-dimensional structure), local recurrence is unlikely, but the tissue in the conserved breast(s) remains at risk. Much of this information comes from follow-up of women with excision of DCIS, which is covered elsewhere in this volume.

REFERENCES

1. Betsill, Jr. WL, Rosen PP, Lieberman PH, et al. Intraductal carcinoma. Long-term follow-up after treatment by biopsy alone. *JAMA* 1978;239:1863–1867.
2. Page DL, Dupont WD, Rogers LW, et al. Intraductal carcinoma of the breast: follow-up after biopsy only. *Cancer* 1982;49:751–758.
3. Page DL, Dupont WD, Rogers LW, et al. Continued local recurrence of carcinoma 15–25 years after a diagnosis of low grade ductal carcinoma in situ of the breast treated only by biopsy. *Cancer* 1995;76:1197–1200.
4. Silverstein MJ, Lagios MD, Groshen S, et al. The influence of margin width on local control of ductal carcinoma in situ of the breast. *N Engl J Med* 1999;340:1455–1461.
5. Lagios MD. Heterogeneity of ductal carcinoma in situ of the breast. *J Cell Biochem* 1993;53:49–52.
6. Lagios MD, Margolin FR, Westdahl PR, et al. Mammographically detected duct carcinoma in situ. *Cancer* 1989;63:618–624.
7. Page DL, Rogers LW. Combined histologic and cytologic criteria for the diagnosis of mammary atypical ductal hyperplasia. *Hum Pathol* 1992;23:1095–1097.
8. Page DL, Dupont WD, Rogers LW, et al. Atypical hyperplastic lesions of the female breast. A long follow-up study. *Cancer* 1985;55:2698–2708.
9. Schnitt SJ, Connolly JL, Tavassoli FA, et al. Interobserver reproducibility in the diagnosis of ductal proliferative breast lesions using standardized criteria. *Am J Surg Pathol* 1992;16:1133–1143.
10. London SJ, Connolly JL, Schnitt SJ, et al. A prospective study of benign breast disease and risk of breast cancer. *JAMA* 1992;267:941–944.
11. Palli D, Rosselli del Turco M, Simoncini R, et al. Benign breast disease and breast cancer: A case-control study in a cohort in Italy. *Int J Cancer* 1991;47:703–706.
12. Marshall LM, Hunter DJ, Connolly JL, et al. Risk of breast cancer associated with atypical hyperplasia of lobular and ductal types. *Cancer Epidemiol Biomarkers Prev* 1997;6:297–301.
13. Dupont WD, Page DL. Risk factors for breast cancer in women with proliferative breast disease. *N Engl J Med* 1985;312:146–151.
14. Dupont WD, Parl FF, Hartmann WH, et al. Breast cancer risk associated with proliferative breast disease and atypical hyperplasia. *Cancer* 1993;71:1258–1265.
15. Fitzgibbons PL, Henson DE, Hutter RV. Benign breast changes and the risk for subsequent breast cancer: An update of the 1985 consensus statement. Cancer Committee of the College of American Pathologists. *Arch Pathol Lab Med* 1998;122:1053–1055.
16. Page DL, Jensen RA, Simpson JF. Premalignant and malignant disease of the breast: the roles of the pathologist. *Mod Pathol* 1998;11:120–128.
17. Page DL, Simpson JF. Ductal carcinoma in situ—the focus for prevention, screening, and breast conservation in breast cancer. *N Engl J Med* 1999;340:1499–1500.
18. Tavassoli FA, Norris HJ. A comparison of the results of long-term follow-up for atypical intraductal hyperplasia and intraductal hyperplasia of the breast. *Cancer* 1990;65:518–529.
19. Bijker N, Peterse JL, Duchateau L, et al. Histological type and marker expression of the primary tumour compared with its local recurrence after breast-conserving therapy for ductal carcinoma in situ. *Br J Cancer* 2001;84:539–544.
20. Goldstein NS, Murphy T. Intraductal carcinoma associated with invasive carcinoma of the breast. A comparison of the two lesions with implications for intraductal carcinoma classification systems. *Am J Clin Pathol* 1996;106:312–318.
21. Lewis D, Geschickter CF. Comedo carcinomas of the breast. *Arch Surg* 1938;36:225–244.
22. Carter D, Smith RR. Carcinoma in situ of the breast. *Cancer* 1977;40:1189–1193.
23. Rosen PP, Senie R, Schottenfeld D, et al. Noninvasive breast carcinoma: frequency of unsuspected invasion and implications for treatment. *Ann Surg* 1979;189:377–382.
24. Holland R, Hendriks J, Verbeek ALM, et al. Extent, distribution, and mammographic/histological correlations of breast ductal carcinoma in situ. *Lancet* 1990;335:519–522.
25. Lagios MD, Westdahl PR, Margolin FR, et al. Duct carcinoma in situ. Relationship of extent of noninvasive disease to the frequency of occult invasion, multicentricity, lymph node metastases, and short-term treatment failures. *Cancer* 1982;50:1309–1314.
26. Page DL. Breast disease in the 1990s: patchwork quilt and growth industry. *Am J Clin Pathol* 1993;99:225–226.
27. Johnson JE, Dutt PL, Page DL. Extent and multicentricity of in situ and invasive carcinoma. In: Bland KI, Copeland, III EM, eds. *The Breast: Comprehensive Management of Benign and Malignant Diseases*, 2nd ed. Philadelphia: WB Saunders, 1998:296–306.
28. Andersen J, Nielsen M, Christensen L. New aspects of the natural history of in situ and invasive carcinoma in the female breast. Results from autopsy investigations. *Verh Dtsch Ges Pathol* 1985;69:88–95.
29. Andersen J, Nielsen M, Christensen L, et al. The significance of the frequency and occurrence of breast cancer for treatment. Essential aspects of new Danish studies of the natural history of breast cancer. *Acta Chir Belg* 1987;87:103–107.
30. Nielsen M, Jensen J, Andersen J. Precancerous and cancerous breast lesions during lifetime and at autopsy. A study of 83 women. *Cancer* 1984;54:612–615.
31. Nielsen M, Christensen L, Andersen J. Contralateral cancerous breast lesions in women with clinical invasive breast carcinoma. *Cancer* 1986;57:897–903.
32. Nielsen M. Autopsy studies of the occurrence of cancerous, atypical and benign epithelial lesions in the female breast. *APMIS Suppl* 1989;10:1–56.
33. Nielsen M, Thomsen JL, Primdahl S, et al. Breast cancer and atypia among young and middle-aged women: a study of 110 medicolegal autopsies. *Br J Cancer* 1987;56:814–819.
34. Bartow SA, Pathak DR, Black WC, et al. Prevalence of benign, atypical, and malignant breast lesions in populations at different risk for breast cancer. A forensic autopsy study. *Cancer* 1987; 60: 2751–2760.
35. Bartow SA, Pathak DR, Mettler FA. Radiographic microcalcification and parenchymal patterns as indicators of histologic "high-risk" benign breast disease. *Cancer* 1990;66:1721–1725.
36. Wellings SR, Jensen HM, Marcum RG. An atlas of subgross pathology of the human breast with special reference to possible precancerous lesions. *J Natl Cancer Inst* 1975;55:231–273.

4

THE EPIDEMIOLOGY OF BREAST CARCINOMA IN SITU

LESLIE BERNSTEIN

Interest in the epidemiology of breast carcinoma in situ (CIS) has increased substantially in the past 10 years. Although breast CIS was first described in the 1930s (1), it remained a relatively rare diagnosis until the 1980s (2). Population-based cancer registries located throughout the world provide information on the growing incidence of this disease. The "epidemic" of breast CIS over the past two decades, observed throughout the United States and in Europe, has paralleled the increasing availability of mammographic screening (3); this raises the question of whether most of these additional diagnoses are a different biologic entity, i.e., an artifact, of increased screening in the population or are true precursors of invasive disease. What we know about risk factors for breast CIS is based almost entirely on studies of patients diagnosed in the 1980s and 1990s. Thus, these risk factor profiles may be influenced by the inclusion of screening-detected patients who might not have been clinically diagnosed with breast cancer during their lifetimes.

INCIDENCE RATES OF BREAST CARCINOMA IN SITU

Progressive increases in the incidence rates of breast CIS have been observed throughout the Western world since the 1980s (2,4–9). In the United States, the incidence rates reported for the nine Surveillance Epidemiology and End Results registries (10) show that among women under age 50 years, breast CIS incidence rates increased 146% for white women and 283% for black women between 1983 and 1997. For older women (aged 50 years or older), the percentage increases were even greater, with incidence rates increasing 308% among white women and 349% among black women. Although increases in incidence have also been observed for invasive breast cancer during this same period, these have been smaller and primarily confined to stage I disease. In 1997, breast CIS accounted for 16.4% of all breast cancers diagnosed among white women and 18.6% of

all breast cancers diagnosed among black women in Surveillance Epidemiology and End Results registry regions (10). Where data have been reported separately by histologic subtype of breast CIS, the increases in incidence are substantially greater for ductal CIS (DCIS) than for lobular CIS (LCIS) (2,4,6–9).

Los Angeles County, CA, has the most ethnically diverse population of any county in the United States; breast CIS incidence rates for Los Angeles County demonstrate broad variation by racial/ethnic group. Population-based cancer incidence registration was initiated in Los Angeles County in 1992. The marked temporal increase in DCIS in Los Angeles County is illustrated in Figure 4.1 in relation to invasive breast cancer and LCIS. Overall, annual age-adjusted incidence rates (standardized to the 1970 U.S. population) increased nearly sevenfold from 2.5 per 100,000 women in 1972 to 16.7 per 100,000 women in 1998. Between 1984 and 1989, the age-adjusted incidence rate for DCIS doubled from 5.1 to 10.2 per 100,000 women. Rates declined in 1989, but then increased 30% during the next 2 years. DCIS rates remained relatively stable during the early 1990s when the age-adjusted incidence rate was approximately 12 per 100,000 women. Incidence rates then increased 38% between 1994 and 1998. A threefold increase in LCIS incidence occurred between 1972 to 1998 with rates increasing from 0.8 to 2.4 per 100,000 women. Most of this increase occurred during the mid-1980s, and Los Angeles County incidence rates appear to have reached a plateau in recent years. During this same time frame, invasive breast cancer incidence rates increased 20% from 86.8 per 100,000 women in 1972 to 112.1 per 100,000 women in 1998.

The age-specific patterns of incidence for Los Angeles County for the 27-year period 1972 to 1998 are shown in Figure 4.2. DCIS rates peak at ages 70 to 74 years, whereas LCIS rates peak at ages 45 to 49 years. The age-specific patterns of DCIS incidence have changed over time and in the 1990s. The incidence patterns reflect a bimodal distribution with peak rates among women 50 to 59 years as well as women 70 to 74 years of age, suggesting a larger contribu-

Rate/100,000

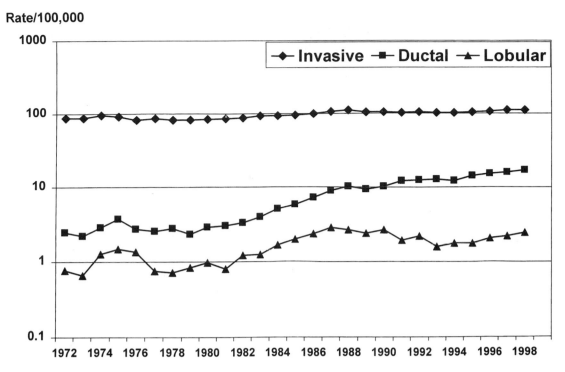

FIGURE 4.1. Annual age-adjusted incidence rates of invasive breast cancer, ductal carcinoma in situ, and lobular carcinoma in situ per 100,000 women in Los Angeles County, CA, from 1972 through 1998. Rates include women of all racial/ethnic groups. Rates are standardized to the 1970 U.S. population.

Rate/100,000

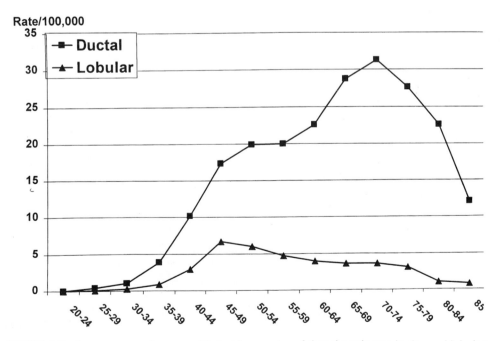

FIGURE 4.2. Average annual age-specific incidence rates of ductal carcinoma in situ and lobular carcinoma in situ per 100,000 women in Los Angeles County, CA, over the period 1972 to 1998. Rates include women of all racial/ethnic groups.

TABLE 4.1. AVERAGE ANNUAL AGE-ADJUSTED INCIDENCE RATES OF BREAST CARCINOMA IN SITU (CIS) AND INVASIVE BREAST CANCER AMONG WOMEN RESIDING IN LOS ANGELES COUNTY, CA, ALL RACIAL/ETHNIC GROUPS COMBINED (RATES STANDARDIZED TO THE 1970 U.S. POPULATION)

Period	Breast CIS	Invasive Breast Cancer	% Breast CIS
1972–1981	3.8	86.1	4.2
1982–1986	6.8	94.0	6.8
1987–1991	13.0	104.7	11.0
1992–1996	15.3	103.3	12.9
1997–1998	19.7	111.5	15.0

tion of tumors detected by mammographic screening. Based on Los Angeles County incidence rates, the contribution of breast CIS to the overall burden of breast cancer has increased over the past 27 years, from 4% of the overall rate in the time period 1972 through 1981 to more than 15% of the rate in the period 1997 to 1998 (Table 4.1).

Incidence rates of invasive and in situ breast cancer vary substantially by ethnic groups in Los Angeles (Fig. 4.3). Non-Hispanic white women have the highest age-adjusted incidence rates of invasive breast cancer, DCIS, and LCIS (110.9, 8.8, and 2.3 per 100,000 women, respectively). Al-

though black women have the second highest incidence rates of invasive breast cancer and LCIS (88.0 and 0.9 per 100,000 women, respectively), their incidence rates of DCIS (7.2 per 100,000 women) are slightly lower than those of Japanese women (7.6 per 100,000 women).

MAMMOGRAPHY

Generally, the increasing incidence in breast CIS (and particularly DCIS) is attributed to increased use of screening mammography (2,3). During the 1980s, the number of mammography machines available in the United States grew exponentially from only 134 in 1982 to a projected 10,000 in 1990 (11). Most women have now had at least one mammogram; a Behavioral Risk Factor Surveillance System report indicates that the percentage of U.S. women aged 40 years or older who have had at least one mammogram increased from 64% to 84% in the relatively short period between 1989 and 1997 (12).

Breast cancer screening programs report diagnosing a greater proportion of DCIS relative to invasive breast cancer than would be expected based on the percentages of each type of tumor ascertained by population-based cancer registries. For example, among asymptomatic women with no palpable lesion undergoing their first screening mammo-

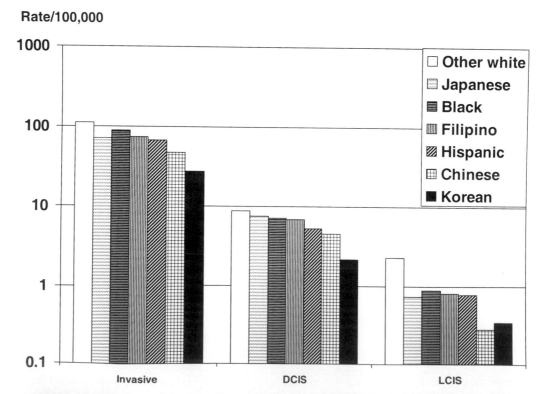

FIGURE 4.3. Average annual age-adjusted incidence rates of invasive breast cancer, ductal carcinoma in situ (DCIS) and lobular carcinoma in situ (LCIS) per 100,000 women in Los Angeles County, CA, classified by racial/ethnic subgroup, over the period 1972 to 1998. Rates are standardized to the 1970 U.S. population.

gram in a San Francisco–based breast screening program from 1985 through 1997, nearly 30% of the breast cancers detected among women aged 40 years or older were DCIS (3). A population-based study of breast cancer among women under age 45 years found that nearly 60% of women with breast CIS had their tumor detected by routine mammogram compared with only 18% of those with localized invasive breast cancer and 8% of those with regional disease or distant metastases (13). Even among low-risk Asian women, the yield of DCIS in screening programs is relatively high. DCIS comprised 26% of the breast cancers diagnosed among primarily Chinese women aged 50 years or older in a screening program in Singapore (14).

Nevertheless, it has been suggested that mammography alone does not account for all the increase in the incidence rates observed for breast CIS. Data from the metropolitan Atlanta Surveillance Epidemiology and End Results registry for the years 1979 through 1986 show that asymptomatic tumors (those detected solely by mammography) accounted for only 25% to 40% of the increase in incidence observed in that geographic area (15). However, these statistics are not likely representative of the incidence of screening-detected tumors in the United States in the 1990s.

Some additional data are available from the Tuscany (Italy) cancer registry where mammography screening by invitation has been underway since the 1970s (4). This population-based cancer registry classifies all patients newly diagnosed with breast CIS according to whether they were screen detected. Among women aged 50 to 69 years diagnosed with breast CIS from 1985 through 1995, 69% of the increase in breast CIS incidence (a 3.8-fold increase in incidence rates) can be attributed directly to mammographic screening.

The rapid increase in incidence of DCIS and the fact that screening mammography appears to be preferentially detecting DCIS raise some important questions about this epidemic. Would some DCIS remain undetected throughout women's lifetimes in the absence of screening? If so, how would we differentiate these lesions from those that will progress if left untreated? Do pathologists agree on the diagnosis of breast CIS or is there some degree of overdiagnosis? Certainly one illustration of the variation in diagnosis of DCIS comes from reliability studies or panel studies. For example, one carefully designed study of six experienced pathologists showed good agreement on the absence of DCIS, but poor agreement on its presence (complete agreement on only two of 10 cases in which at least one of the six pathologists diagnosed DCIS) (16). Some of the issues identified in terms of pathologic diagnosis of DCIS are the difficulties in separating low-grade DCIS from atypical intraductal hyperplasia and the accurate assessment of size or extent of DCIS (17). Because DCIS is a biologically and morphologically heterogeneous disease, it has been proposed that intraductal proliferative lesions (from intraductal hyperplasia to DCIS) be classified as mammary intraepithe-lial neoplasia, ductal type or as ductal intraepithelial neoplasia (17).

AUTOPSY SERIES

Autopsy series can provide some information on the prevalence of breast CIS in the female population that has existed undetected during women's lives. Results of these studies must be considered with caution, however. The selection of who undergoes an autopsy and whether selection criteria for autopsy change over time are potential sources of bias. The degree to which the pathologists involved in these studies scrutinize the breast in conducting autopsies will vary, presenting the possibility of detection bias in some series. The number of slides examined per breast in published autopsy series varies widely (18).

We might expect that the prevalence of undiagnosed breast cancer would decrease as the prevalence of mammographically screened women in the population has increased. Conversely, it is possible that autopsied women are not as likely to have undergone screening mammography. Welch and Black (18) reviewed reports of hospital-based and forensic autopsy series of women who had not been diagnosed with breast cancer during their lifetimes and summarized seven reports published between 1973 and 1987. In these studies, the median prevalence of undiagnosed invasive breast cancer was 1.3% (ranging from none to 1.8% observed) and that of undiagnosed DCIS was 8.9% (ranging from none to 14.7% observed). Three of the seven studies provided information on the prevalence of DCIS among women in the age range most likely to have been screened (40 to 70 years of age). For these women, the prevalence of DCIS ranged from 10% (in one study of women who were 50 to 70 years of age) to 39% (another study of women who were 40 to 49 years of age). With the exception of the one study with no DCIS identified conducted in 1987, the percentages of undiagnosed DCIS identified in autopsy series have increased over time. These results suggest that much CIS remains undiagnosed and that rates will continue to increase with increased usage of mammography and improvements in imaging technology.

NATURAL HISTORY OF BREAST CARCINOMA IN SITU

Early diagnosis of breast CIS by mammography would be expected to result in low rates of recurrence and death either because most of the in situ carcinomas that mammography detects are cancers that are clinically insignificant or biologically benign or because early treatment provides substantial protection against recurrence, progression, and death. Recurrence rates for DCIS will, of course, be affected by the type of treatment a woman receives; although based on clinical trial data, overall survival should be comparable irrespective of whether treatment is mastectomy or breast-conserving surgery with or without radiation and with or without tamoxifen therapy (19,20).

Two studies of women who were originally diagnosed as having benign breast disease on biopsy but who were found to have breast CIS at a later pathology review provide some information on the natural history of breast CIS. Twenty-eight women originally thought to have benign breast disease during the period 1950 through 1968 were later determined to have had small, noncomedo DCIS on re-review (21). These women have now been followed-up for more than 30 years. Seven developed invasive breast cancer in the same quadrant of the same breast as the DCIS occurrence within 10 years of the original DCIS diagnosis. Two women experienced invasive recurrences that were diagnosed 20 to 30 years after the initial excision; one patient had a recurrence of her DCIS 25 years later. In this series of patients, the overall risk of invasive disease was ninefold greater than that of women in the general population. Treatment by today's standards would likely have reduced the risk of invasive disease; however, this study confirms that even low-grade DCIS can be a precursor to invasive breast cancer. Similarly, among 80 patients with DCIS from Northern Italy who were followed-up for an average of 17.5 years, 11% developed ipsilateral invasive breast cancer and 5% developed ipsilateral DCIS (22). In addition, two contralateral invasive breast cancers and one contralateral DCIS were diagnosed. All these women had originally been diagnosed with benign breast disease on biopsy between 1964 and 1976; only two had comedo DCIS, a more frequent diagnosis in recent series (see below).

Boyages and colleagues (23) conducted a meta-analysis of the clinical literature on localized recurrence rates after DCIS treatment, comparing patients treated by breast-conserving surgery without radiation, those treated by breast-conserving surgery with radiation, and those treated by mastectomy. Women treated by breast-conserving surgery alone had a 22.5% recurrence rate, whereas the recurrence rate for those also given radiation was substantially lower (8.9%). For both these groups, approximately half of the recurrences were invasive. Among women treated by mastectomy alone, the recurrence rate was only 1.4%. High-grade tumors with necrosis, tumors with comedo features, and tumors with close or positive surgical margins were most predictive of a recurrence among women treated with breast-conserving surgery.

Data from the National Surgical Adjuvant Breast and Bowel Project (NSABP) randomized clinical trial of lumpectomy with and without radiation as a treatment for DCIS provide more recent information on recurrence for patients who were likely diagnosed by screening mammography (19). Compared with patients treated with surgical excision and radiation, those treated by excision only were significantly more likely to experience local recurrence or a

diagnosis of invasive breast cancer. In the patients treated only by surgical excision, the rate of localized recurrence after 8 years of follow-up was 27% versus 12% among those treated with surgery and radiation.

Population-based studies confirm the findings of clinical studies. Habel and colleagues evaluated the risk of recurrence among women diagnosed with DCIS who were treated with breast-conserving surgery (24) and the risk of contralateral breast cancer among all women diagnosed with breast CIS (25). Both studies were conducted in western Washington State. Approximately 15% of the 709 women comprising the cohort of women with DCIS who were treated with breast-conserving surgery experienced a recurrence within 5 years of diagnosis and 31% experienced a recurrence within 10 years (24). The risk of an invasive recurrence within 10 years of diagnosis was 8%, and the probability of dying of an invasive recurrence was 0.6%. Predictors of recurrence were tumor size (1.5+ cm tumor), comedo subtype, being premenopausal, and being obese. Others have shown that younger age (younger than 45 years) at diagnosis is associated with greater recurrence risk (26) and have attributed this to smaller excision volumes, possibly because of cosmetic concerns of younger women, and a greater likelihood that the DCIS of younger women is of high nuclear grade and has necrosis (27). High nuclear grade and necrosis in patients with DCIS are associated with estrogen receptor negativity, overexpression of HER-2/*neu* and p53 (28–30).

Habel and colleagues (25) also assessed the risk of contralateral breast cancer among 1,929 women with a first primary DCIS and 282 women with a first primary LCIS who had been diagnosed between 1973 and 1993. Twenty-nine women were diagnosed with breast CIS in their contralateral breast after their initial diagnosis, and 66 were diagnosed with a contralateral invasive breast cancer. Overall, the rate of contralateral CIS after primary breast CIS was exceptionally high relative to population rates [relative risk (RR) = 7.2 after DCIS and RR = 36.9 after LCIS] with the risk highest during the first year after the primary diagnosis. The RR of invasive disease was somewhat elevated (RR = 1.8 after DCIS and RR = 3.0 after LCIS), with the risk estimates fairly stable over time.

Franceschi and colleagues (31) evaluated the risk of invasive breast cancer after the diagnosis of breast CIS in a large population-based series of women in Switzerland who were initially diagnosed between 1977 and 1994. The risk of invasive breast cancer was seven times greater among women with prior breast CIS than would be predicted by prevailing breast cancer incidence rates. The cumulative incidence of invasive breast cancer was 24% after 15 years of follow-up. Risk was similarly elevated for women older and younger than 55 years of age. The risk when the first primary was LCIS was similar to that found when the first primary was DCIS, and the histology of the subsequent invasive cancer was usually the same as the CIS. It is noteworthy that in this population, mastectomy rates among patients with breast CIS were substantially lower than those reported by studies of U.S. populations (2,24) and that the subsequent invasive cancers were more likely to occur in the ipsilateral, rather than the contralateral, breast.

Ernster and colleagues (32) assessed mortality among women aged 40 and older who had been diagnosed with DCIS from 1978 through 1989 using data from the Surveillance Epidemiology and End Results registry program. The risk of dying from DCIS within 10 years of the woman's diagnosis was extremely low. Furthermore, women diagnosed from 1984 to 1989 were less likely to have died of their cancer than those diagnosed from 1978 to 1983, when the prevalence of screening mammography was low. The cumulative percentages of women who died of their disease at 5 years were 1.5% for the earlier period and 0.7% for the later period. Percentages at 10 years were 3.4% for the period 1978 through 1983 and 1.9% for the period 1984 through 1989.

It is clear that survival statistics for more recently diagnosed cases are more favorable than those reported historically and that breast CIS is rarely a fatal disease. Yet recurrence rates and rates of contralateral breast cancer are not negligible, and women with breast CIS have a greater risk of developing invasive disease than the population at large. What is most urgent at this time is finding a means for identifying those women who have the greatest risk of recurrence, progression, or contralateral diagnosis. Currently, several large epidemiologic studies are underway to seek specific biomarkers in tumor tissue as sensitive markers of future disease risk (33).

EPIDEMIOLOGIC STUDIES OF RISK FACTORS FOR BREAST CARCINOMA IN SITU

Fairly well accepted risk factors for invasive breast cancer include increasing age, white or black race, history of benign breast disease, first-degree family history of breast cancer (mother, sister, or daughter), early age at menarche, and late age at menopause, nulliparity or late age at first term pregnancy, weight gain during adulthood or high body mass index (for risk of postmenopausal women), exposure to high-dose ionizing radiation, and alcohol consumption of at least one drink per day (34). Other factors that affect breast cancer risk include a sedentary lifestyle, use of hormone replacement therapy (estrogen regimens or estrogen plus progestin regimens), and among parous women, not having breast-fed for a sufficient amount of time. Most of these risk factors for breast cancer, such as ages at menarche and menopause, pregnancy and lactation history, postmenopausal obesity or weight gain as an adult, use of exogenous hormones, alcohol intake, and physical activity can be interpreted as representing measures of the cumulative exposure of the breast to estrogen and progesterone

(35–39). The actions of the ovarian hormones estradiol and progesterone and their exogenous formulations (used in combination oral contraceptives and hormone replacement therapy) on the breast do not appear to be genotoxic but do affect the rate of cell division (40,41). Estrogen stimulates ductal growth and increases cell proliferation rates, which can increase the likelihood of a random genetic error. Progesterone stimulates alveolar growth and has proliferative effects. According to this cell proliferation model, somatic mutations that occur during cell division can lead to a malignant change and the eventual development of a detectable breast cancer (41). Whether this model holds for screen-detected breast CIS is uncertain.

If breast CIS is a precursor to the development invasive disease, risk factors for invasive disease should be observed as risk factors for in situ disease. Relative to the large number of epidemiologic studies of invasive breast cancer that have been conducted, the number of studies specifically reporting results for breast CIS is quite small. The descriptive characteristics of studies of breast CIS are shown in Table 4.2. Most of these studies have relatively small sample sizes, and this results in reduced statistical power to detect relationships. Nearly all include patients diagnosed in the years since mammography became widely available, and, thus, comparisons should take into account the screening histories of participants (13,42). Few have systematically examined the majority of currently accepted risk factors for invasive breast cancer. Table 4.3 summarizes the results of the currently available studies, and these are summarized below by risk factor.

Family History

Women with a family history of breast cancer may have a high risk because of a familial inherited predisposition to breast cancer (such as inherited mutations in the *BRCA1* or *BRCA2* genes); their high risk may not be genetic in origin, however, and may also arise because family members share risk factors for breast cancer. In studies of invasive breast cancer, women with a first-degree family history of breast cancer (a positive history in a mother, sister, or daughter) have a twofold or greater increase in breast cancer risk (34). The risk increases as the number of affected family members increases and is particularly high when family member(s) have been diagnosed at a young age (in their 30s and 40s). Among those studies that have reported results related to the risk of breast CIS associated with a positive family history of breast cancer, all find that risk is greater among women with a first-degree family history of breast cancer, with risk estimates ranging from 1.7 to 2.7 (13,42–46). Whether the increased risk of breast CIS associated with family history is owing to genetic factors or shared exposures to other breast cancer risk factors is uncertain because women with a positive family history clearly comprise a group that is more likely to undergo regular mammographic screening.

TABLE 4.2. CHARACTERISTICS OF EPIDEMIOLOGIC STUDIES EVALUATING RISK FACTORS FOR BREAST CARCINOMA IN SITU

Study	Type of Study	Study Population	Ages of Subjects (yr)	No. of Cases/Controls	Dates of Diagnosis
Brinton et al., 1983 (43)	Case-control study nested within the BCDDP	Screening cohort	Not stated	199/1,250	1973–1977
Brinton et al., 1986 (63)	Case-control study nested within the BCDDP (extends Brinton et al., 1983)	Screening cohort: white women with natural or surgical menopause	Not stated	254/2,258	1973–1980
Schairer et al., 1994 (64)	Follow-up of women in the BCDDP who participated in annual interviews from 1980 to 1986 and an additional questionnaire	Screening cohort of postmeno pausal women with known age at menopause	Not stated	152 cases	1980–1989
Stanford et al., 1995 (65)	Population-based, case-control study	American women	50–64	87/492	1988–1990
Longnecker et al., 1996 (42)	Two population-based, case-control studies	Young women (I), older women (II), American white women	I, ≤40; II, 55–64	I, 68/724; II, 165/1,479	I, 1983–1988; II, 1987–1989
Weiss et al., 1996 (13)	Population-based, case-control study	American women, all races	20–44	228/1,505	1990–1992
Kerlikowske et al., 1997 (44)	Screening cohort	American women	≥30	102/39,177	1985–1995
Lambe et al., 1998 (49)	Nested case-control study linking population registries on births and cancer	Swedish women	<66	1,368	1960–1990
Henrich et al., 1998 (66)	Case-control study nested within screening cohort	Postmenopausal women	≥45	32/545	1987–1992
Gapstur et al., 1999 (45)	Cohort study	Random sample of 37,105 postmeno pausal women	55–69	175	1986–1996
Schairer et al., 1999 (58)	Follow-up of women in the BCDDP who participated in annual interviews from 1980 to 1986 and additional questionnaires (extends Schairer et al., 1994)	Screening cohort. postmenopausal women		255	1980–1995
Ross et al., 2000 (59)	Case-control study: 3 phases (includes some but not all subjects in Longnecker et al., 1996)	Older postmeno pausal women	1, 55–64; 2, 55–69; 3, 55–72	Total 186	1, 1987–1989; 2, 1992; 3, 1995–1996
Trentham-Dietz et al., 2000 (46)	Population-based, case-control study	American women	<75	301/3,789	1988–1990

BCDDP, Breast Cancer Demonstration Project.

TABLE 4.3. EPIDEMIOLOGIC RISK FACTORS* FOR BREAST CARCINOMA IN SITU

Study	Dates of Diagnosis	Factors Predicting Risk	Factors Not Associated With Risk
Brinton et al., 1983 (43)	1973–1977	First-degree family history of breast cancer (yes vs. no, OR = 1.7), age at first birth (≥30 vs. <20, OR = 2.7),† parity (nulliparous vs. <20 at first birth, OR = 2.4), prior breast biopsy (yes vs. no, OR = 2.1), no. of biopsies (≥2 vs. none, OR = 2.3)†	Age at menarche, type of menopause (natural, surgical, hysterectomy only), body mass index (kg/m²), height, weight, education and income, marital status
Brinton et al., 1986 (63)	1973–1980	Estrogen replacement therapy (ERT) (10+ yr vs. none, OR = 1.9)†	
Schairer et al., 1994 (64)	1980–1989	Estrogen plus progestin (E + P) use (ever use vs. no use of E + P or ERT alone, RR = 2.3), current/past E + P use (current vs. no use of ERT or E + P, RR = 2.4; past vs. no use of E or E + P, RR = 2.3), ERT (10+ yr use vs. no use of ERT alone or E + P, RR = 2.0),† current ERT use (vs. no use of E or E + P, RR = 1.8)†	Past ERT (vs. no use of E or E + P)
Stanford et al., 1995 (65)	1988–1990		ERT, E + P therapy
Longnecker et al., 1996 (42)	I, 1983–1988	Women ≤40 yrs (premenopausal): first-degree family history of breast cancer (yes vs. no, OR = 2.7), age at menarche (OR = 0.74/yr increase),† history of benign breast disease (yes vs. no, OR = 2.4), body mass index (kg/m²) (0.92 per kg/m², OR = 0.92)†	No. of full-term pregnancies, age at first full-term pregnancy
	II, 1987–1989	Women 55–64 yr (postmenopausal): first-degree family history of breast cancer (yes vs. no, OR = 2.1), history of benign breast disease (yes vs. no, OR = 1.5), parity (per full-term pregnancy, OR = 0.78),† age at menopause (55+ vs. <45, OR = 2.9, OR = 1.06 per yr increase in age)†	Age at menarche, body mass index (kg/m²), age at first full-term pregnancy, ever use ERT, ever use hormone replacement therapy
Weiss et al., 1996 (13)	1990–1992	First-degree family history of breast cancer (yes vs. no, OR = 2.5; both mother and sister, OR = 6.9), prior breast biopsy (yes vs. no, OR = 2.0), race (black vs. white, OR = 1.8), nulliparous (vs. parous, OR = 2.1), body mass index (kg/m²)(≥29 vs. <22, OR = 0.45)†	Age at menarche, no. of full-term births (trend is of borderline significance), age at first full-term birth, years of breast feeding, time since last full-term birth, alcohol intake (average drinks/week), education
Kerlikowski et al., 1997 (44)	1985–1995	DCIS: 30–49 yr: age (per 10-yr increase, OR = 2.3), first-degree family history of breast cancer (yes vs. no, OR = 2.4), body mass index (kg/m²) (≤25 vs. <25, OR = 0.4), presence of a palpable mass (yes vs. no, OR = 2.0)	Early menarche (<12 vs. ≥12 yr), nulliparous or ≥30 yr at birth of first child, prior breast surgery
		DCIS: 50+ yr: first-degree family history of breast cancer (yes vs. no, OR = 2.2), nulliparous or ≥30 yr at birth of first child (yes vs. no, OR = 2.3)	Age (per 10-yr increase), early menarche (<12 vs. ≥12 yr), prior breast surgery, body mass index (kg/m²) (≤25 vs. <25), hysterectomy, palpable mass

(continues)

TABLE 4.3. (CONTINUED)

Study	Dates of Diagnosis	Factors Predicting Risk	Factors Not Associated With Risk
Lambe et al., 1998 (49)	1960–1990	Parous (vs. nulliparous, OR = 0.76), no. of livebirths (4 vs. 1, OR = 0.8, 5+ vs. 1, OR = 0.5)†	Age at first birth (trend is of borderline significance)
Henrich et al., 1998 (66)	1987–1992		ERT
Gapstur et al., 1999 (45)	1986–1996	DCIS: First-degree family history of breast cancer (yes vs. no, RR = 2.1), age at first birth (≥30 vs. <20 yr,	Hormone replacement therapy, body mass index DCIS: (current and at age 18 yr), RR = 1.9) waist-to-hip ratio, age at menarche, age at menopause, type of menopause, alcohol intake
Schairer et al., 1999 (58)	1980–1995		ERT, E + P therapy
Ross et al., 2000 (59)	3 periods: 1987–1989, 1992, 1994–1995	ERT (per 5 yr of use, OR = 1.4),† E + P (per 5 yr of use, OR = 1.4),†	
Trentham-Dietz et al., 2000 (46)	1988–1990	First-degree family history of breast cancer (yes vs. no, OR = 2.7), biopsy for benign breast disease (yes vs. no, OR = 2.2), no. of births (per livebirth, OR = 0.91),† alcohol intake (<183 g/wk vs. none, OR = 2.3), postmenopausal hormone use (ever vs. never, OR = 1.9, trend in duration of use not statistically significant)	Age at menarche, age at first birth, age at menopause, education, physical activity in early adulthood, body mass index (kg/m²), duration of lactation, daily β-carotene intake, oral contraceptive use

*Factors predicting risk are those for which the reported 95% confidence limits for the odds ratios (OR) or the relative risks (RR) exclude the value 1.0 or a two-sided test for linear trend, which assesses a dose-response effect with increasing level of exposure, is statistically significant.
†Indicates a statistically significant test for trend in risk with increasing level of exposure.
DCIS, ductal carcinoma in situ.

Benign Breast Disease and Prior Breast Biopsy

Women with biopsy-confirmed benign breast disease have somewhat elevated risk for subsequent breast cancer. The magnitude of these increased risks ranges from approximately 2 for proliferative disease without atypia to a range of 3 to 5 for atypical hyperplasia (34). A history of benign breast disease or a prior breast biopsy is also associated with an increased risk of breast CIS in most studies considering this risk factor (13,42,43,46). In one study, a history of breast surgery was not associated with a significantly elevated DCIS risk (44); the question used in this study was not specific for previous biopsies, however. In the positive studies, the odds ratios range from 1.5 to 2.4. Within the context of breast CIS epidemiology, the differences in breast biopsy rates between cases and controls may also represent a difference in the intensity of surveillance for breast cancer being applied to the two groups of women.

Reproductive Characteristics

Reproductive characteristics form a major category of risk factors for invasive breast cancer. Early age at menarche is generally associated with a greater risk of breast cancer, with the risk declining 10% to 20% with each year that menar-che is delayed (47). Epidemiologic studies have consistently demonstrated that late age at menopause is associated with greater breast cancer risk (47). Earlier menopause represents a shorter time period of exposure to ovulatory menstrual cycles. Among women whose menstrual periods stop naturally, breast cancer risk is approximately two times greater for those with a last menstrual period at age 55 years or later than for those whose last period occurred at age 45 or younger (48). For women older than 40 years of age, nulliparity or advanced age at first-term pregnancy and few term pregnancies are associated with small increases in the risk of invasive breast cancer (47).

With the exception of the study of Longnecker and colleagues (42) of women aged 40 or younger, age at menarche was not related to the risk of breast CIS in any of the studies that examined it as a potential risk factor (13,42–46). The effects of age at menopause has only been examined in three studies (Table 4.3) (42,45,46). Two of these found no effect on breast CIS risk (45,46); however, Longnecker and colleagues noted a 6% increase in risk with each year that menopause was delayed. Two studies reported on type of menopause, finding no effect on breast CIS risk (43,45).

Different aspects of pregnancy history were reported in the studies described in Tables 4.2 and 4.3. Results for age at first full-term pregnancy (or first livebirth) were inconsistent; however, the ages of the women in these studies will be an important modifier of risk because the immediate effect of a pregnancy is to increase breast cancer risk, whereas a reduction in risk occurs over the longer term. Thus, in three studies that included primarily older women, older age at first term pregnancy was associated with approximately a twofold increase in breast cancer risk (43–45). In the report by Longnecker and colleagues (42), however, age at first full-term pregnancy was unassociated with the risk of breast CIS of younger (40 years or younger) or older (55 to 64 years old) women. Similarly, no effect of age at first term pregnancy was observed in the studies of Weiss et al. (13) or Trentham-Dietz et al. (46).

Lambe and colleagues (49) linked records from the Swedish Cancer Registry to those of the Swedish Fertility Registry and observed a 24% reduction in risk of breast CIS for women who had at least one birth. Additional births after the first added to this protection. Women who had at least five births had a 50% lower risk of breast CIS than those who had only one birth. Once the number of births was taken into account, only a small increase in risk was associated with advanced age at first birth. Breast CIS risk was 42% greater among women who were 35 years or older when having their first child than among those who were under age 20 years. The trend in risk associated with increasing age at first birth was of borderline statistical significance.

Other studies also show differences by parity status. Although age at first term pregnancy was not associated with breast CIS risk in the study by Weiss et al., nulliparous women had twofold greater risk than parous women (13). Two studies showed that increasing the number of births resulted in progressively lower estimates of risk for breast CIS (42,46).

Body Mass Index

Two aspects of body mass index, obesity, and weight gain as an adult are associated with higher invasive breast cancer risk among postmenopausal women (50,51). Most studies report RR of 1.5 to 2.0 for comparisons of the most obese (or largest weight gain) to the thinnest women (or those with little or no weight gain). The increased risk in heavy postmenopausal women can be attributed to higher levels of circulating estrogen in these women because the main source of endogenous estrogen after menopause is the conversion of the androgen precursor androstenedione to estrone in adipose tissue (52). In contrast to the effects of obesity on postmenopausal women, heavy body weight is associated with a 10% to 30% reduction in breast cancer risk in premenopausal women (53). Among premenopausal women, the effect of obesity on nonovarian estrogen production is likely the same as that among postmenopausal women, but this production adds only a small increment to the high blood levels produced by the ovary during ovulatory menstrual cycles. In addition, obese premenopausal women frequently experience anovulatory menstrual cycles

so that the slightly lower breast cancer risk of obese premenopausal women may be the result of their experiencing fewer ovulatory cycles (54).

The effects of body mass index on the risk of breast CIS were in the expected direction in the studies that included only younger (primarily premenopausal) women, with the risk reduced among larger (or more obese) women (13,42,44). Surprisingly, no effect of body mass index on breast CIS risk was observed among studies of primarily older (postmenopausal) women (42–46).

Hormone Replacement Therapy

Estrogen replacement therapy was initially used for menopausal symptoms until it was linked to the increasing risk of endometrial cancer (55). Most studies with sufficiently large numbers of women who have long-term exposure (10+ years) to estrogen replacement therapy find a modest increase in invasive breast cancer risk among exposed women with the risk increasing approximately 3% per year of use (56). Among studies conducted in the United States where the use of conjugated equine estrogens is the norm, breast cancer risk increases approximately 2.2% per year of use of a standard dose regimen (0.625 mg per day). This translates into increases in risk of 10% after 5 years, 20% after 10 years, and 40% after 15 years of use. Combined hormone replacement therapy regimens add a progestin to the estrogen regimen so that the endometrium will be protected. In these combined regimens, progestins may enhance the proliferative effects of estrogen, and they appear to increase invasive breast cancer risk substantially. Three large-scale population-based epidemiologic studies have recently been published (57–59). These studies show that adding a progestin to the estrogen regimen changes the increase in breast cancer risk after 5 years of use from 10% (on estrogen alone) to 30% (for estrogen plus a progestin).

Studies of hormone replacement therapy have shown that women using such therapy have a better prognosis after the diagnosis of breast cancer (60–62). Thus, we might expect that the association with breast CIS would be stronger than that observed for invasive breast cancer. Furthermore, it is likely that women using hormone replacement therapy are subject to greater medical surveillance than nonusers. Nevertheless, nine references cited in Tables 4.2 and 4.3 have published evaluations of the risk of breast CIS associated with the use of menopausal hormones, and no consistent relationship emerges.

In the earliest report based on the Breast Cancer Detection and Demonstration Project, Brinton and colleagues (63) showed that 10 or more years of use of estrogen replacement therapy was associated with a substantial, 90% increase in breast cancer risk. Schairer and colleagues (64) later used other women from this cohort (and excluded the cases included in Brinton's publication) to examine in greater detail the effects of both estrogen replacement therapy and combined estrogen and progestin therapy. They noted an increase in breast CIS risk with 10 or more years of estrogen replacement therapy, an effect similar to that observed by Brinton and colleagues. This increase in risk was restricted to women who were classified as current users. Risk was also substantially elevated among women who used the combined (estrogen plus progestin) regimen, with both current and past users at similar levels of elevated risk. The most recent publication from the Breast Cancer Detection and Demonstration Project cohort (58), which builds on the 1994 paper by Schairer and colleagues (64), adding 103 additional breast CIS cases, does not provide detailed results for breast CIS but states that neither the estrogen regimen nor the combined regimen was associated with risk of breast CIS. Thus, relatively strong results appear to have become reversed with time.

The papers by Longnecker and colleagues (42) and Ross and colleagues (59) also provide some inconsistent results. These two reports share some cases and controls in common, although the overlap is not as extensive as that of Schairer et al. papers. In the initial report, Longnecker and colleagues (42) analyzed only ever versus never use of estrogen replacement therapy and combined hormone replacement therapy. They found a marginally significant 60% increase in breast CIS risk associated with ever having used estrogen replacement therapy, but no significant increase in risk associated with ever using combined therapy. Ross and colleagues (59), however, showed that both estrogen replacement therapy and combined estrogen plus progestin therapy were associated with a 40% increase in breast CIS risk for each 5 years of use. Other studies showed no effect of replacement hormones on breast CIS risk (45,46,65,66), although one did find a significant effect of ever use (46).

Other Risk Factors

No consistent evaluation of other breast cancer risk factors appears in the epidemiologic literature on breast CIS. Education does not appear to be strongly associated with risk, although in each of the studies that examined risk associated with educational attainment, some subgroups showed greater risks than others did. Alcohol intake was associated with increased risk of breast CIS in one (46) of two studies that evaluated this effect (13,46). The negative study (13) was limited to younger women, whereas studies showing a marked effect of alcohol intake on the risk of invasive disease have primarily demonstrated an increase risk for older women (67).

CONCLUSIONS

In the future, with the greater adherence of women to recommendations for mammographic screening, we can expect that rates of DCIS will continue to increase. Currently, we

know little about factors that predict risk of breast CIS and particularly those that differentiate between DCIS and LCIS. Both family history and history of benign breast disease or breast biopsy can identify subgroups at high risk of breast CIS, but their relationship to breast CIS may, in part, be an artifact because they also identify women who undergo more intensive surveillance for breast cancer. Some aspects of pregnancy history appear linked to breast CIS risk. No clear picture emerges for other breast cancer risk factors. One can conjecture that the lack of an effect of obesity on breast CIS risk may be owing to poorer adherence to screening guidelines of heavier women or to greater difficulty in imaging the breasts of such women. Another possibility, however, is that the breast cancers of obese women proceed through stages of development more rapidly; this latter possibility is consistent with the poorer prognosis of obese women diagnosed with invasive breast cancer.

In the future, molecular characterization of DCIS may help us to determine which tumors are truly at risk of progressing to invasive disease or of recurring. This information can also be applied to epidemiologic studies and should help to clarify the conflicting findings for many risk factors. Molecular epidemiology will offer additional insight into the causes of breast CIS. As we learn more about polymorphisms in genes involved in hormone metabolism and transport, DNA repair, and carcinogen metabolism, we will be able to identify subgroups of women who are at increased risk of breast cancer.

ACKNOWLEDGMENTS

Cancer incidence data were collected under a subcontract with the Public Health Institute, Berkeley, CA, which manages the regional contracts for the California Cancer Registry. The subcontract is supported by the California Department of Health Services as part of its statewide cancer-reporting program, as mandated by Health and Safety Code Sections 103875 and 103885. Support was also provided by Public Health Service contract N01CN67010 and grant CA17054 from the National Cancer Institute, National Institutes of Health, Department of Health and Human Services and grant DAMD 17-96-1-6156, U.S. Army Medical Research and Development Command.

REFERENCES

1. Broders AC. Carcinoma in situ contrasted with penetrating epithelium. *JAMA* 1932;99:1670–1674.
2. Ernster VL, Barclay J, Kerlikowske K, et al. Incidence of and treatment for ductal carcinoma in situ of the breast. *JAMA* 1996;275:913–918.
3. Ernster VL, Barclay J. Increases in ductal carcinoma in situ (DCIS) of the breast in relation to mammography: a dilemma. *Monogr Natl Cancer Inst* 1997;22:151–156.

4. Barchielli A, Paci E, Giorgi D. Recent trends of in situ carcinoma of the breast and mammographic screening in the Florence area, Italy. *Cancer Causes Control* 1999;10:313–317.

5. Adams-Cameron M, Gilliland FD, Hunt WC, et al. Trends in incidence and treatment for ductal carcinoma in situ in Hispanic, American Indian and non-Hispanic white women in New Mexico, 1973–1994. *Cancer* 1999;85:1084–1090.

6. Levi F, Te VC, Randimbison L, et al. Trends of in situ carcinoma of the breast in Vaud, Switzerland. *Eur J Cancer* 1997;33:903–906.

7. Simon MS, Lemanne D, Schwartz AG, et al. Recent trends in the incidence of in situ and invasive breast cancer in the Detroit metropolitan area (1975–1988). *Cancer* 1993;71:769–774.

8. Choi WS, Parker BA, Pierce JP, et al. Regional differences in the incidence and treatment of carcinoma in situ of the breast. *Cancer Epidemiol Biomarkers Prev* 1996;5:317–320.

9. Zheng T, Holford TR, Chen Y, et al. Time trend of female breast carcinoma *in situ* by race and histology in Connecticut, USA. *Eur J Cancer* 1997;33:96–100.

10. Ries LAG, Eisner MP, Kosary CL, et al., eds. *SEER cancer statistics review, 1973–1997*. (NIH pub. no. 00-2789) Bethesda, MD: National Cancer Institute, 2000.

11. Brown ML, Kessler LG, Rueter FG. Is the supply of mammography machines outstripping need and demand? An economic analysis. *Ann Intern Med* 1990;113:547–552.

12. Blackman DK, Bennett EM, Miller DS. Trends in self-reported use of mammograms (1989–1997) and Papanicolaou tests (1991–1997)—Behavioral Risk Factor Surveillance System. CDC surveillance summaries, October 8, 1999. *Morb Mortal Wkly Rep* 1999;48:1–22.

13. Weiss HA, Brinton LA, Brogan D, et al. Epidemiology of *in situ* and invasive breast cancer in women aged under 45. *Br J Cancer* 1996;73:1298–1305.

14. Ng EH, Ng FC, Tan PH, et al. Results of intermediate measures from a population-based, randomized trial of mammographic screening prevalence and detection of breast carcinoma among Asian women: The Singapore Breast Screening Project. *Cancer* 1998;82:1521–1528.

15. Liff JM, Sung JF, Chow WH, et al. Does increased detection account for the rising incidence of breast cancer? *Am J Publ Health* 1991;81:462–465.

16. Schnitt SJ, Connolly JL, Tavassoli FA, et al. Interobserver reproducibility in the diagnosis of ductal proliferative breast lesions using standardized criteria. *Am J Surg Pathol* 1992;16:1133–1143.

17. Tavassoli FA. Ductal carcinoma in situ: introduction of the concept of ductal intraepithelial neoplasia. *Mod Pathol* 1998;11:140–154.

18. Welch HG, Black WC. Using autopsy series to estimate the disease "reservoir" for ductal carcinoma in situ of the breast: how much more breast cancer can we find. *Ann Intern Med* 1997;127:1023–1028.

19. Fisher B, Dignam J, Wolmark N, et al. Lumpectomy and radiation therapy for the treatment of intraductal breast cancer: findings from National Surgical Adjuvant Breast and Bowel Project B-17. *J Clin Oncol* 1998;16:441–452.

20. Fisher B, Dignam J, Wolmark N, et al. Tamoxifen in treatment of intraductal breast cancer: National Surgical Adjuvant Breast and Bowel Project B-24 randomised controlled trial. *Lancet* 1999;353:1993–2000.

21. Page DL, Dupont WD, Rogers LW, et al. Continued local recurrence of carcinoma 15–25 years after diagnosis of low grade ductal carcinoma in situ of the breast treated only by biopsy. *Cancer* 1995;78:1197–1200.

22. Eusebi V, Feudale E, Foschini MP, et al. Long-term follow-up of in situ carcinoma of the breast. *Semin Diagn Pathol* 1994;11:223–235.

23. Boyages J, Delaney G, Taylor R. Predictors of local recurrence after treatment of ductal carcinoma in situ. *Cancer* 1998;85:616–628.

24. Habel LA, Daling JR, Newcomb PA, et al. Risk of recurrence after ductal carcinoma *in situ* of the breast. *Cancer Epidemiol Biomarkers Prev* 1998;7:689–696.

25. Habel LA, Moe RE, Daling JR, et al. Risk of contralateral breast cancer among women with carcinoma *in situ* of the breast. *Ann Surg* 1997;225:69–75.

26. Vicini FA, Kestin LL, Goldstein NS, et al. Impact of young age on outcome in patients with ductal carcinoma-*in-situ* treated with breast conserving surgery. *J Clin Oncol* 2000;18:296–306.

27. Goldstein NS, Vicini FA, Kestin LL, et al. Differences in the pathologic features of ductal carcinoma *in situ* of the breast based on patient age. *Cancer* 2000;88:2553–2560.

28. Bobrow LG, Happerfield LC, Gregory WM, et al. The classification of ductal carcinoma in situ and its association with biological markers. *Semin Diagn Pathol* 1994;11:199–207.

29. Leal CB, Schmitt FC, Bento MJ, et al. Ductal carcinoma in situ of the breast. Histologic categorization and its relationship to ploidy and immunohistochemical expression of hormone receptors, p53, and c-erbB-2 protein. *Cancer* 1995;75:2123–2131.

30. Poller DN, Snead DR, Roberts EC, et al. Oestrogen receptor expression in ductal carcinoma in situ of the breast: relationship to flow cytometric analysis of DNA and expression of the c-erbB-2 oncoprotein. *Br J Cancer* 1993;68:156–161.

31. Franceschi S, Levi F, LaVecchia C, et al. Second cancers following in situ carcinoma of the breast. *Int J Cancer* 1998;77:392–395.

32. Ernster VL, Barclay J, Kerlikowske K, et al. Mortality among women with ductal carcinoma in situ of the breast in the population-based Surveillance, Epidemiology, and End Results program. *Arch Intern Med* 2000;160:953–958.

33. Millikan R, Dressler L, Geradts J, et al. The need for epidemiologic studies of *in-situ* carcinoma of the breast. *Breast Cancer Res Treat* 1995;35:65–77.

34. Kelsey JL, Bernstein L. Epidemiology and prevention of breast cancer. *Annu Rev Publ Health* 1996;17:47–67.

35. Bernstein L, Ross RK, Lobo RA, et al. The effects of moderate physical activity on menstrual cycle patterns in adolescence: implications for breast cancer prevention. *Br J Cancer* 1987;55:681–685.

36. Henderson BE, Ross RK, Bernstein L. Estrogens as a cause of human cancer: The Richard and Hinda Rosenthal Foundation Award Lecture. *Cancer Res* 1988;48:246–253.

37. Bernstein L, Ross RK, Henderson BE. Prospects for the primary prevention of breast cancer. *Am J Epidemiol* 1992;135:142–152.

38. Bernstein L, Ross RK. Hormones and breast cancer. *Epidemiol Rev* 1993;15:48–65.

39. Gill J. The effects of moderate alcohol consumption on female hormone levels and reproductive function. *Alcohol Alcoholism* 2000; 35:417–423.

40. Preston-Martin S, Pike MC, Ross RK, et al. Increased cell division as a cause of human cancer. *Cancer Res* 1990;50:7415–7421.

41. Henderson BE, Feigelson HS. Hormonal carcinogenesis. *Carcinogenesis* 2000;21:427–433.

42. Longnecker MP, Bernstein L, Paganini-Hill A, et al. Risk factors for in situ breast cancer. *Cancer Epidemiol Biomarkers Prev* 1996; 5:961–965.

43. Brinton LA, Hoover R, Fraumeni JFJ. Epidemiology of minimal breast cancer. *JAMA* 1983;249:483–487.

44. Kerlikowske K, Barclay J, Grady D, et al. Comparison of risk factors for ductal carcinoma in situ and invasive breast cancer. *J Natl Cancer Inst* 1997;89:77–82.

45. Gapstur SM, Morrow M, Sellers TA. Hormone replacement therapy and risk of breast cancer with a favorable histology: Re-

sults of the Iowa Women's Health Study. *JAMA* 1999;281:2091–2097.

46. Trentham-Dietz A, Newcomb PA, Storer BE, et al. Risk factors for carcinoma in situ of the breast. *Cancer Epidemiol Biomarkers Prev* 2000;9:697–703.

47. Henderson BE, Pike MC, Bernstein L, et al. Breast cancer. In: Schottenfeld D, Fraumeni Jr J, eds. *Cancer epidemiology and prevention*, 2nd ed. Philadelphia: WB Saunders, 1996:1022–1039.

48. Trichopoulos D, MacMahon B, Cole P. The menopause and breast cancer risk. *J Natl Cancer Inst* 1972;48:605–613.

49. Lambe M, Hsieh CC, Tsaih SW, et al. Parity, age at first birth and the risk of carcinoma in situ of the breast. *Int J Cancer* 1998; 77:330–332.

50. Hunter DJ, Willett WC. Diet, body size, and breast cancer. *Epidemiol Rev* 1993;15:110–132.

51. Huang Z, Hankinson SE, Colditz GA, et al. Dual effects of weight and weight gain on breast cancer risk. *JAMA* 1997;278: 1407–1411.

52. Siiteri PK, MacDonald PC. Role of extraglandular estrogen in human endocrinology. In: Geiger SR, Astwood EB, Greep RO, eds. *Handbook of physiology*. Washington, DC: American Physiological Society, 1973:615–629.

53. Ursin G, Longnecker MP, Haile RW, et al. A meta-analysis of body mass index and risk of premenopausal breast cancer. *Epidemiology* 1995;6:137–141.

54. Pike MC. Reducing cancer risk in women through lifestyle-mediated changes in hormone levels. *Cancer Detect Prev* 1990;14: 595–607.

55. Grady D, Gebretsadik T, Kerlikowske K, et al. Hormone replacement therapy and endometrial cancer risk: a meta-analysis. *Obstet Gynecol* 1995;85:304–313.

56. Pike MC, Bernstein L, Spicer DV. The relationship of exogenous hormones to breast cancer risk. In: Niederhuber J, ed. *Current therapy in oncology*. St. Louis: Mosby, 1993:292–303.

57. Magnusson C, Baron JA, Correia N, et al. Breast-cancer risk following long-term oestrogen- and oestrogen-progestin-replacement therapy. *Int J Cancer* 1999;81:339–344.

58. Schairer C, Lubin J, Troisi R, et al. Menopausal estrogen and estrogen-progestin replacement therapy and breast cancer risk. *JAMA* 2000;283:485–491.

59. Ross RK, Paganini-Hill A, Wan PC, et al. Effect of hormone replacement therapy on breast cancer risk: estrogen versus estrogen plus progestin. *J Natl Cancer Inst* 2000;92:328–332.

60. Bergkvist L, Adami HO, Persson I, et al. Prognosis after breast cancer diagnosis in women exposed to estrogen and estrogen-progestogen replacement therapy. *Am J Epidemiol* 1989;130:221–228.

61. Grodstein F, Stampfer MJ, Colditz GA, et al. Postmenopausal hormone therapy and mortality. *N Engl J Med* 1997;336:1769–1775.

62. Holli K, Isola J, Cuzick J. Low biologic aggressiveness in breast cancer in women using hormone replacement therapy. *J Clin Oncol* 1998;16:3115–3120.

63. Brinton LA, Hoover R, Fraumeni Jr JF. Menopausal oestrogens and breast cancer risk: an expanded case-control study. *Br J Cancer* 1986;54:825–832.

64. Schairer C, Byrne C, Keyl PM, et al. Menopausal estrogen and estrogen-progestin replacement therapy and risk of breast cancer (United States). *Cancer Causes Control* 1994;5:491–500.

65. Stanford JL, Weiss NS, Voigt LF, et al. Combined estrogen and progestin hormone replacement therapy in relation to risk of breast cancer in middle-aged women. *JAMA* 1995;274:137–142.

66. Henrich JB, Kornguth PJ, Viscoli CM, et al. Postmenopausal estrogen use and invasive versus in situ breast cancer risk. *J Clin Oncol* 1998;51:1277–1283.

67. Longnecker MP. Alcoholic beverage consumption in relation to risk of breast cancer: meta-analysis and review. *Cancer Causes Control* 1994;5:73–82.

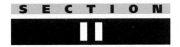

CARCINOGENESIS AND BIOLOGY

5

BIOLOGIC CHARACTERISTICS OF DUCTAL CARCINOMA IN SITU

D. CRAIG ALLRED

Ductal carcinoma in situ (DCIS) is important as the major precursor of invasive breast cancer (IBC). This premise is indirectly supported by several converging lines of epidemiologic, pathologic, and, most recently, biologic evidence. For example, patients with DCIS treated by biopsy alone are at tenfold increased risk for developing IBC (1,2). In patients with DCIS treated by lumpectomy, it is fairly common for IBC to develop at the site of original surgery (3–5). DCIS is 15 to 20 times more common in breasts with synchronous IBC than in breasts from the random population (6–9), and synchronous lesions are histologically very similar (6). Perhaps the most compelling evidence of a precursor-product relationship between DCIS and IBC comes from recent studies showing that they share identical genetic abnormalities, such as loss of tumor suppressor genes and amplification of oncogenes (10).

Before mammography, most DCIS were large and palpable and collectively accounted for less than 5% of all newly diagnosed breast cancers (11,12). Mammography, because of its ability to identify microcalcifications in small nonpalpable lesions, dramatically increased the incidence of detection, and now DCIS accounts for as many as 20% of new breast cancers (11–14). Until recently, regardless of how they were detected, DCIS was usually treated by mastectomy, resulting in cure rates approaching 100% (11,15). Now many DCIS are managed by breast-conserving surgery or lumpectomy, primarily because of the relative success of treating IBC in this manner. In early studies, however, DCIS treated by lumpectomy alone showed local recurrence rates greater than 25% in some series, and, even more troubling, half the recurrences were IBC (16–20). More recently, radiation and hormonal therapy have been used in conjunction with lumpectomy, and these adjuvant modalities reduced the rate of local recurrence to less than 10% (15,20–22).

Thus, there is the dilemma of encountering ever more frequently a nonlethal and potentially curable disease whose treatment is imperfect, controversial, and still evolving. Clearly, the best approach would be to prevent the development of DCIS in the first place, and effective strategies will most likely target the biologic abnormalities underlying its development. Short of prevention, it would also be helpful to identify DCIS with a particularly high probability of progressing to IBC, which might then be treated more aggressively. Our incomplete understanding of the biologic alterations responsible for the development of DCIS and its progression to IBC is a major obstacle to prevention and prognostication, although this is a very active area of research. There have been more than 1,000 articles in the medical literature during the past decade alone dealing with DCIS, many of them biologic in nature. This chapter briefly reviews some of the biologic features of DCIS that have been studied most comprehensively or appear to be particularly important.

GROWTH (PROLIFERATION AND APOPTOSIS)

All breast cancers, including DCIS, are thought to arise from stem cells in normal terminal duct lobular units (TDLUs). On a microscopic scale, DCIS are mass lesions that expand TDLUs and proximal ducts to many times their normal size, which, given enough time, can eventually result in a palpable tumor that is centimeters in diameter. Many studies, using a variety of techniques, have measured the rates of proliferation in TDLUs (23–33) and DCIS (23,33–42) (Table 5.1 and Fig. 5.1A,B). Proliferation in TDLUs averaged only approximately 2% overall. In premenopausal women, the rate fluctuates with the menstrual cycle and is twofold higher in the luteal than the follicular phase (29). The association between hormonal status and proliferation emphasizes the importance of estrogen and progesterone as mitogens for normal breast epithelium (43). Proliferation averaged approximately 5% in histologically low-grade, noncomedo DCIS compared with 25% in high-grade, comedo lesions. However, the widespread practice of simply dichotomizing DCIS into noncomedo and comedo

TABLE 5.1. AVERAGE (APPROXIMATE) PHENOTYPES OF IMPORTANT BIOLOGIC CHARACTERISTICS OF NORMAL TERMINAL DUCT LOBULAR UNITS (TDLUS) AND DUCTAL CARCINOMA IN SITU (DCIS) STRATIFIED BY HISTOLOGIC GRADE

Biomarker Phenotype	Normal TDLUs (%)	Low-Grade DCIS (%)	Intermediate-Grade DCIS (%)	High-Grade DCIS (%)
Proliferation (% proliferating cells)	2	5	15	25
Apoptosis (% apoptosing cells)	0.5?	0.5?	?	>5
Estrogen receptor (% expressing cases)	>90	>90	75	25
erbB2 Oncogene (% abnormal cases)	0	5	30	70
p53 Tumor suppressor gene (% abnormal cases)	0	5	25	50

subtypes is misleading in the sense that, similar to IBC, DCIS shows tremendous histologic diversity along a continuum ranging from very well to very poorly differentiated, and grading systems have been developed that more accurately convey this diversity (44). Proliferation is proportional to differentiation along this histologic continuum with rates averaging as low as 1% in the lowest grade to more than 70% in the highest grade lesions.

The overall growth of DCIS can be viewed simplistically as a balance between cell proliferation and cell death. On average, the cells in DCIS proliferate faster than normal cells in TDLUs, contributing to their positive growth imbalance. Much less is known about cell death or apoptosis (Table 5.1). One preliminary study reported rates of apoptosis averaging approximately 0.5% in TDLUs and low-grade DCIS (45) compared with more than 5% in high-grade lesions (45–48). Even though the rate of cell death in comedo DCIS is very high, they are rapidly growing lesions that can attain large size, suggesting that the relationship or balance between proliferation and apoptosis may not always be accurately portrayed by the static methods used to measure these dynamic processes.

Progressive growth in DCIS must result from alterations of normal growth-regulating mechanisms. Some of the most important, or at least best understood, involve hormones such as estrogen and its receptor, oncogenes such as erbB2, and tumor suppressor genes such as p53, which are dis-

cussed in more detail in the following sections. However, recent studies confirm the involvement of many additional factors and pathways worth mentioning briefly here. For example, it appears that activation of cyclin D1 through gene amplification and/or overexpression is a specific defect in DCIS compared with normal epithelium or atypical ductal hyperplasia, which is thought to be a direct precursor of DCIS (49–51). Other cell-cycle regulating molecules also appear to be up-regulated in subsets of DCIS, including p16, which is an important inhibitor of cyclin-dependent kinases (42). For progressive growth, cells must become "immortal," which requires continual telomerase activity, and recent studies have shown markedly increased telomerase activity in DCIS compared with normal cells (52). Decreased expression of transforming growth factor-β receptor II, a receptor for the transforming growth factor-β family of growth-suppressing factors, is associated with rapid proliferation in high-grade DCIS, suggesting that alterations of growth factor pathways are also important in the development and progression of DCIS (53). Paracrine growth factors derived from fibroblasts from breast cancers, but not normal breasts, appear necessary to support the sustained growth of the human breast cell line MCF10A *in vitro*, and this cell line can produce DCIS-like lesions in xenograft models (54). There are undoubtedly many other biologic alterations contributing to the growth and progression of DCIS yet to be discovered.

FIGURE 5.1. Representative examples of important biologic characteristics of ductal carcinoma in situ (DCIS) as assessed by immunohistochemistry, including cell proliferation (using the Ki67 proliferation–associated antibody),[1] estrogen receptor (ER),[2] the erbB2 oncogene,[3] and the p53 tumor suppressor gene.[4] Proliferation is usually quite low in low-grade, noncomedo DCIS **(A)** but very high in high-grade, comedo lesions **(B)**. Nearly all low-grade DCIS express high levels of estrogen receptor in the majority of cells **(C)**, whereas most high-grade DCIS show no expression **(D)**. Overexpression of erbB2 is usually associated with gene amplification. Most noncomedo DCIS show no evidence of overexpression **(E)**, but it is very common in comedo lesions **(F)**. Similar to erbB2, most low-grade DCIS have a normal p53 status **(G)**, but the gene is mutated commonly in high-grade lesions **(H)** (200× magnification). [1]Proliferating cells show a dark nuclear signal. [2]ER-positive cells show a dark nuclear signal. [3]erbB2 overexpressing cells show a dark signal at the surface membrane. [4]A dark nuclear signal represents accumulation of mutated and inactive p53 protein.

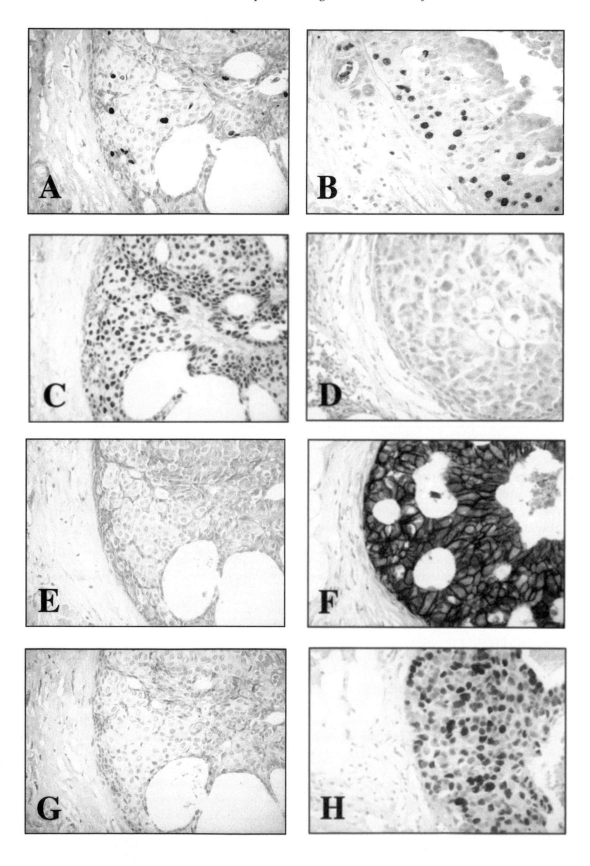

TABLE 5.2. GENERAL CHROMOSOMAL LOCATIONS OF ALLELIC IMBALANCES IN DUCTAL CARCINOMA IN SITU FROM STUDIES ASSESSING LOSS OF HETEROZYGOSITY AND COMPARATIVE GENOMIC HYBRIDIZATION

Chromosome	Losses	Gains	Chromosome	Losses	Gains
1p	x		13p		
1q	x	x	13q	x	
2p	x		14p		
2q	x		14q	x	
3p	x	x	15p		
3q	x	x	15q	x	x
4p	x		16p	x	x
4q	x		16q	x	
5p			17p	x	
5q			17q	x	x
6p	x	x	18p		
6q	x	x	18q	x	
7p	x		19p		
7q	x		19q		x
8p	x		20p		x
8q	x	x	20q		x
9p	x		21p		
9q			21q	x	
10p		x	22p		
10q			22q	x	x
11p	x		Xp		
11q	x		Xq		x
12p	x		Yp		
12q		x	Yq		

x indicates loss or gain.

ESTROGEN AND ESTROGEN RECEPTOR

Estrogen, mediated through estrogen receptor (ER), plays a central role in regulating the growth and differentiation of normal breast epithelium (43,55). It stimulates cell proliferation and regulates the expression of other genes including progesterone receptor. Progesterone receptor then mediates the mitogenic effect of progesterone, further stimulating proliferation (43,55). Many additional factors collectively referred to as coactivators and corepressors have been discovered recently that appear to modulate the functions of these hormones and receptors including their mitogenic activity (56).

Many studies have assessed ER expression in normal TDLUs (29,31,33,57–59) and DCIS (33,37–40,60–71) (Table 5.1 and Fig. 5.1C,D). Most were immunohistochemical studies focusing presumably on ERα, although the potential cross-reactivity for ERβ of all the different antibodies used in these studies is not entirely clear. Mindful of this qualification, studies of normal TDLUs reported that more than 90% express ER, but in a minority of cells for all ages combined, averaged approximately 30%. In premenopausal women, the proportion of ER-positive cells in TDLUs varies with the menstrual cycle, being twice as high during the follicular than the luteal phase (59). Proliferation in TDLUs peaks during the luteal phase (29), suggesting that the mitogenic effect of estrogen may be partially delayed or indirect and mediated by downstream interactions such as that between progesterone and PR. The proportion of ER-positive cells in TDLUs in postmenopausal women is relatively high and stable in the absence of hormone replacement therapy (33).

Collectively, approximately 75% of DCIS express ER, but, like proliferation and many other biologic characteristics, expression varies with histologic differentiation. It is highest in low-grade, noncomedo lesions in which more than 90% show high levels of expression in nearly all cells (Fig. 5.1C). Approximately 75% of intermediate-grade DCIS also express high levels of ER in the majority of cells. Only 25% of high-grade, comedo DCIS express ER and even then in a minority of cells usually. ER is not expressed in approximately 25% of DCIS overall, and, as indicated, these are predominantly high-grade lesions (Fig. 5.1D). There is a recent preliminary study suggesting that the expression of ERβ in DCIS is very similar to that of ERα (72).

Prolonged estrogen exposure is an important risk factor for developing breast cancer, including DCIS, perhaps by allowing random genetic alterations to accumulate in cells continually stimulated to proliferate (55). The very high levels of ER observed in the majority of DCIS (predominantly low- and intermediate-grade lesions) may contribute to their increased proliferation relative to normal cells by allowing them to respond more effectively to any level of estrogen, even the low concentrations observed in postmenopausal women (33). This notion is supported experimentally by studies showing that estrogen greatly accelerates the growth of ER-positive DCIS xenografts, whereas the growth of ER-negative implants is unaffected (73). In addition to increased levels of expression, however, there may be other alterations of ER resulting in increased growth. For example, most of the dividing epithelium in normal breast appears to be ER negative, whereas both ER-negative and ER-positive cells proliferate in DCIS, suggesting that the hormonal regulation of growth is disrupted at this relatively early stage of tumor development (70,74,75). As another example, one recent study measured proliferation in TDLUs and DCIS from the same breasts in a large number of patients stratified by menopausal status (33). Proliferation rates in TDLUs were nearly threefold higher in premenopausal compared with postmenopausal women, consistent with the expected mitogenic effect of estrogen in normal cells. In contrast, the difference in proliferation in DCIS stratified by menopausal status was less than half that of normal cells, again demonstrating that the hormonal regulation of proliferation in these lesions is fundamentally abnormal. Another interesting recent study found a somatic mutation in the ERα gene in 30% of hyperplastic breast lesions, which, when transfected into breast cancer cell lines, showed much higher transcriptional activity and proliferation than wild-type ER at very low concentrations of estrogen such as seen in postmenopausal women (76). The mutated ER also showed markedly increased binding to the coactivator TIF-2, which may partially explain its increased functional responsiveness to estrogen. Whatever the mechanisms, the hypersensitivity to estrogen associated with this mutation may play a very important role in the early development and progression of all premalignant breast diseases including DCIS.

The ER status of DCIS may eventually be useful clinically as a biomarker to predict the ability of adjuvant hormonal therapies such as tamoxifen to reduce the risk of local recurrence in patients treated with breast-conserving surgery, just as it has been used for more than a decade in patients with fully developed IBC. Although it is very likely that the ER status of DCIS will correlate with recurrence, formal scientific demonstration of this is lacking pending the results of ongoing studies assessing ER in DCIS from randomized clinical trials treating patients with lumpectomy followed by tamoxifen such as NSABP B-24.

ONCOGENES (ERBB2)

erbB2 (also known as HER-2/neu) is the most thoroughly studied biomarker in DCIS. The gene for erbB2 resides on chromosome 17q21 and encodes a 185-kd transmembrane oncoprotein protein with intracellular tyrosine kinase activity (77). It is classified as a type 1 growth factor receptor owing to structural homology shared with other members of this family. There do not appear to be any ligands specific for erbB2 alone, but it forms heterodimeric receptor complexes with c-erbB-3 and c-erbB-4, which have high affinity for several ligands including heregulin, and ligand binding promotes cellular differentiation including the expression of adhesion molecules in breast cancer cell lines (78). erbB2 is amplified and/or overexpressed in approximately 20% of IBCs and these abnormalities are associated with increased proliferation, poor clinical outcome, and altered responsiveness to various types of adjuvant therapies (79). erbB2 may also promote cell motility (80,81), which could contribute to the ability of tumor cells overexpressing erbB2 to invade and metastasize.

Many studies have evaluated erbB2 in normal breast (82,83) and DCIS (35,37,38,40,41,66,68,69,71,83–96) (Table 5.1 and Fig. 5.1E,F). Nearly all used immunohistochemistry to detect overexpression of the oncoprotein, which is highly correlated with gene amplification (97). Overexpression has not been observed in normal TDLUs. In DCIS, the average rates of amplification or overexpression were approximately 5% in low-grade, 30% in intermediate-grade, and 70% in high-grade lesions. The overall rate in all DCIS combined is approximately 40%.

Just how alterations of erbB2 contribute to the development and progression of DCIS is unclear. Normal breast epithelium and early premalignant breast lesions (e.g., typical and atypical hyperplasias) have shown no convincing evidence of overexpression (83,98). In contrast, the overall incidence of overexpression is relatively high in DCIS, suggesting that activation of erbB2 is an important early event in malignant transformation leading to a substantial proportion of in situ disease. In particular, the increased proliferation and enhanced cell motility associated with amplified/overexpressed erbB2 might both contribute to the development and progression of DCIS (98). Paradoxically, the overall rate of erbB2 overexpression is much lower in IBC than in DCIS, suggesting that expression discontinues in a significant proportion of DCIS as they progress to invasive disease or, alternatively, that a substantial subset of IBCs arise *de novo* by mechanisms that are independent of erbB2 (83,98).

Assessment of erbB2 status could conceivably become a prognostic factor in the clinical management of patients with DCIS in the sense that any marker associated with an aggressive biologic phenotype might be used alone or in combination with other factors to help make treatment decisions. Currently, however, there are no data to support its routine use in this setting. The predictive implications of erbB2 in DCIS are also obscure, just as they are in IBC in which studies suggest that overexpression confers resistance to certain cytotoxic drugs and sensitivity to others (79). Although it is unlikely that cytotoxic chemotherapy will ever be used in patients with DCIS as chemoprevention against IBC, overexpression of erbB2 may still influence the response to more benign compounds that might be considered in future chemoprevention trials.

TUMOR SUPPRESSOR GENES (P53)

The p53 tumor suppressor gene has also been studied extensively in normal TDLUs (99–102) and DCIS (35,37–41,66–68,89,93,95,101–109) (Table 5.1 and Fig. 5.1G,H). Located on chromosome 17p13, it encodes a 53-kd nuclear phosphoprotein with several important functions including regulation of the cell cycle and programmed cell death (110). Mutated p53 is very common in many types of human cancers (111,112). Most are missense point mutations resulting in an inactive protein with a prolonged half-life that accumulates to very high levels in the cell nucleus (99,113), and, thus, measuring protein levels is a relatively easy and accurate surrogate assay for detecting mutations. Most studies of breast used immunohistochemistry to assess p53 status and showed that 30% to 40% of IBCs are abnormal and that an abnormal phenotype is associated with many other aggressive biologic features and poor clinical outcome (114).

With the exception of morphologically normal breast epithelium in patients with Li-Fraumeni cancer syndrome who have inherited mutations (115), the p53 gene is not mutated or significantly overexpressed in normal TDLUs. In DCIS, alterations of p53 correlate with histologic differentiation. The average proportions of abnormal cases is approximately 5% in low-grade, 20% in intermediate-grade, and 50% in high-grade lesions. The overall average is approximately 25%, approaching that in IBC.

Mutations that inactivate p53 probably contribute to the development and progression of DCIS by the same mechanisms that are thought to be operating in IBC. In replicating cells, particularly when there has been recent DNA damage (e.g., as may happen with ionizing radiation), the level of wild-type p53 protein increases, influencing several cellular functions through the binding of this protein to a number of transcriptional targets. One of these target genes, p21/WAF1, encodes a protein that inhibits cyclin-dependent kinases and DNA polymerase. This arrests replicating cells in the G1 phase of the cell cycle, which presumably allows time for DNA repair, providing a mechanism for maintaining genomic integrity. Loss of p53 function eliminates this G1 checkpoint, interfering with DNA repair and leading to replication of a damaged template during S phase. The result is increased proliferation and genomic instability, leading to clonal expansion and accelerated accumulation of other genetic defects that contribute to neoplastic progression. Normal p53 also appears to be essential for initiating apoptosis, and mutations of p53 might also contribute to clonal expansion by inhibiting cell death (110,116), particularly in hypoxic settings common to tumor cells (117).

There is currently no clinical role for p53 as a prognostic factor in DCIS, although future studies may show that lesions with mutated p53 are threatening enough to warrant relatively aggressive therapy. The predictive implications of p53 in DCIS are also unclear at this time, just as they are in IBC. Although several primarily *in vitro* studies suggest that inactivated p53 may result in resistance to radiotherapy or chemotherapy by inhibiting apoptosis in some types of cells (118–120), the results of studies in clinical breast cancer are ambiguous (121–126).

INVASION-RELATED BIOLOGY

DCIS alone is a harmless disease, but because of its potential to progress to IBC, it must be treated once diagnosed. However, it appears that not all DCIS progress to IBC and those that do vary greatly in the time it takes (22). The treatment of patients with DCIS could be improved by being able to predict invasive potential and matching the aggressiveness of therapy to the risk of progression. For example, small lesions that are unlikely to progress might be adequately managed by breast-conserving surgery alone, whereas large lesions at high risk might benefit from more comprehensive surgery such as mastectomy and adjuvant modalities such as radiation or hormonal therapy. The problem is that DCIS with different capacities for progression may look alike under the microscope, so prognostication will require a thorough understanding of the underlying and histologically silent biologic alterations responsible for invasion. On a simplistic level, the progression of DCIS to IBC is a multistep process involving reduced or at least dynamically changing adhesion between tumor cells and the acquisition of the abilities to degrade and migrate across the basement membrane and through the extracellular matrix. Insights into each of these areas have been gained recently.

For example, the expression of E-cadherin, an important epithelial adhesion molecule, has been demonstrated to decrease on the continuum of normal cells to low-grade DCIS, to high-grade DCIS, to IBC (127). Expression of desmoplakin, a glycoprotein involved in the formation of intercellular attachments referred to a desmosomes, is also decreased in DCIS relative to normal cells, and even further in IBC relative to DCIS (128). Gap junctions are attachments involved in intercellular communication that may have tumor suppressor functions. The gap junction proteins connexin 26 and connexin 43 are expressed at very high levels in IBC relative to DCIS and normal epithelium, suggesting that increased intercellular communication may be required for invasion (129).

DCIS, by definition, are transformed breast epithelial cells still residing within ducts and lobules, anatomic compartments that are surrounded by a continuous layer of myoepithelial cells (MECs) lying on an intact basement membrane. MECs have been shown to actively suppress the invasion of breast cancer cell lines *in vitro* by paracrine mechanisms involving maspin, which is highly expressed in MECs (130). MECs also appear to have antiproliferative effects on benign and malignant breast epithelium (131). MECs and basement membrane are normal barriers that are lacking in areas of invasion arising from DCIS (132).

Considerable evidence also points to the involvement of several enzyme systems in the active degradation and remodeling of basement membrane and extracellular matrix as DCIS becomes invasive. These include several extracellular matrix metalloproteinases such as metalloproteinase 1 (133), metalloproteinase 2 (133), and metalloproteinase 9 (134). Urokinase plasminogen activator and its receptor (UPAR) (135), members of another extracellular enzyme system, are increased in IBC relative to DCIS relative to normal cells, particularly in DCIS known to progress and recur as invasive disease (135).

Several mechanisms appear to increase the motility of cells as DCIS becomes invasive. Thymosin β15 is an intracellular protein that inhibits actin polymerization, increasing cell motility, and its expression is elevated in DCIS relative to normal (136). Gelsolin is another actin-binding protein involved in cell motility that dramatically decreases on the continuum of normal to DCIS to IBC (137). Scatter factor, also known as hepatocyte growth factor, is a cytokine that stimulates epithelial cell motility and invasion. Its receptor, a transmembrane tyrosine kinase, is encoded by the c-met proto-oncogene and the expression of both increases dramatically in IBC relative to DCIS relative to normal cells (138). Tenascin-c is an extracellular matrix glycoprotein that is expressed in areas of epithelial-mesenchymal interaction during fetal development and in neoplasia. It may have antiadhesive properties and thus increase cell motility and invasion. Its expression is markedly increased at the stromal-epithelial interface of DCIS compared with normal epithelium and in DCIS from cancerous (i.e., containing synchronous IBC) compared with noncancerous breasts, supporting the idea that it is also involved in tumor progression and invasion (139,140). Clearly, invasion is a complex process and much remains to be learned.

GENETIC STUDIES (ALLELIC IMBALANCE)

There has been an enormous amount of research in the past two decades focusing on identifying the genetic alterations underlying IBC. These studies benefited greatly from the abundance and availability of relatively large fresh-frozen clinical samples, in addition to many cell lines and animal models. In contrast, until very recently, there were few if any cell lines or animal models of DCIS, and the clinical samples available were small and usually limited to formalin-fixed, paraffin-embedded material. Because of these and other technical limitations, much less is known about the molecular genetics of DCIS than of IBC. Most studies of DCIS so far have looked at genes that were first discovered as important in fully developed IBC, which is a reasonable strategy in the sense that precursor lesions should contain some of the same defects.

The most comprehensive genetic studies of DCIS are those assessing allelic imbalance (AI) by loss of heterozygosity (LOH) or comparative genomic hybridization (CGH), methods that identify the general chromosomal locations of nonfunctional tumor suppressor genes (through losses) or amplified oncogenes (through gains). Collectively, the results of these studies demonstrate that the genetic alterations in DCIS are highly complex, rivaling those in IBC. Recent studies using high-resolution serial analysis of gene expression confirm the tremendous genetic diversity in DCIS and suggest that early defects affecting DNA repair may be especially common and important by promoting a mutator phenotype and thus accelerating the accumulation of additional alterations (141).

Nearly all DCIS showed at least one AI among the more than 200 genetic loci on 22 chromosomes studied so far (10,42,142–167) (Table 5.2). In fact, imbalances have been identified on every human chromosome except 5 and Y to date. Individual DCIS typically contain several synchronous AIs, especially high-grade DCIS, which in some studies showed as many as eight in a single lesion (10,161). Not surprisingly, the same loci that appear to be important in IBC also appear to be involved in DCIS. The highest rates of AI in DCIS approached 80% and involved loci on chromosomes 16q, 17p, and 17q, suggesting that altered genes in these regions may be particularly important in the development of DCIS (10,142,145–148).

Studies of AI in DCIS from breasts with synchronous IBC provide compelling, if not surprising, evidence of their evolutionary relatedness as precursor and product. In one recent study evaluating LOH at 15 loci on 10 chromosomes, 85% of DCIS shared identical AI phenotypes with adjacent IBC, and the sharing usually involved several loci (10), an observation that has been confirmed by many other studies (146–148,157,163,168). Synchronous DCIS and IBC may occasionally also show distinct AIs, suggesting that there may be divergent aspects to their evolution (10,148). An interesting recent study by Deng and colleagues (169) noted that histologically normal TDLUs shared LOH for markers on 3p, 11p, and 17p with closely adjacent IBC, whereas TDLUs farther away in the same breast did not, suggesting that even normal-appearing epithelium may have genotypic abnormalities associated with an elevated risk for developing breast cancer. Another fascinating recent study demonstrated LOH in stromal cells adjacent to DCIS and IBC, and some losses were shared with the cancers, suggesting that breast cancers may evolve as an ecosystem of interacting alterations in many types of cells (170).

Studies of LOH, comparative genomic hybridization, and many other methodologies over the past decade provide crude but compelling evidence that IBC evolves from DCIS by highly diverse genetic and epigenetic mechanisms. Perhaps future studies will provide more detailed information about specific mechanisms that can be targeted to prevent the development and progression of DCIS. Progress in the past has been hampered by a reliance on correlative studies of small archival clinical samples that are difficult to obtain and a lack of appropriate cell lines and animal models to support mechanistic studies. Fortunately, cell lines and animal models are beginning to emerge to support the studies necessary for more fundamental progress (171), such as the MCF10AT cell line, which can mimic certain aspects of DCIS in mouse xenografts (172,173). Additional progress can be expected from the use of new technologies such as laser-capture microdissection and cDNA expression microarrays, which, when combined, allow thousands of genes to be studied in a few hundred cells from small lesions such as DCIS. One preliminary study using this technology has already identified a large number of new genes as potentially important in the progression from normal cells to DCIS (174).

SUMMARY

DCIS is being encountered much more frequently because of screening mammography. Epidemiologic, pathologic, and more recent genetic studies confirm that most IBCs arise from preexisting DCIS. Thus, if DCIS can be treated successfully, or prevented from developing, the incidence of potentially lethal IBC will also be reduced. The prevention of DCIS will almost certainly be based on understanding and targeting the genetic and epigenetic alterations leading to its development and progression. Unfortunately, very little is known about this biology. What is known demonstrates that DCIS possesses many of the same abnormalities found in IBC. Certain alterations appear to play particularly important roles in DCIS such as overexpression and perhaps mutation of ER, amplification and overexpression of erbB2, and mutation of p53. Other studies assessing AI, however, emphasize that many other important genetic defects are yet to be discovered. The identification and characterization of these alterations should increase greatly in the near future with the emergence of new cell lines and animal models of DCIS and new high throughput technologies to study them.

ACKNOWLEDGMENT

This work was supported by grants NIH PO1 CA 30195 and NIH P50 CA 58183.

REFERENCES

1. Bestill Jr WL, Rosen PP, Lieberman PH, et al. Intraductal carcinoma. Long-term follow-up after treatment by biopsy alone. *JAMA* 1978;239:1863–1867.
2. Page DL, Dupont WD, Rogers LW, et al. Continued local recurrence of carcinoma 15–25 years after a diagnosis of low grade ductal carcinoma in situ of the breast treated only by biopsy. *Cancer* 1995;76:1197–200.
3. Silverstein MJ, Lagios MD, Groshen S, et al. The influence of margin width on local control of ductal carcinoma in situ of the breast. *N Engl J Med* 1999;340:1455–1461.
4. van Dogen JA, Voogd AC, Fentiman IS, et al. Long-term results of a randomized trial comparing breast-conserving therapy with mastectomy: European Organization for Research and Treatment of Cancer 10801 trial. *J Natl Cancer Inst* 2000;92:1143–1150.
5. BijKer N, Peterse JL, Duchateau L, et al. Risk factors for recurrence and metastasis after breast-conserving therapy for ductal carcinoma-in-situ: analysis of European Organization for Research and Treatment of Cancer Trial 10853. *J Clin Oncol* 2001;19:2263–2271.
6. Wellings RR, Jensen HM. On the origin and progression of ductal carcinoma in the human breast. *J Natl Cancer Inst* 1973; 50:1111–1118.
7. Wellings SR, Jensen HM, Marcum RG. An atlas of subgross pathology of the human breast with special reference to possible precancerous lesions. *J Natl Cancer Inst* 1975;55:231–243.
8. Alpers CE, Wellings SR. The prevalence of carcinoma in situ in normal and cancer-associated breasts. *Human Pathol* 1985;16: 796–807.
9. Bartow SA, Pathak DR, Black WC, et al. Prevalence of benign, atypical, and malignant breast lesions in populations at different risk for breast cancer. A forensic autopsy study. *Cancer* 1987;60: 2751–2760.
10. O'Connell P, Pekkel V, Fuqua SAW, et al. Analysis of loss of heterozygosity in 399 premalignant breast lesions at 15 genetic loci. *J Natl Cancer Inst* 1998;90:697–703.
11. Schnitt SF, Sile W, Sadowsky NL, et al. Ductal carcinoma in situ (intraductal carcinoma) of the breast. *N Engl J Med* 1988; 318:898–903.
12. Osteen R, Cady B, Chimel J. National survey of carcinoma of the breast by the Commission on Cancer. *J Am Coll Surg* 1994; 178:213–219.
13. Ernster VL, Barclay J, Kerlikowske K, et al. Incidence of and treatment for ductal carcinoma in situ of the breast. *JAMA* 1996;275:913–918.
14. Ernster VL, Barclay J. Increases in ductal carcinoma in situ (DCIS) of the breast in relation to mammography: a dilemma. *J Natl Cancer Inst Monogr* 1997:151–156.
15. Silverstein MJ, Barth A, Poller DN, et al. Ten-year results comparing mastectomy to excision and radiation therapy for ductal carcinoma in situ of the breast. *Eur J Cancer* 1995;31A:1425–1427.
16. Baird RM, Worth A, Hislop G. Recurrence after lumpectomy for comedo-type intraductal carcinoma of the breast. *Am J Surg* 1990;159:479–481.
17. Fisher ER, Leeming R, Anderson S, et al. Conservative management of intraductal carcinoma (DCIS) of the breast. *J Surg Oncol* 1991;47:139–147.
18. Silverstein MJ, Cohlan BF, Gierson ED, et al. Duct carcinoma in situ: 227 cases without microinvasion. *Eur J Cancer* 1992;28: 630–634.
19. Fisher ER, Sass R, Fisher B, et al. Pathologic findings from the National Surgical Adjuvant Breast Project (Protocol 6) I. Intraductal Carcinoma (DCIS). *Cancer* 1986;57:197–208.
20. Fisher B, Costantino J, Redmond C, et al. Lumpectomy compared with lumpectomy and radiation therapy for the treatment of intraductal breast cancer. *N Engl J Med* 1993;328:1581–1586.
21. Warneke J, Grossklaus D, Davis J, et al. Influence of local treatment on the recurrence rate of ductal carcinoma in situ. *J Am Coll Surg* 1995;180:683–688.

22. Solin LJ, Kurtz J, Forquet A, et al. Fifteen-year results of breast-conserving surgery and definitive breast irradiation for the treatment of ductal carcinoma in situ of the breast. *J Clin Oncol* 1996;14:754–763.

23. Meyer JS. Cell proliferation in normal human breast ducts, fibroadenomas, and other ductal hyperplasias measured by nuclear labeling with tritiated thymidine. *Hum Pathol* 1977;8:67–81.

24. Ferguson DJP, Anderson TJ. Morphological evaluation of cell turnover in relation to the menstrual cycle in the "resting" human breast. *Br J Cancer* 1981;44:177–181.

25. Joshi K, Smith JA, Perusinghe N, et al. Cell proliferation in the human mammary epithelium: differential contribution by epithelial and myoepithelial cells. *Am J Pathol* 1986;124:199–206.

26. Longacre TA, Bartow SA. A correlative morphologic study of human breast and endometrium in the menstrual cycle. *Am J Surg Pathol* 1986;10:382–393.

27. Russo J, Calaf GRL, Russo IH. Influence of age and gland topography on cell kinetics of normal breast tissue. *J Natl Cancer Inst* 1987;78:413–418.

28. Going JJ, Anderson TJ, Battersby S, et al. Proliferative and secretory activity in human breast during natural and artificial cycles. *Am J Pathol* 1988;130:193–204.

29. Potten CS, Watson RJ, Williams GT, et al. The effect of age and menstrual cycle upon proliferative activity of the normal human breast. *Br J Cancer* 1988;58:163–170.

30. Kamel OW, Franklin WA, Ringus JC, et al. Thymidine labeling index and Ki-67 growth fraction in lesions of the breast. *Am J Pathol* 1989;134:107–113.

31. Schmitt FC. Multistep progression from an oestrogen-dependent growth towards an autonomous growth in breast carcinogenesis. *Eur J Cancer* 1995;31A:2049–2052.

32. Visscher DW, Gingrich DS, Buckley J, et al. Cell cycle analysis of normal, atrophic, and hyperplastic breast epithelium using two-color multiparametric flow cytometry. *Anal Cell Pathol* 1996;12:115–124.

33. Mohsin SK, Hilsenbeck SG, Allred DC. Estrogen receptors and growth control in premalignant breast disease. *Mod Pathol* 2000:28A(#145).

34. Locker AP, Horrocks C, Gilmour AS, et al. Flow cytometric and histological analysis of ductal carcinoma in situ of the breast. *Br J Surg* 1990;77:564–567.

35. Bobrow LG, Happerfield LC, Gregory WM, et al. The classification of ductal carcinoma in situ and its association with biological markers. *Semin Diagn Pathol* 1994;11:199–207.

36. Poller DN, Silverstein MJ, Galea M, et al. Ductal carcinoma in situ of the breast: a proposal for a new simplified histological classification association between cellular proliferation and c-erbB-2 protein expression. *Mod Pathol* 1994;7:257–262.

37. Zafrani B, Leroyer A, Fourquet A, et al. Mammographically detected ductal in situ carcinoma of the breast analyzed with a new classification. A study of 127 cases: correlation with estrogen and progesterone receptors, p53, and c-erbB-2 proteins, and proliferative activity. *Semin Diagn Pathol* 1994;11:208–214.

38. Albonico G, Querzoli P, Feretti S, et al. Biophenotypes of breast carcinoma in situ defined by image analysis of biological parameters. *Pathol Res Pract* 1996;192:117–123.

39. Moreno A, Lloveras B, Figueras A, et al. Ductal carcinoma in situ of the breast: correlation between histologic classifications and biologic markers. *Mod Pathol* 1997;10:1088–1092.

40. Rudas M, Neumayer R, Gnant MFX, et al. p53 protein expression, cell proliferation and steroid hormone receptors in ductal and lobular in situ carcinomas of the breast. *Eur J Cancer* 1997;33:39–44.

41. Mack L, Kerkvliet N, Doig G, et al. Relationship of a new histological categorization of ductal carcinoma in situ of the breast

with size and the immunohistochemical expression of p53, c-erbB2, bcl-2, and Ki67. *Hum Pathol* 1997;28:974–979.

42. Marsh KL, Varley JM. Frequent alterations of cell cycle regulators in early-stage breast lesions as detected by immunohistochemistry. *Br J Cancer* 1998;77:1460–1468.

43. Pike MC, Spicer DV, Dahmoush L, et al. Estrogens, progestins, normal breast cell proliferation, and breast cancer risk. *Epidemiol Rev* 1993;15:17–35.

44. Shoker BS, Sloane JP. DCIS grading schemes and clinical implications. *Histopathology* 1999;35:393–400.

45. Prosser J, Hilsenbeck SG, Fuqua SAW, et al. Cell turnover (proliferation and apoptosis) in normal epithelium and premalignant lesions in the same breast. *Lab Invest* 1997;76:119.

46. Bodis S, Siziopikou KP, Schitt SJ, et al. Extensive apoptosis in ductal carcinoma in situ of the breast. *Cancer* 1996;77:1831–1835.

47. Harn HJ, Shen KL, Yueh KC, et al. Apoptosis occurs more frequently in intraductal carcinoma than in infiltrating duct carcinoma of human breast cancer and correlates with altered p53 expression: detected by terminal-deoxynucleotidyl-transferase-mediated dUTP-FITC nick end labeling (TUNEL). *Histopathology* 1997;31:534–539.

48. Mommers ECM, van Diest PJ, Leonhart AM, et al. Balance of cell proliferation and apoptosis in breast carcinogenesis. *Breast Cancer Res Treat* 1999;58:163–169.

49. Weinstat-Saslow D, Merino MJ, Manrow RE, et al. Overexpression of cyclin D mRNA distinguishes invasive and in situ breast carcinomas from non-malignant lesions. *Nat Med* 1995;1:1257–1269.

50. Simpson JF, Quan DE, O'Malley F, et al. Amplification of CCND1 and expression of its protein product, cyclin D1, in ductal carcinoma in situ of the breast. *Am J Pathol* 1997;151:161–168.

51. Zhou Q, Hopp T, Fuqua SA, et al. Cyclin D1 in breast premalignancy and early breast cancer: implications for prevention and treatment. *Cancer Lett* 2001;162:3–17.

52. Shpitz B, Zimlichman S, Zemer R, et al. Telomerase activity in ductal carcinoma in situ of the breast. *Breast Cancer Res Treat* 1999;58:65–69.

53. Gobbi H, Arteaga CL, Jensen RA, et al. Loss of expression of transforming growth factor beta type II receptor correlates with high tumour grade in human breast in-situ and invasive carcinomas. *Histopathology* 2000;36:168–177.

54. Shekhar MPV, Werdell J, Santner SJ, et al. Breast stroma plays a dominant regulatory role in breast epithelial growth and differentiation: Implications for tumor development and progression. *Cancer Res* 2001;61:1320–1326.

55. Henderson BE, Ross R, Bernstein L. Estrogens as a cause of human cancer: the Richard and Hindau Rosenthal Foundation Award Lecture. *Cancer Res* 1988;48:246–253.

56. Horwitz KB, Jackson TA, Bain DL, et al. Nuclear receptor coactivators and corepressors. *Mol Endocrinol* 1996;10:1167–1177.

57. Allegra JC, Lippman ME, Green L, et al. Estrogen receptor values in patients with benign breast disease. *Cancer* 1979;44: 228–231.

58. Peterson OW, Hoyer PE, van Deurs B. Frequency and distribution of estrogen receptor-positive cells in normal, nonlactating human breast tissue. *J Natl Cancer Inst* 1986;77:343–349.

59. Ricketts D, Turnbull L, Tyall G, et al. Estrogen and progesterone receptors in the normal female breast. *Cancer Res* 1991;51:1817–1822.

60. Giri DD, Dundas AC, Nottingham JF, et al. Oestrogen receptors in benign epithelial lesions and intraduct carcinomas of the breast: an immunohistological study. *Histopathology* 1989;15:575–584.

61. Helin HJ, Helle MJ, Kallioneimi OP, et al. Immunohistochemical determination of estrogen and progesterone receptors in hu-

man breast carcinoma: correlation with histopathology and DNA flow cytometry. *Cancer* 1989;63:1761–1767.

62. Barnes R, Masood S. Potential value of hormone receptor assay in carcinoma in situ of breast. *Am J Clin Pathol* 1990;94:533–537.

63. Pallis L, Wilking N, Cedermark B, et al. Receptors for estrogen and progesterone in breast carcinoma in situ. *Anticancer Res* 1992;12:2113–2115.

64. Poller DN, Snead DRJ, Roberts EC, et al. Oestrogen receptor expression in ductal carcinoma in situ of the breast: relationship to flow cytometric analysis of DNA and expression of the c-erbB-2 oncoprotein. *Br J Cancer* 1993;68:156–161.

65. Chaudhuri B, Crist KA, Mucci S, et al. Distribution of estrogen receptor in ductal carcinoma in situ of the breast. *Surgery* 1993;113:134–137.

66. Leal CB, Schmitt FC, Bento MJ, et al. Ductal carcinoma in situ of the breast. Histologic categorization and its relationship to ploidy and immunohistochemical expression of hormone receptors, p53, and c-erbB-2 protein. *Cancer* 1995;75:2123–2131.

67. Bose S, Lesser ML, Norton L, et al. Immunophenotype of intraductal carcinoma. *Arch Pathol Lab Med* 1996;120:81–85.

68. Berardo M, Hilsenbeck SG, Allred DC. Histological grading of noninvasive breast cancer and its relationship to biological features. *Lab Invest* 1996;74[15A]:68.

69. Karayiannakis AJ, Bastounis EA, Chatziganni EB, et al. Immunohistochemical detection of oestrogen receptors in ductal carcinoma in situ of the breast. *Eur J Surg Oncol* 1996;22:578–582.

70. Shocker BS, Jarvis C, Clarke RB, et al. Estrogen receptor-positive proliferating cells in the normal and precancerous breast. *Am J Pathol* 1999;155:1811–1815.

71. Claus EB, Chu P, Howe CL, et al. Pathobiologic findings in DCIS of the breast: morphologic features, angiogenesis, HER-2/neu and hormone receptors. *Exp Mol Pathol* 2001;70:303–316.

72. Roger P, Sahla ME, Makela S, et al. Decreased expression of estrogen receptor beta protein in proliferative preinvasive mammary tumors. *Cancer Res* 2001;61:2537–2541.

73. Holland PA, Knox WF, Potten CS, et al. Assessment of hormone dependence of comedo ductal carcinoma in situ of the breast. *J Natl Cancer Inst* 1997;89:1059–1065.

74. Clarke RB, Howell A, Potten CS, et al. Dissociation between steroid receptor expression and cell proliferation in the human breast. *Cancer Res* 1997;57:4987–4991.

75. Shocker BS, Jarvis C, Clarke RB, et al. Abnormal regulation of the oestrogen receptor in benign breast lesions. *J Clin Pathol* 2000;53:778–783.

76. Fuqua SAW, Witschke C, Zhang ZX, et al. A hypersensitivity estrogen receptor alpha mutation in premalignant breast lesions. *Cancer Res* 2000;60:4026–4029.

77. Rajkulmar T, Gullick J. The type 1 growth factor receptors in human breast cancer. *Breast Cancer Res Treat* 1994;29:3–9.

78. Lupu R, Cardilla M, Harris L, et al. Interaction between erbB-receptors and heregulin in breast cancer tumor progression and drug resistance. *Semin Cancer Biol* 1995;6:135–145.

79. DiGiovanna MP. Clinical significance of HER-2/neu overexpression. *PPO Updates* 1999;13(9, 10):1–10; 1–14.

80. De Potter CR, Quatacker J. The p185/erbB2 protein is localized on cell organelles involved in cell motility. *Clin Exp Metastasis* 1993;11:453–461.

81. De Potter CR. The neu-oncogene: more than a prognostic factor? *Hum Pathol* 1994;25:1264–1268.

82. De Potter CR, van Daele S, van de Vijer MJ, et al. The expression of the neu oncogene product in breast lesions and in normal fetal and adult human tissues. *Histopathology* 1989;15:351–362.

83. Allred DC, Clark GM, Molina R, et al. Overexpression of HER-2/neu and its relationship with other prognostic factors change during the progression of in situ to invasive breast cancer. *Hum Pathol* 1992;23:974–979.

84. van de Vijer MJ, Peterse JL, Mooi WJ, et al. neu-Protein overexpression in breast cancer. Association with comedo-type ductal carcinoma in situ and limited prognostic value in stage II breast cancer. *N Engl J Med* 1988;319:1239–1245.

85. Bartkova J, Barnes DM, Millis RR, et al. Immunohistochemical demonstration of c-erbB-2 protein in mammary ductal carcinoma in situ. *Hum Pathol* 1990;21:1164–1167.

86. Lodato RF, Maguire Jr HC, Greene MI, et al. Immunohistochemical evaluation of c-erbB-2 oncogene expression in ductal carcinoma in situ and atypical ductal hyperplasia of the breast. *Mod Pathol* 1990;3:449–454.

87. Ramachandra S, Machin L, Ashley S, et al. Immunohistochemical distribution of c-erbB-2 in in situ breast carcinoma: a detailed morphological analysis. *J Pathol* 1990;161:7–14.

88. Barnes DM, Meyer JS, Gonzalez JG, et al. Relationship between c-erbB-2 immunoreactivity and thymidine labeling index in breast carcinoma in situ. *Breast Cancer Res Treat* 1991;18:11–17.

89. Walker RA, Dearing SJ, Lane DP, et al. Expression of p53 protein in infiltrating and in-situ breast carcinomas. *J Pathol* 1991;165:203–211.

90. Barnes DM, Bartkova J, Camplejohn RS, et al. Overexpression of the c-erbB-2 oncoprotein: why does this occur more frequently in ductal carcinoma in situ than in invasive mammary carcinoma and is this of prognostic significance? *Eur J Cancer* 1992;28:644–648.

91. Schimmelpenning H, Eriksson ET, Pallis L, et al. Immunohistochemical c-erbB-2 proto-oncogene expression and nuclear DNA content in human mammary carcinoma in situ. *Am J Clin Pathol* 1992;97[Suppl]:S48–S52.

92. Somerville JE, Clarke LA, Biggart JD. c-erbB-2 overexpression and histological type of in situ and invasive breast carcinomas. *J Clin Pathol* 1992;45:16–20.

93. Tsuda H, Iwaya K, Fukutomi T, et al. P53 mutations and c-erbB-2 amplification in intraductal and invasive breast carcinomas of high histologic grade. *Jpn J Cancer Res* 1993;84:394–401.

94. De Potter CR, Schelfhout A-M, Verbeeck P, et al. neu-Overexpression correlates with extent of disease in large cell ductal carcinoma in situ of the breast. *Hum Pathol* 1995;26:601–606.

95. Kanthan R, Xiang J, Magliocco AM. p53, ErbB2, and TAG-72 expression in the spectrum of ductal carcinoma in situ of the breast classified by the Van Nuys system. *Arch Pathol Lab Med* 2000;124:234–239.

96. Ottensen GL, Christensen IJ, Larsen JK, et al. Carcinoma in situ of the breast: correlation of histopathology to immunohistochemical markers and DNA ploidy. *Breast Cancer Res Treat* 2000;60:219–226.

97. Venter DJ, Tuzi NL, Kumar S, et al. Overexpression of the c-erbB-2 oncoprotein in human breast carcinomas: immunohistological assessment correlates with gene amplification. *Lancet* 1987;2:69–72.

98. De Potter CR, Schelfheut AM. The neu-protein and breast cancer. *Virchows Arch* 1995;426:107–115.

99. Bartek J, Iggo R, Gannon J, et al. Genetic and immunochemical analysis of mutant p53 in human breast cancer cell lines. *Oncogene* 1990;5:893–899.

100. Davidoff AM, Kerns B-JM, Pence JC, et al. p53 alterations in all stages of breast cancer. *J Surg Oncol* 1991;48:260–267.

101. Eriksson ET, Schimmelpenning H, Aspenblad U, et al. Immunohistochemical expression of the mutant p53 protein and nuclear DNA content during the transition from benign to malignant breast disease. *Hum Pathol* 1994;25:1228–1233.

102. Rajan PB, Scott DJ, Perry RH, et al. p53 protein expression in ductal carcinoma in situ (DCIS) of the breast. *Breast Cancer Res Treat* 1997;42:283–290.

103. Poller DN, Roberts EC, Bell JA, et al. p53 protein expression in mammary ductal carcinoma in situ: relationship to immunohistochemical expression of estrogen receptor and c-erbB-2 protein. *Hum Pathol* 1993;24:463–468.

104. O'Malley FP, Vnencak-Jones CL, et al. p53 mutations are confined to the comedo type ductal carcinoma in situ of the breast: immunohistochemical and sequencing data. *Lab Invest* 1994; 71:67–72.

105. Schmitt FC, Leal D, Lopes C. p53 protein expression and nuclear DNA content in breast intraductal proliferations. *J Pathol* 1995;176:233–241.

106. Chitemere M, Andersen TI, Hom R, et al. TP53 alterations atypical ductal hyperplasia and ductal carcinoma in situ of the breast. *Breast Cancer Res Treat* 1996;41:103–109.

107. Siziopikou KP, Prioleau JE, Harris JR, et al. Bcl-2 expression in the spectrum of preinvasive breast lesions. *Cancer* 1996;77:499– 506.

108. Lukas J, Press MF. p53 mutations and expression in breast carcinoma in situ. *Am J Pathol* 2000;156:183–191.

109. Siziopikou KP, Schnitt SJ. MIB-1 proliferation index in ductal carcinoma in situ of the breast: relationship to the expression of the apoptosis-regulating proteins bcl-2 and p53. *Breast J* 2000; 6(6):400–406.

110. Shimamura A, Fisher DE. Minireview. P53 in life and death. *Clin Cancer Res* 1996;2:435–440.

111. Harris CC, Hollstein M. Clinical implications of the p53 tumor-suppressor gene. *N Engl J Med* 1993;329:1318–1327.

112. Chang F, Syrjanen S, Syrjanen K. Implications of the p53 tumor-suppressor gene in clinical oncology. *J Clin Oncol* 1995;13: 1009–1022.

113. Davidoff AM, Humphrey PA, Iglehart JD, et al. Genetic basis for p53 overexpression in human breast cancer. *Proc Natl Acad Sci U S A* 1991;88:5006–5010.

114. Allred DC, Elledge R, Clark GM, et al. The p53 tumor suppressor gene in human breast cancer. In: Dickson RB, Lippman ME, eds. *Mammary tumorigenesis and malignant progression.* Boston: Kluwer Academic Publishers, 1994:63–77.

115. Barnes DM, Hanby AM, Gillett CE, et al. Abnormal expression of wild type p53 protein in normal cells of a cancer family patient. *Lancet* 1992;340:259–263.

116. Osborne BA, Schwartz LM. Essential genes that regulate apoptosis. *Trends Cell Biol* 1994;4:393–398.

117. Graeber TG, Osmanina C, Jacks T. Hypoxia-mediated selection of cells with diminished apoptotic potential in solid tumours. *Nature* 1996;379:88–91.

118. Clarke AR, Purdie CA, Harrison DJ, et al. Thymocyte apoptosis induced by p53-dependent and independent pathways. *Nature* 1993;362:849–852.

119. Lowe SW, Schmitt EM, Smith SW, et al. p53 is required for radiation-induced apoptosis in mouse thymocytes. *Nature* 1993; 362:847–849.

120. Lowe SW, Ruley HE, Jacks T, et al. p53-dependent apoptosis modulates the cytotoxicity of anticancer agents. *Cell* 1993;74: 957–967.

121. Fan S, Smith ML, Rivet II DJ, et al. Disruption of p53 function sensitizes breast cancer MCF-7 cells to cisplatin and pentoxifylline. *Cancer Res* 1995;55:1649–1654.

122. Shao Z-M, Dawson MI, Li XS, et al. p53 independent G0/G1 arrest and apoptosis induced by a novel retinoid in human breast cancer cells. *Oncogene* 1995;11:493–504.

123. Jansson T, Inganas M, Sjogren S, et al. p53 status predicts survival in breast cancer patients treated with or without postoperative radiotherapy: a novel hypothesis based on clinical findings. *J Clin Oncol* 1995;13:2745–2751.

124. Stal O, Skoog L, Rutqvist LE, et al. S-phase fraction and survival benefit from adjuvant chemotherapy or radiotherapy of breast cancer. *Br J Cancer* 1994;70:1258–1262.

125. Elledge RM, Gray R, Mansour E, et al. Accumulation of p53 protein as a possible predictor of response to adjuvant combination chemotherapy with cyclophosphamide, methotrexate, fluorouracil, and prednisone for breast cancer. *J Natl Cancer Inst* 1995;87:1254–1256.

126. Jacquemier J, Moles JP, Penault-Llorca F, et al. p53 immunohistochemical analysis in breast cancer with four monoclonal antibodies: comparison of staining and PCR-SSCP results. *Br J Cancer* 1994;69:846–852.

127. Gupta SK, Douglas-Jones AG, Jasani B, et al. E-cadherin (E-cad) expression in duct carcinoma in situ (DCIS) of the breast. *Virchows Arch* 1997;430:23–28.

128. Davies EL, Gee JMW, Cochrane RA, et al. The immunohistochemical expression of desmoplakin and its role in vivo in the progression and metastasis of breast cancer. *Eur J Cancer* 1999; 35:902–907.

129. Jamieson S, Going JJ, D'arcy R, et al. Expression of gap junction proteins connexin 26 and connexin 43 in normal human breast and breast tumours. *J Pathol* 1998;184:37–43.

130. Sternlicht MD, Kedeshian P, Shao P, et al. The human myoepithelial cell is a natural tumor suppressor. *Clin Cancer Res* 1997; 3:1949–1958.

131. Shao ZM, Nguyen M, Alpaugh ML, et al. The human myoepithelial cell exerts antiproliferative effects on breast carcinoma cells characterized by p21 induction, G2/M arrest, and apoptosis. *Exp Cell Res* 1998;241:394–403.

132. Damiani S, Ludvikova M, Tomasic G, et al. Myoepithelial cells and basal lamina in poorly differentiated in situ duct carcinoma of the breast. *Virchows Arch* 1999;434:227–234.

133. Brummer O, Athar S, Ricthdorf L, et al. Matrix-metalloproteinases 1, 2 and 3 and their tissue inhibitors 1 and 2 in benign and malignant breast lesions: an in situ hybridization study. *Virchows Arch* 1999;435:566–573.

134. Rha SY, Kim JH, Roh JK, et al. Sequential production and activation of matrix-metalloproteinase-9 (MMP-9) with breast cancer progression. *Breast Cancer Res Treat* 1997;43:175–181.

135. Guyton DP, Evans DM, Sloan-Stakleff KD. Urokinase plasminogen activator receptor (uPAR): a potential indicator of invasion in situ breast cancer. *Breast J* 2000;6:130 136.

136. Gold JS, Bao L, Ghoussoub RAD, et al. Localization and quantitation of expression of the cell motility-related protein thymosin b15 in human breast tissue. *Mod Pathol* 1997;10(11): 1106–1112.

137. Winston JS, Asch HL, Zhang PJ, et al. Down regulation of gelsolin correlates with the progression to breast carcinoma. *Breast Cancer Res Treat* 2001;65:11–21.

138. Jin L, Fuchs A, Schnitt SJ, et al. Expression of scatter factor and c-met receptor in benign and malignant breast tissue. *Cancer* 1997;79:749–760.

139. Jahkola T, Toivonen T, Nordling S, et al. Expression of tenascin-c in intraductal carcinoma of human breast: relationship to invasion. *Eur J Cancer* 1998;34:1687–1692.

140. Iskaros BE, Sison CP, Hajdu SI. Tenascin patterns of expression in ductal carcinoma in situ of the breast. *Ann Clin Lab Sci* 2000; 30:266–271.

141. Shen C-Y, Yu J-C, Lo Y-L, et al. Genome-wide search for loss of heterozygosity using laser capture microdissected tissue of breast carcinoma: an implication for mutator phenotype and breast cancer pathogenesis. *Cancer Res* 2000;60:3884–3892.

142. Radford DM, Fair K, Thompson AM, et al. Allelic loss on chromosome 17 in ductal carcinoma in situ of the breast. *Cancer Res* 1993;53:2947–2950.

143. O'Connell P, Pekkel V, Fuqua S, et al. Molecular genetic stud-

ies of early breast cancer evolution. *Breast Cancer Res Treat* 1994; 32:5–12.

144. Munn KE, Walker RA, Varley JM. Frequent alterations of chromosome 1 in ductal carcinoma in situ of the breast. *Oncogene* 1995;10:1653–1657.

145. Aldaz CM, Chen T, Sahin A, et al. Comparative allelotype of in situ and invasive human breast cancer: high frequency of microsatellite instability in lobular breast carcinomas. *Cancer Res* 1995;55:3976–3981.

146. Radford DM, Fair KL, Phillips NJ, et al. Allelotyping of ductal carcinoma in situ of the breast: deletion of loci on 8p, 13q, 16q, 17p and 17q. *Cancer Res* 1995;55:3399–3405.

147. Stratton MR, Collins N, Lakhani SR, et al. Loss of heterozygosity in ductal carcinoma in situ of the breast. *J Pathol* 1995;175: 195–201.

148. Fujii H, Marsh C, Cairns P, et al. Genetic divergence in the clonal evolution of breast cancer. *Cancer Res* 1996;56:1493– 1497.

149. Fujii H, Szumel R, Marsh C, et al. Genetic progression, histologic grade, and allelic loss in ductal carcinoma in situ of the breast. *Cancer Res* 1996;56:5260–5265.

150. Man S, Ellis IO, Sibbering M, et al. High levels of allele loss at the FHIT and ATM genes in non-comedo ductal carcinoma in situ and grade I tubular invasive breast cancers. *Cancer Res* 1996; 56:5484–5489.

151. Chen T, Sahin A, Aldaz CM. Deletion map of chromosome 16q in ductal carcinoma in situ of the breast: refining a putative tumor suppressor gene region. *Cancer Res* 1996;56:5605–5609.

152. James LA, Mitchell ELD, Menasce L, et al. Comparative genomic hybridization of ductal carcinoma in situ of the breast: identification of regions of DNA amplification and deletion in common with invasive breast carcinoma. *Oncogene* 1997;14: 1059–1065.

153. Lininger RA, Fujii H, Man Y-G, et al. Comparison of loss of heterozygosity in primary and recurrent ductal carcinoma in situ of the breast. *Mod Pathol* 1998;11:1151–1159.

154. Marsh KL, Varley JM. Loss of heterozygosity at chromosome 9p in ductal carcinoma in situ and invasive carcinoma of the breast. *Br J Cancer* 1998;77:1439–1447.

155. Anbazhagan R, Fujii H, Gabrielson E. Allelic loss of chromosomal arm 8p in breast cancer progression. *Am J Pathol* 1998;152: 815–819.

156. Fabre A, McCann AH, O'Shea D, et al. Loss of heterozygosity of the Wilms' tumor suppressor gene (WT1) in in situ and invasive breast carcinoma. *Hum Pathol* 1999;30:661–665.

157. Amari M, Suzuki A, Moriya T, et al. LOH analyses of premalignant and malignant lesions of human breast: frequent LOH in 8p, 16q, and 17q in atypical ductal hyperplasia. *Oncol Rep* 1999;6:1277–1280.

158. Moore E, Manger H, Coyne J, et al. Widespread chromosomal abnormalities in high-grade ductal carcinoma in situ of the breast. Comparative genomic hybridization study of pure high-grade DCIS. *J Pathol* 1999;187:403–409.

159. Buerger H, Otterbach F, Simon R, et al. Comparative genomic hybridization of ductal carcinoma of the breast - evidence of multiple genetic pathways. *J Pathol* 1999;187:396–402.

160. Vos CBJ, ter Haar NT, Rosenberg C, et al. Genetic alterations on chromosome 16 and 17 are important features of ductal carcinoma in situ of the breast and are associated with histologic type. *Br J Cancer* 1999;81:1410–1418.

161. Waldman FM, DeVries S, Chew KL, et al. Chromosomal alterations in ductal carcinomas in situ and their in situ recurrences. *J Natl Cancer Inst* 2000;92:313–320.

162. Marinho AF, Botelho M, Schmitt FC. Evaluation of numerical abnormalities of chromosomes 1 and 17 in proliferative epithelial breast lesions using fluorescence in situ hybridization. *Pathol Res Pract* 2000;196:227–233.

163. Aubele MM, Cummings MC, Mattis A, et al. Accumulation of chromosomal imbalances from intraductal proliferative lesions to adjacent in situ and invasive ductal breast cancer. *Diagn Mol Pathol* 2000;9:14–19.

164. Fiche M, Avet-Loiseau H, Maugard CM, et al. Gene amplifications detected by fluorescence in situ hybridization in pure intraductal breast carcinomas: relation to morphology, cell proliferation and expression of breast cancer-related genes. *Int J Cancer* 2000;89:403–410.

165. Cummings MC, Aubele M, Mattis A, et al. Increasing chromosome 1 copy number parallels histological progression in breast carcinogenesis. *Br J Cancer* 2000;82:1204–1210.

166. Glockner S, Lehmann U, Wilke N, et al. Amplification of growth regulatory genes in intraductal breast cancer is associated with higher nuclear grade but not with the progression to invasiveness. *Lab Invest* 2001;81:565–571.

167. Maitra A, Wistuba II, Washington C, et al. High-resolution chromosome 3p allelotyping of breast carcinomas and precursor lesions demonstrates frequent loss of heterozygosity and a discontinuous pattern of allele loss. *Am J Pathol* 2001;159:119–130.

168. Zhuang Z, Merino MJ, Chuaqua R, et al. Identical allelic loss on chromosome 11q13 in microdissected in situ and invasive human breast cancer. *Cancer Res* 1995;55:467–471.

169. Deng G, Lu Y, Zlotnikov G, et al. Loss of heterozygosity in normal tissue adjacent to breast carcinomas. *Science* 1996;274: 2057–2059.

170. Moinfar F, Man YG, Arnould L, et al. Concurrent and independent genetic alterations in the stromal and epithelial cells of mammary carcinoma: implications for tumorigenesis. *Cancer Res* 2000;60:2562–2566.

171. Allred DC, Medina D. Introduction: models of premalignant breast disease. *J Mammary Gland Biol Neoplasia* 2000;5:339–340.

172. Dawson PJ, Wolman SR, Tait L, et al. MCF10AT: a model for the evolution of cancer from proliferative breast disease. *Am J Pathol* 1996;148:313–319.

173. Shekhar MPV, Nangia-Makker P, Wolman SR, et al. Direct action of estrogen on sequence of progression of human preneoplastic breast disease. *Am J Pathol* 1998;152:1129–1132.

174. Luzzi V, Holtschlag V, Watson MA. Expression profiling of ductal carcinoma in situ by laser capture microdissection and high-density oligonucleotide arrays. *Am J Pathol* 2001;158: 2005–2010.

PROGNOSTIC FACTORS IN DUCTAL CARCINOMA IN SITU

PETER M. RAVDIN

Why might the measurement of prognostic factors be of value in the ductal carcinoma in situ (DCIS) form of breast cancer? There are the immediately practical issues of defining subsets of women most likely to have local recurrence after conservative therapy and then predicting in which subsets of women are specific forms of therapy such as radiation or tamoxifen most likely to reduce the risk of recurrence. Finally, these studies might lead to a deeper insight into the evolution of breast cancer (1). Understanding the evolution of breast cancer has obvious implications in breast cancer prevention and perhaps in the treatment of invasive breast cancers.

The use of biomarkers in the prognostic assessment and treatment selection of patients with DCIS remains an area in which definitive work has not yet been done. This is reflected in the fact that the major consensus conference guidelines do not yet recommend the use of laboratory-derived biomarkers for clinical decision making (2). Such a use may be on the immediate horizon, however, with the completion of three large randomized trials. In the National Surgical Adjuvant Breast Project B-17 (3) and European Organization for Research and Treatment of Cancer trial 10853 (4), patients were randomized as local resection alone or local resection plus radiation therapy. Papers detailing the risk of recurrence as correlated with demographic and pathologic tumor–related variables have appeared from these trials (5–7). Reports from these studies detailing the risk of recurrence as correlated with biomarkers are awaited. In the National Surgical Adjuvant Breast Project B-24, patients were randomized as local resection plus radiation therapy and local resection plus radiation therapy plus tamoxifen. This study showed that tamoxifen further reduces the risk of recurrence (8). The question of whether there are particular subsets of patients with DCIS (patients with estrogen receptor–positive or progesterone receptor–positive disease who particularly benefit from adjuvant tamoxifen will be addressed in the correlative studies done as part of this trial, but at this time nothing has not been reported.

Thus, at present, the large randomized studies required to help identify the risk factors for recurrence and to assess the value of radiation therapy and tamoxifen to reduce that risk have been completed, but the correlative studies with biomarkers have not. There is reason to believe, however, that such studies have the potential in the future to improve treatment planning for patients with DCIS. This optimism is based on a strong correlation between pathologic variables that are known to be predictive of recurrence and several biomarkers. This correlation makes it likely that biomarkers will have prognostic significance, and as we understand predictors of response to radiation and tamoxifen, these insights will be translated and validated for use in DCIS.

SPECIAL CHALLENGES IN CORRELATIVE STUDIES IN DUCTAL CARCINOMA IN SITU

Compared with the extensive literature on prognostic factors in invasive breast cancer, relatively little has been written about prognostic factors in DCIS. Workers in this field have faced several difficulties. (i) Until recently, DCIS has been a relatively uncommon lesion, so that very few centers had large numbers of cases and few cooperative group studies were undertaken. (ii) Because no prognostic factor was of known utility in the treatment of DCIS, tissue was not routinely analyzed for prognostic factors or prospectively stored for these studies. (iii) Because even after conservative therapy, local recurrence rates are low (and distant recurrence rates essentially zero), large numbers of patients must be included in studies to obtain any reasonable statistical power for finding correlations with clinical outcome. Taken together, these problems have slowed research on prognostic factors in DCIS, but this situation has changed with DCIS becoming more common, and large prospective studies having been completed.

Another special problem in research in DCIS is the definition of recurrence. This is because there are three types of recurrences in patients with DCIS. The one of greatest in-

TABLE 6.1. SOME OF THE CHARACTERISTICS OF TRIALS WITH PATHOLOGIC AND CLINICAL CORRELATIONS

Trial or Study	n	Follow-Up (yr)	Treatment	Correlates with Recurrence (Multivariate)
Ottesen et al. (11)	275	10	Local resection	Comedonecrosis, size
Silverstein et al. (12)	333	6.5	Various	Comedonecrosis, margins, size
NSABP B-17 (3)	814	8	Local resection ± radiation therapy	Comedonecrosis, margins
EORTC (4)	1,010	5.4	Local resection ± radiation therapy	Poorly differentiation, size, age
NSABP B-24 (6)	1,804	5	Local resection + radiation therapy ± tamoxifen	Comedonecrosis, margins, age

terest is ipsilateral breast cancer recurrence representing residual tumor. It is this type of recurrence that local radiation therapy in particular is meant to control. Studies of chromosomal changes and at least one pathologic correlative and biomarker study (9) suggest that most, but not all, ipsilateral breast cancer recurrences are clonally related to the primary DCIS. The third type of recurrence in DCIS studies is contralateral recurrence. This type of recurrence is of interest but not of great relevance in therapeutic studies of local control of DCIS with surgery and radiation, and in general these events are excluded from these analyses.

Most of the biomarker studies have reported correlations of the biomarkers with pathologic variables rather than relapse. As noted previously, this is because most studies have only modest numbers of patients, modest number of events, and low statistical power to investigate correlations of the markers with the end point of ipsilateral breast relapse. Table 6.1 lists the larger studies that will eventually lead to the definitive insights as the value of biomarkers. Small studies of fewer than 100 patients may be useful for examining the correlations between biomarkers and pathologic variables but are not of value in studies of correlations with recurrence. Failure of such studies to find expected correlations is not surprising given their low statistical power, for example, a study of 49 cases failing to find useful biomarker correlations with outcome (10).

HOW HISTOPATHOLOGIC VARIABLES CORRELATE WITH OUTCOME

As shown in Table 6.1, the prognostically more troubling cases of DCIS (in terms of probability of recurrence after breast-conserving therapy), seem to be in general more often associated with comedonecrosis and comedo subtype and poor differentiation. At the very least, prognostic factors that correlate with these variables should have a good chance to be predictors of unfavorable outcome. This might suggest that those markers associated with a poor nuclear grade in invasive carcinomas such as aneuploidy might be predictive of poor outcome. In addition, because the comedo subtype is associated with a high mitotic index and necrosis, it might be expected that prognostic markers associated with a high proliferative rate, such as a high S phase, or with increased cell death, such as measures of apoptosis, might also be pre-

dictive of DCIS treatment failure. Markers for these features as well as p53, receptors for sex steroids and peptide hormones, markers for angiogenesis, and several other features have been measured in DCIS specimens. Understanding the incidence and level of expression of these prognostic factors in DCIS and how these prognostic factors correlate with the histopathologic variables provides information crucial for designing the studies that will explore the impact of prognostic factors on the clinical outcome of patients with DCIS.

MEASURES OF DNA CONTENT

If breast cancers evolve through hyperplastic stages to DCIS and then to invasive cancers and along this path acquire an increasing number of genomic abnormalities, then one might expect DNA content to become increasingly abnormal during this process. In fact, measures of DNA content show that hyperplasias are usually diploid, whereas DCIS is more often aneuploid. This difference in the percentage of cases with abnormal DNA content is consistent with the view that hyperplastic lesions evolve into DCIS, and the DCIS lesion often have major abnormalities in their genomic makeup. For example, Eriksson et al. (13) found that more than 50% of cases of DCIS were aneuploid. This work is consistent with the work of others. It is perhaps not surprising that the comedo form of DCIS (which generally has a high nuclear grade) is particularly likely to be aneuploid (13–15).

Studies of concordance of DNA content in noninvasive (DCIS) and invasive components of the same tumor allow insights into the evolution of breast cancers. Iglehart et al. (16) reported a near-perfect concordance in the DNA index between invasive and noninvasive components of tumors. Concordance was good but not as striking in an initial set of 30 samples with both invasive and noninvasive components within single tumors from the National Surgical Adjuvant Breast Project B-17 (17) and another set of 30 samples reported from Brazil (6) in which the concordance rate was 80%. These observations are consistent with the view that major changes in DNA content occur often but not always during the evolution of breast cancers and are not necessary for the transition from noninvasive to invasive forms.

The clinical application of this information about DNA content is as yet uncertain given that the completed studies did not directly correlate DNA content with the probability of relapse after conservative local therapy or other clinically relevant outcomes.

MEASURES OF PROLIFERATIVE RATE

For invasive cancers, measures of proliferative rate correlate with the risk of early relapse and death (18). It might also be expected that more rapidly proliferative premalignant lesions would evolve more quickly and would be particularly dangerous after acquiring the malignant phenotype. Measures of proliferative rate would therefore be of particular interest.

A strong correlation between the histologic subtype of DCIS and the proliferative rate has been demonstrated by several methodologies. Comedo DCIS and high-grade DCIS have a higher proliferative rate as measured by flow cytometry (19) and Ki67 (14). A generalized aberration control of cell death in high-grade DCIS lesions is suggested by the fact that apoptosis rates are higher in high-grade DCIS lesions than in low-grade lesions (20). This suggests that such measures might be used to help decide which local therapies might be most appropriate for individual patients with DCIS, given that high-grade DCIS lesions are more likely to recur after breast-conserving therapy. Studies to confirm this indirect inference, however, have not yet been done, and it is not yet clear that there are any real advantages to laboratory-based biomarker determinations versus histologic subtyping and grading.

STEROID HORMONE RECEPTOR STATUS (ESTROGEN AND PROGESTERONE RECEPTORS)

If the evolution of breast cancers could be arrested at the preinvasive DCIS stage, then the potentially lethal invasive form of the disease could be prevented. Because relatively nontoxic forms of therapy based on the manipulation of the hormonal milieu are available, it is logical to ask whether these forms of therapy might be effective in preventing progression beyond the premalignant stages of breast neoplasia such as DCIS. Because hormonal therapies are thought to be mediated by the estrogen receptor and the progesterone receptor, an important question in developing prevention strategies is whether DCIS lesions express these receptors.

Several investigators have addressed the incidence of estrogen receptor and progesterone receptor in premalignant lesions and in correlation with other pathologic variables (14,21–25). Overall, approximately one-half of the DCIS lesions express estrogen receptor and/or progesterone receptor. There also seems to be a correlation between the DCIS subtype and steroid hormone receptor, with comedo forms of DCIS less likely to express estrogen receptor or progesterone receptor.

There are no immediate clinical applications of this information. These observations, however, suggest that prevention strategies based on such agents as tamoxifen might block progression of only approximately one-half of evolving cancers, which seems consistent with current observations suggesting that tamoxifen reduces the incidence of second primary breast cancers by approximately half (26). The National Surgical Adjuvant Breast Project trial B-24 shows that tamoxifen clearly plays a role in preventing local recurrence in patients with DCIS after breast-conserving therapy (8). The steroid receptor expression in the specimens from this trial will be crucial to the trial's interpretation. The trial has reported that there is no apparent difference in effectiveness of tamoxifen in the patients with or without comedonecrosis (31% versus 23% reduction in ipsilateral recurrence). This result runs counter to the expectation that tamoxifen would be more effective in the group without comedonecrosis, which presumably in this study expressed more estrogen receptor, but definitive interpretation awaits actual estrogen receptor determination.

C-ERBB-2 IN DUCTAL CARCINOMA IN SITU

c-erbB-2 is often expressed in DCIS. Like many of the other prognostic factors, it is more frequently expressed in higher grade DCIS lesions. Also, like other prognostic factors, its clinical utility for decision making in DCIS is uncertain because studies have so far correlated c-erbB-2 expression with pathologic variables but not with clinical outcome. A possible future use is suggested by the work of De Potter et al. (27) in which the extent of disease was correlated with c-erbB-2 expression. This might suggest that future studies could show that c-erbB-2–positive DCIS lesions would be more likely to recur after local resection.

One of the interesting aspects of c-erbB-2 expression in DCIS is that it seems to occur more frequently than in invasive cancers. This seems to be somewhat paradoxical, in that if clonal evolution of tumors involves an increasing expression of abnormalities and if overexpression of c-erbB-2 is one of the abnormalities associated with evolution to a more aggressive phenotype, then one would expect c-erbB-2 expression to be more common in invasive carcinomas than in DCIS.

One of the groups to directly address this question, based at Guy's Hospital in London, has produced three studies of expression of c-erbB-2 (28). One of these was in pure DCIS, one with the majority of tumors containing a small invasive component, and one in pure invasive carcinoma. The rate of c-erbB-2 overexpression was 61% in the pure DCIS study, 31% in the mixed cases, and 26% in the invasive cases. They reported that when they specifically looked at cases with larger nuclei, these cases had significantly higher rates of erbB-2 cover expression than those with small nuclei. In pure DCIS cases, the rate of DCIS expression in cases with larger nuclei was 90%, but in cases of DCIS with an infiltrating component, the rate of c-erbB-2 overexpression was only 45%. Tumors in these studies that had both DCIS and infiltrating components showed a concordance of staining for c-erbB-2 of 98% (113 of 115, 31 with positive staining). A hypothesis advanced by this group to explain their data is that tumors that have the shortest DCIS stage are those that have high proliferative rates but do not express c-erbB-2. These tumors would therefore be underrepresented in studies of DCIS but would be the major contributors to the development of invasive carcinoma.

Results consistent with this hypothesis were reported by Allred et al. (29), who found perfect concordance in c-erbB-2 expression between invasive and noninvasive components of the same lesion and rates of c-erbB-2 positively of 56% in cases of pure DCIS, 22% in invasive cases with an intraductal component, and 11% in purely invasive carcinomas The basic observation of good concordance in c-erbB-2 expression between the invasive and noninvasive components of a tumor is further supported by Iglehart et al. (16). Taken together, these results suggest that DCIS lesions may not all lie along a simple single evolutionary path leading to invasive breast cancers. Perhaps some DCIS phenotypes do not often evolve into invasive breast cancers and are thus overrepresented in DCIS and underrepresented in invasive breast cancers.

P53 EXPRESSION IN DUCTAL CARCINOMA IN SITU

The incidence of aberrant expression of p53 in DCIS lesions has been examined in several studies (30). In these studies, a striking pattern emerges, with p53 rarely expressed in low-grade DCIS but much more frequently expressed in high-grade DCIS. There are no studies that specifically address the issue of whether p53 predicts risk of relapse in patients with DCIS or the risk of progression to invasive cancer, although it might be indirectly inferred that aberrant p53 expression in DCIS would be associated with an increased risk of local recurrence. Nevertheless, p53 expression cannot yet be used to make clinical decisions about the treatment of DCIS, although it must be considered a very promising candidate biomarker for such studies.

Studies of the role of p53 in the evolution of breast cancer may also provide important insights. p53 has been shown to be abnormal in less than 10% of the cases of atypical hyperplasia but more frequently in DCIS and in invasive cancers (31–34). Thus, development of abnormal expression of p53 may play a role in the progression of some premalignant lesions to DCIS. The high levels of concordance between p53 expression in the invasive and noninva-

sive components of the same tumors show that the acquisition of abnormalities in p53 is not commonly an event causing DCIS to progress to an invasive phenotype, but neither is there a similar paradoxical increased incidence of expression of p53 in DCIS relative to invasive breast cancer as there is for c-erbB-2.

DISCUSSION

Depending on the context, there are actually two very different meanings for a poor prognosis for a DCIS lesion. In the most widely used context, it means having a high risk for local recurrence if managed by conservative local measures (less than a modified radical mastectomy). In the context of primary breast cancer prevention, it means having a high probability for evolution to a breast cancer capable of developing an invasive and metastatic character.

These two definitions have quite different implications. For example, one hypothesis might be that some forms of comedo DCIS that are c-erbB-2 overexpressors actually have only modest rates of evolution to invasive phenotypes but are dangerous because of their ability to widely disseminate mechanically through the breast ductal system and are thus not easily managed by breast-sparing surgery. Ancillary studies to trials such as NSABP B-24 will allow better understanding of how prognostic factors can be used to predict clinical outcome for women with DCIS and how some types of lesions may be susceptible to arrest of their usual evolution. Nevertheless, at this time there are no established clinical prognostic factors in DCIS other than histopathologic variables currently in use.

REFERENCES

1. Allred DC, Mohsin SK, Fuqua SA. Histological and biological evolution of human premalignant breast disease. *Endocr Relat Cancer* 2001;8:47–61.
2. Schwartz GF, Solin LJ, Olivotto IA, et al. Consensus Conference on the Treatment of In Situ Ductal Carcinoma of the Breast, April 22–25, 1999. *Cancer* 2000;88:946–54.
3. Fisher B, Constantino J, Redmond C, et al. Lumpectomy compared with lumpectomy and radiation therapy for the treatment of Intraductal breast cancer. *N Engl J Med* 1993;328:1581–1586.
4. Julien JP, Bijker N, Fentiman IS. Radiotherapy in breast conserving treatment for ductal carcinoma in situ: first results of the EORTC randomized trial 10853. *Lancet* 2000;355:528–533.
5. Fisher ER, Costantino J, Fisher B, et al. Pathologic findings from the National Surgical Adjuvant Breast Project (NSABP) Protocol B-17. Intraductal carcinoma (ductal carcinoma in situ). *Cancer* 1995;75:1310–1319.
6. Fisher ER, Dignam J, Tan-Chiu E, et al. Pathologic findings from the National Surgical Adjuvant Breast Project (NSABP) eight-year update of Protocol B-17: intraductal carcinoma. *Cancer* 1999;86:375–377.
7. Bijker N, Peterse JL, Duchateau L, et al. Risk factors for recurrence and metastasis after breast-conserving therapy for ductal carcinoma-in-situ: analysis of European Organization for Re-

search and Treatment of Cancer Trial 10853. *J Clin Oncol* 2001; 19:2263–2271.

8. Fisher B, Dignam J, Wolmark N, et al. Tamoxifen in treatment of intraductal breast cancer: National Surgical Adjuvant Breast and Bowel Project B-24 randomised controlled trial. *Lancet* 2000;353:1993–2000.

9. Bijker N, Peterse JL, Duchateau L, et al. Histological type and marker expression of the primary tumour compared with its local recurrence after breast-conserving therapy for ductal carcinoma in situ. *Br J Cancer* 2001;84:539–544.

10. Perin T, Canzonieri V, Massarut S, et al. Immunochemical evaluation of multiple biological markers in ductal carcinoma in situ of the breast. *Eur J Cancer* 1996;32A:1148–1155.

11. Ottesen GL, Graversen HP, Blichert-Toft M, et al. Carcinoma in situ of the female breast. 10 year follow-up results of a prospective nationwide study. *Breast Cancer Res Treat* 2000;62:197–210.

12. Silverstein MJ, Lagios MD, Craig PH, et al. A prognostic index for ductal carcinoma in situ of the breast. *Cancer* 1996;77:2267–2274.

13. Eriksson ET, Schimmelpenning H, Aspenblad U, et al. Immunohistochemical expression of the mutant p53 protein and nuclear DNA content during the transition from benign to malignant breast disease. *Hum Pathol* 1994;25:1228–1233.

14. Ringberg A, Anagnostaki L, Anderson H, et al. Cell biological factors in ductal carcinoma in situ (DCIS) of the breast-relationship to ipsilateral local recurrence and histopathological characteristics. *Eur J Cancer* 2001;37:1514–1522.

15. Visscher D, Jimenez RE, Grayson M 3rd, et al. Histopathologic analysis of chromosome aneuploidy in ductal carcinoma in situ. *Hum Pathol* 2000;31:201–207.

16. Iglehart JD, Kems BJ, Huper G, et al. Maintenance of DNA content and erbB-2 alterations in intraductal and invasive phases of mammary cancer. *Breast Cancer Res Treat* 1995;34:253–263.

17. Fisher ER, Siderits R. Value of cytometric analysis for distinction of intraductal carcinoma of the breast. *Breast Cancer Res Treat* 1992;21:165–172.

18. Hedely DW, Clark GM, Cornelisse CJ, et al. Consensus review of the clinical utility of DNA cytometry in carcinoma of the breast. *Breast Cancer Res Treat* 1994;28:52–60.

19. Stomper PC, DeBloom JR 2nd, Winston JS, et al. Flow cytometric DNA analysis of specimen mammography-guided fine-needle aspirates of ductal carcinoma in situ. *J Exp Clin Cancer Res* 2000;19:309–315.

20. Gandhi A, Holland PA, Knox WF, et al. Evidence of significant apoptosis in poorly differentiated ductal carcinoma in situ of the breast. *Br J Cancer* 1998;78:788–794.

21. Zofrani B, Leroyer A, Fourquet A, et al. Mammographically-detected ductal in situ carcinoma of the breast analyzed with a new classification. A study of 127 cases: correlation with estrogen and progesterone receptors, p53 and c-erbB-2 proteins and proliferative activity. *Semin Diagn Pathol* 1994;11:208–214.

22. Chaudhuri B, Crist KA, Mucci S, et al. Distribution of estrogen receptor in ductal carcinoma in situ of the breast. *Surgery* 1993; 113:134–137.

23. Pallis L, Wilking N, Cedermark B, et al. Receptors for estrogen and progesterone in breast carcinoma in situ. *Anticancer Res* 1992;12:2113–2115.

24. Poller DN, Roberts EC, Bell JA, et al. P53 protein expression in mammary ductal carcinoma in situ: relationship to immunohistochemical expression of estrogen receptor and c-erbB-2 protein. *Hum Pathol* 1993;24:463–468.

25. Claus EB, Chu P, Howe CL, et al. Pathobiologic findings in DCIS of the breast: morphologic features, angiogenesis, HER-2/neu and hormone receptors. *Exp Mol Pathol* 2001;70:303–316.

26. Anonymous. Tamoxifen for early breast cancer: an overview of randomised trials. Early Breast Cancer Trialists' Collaborative Group. *Lancet* 1998;351:1451–1467.

27. De Potter CR, Schelfout AM, Verbeeck P, et al. Neu overexpression correlates with extent of disease in large cell ductal carcinoma in situ of the breast. *Hum Pathol* 1995;26:601–606.

28. Barnes DM, Bartkova J, Camplejohn RS, et al. Overexpression of the c-erbB-2 oncoprotein: why does this occur more invasive mammary carcinoma and is this of prognostic significance? *Eur J Cancer* 1992;28:644–648.

29. Allred DC, Clark GM, Molina R, et al. Overexpression of HER-2/neu and its relationship with other prognostic factors change during the progression of in situ to invasive breast cancer. *Hum Pathol* 1992;23:974–979.

30. Rajan PB, Scott DJ, Perry RH, et al. P53 expression in ductal carcinoma in situ (DCIS) of the breast. *Breast Cancer Res Treat* 1997; 42:283–290.

31. Umekita Y, Takasaki T, Yoshida H. Expression of p53 protein in benign epithelial hyperplasia, atypical ductal hyperplasia, non-invasive and invasive mammary carcinoma: an immunohistochemical study. *Virchows Arch* 1994;424:491–494.

32. Tsuda H, Iwaya K, Fukutomi T, et al. p53 mutations and c-erbB-2 amplification in intraductal and invasive breast carcinomas of high histologic grade. *Jpn J Cancer Res* 1993;84:394–401.

33. Schmitt FC, Leal C, Lopes C. p53 protein expression and nuclear DNA content in breast intraductal proliferations. *J Pathol* 1995; 176:233–241.

34. Eriksson ET, Schimmelpenning H, Aspenblad U, et al. Immunohistochemical expression of the mutant p53 protein and nuclear DNA content during the transition from benign to malignant breast disease. *Hum Pathol* 1994;25:1228–1233.

HER-2/*NEU* GENE AMPLIFICATION AND OVEREXPRESSION IN DUCTAL CARCINOMA IN SITU

ISABELL A. SCHMITT
MICHAEL F. PRESS

The human epidermal growth factor receptor type 2, referred to as HER-2, is the human homolog of the rodent *neu* oncogene. This gene, referred to here as the HER-2/*neu* gene, is also known as the c-*erb* B-2 gene. It encodes a membrane receptor protein that is a member of the epidermal growth factor receptor family. The protein product is a 185,000-kd protein (p185$^{HER-2/neu}$) with extracellular, transmembrane, tyrosine kinase, and autophosphorylation domains. Although the extracellular domains of the other family members (HER-1, HER-3, and HER-4) are known to bind specific peptide ligands, the extracellular domain of p185$^{HER-2/neu}$ does not bind any known ligand and HER-2/*neu* is, therefore, considered to encode an orphan receptor. Epidermal growth factor (EGF) receptor family members are activated through interactions with their respective ligands and formation of either receptor homodimers or heterodimers. p185$^{HER-2/neu}$ is the promiscuous member of the family forming heterodimers with each of the other family members. While HER-2/*neu* does not bind any ligand, HER-3 lacks tyrosine kinase activity. HER-2/*neu*, conversely, appears to have the strongest tyrosine kinase activity among the family members. Therefore, HER-2 can be activated by various EGF family ligands through heterodimerization (1,2). This heterodimerization activates strong tyrosine kinase activity, especially as part of HER2-HER3 heterodimers. Activation of the EGF family of receptors including HER-2/*neu* results in the initiation of a phosphorylation signal transduction cascade. Signal transduction by EGF receptor family members results in changes of biologic activity in the cell. For example, HER-2/*neu* activation results in an increased rate of DNA synthesis, increased cell migration, and synthesis of angiogenesis growth factors.

TUMOR BIOLOGY

In 1987, the HER-2/*neu* oncogene was first identified as having an increase in copy number in approximately 20%

to 30% of invasive breast cancers (3). This increase in gene copy number, usually in the form of tandem repeats in homogeneous staining regions of chromosomes or extrachromosomal double minute chromosomes, is referred to as gene amplification. HER-2/*neu* gene amplification was correlated with poor clinical outcome among women with node-positive breast cancer (3). Initially, the observation of HER-2/*neu* gene amplification was viewed by some as an interesting marker gene alteration of poor clinical outcome, but questions were raised about the relationship of the genetic alteration to the disease process. Subsequent work demonstrated that the HER-2/*neu* gene was not only amplified in human breast cancers but had an increased level of expression, referred to as overexpression, in these cancers proportionate to the level of amplification (4,5). In addition, HER-2/*neu* overexpression in transfected cell lines showed a transformed phenotype (6,7), and treatment of cell lines having HER-2/*neu* overexpression with monoclonal antibody to the extracellular domain of HER-2/*neu* resulted in arrest of cell proliferation, reversing the malignant phenotype (8). Transgenic mice containing either the mouse *neu* oncogene or the human HER-2/*neu* homolog as transgene behind a mouse mammary tumor virus promoter developed breast cancer (9,10).

Considerable circumstantial evidence suggests that HER-2/*neu* gene amplification and overexpression plays a similarly important role in the biology of selected human cancers, especially breast cancer. For example, clinical trials of Herceptin, a recombinant, humanized anti-HER-2/*neu* antibody, in women with metastatic HER-2/*neu*-overexpressing breast cancer have demonstrated both complete and partial remissions of metastatic breast cancer (11–13). Therefore, the accumulated direct and indirect evidence strongly indicates that HER-2/*neu* amplification/overexpression plays an important pathogenetic role in the disease process.

CLINICAL BACKGROUND INFORMATION

Although at times disputed, HER-2/*neu* gene amplification and overexpression have been shown to be markers of poor prognosis in both node-negative (14–26) and node-positive (4,16) invasive breast cancer. Although not confirmed by all investigators, women whose invasive breast cancers have HER-2/*neu* gene amplification and overexpression experience a shorter disease-free interval and a shorter overall survival (4,14,26). The differences in conclusions about HER-2/*neu* as a prognostic marker are at least partially related to such study design problems as inadequate sample size (16) and poorly characterized methods of HER-2/*neu* evaluation (27).

HER-2/*neu* amplification and overexpression in invasive breast cancer are considered a predictor of responsiveness to various forms of therapy. Overexpression has been associated with a lack of responsiveness to cyclophosphamide, methotrexate, and 5-fluorouracil chemotherapy (21,23,28) and an increased responsiveness to adriamycin chemotherapy (29,30). Women whose breast cancers have HER-2/*neu* overexpression are reported to be less likely to respond to antihormonal therapy with tamoxifen (31–33). Most importantly, responsiveness to Herceptin immunotherapy is observed almost exclusively in women whose breast cancers have HER-2/*neu* gene amplification and overexpression (13). However, differences in the accuracy of HER-2/*neu* assay methods used in these investigations have probably been an important problem confounding interpretation of the results in these clinical trials (13,27).

METHODS OF HER-2/*NEU* ANALYSIS

Immunohistochemistry has been the most frequently used method to analyze HER-2/*neu* alterations. This method has a number of advantages as an analytical technique. Immunohistochemistry is widely available, light microscopy-based, relatively simple and short to perform, a familiar method for pathologists, reasonably inexpensive, and approved by the U.S. Food and Drug Administration for Herceptin eligibility selection. However, this method also has several important disadvantages. The antibodies used for immunohistochemistry show variable sensitivity and specificity when used in paraffin-embedded tissues (27,34). Immunoreactivity of anti-HER-2/*neu* antibodies is affected by tissue-processing artifacts such as fixative used (35–37) and fixation time. In addition, antigen retrieval affects the immunostaining in a variable fashion, which has not been assessed for this antigen. Finally, the scoring systems used in the literature are based on subjective evaluation of the amount of immunostaining and have low interobserver concordance. These problems with immunohistochemistry as an analytical method are probably at least partially responsible for the substantial differences reported in HER-2/*neu*

overexpression in different studies of both invasive breast carcinomas and ductal carcinoma in situ (DCIS) (Table 7.1, Fig. 7.1B, C).

Because DNA is more stable than protein, analysis of HER-2/*neu* gene amplification is expected to provide more consistent results between specimens and laboratories. Polymerase chain reaction (PCR) has been used to demonstrate increased HER-2/*neu* PCR product relative to control genes on chromosome 17 in human breast cancers and DCIS (38–40). Although PCR analyses have the advantage of being a DNA-based method, the assessment of the result is primarily by visual inspection of PCR products on a gel after more than 30 cycles of PCR amplification (38,39). Although this approach has some advantages over immunohistochemistry, it does not permit a cell-by-cell assessment of status and is subjectively evaluated. In addition, PCR has been used in few studies of HER-2/*neu* gene amplification of invasive breast cancers and has achieved relatively limited acceptance as a method for assessment of HER-2/*neu* status.

Another DNA-based assay method for HER-2/*neu* gene amplification is fluorescence *in situ* hybridization (FISH). FISH has been used to analyze HER-2/*neu* gene amplification in a number of studies of invasive breast cancer (15,37,41), and this method has been shown to be both sensitive and specific for HER-2/*neu* gene amplification compared with Southern hybridization (15). FISH combines tissue morphology with molecular biology to localize individual copies of the HER-2/*neu* gene within tumor cell nuclei (Fig. 7.1D). This approach permits counting the number of gene copies to determine whether they are increased (amplified). The HER-2/*neu* gene copy level for a breast cancer can either be expressed as an average number of copies per tumor cell nucleus or a ratio relative to an internal control gene located on the same chromosome such as chromosome 17 centromere. The latter approach has some advantages because it corrects for tissue-sectioning artifacts and because it corrects for chromosome 17 aneusomy, ensuring that amplification and not aneuploidy is responsible for the increased gene copy number (Fig. 7.1D).

FISH has several advantages as an analytical technique. It has standardized thresholds established for gene amplification, low interlaboratory variability, and high precision (34) and strongly predicts responsiveness to Herceptin therapy (13). Conversely, there are some disadvantages to FISH as an analytical technique for determining HER-2/*neu* status. Fluorescence microscopy is required. Fewer laboratories are performing FISH, and, therefore, pathologists are generally less familiar with this technique and resistant to adopting it. The procedure requires more time and slightly more expertise. It is more expensive to perform and U.S. Food and Drug Administration approval does not yet include an indication for Herceptin, although this is currently pending. To date, no studies of breast carcinoma in situ have been reported using this technique.

TABLE 7.1. SUMMARY OF STUDIES CHARACTERIZING HER-2/NEU IN DUCTAL CARCINOMA IN SITU

Author	Patient Cases (n)	Method of Analysis	Overall Frequency	Frequency in Comedocas (or High-Grade DCIS)	Frequency in Non-comedocas (or Low-Grade)	P-Value	Comment
Van de Vijver, 1988 (53)	45	IHC (3B5)	19/45 (42%)	19/29 (66%)	0/16 (0%)	0.0005	
Gusterson, 1988 (47)	74	IHC (21N)	33/74 (44%)				5/6 (83%) cases of Paget's disease with HER-2/neu positivity.
McCann, 1991 (48)	11	IHC (21N)	7/11 (64%)	7/7 (100%)			Concordance between HER-2/neu in DCIS and IDC. IDC 14% and IDC with DCIS 28% HER-2 positive. No inverse correlation with ER.
Schimmelpenning, 1992 (56)	107	IHC (OA-11-854)	51/107 (48%)	31/36 (86%)	20/71 (28%)		HER2 positive in 3 Paget's disease cases and in 30% of diploid and 58% of aneuploid DCIS.
Somerville, 1992 (52)	48	IHC (pAb1, ICR 12)	22/48 (46%)	18/25 (72%)	4/23 (17%)	0.05	
Maguire, 1992 (55)	25	IHC (OM-11-952)	10/25 (40%)	10/13 (78%)	0/12 (0%)		Concordance between HER-2/neu in DCIS and IDC.

(continues)

Study	N	Method			p value	Comments
Liu, 1992 (38)	27	Differential PCR IHC (OA-11-854)	13/27 (48%)			Concordance between HER-2/neu in DCIS and IDC. IDC 21% HER2 positive.
Allred, 1992 (43)	59	IHC (21N)	33/59 (56%)	30/39 (77%)		Concordance between HER-2/neu in DCIS and IDC. HER2-positivity in DCIS (56%), IDC with >10% DCIS (22%) and IDC alone (11%) (p < 0.0001).
Poller, 1993 (69)	116	IHC (21N)	60/116 (52%)			HER-2/neu inversely associated with ER expression (p < 0.01); no assoc. with p53.
Zafrani, 1994 (73)	95	IHC (DAKO)	54/95 (57%)	36/41 (88%)	0.0001	HER-2/neu correlated with calcifications, ductal distribution of calcifications, granular calcifications and rod-shaped calcifications in mammograms.
Evans, 1994 (50)	175	IHC (21N)	87/175 (50%)	37/53 (69%) 50/122 (41%)		
Leal, 1994 (46)	40	IHC (DAKO)	18/40 (45%)	11/13 (85%) 3 22/50 (44%) VN +2 7/27 (23%) VN 1	0.00002	Van Nuys histologic classification used.
Silverstein, 1995 (60)	144	IHC (R-60)	41/144 (28%)	19/94 (20%)	0.05	

(continues)

TABLE 7.1. CONTINUED

Author	Patient Cases (n)	Method of Analysis	Overall Frequency	Frequency in Comedocas (or High-Grade DCIS)	Frequency in Non-comedocas (or Low-Grade)	P-Value	Comment
De Potter, 1995 (54)	75	IHC (3B5)	24/75 (32%)	11/26 (42%)	13/49 (27%)		HER-2/neu expression correlated with larger extent of DCIS lesions and cytologically large cell DCIS (p < 0.05).
Iglehart, 1995 (44)	10	IHC (pAb) and Image Analysis	6/10 (60%)	4/6 (67%)	2/4 (50%)		Concordance between HER-2/neu in DCIS and IDC.
Bobrow, 1995* (49)	105	IHC (21N)	47/105 (45%)	30/43 (70%)	17/62 (27%)	0.0001	HER-2/neu correlated with proliferation index and p53, and inversely with PR.
Bose, 1996 (74)	40	IHC (R60 pAb)	20/40 (50%)	11/13 (85%)	9/27 (33%)	0.006	7/7 (100%) of Paget's disease cases positive for HER-2/neu
Mack, 1997 (89)	70	IHC (CB 11)	Not described	Not described	Not described	0.007	Semiquantitative Scoring system

(continues)

Study	n	Method				p-value	Comments
Querzoli, 1998 (51)	84	IHC (pAb-1)	27/84 (32%)	20/28 (73%)	7/56 (13%)	0.001	Concordance between HER-2/neu in DCIS and IDC.
Tsuda, 1998 (59)	11	IHC (rabbit pAb)	2/11 (18%)	2/2 (100%)	0/9 (0%)		
Ho, 2000 (39)	30	Differential PCR	12/30 (40%)	9/13 (69%)	3/17 (18%)	0.008	HER-2/neu expression correlated with higher nuclear grade and microvessel density but inversely correlated with ER/PR expression.
Claus, 2001 (45)	191	IHC (3B5)	54/191 (28%)	12/24 (50%)	42/167 (25%)	0.01	
Glockner, 2001** (40)	37	Quantitative real-time PCR	12/37 (33%)	11/27 (40%)	1/10 (10%)	0.02	Van Nuys (VN3) histologic grading used. Concordance between HER-2/neu in DCIS and invasive carcinomas from same case.
Mommers, 2001 (57)	61	IHC (Dutch Ab)	13/61 (21%)	12/37 (32%)	1/24 (4%)	0.01	Concordance between HER-2/neu in DCIS and IDC.
Totals:	**1680**		**655/1610**	**343/525 (65.3%)**	**216/864 (25.0%)**	**(40.7%)**	

IHC, immunohistochemistry; PCR, polymerase chain reaction; IDC, invasive ductal carcinoma; DCIS, ductal carcinoma in situ.
*The same 105 cases were reported separately in another paper (90).
**The results from the same 83 cases were described in a previous paper by the same authors (Glockner et al. 2000) (58).

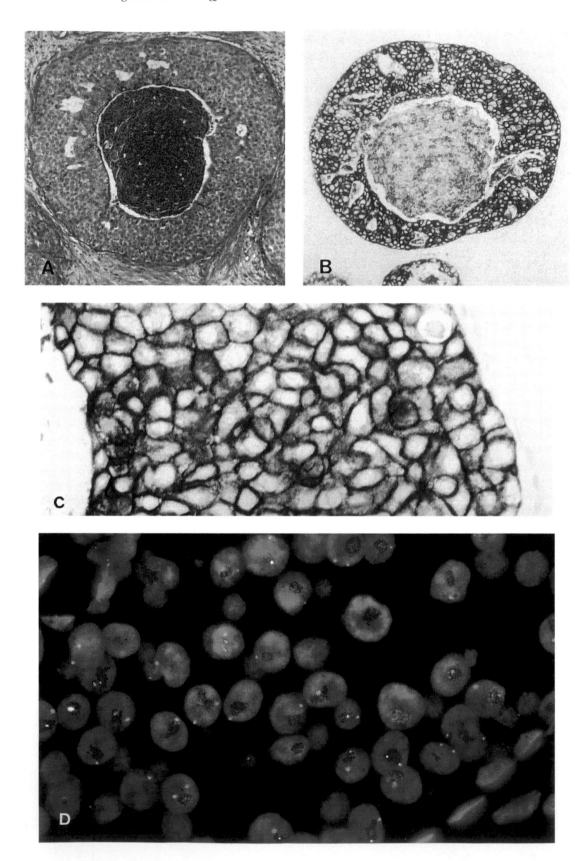

HER-2/*NEU* GENE AMPLIFICATION AND OVEREXPRESSION IN DUCTAL CARCINOMA IN SITU

Some have suggested that HER-2/*neu* amplification and overexpression are not strongly correlated with disease outcome because the alteration develops late in the disease process and is prognostically important in large but not small breast cancers (42). However, studies by various investigators have shown HER-2/*neu* amplification and/or overexpression in DCIS (Table 7.1), suggesting that, at least in some proportion of breast cancers, the alteration develops early in the disease process, i.e., before invasion of the surrounding breast tissue. Others have speculated that HER-2/*neu* plays a more important role in initiation of the early DCIS lesions than in progression of ductal carcinomas after invasion (43).

Since 1988, several groups have studied HER-2/*neu* in DCIS as a means of assessing the role of HER-2/*neu* in breast carcinogenesis (Table 7.1). HER-2/*neu* alterations were evaluated in as few as 10 (44) and as many as 191 (45) DCIS cases. These studies of DCIS not only show considerable variation in study size but vary substantially with regard to method of assessing HER-2/*neu* status. Although the majority of the studies used immunohistochemical assays to assess HER-2/*neu*, they varied with regard to anti-HER-2/*neu* antibodies used. These studies used "the antibody from DAKO" (46), the 21N polyclonal rabbit antibody (23,43,47–50), a rabbit polyclonal antibody Ab-1 from Triton Biosciences, Inc. (51,52), 3B5 monoclonal antibody (45,53,54), antibody OM-11-952 (55), antibody OA-11-854 (38,56), and other antibodies not further specified but provided by organizations such as the Dutch Cancer Institute (57) and Cell Analysis Systems, Inc. (44). In addition, the studies summarized in Table 7.1 varied with regard to use of antigen retrieval, antibody detection systems, and subjective method for scoring of specimen immunostaining.

Three groups evaluated HER-2/*neu* gene amplification in DCIS. All three studies used PCR to characterize HER-2/*neu* gene amplification (38,39,58). Only one study correlated HER-2/*neu* gene amplification with overexpression of HER-2/neu protein determined by immunohistochemistry (38). One group used computerized image analysis to score HER-2/*neu* immunostaining and to provide a more objective assessment of HER-2/*neu* expression (44). The inconsistencies between the different studies make direct comparisons difficult.

Several studies have compared the HER-2/*neu* status in DCIS with the status in invasive breast cancer and normal tissue and attempted to establish a model of HER-2/*neu* alterations in early breast tumorigenesis. The prevalence of HER-2/*neu* overexpression by immunohistochemical staining is higher in DCIS generally than it is overall among invasive breast carcinomas (Table 7.1). The higher prevalence of HER-2/*neu* overexpression among DCIS than among invasive breast carcinomas could be explained by any of several hypotheses: (i) HER-2/*neu* overexpression may be lost during progression of an intraductal carcinoma to an invasive carcinoma (43), (ii) invasive carcinomas may arise more commonly from noncomedocarcinomas that have a lower prevalence of HER-2/*neu* overexpression, (iii) the relative spectrum of DCIS subtypes observed in the overall population may differ from that observed in the population coming to surgical attention as DCIS owing to mammography or other selection bias, (iv) some invasive carcinomas may be invasive from their origin without going through an in situ phase or may go through a relatively short in situ phase (38), or (v) the observation may be an artifact of the processing or interpreting of HER-2/*neu* immunostaining in DCIS compared with invasive breast cancers. The first of these possibilities is unlikely because HER-2/*neu* status of invasive and in situ components of the same breast cancer are nearly always the same (44,48,55,57,59). The second possibility appears to be also unlikely because comedocarcinomas, not noncomedocarcinomas, are most often associated with recurrent or invasive disease after surgical removal. Regarding the third possibility, most published series of invasive breast cancers contain both invasive ductal carcinomas and invasive lobular carcinomas. Invasive lobular carcinomas may

FIGURE 7.1. HER-2/*neu* gene amplification and overexpression in a high-grade, large-cell comedocarcinoma ductal carcinoma in situ (DCIS) lesion. **A:** Histologic section of an intraductal comedocarcinoma stained with hematoxylin and eosin. Necrotic debris occupies the center of the duct lumen surrounded by high-grade DCIS tumor cells (magnification 400×). **B:** Photomicrograph of a serial section prepared from the comedocarcinoma illustrated in **A** shows immunostaining for HER-2/*neu* protein in tumor cells of the comedocarcinoma. 10H8 anti-HER-2/*neu* monoclonal antibody (magnification 400×). **C:** Photomicrograph of comedocarcinoma shown in **B** demonstrating membrane immunostaining for HER-2/*neu* protein in tumor cells. 10H8 anti-HER-2/*neu* monoclonal antibody (magnification 2,400×). **D:** Fluorescence in situ hybridization for HER-2/*neu* gene (red) and chromosome 17 centromere (green) prepared with a serial section from the comedocarcinoma shown in **A–C**. Each DCIS tumor cell nucleus contains multiple copies of the HER-2/*neu* gene shown as red fluorescence signals. This DCIS comedocarcinoma had an average of 19.33 HER-2/*neu* gene copies and 1.95 chromosome 17 centromeres per tumor cell nucleus. The ratio was 9.91 HER-2/*neu* gene-to-chromosome 17 centromere copies per tumor cell nucleus indicating HER-2/*neu* gene amplification (≥2.0 HER-2/*neu* gene-to-chromosome 17 centromere copies per tumor cell nucleus is an amplified ratio).

comprise 10% or more of the study cohort and seldom have HER-2/*neu* amplification or overexpression. This may be a factor in the apparent discrepancy between HER-2/*neu* positivity in breast carcinoma in situ and invasive breast cancer. The fourth and fifth possibilities are also potential explanations for the observation that HER-2/*neu* overexpression by immunohistochemistry is identified more frequently in DCIS than in invasive breast cancer. Additional studies are needed for resolution of this issue.

In an early study of HER-2/*neu* immunostaining in 45 DCIS cases, 42% (19 of 45) showed positive membrane staining among only the large-cell, comedo subtype (53). Subsequent studies have supported the high prevalence of HER-2/*neu* overexpression in comedocarcinomas or high-grade lesions compared with other subtypes of intraductal carcinomas (Table 7.1). Various histomorphologic classifications have been used. Some studies of DCIS have used pathologic classifications with comedocarcinoma, solid, cribriform, micropapillary, papillary, or mixed intraductal carcinomas (46). Others have used cytologic criteria such as the Van Nuys classification based on nuclear grade and the presence or absence of necrosis to separate DCIS into high-, intermediate-, and low-grade lesions (60). However, the aggregate of data confirms that high-grade DCIS lesions are significantly more likely to have HER-2/*neu* overexpression than are low-grade DCIS lesions (Table 7.1). Overall, HER-2/*neu* has been characterized in more than 1,600 DCIS, with approximately 41% of these DCIS showing overexpression and/or amplification. Among those lesions classified as comedocarcinomas or high-grade, large cell DCIS, approximately 65% show overexpression and/or amplification, whereas those DCIS lesions classified as noncomedocarcinomas or low-grade, small-cell lesions show overexpression and/or amplification in approximately 25% of cases (Table 7.1). In contrast, only 20% to 30% of invasive breast carcinomas are HER-2/*neu* amplified overexpressors (3–5,14,16–18,21,24,25,61,62).

CORRELATION OF HER-2/*NEU* STATUS WITH ESTROGEN RECEPTOR AND PROGESTERONE RECEPTOR STATUS

Estrogen receptor (ER) and progesterone receptor (PR) are ligand-activated nuclear transcription proteins with sequence-specific regulatory activity. Two ER proteins, α and β, have been identified (63–65). However, only ERα, the classical estrogen receptor, appears to be functionally important in breast cancer (66). ER recruits coactivator proteins, and together they function as a complex to regulate the effect of estrogens in peripheral tissue (67). Estrogens stimulate tumor growth through ER activation. ER is expressed in 50% to 80% of breast cancers depending on patient age (68). The presence of ER and PR in invasive breast

cancer is correlated with a longer disease-free interval, longer overall survival, and increased responsiveness to hormonal therapies.

ER is expressed in approximately 30% to 80% of DCIS cases. These ER-positive DCIS are usually low-grade, noncomedo histologic types with small cell size and a higher S-phase fraction (69). An inverse correlation has been observed between ER and PR expression and HER-2/*neu* overexpression in both invasive breast cancer and DCIS (70–72). Three different studies of DCIS show a significant inverse correlation between ER-positive/PR-positive status and HER-2/*neu* overexpression ($p = 0.002$, $p < 0.01$, and $p < 0.01$) (43,45,69). Other studies of biologic markers in DCIS do not correlate ER/PR status with HER-2/*neu* status but find inverse correlations between necrosis and positive ER/PR status (73) or significant correlations between comedo subtype and HER-2/*neu* overexpression (74). Poor differentiation and necrosis have been inversely correlated with positive PR and directly correlated with the presence of HER-2/*neu* overexpression (49). Although an inverse correlation between HER-2/*neu* overexpression and positive ER/PR status is not analyzed in these papers, it is possible that such a correlation might have been found had it been evaluated. One study finds no significant relationship between ER status and HER-2/*neu* status (48).

CORRELATION OF HER-2/*NEU* STATUS AND *P53* STATUS

p53 is a tumor suppressor gene located on the short arm of chromosome 17 that is frequently mutated and/or overexpressed in human invasive and intraductal breast cancer (39,46,49,51,57,60,73–80). Accumulation or overexpression of p53 protein in the cell nucleus is correlated with underlying *p53* mutations (80). In the studies summarized in Table 7.1, *p53* overexpression is noted in 12% to 40% of cases (39,46,49,51,57,60,73,74,79). Two of these studies show a correlation between HER-2/*neu* membrane staining and *p53* immunostaining (49,57). *p53* overexpression is associated with large-cell DCIS (79), comedo histology (46,73,74), and the presence of necrosis (79). HER-2/*neu* is also associated with large-cell DCIS (52,53), comedo histology (47,51,52,73,74), and the presence of necrosis (73). One study does not find a correlation between HER-2/*neu* amplification and *p53* mutations (39).

HER-2/*NEU* AND DNA PLOIDY AND ANGIOGENESIS

During cancer progression, DNA aberrations accumulate and cells often become nondiploid or aneuploid. Diploid DNA content assessed by DNA flow cytometry is normal.

Cancer cells with abnormal DNA content or a nondiploid amount of DNA are aneuploid. DNA ploidy is a frequently characterized prognostic factor for breast cancer (81). Nondiploid DNA content of invasive breast cancers is correlated with shorter disease-free and overall patient survival (82,83). A positive correlation between HER-2/neu overexpression and aneuploidy is described in invasive breast cancers (84). It is not known whether aneuploidy is an important biologic marker in DCIS. Aneuploidy has been detected in more than 50% of DCIS cases (85–88). In the studies listed in Table 7.1, one group detects a positive association between aneuploidy and HER-2/neu positivity in DCIS that is maintained in invasive disease (44). In one study, HER-2/neu staining has been reported in 11 of 37 (29.7%) diploid DCIS tumors and in 40 of 69 (58%) aneuploid DCIS tumors (56). Two others detect aneuploidy in 39% to 77% of DCIS without assessing a correlation between HER-2/neu status and aneuploidy (46,69).

Angiogenesis is essential for breast carcinoma invasion beyond breast ducts. In one study analyzing angiogenesis and HER-2/neu status in DCIS, HER-2/neu overexpression has been positively correlated with periductal vascularization (45). This result confirms an earlier study detecting a pronounced, but not statistically significant, periductal angiogenic pattern associated with the comedo DCIS subtype (74).

CLINICAL ASSOCIATIONS WITH HER-2/*NEU* STATUS IN DUCTAL CARCINOMA IN SITU

HER-2/neu overexpression has been associated with increased cell motility and has been localized to portions of the cell membrane actively engaged in cell migration (54). Therefore, De Potter et al. (54) hypothesized that HER-2/neu overexpression in DCIS could enhance cell motility and increase the spread of HER-2/neu-overexpressing DCIS tumor cells throughout the ductal system of the breast, which would result in more extensive disease. These investigators found that HER-2/neu overexpression in DCIS was associated with larger diameter DCIS (54). They also found a highly significant relationship between HER-2/neu overexpression, extent of DCIS, and cell type. Among those cases studied, only four of 23 (17%) HER-2/neu-positive DCIS were smaller than 10 mm in diameter, whereas 35 of 52 (67%) HER-2/neu-negative DCIS were smaller than 10 mm in diameter. This hypothesis of HER-2/neu overexpression leading to increased tumor cell motility is also consistent with the observation that the breast carcinoma cells found in the skin with Paget's disease have HER-2/neu overexpression in more than 90% of the cases (47,56,74).

The mammographic features of HER-2/neu-positive and HER-2/neu-negative DCIS are significantly different from one another (50). The presence of calcifications, intraductal distribution of calcifications, rod-shaped calcifications, and granular calcifications are seen more commonly in HER-2/neu-positive DCIS, whereas abnormal mammograms without calcifications are seen more commonly in HER-2/neu-negative disease (50).

The role of HER-2/neu in the clinical management of DCIS is still not clearly defined. HER-2/neu overexpression has been associated with unfavorable pathobiologic characteristics, such as comedo histologic type, high nuclear grade, and high proliferative activity. High-grade DCIS lesions are known to have a higher rate of recurrent and invasive disease. Although these associations have led many authors to suggest that DCIS lesions with overexpression of HER-2/neu are biologically more aggressive, few studies have addressed this issue and no studies have demonstrated the clinical utility of HER-2/neu analysis in DCIS. This could be related to the relatively small number of DCIS study cases with long-term clinical follow-up and the low rate of recurrent and invasive disease associated with treated DCIS. A large population size would be required to achieve sufficient statistical power to demonstrate a worse clinical outcome for women with HER-2/neu overexpressing DCIS.

ACKNOWLEDGMENT

Supported by grants from the National Cancer Institute (CA48780) and U.S. Army Medical Research & Development Command (DAMD17-96-1-6156).

REFERENCES

1. Alroy I, Yarden Y. The erbB signaling network in embryogenesis and oncogenesis: signal diversification through combinatorial ligand-receptor interactions. *FEBS Lett* 1997;410:83–86.
2. Tzahar E, Waterman H, Chen X, et al. A hierarchical network of interreceptor interactions determines signal transduction by neu differentiation factor/neuregulin and epidermal growth factor. *Mol Cell Biol* 1996;16:5276–5287.
3. Slamon D, Clark G, Wong S, et al. Human breast cancer: correlation of relapse and survival with amplification of the HER-2/neu oncogene. *Science* 1987;235:177–182.
4. Slamon D, Godolphin W, Jones L, et al. Studies of the HER-2/neu proto-oncogene in human breast and ovarian cancer. *Science* 1989;244:707–712.
5. Slamon D, Press M, Godolphin W, et al. Studies of the HER-2/neu proto-oncogene in human breast cancer. *Cancer Cells* 1989; 7:371–380.
6. DiFiore P, Pierce J, Kraus M, et al. erb B-2 is a potent oncogene when overexpressed in NIH/3T3 cells. *Science* 1987;237:178–182.
7. Chazin V, Kaleko M, Miller A, et al. Transformation mediated by the human HER-2 gene independent of the epidermal growth factor receptor. *Oncogene* 1992;7:1859–1866.
8. Pietras R, Pegram M, Finn R, et al. Remission of human breast cancer xenografts on therapy with humanized monoclonal anti-

body to HER-2 receptor and DNA-reactive drugs. *Oncogene* 1998;17:2235–2249.

9. Muller W, Sinn E, Pattengale P, et al. Single-step induction of mammary adenocarcinoma in transgenic mice bearing the activated c-*neu* oncogene. *Cell* 1988;54:105–115.

10. Guy C, Webster M, Schaller M, et al. Expression of the *neu* protooncogene in the mammary epithelium of transgenic mice induces metastatic disease. *Proc Natl Acad Sci U S A* 1992;89: 10578–10582.

11. Cobleigh M, Vogel C, Tripathy D, et al. Multinational study of the efficacy and safety of humanized anti-HER2 monoclonal antibody in women who have HER2-overexpressing metastatic breast cancer that has progressed after chemotherapy for metastatic disease. *J Clin Oncol* 1999;17:2639–2648.

12. Slamon D, Leyland-Jones B, Shak S, et al. Use of chemotherapy plus a monoclonal antibody against HER2 for metastatic breast cancer that overexpresses HER2. *N Engl J Med* 2001;344:783–792.

13. Vogel C, Cobleigh M, Tripathy D, et al. Efficacy and safety of trastuzumab (Herceptin) as a single agent in first-line treatment of HER2-overexpressing metastatic breast cancer. *J Clin Oncol* 2002;20:719–726.

14. Press M, Pike M, Chazin, V, et al. HER-2/*neu* expression in node-negative breast cancers: direct tissue quantitation by computerized image analysis and association of overexpression with increased risk of recurrent disease. *Cancer Res* 1993;53:4960–4970.

15. Press M, Bernstein L, Thomas P, et al. HER-2/*neu* gene amplification by fluorescence *in situ* hybridization: evaluation of archival specimens and utility as a marker of poor prognosis in node-negative invasive breast carcinomas. *J Clin Oncol* 1997;15:2894–2904.

16. Gullick W, Love S, Wright C, et al. c-*erb* B-2 protein over-expression in breast cancer is a risk factor in patients with involved and uninvolved lymph nodes. *Br J Cancer* 1991;63:434–438.

17. Winstanley J, Cooke T, Murray G, et al. The long term prognostic significance of c-*erb* B-2 in primary breast cancer. *Br J Cancer* 1991;63:447–450.

18. Kallioniemi O-P, Holli K, Visakorpi T, et al. Association of c-*erb* B-2 oncogene overexpression with high rate of cell proliferation, increased risk for visceral metastasis and poor long-term survival in breast cancer. *Int J Cancer* 1991;49:650–655.

19. Ro J, El-Naggar A, Ro J, et al. c-*erb* B-2 amplification in node-negative breast cancer. *Cancer Res* 1989;49:6941–6944.

20. Giampietro G, Gullick W, Bevilacqua P, et al. Human breast cancer: prognostic significance of the c-*erb* B-2 oncoprotein compared with epidermal growth factor receptor, DNA ploidy, and conventional pathologic features. *J Clin Oncol* 1992;10:686–695.

21. Gusterson B, Gelber R, Goldhirsch A, et al. Prognostic importance of c-*erb*B-2 expression in breast cancer. International (Ludwig) Breast Cancer Study Group. *J Clin Oncol* 1992;10:1049–1056.

22. Paterson M, Dietrich K, Danyluk J, et al. Correlation between c-*erb* B-2 amplification and risk of early relapse in node-negative breast cancer. *Cancer Res* 1991;51:556–567.

23. Allred D, Lark G, Tandon A, et al. HER-2/*neu* in node-negative breast cancer: prognostic significance of overexpression influenced by the presence of *in situ* carcinoma. *J Clin Oncol* 1992;10: 599–605.

24. Paik S, Hazan R, Fisher E, et al. Pathologic findings from the National Surgical Adjuvant Breast and Bowel Project: prognostic significance of *erb* B-2 protein overexpression in primary breast cancer. *J Clin Oncol* 1990;8:103–112.

25. Wright C, Angus B, Nicholson S, et al. Expression of c-*erb* B-2 oncoprotein: a prognostic indicator in human breast cancer. *Cancer Res* 1989;49:2087–2090.

26. Rilke F, Colnaghi M, Cascinelli N, et al. Prognostic significance of HER-2/*neu* expression in breast cancer and its relationship to other prognostic factors. *Int J Cancer* 1991;49:44–49.

27. Press M, Hung G, Godolphin W, et al. Sensitivity of HER-2/*neu* antibodies in archival tissue samples: potential source of error in immunohistochemical studies of expression. *Cancer Res* 1994;54: 2771–2777.

28. Tetu B, Brisson J, Plante V, et al. p53 and c-*erb* B-2 as markers of resistance to adjuvant chemotherapy in breast cancer. *Mod Pathol* 1998;11:823–830.

29. Thor A, Berry D, Budman D, et al. *erb* B-2, p53, and efficacy of adjuvant therapy in lymph node-positive breast cancer. *J Natl Cancer Inst* 1998;90:1346–1360.

30. Muss H, Thor A, Berry D, et al. c*erb* B-2 expression and response to adjuvant therapy in women with node-positive early breast cancer. *N Engl J Med* 1994;330:1260–1266.

31. Wright C, Nicholson S, Angus B, et al. Relationship between c-*erb* B-2 protein product expression and response to endocrine therapy in advanced breast cancer. *Br J Cancer* 1992;65:118–121.

32. Carlomagno C, Perrone F, Gallo C, et al. c-*erb* B2 overexpression decreases the benefit of adjuvant tamoxifen in early-stage breast cancer without axillary lymph node metastases. *J Clin Oncol* 1996;14:2702–2708.

33. Borg A, Baldetorp B, Ferno M, et al. *erb* B2 amplification is associated with tamoxifen resistance in steroid-receptor positive breast cancer. *Cancer Lett* 1994;81:137–144.

34. Press M, Slamon D, Flom K, et al. Evaluation of HER-2/*neu* gene amplification and overexpression: comparison of frequently used assay methods in a molecularly characterized cohort of breast cancer specimens. *J Clin Oncol* (*in press*) 2002.

35. Penault-Llorca F, Adelaide J, Houvenaeghel G, et al. Optimization of immunohistochemical detection of ERBB2 in human breast cancer: impact of fixation. *J Pathol* 1994;173: 65–75.

36. Roche P, Ingle J. Increased HER2 with U.S. Food and Drug Administration-approved antibody. *J Clin Oncol* 1999;l17:434.

37. Jacobs T, Gown A, Yaziji H, et al. Specificity of HercepTest in determining HER-2/*neu* status of breast cancers using the United States Food and Drug Administration-approved scoring system. *J Clin Oncol* 1999;17:1983–1987.

38. Liu E, Thor A, He M, et al. The HER2 (c-*erb* B-2) oncogene is frequently amplified in *in situ* carcinomas of the breast. *Oncogene* 1992;7:1027–1032.

39. Ho G, Calvano J, Bisogna M, et al. In microdissected ductal carcinoma *in situ*, HER-2/*neu* amplification, but not p53 mutation, is associated with high nuclear grade and comedo histology. *Am Cancer Soc* 2000;89:2153–2160.

40. Glockner S, Lehmann U, Wilke N, et al. Amplification of growth regulatory genes in intraductal breast cancer is associated with higher nuclear grade but not with the progression to invasiveness. *Lab Invest* 2001;81:565–571.

41. Jacobs T, Gown A, Yaziji H, et al. Comparison of fluorescence *in situ* hybridization and immunohistochemistry for the evaluation of HER-2/*neu* in breast cancer. *J Clin Oncol* 1999;17:1974–1982.

42. Thor A, Schwartz L, Koerner F, et al. Analysis of c-*erb* B-2 expression in breast carcinomas with clinical follow-up. *Cancer Res* 1989;49:7147–7152.

43. Allred D, Clark G, Molina R, et al. Overexpression of HER-2/*neu* and its relationship with other prognostic factors change during the progression of *in situ* to invasive breast cancer. *Hum Pathol* 1992;23:974–979.

44. Iglehart J, Kerns B-J, Huper G, et al. Maintenance of DNA content and *erb* B-2 alterations in intraductal and invasive phases of mammary cancer. *Breast Cancer Res Treat* 1995;34:253–263.

45. Claus E, Chu P, Howe C, et al. Pathobiologic findings in DCIS of the breast: morphologic features, angiogenesis, HER-2/*neu* and hormone receptors. *Exp Mol Pathol* 2001;70:303–316.

46. Leal C, Schmitt F, Bento M, et al. Ductal carcinoma *in situ* of the breast: Histologic categorization and its relationship to ploidy and immunohistochemical expression of hormone receptors, p53, and c-erb B-2 protein. *Cancer* 1995;75:2123–2131.

47. Gusterson B, Machin L, Gullick W, et al. Immunohistochemical distribution of *c-erb* B-2 in infiltrating and *in situ* breast cancer. *Int J Cancer* 1988;42:842–845.

48. McCann A, Dervan P, O'Regan M, et al. Prognostic significance of c-erb B-2 and estrogen receptor status in human breast cancer. *Cancer Res* 1991;51:3296–3303.

49. Bobrow L, Happerfield L, Gregory W, et al. Ductal carcinoma *in situ*: assessment of necrosis and nuclear morphology and their association with biological markers. *J Pathol* 1995;176:333–341.

50. Evans A, Pinder SE, Ellis I, et al. Correlations between the mammographic features of ductal carcinoma *in situ* (DCIS) and c-erb B-2 oncogene expression. *Clin Radiol* 1994;49:559–562.

51. Querzoli P, Albonico G, Ferretti S, et al. Modulation of biomarkers in minimal breast carcinoma—a model for human breast carcinoma progression. *Am Cancer Soc* 1998;83:89–97.

52. Somerville J, Clarke L, Biggart J. c-erb B-2 overexpression and histological type of *in situ* and invasive breast carcinoma. *J Clin Pathol* 1992;45:16–20.

53. Van de Vijver M, Peterse J, Mooi W, et al. *neu*-protein overexpression in breast cancer. Association with comedo-type ductal carcinoma *in situ* and limited prognostic value in stage II breast cancer. *N Engl J Med* 1988;319:1239–1245.

54. De Potter C, Schelfhout A-M, Verbeeck P, et al. *neu* overexpression correlates with extent of disease in large cell ductal carcinoma *in situ* of the breast. *Hum Pathol* 1995;26:601–606.

55. Maguire HJ, Hellman M, Greene M, et al. Expression of c-erb B-2 in *in situ* and in adjacent invasive ductal adenocarcinomas of the female breast. *Pathobiology* 1992;60:117–121.

56. Schimmelpenning H, Eriksson E, Falkmer U, et al. Expression of the c-erb B-2 proto-oncogene product and nuclear DNA content in benign and malignant human breast parenchyma. *Virchows Arch* 1992;420:433–440.

57. Mommers E, Leonhart, A, Falix F, et al. Similarity in expression of cell cycle proteins between *in situ* and invasive ductal breast lesions of same differentiation grade. *J Pathol* 2001;194:327–333.

58. Glockner S, Lehmann U, Wilke N, et al. Detection of gene amplification in intraductal and infiltrating breast cancer by laser-assisted microdissection and quantitative real-time PCR. *Pathobiology* 2000;68:173–179.

59. Tsuda H, Hirohashi S. Multiple developmental pathways of highly aggressive breast cancers disclosed by comparison of histological grades and c-erb B-2 expression patterns in both the noninvasive and invasive portions. *Pathol Int* 1998;48:518–525.

60. Silverstein M, Poller D, Waisman J, et al. Prognostic classification of breast ductal carcinoma-in-situ. *Lancet* 1995;345:1154–1157.

61. Tetu B, Brisson J. Prognostic significance of HER-2/neu oncoprotein expression in node-positive breast cancer: the influence of the pattern of immunostaining and adjuvant therapy. *Cancer* 1994;73:2359–2365.

62. O'Reilly S, Barnes D, Camplejohn R, et al. The relationship between c-erb B-2 expression, S-phase fraction and prognosis in breast cancer. *Br J Cancer* 1991;63:444–446.

63. Kuiper G, Enmark E, Pelto-Huikko P, et al. Cloning of a novel estrogen receptor expressed in rat prostate and ovary. *Proc Natl Acad Sci U S A* 1996;93:5925–5930.

64. Kuiper G, Carlsson B, Grandien K, et al. Comparison of the ligand binding specificity and transcript tissue distribution of estrogen receptors α and β. *Endocrinology* 1997;138:863–870.

65. Mosselman S, Polman J, Dijkema R. ERβ: identification and characterization of a novel human estrogen receptor. *FEBS Lett* 1996;392:49–53.

66. Cullen R, Maguire T, McDermott E, et al. Studies of oestrogen receptor-alpha and -beta mRNA in breast cancer. *Eur J Cancer* 2001;37:1118–1122.

67. Glass G, Rose D, Rosenfeld M. Nuclear receptor coactivators. *Curr Opin Cell Biol* 1997;9:222–232.

68. Clark G, Osborne C, McGuire W. Correlations between estrogen receptor, progesterone receptor, and patient characteristics in human breast cancer. *J Clin Oncol* 1984;2:1102–1109.

69. Poller D, Snead D, Roberts E, et al. Oestrogen receptor expression in ductal carcinoma *in situ* of the breast: relationship to flow cytometric analysis of DNA and expression of the c-erb B-2 oncoprotein. *Br J Cancer* 1993;68:156–161.

70. Ciocca D, Fujimura F, Tandon A. Correlation of HER-2/neu amplification with expression and with other prognostic factors in 1103 breast cancers. *J Natl Cancer Inst* 1992;84:1279–1282.

71. Bacus S, Chin D, Yarden Y, et al. Type I receptor tyrosine kinases are differentially phosphorylated in mammary carcinoma and differentially associated with steroid receptors. *Am J Pathol* 1996;148:549–581.

72. DiGiovanna M, Carter D, Flynn S, et al. Functional assay for HER-2/neu demonstrates active signaling in a minority of HER-2/neu-overexpressing invasive human breast tumours. *Br J Cancer* 1996;74:802–806.

73. Zafrani B, Leroyer A, Fourquet A, et al. Mammographically-detected ductal *in situ* carcinoma of the breast analyzed with a new classification. A study of 127 cases: correlation with estrogen and progesterone receptors, p53 and c-erbB-2 proteins, and proliferative activity. *Semin Diagn Pathol* 1994;11:208–214.

74. Bose S, Lesser M, Norton L, et al. Immunophenotype of intraductal carcinoma. *Arch Pathol Lab Med* 1996;120:81–85.

75. Eyfjord J, Thorlacius S, Steinarsdottir M, et al. P53 abnormalities and genomic instability in primary human breast carcinomas. *Cancer Res* 1995;55:646–651.

76. Harris A. P53 expression in human breast cancer. 1992;59:69–88.

77. Harris C, Hollstein M. Clinical implications of the p53 tumor suppressor gene. *N Engl J Med* 1993;329:1318–1327.

78. Barnes D, Dublin E, Fisher C, et al. Immunohistochemical detection of p53 protein in mammary carcinoma: an important independent indicator of prognosis? *Hum Pathol* 1993;24:468–476.

79. Poller D, Roberts E, Bell J, et al. P53 protein expression in mammary ductal carcinoma *in situ*: relationship to immunohistochemical expression of estrogen receptor and c-erbB-2 protein. *Hum Pathol* 1993;24:463–468.

80. Lukas J, Niu N, Press M. P53 mutations and expression in breast carcinoma *in situ*. *Am J Pathol* 2000;156:183–191.

81. Mansour E, Ravdin P, Dressler L. Prognostic factors in early breast carcinoma. *Cancer* 1994;74:381–400.

82. Dressler L. Are DNA flow cytometry measurements providing useful information in the management of nodes positive early breast cancer. *Cancer Invest* 1993;10:477–486.

83. Hedley D, Clark G, Cornelisse C, et al. Consensus review of the clinical utility of DNA cytometry in carcinoma of the breast. *Cytometry* 1993;14:482–485.

84. Revillion F, Bonneterre J, Peyrat J. ERBB2 oncogene in human breast cancer and its clinical significance. *Eur J Cancer* 1998;34:791–808.

85. Bacus S, Bacus J, Slamon D, et al. HER-2/neu oncogene expression and DNA ploidy analysis in breast cancer. *Arch Pathol Lab Med* 1990;114:164–169.

86. Eriksson F, Schimmelpenning H, Aspenblad U, et al. Immunohistochemical expression of the mutant p53 protein and nuclear DNA content during the transition from benign to malignant breast disease. *Hum Pathol* 1994;25:1228–1232.

87. Ottesen G, Christensen L, Larsen J, et al. DNA analysis of *in situ* ductal carcinoma of the breast via flow cytometry. *Cytometry* 1995;22:168–176.

88. Fisher E, Siderits R. Value of cytometric analysis for distinction of intraductal carcinoma of the breast. *Breast Cancer Res Treat* 1992;21:165–172.

89. Mack L, Kerkvliet N, Doig G, et al. Relationship of a new histological categorization of ductal carcinoma *in situ* of the breast with size and the immunohistochemical expression of p53, c-*erb* B2, bcl-2, and ki-67. *Hum Pathol* 1997;28:974–979.

90. Bobrow L, Happerfield L, Gregory W, et al. The classification of ductal carcinoma *in situ* and its association with biological markers. *Semin Diagn Pathol* 1994;11:199–207.

8

NEW INSIGHTS INTO THE PATHOGENESIS OF IN SITU CARCINOMAS OF THE BREAST BY MEANS OF COMPARATIVE GENOMIC HYBRIDIZATION

HORST BÜRGER
WERNER BÖCKER

HISTORICAL AND TECHNICAL BACKGROUND

Breast carcinogenesis is caused and reflected by an accumulation of genetic changes, some of which can be made be visible using chromosomal banding techniques and light microscopy. Nevertheless, most of these alterations can only be detected by means of modern molecular biologic techniques.

With the introduction of the common G banding for the identification of chromosomes or chromosomal breakpoints in hematologic and solid tumors, a technique was created that for the first time allowed a detailed overview of chromosomal alterations within a given tumor (1). The protocols and theory behind this technique seemed very convincing, although its drawbacks and disadvantages were equally obvious. Concerning solid tumors, the low success rate (20% and below) of gaining metaphase chromosomes was especially disappointing because it questioned the cytogenetic results. This problem is further enhanced by short-time culture of tumor cells, which opens the possibility of selecting special tumor clones. In addition, this technique requires fresh and unfixed tissue unsuitable for further pathologic evaluation, which, of course, is the basic indication for an invasive breast biopsy. As a result, small or even minuscule specimens gained in standard diagnostic procedures cannot be investigated with this technique.

Other techniques, such as polymerase chain reaction-based microsatellite analysis or fluorescence in situ hybridization circumvent these problems because they can be applied in cases in which only a few hundred, or even fewer, cells have been obtained. In contrast to conventional cytogenetics, the resolution of these techniques is dramatically higher so that single genes or defined genetic sequences can

be recognized. Unfortunately, it is virtually impossible to obtain an overview of all the genetic changes in a given tumorous lesion with these techniques unless a considerable and time-consuming effort is made. Against this background, their use as simple screening techniques cannot be recommended.

In 1992, a new fluorescence in situ hybridization-based technique called comparative genomic hybridization (CGH) was first described, which offered a rapid and reliable technique for the detection of all unbalanced chromosomal alterations within a given tumor (2,3). The number of studies using CGH has grown steadily since then and yielded exciting insights into the pathogenesis of breast cancer.

THE COMPARATIVE GENOMIC HYBRIDIZATION METHOD

For CGH, total test (tumor) DNA and reference DNA (the latter from a healthy person) is labeled with biotinylated and digoxigenated deoxyuridine 5-triphosphate, respectively. Both DNAs are hybridized simultaneously to normal metaphase spreads in the presence of unlabeled Cot-1 DNA that inhibits unintended binding of the labeled DNA to the centromeric and heterochromatic regions of the chromosomes. The adequate amount of test and reference DNA then competes for hybridization on a given chromosomal locus. After hybridization, test and reference DNA is detected with avidin-bound fluorescein isothiocyanate (green fluorescence) and rhodamine-bound antidigoxigenin (red fluorescence). The overall intensity of the reaction is a result of increased or decreased hybridization of fitting DNA sequences. Gained and lost genetic material of the test DNA

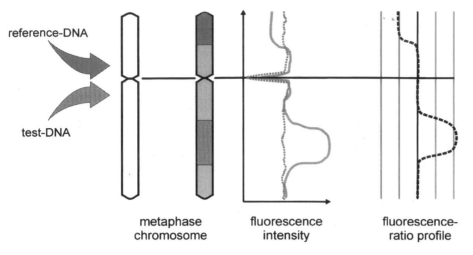

reference-DNA

test-DNA

metaphase
chromosome

fluorescence
intensity

fluorescence-
ratio profile

FIGURE 8.1. Schematic drawing of the principles of comparative genomic hybridization. Equal amounts of fluorescent dye-labeled tumor and reference DNA are cohybridized on normal metaphase chromosomes of human lymphocytes. Differences in DNA concentrations of distinct chromosomal regions result in varying fluorescence intensity finally transferred to a fluorescence ratio profile by specialized software.

compared with normal reference DNA appears as pronounced or reduced fluorescence intensity on the hybridized chromosomes. The red and green fluorescence signals of each chromosome are measured by a digital image analysis system. A special software integrates fluorescence intensities along the chromosomal axis, subtracts local background, and calculates the green-to-red fluorescence ratio for each chromosomal locus, which reflects the relative copy numbers of the homologous sequences contained in the compared DNA samples. Disomic sequences of the tumor and reference DNA therefore lead to a fluorescence ratio of 2:2 (= 1), whereas trisomic chromosomal areas result in a ratio of 3:2 (= 1.5) and monosomy in a ratio of 1:2 (= 0.5). Under laboratory conditions, these thresholds may shift owing to contamination of the test DNA with normal cells. This procedure is based on previous karyotyping of the metaphase chromosomes, which therefore are counterstained with 4,6-diamidino-2-phenylindole. A schematic drawing is given in Figure 8.1.

The major advantage is that CGH can be performed with fresh frozen and with formalin-fixed and paraffin-embedded tissues and therefore allows the investigation of large, morphologically well-defined tumor series. Nevertheless, it is evident that CGH does not give any information about the DNA ploidy status of a tumor and cannot detect balanced chromosomal translocations. Therefore, this new technique does not replace other modern molecular genetic methods or classical cytogenetics; rather, it has to be regarded as a highly valuable supplement to these techniques.

COMPARATIVE GENOMIC HYBRIDIZATION AND INVASIVE BREAST CANCER

The impact of CGH became evident when Kallioniemi et al. (4) published the first study in which 26 genomic regions were mapped as affected by increased DNA copy numbers. Until then, it was largely unknown that some of these were

even involved in the development of breast cancer. In particular, the chromosomal regions 17q22–24 and 20q13 attracted further attention because they show elevated frequency rates of chromosomal high-level gains, which are indicative of gene amplifications. The usefulness of this new approach for the detection of gene amplifications was further substantiated by comparing it with established methods such as Southern blot (5). Moreover, comparison of CGH data with common chromosome banding techniques demonstrated that tumors with homogeneously staining regions indicative of gene amplifications revealed such amplifications on CGH almost without any exception (6). In contrast, conventional cytogenetic data have reproducibility rates that generally amount to no more than 50% of all cases. The underlying reason might be seen in growth advantages of single tumor cell clones in cell culture. Conversely, intratumoral genetic heterogeneity cannot be detected by means of CGH, which only reveals the average of all unbalanced genetic alterations (7).

Nevertheless, the complexity of genetic changes in breast cancer found at the CGH level, with tens of Mb involved in high-level gains, was unexpected and gave rise to the hypothesis that multiply affected genes in a given region are a characteristic feature of genetic instability in tumor progression (4). In addition, it could be shown that defined, established breast cancer cell lines share the most common genetic changes of primary breast cancer and therefore are reliable tools in breast cancer research that seek to identify a kind of cytogenetic single-tumor specific fingerprint (4,8,9).

Further studies in the following years dealt with well-known clinical problems. The treatment of node-negative breast cancer still represents a particularly urgent one and the availability of reproducible, independent prognostic markers would definitely allow treatment protocols that are more precisely patient-tailored. Gains of chromosomal material of 8q and 20q13, as well as an elevated number of genetic alterations, were found to be associated with a worsened prognosis, an early tumor relapse (10), and poor prognostic morphometric parameters, such as the DNA ploidy index, tumor cell size, and proliferation rate (11,12). The association of specific genetic changes with high telomerase activity as a marker of a worsened prognosis highlighted the capability of CGH in defining chromosomal regions important in breast carcinogenesis (13). Investigations concentrating on special clinical subgroups such as BRCA1 and 2 mutation carriers of female and male breast cancer patients or patients with hypodiploid breast cancer could clearly demonstrate the existence of different genetic subgroups, which point to divergent molecular biologic mechanisms in breast carcinogenesis (14–16). These data raised some doubt regarding the widespread view of a purely serial progression of breast cancer. In particular, studies investigating the problem of distant, synchronous, and metachronous metastases, e.g., lymph node metastases, did not reveal any association of such lesions with the accumulation of distinct genetic alterations generally associated with invasive growth properties (17). Rather, it became evident that the step to metastatic disease seems to be determined by events that occur at a very early stage in breast cancer evolution and are therefore not necessarily mirrored on the cytogenetic level (18). Only very few studies dealt with the problem of the phenotype-genotype relationship. Lobular invasive carcinomas were the only ones shown to be associated with losses of the long arm of chromosome 16 (19–21).

To date, a multitude of further CGH studies pieced together the details of a characteristic, highly elaborate, and reproducible pattern of cytogenetic changes in more than 900 invasive breast cancer cases. It was noteworthy to what extent these results coincided. The comprehensive results of 17 CGH studies (4,5,10–12,14–17,19,20,22–26) drawing on selected and unselected breast cancer cases are summarized in Figure 8.2. Irrespective of the fact that almost all chromosomal regions are affected by chromosomal changes, distinct regions have evolved that show a significantly elevated frequency of gains and losses, as expected by chance pointing to the importance of these regions in breast carcinogenesis.

COMPARATIVE GENOMIC HYBRIDIZATION AND DUCTAL CARCINOMA IN SITU

Based on these results, a comparison of CGH data derived from ductal carcinoma in situ (DCIS) allowed a preliminary indirect judgment about the true relationship of invasive breast cancer and DCIS as its proposed and suspected ultimate precursor. Studies focusing on that issue could clearly demonstrate that almost all DCIS cases shared a high degree of cytogenetic homology with invasive breast cancer. This finding substantiated the hypothesis that the most common genetic changes of invasive carcinoma already take place on the in situ carcinoma level, and, therefore, the genetic heterogeneity of invasive breast cancer is fully developed in DCIS as a genetically far advanced lesion (27–30). The direct comparison of DCIS and its invasive counterpart in one patient emphasized this hypothesis (31). In addition, CGH analysis also demonstrated an intratumoral cytogenetic heterogeneity already present in in situ carcinomas (27,32,33) that had previously been described using microsatellite analysis (34). This is not only of tumor biologic and theoretical importance, but it also tremendously complicates the definition of genetic markers associated with or causing invasive growth properties. Generally speaking, it cannot be overlooked that the presence of a distinct genetic alteration in invasive breast cancer and the lack of this alteration in an as-

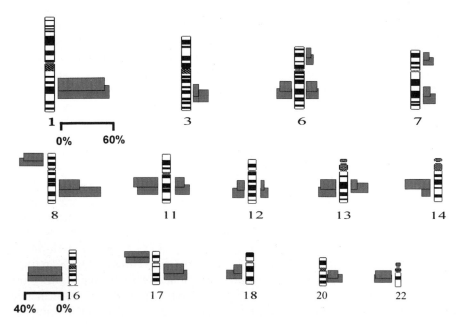

FIGURE 8.2. Summary of more than 900 invasive breast cancer cases analyzed by comparative genomic hybridization (CGH) in contrast to CGH data obtained from ductal carcinoma in situ. Bars on the left side of the chromosome ideogram represent losses of the respective chromosomal arm, bars on the right side gains. Invasive breast cancers are depicted in red and ductal carcinoma in situ cases in green. References are given in the text.

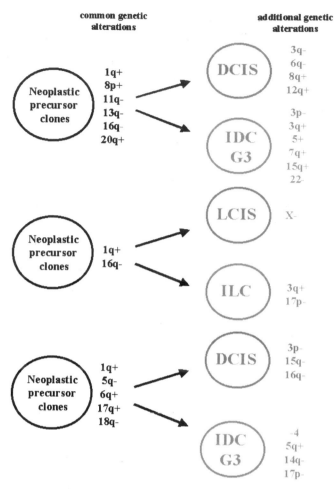

FIGURE 8.3. Lines of cytogenetic evolution in pairs of in situ carcinomas and invasive breast cancers in the same patient. Neoplastic precursor clones, which share a number of cytogenetic alterations, progress toward an invasive or an in situ carcinoma, both with additional, but often different genetic, alterations. It is obvious that the stage of invasion is not characterized by a stepwise accumulation of distinct chromosomal alterations. This model gives indirect evidence of an intratumoral heterogeneity already present in in situ carcinomas.

sociated carcinoma in situ in the same patient merely reflects an early intratumoral (intra-DCIS) genetic heterogeneity rather than being a marker of invasive growth (32). Examples are given in Figure 8.3.

PHENOTYPE-GENOTYPE CORRELATIONS IN DUCTAL CARCINOMA IN SITU

A multitude of pathomorphologic classification systems reflects the broad intra- and interindividual morphologic heterogeneity in the diagnosis of preinvasive breast cancer. The architectural pattern, nuclear size, and absence or presence of necrosis were considered the most important parameters in the classification of DCIS. Interestingly, parameters of tumor proliferation as one of the strongest morphology-based prognostic parameters in invasive breast cancer were not included in any of these classification systems.

The most commonly used protocols proposed three classes of DCIS, and in all these classification systems, the extreme ends could be defined with a high degree of reproducibility (35,36). The weakness shared by all these classification systems is the very low reproducibility in the intermediate groups (37), some reflecting a relationship with DCIS of poor differentiation and some characteristics of highly differentiated DCIS. Nevertheless, these classification systems try to correlate morphology with underlying biologic features and thus are the basis for assessing the clinical significance associated with these lesions. Definition of the genetic alterations might help us to reach somewhat firmer ground in view of the biologic (35) and clinical diversity (36) of these tumors.

Regarding the formal pathogenesis of DCIS, it was widely accepted that DCIS evolves from ductal hyperplasia via atypical ductal hyperplasia, followed by a stepwise dedifferentiation from well- to poorly differentiated DCIS. This interpretation was mainly based on epidemiologic data (38) but was also supported by morphometric, immunohistochemical, and genetic findings (39–42). Once the DCIS stage was reached, further progression was seen as a stepwise morphologic dedifferentiation, which was equally reflected in the gradual accumulation of genetic alterations from DCIS with low nuclear grade to DCIS with high nuclear grade and comedonecrosis.

CGH analysis raised doubts concerning the simple transferability of these epidemiologic data to the cytogenetic level. In a (first published and later enlarged) series (29,43) of up-to-date 51 cases of DCIS were analyzed, which, in terms of the European Organization for Research and Treatment of Cancer guidelines and with reference to the protocols proposed by Holland et al. (35), were representative of the entire morphologic range of DCIS subgroups. Figure 8.4 provides an overview of all the genetic changes detected. Based on quantitative changes alone, the stepwise accumulation of genetic alterations, as shown in Figure 8.5, might support the concept of serial progression. The qualitative genetic aberrations seen in this series, however, gave evidence of distinct pathways in the evolution of DCIS. These main genetic pathways also proved to be characteristic of one of the morphologically different subgroups of DCIS. Tumors at the highly differentiated end of the morphologic spectrum including a subset of intermediately differentiated DCIS were characterized by a loss of genetic material of 16q, with the shortest region of overlap located on 16q22–24. A strong argument in favor of the progression of well toward intermediately differentiated DCIS might be the increase in the average number of genetic aberrations per case from 2.5 to 5.5 in well-differentiated and intermediately differentiated DCIS, respectively. Additionally, this is supported by significantly increased rates of 1q gains and 11q losses in intermediately differentiated DCIS. Poorly differentiated DCIS differed

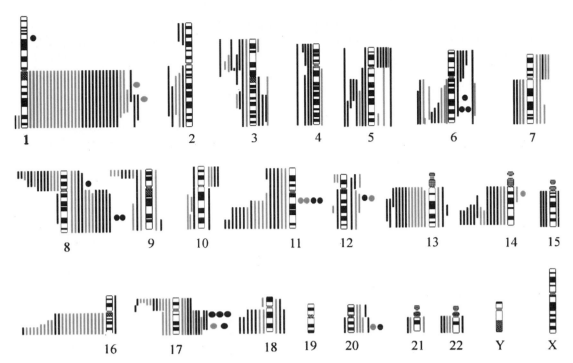

FIGURE 8.4. CGH analysis of 51 cases of DCIS. Summary of all chromosomal imbalances detected by CGH in well-, intermediately, and poorly differentiated ductal carcinoma in situ (DCIS). The vertical lines on the left side of the chromosome ideograms indicate losses and those on the right side indicate gains of genetic material in the tumor DNA. Each line illustrates the region of the chromosome affected in one tumor. Well-differentiated DCIS is depicted in red, intermediately differentiated DCIS in green, and poorly differentiated DCIS in black. Amplifications are represented by thick points. The chromosomal regions 1p, 16p, and 19 were excluded from analysis.

from the other subgroups both in quantitative and qualitative terms. Thus, poorly differentiated DCIS revealed a reduced rate of losses of 16q and an increase of 17q gains compared with well and intermediately differentiated DCIS. Furthermore, it disclosed a larger number of amplifications. Specific chromosomal loci involved in amplifications in this subgroup included 17q12, 14q22–24, 20q13, and 11q13. In summary,

there are strong lines of evidence in favor of poorly differentiated DCIS representing a second pathway rather than being the final stage in the evolution of DCIS via well-differentiated DCIS. Such a conclusion has also been proposed by other authors drawing on immunohistochemistry and morphometric measurements (41,44). A subgroup of intermediately differentiated DCIS, however, shared genetic amplifications with

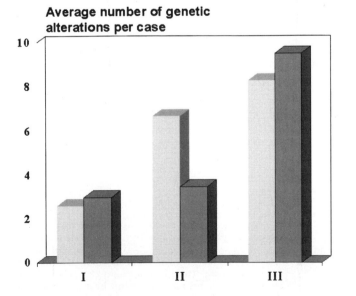

Average number of genetic alterations per case

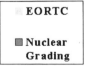

FIGURE 8.5. Correlation of the average number of genetic alterations per case with different morphologic classification systems. A stepwise increase in the average number of genetic alterations can be detected with both approaches. The highest degree of discordance is revealed in the intermediate subgroup.

poorly differentiated DCIS in the chromosomal band 11q13. Therefore, it might be suggested, although it cannot be proved, that a small number of poorly differentiated DCIS may develop via intermediately differentiated DCIS. The important tumor type specific role of 16q losses and 17q gains could be confirmed by another independent group using CGH and microsatellite analysis based on a very stringently classified DCIS collective (30). Other studies focusing on poorly differentiated, comedo-type DCIS at least showed a low frequency of 16q losses in these tumors (28,33,45).

If the claim is that of a fundamental role of 16q losses in the pathogenesis of a subgroup of preinvasive breast cancer, such an effect has to be shown to be reproducible, irrespective of the classification protocol chosen. The reclassification of the above-mentioned series of preinvasive tumors chosen with reference to a grading system based exclusively on cytonuclear features (46) confirmed this hypothesis, as shown in Figure 8.6. Although 100% of low nuclear grade DCIS showed a 16q loss, the same feature could be demonstrated with a somewhat lower ratio for intermediate and high nuclear grade DCIS, clearly pointing to an underlying biologic principle.

The reclassification of these DCIS cases with reference to exclusively nuclear parameters (46) also revealed that low and intermediate nuclear grade DCIS did not differ significantly in the average number of genetic alterations per case. This might be interpreted as a biologic rationale for deciding in favor of a two-tiered grading system that merely distinguishes between low and high nuclear grade DCIS, as proposed in the Van Nuys Prognostic Index (36).

INDEPENDENT LINES OF EVIDENCE FOR THE EXISTENCE OF MULTIPLE CYTOGENETIC PATHWAYS IN DUCTAL CARCINOMA IN SITU

Although it was highly unlikely that all these genotype-phenotype correlations were owing to simple grading or classification errors, further studies drawing on grading-indepen-

dent morphometric parameters were undertaken. There are several lines of evidence that independently support the theory of different cytogenetic pathways (43).

- Subdividing all DCIS according to their degree of genetic instability in terms of the number of genetic alterations per case showed an increasing frequency of almost all genetic alterations, with the exception of the rate of 16q losses, which remained constant and ultimately decreased in genetically far advanced tumors with 11 to 15 alterations per case. Under the assumption of a stepwise genetic dedifferentiation involving all genetic loci in random and nonrandom fashion, the distribution of 16q losses in this context is surprising and might be seen as a case in point against a purely serial progression in the carcinogenesis of DCIS.

- Correlating the absence and presence of necrosis as one parameter of DCIS classification with specific genetic alterations resulted in no more than two alterations gaining statistical significance. Losses of 16q were detected with greater frequency in DCIS without necrosis, whereas 17q gains were seen exclusively in DCIS with necrosis.

- Tumors with a 16q loss revealed significantly lower mitotic and apoptotic activity. In contrast, tumors with a loss of 8p and gains of 6q and 8q showed opposite results.

- Tumors with gains of 6q, 8q, and 17q displayed a higher rate of amplifications and an average number of chromosomal alterations.

It became obvious that distinct chromosomal alterations were associated with important biologic and pathomorphologic features used for the classification of DCIS. When these new data were integrated into existing paradigms, it became increasingly evident that the proposed cytogenetic pathways of DCIS could be reproduced by several independent methods.

Therefore, the evolution of DCIS, as defined according to the classification system by Holland et al. (35), might indeed be characterized by a sequential progression cascade in rare cases, but for the majority, the tumor progression seems to be shaped by parallel pathways (29,30). The concept of

16q-losses and differentiation

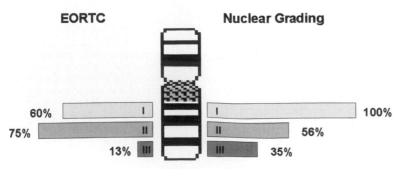

FIGURE 8.6. Distribution of the frequency of 16q losses in morphologic classification systems of ductal carcinoma in situ (DCIS). Whereas the two higher differentiated DCIS subgroups in both classification systems revealed 16q losses in 56% to 100%, the poorly differentiated, high-grade DCIS revealed significantly fewer 16q losses. The distinguishing character of 16q losses seems to be an underlying biologic principle rather than a classification-dependent phenomenon.

nonobligate tumor dedifferentiation is further substantiated by the fact that DCIS recurrences generally have a similar phenotype and an almost identical genotype with their original tumors (47).

In view of the above-mentioned phenotype-genotype correlation, it is more sensible to devise concepts and parameters that lend themselves to the definition of a two-tiered classification system, which more accurately reflects the underlying genetic mechanisms. A revision of the existing classification systems that takes into account those biologic data is therefore urgently needed to improve diagnostic reproducibility. Against the background of these findings, the inclusion of necrosis as a major distinguishing parameter in one tumor subgroup seems questionable.

CYTOGENETIC MARKERS FOR THE AGGRESSIVENESS OF DUCTAL CARCINOMA IN SITU

Comparing DCIS with and without an invasive component, three genetic events were generally associated with the absence or presence of invasiveness. Earlier studies described the loss of heterozygosity of 11q13 predominantly in DCIS with an associated invasive component (48), whereas CGH characterized the amplification of 11q13 as the underlying mechanism of this finding in this DCIS subgroup (29) but as equally in invasive breast cancer (22). In lobular carcinoma in situ (LCIS), gains of 1q were significantly rarer than in invasive lobular carcinoma, whereas the gain of 6q material was significantly more prevalent in LCIS without associated invasive lobular carcinoma. This might be interpreted as caused by potentially different genetic mechanisms associated with invasion in lobular and otherwise differentiated breast cancers (25). In contrast, losses of 14q and gains of Xq have been described as associated with intraductal (e.g., intralobular) growth (27,29), therefore defining clinically less aggressive DCIS/LCIS. The genes involved in this protective role have not yet been elucidated. Interestingly, the important role of genes residing on 14q could further be confirmed in cases of lymph node-negative breast cancer (49). The use of constantly improved high-resolution techniques might one day allow the characterization of putative candidate genes as the targets of future diagnosis and treatment because definition of other than clinical markers for the characterization of high-risk patients with DCIS is urgently needed for an individualized treatment.

ARE THESE PHENOTYPE-GENOTYPE CORRELATIONS MIRRORED IN INVASIVE BREAST CANCER?

Looking back to the beginnings of CGH studies of DCIS with the overwhelming evidence of DCIS as ultimate pre-

cursor of invasive breast cancer in mind, it might be expected that such a cytogenetic and morphologic dichotomy is retained and reflected in invasive breast cancer. Purely pathomorphologic observations revealed an association of special morphologic subtypes of invasive breast cancer with distinct DCIS subtypes (35). Comparing tubular and tubulolobular invasive carcinomas of the breast with well-differentiated DCIS, a strikingly similar cytogenetic pattern in terms of the degree of genetic instability and the rate of 16q losses and gene amplifications was detected (20). Similar results were obtained for ductal invasive G1 carcinomas (23,26). At the other end of the morphologic differentiation spectrum, poorly differentiated DCIS revealed a high degree of genetic homology with ductal invasive G3 carcinomas (20). The analysis of ductal invasive G2 carcinomas with elaborate genetic and morphometric techniques yields a highly heterogeneous picture of this subgroup, which might mirror the fact that the lesions evolved along two distinct pathways (50). In other words, the ostensible genetic progression demonstrated by several groups turned out to be a morphologic and genetic mixture of two quite different subgroups of invasive breast cancer (12,22,24).

DUCTAL CARCINOMA IN SITU AND LOBULAR DIFFERENTIATED PRENEOPLASTIC LESIONS

Despite the highly controversial results regarding 16q losses in the pathogenesis and prognosis of breast cancer, their role in the development of lobular differentiated precursor or indicator lesions of invasive breast cancer is beyond doubt. Microsatellite and mutation analysis could demonstrate the important role of E-cadherin in the typical morphology of these lesions (51,52). The major difference between ductal and lobular cancer has to be seen in the expression pattern of E-cadherin, which is almost completely absent in lobular invasive carcinoma and LCIS (53–55).

Only a few LCIS have been investigated by means of CGH so far and revealed highly reproducible results concerning quantitative and qualitative genetic features (25,32). As already demonstrated for lobular invasive carcinoma, the loss of 16q was a major characteristic of this unique variation with a very low number of genetic alterations per case. The impact of these results has been:

- For many years, LCIS has been exclusively defined as an indicator lesion of an increased risk to develop breast cancer in either breast, irrespective of the breast biopsied. The finding of gross cytogenetic alterations, for many a sign of potential malignancy, will render this interpretation more plausible. The fact that those lesions revealed a vastly overlapping genetic pattern with lobular invasive breast cancer as well as with well-differentiated or non-high-grade DCIS characterizes them as direct precursor lesions of at least lobular invasive breast cancer. This hypothesis is of considerable impact but has yet to be proven by extended follow-up studies. It is already obvious, however, that these molecular pathologic investigations will change the treatment modalities of LCIS considerably. In view of those results, the radically different treatment protocols for LCIS and well-differentiated DCIS seem at least questionable. Nevertheless, identical results concerning bilateral LCIS within one patient (25) also suggest the possibility that this typical growth pattern might be caused by a genetic mechanism, a widespread phenomenon in breast tissue.

■ Support for a related biologic and potentially clinical role of LCIS and subgroups of DCIS comes from clinicopathologic studies. Morphologically, the differential diagnosis of DCIS and LCIS might be very complicated and suggests a close relationship between the two lesions. From an epidemiologic point of view, it is of interest that in 15% to 25% of cases with DCIS, invasive lobular carcinoma is associated and vice versa. Moreover, the same percentage of patients diagnosed with LCIS will develop an invasive carcinoma of the ductal subtype over the next 15 to 20 years. The putative relationship between those preinvasive subtypes is nevertheless a matter of debate (25,56). So far, no direct comparison of DCIS and LCIS within the same patient has been performed using CGH. The close relationship between LCIS and well-differentiated DCIS has been mentioned before, but the hypothesis of a common genotype and different phenotypes has been supported by at least one study. Investigating rare

breast cancer cases with an intermediately differentiated DCIS component and associated LCIS within the same patient, a high or even complete genetic homology could be demonstrated. This would fit into the proposed cytogenetic and morphologically based progression model of invasive breast cancer and its ultimate precursor lesions (32). Therefore, we regard LCIS and well-differentiated DCIS as different phenotypes of a common genotype with the loss of E-cadherin expression as the major distinguishing hallmark in the differential diagnosis of LCIS and well-differentiated DCIS.

In summary, the introduction of CGH as a routine research tool has enabled new, exciting insights into the pathogenesis of in situ and invasive carcinomas of the breast and led to the proposal of a new morphology-based cytogenetic progression model of invasive breast cancer with the loss of 16q material as a major distinguishing feature, as shown in Figure 8.7. Further clinicopathologic studies are needed to show to what extent those chromosomal alterations will acquire clinical significance in terms of tumor recurrence and prognosis, as has been shown for invasive breast cancer (10). Based on the genetic results, this holds also true for LCIS and well-differentiated DCIS. The treatment modalities for these premalignant tumor entities might be altered along the lines of either paying greater attention to LCIS or using less aggressive treatment for well-differentiated DCIS.

We are left with a host of open questions that need to be explored in future research projects. CGH studies of DCIS

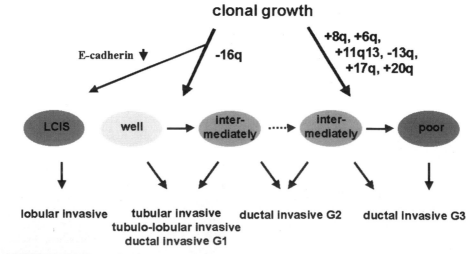

FIGURE 8.7. Proposal of an extended morphologically based cytogenetic progression model of in situ carcinomas of the breast and invasive breast cancer. The loss of 16q material represents an early chromosomal event in a subgroup of highly differentiated ductal carcinoma in situ (DCIS) and lobular carcinoma in situ (LCIS). Although the loss of the E-cadherin expression probably accounts for the typical morphology of LCIS, less is known about the factors responsible for the different phenotypes in well- and intermediately differentiated DCIS. In contrast, a subgroup of intermediately and poorly differentiated DCIS is characterized by many genetic alterations, some of which can be associated with typical morphologic characteristics. The step toward invasion is not reflected on a cytogenetic level; nevertheless, the previously mentioned phenotype-genotype correlation can also be detected in subgroups of invasive breast cancer.

could convincingly demonstrate the role of this lesion as the ultimate precursor of invasive breast cancer, thus requiring much medical attention. In contrast, little is known about lesions such as ductal hyperplasia of the usual type, atypical ductal hyperplasia, papillomas, radial scars, or scleradenosis, all associated with an increased risk of breast cancer. Our knowledge about breast carcinogenesis will definitely increase if we know at which step distinct genetic alterations occur in the course of breast cancer development.

Pilot studies of more than 40 benign proliferative breast lesions such as ductal hyperplasias of the usual type and papillomas revealed no evidence that unbalanced chromosomal alterations are present in these lesions (57). Given the assumption that ductal hyperplasia is a precursor lesion of DCIS, one might have expected at least some recurring genetic events in ductal hyperplasia. Therefore, the acquisition of unbalanced genetic alterations seems to reflect, if not cause, the transition from a hyperplastic lesion to an in situ carcinoma. Elucidating the underlying biologic cell disturbances that will ultimately result in uneven chromosomal distribution will open new horizons for breast cancer prevention.

No matter how fundamental the insights provided by CGH are, modern, high-resolution techniques such as microarray CGH and microarray expression analysis (58,59) will gradually replace conventional CGH and give a more detailed and individualized impression of in situ and invasive breast cancer.

REFERENCES

1. Seabright M. A rapid banding technique for human chromosomes. *Lancet* 1971;2:971–972.
2. Kallioniemi A, Kallioniemi OP, Sudar D, et al. Comparative genomic hybridization for molecular cytogenetic analysis of solid tumours. *Science* 1992;258:818–821.
3. du Manoir S, Speicher MR, Joos S, et al. Detection of complete and partial chromosome gains and losses by comparative genomic in situ hybridization. *Hum Genet* 1993;90:590–610.
4. Kallioniemi A, Kallioniemi OP, Piper J, et al. Detection and mapping of amplified DNA sequences in breast cancer by comparative genomic hybridization. *Proc Natl Acad Sci U S A* 1994;91:2156–2160.
5. Courjal F, Theillet C. Comparative genomic hybridization analysis of breast tumors with predetermined profiles of DNA amplification. *Cancer Res* 1997;57:4368–4377.
6. Muleris M, Almeida A, Gerbault SM, et al. Detection of DNA amplification in 17 primary breast carcinomas with homogeneously staining regions by a modified comparative genomic hybridization technique. *Genes Chromosomes Cancer* 1994;10:160–170.
7. Persson K, Pandis N, Mertens F, et al. Chromosomal aberrations in breast cancer: a comparison between cytogenetics and comparative genomic hybridization. *Genes Chromosomes Cancer* 1999;25:115–122.
8. Forozan F, Mahlamaki EH, Monni O, et al. Comparative genomic hybridization analysis of 38 breast cancer cell lines: a basis for interpreting complementary DNA microarray data. *Cancer Res* 2000;60:4519–4525.
9. Forozan F, Veldman R, Ammermann CW, et al. Molecular cytogenetic analysis of 11 new breast cancer cell lines. *Br J Cancer* 1999;81:1328–1334.
10. Isola JJ, Kallioniemi OP, Chu LW, et al. Genetic aberrations detected by comparative genomic hybridization predict outcome in node-negative breast cancer. *Am J Pathol* 1995;147:905–911.
11. Ried T, Just KE, Holtgreve GH, et al. Comparative genomic hybridization of formalin-fixed, paraffin-embedded breast tumors reveals different patterns of chromosomal gains and losses in fibroadenomas and diploid and aneuploid carcinomas. *Cancer Res* 1995;55:5415–5423.
12. Hermsen MAJA, Baak JP, Meijer GA, et al. Genetic analysis of 53 lymph node-negative breast carcinomas by CGH and relation to clinical, pathological, morphometric, and DNA cytometric prognostic factors. *J Pathol* 1998;186:356–362.
13. Loveday RL, Greenman J, Drew PJ, et al. Genetic changes associated with telomerase activity in breast cancer. *Int J Cancer* 1999;84:516–520.
14. Tirkkonen M, Johannsson O, Agnarsson BA, et al. Distinct somatic genetic changes associated with tumor progression in carriers of BRCA1 and BRCA2 germ-line mutations. *Cancer Res* 1997;57:1222–1227.
15. Tirkkonen M, Kainu T, Loman N, et al. Somatic genetic alterations in BRCA2-associated and sporadic male breast cancer. *Genes Chromosomes Cancer* 1999;24:56–61.
16. Tanner MM, Karhu RA, Nupponen NN, et al. Genetic aberrations in hypodiploid breast cancer: frequent loss of chromosome 4 and amplification of cyclin D1 oncogene. *Am J Pathol* 1998;153:191–199.
17. Nishizaki T, DeVries S, Chew K, et al. Genetic alterations in primary breast cancers and their metastases: direct comparison using modified comparative genomic hybridization. *Genes Chromosomes Cancer* 1997;19:267–272.
18. Kuukasjarvi T, Karhu R, Tanner M, et al. Genetic heterogeneity and clonal evolution underlying development of asynchronous metastasis in human breast cancer. *Cancer Res* 1997;57:1597–1604.
19. Nishizaki T, Chew K, Chu L, et al. Genetic alterations in lobular breast cancer by comparative genomic hybridization. *Int J Cancer* 1997;74:513–517.
20. Buerger H, Otterbach F, Simon R, et al. Different genetic pathways in the evolution of invasive breast cancer are associated with distinct morphological subtypes. *J Pathol* 1999;189:521–526.
21. Günther K, Merkelbach-Kruse S, Amo-Takyi BK, et al. Differences in genetic alterations between primary lobular and ductal breast cancers detected by comparative genomic hybridization. *J Pathol* 2001;193:40–47.
22. Tirkkonen M, Tanner M, Karhu R, et al. Molecular cytogenetics of primary breast cancer by CGH. *Genes Chromosomes Cancer* 1998;21:177–184.
23. Richard F, Pacyna GM, Schlegel H, et al. Patterns of chromosomal imbalances in invasive breast cancer. *Int J Cancer* 2000;89:305–310.
24. Schwendel A, Richard F, Langreck H, et al. Chromosome alterations in breast carcinomas: frequent involvement of DNA losses including chromosomes 4q and 21q. *Br J Cancer* 1998;78:806–811.
25. Lu YJ, Osin P, Lakhani SR, et al. Comparative genomic hybridization analysis of lobular carcinoma in situ and atypical lobular hyperplasia and potential roles for gains and losses of genetic material in breast neoplasia. *Cancer Res* 1998;58:4721–4727.
26. Roylance R, Gorman P, Harris W, et al. Comparative genomic hybridization of breast tumours stratified by histological grade reveals new insights into the biological progression of breast cancer. *Cancer Res* 1999;59:1433–1436.
27. Kuukasjarvi T, Tanner M, Pennanen S, et al. Genetic changes in

intraductal breast cancer detected by comparative genomic hybridization. *Am J Pathol* 1997;150:1465–1471.

28. James LA, Mitchell EL, Menasce L, et al. Comparative genomic hybridization of ductal carcinoma in situ of the breast: identification of regions of DNA amplification and deletion in common with invasive breast carcinoma. *Oncogene* 1997;14:1059–1065.

29. Buerger H, Otterbach F, Simon R, et al. Comparative genomic hybridization of ductal carcinoma in situ of the breast- evidence of multiple genetic pathways. *J Pathol* 1999;187:396–402.

30. Vos CB, Rosenberg C, Peterse JL, et al. Genetic alterations on chromosome 16 and 17 are important features of ductal carcinoma in situ of the breast and are associated with histologic type. *Br J Cancer* 2000;81:1410–1418.

31. Aubele M, Mattis A, Zitzelsberger H, et al. Extensive ductal carcinoma in situ with small foci of invasive ductal carcinoma: Evidence of genetic resemblance by CGH. *Int J Cancer* 2000;85:82–86.

32. Buerger H, Simon R, Schaefer KL, et al. Genetic relationship of lobular carcinoma *in situ*, ductal carcinoma *in situ* and associated invasive carcinoma of the breast. *Mol Pathol* 2000;53:118–121.

33. Aubele M, Cummings M, Mattis A, et al. Accumulation of chromosomal imbalances from intraductal proliferative lesions to adjacent in situ and invasive ductal breast cancer. *Diagn Mol Pathol* 2000;9:14–19.

34. Fujii H, Marsh C, Cairns P, et al. Genetic divergence in the clonal evolution of breast cancer. *Cancer Res* 1996;56:1493–1497.

35. Holland R, Peterse JL, Millis RR, et al. Ductal carcinoma in situ: a proposal for a new classification. *Semin Diagn Pathol* 1994;11:167–180.

36. Silverstein MJ, Poller DN, Waisman JR, et al. Prognostic classification of breast ductal carcinoma-in-situ. *Lancet* 1995;345:1154–1157.

37. Sloane JP, Amendoeira I, Apostolikas N, et al. Consistency achieved by 23 European pathologists in categorizing ductal carcinoma in situ of the breast using five classifications. European Commission Working Group on Breast Screening Pathology. *Hum Pathol* 1998;29:1056–1062.

38. Dupont WD, Page DL. Risk factors for breast cancer in women with proliferative breast disease. *J Natl Cancer Inst* 1981;312:146–151.

39. Viacava P, Naccarato A, Bevilacqua G. Different proliferative patterns characterize different preinvasive breast lesions. *J Pathol* 1999;188:245–251.

40. Mommers E, Poulin N, Sangulin J, et al. Nuclear cytometric changes in breast carcinogenesis. *J Pathol* 2001;193:33–39.

41. Mommers E, van Diest PJ, Leonhart AM, et al. Balance of apoptosis and proliferation in the progression of pre-invasive breast lesions. *Breast Cancer Res Treat* 1999;58:163–169.

42. O'Connell P, Pekkel V, Fuqua SA, et al. Analysis of loss of heterozygosity in 399 premalignant breast lesions at 15 genetic loci. *J Natl Cancer Inst* 1998;90:697–703.

43. Buerger H, Mommers E, Littmann R, et al. Correlation of morphologic and cytogenetic parameters of genetic instability with chromosomal alterations in in situ carcinomas of the breast. *Am J Clin Pathol* 2000;114:854–859.

44. Zafrani B, Leroyer A, Fourquet A. Mammographically detected ductal in situ carcinomas of the breast analyzed with a new classification. A study of 127 cases: correlation with estrogen and progesterone receptors, p53, and c-erB-2 proteins, and proliferative activity. *Semin Diagn Pathol* 1994;11:208–214.

45. Moore E, Magee H, Coyne J, et al. Widespread chromosomal abnormalities in high-grade ductal carcinoma in situ of the breast. Comparative genomic hybridization study of pure high-grade DCIS. *J Pathol* 1999;187:403–409.

46. Silverstein MJ, Craig PH, Lagios MD, et al. Developing a prognostic index for ductal carcinoma in situ of the breast. Are we there yet? [letter; comment]. *Cancer* 1996;78:1138–1140.

47. Waldman F, DeVries S, Chew K, et al. Chromosomal alterations in ductal carcinomas in situ and their in situ recurrences. *J Natl Cancer Inst* 2000;92:323–330.

48. Chuaqui RF, Zhuang Z, Emmert BM, et al. Analysis of loss of heterozygosity on chromosome 11q13 in atypical ductal hyperplasia and in situ carcinoma of the breast. *Am J Pathol* 1997;150:297–303.

49. O'Connell P, Fischbach K, Hilsenbeck SG, et al. Loss of heterozygosity at D14S62 and metastatic potential of breast cancer. *J Natl Cancer Inst* 1999;91:1391–1397.

50. Buerger H, Mommers E, Littmann R, et al. Ductal invasive G2 and G3 carcinomas of the breast are the end stages of at least two different lines of genetic evolution. *J Pathol* 2001;194:165–170.

51. Berx G, Cleton JA, Strumane K, et al. E-cadherin is inactivated in a majority of invasive human lobular breast cancers by truncation mutations throughout its extracellular domain. *Oncogene* 1996;13:1919–1925.

52. Berx G, Cleton JA, Nollet F, et al. E-cadherin is a tumour/invasion suppressor gene mutated in human lobular breast cancers. *EMBO J* 1995;14:6107–6115.

53. De-Leeuw WJ, Berx G, Vos CB, et al. Simultaneous loss of E-cadherin and catenins in invasive lobular breast cancer and lobular carcinoma in situ. *J Pathol* 1997;183:404–411.

54. Moll R, Mitze M, Frixen UH, et al. Differential loss of E-cadherin expression in infiltrating ductal and lobular breast carcinomas. *Am J Pathol* 1993;143:1731–1742.

55. Bankfalvi A, Terpe H-J, Breukelmann D, et al. Immunophenotypic and prognostic analysis of E-cadherin (E-Cad) and B-catenin (B-Cat) expression during breast carcinogenesis and tumour progression: a comparative study with CD44. *Histopathology* 1999;34:25–34.

56. Lakhani SR. The transition from hyperplasia to invasive carcinoma of the breast. *J Pathol* 1999;187:272–278.

57. Boecker W, Buerger H, Schmitz K, et al. Ductal epithelial proliferations of the breast: a histological continuum? Comparative genomic hybridization and high-molecular cytokeratin expression patterns. *J Pathol* 2001;195:415–421.

58. Pinkel D, Segraves R, Sudar D, et al. High resolution analysis of DNA copy number variation using comparative genomic hybridization to microarrays. *Nat Genet* 1998;20:207–211.

59. Albertson DG, Ylstra B, Segraves R, et al. Quantitative mapping of amplicon structure by array CGH identifies CYP24 as a candidate oncogene. *Nat Genet* 2000;25:144–146.

9

MODEL SYSTEMS FOR DUCTAL CARCINOMA IN SITU

NIGEL J. BUNDRED

Until the advent of screening mammography, ductal carcinoma in situ (DCIS) was an unusual diagnosis and treatment largely consisted of mastectomy. Earlier detection by mammography has led to up to 30% of breast cancers detected being in situ cancer (1,2). Greater use of breast-conserving surgery and interest in preventing breast cancer development by intervention with antiestrogens or other drugs have led to increasing interest in the mechanism underlying the development of ductal carcinoma in situ (3,4).

Although primary culture of human mammary epithelial cells (HMECs) is well documented (5,6), at present, culture of in situ or invasive cancer is difficult. HMECs are estrogen receptor (ER) negative and respond to epidermal growth factor and insulin-like growth factor with increased proliferation (5,6). In contrast, 10% to 15% of cells in the normal breast contain estrogen receptor, and 40% to 70% of DCIS express ER (7). At least 50% of DCIS lesions are ER negative, particularly grade III lesions. Thus, while ER positive DCIS growth might be expected to be under hormonal control, little is known about growth control of ER-DCIS.

To study the growth of early proliferative breast lesions, three groups of animal models have been developed over the last ten years:

(i) Transgenic mice models
(ii) Cell line xenograft models, and
(iii) Human DCIS xenograft models.

Our knowledge of DCIS has been enhanced by the use of molecular biology to study the changes seen in these models together with therapeutic manipulation, which allows us to study potential novel therapies.

TRANSGENIC MICE MODELS

The development of transgenic mice models has allowed understanding of the principles underlying transformation and cancer development in rodents (8,9).

In general, approximately 10% of transgenic mice that overexpress transforming growth factor-α (TGFα) develop alveolar hyperplasia and, eventually, unifocal tumor formation (9). Overexpression of CerbB2 oncogene/Neu protein in transgenic mice breast leads to hyperplasia and tumor formation in 35% of mice (10,11). Crossbreeding TGFα transgenic mice with Neu/CerbB2 mice leads to bitransgenic mice with a 95% multifocal tumor development by 5 months (10). Thus, expression of two genes in the type 1 tyrosine kinase growth factor family enhances tumor development. Likewise, bi-transgenic TGFα/Cmyc mice develop poorly differentiated tumors that produce lung metastases, while single transgenic mice for either gene have a low incidence of tumor formation. This suggests that TGFα, which pushes cells into the cell cycle and increases proliferation, leads to cancer formation when combined with other genetic alterations (10).

Instead of overexpressing genes in all body organs, mammary-targeted overexpression can be used; a mouse mammary tumor virus (MMTV) or whey acidic protein (WAP) promoter is commonly used to direct gene expression to the mammary gland (8,9). These promoters are dependent on the mice becoming pregnant, in contrast to the situation in humans where pregnancy is protective. An alternative promoter is the prostate steroid binding protein (PSBP), which has been used to direct SV40 large T-antigen to the prostate and breast epithelium (8).

Targeting of SV40 T-antigen to the mammary epithelium using either BSPB (8) or WAP (12) promotion leads to tumorigenesis in 100% of mice by 8 to 9 months. These mice have either p53 or retinoblastoma protein (or both) inactivated in their mammary epithelium, and develop proliferative breast disease, followed by in situ breast cancer, and eventually invasive disease. These models demonstrate that multistep progression is essential for mammary tumor progression. In the stage of proliferative disease/DCIS, amplification of kiRas, mRNA, and protein is associated with increased mitogen-activated protein kinase (MAPK) activity (8,12), and mice lacking one allele of kiRas have retarded tumor development (8). The process of tumor development may not occur synchronously in each breast, so each mouse may harbor an invasive cancer in one of its mammary glands while other glands harbor DCIS or atypical hyperplasia.

Loss of apoptosis also appears to be important in tumor development in these mice models. As in humans, a low apoptotic and proliferative rate is present in the epithelium of normal breast. As in the human breast, the development of ductal carcinoma in situ is associated with a rise in epithelial proliferation and apoptosis (from 1% to 13% apoptotic index) (8). Subsequent development of invasive tumors is associated with loss of apoptosis but increased epithelial proliferation continues. Increased apoptosis in the DCIS stage of this model is associated with elevated expression of bax, a pro-apoptotic gene. Mice transgenically lacking bax develop invasive tumors significantly earlier (8). These T-antigen expressing transgenic mice provide a useful model to assess chemoprevention agents; both 9cis retinoic acid and difluoromethylornithine have already been shown to reduce the incidence of multifocality of tumor growth in these models (8,12).

XENOGRAFT MODELS

The first described xenograft model originated at the Michigan Cancer Foundation from a series of cell lines derived from fibrocystic disease epithelium. The Human MCF10 cell line does not form tumors in nude mice, but when transfected with mutated H ras gene, tumors develop after injection into immunosuppressed mice with a latency period of approximately 1 year (13). Several of these tumors exhibit morphologic similarity reminiscent of intraduct carcinoma in situ. The problem with the model lies in the long latency period and the unpredictability of development of DCIS or invasive malignancy; but the longitudinal nature of the model means that it can be used to study possible chemoprevention agents.

HUMAN DUCTAL CARCINOMA IN SITU XENOGRAFT MODEL

The use of normal breast xenografts implanted into athymic nude mice demonstrated that over 95% could be retrieved and study made of the factors inducing epithelial proliferation. Estrogen increased epithelial proliferation and induced progesterone receptor expression, whereas progesterone had no effect (14). This encouraged us to believe we would be able to do the same experiments with human DCIS tissue. We subsequently implanted 2 × 1 × 1 mm xenografts of breast tissue taken from microcalcification areas associated with ductal carcinoma in situ in women undergoing mastectomy (15). Approximately one-third of the xenografts

taken from mammographic microcalcification areas containing histologically verified ductal carcinoma in situ prior to implantation and subsequently 33% of all xenografts retrieved from the animals contained foci of DCIS, and retrieval of DCIS was 92% of that expected (range 33% to 203%). The majority (70%) of DCIS identified by mammographic microcalcification was estrogen receptor–negative and expressed CerbB2 oncoprotein and epidermal growth factor receptor (EGFR).

Initial experiments demonstrated that viable xenografts containing DCIS could be obtained with DCIS survival 83% at 56 days in the mice. No changes in architecture of the DCIS were seen. To determine the role of estrogen in DCIS proliferation and survival, half of the mice in each experiment had an estradiol implant, which gave a level of estradiol in the mice of 1,400 pmol/L compared with levels of 125 pmol/L in unsupplemented mice. In estrogen receptor–positive DCIS, a significant increase in epithelial proliferation and apoptosis was seen in xenografts stimulated by estrogen, whereas no change in proliferation or apoptosis was seen in estrogen receptor–negative DCIS (Fig. 9.1). Subsequently, we used the pure antiestrogen Faslodex (16) to test whether antiestrogens could inhibit epithelial proliferation and induce apoptosis.

STUDIES WITH ANTIESTROGEN THERAPY

ER-negative DCIS had a significantly elevated proliferation rate of 20.6% (95% CI, 18.5% to 22.9%) compared with that of ER-positive DCIS at 3.1% (95% CI, 2.2% to 4.2%, $p < 0.001$) (16). Similarly, increased apoptosis was seen in ER-negative DCIS lesions, at 1.45% (95% CI, 1.21% to 1.77%) compared with 0.32% (95% CI, 0.22% to 0.45%, $p < 0.01$) in ER-positive DCIS. ER-positive DCIS showed a rise in epithelial proliferation and apoptosis as expected after 14 days of estrogen therapy, whereas ER-positive DCIS xenografts exposed to the antiestrogen Faslodex showed a rise in apoptosis but no significant change in proliferation (16) (Fig. 9.2). The antiestrogen effects of Faslodex on ER-positive DCIS xenografts were confirmed by immunohistochemical assessment of progesterone receptor in the xenografts. Compared with controls, Faslodex significantly inhibited expression of the progesterone receptor (an estrogen-regulated protein) in the ER-positive DCIS treated with the dose. Progesterone receptor protein expression was 40% (95% CI, 32% to 48%) in day-0 ER-positive xenografts, and 47% (95% CI, 42% to 52%) after 28 days of estrogen treatment, but fell to 18% (17.4% to 18.2%, $p < 0.001$) after treatment with Faslodex for 28 days (16). It was thus apparent that ER-positive DCIS proliferates under hormonal influences and responds to antiestrogen therapy, whereas ER-negative DCIS is estrogen independent.

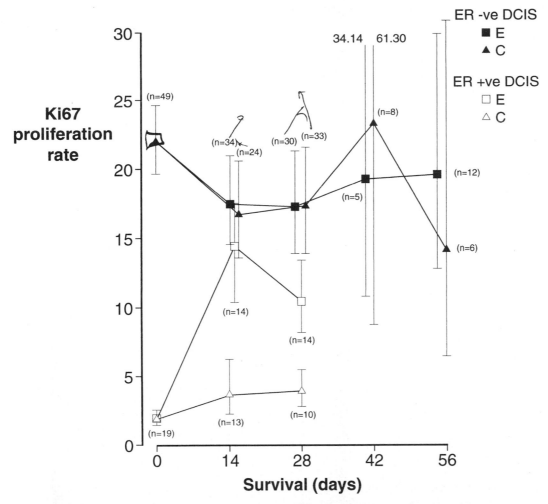

FIGURE 9.1. Epithelial proliferation in estrogen receptor (ER)-negative comedo ductal carcinoma in situ (DCIS) *(black squares)* and ER-positive noncomedo DCIS *(open squares)*. Proliferation was assessed by the immunohistochemical staining of Ki67, and the data are presented as mean values with 95% confidence intervals. Mice implanted with either comedo or noncomedo DCIS were given estrogen *(E)* or control *(C)* implants. Foci of DCIS were identified histologically in 302 (22%) of 1,355 day-0 grants. At day 0, Ki67 proliferation rates were significantly higher in the 10 ER-negative DCIS cases (n=49 grafts) compared with the three ER-positive DCIS cases (n=19 grafts). No change in epithelial proliferation in the ER-negative DCIS was seen with time or with estrogen supplementation. In contrast, DCIS implanted from three cases of ER-positive DCIS was significantly stimulated to proliferate by estrogen supplementation, and showed increased proliferation rates at days 14 and 28. In the ER-positive DCIS implanted into control mice, a significant elevation of proliferation rate occurred, but the proliferation rate in control-treated mice was significantly lower at both days 14 and 28 than in the estrogen-treated mice. From Holland *J Natl Cancer Inst*, with permission.

RELEVANCE OF DUCTAL CARCINOMA IN SITU MODEL FINDINGS TO THE CLINICAL SITUATION

Two studies have randomized patients to adjuvant tamoxifen or placebo after surgical therapy. The NSABP-24 study, which randomized women after breast-conserving surgery and radiotherapy, demonstrated a 40% reduction in breast cancer events on tamoxifen. A reduced incidence of ipsilateral invasive cancer but no reduction in ipsilateral DCIS was seen in the trial. Additionally, a halving of contralateral breast cancer was seen. Approximately one-third of the women in this trial were under 50 years of age, and the majority of tamoxifen's benefit was found in this age group (20).

In the UK DCIS trial, which consisted predominantly (93%) of women aged 50 or over, the four-way randomization was with radiotherapy and tamoxifen or either intervention as possible options. In this trial, tamoxifen had no significant benefit if radiotherapy was given, although a small nonsignificant benefit was seen from tamoxifen therapy in the absence of radiotherapy (W. D. George, personal

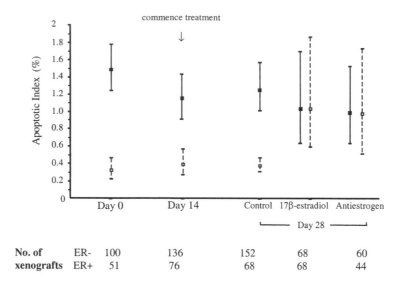

| No. of | ER- | 100 | 136 | 152 | 68 | 60 |
| xenografts | ER+ | 51 | 76 | 68 | 68 | 44 |

FIGURE 9.2. Apoptotic cell death in estrogen receptor (ER)-negative *(solid symbols, solid line)* and ER-positive *(open symbols, dotted line)* ductal carcinoma in situ (DCIS). Apoptosis was assessed by morphologic assessment of H&E sections of xenografts retrieved from mice exposed to 17β-estrodiol, antiestrogen, or a control vehicle oil. An apoptotic index was calculated by noting the number of cells showing morphologic evidence of apoptotic cell death (see Kerr et al., 1994) as a percentage of total number of cells counted in each retrieved xenograft containing DCIS. Results are presented as geometric mean values with their 95% confidence intervals. The number of xenografts used for each time point is presented adjacent to each error bar. At day 0, ER-negative DCIS displays a much higher apoptotic index than ER-positive DCIS. In both subtypes, the apoptotic index does not change significantly in the 14-day pretreatment period. Treatment commenced on day 14. Hormonal manipulation of ER-negative DCIS had no effect on apoptotic cell death compared with control or pretreatment xenografts. ER-positive DCIS displayed a significant rise in cell death when exposed to 17β-estradiol or antiestrogen therapy. From *Cancer Res* 2000:60:4284–4288, with permission.

communication, 2001). Thus, the value of adjuvant tamoxifen in women over 50 years of age treated for DCIS is unclear, although it would appear to be beneficial in younger women.

The mechanism by which tamoxifen reduces recurrent ipsilateral invasive cancer in younger women may relate to its effects preventing cancer in the breast by inhibiting the effect of endogenous estrogen on the breast rather than direct effects on DCIS.

GROWTH FACTOR INFLUENCES IN ESTROGEN RECEPTOR–NEGATIVE DUCTAL CARCINOMA IN SITU

Estrogen receptor–negative DCIS has been shown to express type 1 tyrosine kinase growth factor receptors of the Cerb family (17–21). Epidermal growth factor receptor (EGFR/CerbB1) and CerbB2 both have an extra cellular receptor–binding domain, and on attachment of ligands to these receptors, the receptors dimerize with either another similar receptor (homodimerization) or with another member of the same receptor family (heterodimerization) (22). No known ligand for CerbB2 has yet been identified. Dimerization of receptors results in tyrosine kinase autophosphorylation, which then activates a number of potential different intracellular signaling pathways (Fig. 9.3), including RAS protein and the MAPK signaling pathways that lead to cell proliferation and apoptosis prevention (23–27).

Epidermal growth factor receptor is a 170 kd transmembrane glycoprotein that is found on many epithelial cells (21). It is activated by at least six ligands, including EGF, transforming growth factor-α (TGFα), and amphiregulin (21–24). Overexpression of EGFR in mammary epithelium is associated with increased development of mammary tumors (10–25). Recent studies on the normal breast epithelium indicates that only 5% to 10% of cells express steroid hormone receptors, and the fraction of cells that divide and undergo mitosis are not steroid hormone receptor–positive (7). Since human primary mammary epithelial cell culture produces ER-negative cells that respond to epidermal growth factor and insulin-like growth factor (IGF), it is likely that growth in the breast is largely controlled by stimulation of these two growth factor receptors (5,6). Stimulation of the IGF receptor leads to release of TGFα from the cell, which transactivates the EGFR in the same cell in an autocrine manner (28). Thus, accumulating evidence demonstrates that the EGFR is the main receptor pathway associated with epithelial proliferation in the human breast (21). CerbB2 (also called Her2 and Neu) is a 185 kd transmembrane tyrosine kinase with considerable homology to EGFR, although

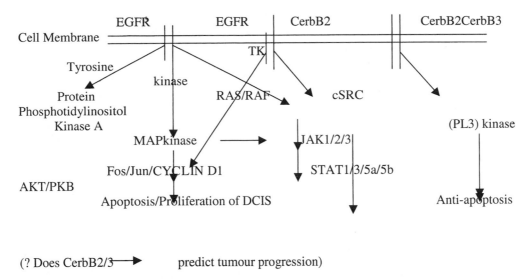

FIGURE 9.3. Type 1 tyrosine kinase receptor signaling. Epidermal growth factor receptor, CerbB2, CerbB3, and CerbB4 can all heterodimerize to produce cell growth or apoptosis signals.

a ligand for CerbB2 has not been identified. Instead, the presence of CerbB2 may allow more frequent formation of CerbB1 and CerbB2 heterodimers with augmentation of EGFR cell surface signaling into RAS-MAPK pathways, leading to increased proliferation (22–26).

Heterodimerization of CerbB2 with CerbB3 is also a possible explanation. Muller et al. (10,11) have studied tumors developing in mouse mammary glands from mice containing activated CerbB2 oncogenes. Tumor progression in these mice was associated with elevated levels of phosphorylated CerbB2 and CerbB3. Additionally, a series of primary breast tumors studied by the same group found frequent coexpression of transcripts for both CerbB2 and CerbB3 (11).

Thus, metastasis may result from CerbB2/CerbB3 heterodimers, although the low expression of CerbB2 in normal breast suggests development of DCIS must involve CerbB1/EGFR rather than CerbB2 (21).

Several investigators have reported a relationship between overexpression (amplification) of CerbB2 or expression of EGFR and a poor prognosis in women with breast cancer (24).

CerbB2 antibody therapy (Herceptin) has been shown to produce tumor responses in women with metastatic breast cancer (29), and tyrosine kinase inhibitors of the EGFR inhibit proliferation and/or induce apoptosis *in vitro* and *in vivo* in breast, ovary, lung, colon, and gastric cell lines (30–31).

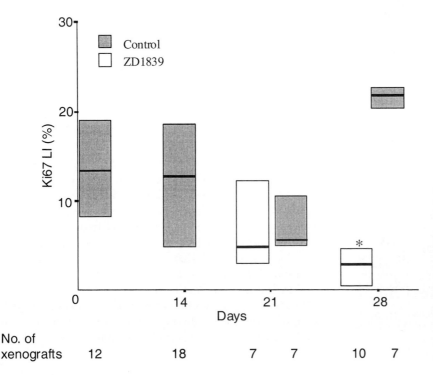

| No. of xenografts | 12 | 18 | 7 | 7 | 10 | 7 |

FIGURE 9.4. ZD1839 or vehicle was given from day 14 onward. Values for days 0 and 14 are from untreated mice. A significant decrease in proliferation (Ki67 LI) in the ZD1839 group was seen following 14 days of treatment (day 28, $p <$ 0.01 versus control, Mann-Whitney test). Numbers in parentheses represent the number of observations seen for that particular time point and for that group. Median values are shown as thick horizontal lines, boxes represent interquartile range. From Chan KC, Gandhi A, Slamon DJ, et al. Blockade of growth factor receptors in ductal carcinoma in situ inhibition epithelial proliferation. *Br J Surg* 2001;88:412–418, with permission.

Therefore, we then studied the effect of CerbB2 monoclonal antibody therapy and EGFR tyrosine kinase inhibition on epithelial proliferation and apoptosis in DCIS.

BLOCKADE OF GROWTH FACTOR RECEPTORS IN DUCTAL CARCINOMA IN SITU INHIBITS EPITHELIAL PROLIFERATION

Using antibodies to CerbB2 and EGFR, we studied expression in DCIS of varying grades. All DCIS specimens expressed epidermal growth factor receptor (EGFR), and 70% of DCIS studied were CerbB2-positive (32) (Fig. 9.5).

We therefore studied the effect of 4D5 monoclonal antibody directed against an extracellular domain of CerbB2. Positive control experiments with SKOV3 ovarian cancer cells implanted into athymic nude mice and allowed to form tumors were performed, and this demonstrated significant tumor growth inhibition with 4D5 monoclonal antibody injected intraperitoneally (32). In seven DCIS experiments using 4D5 monoclonal antibody, five cases were immunohistochemically CerbB2-positive, and all seven were estrogen receptor–negative. After 28 days treatment of DCIS with anti-CerbB2 monoclonal antibody, the LI was 24.5

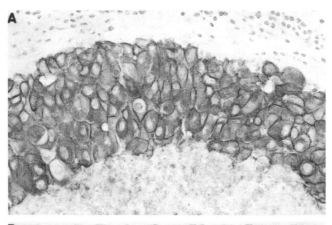

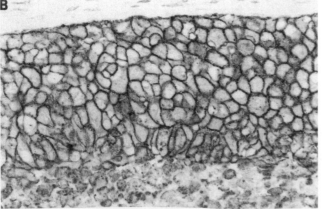

FIGURE 9.5. Photomicrographs of sections of ductal carcinoma in situ stained immunohistochemically for **(A)** CerbB2 membrane receptor and **(B)** epidermal growth factor receptor.

(IQR 11.6 to 36.8) compared with 19.9 (15.0 to 35.2) in control patients (32). No effect on epithelial proliferation or apoptosis was seen with 4D5 CerbB2 monoclonal antibody in DCIS xenografts (32). The lack of response may relate to the use of large monoclonal antibodies (such as 4D5), since we have previously shown that large molecules do not easily penetrate the DCIS basement membrane (15). Alternatively, as suggested by others, CerbB2 oncoprotein may not be the main receptor driving epithelial proliferation in DCIS (17) (Fig. 9.4).

We then used a novel epidermal growth factor tyrosine kinase inhibitor (Iressa) that selectively blocks the tyrosine kinase of the EGFR at an IC_{50} of 0.05 μM (compared with inhibition of CerbB2 at 1.2 to 3.7 μM and KDR at 3.7 to 37 μM). All other kinase assays showed no inhibition with Iressa (30). Out of 13 DCIS experiments, the majority (11) contained EGFR-positive DCIS (10 were also CerbB2-positive), while two were EGFR-negative by immunohistochemical staining.

Statistical analysis was made with nesting of samples within patients using appropriate repeated measures analysis of variance models. Comparisons between Iressa and control samples were made within patients. Geometric mean LI and AI was higher in ER-negative/EGFR-positive DCIS than ER-positive/EGFR-positive DCIS. A significant fall in proliferation was seen in Iressa-treated DCIS compared with controls at days 21, 28, and 42, with a geometric mean proliferation at day 42 of 11.0% (IQR 10.8 to11.8) versus 13.1% (IQR 12.0 to 14.8, $p = 0.01$) in the controls. Apoptotic index rose at day 21, but fell back to control levels thereafter.

Additionally, compared with controls, expression of autophosphorylated activated EGFR and MAPK levels were significantly inhibited in Iressa-treated DCIS when assessed using immunohistochemistry.

Clearly, EGFR inhibition lowers proliferation in DCIS, although a clear dose-response interaction was seen, with higher doses being more effective ($p < 0.0035$), indicating part of the action may occur via inhibition of CerbB2 autophosphorylation (EGFR-CerbB2 heterodimerization activating CerbB2 Tyrosine Kinase intracellularly). An alternative explanation is that whereas levels of EGF, TGF, and the other related ligands that stimulate EGFR are low in normal breast, an increased expression of EGF-like ligands are seen in DCIS and invasive cancer, which compete with Iressa for receptor binding. Despite the fact that EGFR is expressed in many tissues, no toxic signs were seen in the mice treated. In phase I and II clinical trials of Iressa, the only side effects frequently seen have been a low-grade acne and mild diarrhea in 10% of cases, both of which settled on cessation of therapy.

The finding of a correlation between MAPK expression and epithelial proliferation rate indicates that MAPK signaling is important in mediating cell proliferation in DCIS. It implies that therapeutic agents that inhibit the EGFR →

RAS → MAPK pathway will reduce proliferation in DCIS and ER-negative invasive tumors.

EFFECTS OF EPIDERMAL GROWTH FACTOR RECEPTOR INHIBITION ON NORMAL BREAST EPITHELIUM

An additional finding was the marked inhibition of epithelial proliferation in normal breast tissue in the presence or absence of estrogen.

Increased apoptosis was also seen in the normal breast epithelium after 7 days of therapy. This finding underscores the importance of the epidermal growth factor receptor in controlling proliferation in the breast, and indicates the potential for chemoprevention of breast cancer with these novel agents.

CONCLUSION

The expression and function of EGFR in normal breast and DCIS indicates that the major growth-modulating receptor in murine and human breast is the EGFR. Inhibition of the EGFR in xenograft models inhibits epithelial proliferation. Indeed, Robertson et al. (17) quantitated EGFR and CerbB2 in normal breast and breast cancer, and found that all normal breast tissue expressed EGFR and that expression of EGFR in tumors correlated directly with bromodeoxyuridine labeling index (a surrogate measure of epithelial proliferation). Gompel et al. (21) also found wide expression of EGFR in normal breast tissue, whereas CerbB2 was rarely present. Although EGFR is down-regulated in the majority of invasive breast cancers and CerbB2 is overexpressed in only 30% invasive cancers, both EGFR and CerbB2 are expressed in estrogen receptor–negative DCIS, and EGFR is expressed in the majority of estrogen receptor–positive DCIS. Evidence supports interaction of EGFR and CerbB2 in the formation of heterodimers facilitating receptor signaling, and the presence of increased TGFα/EGF and other ligands in DCIS combined with expression of both receptors explains the markedly increased proliferation and apoptosis seen in ER-negative DCIS.

The preclinical studies described on human DCIS xenografted into nude mice suggest a potential role for novel agents that inhibit intracellular signal transduction pathways. EGFR tyrosine kinase inhibitors, RAS farnesylation transferase inhibitors, and MAPK inhibitors may all potentially be active in DCIS.

Response of DCIS to these novel agents needs to be evaluated in phase III clinical trials after diagnostic biopsy of DCIS by wide bore needle, accompanied by study of the effect of the agent on DCIS proliferation and apoptosis against placebo therapy during the period between diagnosis and surgical treatment. This allows drug efficacy to be demonstrated in a short-term study, prior to testing it in a long-term adjuvant study. Alternatively, such drugs could be used in longer-term studies as chemopreventative agents in women with DCIS or LCIS.

We have reached a new exciting phase in our understanding of DCIS growth, and the next decade will potentially see major advances in our understanding of breast carcinogenesis and the prevention of DCIS progressing to invasive cancer.

REFERENCES

1. National Center for Health Statistics. See cancer statistics review, 1973–1995 1998; Bethesda, MD: US National Cancer Institute, 1998.
2. Ernster VL, Barclay J, Kerlikowske K, et al. Incidence of and treatment for ductal carcinoma in situ of the breast. *JAMA* 1996;275:913–918.
3. Fisher B, Costantino JP, Wickerham DL, et al. Tamoxifen for prevention of breast cancer: report of the National Surgical Adjuvant Breast and Bowel Project P-1 Study. *J Natl Cancer Inst* 1998;90:1371–1388.
4. Ettinger B, Black DM, Mitlak BH, et al. Reduction of vertebral fracture risk in postmenopausal women with osteoporosis treated with raloxifene: results from a 3-year randomized clinical trial. Multiple Outcomes of Raloxifene Evaluation (MORE) Investigators. *JAMA* 1999;282:637–645.
5. Price P, Sinnett HD, Gusterson B, et al. Duct carcinoma in situ: predictors of local recurrence and progression in patients treated by surgery alone. *Br J Cancer* 1990;61:869–872.
6. Silverstein MJ. Ductal carcinoma in situ of the breast. *BMJ* 1998;317:734–739.
7. Clarke RB, Howell A, Potten CS, et al. Dissociation between steroid receptor expression and cell proliferation in the human breast. *Cancer Res* 1997;57(22):4987–4991.
8. Green JE, Shibata MA, Yoshidome K, et al. The C3(1)/SV40 T-antigen transgenic mouse model of mammary cancer: ductal epithelial cell targeting with multistage progression to carcinoma. *Oncogene* 2000;19:1020–1027.
9. Coffey RJ, Meise KS, Matsui Y, et al. Acceleration of mammary neoplasia in transforming growth factor and transgenic mice by 7,12 Dimethylbentanthiacene. *Cancer Res* 1994;54:1678–1683.
10. Dankort DL, Muller WJ. Signal transduction in mammary tumorigenesis: a transgenic prospective. *Oncogene* 2000;19:1038–1044.
11. Siegel PM, Ryan ED, Cardiff RD, et al. Elevated expression of activated forms of Neu/erbB2 and erbB3 are involved in the induction of mammary tumors in transgenic mice. *EMBO J* 1999;18:2149–2164.
12. Schultze-Garg C, Kohler J, Goeht A, et al. A transgenic mouse model for the ductal carcinoma in situ (DCIS) of the mammary gland. *Oncogene* 2000;19:1028–1037.
13. Miller FR, Soule HD, Tait L, et al. Xenograft model of progressive human proliferative breast disease. *J Natl Cancer Inst* 1993;85:1725–1732.
14. Laidlaw IJ, Clarke RB, Howell A, et al. The proliferation of normal human breast tissue implanted into athymic nude mice is stimulated by estrogen but not by progesterone. *Endocrinology* 1995;136:164–171.
15. Holland PA, Knox WF, Potten CS, et al. Assessment of hormone dependence of comedo ductal carcinoma in situ of the breast. *J Natl Cancer Inst* 1997;89:1059–1065.

16. Gandhi A, Holland PA, Knox WF, et al. Effects of a pure anti-estrogen on apoptosis and proliferation within human breast ductal carcinoma in situ. *Cancer Res* 2000;60:4284–4288.
17. Robertson KW, Reeves JR, Smith G, et al. Quantitative estimation of epidermal growth factor receptor and CerbB-2 in human breast cancer. *Cancer Res* 1996;56:3823–3830.
18. Pavelic ZP, Pavelic L, Lower EE, et al. Cmyc, CerbB-2, and Ki-67 expression in normal breast tissue and in invasive and noninvasive breast carcinoma. *Cancer Res* 1992;52:2597–2602.
19. Hanna W, Kahn HJ, Andrulis I, et al. Distribution and patterns of staining of Neu oncogene product in benign and malignant breast diseases. *Mod Pathol* 1990;3:455–461.
20. Fisher B, Dignam J, Wolmak N, et al. Tamoxifen in treatment of intraduct breast cancer. National Surgical Adjuvant Breast and Bowel Project B24 randomised controlled trial. Lancet 1999; 353:1993–2000.
21. Gompel A, Martin A, Simon P, et al. Epidermal growth factor receptor and CerbB2 expression in normal breast tissue during the menstrual cycle. *Breast Cancer Res Treat* 1996;38:227–235.
22. Wells A. EGF receptor. *Int J Biochem Cell Biol* 1999;31:637–643.
23. Ullrich A, Schlessinger J. Signal transduction by receptors with tyrosine kinase activity. *Cell* 1990;61:203–212.
24. Saloman DS, Brandt R, Ciardiello F, et al. Epidermal growth factor-related peptides and their receptors in human malignancies. *Crit Rev Oncol Hematol* 1995;19:183–232.
25. Muthuswamy SK, Siegal PM, Dankort DL, et al. Mammary tumors expressing the Neu protooncogene possess elevated c-src tyrosine kinase activity. *Mol Cell Biol* 1994;14:739.
26. Dougall WC, Qian X, Greene MI. Interaction of the Neu/p185 and EGF receptor tyrosine kinases: implications for cellular transformation and tumor therapy. *J Cell Biochem* 1993;53:61–73.
27. Baselga J, Mendelsohn J. Type I receptor tyrosine kinases as targets for therapy in breast cancer. *J Mammary Gland Biol Neoplasia* 1997;2:165–174.
28. Roudabush FL, Pierce KL, Maudsley S, et al. Transactivation of the EGFR receptor mediates IGF-1 stimulated Shc phosphorylation and erk1/2 activation in Cos-7 cells. *J Biol Chem* 2000;275: 22583–22589.
29. Cobleigh MA, Vogel CL, Tripathy D, et al. Multinational study of the efficacy and safety of humanized anti-Her2 monoclonal antibody in women who have Her2-overexpressing metastatic breast cancer. *J Clin Oncol* 1999,17:2639–2648.
30. Baselga J, Ranson M, Averbuch S. A pharmacokinetic/pharmacodynamic trial of ZD1839 (Iressa), a novel oral EGFR tyrosine kinase inhibitor, in patients with 5 selected tumor types (a phase I/II trial of continuous once daily treatment). *Clin Cancer Res* 1999;5:3735S,abs29.
31. Woodburn JR, Morris CQ, Kelly H, et al. EGF receptor tyrosine kinase inhibitors as anti-cancer agents–preclinical and early clinical profile of ZD1839. *Cell Mol Biol Lett* 1998;3:348–349.
32. Chan KC, Gandhi A, Slamon DJ, et al. Blockade of growth factor receptors in ductal carcinoma in situ inhibition epithelial proliferation. *Br J Surg* 2001;88:412–418.

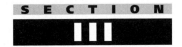

DETECTION AND EVALUATION

10

MAMMOGRAPHIC APPEARANCES OF IN SITU CARCINOMAS

LÁSZÓ TABÁR
ADEL GAD
WARD C. PARSONS
DAVID B. NEELAND

The term ductal carcinoma in situ (DCIS) is a convenient, simplified description of many different breast malignancies with one major common characteristic: proliferating cells confined by an intact basement membrane. "Recent studies have clearly suggested that DCIS is not a single disease. Rather, this term encompasses a diverse group of lesions that differ with regard to their clinical presentation from mammographic features, extent and distribution within the breast, histologic characteristics, and biologic markers" (1).

Since the mammographic image is a representation of the underlying histology, it is understandable that the mammographic images of the different diseases that we call DCIS can vary substantially (Fig. 10.1).

Rather than simplifying the histologic reporting of these different diseases by using the generic term ductal carcinoma in situ (DCIS, intraductal carcinoma, noninvasive breast cancer, etc.), "we advocate the consistent histopathologic reporting of DCIS by subtypes" (2).

HISTOLOGIC APPEARANCE

1. *Nuclear grade* is a cytologic evaluation of the nuclear features (outline, chromatin distribution, presence or absence of mitoses) of tumor nuclei compared with the nuclei of normal cells. According to Lagios (3), this will distinguish high nuclear grade, intermediate nuclear grade, and low nuclear grade (Fig. 10.2).
2. The most common *growth patterns or architecture of the malignant cells* are solid, micropapillary, and cribriform or any combination of these (Fig. 10.3).
3. The *presence or absence of necrosis* in in situ carcinomas is an important histologic feature (Fig. 10.4).
4. The *presence of calcifications* in in situ carcinomas makes the mammographic detection possible, and the *type of calcifications* helps in the preoperative differential diagnosis (4,5,6,7,8,9) (Fig. 10.5).

CLINICAL PRESENTATIONS AND BIOLOGIC BEHAVIOR

"The different histologic subtypes of DCIS have different biologic behavior" (2). "There is substantial evidence that the comedo or high-grade type of DCIS has great and relatively immediate malignant potential, whereas the low-grade, noncomedo type of DCIS is a precursor lesion with prolonged clinical evolution and lesser commitment to invasion" (12).

MAMMOGRAPHIC APPEARANCE

There is a significant positive correlation between the mammographic appearance and histologic finding.

Between 1977 and 1994, 207 consecutive cases of in situ "ductal" carcinoma were diagnosed at Falun Central Hospital, Sweden. Of these cases, 198 (95%) had abnormalities on the mammogram. Figure 10.6 summarizes the mammographic appearances and their histologic correlation. Of these 198 cases, 88 (44%) had the histologic features that correspond to high nuclear grade cancer in situ (3), or poorly differentiated (14), or Van Nuys group three (15). The remaining 110 cases (56%) corresponded to the combined intermediate and low nuclear grade (3), or moderately and well differentiated (14), or Van Nuys groups two and one (15).

The most valuable mammographic finding in detecting cases in group A was the presence of microcalcifications (85%). The remaining 15% presented as asymmetric density with architectural distortion.

While microcalcifications were also the dominant finding in group B (69%), demonstrating them required meticulous mammographic workup, including microfocus magnification. The detection of the remaining 31% required additional diagnostic tools such as ductography, ultrasound examination, etc.

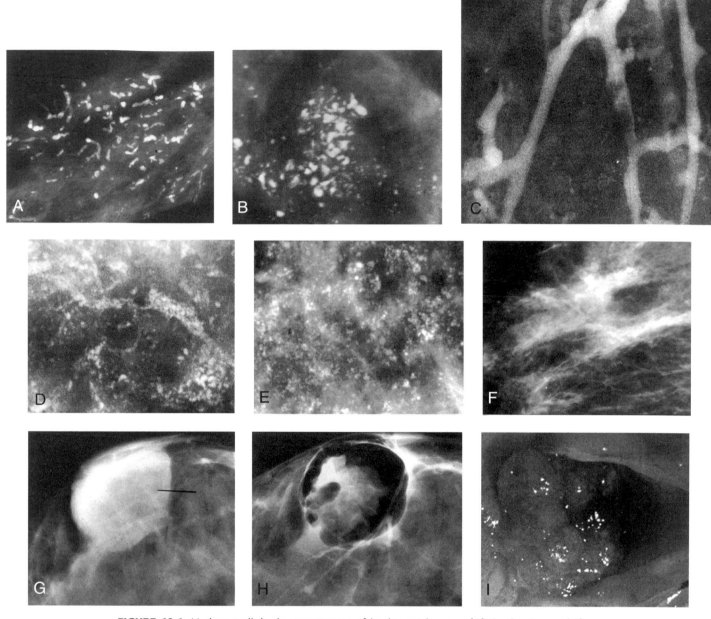

FIGURE 10.1. Various radiologic appearances of in situ carcinomas. **(A)** Casting-type calcifications. **(B)** Crushed stone–like calcifications. **(C)** Galactogram with multiple filling defects. **(D)** Dotted casting-type calcifications. **(E)** Powderish calcifications. **(F)** Asymmetric density with architectural distortion. **(G–I)** Mammogram, pneumocystogram, and operative specimen of a dominant mass.

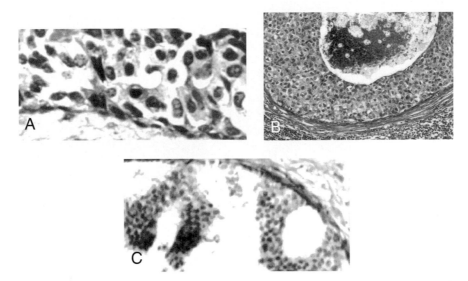

FIGURE 10.2. **A:** High nuclear grade. **(B)** Intermediate nuclear grade. **(C)** Low nuclear grade.

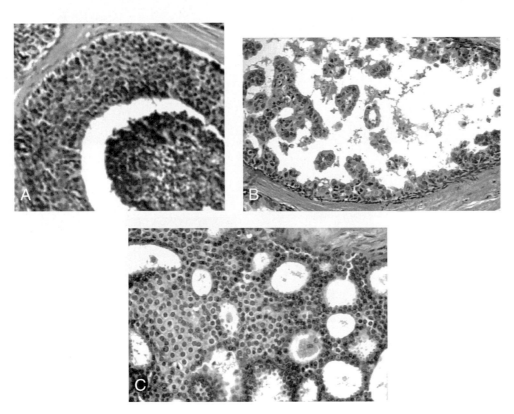

FIGURE 10.3. **A:** Solid cell proliferation. **(B)** Micropapillary growth pattern. **(C)** Cribriform pattern.

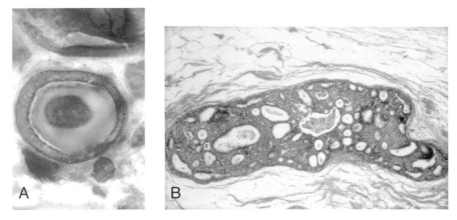

FIGURE 10.4. A: Necrosis present. **(B)** Necrosis absent.

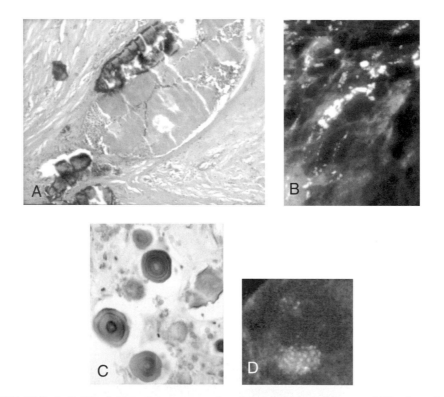

FIGURE 10.5. A–B: Histology and mammography of dystrophic, amorphous calcifications. **(C–D)** Histology and mammography of psammoma body–like, onion ring–like calcifications.

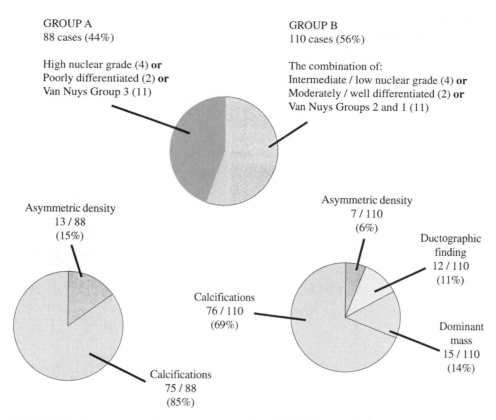

GROUP A
88 cases (44%)

High nuclear grade (4) **or**
Poorly differentiated (2) **or**
Van Nuys Group 3 (11)

GROUP B
110 cases (56%)

The combination of:
Intermediate / low nuclear grade (4) **or**
Moderately / well differentiated (2) **or**
Van Nuys Groups 2 and 1 (11)

Asymmetric density
13 / 88
(15%)

Calcifications
75 / 88
(85%)

Asymmetric density
7 / 110
(6%)

Ductographic
finding
12 / 110
(11%)

Calcifications
76 / 110
(69%)

Dominant
mass
15 / 110
(14%)

FIGURE 10.6. Mammographic appearances and their histologic correlation.

DETAILED ANALYSIS OF THE MAMMOGRAPHIC FINDINGS LEADING TO THE DETECTION OF IN SITU CARCINOMAS

Microcalcifications

151 of 198 cases (76%) were detected by finding microcalcifications. Figure 10.7 shows the frequency of the different types of calcifications.

The morphology and distribution of the calcifications on the mammogram are determined by the histologic features of the underlying disease (4,5,6,7,9). The predominantly high nuclear grade/poorly differentiated in situ carcinomas typically present either with the casting-type or the crushed stone–like calcifications.

Casting-type Calcifications

The *casting-type calcifications* are reliable indicators of high nuclear grade/poorly differentiated in situ carcinoma.

The casting-type calcifications have two different mammographic appearances according to the growth pattern of the high nuclear grade malignant cells. The histologic-mammographic correlation can be summarized as follows.

i. **Casting-type calcifications, fragmented, rod-like (characteristic for cases with solid cell proliferation)** (Figs. 10.8 and 10.9).

Histology
- Poorly differentiated cells, polymorphic, large nuclei with frequent mitoses
- Solid growth pattern
- Significant amount of necrosis
- Amorphous calcifications

Mammography
- Characteristic calcifications
- Fragmented, rod-like, irregular, dense, casting-type
- Scattered within a large part of the lobe, since they are confined to the distended ducts and their branches

ii. **Casting-type calcifications, snake skin–like (characteristic for cases with predominantly micropapillary cell proliferation)** (Figs. 10.10 and 10.11).

Histology
- poorly differentiated cells, polymorphic, large nuclei with frequent mitoses
- Various growth pattern: micropapillary and solid
- Necrosis present
- Amorphous calcifications

Mammography
Characteristic calcifications:
- Dotted casting-type, snake skin–like
- Scattered, outlining most of the lobe

GROUP A
75 of 88 cases (85%)

High nuclear grade / poorly differentiated

GROUP B
76 of 110 cases (69%)

The combination of:
Intermediate / low nuclear grade -
moderately / well differentiated

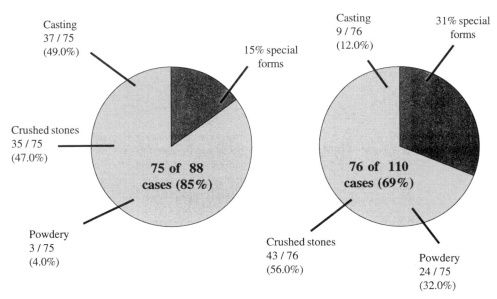

Casting
37 / 75
(49.0%)

15% special
forms

Crushed stones
35 / 75
(47.0%)

**75 of 88
cases (85%)**

Powdery
3 / 75
(4.0%)

Casting
9 / 76
(12.0%)

31% special
forms

**76 of 110
cases (69%)**

Crushed stones
43 / 76
(56.0%)

Powdery
24 / 75
(32.0%)

FIGURE 10.7. The frequency of different types of calcification.

Crushed Stone–like Calcifications

The *crushed stone–like calcifications* are the most common type seen in the intermediate/moderately differentiated in situ carcinoma. They are also frequent markers for high nuclear grade/poorly differentiated in situ carcinoma. The histologic-mammographic correlation can be summarized as follows (Figs. 10.12, 10.13 and 10.14).

Histology
- High, intermediate, or low nuclear grade cells
- Any growth pattern, although solid is most common
- Amorphous calcifications localized within distended lobules

Mammography
- Single or multiple clusters, since they are confined to distended lobules
- The microcalcifications are distinguishable as individual particles
- The shape calcifications can be described as crushed stone/broken needle/arrowhead/spear head–like or coarse granular type. A few casting-type calcification among these amorphous calcifications

Powdery Calcifications

The *powdery calcifications* primarily represent low nuclear grade/well-differentiated carcinoma in situ.

The histologic-mammographic correlation can be summarized as follows (Fig. 10.16).

Histology
- Low nuclear grade cells
- Micropapillary and/or cribriform growth pattern
- No significant necrosis present
- Laminated, onion ring–like calcifications localized within distended lobules

Mammography
- Single or multiple cluster distribution, since they are confined to the distended lobules

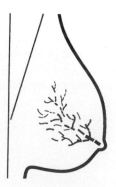

FIGURE 10.8. Schematic drawing of casting-type calcification.

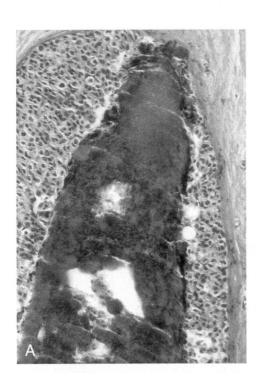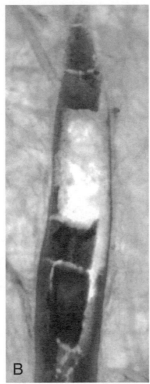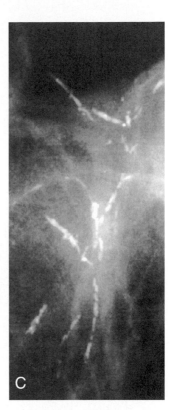

FIGURE 10.9. 70-year-old asymptomatic woman, screening case. Histologic-mammographic correlation of high nuclear grade ductal carcinoma in situ with fragmented, rod-like, casting-type calcifications on the mammogram. **(A)** High nuclear grade/poorly differentiated ductal cancer in situ with necrosis. **(B)** Thick-section histology. **(C)** Microfocus magnification mammography.

■ The microcalcifications are not distinguishable as individual particles. The powdery calcifications give a cotton ball–like appearance

Differential Diagnostic Problems

The powderish, multiple cluster microcalcifications in low nuclear grade/well-differentiated cancer in situ may be indistinguishable mammographically from those seen in sclerosing adenosis with or without atypia (Fig. 10.17). Since the powderish calcifications are frequently located in sclerosing adenosis adjacent to mammographically occult can-

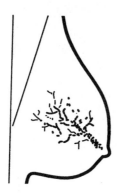

FIGURE 10.10. Schematic drawing of snake skin-like calcification.

cer in situ, open surgical biopsy is preferred to large core needle biopsy.

Practical Notes Regarding Microcalcifications seen on the Mammogram

■ Malignant cells are histologically present beyond the mammographically detectable calcifications. The size discrepancy is usually greater in low nuclear grade/well-differentiated in situ carcinoma than in the high nuclear grade/poorly differentiated types. This has practical implications for obtaining clear margins at surgical excision.

■ In high nuclear grade/poorly differentiated in situ carcinoma, and also in intermediate/moderately differentiated in situ cases, there is an intimate relationship between the calcifications and the malignant cells producing them. Thus, accurate targeting of calcifications is essential when performing fine needle aspiration biopsy or large core needle biopsy.

■ Casting-type calcifications have to be differentiated from plasma cell mastitis–type calcifications. When the branching/casting-type calcifications are unilateral and focal, they most likely represent a high nuclear grade/poorly differentiated in situ carcinoma (Fig. 10.18).

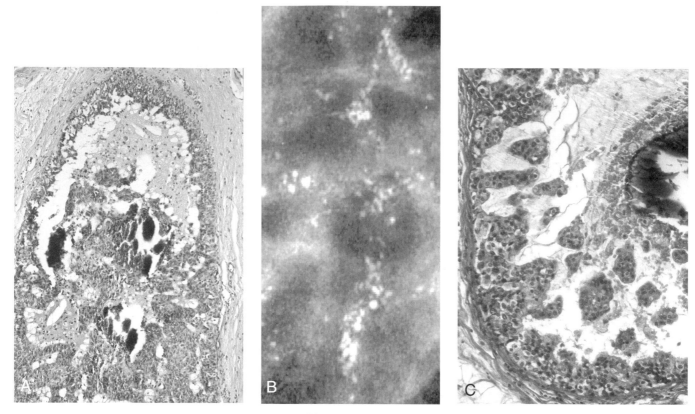

FIGURE 10.11. Histologic-mammographic correlation of high nuclear grade/poorly differenti-ated ductal carcinoma in situ with dotted casting-type calcifications on the mammogram. Histol-ogy shows predominantly micropapillary growth pattern. **(A)** High nuclear grade carcinoma in situ with dotted amorphous calcifications. **(B)** Microfocus magnification of dotted casting-type calcifications. **(C)** High nuclear grade, micropapillary carcinoma in situ with amorphous calcifica-tions.

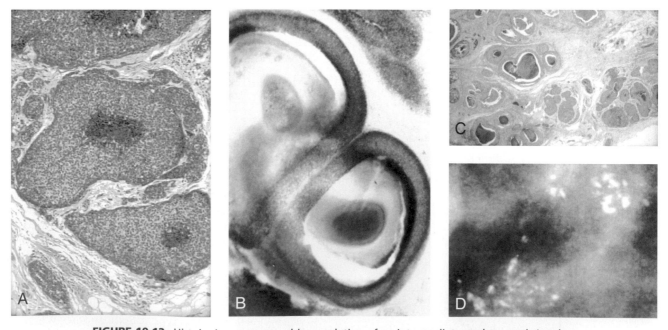

FIGURE 10.12. Histologic-mammographic correlation of an intermediate nuclear grade/moder-ately differentiated ductal carcinoma in situ case. **(A)** Histology: solid cell proliferation with necro-sis. **(B)** Three-dimensional histology with central necrosis and amorphous calcifications. **(C)** His-tology: solid cell proliferation with necrosis. **(D)** Multiple cluster crushed stone–like calcifications.

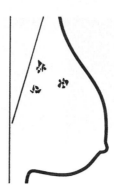

FIGURE 10.13. Schematic drawing of multiple-cluster, crushed stone-like calcifications.

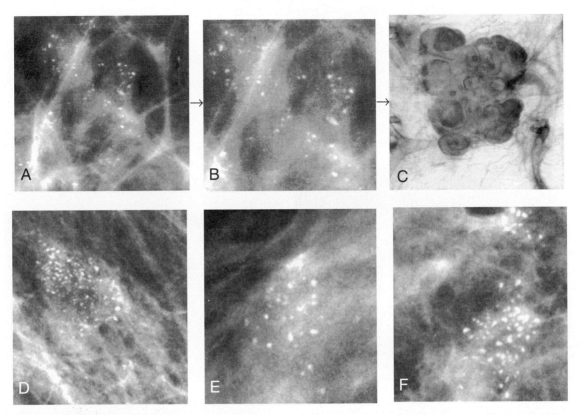

FIGURE 10.14. Examples of multiple cluster, crushed stone–like calcifications in intermediate nuclear grade/moderately differentiated ductal carcinoma in situ cases. **(A)** Detail of mammogram without magnification. **(B)** Microfocus magnification. **(C)** Three-dimensional histology of one terminal duct lobular unit distended by cancer. **(D–F)** Microfocus magnification images of crushed stone–like calcifications.

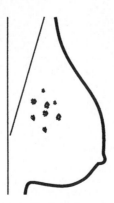

FIGURE 10.15. Schematic drawing of multiple-cluster, powdery/cotton ball-like calcifications.

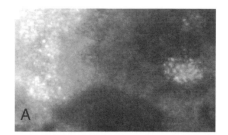
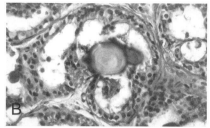

FIGURE 10.16. A: Multiple cluster powdery/cotton ball–like calcifications. **(B)** Histology: low nuclear grade/well-differentiated cancer in situ.

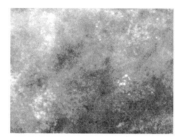

FIGURE 10.17. Multiple cluster powdery calcifications. Histology: sclerosing adenosis.

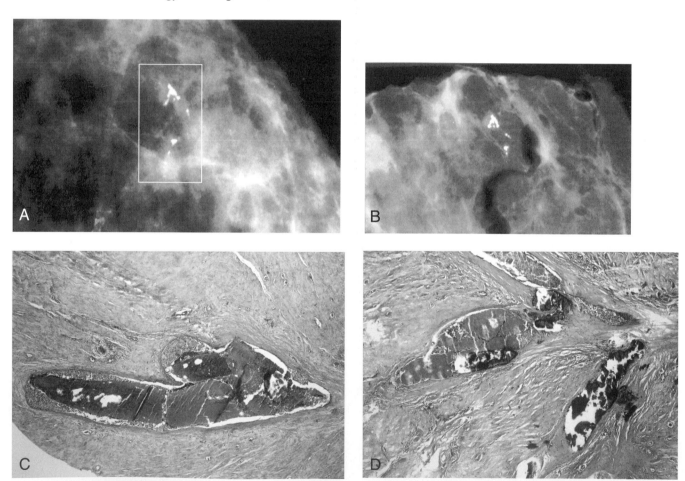

FIGURE 10.18. 67-year-old woman with screen-detected unilateral, focal, casting-type calcifications, representing high nuclear grade/poorly differentiated ductal carcinoma in situ. **(A)** Cranion-caudal projection microfocus magnification. **(B)** Specimen x-ray film. **(C–D)** Histology: high nuclear grade/poorly differentiated cancer in situ with extensive necrosis.

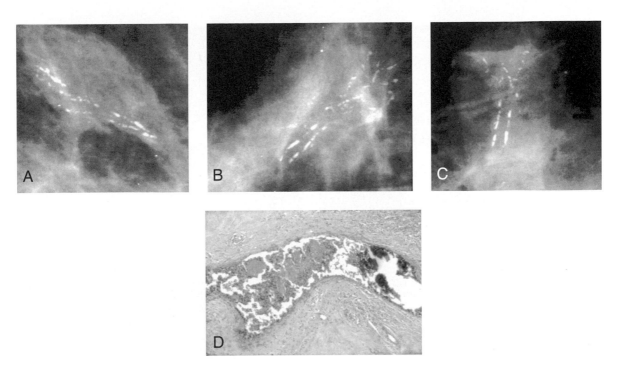

FIGURE 10.19. 63-year-old, asymptomatic woman, screening case. **(A)** Medio-lateral oblique magnification shows casting-type calcifications characteristic for high nuclear grade cancer in situ. **(B)** CC magnification. **(C)** Specimen x-ray film demonstrates the calcifications at the surgical margin. **(D)** Histology: high nuclear grade carcinoma in situ with free margins (unlikely according to the specimen x-ray film).

- Therapeutic failure frequently occurs in high nuclear grade/poorly differentiated in situ carcinomas. The possible "recurrence" at the site of excision will be a short-term event (2 to 3 years following surgery). Postoperative irradiation usually cannot compensate for incomplete surgical excision (Figs. 10.19 and 10.20). Follow-up: Postoperative irradiation. "Recurrence" at the site of biopsy (Fig. 10.20).
- Usually a large part of the lobe is involved due to the extensive proliferation of the malignant cells in high nuclear grade/poorly differentiated in situ carcinoma, resulting in a segmental distribution. It is often difficult to obtain clear margins with acceptable results. (Fig. 10.21).
- Specimen x-ray is mandatory to ensure that the suspected calcifications have been removed. Immediate confirmation with specimen radiography is preferable to early postoperative mammography (Fig. 10.22).
- Preferably, the pathologist should slice the specimen and obtain microfocus specimen x-rays of the tissue slices in order to localize the areas of concern.
- x-ray of the paraffin blocks may be necessary to locate the mammographically suspicious calcifications (Fig. 10.23).

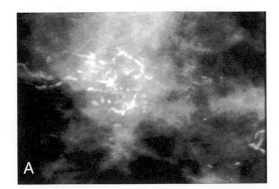
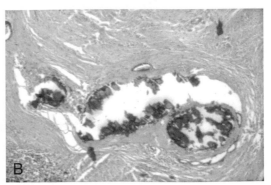

FIGURE 10.20. A: Microfocus magnification 23 months following surgery and irradiation. **(B)** Histology: in situ carcinoma, similar to initial biopsy.

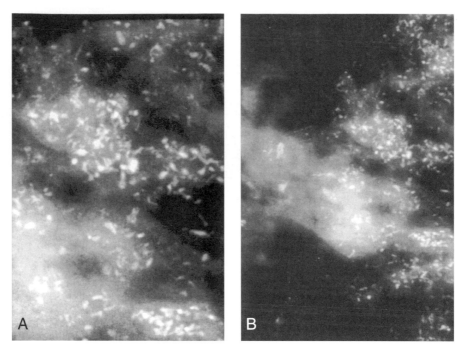

FIGURE 10.21. 7 × 8 cm area with casting-type calcifications.

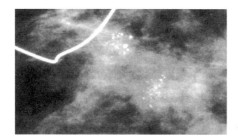

FIGURE 10.22. Microfocus magnification of specimen.

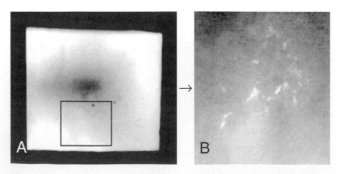

FIGURE 10.23. A: x-ray film of the paraffin block. **(B)** Microfocus magnification image of the paraffin block.

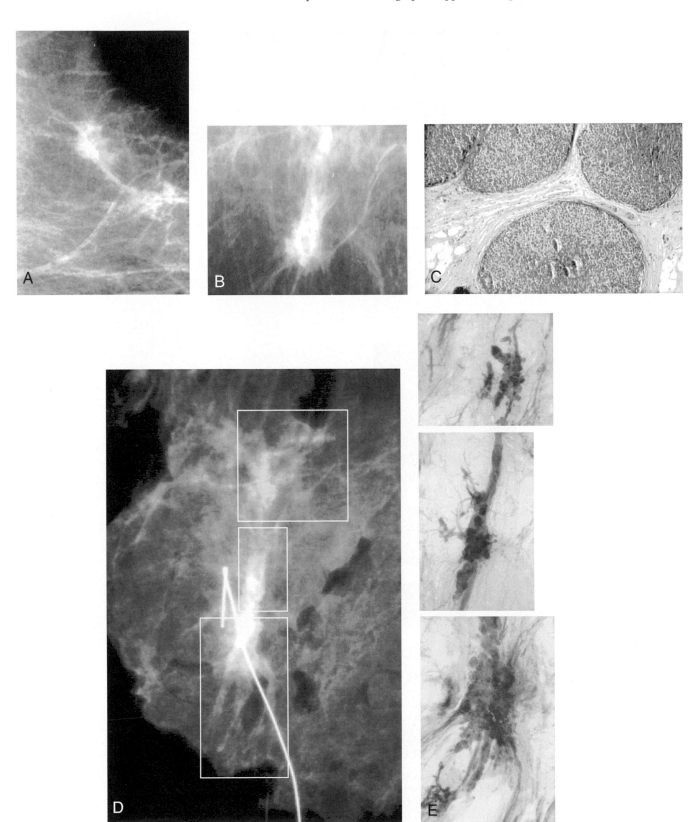

FIGURE 10.24. Example of asymmetric density with architectural distortion seen in a 70-year-old asymptomatic woman. **(A)** Detail of the left MLO projection. **(B)** Microfocus magnification. **(C)** Histology: low nuclear grade/well-differentiated cancer in situ. **(D)** Specimen x-ray film. **(E)** Thick section histology.

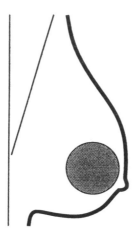

FIGURE 10.25. Schematic drawing of solitary circular/oval-shaped mass.

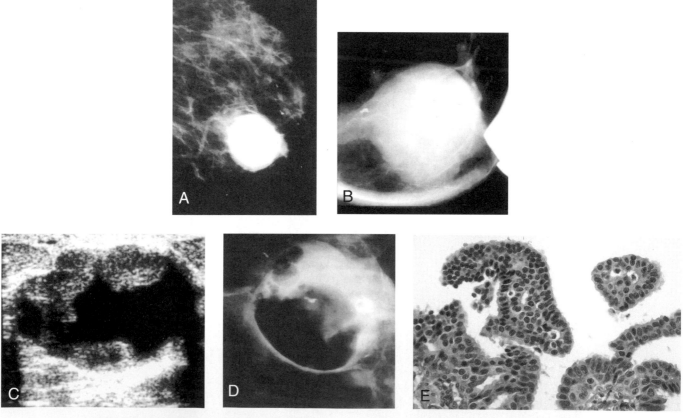

FIGURE 10.26. Example of intracystic papillary carcinoma presenting as a solitary mass in a 75-year-old woman. **(A)** MLO projection. **(B)** Microfocus magnification. **(C)** Ultrasound image. **(D)** Pneumocystogram. **(E)** Histology: intracystic papillary carcinoma.

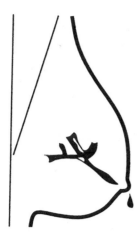

FIGURE 10.27. Schematic drawing of ductal filling defects and/or ductal amputations seen with galactography.

Asymmetric Density with Architectural Distortion with or without Demonstrable Microcalcifications

Asymmetric density with architectural distortion is one of the atypical mammographic appearances leading to the detection of carcinoma in situ (16) (Fig. 10.24).

In our material, this was the mammographic sign of high nuclear grade/poorly differentiated in situ carcinoma in 15% of the cases and in 6% of the combined low-intermediate nuclear grade/well-moderately differentiated in situ cases.

The unilateral asymmetric density with architectural distortion is usually localized to one lobe. Using microfocus magnification, one can often demonstrate otherwise occult microcalcifications. The density on the mammogram may correspond to desmoplastic reaction, radial scar, or focal fibrocystic change at histologic examination.

Solitary or Multiple Circular/Oval Shaped Masses

This mammographic finding occurred in 14% of all combined low-intermediate/well-moderately differentiated in situ carcinoma cases. Histologic examination showed either intracystic papillary carcinoma or multiple in situ papillary carcinomas. This presentation did not occur among the high nuclear grade/poorly differentiated cases (Figs. 10.25 and 10.26).

Ductal Filling Defects and/or Ductal Amputations seen with Galactography

When the only clinical symptom is serous or bloody nipple discharge, galactography is the diagnostic procedure of choice. Preoperative localization with methylene blue will outline the affected duct.

Of the combined low-intermediate/well-moderately differentiated in situ carcinoma cases, 11% presented with serous or bloody nipple discharge. This lead to the galactographic demonstration of intraductal filling defects and/or amputations (Figs. 10.27 and 10.28).

OVERVIEW OF HISTOLOGIC-MAMMOGRAPHIC CORRELATION OF IN SITU CARCINOMA CASES

The results of histologic-mammographic correlation of 198 in situ carcinoma cases diagnosed between 1977 and 1994 in Kopparberg county, Sweden are summarized on Figures 10.29 and 10.30. During the same period, an additional nine cases were found at histology, unrelated to mammographic findings, or did not have mammography.

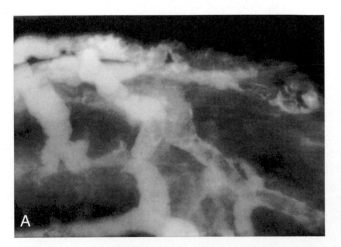
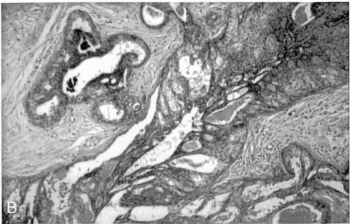

FIGURE 10.28. 41-year-old woman with serous nipple discharge. **(A)** Multiple filling defects on the galactogram. **(B)** Histology: low nuclear grade/well-differentiated ductal carcinoma in situ.

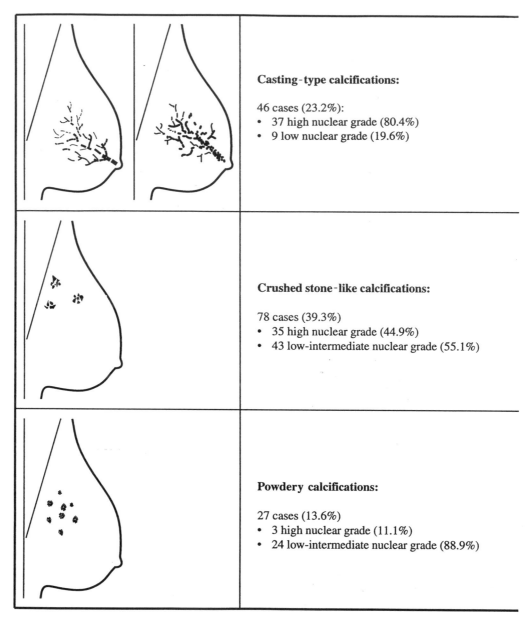

Casting-type calcifications:

46 cases (23.2%):
- 37 high nuclear grade (80.4%)
- 9 low nuclear grade (19.6%)

Crushed stone-like calcifications:

78 cases (39.3%)
- 35 high nuclear grade (44.9%)
- 43 low-intermediate nuclear grade (55.1%)

Powdery calcifications:

27 cases (13.6%)
- 3 high nuclear grade (11.1%)
- 24 low-intermediate nuclear grade (88.9%)

FIGURE 10.29. Schematic representation of different type calcifications seen in in situ carcinomas.

Microcalcifications were the most frequent findings on the mammogram in detecting in situ carcinomas (76%). Casting-type calcifications are most often associated with high nuclear grade/poorly differentiated in situ carcinoma, while the powderish, cotton ball–like calcifications represented low nuclear grade/well-differentiated cases. The majority of the calcification cases were crushed stone–like and represented all grades.

The remaining 24% of all in situ carcinomas were demonstrated by asymmetric density with architectural distortion, or by finding solitary or multiple circular/oval masses, or by performing galactography. This shows that demonstrating as many in situ carcinoma cases as possible requires not only meticulous workup with mammographic examination, but also the use of ultrasound and galactography.

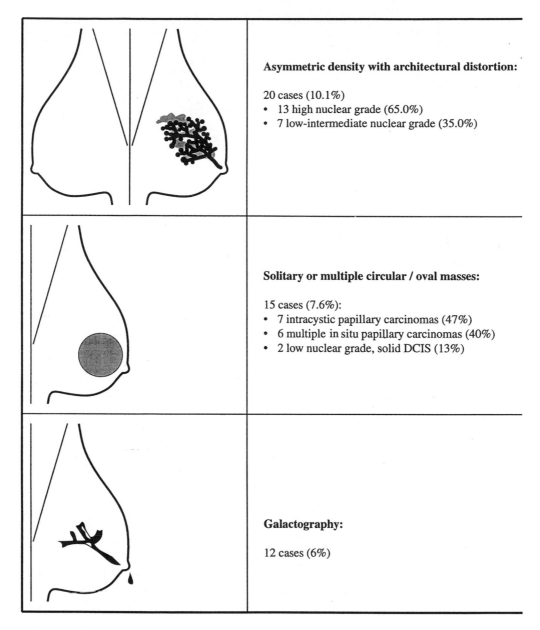

Asymmetric density with architectural distortion:

20 cases (10.1%)
- 13 high nuclear grade (65.0%)
- 7 low-intermediate nuclear grade (35.0%)

Solitary or multiple circular / oval masses:

15 cases (7.6%):
- 7 intracystic papillary carcinomas (47%)
- 6 multiple in situ papillary carcinomas (40%)
- 2 low nuclear grade, solid DCIS (13%)

Galactography:

12 cases (6%)

FIGURE 10.30. Atypical mammographic appearances of in situ carcinomas.

REFERENCES

1. Schnitt SJ, Harris JR, Smith BL. Developing a prognostic index for ductal carcinoma in situ of the breast–are we there yet? *Cancer* 1996;77:2189–2192.
2. Lodato RF, Maguire HC, et al. Immunohistochemical evaluation of c-erbB-2 oncogene expression in ductal carcinoma in situ and atypical ductal hyperplasia of the breast. *Mod Pathol* 1990;4:449–454.
3. Lagios MD. Duct carcinoma in situ. *Surg Clin North Am* 1990;70:853–871.
4. Holland R, Hendriks JHCL. Microcalcifications associated with ductal carcinoma in situ: Mammographic-pathologic correlation. *Semin Diagn Pathol* 1994;11:181–192.
5. Lányi M. *Diagnosis and differential diagnosis of breast calcifications.* New York: Springer-Verlag, 1987.
6. Millis RR, Davis R, Stacey HJ. The detection and significance of calcifications in the breast. A radiologic and pathologic study. *Br J Radiol* 1976;49:12–26.
7. Stomper PC, Connolly JL. Ductal carcinoma in situ of the breast: correlation between mammographic calcification and tumor subtype. *AJR Am J Roentgenol* 1992;159:483–485.
8. Stomper PC, Margolin FR. Ductal carcinoma in situ: The mammographer's perspective. *AJR Am J Roentgenol* 1994;162:585–591.

9. Tabar L, Dean PB. *Teaching atlas of mammography*, 2nd ed. New York: Thieme Medical Publishers, 1985.

10. Lagios MD, Margolin FR, et al. Mammographically detected duct carcinoma in situ. Frequency of local recurrence following tylectomy and prognostic effect of nuclear grade on local recurrence. *Cancer* 1989;63:618–624.

11. Silverstein MJ, Lagios MD, Craig PH, et al. A prognostic index for ductal carcinoma in situ of the breast. *Cancer* 1996;77:2267–2274.

12. Simpson JF, Page DL. Pathology of pre-invasive and excellent-prognosis breast cancer. *Curr Opin Oncol* 1995;7:501–505.

13. Solin LJ, Yeh I, Kurtz J, et al. Ductal carcinoma in situ (intraductal carcinoma) of the breast treated with breast-conserving surgery and definitive irradiation. *Cancer* 1993;71:2532–2542.

14. Holland R, Peterse JL, et al. Ductal carcinoma in situ: a proposal for a new classification. *Semin Diagn Pathol* 1994;11:167–180.

15. Silverstein MJ, Poller DN, Waisman JR, et al. Prognostic classification of breast ductal carcinoma in situ. *Lancet* 1995;345:1154–1157.

16. Ikeda DM, Andersson I. Ductal carcinoma in situ: Atypical mammographic appearances *Radiology* 1989;172:661–666.

11

DUCTAL CARCINOMA IN SITU: A RADIOLOGICAL PERSPECTIVE

EVA RUBIN

Ductal carcinoma in situ (DCIS) is a condition in which knowledge of the radiologic features facilitates pathologic identification and description of extent. An understanding of the pathology is also critical to accurate classification and characterization of the radiographic findings. The explosion in the diagnosis of DCIS over the last few decades is largely a product of the mammographic era (1,2). Not only is more DCIS being diagnosed, but the spectrum of the disease now being found is also substantially different from that described in the past. This makes comparison of current case series with historical reviews complicated and perplexing.

The acronym DCIS lends itself to wordplay. In 1997, Edwin Fisher (3), a pathologist, used the following words to characterize DCIS: "Dilemma, Consternation, Inconsistency, Superficiality." These descriptors focused on the pathologist's difficulty in distinguishing among benign alterations in ductal epithelium, the atypical epithelial hyperplasias, and truly malignant changes. The modifications of ductal epithelium that occur in these conditions are not quantum jumps but rather a continuous spectrum of alterations that may be inconsistently characterized from one pathologist to the next (4).

From the radiologist's perspective, the following words might apply: "Distressing, Complex, Indistinguishable, Subtle." The radiologists' ability to perceive abnormalities of ductal epithelium is largely related to the detection of calcification, an indirect sign at best. DCIS without calcification may not be detectable on mammography, or (even in cases where calcification is identifiable) the extent of disease may be underestimated when portions of the disease contain no radiographically identifiable calcification. In addition, benign processes are responsible for most calcification in the breast and there is considerable overlap in the appearance of calcifications in benign and malignant disease.

Wordplay from the patient standpoint might yield the following adjectives: "Depressed, Confused, Insecure, Scared" (Fig. 11.1). Doubts have been expressed as to whether DCIS should be considered a true malignancy (5,6). However, the facts that recurrences after limited excision almost always occur at the original biopsy site and that

approximately half of these are invasive (7–10) strongly suggest that DCIS has significant malignant potential. Follow-up studies on DCIS inadvertently treated by biopsy only (due to misdiagnosis) (11,12) suggested 39% to 75% risk of invasive cancer in the ipsilateral breast after 10 to 15 years. Whether such high rates would also pertain to prospectively diagnosed, mammographically detected DCIS with detailed presurgical mammographic mapping and appropriate wedge excision is unknown.

Nonetheless, for years patients have been presented with the conundrum that early detection of in situ breast cancers is more likely to result in treatment with mastectomy than is detection of biologically more advanced, but presumably more localized, invasive disease. The lack of consensus as to which alterations constitute true disease, which are truly dangerous to the patient, and how the condition should be treated are truly sources of uncertainty and trepidation for all who encounter this disease.

ANATOMY

DCIS is defined as a pathologic condition in which duct(s) and lobules contain malignant-appearing cells that do not extend beyond the basement membrane on light microscopy (Fig. 11.2). The tumor cells can occupy variable portions of the ductal system of the breast, ranging from a few ducts visible only on microscopy to involvement of an entire ductal system. The volume of breast occupied by a single duct system is highly variable—a fact well known to those who perform ductography (13,14).

The breast contains 15 to 20 lobes and a corresponding number of major ducts culminating at the nipple. (The number of major lactiferous ducts opening onto the nipple may be as few as five to eight, since some ducts join as they near the nipple.) The arborization of a single duct system from nipple to base of the breast defines the size of a lobe. A single duct system (lobe) may span more than one quadrant or may define only a small volume of a single quadrant of the breast. The ductal distribution of DCIS may appear dis-

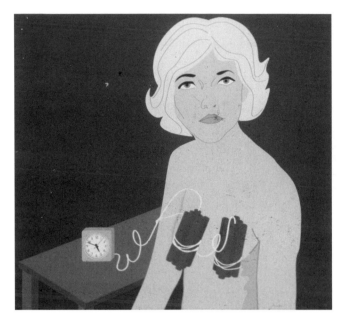

FIGURE 11.1. Ductal Carcinoma in Situ—a patient's perspective. Depressed, Confused, Insecure, Scared.

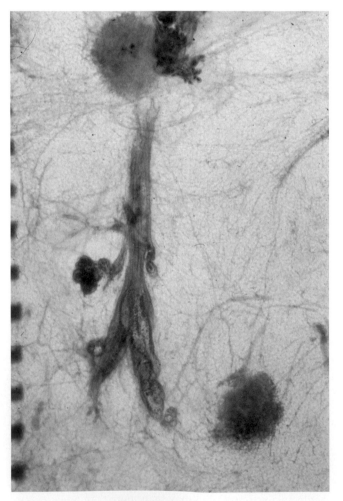

FIGURE 11.2. Three-dimensional histology showing malignant cells within duct and lobules in ductal carcinoma in situ. (Photomicrograph courtesy of Dr. Tibor Tot.)

continuous when examined in cross-section, as is the case in most standard histologic preparations. Thus, it is easy to understand why the disease is so often characterized as multifocal (multiple foci in one quadrant) and multicentric (involving more than one quadrant) (15–18).

Modern studies focusing on mammographically detected DCIS, such as the classic study by Holland et al. (19), indicate that true multifocality and multicentricity are unusual. Holland's study showed DCIS to be confined to one quadrant in two-thirds of cases; multicentric distribution, in which there was discontinuous involvement in opposite but not neighboring quadrants, was seen in only one of his 82 cases. The cases in the Holland study were generally large (5 cm or greater in extent), suggesting that in smaller lesions, multifocality and multicentricity are even more rare.

Classification by histologic subtype is frequently used for characterization of DCIS, and has prognostic significance. The most commonly used classification divides DCIS into solid, cribriform, papillary and micropapillary, and comedo subtypes. The hallmark of DCIS on mammography is the presence of ductally distributed 'casting-type' calcification (Fig. 11.3). Mammographic detection of DCIS is most likely in those cases in which there is calcification within tumor cells or within the intraductal debris produced by tumor cells, i.e., in cases with necrosis.

In Holland's study, 60% of cases were of the predominantly comedo type, and 40% of the predominantly cribriform/micropapillary type. Mammographic extent most closely correlated with histologic extent when the comedo subtype was present. In Holland's original study (19), mammography did not predict histologic subtype with a high degree of accuracy. However, in a follow-up study in which most of the cases were evaluated with magnification views (20), accuracy was improved, although underestimation of extent of disease was still frequent, particularly in low grade (well-differentiated) forms of DCIS, large portions of which may be uncalcified.

A number of recent articles have emphasized the importance of recognizing the heterogeneous nature of DCIS (21) and the inadequacy of current nomenclature for defining appropriate management. While it has become increasingly apparent that many women with a diagnosis of DCIS may be overtreated for their "disease," long-term follow-up studies continue to merit caution in dismissing even low-grade lesions as inconsequential. In an update of the classic Vanderbilt study of low-grade DCIS (misdiagnosed and) treated by biopsy only, Page et al. (22) identified nine recurrences among 28 patients followed for 15 to 25 years, with 78% (7 of 9) progressing to invasive cancer, and five deaths.

A number of new classifications to better match treatment to expected outcome in these patients has been proposed (23–26). One of the most promising of these is the Van Nuys Prognostic Index (VNPI) (27), which combines three significant predictors of local recurrence: tumor size, margin width, and pathologic classification to produce an

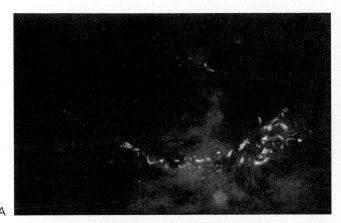
A

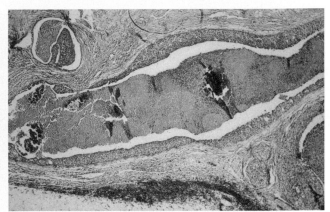
B

FIGURE 11.3. A: Specimen radiograph showing long segment of linearly distributed predominantly linear calcification in a case of comedo-type ductal carcinoma in situ (DCIS). **(B)** Microradiogram of comedo-type DCIS showing duct containing linear calcifications within lumen. Note malignant cells lining duct.

overall score ranging from three to nine. In 333 patients with DCIS treated with breast preservation (at 8 year follow-up), radiation therapy did not appear to significantly affect local recurrence rates in patients with VNPI scores of three or four. In patients with intermediate scores (five, six, or seven), radiotherapy resulted in a 17% reduction in local recurrence, while patients with scores of eight or nine experienced very high local recurrence rates, even with radiotherapy.

MAMMOGRAPHIC FEATURES OF DUCTAL CARCINOMA IN SITU

Ducts are not usually perceived as abnormal unless they are unusually large or distorted (Fig. 11.4), or unless they contain material that differs in opacity from normal ductal content. Thus, abnormalities of ducts are usually identified because of intraductal calcifications, dilatation or distortion of ducts (Fig. 11.5), or periductal reactive changes.

DCIS may be invisible on standard mammograms. Such cases are detected because of palpable thickening, nipple changes of Paget's disease, nipple discharge, or findings on ultrasound or magnetic resonance imaging. In patients presenting with nipple discharge, additional information may be obtained from ultrasound or ductography (Fig. 11.6). Intraductal filling defects, abnormal duct caliber, and amputated segments may be seen.

Cases of DCIS that manifest solely as mass have also been described (28,29). DCIS detected due to soft tissue abnormality without associated calcification represents less than 10% of cases (Fig. 11.7). Most of these "masses" are due to inflammatory or fibrotic reaction associated with the malignant process. In some cases, the soft tissue abnormality may be unrelated to the DCIS, e.g., a fibroadenoma or papilloma containing DCIS. Other masses are intracystic tumors; the subtype in such cases is usually papillary. Spiculation in as-

sociation with DCIS is unusual. Unless another etiology for the distortion (radial scar, sclerosing adenosis, papillomatosis) is found in the pathologic specimen, the presence of an undetected invasive component should be strongly suspected, and review of the histologic sections should be considered.

Most diagnosed cases of DCIS currently are manifest by calcifications identified on a routine screening mammogram. The calcifications leading to the mammographic detection of DCIS are

(i) dystrophic calcifications of necrotic cells and debris within the ductal lumen;

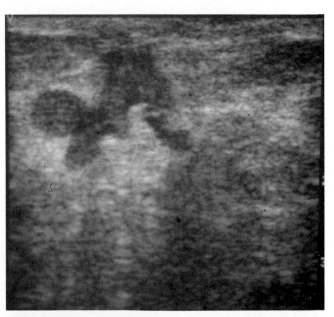

FIGURE 11.4. Ultrasound image showing dilated deformed ducts containing echogenic material representing low-grade ductal carcinoma in situ.

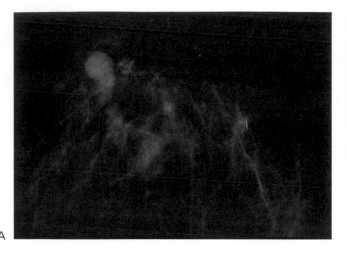

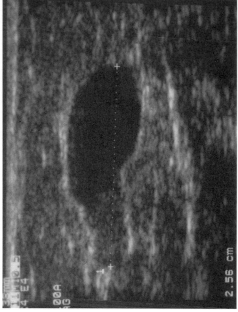

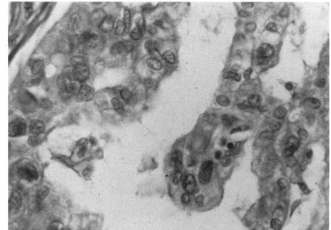

FIGURE 11.5. A: Mammogram showing solitary tubular structure consistent with an enlarged duct. **(B)** Ultrasound image from same patient showing dilated duct. The anterior portion of the duct is fluid-filled; the posterior portion is echo-filled. Excisional biopsy confirmed papillary ductal carcinoma in situ. **(C)** Papillary fronds within distended ducts in a case of papillary ductal carcinoma in situ.

(ii) calcifications of abnormal material produced by the malignant ductal cells; or

(iii) calcifications associated with benign processes, incidentally or etiologically, related to the in situ malignancy.

Because some of the calcific foci leading to the detection of malignant disease are within benign processes, considerable confusion can arise as to which patterns of calcification should be considered suspicious.

The predominant features of DCIS calcifications are

i) pleomorphism, and

ii) linear or segmental distribution.

When both of these features are present, the likelihood of DCIS is very high, and 70% of cases with these characteristics will be of the comedo subtype (30). However, mammographic appearance does not reliably predict either subtype (31) or grade (32).

Breast calcifications correspond in size and shape to the structures that contain them. In understanding the form and distribution of DCIS calcifications, knowledge of the size and shape of the architectural components of the breast is critical. Calcifications occur in the residual lumina of involved ductal structures as well as in the acini of involved lobules. Because the growth pattern of the in situ malignancy is fairly continuous within a ductal segment, distribution is the feature that is often most helpful in ascertaining whether calcifications are more likely malignant or benign.

Benign proliferative disease of the breast, such as sclerosing adenosis, is often diffuse and bilateral. Much of the associated calcification is found in lobules, and the individual calcific foci are uniformly round or punctate and are present in a rosette distribution. Linear distribution is not usually present in these cases. Calcifications associated with malignancy may also have a round or punctate morphology, identical to that seen in benign processes. Such calcifications are more often associated with cribriform patterns of ductal involvement. The piecemeal necrosis seen in ducts involved with cribriform DCIS produces spaces similar in size and shape to those present in a distended lobule. However, benign lobular calcifications do not usually extend linearly along a duct; while malignant ductal processes do. Fortu-

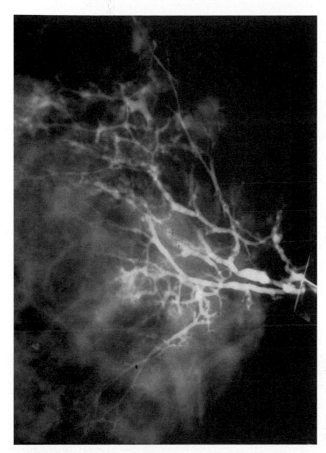

FIGURE 11.6. Ductogram in patient who presented with bloody nipple discharge. The caliber of the ducts is abnormal with alternating areas of constriction and dilatation. Filling defects and amputated segments are also apparent.

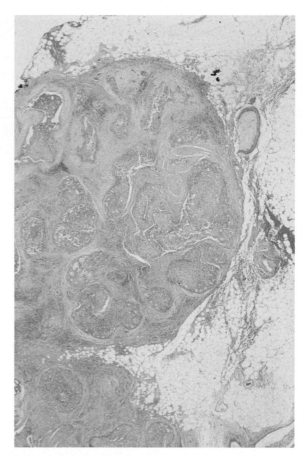

FIGURE 11.7. Nodule approximately 7 mm in size produced by ductal carcinoma in situ. Mammogram showed a well-defined benign-appearing soft tissue nodule with no associated calcification.

nately, the linear or segmental distribution of the calcifications of DCIS provides a clue to their malignant nature, even when the individual calcific particles are round. When the malignancy is very limited in extent, the focus of calcification may appear rounded or oval, and benign-malignant distinction becomes more difficult.

Other features of calcifications, such as size of individual particles, number of particles, extensiveness, and stability are less helpful. Calcifications present in comedocarcinoma may be relatively coarse when they occur in larger ducts (Fig. 11.8). Only one or two casting calcifications may be sufficient to recommend biopsy (Fig. 11.9). DCIS may involve virtually the entire breast (Fig. 11.8). And, finally, calcific debris associated with DCIS may remain stable while mammographically invisible tumor cells continue to grow through the ductal system (Fig. 11.10). Because the growth rate of DCIS is difficult to establish (33) and because growth may not be reflected by change in number or extent of calcification, protocols recommending six-month follow-up (34,35) for indeterminate foci of calcification are not easily validated by clinical data.

Two forms of calcification are classically described in association with DCIS: granular and casting. Tabár's mam-

mography atlas (36) defines granular calcification using the words of Leborgne from his 1953 textbook of mammography, "Calcifications in carcinoma are, generally, tiny, dot-like or somewhat elongated, innumerable and irregularly grouped very close together in an area of the breast, resembling fine grains of salt." These calcifications are usually so

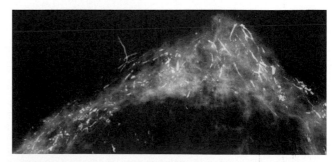

FIGURE 11.8. Extensive ductal carcinoma in situ occupying nearly the entire volume of the breast. Note that as the ducts enlarge as they approach the nipple, the associated calcifications are also large, simply reflecting the larger available luminal size in the involved ducts. The ducts do not arborize normally, coursing laterally rather than toward the nipple in some areas, and there are irregularities in caliber.

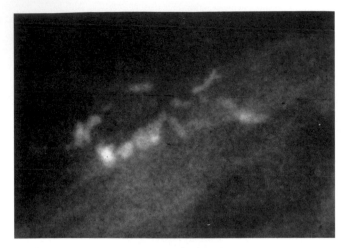

FIGURE 11.9. Highly magnified area from a specimen radiograph showing linear branched calcifications from a case of high-grade ductal carcinoma in situ. The standard mammogram showed only a single V-shaped calcification measuring 3 mm in maximum dimension.

fine (powdery) that individual particles may be difficult to distinguish (Fig. 11.11). They are most often distributed in single or multiple clusters that correspond to distended lobular structures. These calcifications may be indistinguishable from lobular-type calcifications present in benign proliferative diseases of the breast, such as sclerosing adenosis (Fig. 11.12). When associated with DCIS, the tumor is usually of low nuclear grade.

Casting calcifications are defined as those that fill in segments of ducts and occasionally their side-branches. The width of the individual calcifications is determined by the available size of the duct lumen. The calcific fragments differ in density and length. The outline of the calcifications is "highly irregular" due to the irregular nature of the tumor cell proliferation within the duct. Such calcifications often have clefts within them, as opposed to the more continuous appearance of benign intraductal calcifications.

Tabár (36) defines two types of casting calcification,

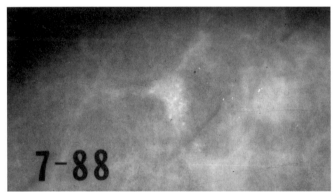

A

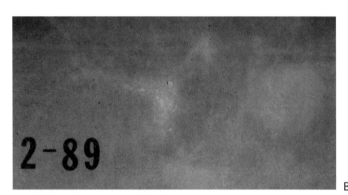

B

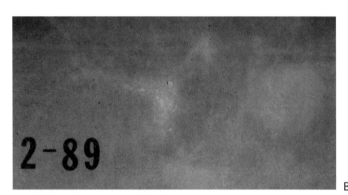

C

FIGURE 11.10. A: Tubular structure containing relatively coarse predominantly rod-shaped calcifications seen on mammogram of a 56-year-old woman who had recently begun hormone replacement therapy. Note well-defined rounded nodule to the right of the calcified area. **(B)** Mammogram seven months later, February 1989, at which time the patient was referred for a second opinion to the University of Alabama at Birmingham (UAB) due to enlargement of the benign-appearing rounded nodule. An ultrasound demonstrated simple cysts. However, the patient was advised to have the area of calcification removed, as, despite its stability, the morphology and distribution of the calcifications suggested malignancy. **(C)** Mammogram performed at UAB one year later, February 1990. The examination is better quality than the examinations illustrated in **(A)** and **(B)**. The calcific focus shows little change. However, posterior to it, an irregular density is seen. In the interim between this examination and the 1989 exam, the patient had returned to her original institution and underwent biopsy of the benign-appearing masses, which were confirmed to be cysts. Biopsy at UAB confirmed high-grade DCIS in the area of the calcific focus with diffuse microinvasion throughout the breast and 36 of 36 nodes positive for carcinoma.

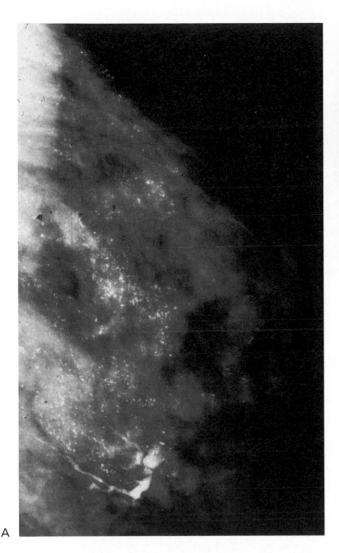

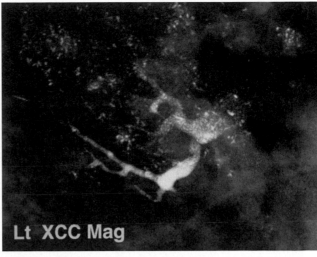

A

FIGURE 11.11. A: Extensive low-grade predominantly cribriform-type ductal carcinoma in situ. **(B)** Detail from **(A)** showing ductally distributed, extremely fine calcifications packing ducts and simulating the appearance of a ductogram.

which differ according to the growth pattern of the tumor cells. These are:

i) fragmented, rod-like calcifications (Fig. 11.3A), most often associated with high-grade solid cell proliferation. The calcifications tend to be dense and relatively large, outlining a variable, and often large, part of the lobe.

ii) snake skin–like calcifications (Fig. 11.11B), most often associated with high-grade micropapillary cell proliferation. These calcifications are individually dot-like, but are linearly distributed, outlining a variable, but often large, part of the lobe.

An intermediate form of calcification, constituting a mixture of amorphous, granular, and occasional casting calcifications has been likened to the appearance of crushed stones or broken needle tips (Fig. 11.13). Unlike granular calcifications, the individual particles are usually distinguishable. These are also distributed in single or multiple clusters corresponding to distended lobules. They may be associated with high, intermediate, or low-grade lesions.

The Tabár descriptors for calcification are certainly more poetic and graphic than those in the lexicon approved by the American College of Radiology (ACR). In the ACR lexicon, there are separate descriptors for morphology (heterogeneous, thin rod-like, etc.) and distribution (grouped, linear, segmental). When combined, these yield designations with the same import as those used by Tabár. Because DCIS is a lobar process, the area containing calcifications is often triangular, with the base of the triangle paralleling the chest wall and the apex extending in the direction of the nipple (Fig. 11.14).

Microcalcifications with an associated mass or density were the indication for biopsy in 30% of 54 cases of DCIS in a series collected by Dershaw (37), and in 10% of 100 cases in a series by Stomper (38). The mass or density may be produced by the outline of a distended duct or ducts, or in some instances may be due to inflammation or fibrosis in the stroma surrounding the involved portions of the ductal system. When extensive, this type of DCIS may be palpable.

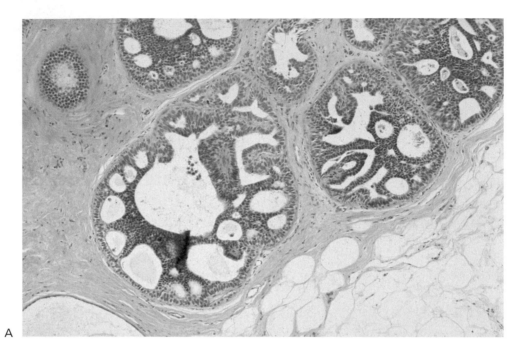

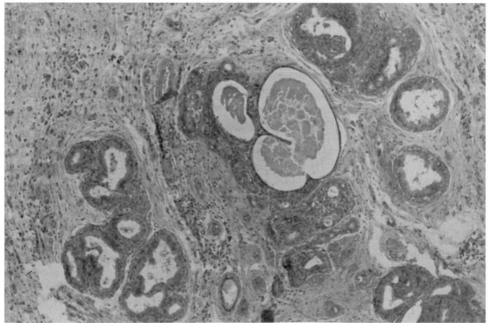

FIGURE 11.12. A: Ducts with cribriform-type ductal carcinoma in situ (DCIS). Note the rounded open spaces in which calcifications form. **(B)** Benign epithelial proliferative change. Note the small rounded spaces; these are similar in size and shape to the spaces present in the cribriform DCIS shown in **(A)**.

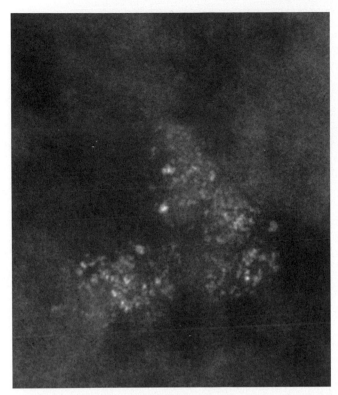

FIGURE 11.13. Highly magnified view of "crushed stone" type calcifications. Mammographic cluster size was approximately 5 mm. The calcifications are heterogeneous, varying in size, shape, and density. They are too numerous to count, but nonetheless are individually distinguishable. Note the triangular shape of the calcific focus.

MAMMOGRAPHIC ASSESSMENT IN SUSPECTED DUCTAL CARCINOMA IN SITU

Once calcifications have been identified on mammography, the mammographer must determine:

i)   whether they are suspicious enough to warrant a recommendation for biopsy,
ii) their location in two planes, and
iii) their extent (39).

The most important tool available for these determinations is magnification. Optimal magnification requires use of a small focal spot. For a magnification factor of 1.5, a true (rather than nominal) focal spot size of 0.2 mm is necessary; for a magnification factor of 2.0, a true focal spot size of 0.1 mm or less is required.

Magnification is accomplished by increasing the distance from the breast to the image receptor. Sharpness is decreased when the distance from object to film is increased; however, the small focal spot and the reduction in scatter produced by the "air gap" compensate for the increased unsharpness that accompanies magnification. Grids are unnecessary, and should not be used for magnification mammography.

Exposure time is considerably longer for (non-digital) magnification views, and radiation doses are consequently

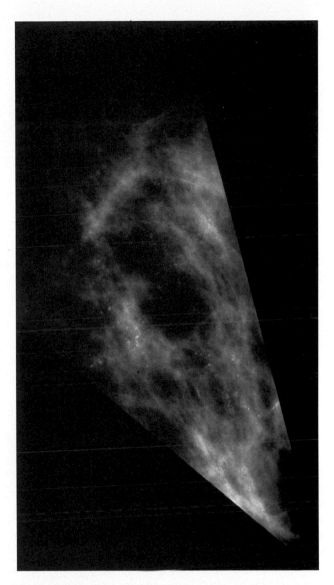

FIGURE 11.14. Malignant calcifications are present in a segmental distribution. If calcifications subtend a triangle with the apex at the nipple and the base at the chest wall, suspicion of ductal carcinoma in situ is raised.

one and a half to three times higher than with standard exposures. When exposure times are very long, patient motion is likely to occur, resulting in blurring of the image (40). Therefore, in situations where motion is predictable, such as uncooperative patients or those with very thick or dense breasts, a non-magnified spot compression view may provide more information than a magnified view.

Other than in the situations described above, magnification can usually be readily accomplished and results in improved resolution. In most cases, more calcification will be apparent on the magnification films than on standard projections, and the form of the individual calcifications will be more apparent. This allows more accurate assessment of the probability of malignancy, and consequently, the need for biopsy.

A decision must be made as to whether a full area magnification should be done or whether a coned spot compression magnification view will be more valuable. Coning down as much as possible reduces scatter and improves detail. However, coning has a number of drawbacks:

i) even expert technologists may have difficulty positioning the region of interest in the smaller spot compression field, thus multiple exposures may be performed before a satisfactory image is obtained with resultant high radiation dose exposure,
ii) motion artifact may be more likely, and
iii) extent of involvement may be underestimated due to the small field of view.

As a rule of thumb, when possible, it is preferable to perform spot compression magnification for the evaluation of noncalcified masses or areas of distortion, and area magnification for evaluation of calcifications. When malignant calcification is strongly suspected, special attention should be devoted to the subareolar area. If there is any suggestion of calcification in this area on the standard films, a separate magnified view should be obtained (unless the nipple is already included on the other magnified view). Magnification views of suspicious calcified areas should be done in two projections whenever possible. If milk-of-calcium is a consideration, one of the projections should be an upright lateral.

With digital techniques, magnification may be obtained without subjecting the patient to an additional radiographic exposure. Current digital technology has lower resolution than film-screen technique. It is not yet clear whether this will prove to be a diagnostic disadvantage.

Once it is established that calcifications are sufficiently suspicious as to merit biopsy, a decision must be made as to whether to perform percutaneous biopsy or proceed directly to surgical excision. In very high (τ 95%) suspicion lesions, an argument can be made that percutaneous sampling simply adds an extra procedure for most patients. On the other hand, percutaneous diagnosis allows patients who elect (or require) mastectomy to bypass excisional biopsy. In addition, a potentially unsightly biopsy scar may be avoided in the patient who undergoes reconstruction after skin sparing mastectomy. Core biopsy also allows patients with high suspicion of multicentric disease or with extensive disease to have the diagnosis confirmed and proceed directly to mastectomy.

Stereotactic core biopsy has proven to be a viable alternative diagnostic method compared with surgical excisional biopsy. However, it does underestimate the presence of invasive carcinoma in at least 16% to 21% of patients when DCIS is diagnosed with a 14-gauge spring-activated biopsy gun (41–43). In one study, seven of 20 cases (35%) of DCIS diagnosed with a 14-gauge automated gun were found to have invasive cancer at surgery, compared with only three of 20 cases (15%) biopsied using an 11-gauge vacuum-assisted device (44).

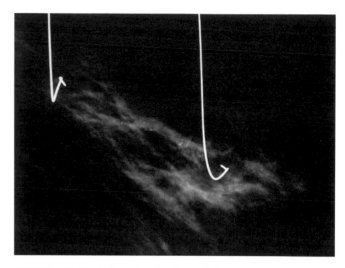

FIGURE 11.15. Linear distribution of ductal carcinoma in situ calcifications bracketed for excisional biopsy. Lumpectomy with negative margins was successfully accomplished.

With the aid of the information provided by the magnification views, the mammographer should be able to optimize the needle localization procedure to assure that appropriate areas are sampled. Localization of two or more sites of calcification may be necessary to confirm suspicion of multicentricity (in cases where percutaneous biopsy has not been performed). When a segment of involvement can be clearly defined mammographically, use of more than one localizing wire is often necessary to aid the surgeon to excise the appropriate wedge of tissue. Linearly distributed calcifications that extend over several centimeters in length may be localized with a freehand approach (Fig. 11.15) that tracks along the axis of the calcifications or, alternatively, with two wires demarcating the anterior and posterior extent of the calcifications. Segmental areas of calcification may require placement of three or more wires.

Because size and, ultimately, margin width (45) are important determinants of local recurrence in conservatively treated DCIS cases, it is imperative for the mammographer to as accurately as possible assess the size and extent of the

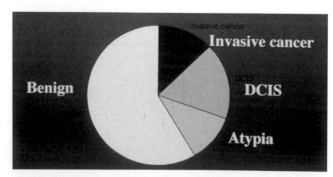

FIGURE 11.16. Graphic showing distribution of pathology in 663 consecutive needle-localized biopsies performed for microcalcification without mass.

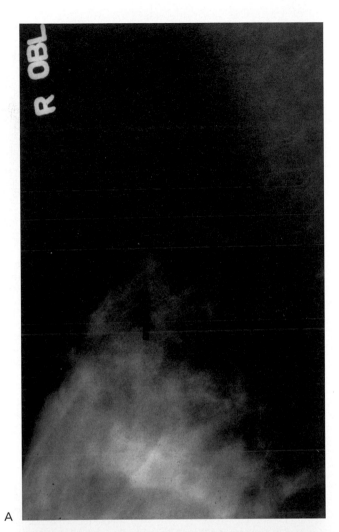

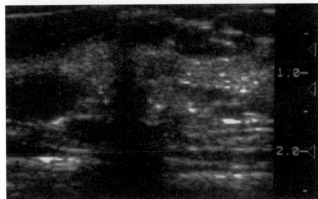

area containing calcification, and to localize the entire area for excision. Since many, if not most, cases currently will have been diagnosed by percutaneous sampling, the objective is no longer to perform a minimal-volume excision, but rather to excise with widely clear margins at the first and, hopefully, only operative procedure. Careful preoperative mammographic assessment, prudent use of core biopsy, and tailoring of the needle localization procedure should pay dividends in avoiding multiple re-excisions and in allowing selection of the appropriate surgical procedure based on the extent of disease present.

EXTENSIVE INTRADUCTAL COMPONENT

In at least 40% of cases of carcinoma manifest as calcification without mass, an invasive focus is present (Fig. 11.16). The occult invasive focus may be identifiable on ultrasound (Fig. 11.17). When there is a predominant feature of non-invasive carcinoma in association with an invasive breast cancer, extensive intraductal component (EIC) is said to be present (Fig. 11.18). Invasive carcinomas may be associated with an EIC in 25% to 30% of cases. EIC is defined as

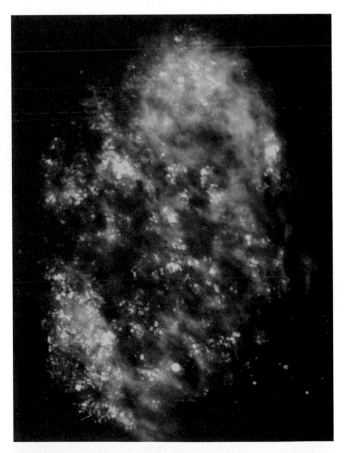

FIGURE 11.17. A: Mediolateral oblique (MLO) view from baseline screening mammogram of a 36-year-old woman showing grouped amorphous calcifications *(arrow)* located within an area of dense tissue. **(B)** Ultrasound image of area in **(A)** shows a 5 mm irregularly marginated solid mass with distal acoustic shadowing. Fine needle biopsy revealed carcinoma. Subsequent excisional biopsy showed invasive cancer.

FIGURE 11.18. MLO view of patient with florid example of extensive intraductal carcinoma associated with a palpable invasive ductal carcinoma. The invasive cancer itself, located at the top of the image, is also heavily calcified.

DCIS either prominently present within the invasive tumor component or extending beyond the invasive margin of the tumor. Data from the Joint Center for Radiation Therapy in Boston suggested an increased risk of recurrence following conservation treatment of invasive breast cancer when an EIC was present (46). Ten-year actuarial risk of recurrence was more than twice as high for patients with an EIC-positive tumor than for those with EIC-negative tumors, 32% versus 14%.

There has been some debate as to whether this difference reflects qualitative differences in tumor biology, such as decreased radiosensitivity of EIC-positive tumors relative to EIC-negative tumors, or whether the difference is quantitative, indicating only that more extensive disease is present in the breast in the case of EIC-positive tumors. If the latter were the case, EIC-positive tumors would require more extensive surgery (quadrantectomy or mastectomy) to obtain clear margins than EIC-negative tumors would. Accurate preoperative mammographic evaluation and margin assessment could significantly improve results. Holland (47) has published data showing that EIC-positive tumors have a larger subclinical burden of tumor than EIC-negative tumors. Whether the presence and extent of an EIC can be accurately assessed by mammography is not yet known.

MAMMOGRAPHIC FOLLOW-UP AFTER CONSERVATION TREATMENT OF DUCTAL CARCINOMA IN SITU

In those treated conservatively, women with DCIS have an increased risk for subsequent development of cancer in the contralateral breast as well as in the ipsilateral breast. In the NSABP B-17 trial (48), local recurrence at 8 years was 12% in patients treated with excision plus radiation compared with 27% in those treated with excision alone. In the Silverstein series recently published in the *New England Journal of Medicine* (45), the mean estimated probability of recurrence at 8 years was only 4% among patients whose margin widths exceeded 10 mm in every direction. Approximately 50% of recurrences in patients with DCIS are invasive (49). Tamoxifen appears to produce a significant reduction in invasive breast cancer in both the ipsilateral and the contralateral breast (50).

These statistics emphasize the need to closely follow patients with DCIS after conservation surgery. Most follow-up protocols involve annual mammography of the contralateral breast and a period of several (1 to 3) years of six-month follow-ups of the patient's ipsilateral breast. The rationale for the early six-month follow-ups is simply to reestablish a stable baseline. Once this has been accomplished, annual follow-up should be resumed. Most recurrences are diagnosed 3 to 5 years after treatment. Magnification views of the lumpectomy site (Fig. 11.19), particularly for those tumors that were manifest by calcification, may be

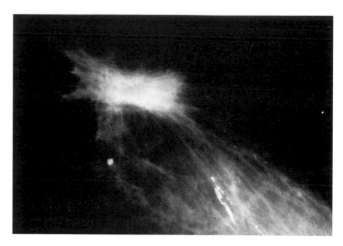

FIGURE 11.19. Detail from magnified MLO view of a patient 18 months post-lumpectomy and radiation therapy for carcinoma. The dense spiculated area is the lumpectomy scar. Below it are three different areas of calcification, all of which had developed since previous post-treatment examinations at 6 and 12 months. On the left, a single coarse round dystrophic calcification is present. In the center of the image, a linear area of relatively coarse calcification is seen anteroinferior to the scar. Coursing toward the nipple is an area of fine linear calcifications. Both of these latter sites represented recurrent ductal carcinoma in situ.

helpful during this risk period to detect recurrence as early as possible.

REFERENCES

1. Surveillance, Epidemiology, and End Results (SEER) Program Public use CD-ROM (1973–1992), Bethesda, MD: National Cancer Institute, DCPC, Surveillance Program, Cancer Statistics Branch; July, 1995.
2. Ernster VL, Barclay J, Kerlikowske K, et al. Incidence of and treatment for ductal carcinoma in situ of the breast. *JAMA* 1996; 275:913–918.
3. Fisher ER. Pathobiological considerations relating to the treatment of intraductal carcinoma (ductal carcinoma in situ) of the breast. *Cancer* 1997;47:52–64.
4. Scott MA, Lagios MD, Axelsson K, et al. Ductal carcinoma in situ of the breast: reproducibility of histological subtype analysis. *Hum Pathol* 1997;28:967–973.
5. Wright CJ. Breast cancer screening: A different look at the evidence. *Surgery* 1986;100:594–598.
6. Ketcham AS, Moffat FL. Vexed surgeons, perplexed patients, and breast cancers which may not be cancer. *Cancer* 1990;65:387–393.
7. Fisher ER, Sass R, Fisher B. Pathologic findings from the National Surgical Adjuvant Breast Project (Protocol 6). I. Intraductal carcinoma (DCIS). *Cancer* 1986;57:197–208.
8. Gump FE, Jicha DL, Ozello L. Ductal carcinoma in situ (DCIS): A revised concept. *Surgery* 1987;102:790–795.
9. Lagios MD, Margolin FR, Westdahl PR. Mammographically detected duct carcinoma in situ: Frequency of local recurrence following tylectomy arid prognostic effect of nuclear grade on local recurrence. *Cancer* 1989;63:618–624.
10. Price P, Sinnett HD, Gusterson B, et al. Ductal carcinoma in situ: Predictors of local recurrence and progression in patients treated by surgery alone. *Br J Cancer* 1990;61:869–872.

11. Betsill WL, Rosen PP, Lieberman PH, et al. Intraductal carcinoma. Long-term follow-up after treatment by biopsy alone. *JAMA* 1978;239:1863–1867.
12. Page DI, Dupont WD, Rogers LW, et al. Intraductal carcinoma of the breast: Follow-up after biopsy only. *Cancer* 1982;49:751–758.
13. Barth V, Prechtel K. *Atlas of Breast Disease*. Philadelphia: B.C. Decker, 1991.
14. Slawson SH, Johnson BA. Ductography: how to and what if? *Radiographics* 2001;21:133–150.
15. Gallager HS, Martin JE. The study of mammary carcinoma by mammography and whole organ sectioning. *Cancer* 1969;23:855–873.
16. Fisher ER, Gregoria R, Redmond C, et al. Pathologic findings from the National Surgical Adjuvant Breast Project (Protocol No. 4): I. Observations concerning the multicentricity of mammary cancer. *Cancer* 1975;35:247–253.
17. Rosen PP, Senie R, Schottenfeld D, et al. Noninvasive breast carcinoma. Frequency of unsuspected invasion and implications for treatment. *Ann Surg* 1979;189:377–382.
18. Fentiman IS, Fagg N, Millis RR, et al. In situ ductal carcinoma of the breast. Implication of disease pattern and treatment. *Eur J Surg Oncol* 1986;12:261–266.
19. Holland R, Hendriks JHCL, Verbeek ALM, et al. Extent, distribution, and mammographic/histological correlations of breast ductal carcinoma in situ. *Lancet* 1990; 335:519–522.
20. Holland R, Hendriks JHCL. Microcalcifications associated with ductal carcinoma in situ: mammographic-pathologic correlation. *Semin Diagn Pathol* 1994;11:181–192.
21. Page DI, Jensen PA. Ductal carcinoma in situ of the breast: understanding the misunderstood stepchild. *JAMA* 1996;275:948–949.
22. Page DL, Dupont WD, Rogers LW, et al. Continued local recurrence of carcinoma 15–25 years after a diagnosis of low grade ductal carcinoma-in-situ of the breast treated only by biopsy. *Cancer* 1995;76:1197–1200.
23. Holland R, Peterse JL, Millis RR, et al. Ductal carcinoma-in-situ: a proposal for a new classification. *Semin Diagn Pathol* 1994;11:167–180.
24. Simpson JF, Page DL. The role of pathology in premalignancy and as a guide for treatment and prognosis in breast cancer. *Semin Oncol* 1996;23:428–435.
25. Douglas-Jones AG, Gupta SK, Attanoos RL, et al. A critical appraisal of six modern classifications of ductal carcinoma in situ (DCIS): correlation with grade of associated invasive carcinoma. *Histopathology* 1996;29:397–409.
26. Patchefsky AS, Schwartz GF, Finkelstein SD, et al. Heterogeneity of intraductal carcinoma of the breast. *Cancer* 1989;63:731–741.
27. Silverstein MJ, Lagios MD, Craig PH, et al. A prognostic index for ductal carcinoma in situ of the breast. *Cancer* 1996;77:2267–2274.
28. Mitnick JS, Roses DF, Harris MN, et al. Circumscribed intraductal carcinoma of the breast. *Radiology* 1989;170:423–425.
29. Ikeda DM, Andersson I. Ductal carcinoma in situ: Atypical mammographic appearances. *Radiology* 1989;172:661–666.
30. Rubin E, Mazur MT, Urist MM, et al. Clinical, radiographic, and pathologic correlation of atypical hyperplasia, ductal carcinoma in situ, and ductal carcinoma in situ with microinvasion. *The Breast* 1993;2:21–26.
31. Stomper PC, Connolly JL. Ductal carcinoma in situ of the breast: Correlation between mammographic calcification and tumor subtype. *AJR Am J Roentgenol* 1992;159:483–485.
32. Dinkel HP, Gassel AM, Tschammler A. Is the appearance of microcalcifications on mammography useful in predicting histological grade of malignancy in ductal cancer in situ? *Br J Radiol* 2000;73:938–944.
33. Thomson JZ, Evans AJ, Pinder SE, et al. Growth pattern of ductal carcinoma in situ (DCIS): a retrospective analysis based on mammographic findings. *Br J Cancer* 2001;85:225–227.
34. Sickles EA. Probably benign breast lesions: when should follow-up be recommended and what is the optimal follow-up protocol? *Radiology* 1999;213:11–14, discussion 19–21.
35. Rubin E. Six-month follow-up: an alternative view. *Radiology* 1999;213:15–18; discussion 19–21.
36. Tabár L, Dean PB. *Teaching atlas of mammography*. New York: Thieme-Stratton, 1983.
37. Dershaw DD, Abramson A, Kinne DW. Ductal carcinoma in situ: Mammographic findings and clinical implications. *Radiology* 1989;170:411–415.
38. Stomper PC, Connolly JL. Ductal carcinoma in situ of the breast: Correlation between mammographic calcification and tumor subtype. *AJR Am J Roentgenol* 1992;159:483–485.
39. Cardenosa G, Mendelson E, Bassett L, et al. Appropriate imaging work-up of breast microcalcifications. American College of Radiology. ACR Appropriateness Criteria. *Radiology* 2000;215:973–980.
40. Sickles EA. Magnification mammography. In: Bassett LW, Gold RH, eds. *Breast Cancer Detection: Mammography and Other Methods in Breast Imaging*. Orlando: Grune & Stratton, 1987:111–117.
41. Jackman RJ, Nowels KW, Shepard MJ, et al. Stereotaxic large-core needle biopsy of 450 nonpalpable breast lesions with surgical correlation in lesions with cancer or atypical hyperplasia. *Radiology* 1994;193:91–95.
42. Liberman L, Dershaw DD, Rosen PP, et al. Stereotaxic core biopsy of breast carcinoma: accuracy of predicting invasion. *Radiology* 1995;194:379–381.
43. Burbank F. Stereotactic breast biopsy of atypical ductal hyperplasia and ductal carcinoma in situ lesions: improved accuracy with directional vacuum-assisted biopsy. *Radiology* 1997;202:843–847.
44. Won B, Reynolds HE, Lazaridis CL, et al. Stereotactic biopsy of ductal carcinoma in situ of the breast using an 11-gauge vacuum-assisted device: persistent underestimation of disease. *AJR Am J Roentgenol* 1999;173:227–229.
45. Silverstein MJ, Lagios MD, Groshen S, et al. The influence of margin width on local control of ductal carcinoma in situ of the breast. *N Engl J Med* 1999;340:1455–1461.
46. Boyages J, Recht A, Connolly JL. Early breast cancer: Predictors of breast recurrence for patients treated with conservative surgery and radiation therapy. *Radiother Oncol* 1990;19:29–41.
47. Holland R, Connolly JL, Getman R, et al. The presence of an extensive intraductal component following a limited excision correlates with prominent residual disease in the remainder of the breast. *J Clin Oncol* 1990;8:113–118.
48. Fisher B, Dignam J, Wolmark N, et al. Lumpectomy compared with lumpectomy and radiation therapy for the treatment of intraductal breast cancer: findings from national surgical adjuvant breast and bowel project B-17. *J Clin Oncol* 1998;16:441–445.
49. Silverstein MJ. Fortnightly review: ductal carcinoma in situ of the breast. *BMJ* 1998;317:734–739.
50. Fisher B, Dignam J, Wolmark N, et al. Tamoxifen in treatment of intraductal breast cancer: National Surgical Adjuvant Breast and Bowel Project B-24 randomised controlled trial. *Lancet* 1999;353:1993–2000.

12

ROLES OF BREAST MAGNETIC RESONANCE IMAGING FOR DUCTAL CARCINOMA IN SITU

STEVEN E. HARMS

Widespread mammographic screening has led to an improved detection of ductal carcinoma in situ (DCIS). Some centers with a large screening population have reported pure DCIS to represent as much as half of breast cancers (1,2). Before mammographic screening, however, pure DCIS accounted for only 2% of breast cancer (3).

Despite the improved detection, mammography has significant shortcomings that limit the optimal treatment of DCIS. Most experts agree that mastectomy for pure DCIS usually is not necessary. Small foci of DCIS may be effectively treated with lumpectomy instead of mastectomy (4). But while mammography can detect DCIS early, the mammographic findings poorly correlate with extent of disease (5,6). And without knowledge of extent, the surgical excision cannot be optimally planned.

At the expense of a poorer cosmetic result, there is a tendency to remove more tissue than necessary in order to avoid positive margins. Taken to the extreme, the attempt to completely excise the DCIS has led some to mastectomy. In other patients, the inability to predict extent by mammography led to a smaller excision than necessary, resulting in positive pathologic margins. This problem is compounded by the tendency of DCIS to extend in a ductal ray rather than expanding in a spherical mass. Repeat surgery is usually performed to obtain clear margins. Neither overtreatment nor under-treatment is a desirable outcome. To avoid these problems, a better definition of disease extent is needed prior to surgery.

Mammographic evaluations of DCIS cannot accurately exclude the presence of infiltrating disease. The treatment of pure DCIS could be different from an infiltrating carcinoma with extensive intraductal component. To help with treatment planning, imaging technology that can accurately exclude infiltrating carcinoma or determine the location of infiltrating disease within a large area of DCIS is needed (7).

Mammographic localization of DCIS is usually performed to identify areas of microcalcification prior to excision. The localization wire is placed in proximity to the calcifications and assumed to be near the center of the lesion (8). Unfortunately, the depiction of DCIS on mammography cannot accurately define extent. Since DCIS usually extends in a ductal ray, a spherical excision will likely lead to positive margins. A better method for localization would be to mark the margins of the DCIS rather than the center of the microcalcifications. But again, inaccuracies in definition of mammographic extent preclude the localization of margins. If an imaging examination could accurately define DCIS extent, a better localization approach would be to mark the margins. The transfer of margin information to the surgeon should lead to better lumpectomies, resulting in both fewer positive margins and better cosmesis.

In many ways, breast magnetic resonance imaging (MRI) answers many of the deficiencies of mammography in the treatment of DCIS. This chapter will discuss some of the challenges for breast MRI and the practical aspects of implementation for the management of DCIS.

TECHNICAL ISSUES

Ductal carcinoma in situ presents some difficult challenges for magnetic resonance (MR) imaging that are not encountered with imaging of neoplasms in other parts of the body. DCIS consists of tumor cells confined to the basement membrane of the duct. DCIS tends to extend along a duct or system of interconnected ducts. By definition, the cancer does not extend into surrounding parenchyma. A region involved by DCIS is also intermixed with normal tissue that surrounds the ducts. Most neoplasms visualized by MRI grow concentrically and are not intermixed with normal parenchyma.

MR images are generated as a series of three dimensional cubes called voxels. A signal intensity of each voxel represents the average of all intensities that fill the voxel. The main problem in the MR imaging of DCIS is the partial filling of a voxel by normal and tumor constituents. Although a voxel that is filled by tumor may be hyperintense, a voxel that is only partially filled with tumor will be averaged with normal intensity parenchyma. This reduction in signal may be enough to render the voxel as isointense with surroundings. This effect is called volume averaging, and is one of the major obstacles to be overcome in the successful MR imaging of DCIS (7).

Volume averaging effects can be reduced by making the voxels smaller, thereby increasing the likelihood for complete filling of the voxel by tumor cells. Voxels have three dimensions. To reduce volume averaging, the optimal voxel dimensions should be nearly symmetrical. A 1 mm voxel volume that is thick in the slice direction will have greater volume averaging effects than a 1 mm cube. Many MR breast images use a high resolution only in the in-plane dimension, which is more pleasing to the eye, but sacrifices resolution in the slice dimension. This decision will make the imaging of DCIS difficult due to volume averaging effects.

A typical rotating delivery of excitation off-resonance (RODEO) image set will have 128 1.2 mm slices with 0.7 mm in-plane resolution (9–11). This selection is an attempt to define cubic voxels to reduce volume averaging effects as much as possible (Fig. 12.1). A common commercially available high-resolution image set will reduce the number of slices to 64, increase the slice thickness to 2 to 3 mm, and reduce the in-plane voxel dimension to around 0.5 to 0.3 mm (12,13,14). The voxels with this data set will approach RODEO voxel volumes but will be elongated by the longer

slice thickness. Although these images will have higher resolution when displayed in plane, there will be greater susceptibility to volume averaging effects due to the thicker slices. A typical dynamic breast MRI will employ lower resolution, rapidly acquired images of both breasts. These images will have a slice thickness of 3 to 5 mm and an in-plane resolution of up to 2.5 mm (15,16). These voxels will have a significantly higher volume and be quite susceptible to volume averaging effects. To compound these effects, the inherent image contrast also is often sacrificed. The dynamic enhancement curves for DCIS are frequently indistinguishable from benign (17,18). For these reasons, it is difficult to detect DCIS on dynamic breast MR images.

Another way to reduce volume averaging effects is to improve lesion contrast. A microcalcification is visualized on a mammogram because of the tremendous contrast with surrounding soft tissues. Even partial filling of a voxel may be sufficient if the tissue has a high enough contrast. Contrast with surrounding tissue is provided most commonly with fat suppression. Fat suppression may be performed with a variety of methods. We prefer the RODEO method, which efficiently eliminates the excitation of a narrow bandwidth of resonance, typically fat, while providing broad excitation of off-resonance signal. Another popular method uses the excitation of a narrow resonance, typically fat, with an inversion recovery pulse and centering the projections for reconstruction space on the fat null. This method is called spacial-spectral inversion recovery (SPECIAL) (12,13,14,18). The SPECIAL method results in reduced contrast due to the intermixing of signals generated off the fat null. Subtraction is another popular method employed typically on low resolution, dynamic MR scans (15–17). Subtraction has an inherently low signal-to-noise ratio, since most of the signal is subtracted away. Many studies employing subtraction have had difficulty in identifying DCIS.

In addition to suppression of fat to improve contrast, the manipulation of ductal tissue contrast may also improve lesion contrast. The most effective method for suppressing ductal tissue signal is the use of magnetization transfer contrast (18,19). Magnetization transfer contrast is produced by the excitation of protein-bound water resonance. Water resonance occupies a broad bandwidth. To avoid overlap with free water resonance, magnetization transfer excitation is typically applied at some distance in bandwidth from free water. High power is used to better enhance the magnetization transfer effect. Most magnetization transfer applications employ an radiofrequencypulse off the free water resonance before the standard sequence. This additional pulse takes time and is more susceptible to the generation of image artifacts. Magnetization transfer effects are integrated into the RODEO process (9). Instead of pulses that are applied far from the water resonance to avoid overlap with the standard excitation, RODEO can excite bound water near the free water resonance, since both are simultaneously

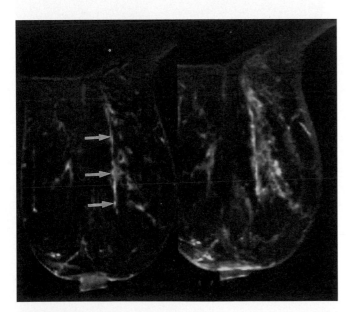

FIGURE 12.1. Volume averaging effects. An axial reformatted post-contrast RODEO image with a section thickness of 0.74 mm *(left)* is compared with the same acquisition using a 5 mm section thickness. The thinner section *(left)* depicts a linear enhancement *(arrows)* typical of ductal carcinoma in situ. The thicker section *(right)* loses the linear enhancement in a background of ductal tissue.

generated. Thus RODEO is a very efficient method for producing magnetization transfer contrast.

A key feature for the characterization of DCIS is the identification of microcalcifications. It is not commonly thought that MRI can visualize microcalcifications. Microcalcifications can produce a small perturbation in the magnetic field due to differences in magnetic susceptibility compared with surrounding tissue. The effect on the magnetic field results in a signal void over a narrow range of frequencies. The extent of this signal void is dependent upon the receiver bandwidth (number of hertz in the frequency-encoded direction). This proportional effect of the signal void will be greater with a smaller receiver bandwidth. On RODEO images, we typically use a bandwidth of 16 kHz. Other methods that depend upon more rf pulses typically use a larger bandwidth of up to 64 kHz to conserve time. This broad bandwidth may preclude the detection of small calcifications. In addition, the signal-to-noise is reduced inversely proportional to the bandwidth.

Motion artifacts can severely impair the visualization of small breast lesions, particularly in the axillary tail. The breast shares a neighborhood with the heart and lungs, some of the greatest artifact producers in the body. One major tool in the fight against motion artifacts is the use of a transmit-receive breast coil. Confining the transmit field to the breast greatly reduces the signal contribution from tissues outside the breast. Unfortunately, most commercially available breast coils are receive-only coils. The body coil is used for the transmitter, resulting in excitation of the entire 48 cm field-of-view contained within the body coil. Another problem with body coil excitation is the need for selective excitation rf pulses. Selective excitation is the combination of an rf pulse matched to a narrow bandwidth of frequencies during the presence of a magnetic field gradient. The result of selective excitation is the spatial definition of a slab of spins within the desired field-of-view. The longer rf excitation in the presence of a gradient increases the susceptibility to motion artifacts. This effect is increased by more rf pulses and longer duration pulses. RODEO does not use a selective excitation. Typical RODEO images can visualize the myocardium of the heart and the axillary tail of the breast without significant artifact. The lack of motion artifacts on the RODEO images improves the detection of axillary and internal mammary lymph nodes (20–22).

IMAGE INTERPRETATION

The interpretation of breast MR images in patients with DCIS is more problematic. As mentioned in the prior section, it is critical to have high-resolution, high-contrast images to avoid volume effects. The dynamic enhancement profiles of DCIS have significant overlap with benign tissue (17,18). Schemes that rely heavily on enhancement profiles will miss most DCIS. In addition, many dynamic breast

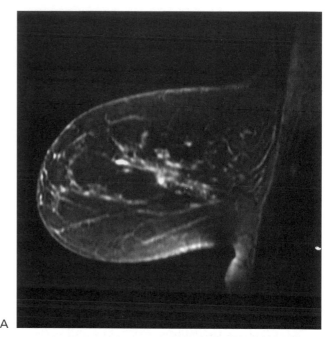

A

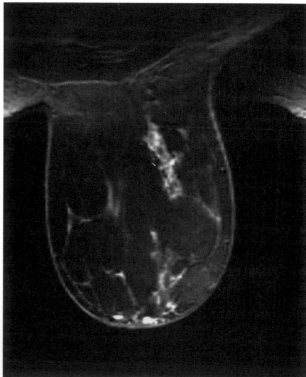

B

FIGURE 12.2. Typical ductal carcinoma in situ morphology. A sagittal post-contrast RODEO image **(A)** depicts clumped enhancement along a ductal ray. The linear nature of the clumped enhancement is better seen on **(B)**, the axial reformatted post-contrast RODEO image.

MRI protocols sacrifice spatial resolution for temporal resolution, which further compounds the problem.

DCIS will usually appear on MR images as a patch of clumped enhancement. It will often follow a ductal ray (Fig. 12.2) and have some linear or branched character. With sequences that use a narrow receiver bandwidth, small foci of

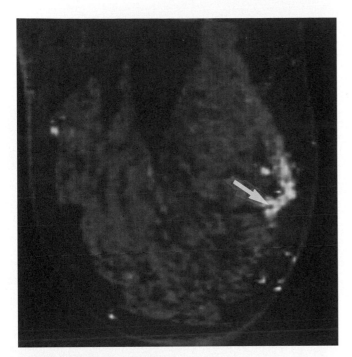

FIGURE 12.3. Microcalcifications on breast magnetic resonance (MR) imaging. This axial reformatted post-contrast RODEO image depicts microcalcifications as small, hypointense foci *(arrow)* intermixed with clumped enhancement. The hypointensity is caused by differences in magnetic susceptibility between calcium and surrounding soft tissue. This effect is best seen on MR images using a narrow receiver bandwidth. Most systems employ wider bandwidths to improve acquisition efficiency, and microcalcifications will often be missed with this approach.

low signal intensity will be intermixed with clumped enhancement (Fig. 12.3). These areas represent microcalcifications. Low signal intensity is due to the differences in magnetic susceptibility of calcification compared with surrounding soft tissue (9).

The presence of spiculation indicates a high potential for invasive disease (Fig. 12.4). Ring enhancement is highly predictive of invasive carcinoma (Fig. 12.5) (13). Surprisingly, even cases of DCIS with microinvasive cells usually exhibit some spiculation (9). It is not likely that breast MRI detects the small amount of microinvasive cells. The MRI appearance of spiculation probably is a prognostic indicator that reflects a more aggressive character for the lesion that histologically is represented as microinvasion. DCIS is often intermixed with invasive carcinoma (5). The distinction of in situ and invasive components may be used to localize or biopsy. The demonstration of extent of associated DCIS is important for surgical planning (Fig. 12.6).

It is important to distinguish DCIS from benign proliferative change. Unfortunately, this cannot always be accomplished, and needle biopsy may be indicated. Some of the key distinguishing features of benign proliferative change will be outlined. Diffuse sand-like or stippled enhancement that involves all the ductal tissue is almost never malignant (Fig. 12.7). Benign proliferative change may be

A
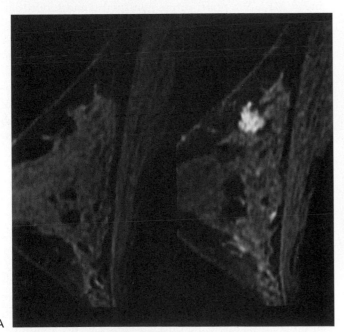

B
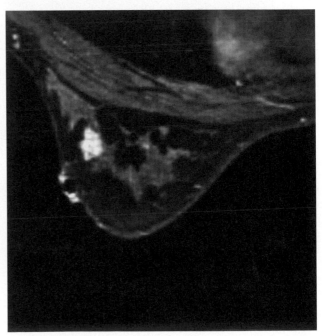

FIGURE 12.4. Ductal carcinoma in situ (DCIS) with microinvasion. Sagittal pre- *(left)* and post-contrast *(right)* RODEO images **(A)** depict an area of abnormal enhancement that is primarily clumped, but with some irregular borders. The axial reformatted post-contrast RODEO image **(B)** depicts an area of spiculation along the border of the lesion. Upon sampling at pathology, DCIS with microinvasion was identified. The magnetic resonance (MR) imaging is not depicting the small focus of abnormal cells. Instead, the MR appearance indicates a more aggressive lesion. In a sense, the MR appearance is a prognostic indicator. All of the cells of the lesion are not seen by the pathologist, but the appearance on some sections indicates a more aggressive lesion. In our experience, we have no cases of pure DCIS with a spiculated appearance.

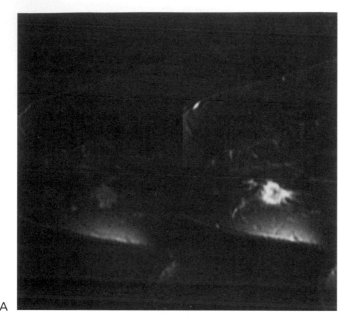

A

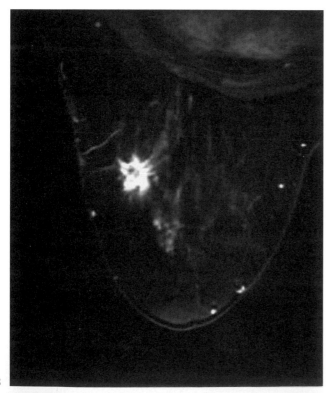

B

FIGURE 12.5. Invasive ductal carcinoma. Sagittal pre- *(left)* and post-contrast *(right)* RODEO images **(A)** show a spiculated, ring-enhancing mass in the lower breast. The axial reformatted post-contrast RODEO image **(B)** further depicts the aggressive morphologic character of this invasive ductal carcinoma. Spiculation and ring enhancement is highly predictive of invasive disease and requires biopsy.

more pronounced in the upper outer quadrant, but similar changes will be seen elsewhere in the breast. Often the stippled enhancement will become more pronounced at the periphery of the ductal tissue near the junction with subcutaneous fat. This effect can be readily distinguished from DCIS, which tends to occupy a region, usually a ductal ray. An occasional pre-menopausal patient will have florid enhancement throughout the breast.

If the opposite breast has a similar behavior, consider the possibility of hormonal stimulation during the menstrual cycle. A repeat scan 7 to 14 days past the start of menses may result in a resolution of the abnormal enhancement. We have also seen one post-menopausal woman with diffuse florid enhancement due to estrogen supplements. The MRI appearance resolved after cessation of hormonal supplements. Any focal, regional, or linear clumped enhancement may be considered a justification for needle biopsy or localization. The positive biopsy rate on these lesions should be expected to be less than for spiculated masses.

Treatment greatly affects the appearance of breast MR images. Tamoxifen therapy significantly reduces the abnormal enhancement seen with benign proliferative changes (23). In fact, breast MR imaging has been proposed as a possible surrogate end point for chemoprevention trials. Chemotherapy significantly reduces abnormal enhancement within the breast. During the course of chemotherapy, however, the water content of the breast increases. Edema is usually not a problem to distinguish from residual tumor on breast MRI. We prefer to use non-spoiled and spoiled images to aid in this distinction. Radiation therapy has been reported to produce false positive enhancement for up to 18 months following treatment. These reports used low resolution, dynamic MR imaging, and we have not found similar problems with RODEO. In our experience, the use of adjuvant or neoadjuvant therapy actually enhances the ability of breast MRI to detect residual disease. A breast MRI with persistent clumped or spiculated enhancement after adjuvant therapy should be considered suspicious.

CLINICAL USES OF BREAST MAGNETIC RESONANCE IMAGING INFORMATION

The determination of disease extent in DCIS is difficult by physical examination, mammography, or ultrasound. Accurate definition of disease extent is critical for optimal excision. Breast MRI has dramatically changed the preoperative local staging of DCIS. If multiple regions of DCIS are seen in different quadrants, a directed biopsy to the additional area may be indicated prior to committing the patient to mastectomy. If patients are indecisive between breast conservation or skin-sparing mastectomy, the MRI information on disease size and extent may be helpful in making this decision.

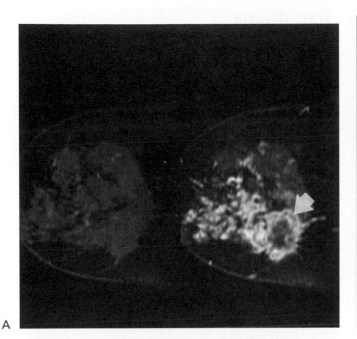
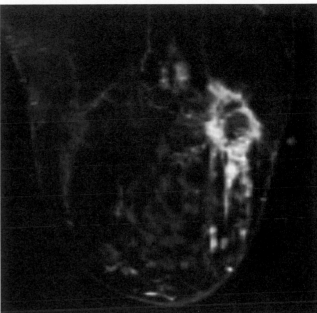

A   B

FIGURE 12.6. Ductal carcinoma in situ (DCIS) with invasive ductal carcinoma. The sagittal pre-*(left)* and post-contrast *(right)* RODEO images **(A)** depict diffuse clumped enhancement typical of DCIS. Toward the posterior aspect of the breast lies a spiculated, ring-enhancing mass *(arrow)* that represents the infiltrating ductal carcinoma. The axial reformatted post-contrast RODEO image **(B)** better depicts the spiculated enhancing mass with rays of DCIS extending anteriorly. Breast magnetic resonance imaging can accurately show regions of infiltrating carcinoma and separate areas of DCIS. This information will be helpful in planning the biopsy and surgical treatment.

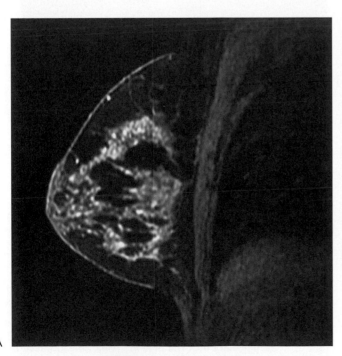
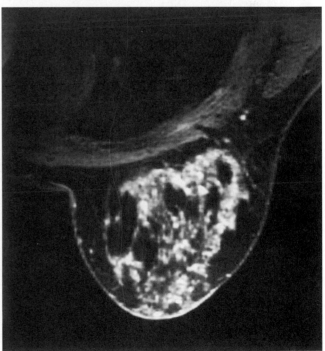

A   B

FIGURE 12.7. Benign proliferative change. The sagittal **(A)** and axial reformatted **(B)** post-contrast RODEO images depict stippled enhancement that is diffusely distributed throughout the ductal tissue. This appearance is typical of benign proliferative change and almost never represents cancer.

The presence of infiltrating disease or microinvasion may be predicted from the MRI appearance (9). This information may help plan the surgical course and identify the area for more detailed pathologic analysis. The proximity of disease to the skin, chest wall, and nipple can be accurately portrayed on breast MRI.

The positive predictive value for lymph nodes is good for breast MRI, but nodal involvement cannot be excluded. A positive node can be predicted by enlargement, enhancement with contrast, and loss of the fatty hilum. Positive nodes can also have a normal morphologic appearance.

STEREOTAXIS

Stereotaxis is an important part of any breast MRI center. If disease is detected on breast MRI that cannot be determined by any other procedure, some method for transferring this spatial information for action is required. One of our more common procedures is the localization of DCIS margins prior to surgery (Fig. 12.8). Another common indication is the needle biopsy of additional disease, where, if malignant, the information would change the surgical approach.

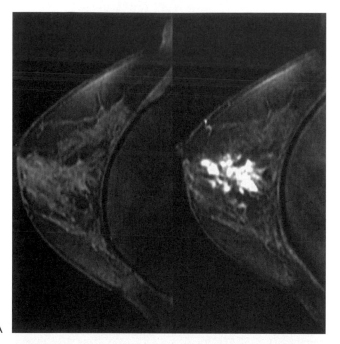

A

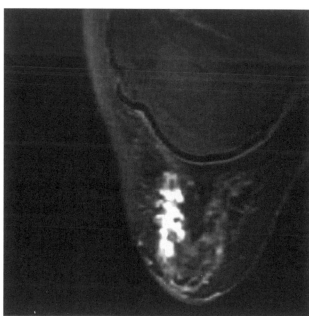

B

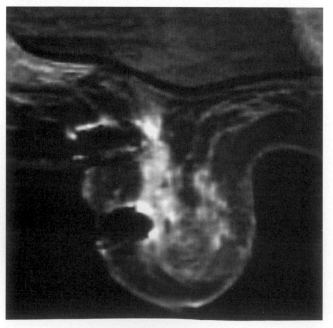

C

FIGURE 12.8. Localization of ductal carcinoma in situ (DCIS). Sagittal pre- *(left)* and post-contrast *(right)* RODEO images **(A)** show a linear band of clumped enhancement along a ductal ray in the lateral aspect of the breast. The axial reformatted post-contrast RODEO image **(B)** depicts the medial-lateral extent of the lesion. Stereotaxic magnetic resonance imaging (MRI) guidance is used to mark the boundaries of the DCIS prior to surgery. The axial reformatted RODEO image after localization wires are placed **(C)** show the anterior and posterior wires as hypointense bands due to the magnetic susceptibility effects of the MRI-compatible wires. Note that the contrast enhancement of the lesion has blended away with the background due to the redistribution of contrast that took place over the time interval of the localization. For this reason, real-time localization in an open MRI system is not feasible for lesions seen only on MRI. Accurate stereotaxis is required, and follow-up images can only confirm MRI coordinate accuracy and not location relative to a lesion.

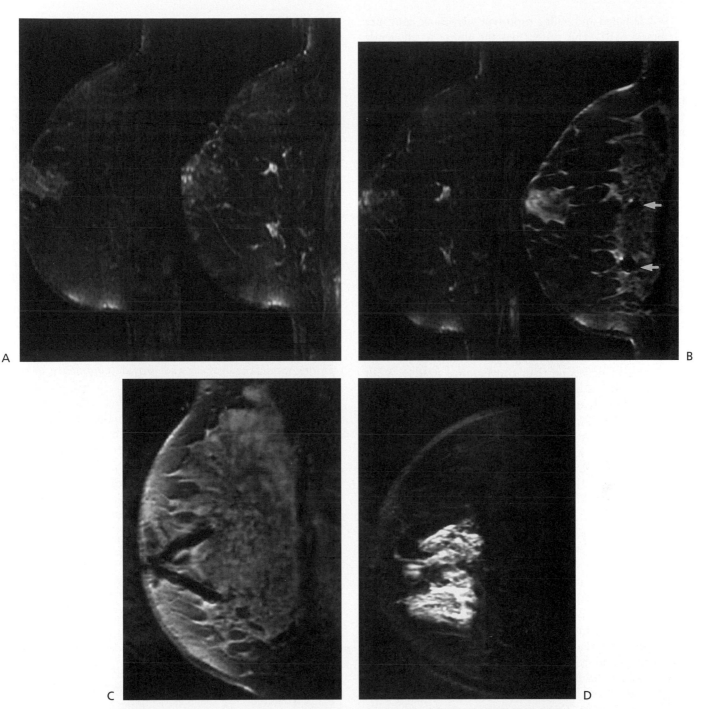

FIGURE 12.9. Hematoma localization. Sagittal pre- *(left)* and post-contrast *(right)* RODEO images **(A)** define two small spiculated enhancing masses *(arrows)* in addition to the lesion seen on mammography. A stereotaxic localization was performed to place magnetic resonance (MR)-compatible 20 gauge needles into the lesions. The hypointense zones *(arrows)* due to magnetic susceptibility effects of the needles is seen *(right)* and compared with the post-contrast RODEO image **(B)**. Our stereotaxic system allows the placement of needles at different angles through the same entry site. Different targets can be hit with a single skin preparation. The axial reformatted RODEO image depicts the needle locations. Instead of placing wire, approximately 2 cc of the patient's blood is instilled into each location. Hyperintense zones are seen on the sagittal RODEO projection image **(D)**.

We designed and built a prototype stereotaxic appliance for breast MRI. This system has the ability to efficiently and accurately target multiple areas for localization. This device has a reproducible accuracy of 2 mm. The breast is held in mild compression by two plates that are drilled throughout with 1 cm diameter holes. The breast protrudes through the holes and provides some lateral stability for the skin. This protrusion has the added advantage of being visualized on MRI. MR images are obtained to identify the lesion, and a hole is selected for access. A line is drawn on the scanner console from the target to the entry site. This line gives information on the depth from the skin and two angles. One angle is in the superior-inferior dimension; the other is in the anterior-posterior dimension. These angles are dialed into two protractors that align a laser light that resides at a distance approximately 2 feet from the patient's breast. The light point is adjusted to where it is centered on the entry site. The skin is prepped and anesthetized. The tip of the needle is placed at the site where the laser light meets the skin. The hub of the needle is then aligned with the tip, and the needle is advanced to the specified distance. MRI-compatible needles are more susceptible to deflection than conventional needles. With this system, it can be determined if the needle is off course by the deflection of the hub off the alignment with the laser light. When aligned, the hub will glow, due to the laser light reflection. If the hub is released and bounces off the beam, it will lose its glow. Correction of the needle alignment can then take place to assure accurate targeting. Multiple needles with greatly different targets can be placed through the same skin entry site.

A better way of marking lesions is needed. The typical MRI-compatible Kopans hookwires are often employed. These wires have several major disadvantages. The wire has restricted movement when pulling out, but the wire is not as restricted for advancing inward. The wire, therefore, can change position. Wires need to be placed just before the patient goes to surgery. Often this arrangement is not convenient for the patient or the radiologist. For these reasons, we developed a different marking system that uses the patient's blood as a marking agent (Fig. 12.9). Needles are placed as if wires were to be deployed. Instead of a wire, we inject approximately 2 cc of the patient's partially clotted blood through the needle. These hematoma localizations can be seen as hyperintense signal on MRI and hypointense signal on sonography. When the surgeon cuts down, the hematoma can be visualized. In the operating room, the coordination of ultrasound detection and visual confirmation can accurately define surgical margins relative to the localization. An added benefit is that the hematoma lasts for several days. MRI localization can take place well before surgery. We often localize for patients having surgery at other hospitals. Patients have even had surgery at out of state facilities after our localization. This approach would not have been practical with hookwire localizations.

SUMMARY

Breast MR imaging provides critical diagnostic information needed to significantly improve the management of DCIS. The extent of disease can be accurately determined and the presence of infiltrating components excluded. Stereotaxic procedures can precisely define the margins for better excision. The exclusion of subclinical residual disease may reduce the need for adjuvant radiation therapy. The use of breast MR imaging may validate the effectiveness of tamoxifen or other hormonal therapies for the reduction of benign proliferative changes. These are major steps toward our goal of more effective treatment with fewer side effects.

All new treatment schemes will require clinical trials for validation. Perhaps our greatest challenge is to implement timely and meaningful trials in an atmosphere of decreasing heath care resources. Many are working in clinical trial groups to integrate breast MR imaging into treatment trials for greater efficiency. Not only could breast MR imaging be validated by this approach, but its specific use in a particular therapy could be investigated. The sharing of imaging and therapy resources would improve greater awareness among clinical colleagues and provide confidence in the quality of local imaging resources.

Many of the tools described in this chapter are not commercially available. We are working to improve access, but breast MR imaging is still not recognized by some major manufacturers as a significant source of referrals. Unfortunately, without sufficient tools, breast MRI utilization cannot grow. Several small companies recently entered the market, however, and we are hopeful that widespread availability of workable devices will soon be available to most institutions.

REFERENCES

1. Silverstein MJ, Gamagami P, Colburn WJ, et al. Nonpalpable breast lesions: diagnosis with slightly over-penetrated screen-film mammography and hook wire-directed biopsy in 1014 cases. *Radiology* 1989;171:633–638.
2. Alexander HR, Candela FC, Dershaw DD, et al. Needle localized mammographic lesions: results and evolving treatment strategy. *Arch Surg* 1990;125:1441–1444.
3. Rosner D, Bedwani RN, Vana J, et al. Noninvasive breast carcinoma: results of a national survey by the American College of Surgeons. *Ann Surg* 1980;192:139–147.
4. Fisher B, Contantino J, Redmond C, et al. Lumpectomy compared with lumpectomy and radiation therapy for the treatment of intraductal breast cancer. *N Engl J Med* 1993;328:1581–1586.
5. Lagios MD, Westdahl PR, Margolin FR, et al. Duct carcinoma in situ: relationship of extent of noninvasive disease to the frequency of occult invasion, multicentricity, lymph node metastases, and short-term treatment failures. *Cancer* 1982;63:619–624.
6. Lagios MD, Margolin FR, Westdahl PR, et al. Mammographically detected duct carcinoma in situ: Frequency of local recurrence following tylectomy and prognostic effect of nuclear grade on local recurrence. *Cancer* 1989;63:618–624.
7. Soderstrom CE, Harms SE, Copit DS, et al. 3D RODEO breast MRI of lesions containing ductal carcinoma in situ. *Radiology* 1996;201:427–432.

8. Meyer JE, Kopans DB, Stomper PC, et al. Occult breast abnormalities: percutaneous preoperative needle localization. *Radiology* 1984;150:335.

9. Harms SE, Flamig DP, Hesley KL, et al. Breast MRI: rotating delivery of excitation off-resonance: clinical experience with pathologic correlations. *Radiology* 1993;187:493–501.

10. Harms SE, Flamig DP, Hesley KL, et al. Magnetic resonance imaging of the breast. *Magn Reson Q* 1992;8:139–155.

11. Harms SE, Flamig DP, Hesley KL, et al. Fat suppressed three-dimensional MR imaging of the breast. *Radiographics* 1993;13: 247–267.

12. Orel SG, Schnall MD, LiVolsi VA, et al. Suspicious breast lesions: MR imaging with radiologic-pathologic correlation. *Radiology* 1994;190:485–493.

13. Nunes LW, Schnall MD, Orel SG, et al. Breast MR imaging: interpretation model. *Radiology* 1997;202:833–841.

14. Orel SG, Mendonca MH, Reynolds C, et al. MR imaging of ductal carcinoma in situ. *Radiology* 1997;202:413–420.

15. Heywang S, Hahn D, Schmidt H, et al. Magnetic resonance imaging of the breast using gadolinium-DTPA. *J Comput Assist Tomogr* 1986;10:199–204.

16. Kaiser WA, Zeitler E. MR imaging of the breast: fast imaging sequences with and without Gd-DTPA. *Radiology* 1989;170:681–686.

17. Kuhl CK, Mielcareck P, Klaschik S, et al. Dynamic breast MR imaging: are signal intensity time course data useful for differential diagnosis of enhancing lesions? *Radiology* 1999;211:101–110.

18. Leong CS, Daniel BL, Herfkens RJ. Characterization of breast lesion morphology with delayed 3DSSMT: an adjunct to dynamic breast MRI. *J Magn Reson Imaging* 2000;11:87–96.

19. Pierce WB, Harms SE, Flamig DP, et al. Gd-DTPA enhanced MR imaging of the breast: a new fat suppressed three-dimensional imaging sequence. *Radiology* 1991;181:757–763.

20. Harms SE, Flamig DP, Hesley KL, et al. Fat suppressed three-dimensional MR imaging of the breast. *Radiographics* 1993;13: 247–267.

21. Harms SE, Flamig DP. Staging of breast cancer with magnetic resonance. *Magn Reson Imaging Clin N Am* 1994;2:273–284.

22. Harms SE, Flamig DP. MR Imaging of the breast. *J Magn Reson Imaging* 1993;3:277–283.

23. Schnall MD, Orel SG, McDermott J, et al. Breast MRI on patients taking tamoxifen. *Proc Intl Soc Magn Reson Med* 1999;7:360.

13

ULTRASOUND OF DUCTAL CARCINOMA IN SITU

A. THOMAS STAVROS

Ultrasound has traditionally and appropriately had a relatively small role in the diagnosis and evaluation of pure ductal carcinoma in situ (DCIS), but its role is expanding. Currently most cases of DCIS are detected because of the presence of microcalcifications on routine screening mammograms. In such cases, the diagnosis of DCIS is made either with stereotactically guided vacuum-assisted biopsy, or by mammographically guided needle localization excisional biopsy, and ultrasound is not usually considered necessary. However, in some cases DCIS causes a nonspecific mammographic abnormality or a palpable lump for which sonography is the best diagnostic tool we have available. In the vast majority of such cases, sonography will show a solid nodule that requires sonographic characterization, or an area that has an appearance very similar to "gray" glandular tissue, fibrocystic change, or benign proliferative disorders such as florid or papillary duct hyperplasia or tumoral adenosis.

When DCIS presents as a solid nodule on sonography, it will be characterized using a battery of multiple findings in a strict algorithmic approach. Breast cancer is far too heterogeneous to be diagnosed by single sonographic findings; therefore, we currently employ a panel of nine individual suspicious sonographic findings with a strict algorithmic approach that enables us to identify malignant solid nodules with greater than 98% sensitivity. A complete discussion of all of the findings, the complete rationale for using them, their histopathologic basis, and the techniques required to demonstrate them are beyond the scope of this chapter. However, the suspicious findings are listed according to the characteristic of the nodule being assessed in Table 13.1 and according to whether the finding is "hard," "soft," or "mixed" in Table 13.2.

Each of the nine findings is sought in each case, and if a single one of the suspicious findings is present, the nodule cannot be characterized as probably benign and must undergo biopsy. Hard findings are primarily manifestations of invasive malignancy, soft findings are primarily manifestations of DCIS or intraductal components of tumor, and mixed findings may be seen with either invasive or in situ malignancy. Soft findings generally have high sensitivity, but low positive predictive values and result in more false positives and biopsies of benign disease. On the other hand, hard findings generally have somewhat lower sensitivity but higher positive predictive values. Reliance upon only hard findings would improve positive predictive value, but would reduce sensitivity for pure DCIS and some cases of invasive tumor that contain DCIS components in the periphery.

Based on the presence or absence of findings, the number of findings, and whether or not the findings are "hard" or "soft," each nodule is assigned to a **Breast Imaging Reporting and Data System (BIRADS) category**. This risk stratification scheme was implemented by the American College of Radiology to help standardize interpretation, reporting, and adjudication of mammography results between radiologists. BIRADS classification has value for both the radiologist and the referring clinician or surgeon because the risk of malignancy and methods of management are well defined within each category. Table 13.3 lists the BIRADS categories and the expected risk of malignancy and generally accepted management for each category.

Table 13.4 shows the actual percentage risk of malignancy in 1,211 solid nodules that were prospectively assigned to BIRADS categories and subsequently underwent biopsy. Note that the actual percentage of malignant nodules falls within the range of expected risks, and that we can successfully stratify solid nodules into risk BIRADS categories with sonography. That means that we can also use standard the BIRADS management algorithms for each of the BIRADS categories.

For solid nodules, there is no BIRADS 1 category. By definition all solid nodules are abnormal, and thus, must be assigned a category of BIRADS 2 or higher. (However, DCIS that has an appearance similar to "gray glandular" tissue might be classified as BIRADS 1 and a false negative sonogram could result.) The only BIRADS 2 (definitively benign) solid breast nodules are lipomas, hamartomas, and sonographically normal-appearing intramammary lymph nodes. Nodules that are thought likely to be benign fibroadenomas or papillomas and meet strict criteria should

TABLE 13.1. NODULE CHARACTERISTICS

Nodule Characteristic	Sonographic Solid Nodule Suspicious Findings
Surface characteristics	Spiculation or thick echogenic halo Angular margins Microlobulation
Shapes	Taller than wide Duct extension Branch pattern
Internal characteristics	Shadowing Hypoechoic echotexture Calcifications

TABLE 13.2. TYPE OF FINDINGS

Type of Finding	Sonographic Solid Nodule Suspicious Findings
Hard finding of invasion	Spiculation or thick echogenic halo Angular margins Shadowing
Intermediate findings invasion or DCIS	Taller than wide Hypoechoic echotexture
Soft finding of pure DCIS or DCIS components	Microlobulation Duct extension Branch pattern Calcifications

be assigned to the BIRADS 3 category (probably benign) with the understanding that up to 2% of these nodules could be malignant. The distinction between BIRADS 2 and 3 is critical. Patients with solid nodules that are classified BIRADS 2 require no additional evaluation and can be returned to routine screening. However, patients with solid nodules that have been classified as BIRADS 3 must be informed that there is up to a 2% chance the nodule could be malignant and must be offered the choice between various types of biopsy and short interval sonographic follow-up. All solid nodules that are characterized into a BIRADS 4a or higher category must obligatorily undergo biopsy. The stratification into categories 4a, 4b, and 5 serves to sharpen our diagnostic skills, helps decide presurgical imaging and biopsy workup, and reveals where improvements in positive predictive value may be possible. Note that in categories 4b (with a 63% risk of malignancy), and category 5 (with a 91% risk of malignancy), there is little need for additional diagnostic imaging (except for staging). The patient needs biopsy. However, in category 4a, where the risk of malignancy is only 10%, ancillary imaging such as sestamibi, contrast-enhanced magnetic resonance imaging (MRI) with the rotating delivery of excitation off-resonance (RODEO) sequence, could potentially be useful (see Chapter 12). It also reveals the category in which the sonographic algorithm might be improved. It is quite possible that dropping or modifying one or two of the suspicious findings could improve the positive predictive value without adversely affecting sensitivity.

The BIRADS risk stratification scheme was developed for mammography, but is also easily adapted to and useful in sonography. We categorize every sonographic finding with one minor modification, which is that we have divided the BIRADS 4 (suspicious) category into two categories—4a (mildly suspicious) and 4b (moderately suspicious). Because the BIRADS 4 category is very large, spanning from 3% to 89% risk of malignancy, we simply divided that category at 50%, the legal definition of "probable." Thus, category 4a carries a risk of malignancy of 3% to 49%, and 4b carries a risk of 50% to 89%. Table 13.3 shows our sonographic BIRADS categories, the expected risk of malignancy, and the actual number and percentage of solid nodules in each category in the last 1,211 nodules that we have characterized that have subsequently undergone biopsy. In assigning a BIRADS category to sonographic solid nodules, the more numerous the suspicious findings and the more hard findings that are present, the higher the BIRADS category that is assigned. For example, a spiculated solid nodule that also has angular margins and that causes an intense acoustic shadow would be characterized as BIRADS 5 and would have a 91% chance of being malignant. Conversely, a nodule that had only a couple of soft findings, such as duct extension and branch pattern, would be assigned to the BIRADS 4a category in which only 10% of nodules are malignant. Biopsy of all of BIRADS 4 solid nodules yields many benign histologic diagnoses. However, most of the pure cases of DCIS that fall into this category contain only soft findings, and not sub-

TABLE 13.3. ACR BIRADS MAMMOGRAPHIC RISK CATEGORIES

BIRADS Category	Description	Risk of Malignancy	Management[a]
0[b]	Incomplete, needs additional evaluation	Uncertain	Diagnostic mamms, ultrasound, bx, etc.
1	Normal	0%	Return to routine screening
2	Benign finding	0%	Return to routine screening
3	Probably benign	≤2%[c]	Patient choice: follow-up vs. bx
4	Suspicious	>2% and <90%	Biopsy
5	Malignant	>90%	Biopsy

TABLE 13.4. PROSPECTIVE CHARACTERIZATION OF 1,211 SOLID NODULES INTO BIRADS CATEGORIES (ALL 1,211 NODULES HAVE UNDERGONE BIOPSY)

BIRADS Category	No. of Nodules Biopsied	No. of Malignant Nodules	Expected Risk of CA	Actual Risk of CA
2	15	0	0%	**0%**
3	231	1	≤2%	**0.4%**
4a	515	52	3%–49%	**10%**
4b	191	118	50%–89%	**62%**
5	259	236	≥90%	**91%**
ALL CATEGORIES	1,211	407		**34%**

No solid nodules can be classified as BIRADS 1. Overall negative to positive biopsy ratio is 2 to 1.

jecting all BIRADS 4a nodules to biopsy would cause misdiagnosis of DCIS in too many cases.

In addition to discussing the sonographic appearance and diagnosis of pure DCIS, we will also discuss the appearance of the DCIS components in mixed invasive and intraductal lesions. It is important to remember that approximately 85% of all invasive ductal (NOS) carcinomas contain varying mixtures of invasive carcinoma and DCIS. In most of these cases, the DCIS components are located predominantly in the periphery of the tumor. The presence of DCIS components in an invasive malignant nodule can be important to the sonographer and surgeon for three reasons:

i)   First, the peripherally located DCIS components of the tumor often determine the surface characteristics and shape of the lesion. Surface characteristics, such as microlobulation, and shapes, such as duct extension and branch pattern, are important sonographic features that facilitate our characterization of solid breast nodules. In some cases (especially in "circumscribed" invasive carcinomas), the DCIS components of tumor cause the only suspicious findings.

ii) Second, the sonographic detection of abnormally distended ducts and lobules extending into surrounding tissues from the periphery of the main nodule suggests the presence of extensive intraductal components. Detection of such components improves our assessment of the true extent of the lesion; may indicate the need for contrast-enhanced MRI "staging;" may guide preoperative core needle or mammotome biopsy mapping of the lesion; has the potential to aid in selecting the type and extent of surgery; and may also help to decrease the incidence of local recurrence.

iii) Finally, the exercise of evaluating the ducts extending centrally and peripherally from the main body of the tumor improves our chances of detecting and appropriately extirpating multifocal lesions. In careful serial sectioning evaluations, these lesions have been shown to represent different foci of invasion that are connected to one another by intraductal components of tumor (DCIS) within a single lesion.

SONOGRAPHY OF PURE DUCTAL CARCINOMA IN SITU

There is little question that mammography is more effective than sonography for detection of pure DCIS in most cases. The reasons are:

i)   that mammography is the primary screening test used in almost all patients in the United States, while ultrasound is used as a diagnostic test in only a small minority of patients; and

ii) that mammography is more effective that sonography at detecting and characterizing the microcalcifications that are present in a majority of patients with DCIS.

Furthermore, there is little reason to perform diagnostic sonography to evaluate BIRADS 4 or 5 calcifications. Needle localization excisional biopsy or stereotactically guided large-core needle or mammotome biopsy will usually be necessary to make the diagnosis regardless of the sonographic findings. However, despite the superiority of mammography in most cases of pure DCIS, it would be incorrect to conclude that sonography is completely incapable of demonstrating DCIS or that it has no role in diagnosing DCIS. There are several specific circumstances in which sonography may be of benefit in the evaluation of patients with DCIS. These include:

i)   evaluation of the 10% of patients in whom DCIS creates nonspecific mammographic soft tissue densities without calcifications;

ii)   evaluation of patients with negative or nonspecific mammograms in whom DCIS creates palpable abnormalities;

iii) evaluation of selected patients with nipple discharge;

iv)   2nd look ultrasound after "staging" MRI;

v)   guiding needle localization of calcifications;

vi)   preoperative percutaneous ductography and/or needle localization of intraductal papillary lesions;

vii) guiding aspiration, core needle biopsy, or needle localization for excisional biopsy of intracystic papillary lesions;

viii) guiding core needle biopsy in the rare cases when stereotactic biopsy is not possible;

ix) assessing lymph nodes in patients with large, bulky, high nuclear grade DCIS lesions in which histologic sampling is more likely to miss microscopic foci of invasion;

x) assessing calcifications prior to biopsy (enticing, but not proven).

These indications will be discussed in greater detail below.

Sonographic Technique

Sonographic demonstration of DCIS can be difficult in many cases, and is most likely to succeed if radial and antiradial scan planes are used instead of relying upon routine longitudinal and transverse planes. We know that normal terminal ducts and lobular units (TDLUs) are demonstrable, so it should not be surprising that it is also possible to sonographically demonstrate ducts and TDLUs that are abnormally distended by DCIS and other benign and malignant processes. However, demonstrating ductal and lobular anatomy requires scanning in planes that are related to breast anatomy, not arbitrary longitudinal and transverse planes. It requires that scan planes be in the long (radial) and short (antiradial) axes of the breast lobes and major mammary ducts, which course in a generally radial fashion away from the nipple (Fig. 13.1).

Sonographic Findings

DCIS represents of spectrum of diseases rather than a single entity. Therefore, it should not be surprising that DCIS may cause a wide spectrum of sonographic findings. These findings vary with the site of origin, nuclear grade, and extent of DCIS. Most cases of DCIS arise *de novo* within the lobules and/or peripheral ducts, and have sonographic features that are those of DCIS, i.e., abnormal enlargement of ducts and lobules. However, a small percentage of DCIS lesions arise within pre-existing benign lesions such as intraductal or intracystic papillomas and radial scars. In such cases, the sonographic findings may reflect of the features of the underlying lesion rather that of the DCIS.

Cases of DCIS that are evaluated with and/or detected by sonography rather than as isolated mammographic calcifications generally represent only a subset of all patients with DCIS. This subset is more likely to be larger than non-palpable cases that present with calcifications as the sole mammographic finding. This subset is also more likely to be of high nuclear grade.

The sonographic findings of DCIS include:

i) abnormal distention of large and/or small ducts and TDLUs,

ii) solid nodules with microlobulation, duct extension, or branch pattern,

iii) intraductal papillary nodules,

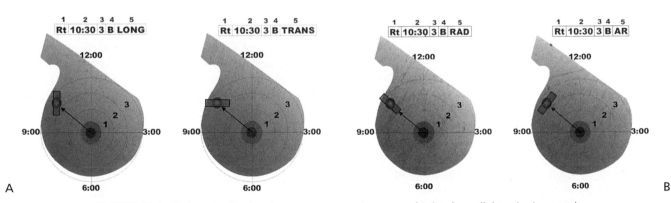

FIGURE 13.1. A: Longitudinal and transverse scan planes are obtained parallel to the long and short axes of the thorax. While such scan planes are very useful in most body parts scanned with ultrasound, they are less useful in the breast than elsewhere. The anatomy planes of the breast are not oriented longitudinally or transversely with respect to the thorax, except exactly in the 12-o'clock, 3-o'clock, 6-o'clock, and 9-o'clock positions. Lesions that lie in the upper outer quadrants of the breast, where most breast tissue and lesions lie at oblique angles to the longitudinal and transverse planes. **(B)** The radial scan plane extends out from the nipple, as would the spoke from the hub of a wheel. The antiradial plane lies at 90° relative to the radial plane. The radial plane is parallel to the longitudinal plane at 6-o'clock and 12-o'clock, and parallel to the transverse plane at exactly 3-o'clock and 9-o'clock. The antiradial plane is parallel to the longitudinal plane at exactly 3-o'clock and 9-o'clock and parallel to the transverse plane at exactly 12-o'clock and 6-o'clock. The major lobar ducts extend out from the nipple in radial fashion. Thus, radial scan planes roughly parallel the long axis of the lobar ducts. The true radial plane is the starting point of lesion assessment. In order to assess the relationship of a lesion to the ductal system, the scan plane may need to be adjusted slightly off the true radial plane because of tortuosity of the central ducts or the location of peripheral lesions in branch ducts.

iv) intracystic papillary lesions,

v) "gray" glandular tissue, or

vi) calcifications within solid nodules or "gray glandular" tissue.

Identifying DCIS at sonography is 3-step process:

i) First, enlargement of the ducts and/or lobules must be detected. This is complicated by the fact that the ducts and lobules are not grossly distended in all cases of DCIS. Most cases of low nuclear grade DCIS and some cases of intermediate nuclear grade DCIS do not grossly distend ducts and lobules.

ii) Second, ducts and lobules that are abnormally distended by DCIS must be distinguished from those that are enlarged by benign processes. Neoplasm is not the only cause of ductal and lobular enlargement. Duct ectasia and benign proliferative disorders, such as florid duct hyperplasia, can enlarge ducts in a fashion that is indistinguishable from DCIS and fibrocystic change. Benign proliferative disorders such as adenosis, florid duct hyperplasia, and papillary apocrine metaplasia can also enlarge lobules in a manner that is sonographically indistinguishable from DCIS.

iii) Finally, some cases of DCIS may develop in pre-existing pathologic structures such as intraductal papillomas or radial scars. Recognizing that DCIS may lie within such lesions is important. In other cases, DCIS attracts attention to itself by becoming encysted. The dominant features of DCIS in such cases will be that of a complex cyst, and the diagnostic difficulty is in distinguishing the relatively uncommon DCIS-containing complex cyst from the innumerable complex cysts that are part of the broad spectrum of fibrocystic change.

The ability of ultrasound to detect abnormally enlarged ducts and lobules and to distinguish them from the enlarged ducts and lobules caused by benign fibrocystic change or benign proliferative disorders depends greatly upon the nuclear grade of the lesion. Enlargement of ducts and lobules and creation of a solid nodule or gray glandular appearance are all more likely to occur to a degree sufficient to cause a palpable lump or mammographic soft tissue opacity when the lesion is high nuclear grade (HNG) DCIS. There are four histologic mechanisms by which DCIS can distend a duct or intralobular ductule:

i) First, solid tumor may expand the duct or ductule.

ii) Second, necrotic debris may distend the lumen of the duct or ductule.

iii) Third, DCIS may incite periductal inflammatory reaction.

iv) Finally, DCIS may incite a periductal desmoplastic response.

All four mechanisms of ductal and/or intralobular ductular enlargement are not necessarily present in all cases. In some cases, only one mechanism is present, while in others two, three, or even all four are present. HNG DCIS is much more likely to enlarge the ducts or ductules by any of these four mechanisms than is low nuclear grade (LNG) DCIS. Of course, intermediate nuclear grade (ING) has an intermediate likelihood of grossly distending ducts and lobules. HNG DCIS does not necessarily always enlarge ducts and lobules enough to be sonographically obvious, and it would be untrue to state that LNG DCIS never does. Gross enlargement of ducts and lobules by DCIS to a degree that is sufficiently detectable sonographically is a simple matter of percentages, and is more likely the higher the nuclear grade and less likely the lower the nuclear grade.

In addition to these four methods of ductal and lobular enlargement, some believe that HNG DCIS creates mammographic soft tissue densities and palpable masses by forming completely new ducts/ductules in addition to enlarging pre-existing ducts and lobules. Based upon the sonographic appearance of some cases of HNG DCIS, we believe there is some validity to this viewpoint. In such cases, the neoplastic ducts appear far too numerous and too closely packed to be caused by tumor growing within pre-existing ducts.

The severity of distention of ducts and lobules (and possible formation of new ducts) is the key to sonographic detection. However, recognition of abnormal neoplastic enlargement is limited in cases where benign fibrocystic change (FCC) and benign proliferative disorders (BPD) such as adenosis, florid or papillary duct hyperplasia, and papillary apocrine metaplasia cause the surrounding non-neoplastic ducts and lobules to be enlarged. Thus, it is the relative size of neoplastic to non-neoplastic ducts and lobules that determines sonographic sensitivity for DCIS. Even though LNG DCIS that does not grossly enlarge ducts and lobules can be resolved and identified sonographically, it cannot necessarily be distinguished from benign causes of ductal and lobular enlargement, which may cause similar or greater degrees of enlargement. Complicating things even further is the highly variable size of normal TDLUs and the highly variable effect that FCC and BPD can have on the size of ducts and lobules. These non-neoplastic TDLUs vary greatly in size not only from patient to patient and from the right breast to the left but from one quadrant to another, and even within the same quadrant. Therefore, to sonographically detect DCIS, the lesion must either create a discrete solid nodule or enlarge ducts and lobules out of proportion to the degree of enlargement of the TDLUs that are most severely affected by FCC or BPD. High nuclear grade DCIS is more likely to make the involved ducts and lobules grossly disproportionate to the surrounding non-neoplastic ducts and TDLUs than is low nuclear grade DCIS. This is why LNG DCIS is more likely to be missed by sonography. The percentage of ING DCIS cases where ducts and lobules are disproportionately enlarged is intermediate between that of HNG and LNG.

The DCIS site of origin may be central (from large ducts or centrally located TDLUs) or peripheral (from TDLUs or peripheral ducts). Peripheral origin is far more common than central origin. Many centrally arising DCIS lesions originate in pre-existing papillomatous lesions.

The two most common sonographic appearances for sonographically visible centrally arising HNG DCIS are:

i) a bulky, solid, hypoechoic mass, and
ii) one or more distended solid ducts extending peripherally from the subareolar region.

When HNG DCIS forms a bulky mass, its long axis is radially oriented and parallel to the long axis of a breast lobe. Such masses are often so long that they exceed the length of most small parts probes, requiring split-screen "combine" images, virtual convex image display, or extended field of view to show the entire long axis of the lesion (Fig. 13.2). The mass is usually hypoechoic and shows evidence of enhanced through transmission (Fig. 13.3). Calcifications are often visible sonographically, although somewhat less frequently than they are mammographically. In many cases, it can be shown than each calcification lies within its own microlobulation that represents an enlarged duct containing central necrosis (Fig. 13.4). The calcifications may lie within a homogeneous nodule, a sheet of gray tissue, or within individual ducts and lobules. Calcifications will be discussed in greater detail later in this chapter. In the short axis or antiradial views, the mass is often heavily microlobulated, es-

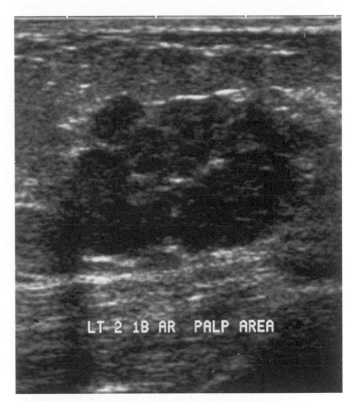

FIGURE 13.3. Most high nuclear grade ductal carcinoma in situ lesions are hypoechoic and demonstrate enhanced through transmission.

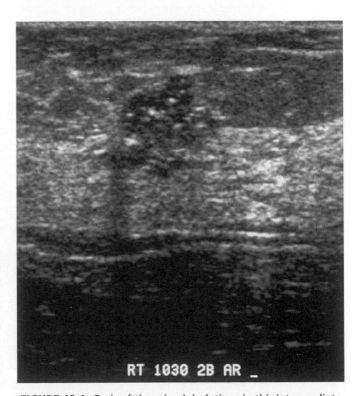

FIGURE 13.4. Each of the microlobulations in this intermediate nuclear grade ductal carcinoma in situ lesion represents a duct distended with tumor. The bright echoes centered within the microlobulations are calcifications within the necrotic debris in the central lumen of the tumor-filled ducts.

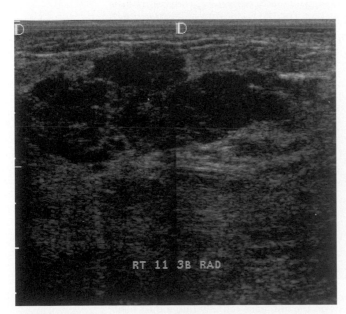

FIGURE 13.2. This bulky high nuclear grade ductal carcinoma in situ lesion is so large that combined split-screen images are necessary to display it. Such lesions are likely to contain areas of microscopic invasion.

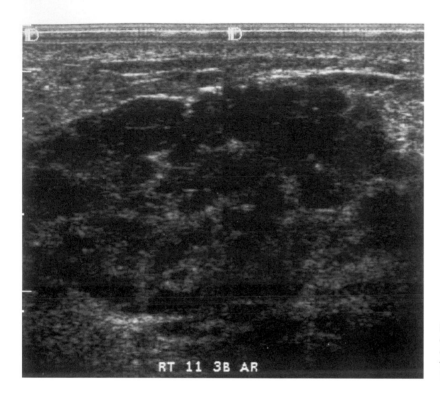

FIGURE 13.5. Microlobulations involve both the center and the surface of this high nuclear grade ductal carcinoma in situ lesion. The microlobulations represent either tumor-filled ducts or cancerized lobules.

pecially near the nipple. The microlobulations not only involve both the surface of the nodule and its interior (Fig. 13.5). Each microlobule represents either a duct or ductule distended with DCIS or a cancerized lobule. The tumor-filled ducts often appear more numerous and closely packed than would be the case if the DCIS were involving only the underlying normal ductal system, suggesting that the tumor forms new ducts as it grows (Fig. 13.6). Color or power Doppler studies usually show these bulky masses to be quite vascular (Fig. 13.7). The increased vascularity is likely caused by a combination of both tumor neovascularity and inflammatory hyperemia. High nuclear grade tumors often

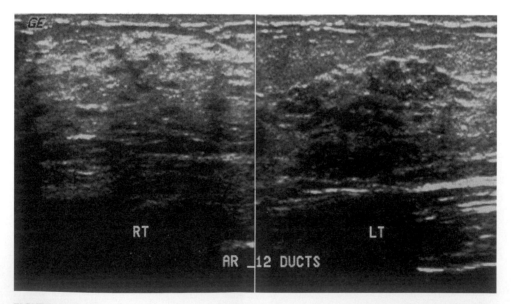

FIGURE 13.6. This split screen of mirror image locations in the 12-o'clock positions of the right and left breast shows innumerable microlobulations on the left, each representing a duct filled with high nuclear grade ductal carcinoma in situ. Many of the ducts contain calcifications within the central debris. The tumor-filled ducts are so numerous compared with the normal ducts on the contralateral side that one would have to question whether the tumor is forming its own ducts rather than merely affecting the underlying ducts.

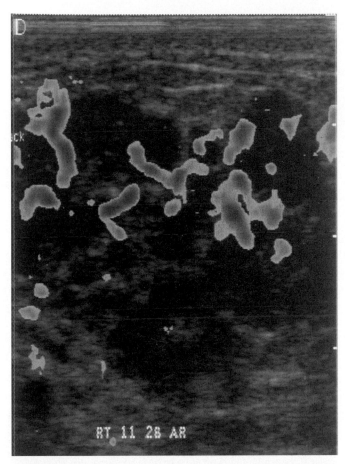

FIGURE 13.7. While low and intermediate nuclear grade ductal carcinoma in situ (DCIS) may not be hypervascular, high nuclear grade DCIS usually is.

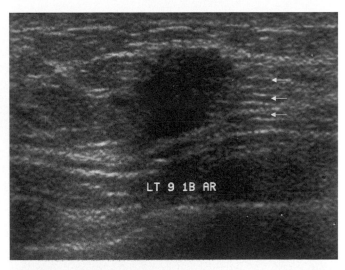

FIGURE 13.8. Spiculations are mammographic findings that have been applied directly to sonography. Spiculation is a "hard" sonographic finding suggesting the presence of invasive malignancy.

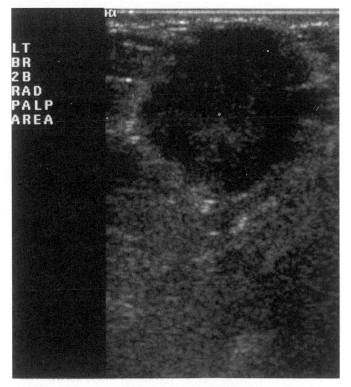

FIGURE 13.9. The thick echogenic halo surrounding this lesion represents spiculations too small to resolve sonographically. Because it represents unresolved spiculations, it, too, is a "hard" sonographic finding suggesting the presence of invasive malignancy.

incite a lymphoblastic or plasmacytic periductal inflammatory response. The mass is obviously suspicious sonographically, and routinely classified as BIRADS 4a, 4b, or 5, thus mandating biopsy. However, one of the chief diagnostic problems is to sonographically determine whether or not there is an invasive component, or whether the lesion is pure DCIS. This is a difficult problem, and is not often sonographically possible with absolute certainty. However, in many cases, the presence of one or more "hard" sonographic findings can suggest the presence of invasive components. Spiculations (Fig. 13.8), a thick, echogenic rim or halo around the mass (Fig. 13.9), angular margins (Fig. 13.10), and/or shadowing (Fig. 13.11) suggest the presence of invasion, but are not absolutely definitive. Evaluation of the points at which Cooper's ligaments intersect the mass can also be helpful, especially if there is evidence of cancerous lobules within the ligament (Figs. 13.10 and 13.11). Any extension of tumor beyond the cancerous lobule must represent invasion, since there are no ducts beyond the lobule (Fig. 13.12). Additionally, sonographic evaluation of the axilla may be helpful in determining whether there is an inva-

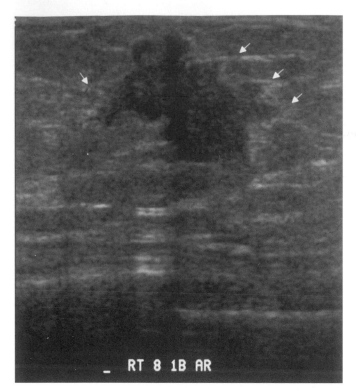

FIGURE 13.10. Angular margins (described in the literature as jagged or irregular margins) is another "hard" sonographic finding suggesting the presence of invasion. Note that the base of Cooper's ligaments *(arrows)* represents a path of low resistance to invasion, and therefore, is a common site for angular margins to occur.

sive component. The presence of an abnormal axillary lymph node implies that the tumor has at least one area of microscopic invasion (Fig. 13.13). In some cases, ultrasound-guided core biopsy of areas suspicious for invasion and/or abnormal-appearing axillary lymph nodes can preoperatively confirm the presence of invasion and/or lymph node metastasis. It is very important that ultrasound-guided biopsy be directed to the precise areas within the nodule that are suspicious for invasion, since random sampling of the tumor is more likely to under diagnose the presence of invasion.

The other sonographic appearance of central HNG DCIS is that of grossly enlarged ducts, particularly subareolar ducts. These ducts appear hypoechoic, and have normal or enhanced through transmission (Fig. 13.14). There may be sonographically visible calcifications within the duct (Fig. 13.15). The tumor often appears to reach the nipple, and it may be difficult to determine with certainty whether the nipple is involved (subclinical Paget's disease), because the portion of the duct deep to the nipple is not well defined due to the fact that it angles steeply away from the transducer, creating a suboptimally steep angle of incidence with the ultrasound beam (Fig. 13.16). There are special maneu-

vers for demonstrating the subareolar ducts and even the duct within the nipple. The extent of duct involvement varies greatly. In some cases, only a single subareolar duct appears enlarged (Fig. 13.17). In other cases, calcifications within a non-distended duct extend into the nipple (Fig. 13.18). Only one lobar subareolar duct is generally involved, but the tumor may extend into multiple branches (Fig. 13.19). In other cases, abnormally distended solid ducts are present throughout an entire quadrant of the breast (Fig. 13.20). The appearance of large, solid subareolar ducts is not specific for DCIS, and can be seen in benign papillomas and in chronic ductal ectasia. Papillomas may assume a very elongated shape, appearing to fill a duct and even its branches (Fig. 13.21). We have also been fooled by chronic ductal ectasia in which debris has layered (Fig. 13.22), or in which chronic periductal mastitis has led to periductal and intraductal fibrosis (Fig. 13.23). Periductal fibrosis in chronic duct ectasia can involve relatively large portions of a breast lobe, and can be indistinguishable from DCIS, distending many ducts' branches within a breast lobe (Fig. 13.24). Ducts involved with chronic ductal ectasia can even have central calcifications that simulate those in DCIS.

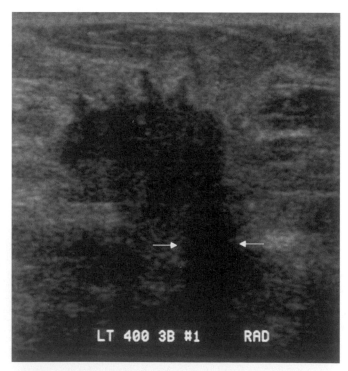

FIGURE 13.11. Complete or partial (as in this case) acoustic shadowing *(arrows)* deep to the lesion suggests a very high component of internal desmoplasia, a "hard" finding suggesting invasive malignancy. While high nuclear grade ductal carcinoma in situ (DCIS) may incite a periductal desmoplastic response, the degree of desmoplasia with pure DCIS is usually inadequate to cause acoustic shadowing. Acoustic shadowing is more typical of low histologic grade invasive malignancy. High-grade invasive ductal carcinomas usually exhibit enhanced through transmission.

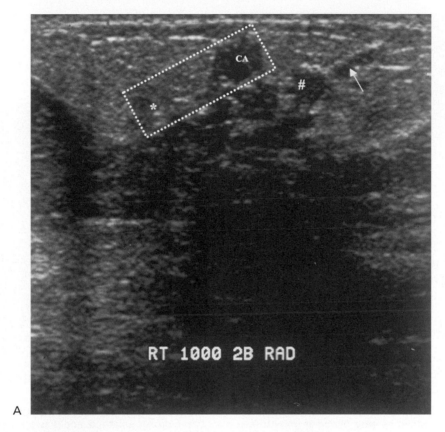

A

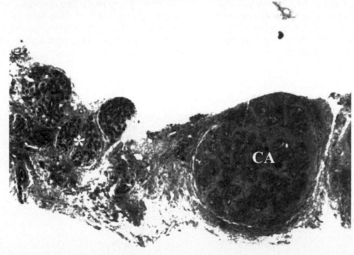

B

FIGURE 13.12. A: This high nuclear grade ductal carcinoma in situ (DCIS) lesion exhibits florid cancerization of lobules. The rectangular box represents the path of the core needle biopsy documenting the cancerized lobules. The large hypoechoic lobule in the upper left part of the box is cancerized *(CA)*. The isoechoic lobule in the lower left aspect of the box *(*)* is histologically normal. Note that there are other cancerized lobules. Beyond one of the additional cancerous lobules is a growth of tumor within Cooper's ligament *(arrow)*. Since there is no ductal system beyond the lobule, this must represent microscopic disease. In fact, after seeing this, we examined the axilla and found an abnormal-appearing lymph node. Lymph node biopsy proved the presence of metastatic carcinoma and the presence of invasion in a lesion that had mistakenly been diagnosed as pure DCIS on random sectioning histologic technique. Resectioning the lumpectomy specimen with serial section technique revealed the small focus of invasion that had initially been missed. While sonography is not by any means "microscopic," a thorough understanding of breast anatomy and growth patterns of DCIS can be remarkably revealing. **(B)** Histologic specimen from core needle biopsy path shown in **(A)**. Note the cancerized lobule *(CA)* and the normal lobule *(*)* that were seen prior to biopsy sonographically.

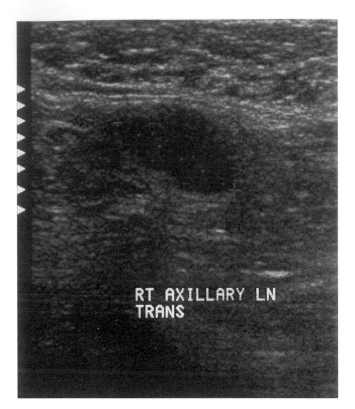

FIGURE 13.13. This axillary lymph node is morphologically abnormal. The axilla was scanned because of tumor growth seen within Cooper's ligament shown in Figure 13.12. Ultrasound-guided core needle biopsy showed metastatic breast carcinoma, indicating that a lesion histologically diagnosed as pure DCIS, in fact, contained an undiagnosed area of invasion. This was confirmed by re-sectioning the lumpectomy specimen.

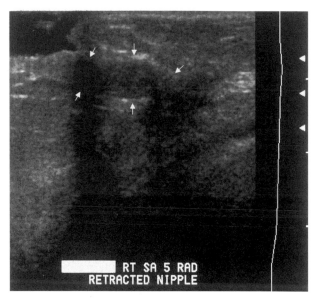

FIGURE 13.14. Central high nuclear grade ductal carcinoma in situ (HNG DCIS) may involve a single subareolar duct that becomes grossly enlarged, and is associated with nipple retraction. The nipple was retracted clinically and also on mammography. As suspected because of nipple retraction, histologic evaluation of the mastectomy specimen revealed high-grade invasive carcinoma with extensive intraductal components rather than pure HNG DCIS.

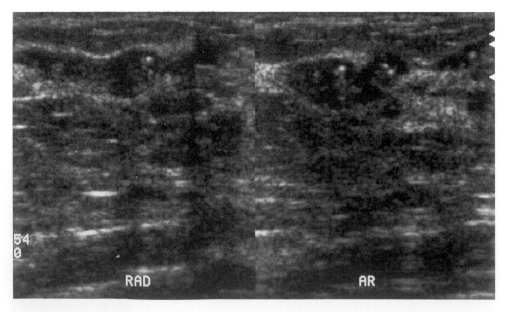

FIGURE 13.15. The central ducts that are enlarged with high nuclear grade ductal carcinoma in situ contain multiple calcifications.

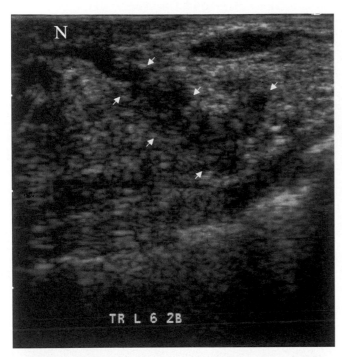

FIGURE 13.16. Because of the oblique angle of the subareolar ducts that are involved with ductal carcinoma in situ *(arrows)*, it may be difficult to determine whether or not the nipple *(N)* is involved.

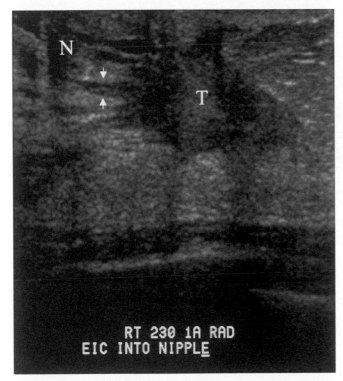

FIGURE 13.17. Two-handed compression technique was used to create a better angle of incidence with the subareolar and intra-nipple ducts, and shows a duct extension of ductal carcinoma in situ (DCIS) extending from the main body of invasive carcinoma *(T)* into the carcinoma into the base of the nipple *(arrow)*. This image was obtained after 6 weeks of induction chemotherapy. The main body of invasive tumor regressed 75% in volume, but the DCIS components of the tumor did not regress. At mastectomy, non-necrotic, apparently viable tumor remained within the ducts in the base of the nipple.

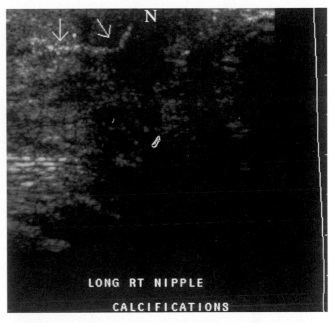

FIGURE 13.18. Sonography shows ductal carcinoma in situ (DCIS) calcifications within a non-distended duct *(arrows)* extending into the nipple *(N)*. This was missed on the routine diagnostic mammogram because of overpenetration of the skin line, but was demonstrable on spot compression mammograms obtained after sonography. Mastectomy showed low and intermediate nuclear grade DCIS extending into the nipple.

In most cases, the secretory calcifications of duct ectasia are well circumscribed linear and branching calcifications that are mammographically definitively benign (Fig. 13.25). Such calcifications can also be sonographically demonstrated within solid appearing, but normal size ducts (Fig. 13.25). However, in some cases, especially when associated with severe periductal fibrosis, the secretory calcifications have a suspicious mammographic appearance (granular, less well-defined and smaller linear forms, pleomorphic) (Fig. 13.26). In such cases, the sonographic appearance is also more suspicious and much more difficult to distinguish from centrally occurring HNG DCIS. Even though the central lumen that contains the calcifications is severely compressed by the surrounding exuberant periductal fibrosis, the sonographic appearance is that of a central calcification within an abnormally enlarged, solid-appearing duct, because sonography is unable to distinguish intraductal tumor from periductal fibrosis (Fig. 13.26). The similarities in the onographic appearance of chronic ductal ectasia and HNG DCIS with comedonecrosis should not be surprising since their gross pathologic appearance is so similar; even the terms used to describe the gross appearance are similar—comedocarcinoma and comedomastitis. Obviously, one would not want to proceed with mastectomy for extensive duct involvement such as this without histologic proof that the lesion is, in fact, DCIS rather than chronic ductal ectasia.

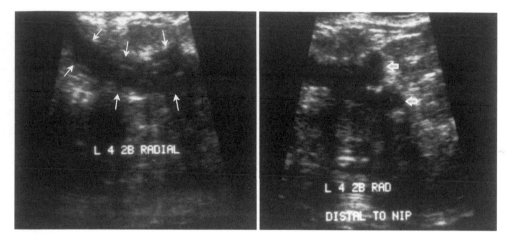

FIGURE 13.19. Centrally located high nuclear grade ductal carcinoma in situ generally involves a single subareolar lobar duct *(small arrows, left image)*, but peripherally may involve many branches *(large arrows, right image)*.

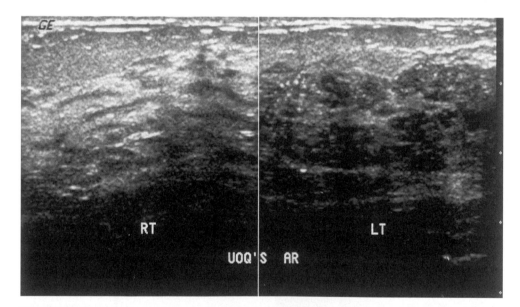

FIGURE 13.20. Ductal carcinoma in situ may involve a whole breast lobe, as in this case. These split-screen images show the upper outer quadrant mirror image locations in the right and left breasts. The ducts in the right breast are normal, but all of the ducts throughout the field of view in the left upper quadrant are abnormally enlarged, and many contain punctate echoes representing central calcifications.

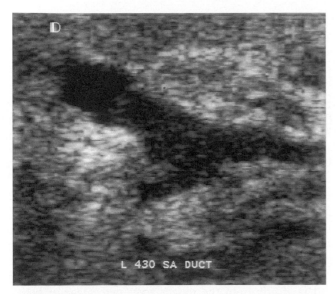

FIGURE 13.21. Large duct papillomas that have elongated along the course of the duct may greatly distend the central duct and even involve branch ducts. The sonographic appearance is indistinguishable from centrally located high nuclear grade ductal carcinoma in situ (DCIS) requiring biopsy. Approximately 6% of such large papillomas contain DCIS, and another 7% contain atypical ductal hyperplasia.

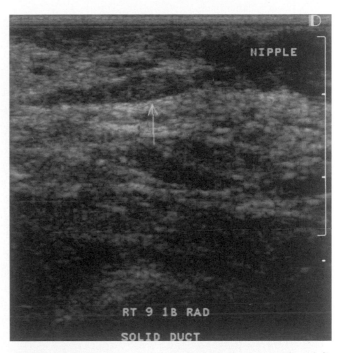

FIGURE 13.23. Chronic duct ectasia with severe periductal fibrosis may be indistinguishable from centrally located high nuclear grade ductal carcinoma in situ. This case required biopsy for diagnosis. The periductal fibrosis had completely compressed the duct lumen and the solid material that appears to lie within the duct actually represents the periductal fibrosis. The duct lumen is so severely compressed by the surrounding fibrosis that it is virtually obliterated and not sonographically visible.

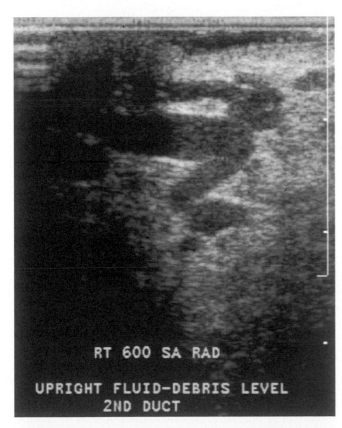

FIGURE 13.22. Chronic duct ectasia that contains a fluid debris level may simulate centrally located HNG DCIS. Ballottement of the duct caused the debris to swirl and move within the duct secretions, allowing the distinction to be made in this case.

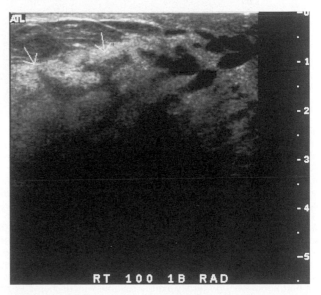

FIGURE 13.24. Chronic duct ectasia and periductal mastitis resulting in periductal fibrosis may involve peripheral ducts as well as central ducts. As is the case for central duct involvement, the sonographic appearance is indistinguishable from that of ductal carcinoma in situ. Both processes may involve an entire lobe.

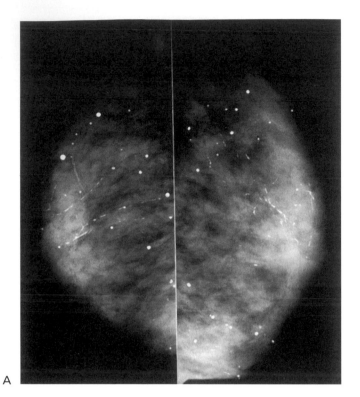

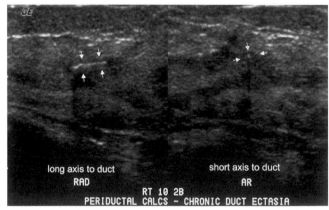

FIGURE 13.25. A: Chronic duct ectasia can lead to secretory calcifications that have a typically benign (BIRADS 2) rod-like appearance mammographically and that should not be confused with suspicious intraductal calcifications that are associated with ductal carcinoma in situ (DCIS). **(B)** The benign secretory calcifications associated with chronic duct ectasia can be demonstrated as bright linear echoes within the duct lumen in long axis images of the duct and punctate echoes within the lumen in images obtained at short axis to the ducts. Note that the duct is mildly, but not grossly distended. This sonographic appearance, however, is not as definitively benign as the mammographic appearance, and is sonographically indistinguishable from the calcifications associated with low or intermediate nuclear grade DCIS. Thus, the mammogram is generally a more reliable way to characterize secretory calcifications. (Note that these calcifications are large and dense enough to cause an acoustic shadow on the short axis image, a finding that could be seen with high nuclear grade DCIS, but would rarely be seen with low nuclear grade DCIS.)

The sonographic appearances of DCIS described above are typically those of HNG DCIS. LNG DCIS is sonographically visible in a much smaller percentage of cases because it is less likely to enlarge ducts and lobules enough for them to be distinguished from FCC and BPD, and because the lack of surrounding enlarged ducts and/or lobules tends to make the punctate echoes of LNG DCIS calcifications difficult to distinguish from the surrounding heterogeneously hyperechoic fibroglandular elements. However, LNG DCIS is sonographically visible in some cases. Most cases of sonographically visible LNG DCIS are secondary and develop within pre-existing benign lesions such as intraductal or intracystic papillomas or within the benign proliferative change that occurs in the periphery of radial scars. *De novo* cases of LNG DCIS are much less likely to be sonographically visible. Thus, the appearance of the smaller percentage of cases where LNG DCIS is sonographically visible differs greatly from the much larger percentage of HNG DCIS that is sonographically visible. The sonographic appearance of HNG DCIS is caused by gross enlargement of ducts and lobules, periductal stromal and inflammatory response, and intraductal calcifications, while the sonographic appearance of LNG DCIS is merely a reflection of the appearance of the pre-existing lesion from which the LNG DCIS arose.

There are two general patterns of sonographic findings for secondary LNG DCIS that arises in a pre-existing lesion—a central pattern and a peripheral pattern. The peripheral pattern reflects origin within the TDLU (most commonly within the periphery of a radial scar or sclerosing adenosis), while the central pattern usually reflects origin within the surface epithelium of pre-existing papillomas. LNG DCIS certainly arises peripherally far more commonly that it arises centrally. However, the more common peripherally arising LNG DCIS is usually detected because of mammographically visible microcalcifications that lead to stereotactically guided vacuum-assisted large-core needle biopsy, and are not routinely sonographically evaluated. On the other hand, the less commonly occurring, centrally arising LNG DCIS develops within pre-existing intraductal papillomas or intracystic papillomas that cause nipple discharge or palpable or mammographic abnormalities for which sonographic evaluation is particularly well-suited. Thus, the sonographically visible LNG DCIS lesions tend to be part of a small central subset of all LNG DCIS lesions. The sonographic appearance of central LNG DCIS is merely that of the intraductal or intracystic papillomas in which the DCIS arose, and is not at all unique to DCIS. The sonographic pattern varies greatly, depending upon the length and width of the underlying papillary lesion, involvement of branches, the distribution of fluid within the ductal system, and the presence or absence of a cyst. The wide range of appearances of centrally arising LNG DCIS and the underlying papillary lesions is shown in Figure

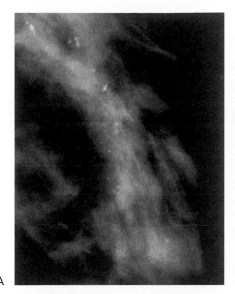 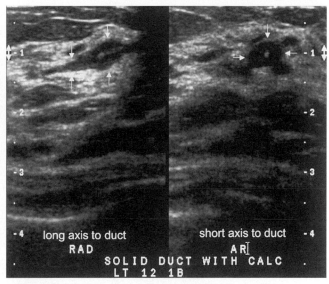

FIGURE 13.26. A: While chronic duct ectasia may lead to classically benign secretory calcifications in many cases, in some cases it may cause calcifications that are granular, less well-defined linear, and pleomorphic forms that are more mammographically suspicious for ductal carcinoma in situ (DCIS). Such calcifications are more commonly seen when there is periductal fibrosis that irregularly compresses the duct lumina, resulting in more irregularly shaped secretory calcifications. **(B)** The calcifications associated with chronic duct ectasia and periductal fibrosis are associated with apparent gross enlargement of the duct, and shorter, more irregular secretory calcifications that lie within the severely compressed duct lumen. The mildly hypoechoic material that appears to enlarge the duct is actually periductal fibrosis that compresses the duct lumen. Despite the vastly different histology from DCIS, the sonographic appearance is absolutely indistinguishable from high nuclear grade DCIS with calcifications developing within central necrosis. Biopsy cannot be avoided. (*RAD*, radial view; *AR*, antiradial view.)

13.27. Lesions that secrete fluid are associated with ectatic ducts or cysts, while lesions that no longer secrete fluid appear as solid nodules. As centrally arising LNG DCIS lesions become large enough to become palpable or to create a mammographic opacity, they usually manifest as an exaggeration of one of the papilloma appearances shown in Figures 13.27, 13.28, and 13.29.

The sonographic appearance of peripherally arising LNG DCIS is not specific for DCIS, but merely reflects sonographic appearance of the underlying benign process from which it arose, usually sclerosing adenosis (Fig. 13.30), florid papillary duct hyperplasia (Fig. 13.31), or radial scar (Fig. 13.32). It is generally impossible to sonographically distinguish LNG DCIS from FCC or BPD, but one subtle difference is that DCIS has a propensity to grossly distend the extralobular terminal duct disproportional to the degree of distention of the lobule (Fig. 13.33).

Limitations of Sonography in Identifying and Diagnosing Ductal Carcinoma in Situ

Even when optimal technique and equipment is used, sonographic diagnosis of DCIS can be very difficult, and may be compromised by several factors that have been previously mentioned.

i) First, DCIS does not always grossly distend ducts and TDLUs. Ducts and TDLUs that are not abnormally enlarged will not be recognized sonographically. LNG DCIS is the least likely to grossly distend ducts and lobules, and therefore, the most likely to be missed sonographically.

ii) Second, DCIS is not the only pathologic process that can enlarge the ducts and TDLUs. Virtually the entire spectrum of fibrocystic change and benign proliferative conditions can enlarge these structures, including fibrocystic change with microcysts, apocrine metaplasia, fibrosclerosis, papillary duct hyperplasia, adenosis, and secretory change. Further complicating matters is the heterogeneous involvement of TDLUs by these benign processes, resulting in highly variable degrees of TDLU enlargement, even within the same lobe of the breast. For this reason, enlarged TDLUs must be interpreted within the context of the anatomy of the rest of the breast. If there is diffuse enlargement of TDLUs throughout both breasts, it must be assumed that similarly enlarged TDLUs in the region of clinical or mammographic interest are enlarged because of fibrocystic change or papillary ductal hyperplasia (based upon sonographic findings alone). On the other hand, if the TDLUs in the area of interest are enlarged out of pro-

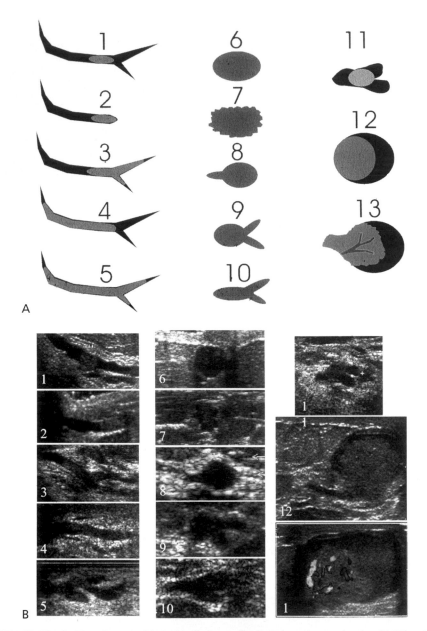

FIGURE 13.27. A: Most low and intermediate grade ductal carcinoma in situ (DCIS) arises peripherally rather than centrally. The uncommon centrally arising DCIS lesion does not have its own sonographic appearance. Rather, the sonographic appearance of centrally arising low or intermediate grade DCIS is usually that of an underlying large duct papilloma within which the DCIS arises. The appearances of central papillary lesions varies greatly, depending upon the length of duct involved, whether or not the duct is expanded, the presence and distribution of fluid within the duct, and whether or not the lesion has become encysted. **(B)** This figure shows the broad spectrum of large duct papillary lesions illustrated in **(A)**.

portion to other TDLUs in the breast, there should be more concern. This is particularly true when the patient is post-menopausal.

iii) Third, diffuse enlargement of larger order, more centrally located ducts may be also caused by benign breast conditions that simulate DCIS, e.g., chronic ductal ectasia and benign papillomas. While most small central papillary lesions are benign papillomas, approximately

6% to 7% represent LNG DCIS, and another 6% to 7% represent atypical duct hyperplasia.

iv) Fourth, calcifications are generally sonographically demonstrable only when they lie within an enlarged duct or TDLU, within the lumen or wall of a cyst, or within a relatively homogeneous isoechoic or hypoechoic nodule. This is especially true of the smaller granular or amorphous calcifications seen in low and inter-

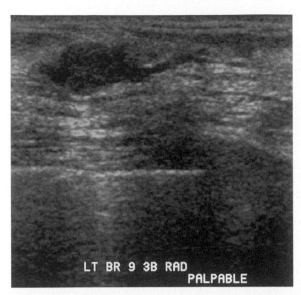

FIGURE 13.28. Large duct papillomas that have undergone malignant changes generally reflect the shape of the lesion in which they arose. This low nuclear grade ductal carcinoma in situ lesion arose within a pre-existing intraductal papilloma and is merely an exaggerated caricature of the papilloma in which it arose. The lesion clearly has a duct extension toward the nipple that is so typical of intraductal papillomas.

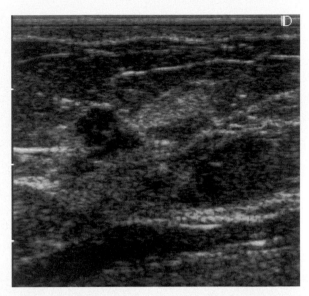

FIGURE 13.30. Small peripherally arising low or intermediate nuclear grade ductal carcinoma in situ (DCIS), like its centrally arising cousins, does not have a unique sonographic appearance. Rather, it usually merely reflects the sonographic appearance of the fibrocystic change (FCC) or benign proliferative disorder in which it arose. Since there is a continuous spectrum from atypical ductal hyperplasia (ADH) to DCIS, the sonographic appearance of ADH also reflects the appearance underlying FCC or benign proliferative disorders. This case was diagnosed as ADH on core needle biopsy, but upgraded to low nuclear grade DCIS at excision. Its sonographic appearance, that of a cluster of disproportionately enlarged lobules, reflects the appearance of the sclerosing adenosis in which it arose.

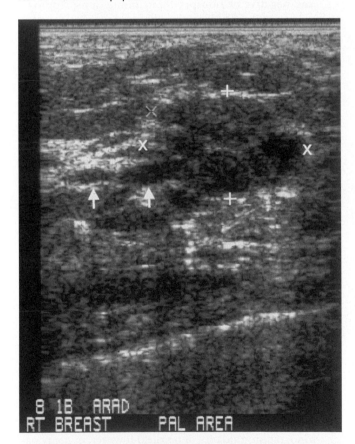

FIGURE 13.29. This markedly microlobulated high nuclear grade ductal carcinoma in situ *(calipers)* arose in a pre-existing papilloma. Note the long duct extension *(arrow)* and the marked expansion of the duct. The degree of microlobulation is far more that would be expected from a benign papillomas and also suggests formation of new ducts by the lesion, as the central duct in which it formed does not have that many branch ducts arising from it.

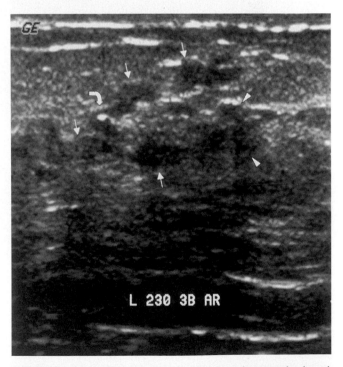

FIGURE 13.31. This case of intermediate nuclear grade ductal carcinoma in situ reflects the sonographic appearance of the florid duct hyperplasia within which it arose. Ducts *(arrows)* and lobules *(arrowheads)* are mildly enlarged, and there is one ductal calcification *(bent arrow)*.

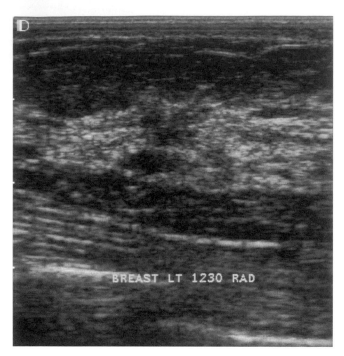

FIGURE 13.32. The sonographic appearance of this low nuclear grade ductal carcinoma in situ reflects that of the radial scar within which it arose. Note the spiculations.

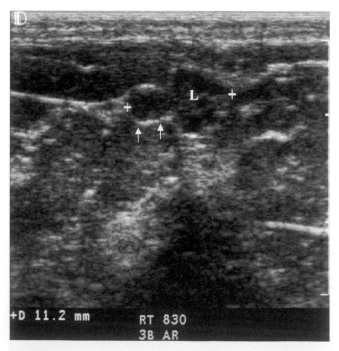

FIGURE 13.33. About the only way to distinguish between benign processes (fibrocystic changes [FCC] or benign proliferative disorders [BPD]) and ductal carcinoma in situ (DCIS) is by the degree of enlargement of the extralobular terminal duct. FCC and BPD tend to affect mainly the lobule, while DCIS is more likely to grossly distend the extralobular terminal duct. This figure shows a lobule enlarged by intermediate nuclear grade DCIS. Note that the extralobular terminal duct *(arrows)* is enlarged out of proportion to the lobule *(L)*

mediate nuclear grade DCIS. Therefore, if there is no nodule and no gross enlargement of the ducts or TD-LUs, the calcifications are unlikely to be sonographically demonstrable. The calcifications that occur with ING DCIS and HNG DCIS tend to be larger. They are also more likely to lie within a hypoechoic mass that creates a dark background against which echogenic calcifications are more sonographically obvious.

Selected Cases of Ductal Carcinoma in Situ where Ultrasound may be of Value

i)   **Evaluation of the 10% of patients who have soft tissue densities without calcifications.** Approximately 10% of patients with DCIS present with a mammographic soft tissue density but no calcifications. Since these lesions are not infiltrative, the mammographic nodules or asymmetric densities are not usually classically spiculated masses. Rather, they are the indistinct or partially obscured nonspecific densities for which sonographic evaluation is ideal.

ii) **Evaluation of patients with palpable abnormalities and negative or nonspecific mammograms.** Approximately 5% of DCIS cases will present with a palpable abnormality. In the small percentage of patients in whom DCIS causes palpable lumps, sonographic evaluation will be of benefit. The principles for evaluation are the same as for any other palpable abnormality, and sonographic evaluation will be to similar to those described for mammographic densities.

iii) **Evaluation of the patient with nipple discharge.** Galactography is generally the procedure of choice for evaluation nipple discharge. However, in most patients, ultrasound is also quite good for this indication. Centrally located intraductal papillary lesions are usually benign intraductal papillomas, but in up to 13% of cases, the papillomas have developed Atypical Dudal Hyperplasia or low nuclear grade DCIS within the surface epithelium.

iv) **Guiding needle localization of calcifications.** Ultrasound can be useful in guiding needle localization for excisional breast biopsy. While mammographic stereotactic guidance rather than sonographic guidance is virtually always performed for large-core needle or mammotome breast biopsy, there are certain advantages to using ultrasound for the needle localization biopsy. Of course, there are many patients with DCIS whose lesions are not sonographically visible, and such patients will require mammographic rather than sonographic guidance of needle. However, in many patients, a nodule, mass, enlarged solid ducts, and/or calcifications are sonographically visible, and ultrasound-guided needle localization is possible (Fig. 13.34). Even the presence of calcifications within the surgical

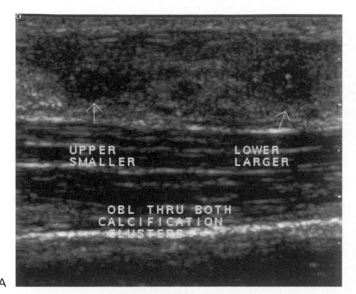
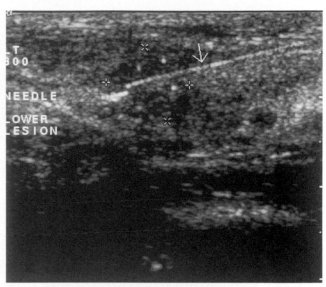

FIGURE 13.34. A: This patient from an outside hospital arrived without the outside mammograms for preoperative needle localization of clustered calcifications. One cluster of calcifications was visible on routine pre-needle localization mammograms. As always, we took a quick look with ultrasound to see if the calcifications were visible, because sonographic localization is quicker and more precise than mammographic localization. The calcifications were visible, but a second group of calcifications *(upper)* that was not evident on the routine mammograms was sonographically visible. Both clusters were localized and both showed low nuclear grade ductal carcinoma in situ. **(B)** Ultrasound-guided needle localization of sonographically visible calcifications is quick and accurate.

specimen can be assessed sonographically. Sometimes sonography shows a positive margin that was not suspected by the specimen radiograph (Fig. 13.35).

In our practice in recent months, the vast majority of needle localizations for microcalcifications have been performed on patients in whom a definitive diagnosis of malignancy has already been established with mammotome biopsy. Even though the calcifications have been removed by vacuum-assisted large-core needle biopsy, a small seroma collects within the mammotomy cavity. The small mammotomy cavity seroma or hematoma remains for a few weeks, and makes an excellent target for sonographic localization (Fig. 13.36).

We usually perform a very brief ultrasound examination prior to beginning any mammographically guided needle localization of calcifications. There are several reasons for performing the needle localization under ultrasound rather than mammographic guidance:

a) First, if the lesion is visible sonographically, targeting is quicker and more precise than with mammographic free-hand guidance. The needle is always precisely placed on the first attempt. Repositioning of the needle is virtually never necessary. Lesions that are definitely sonographically visible are then localized with sonographic guidance. If the lesion is not visible or questionably visible sonographically, mammographic localization is performed as origi-

nally scheduled. Of course, regardless of whether sonographic or mammographic guidance is performed, if the lesion is mammographically visible, a mammogram is performed after wire placement to ensure proper placement. Specimen radiographs are also obtained to ensure appropriate removal of all of the calcifications and the absence of calcifications in the margins of the excised specimen. If the lesion is visible only sonographically, specimen sonography is also possible.

b) Second, during the sonographic localization, it is sometimes apparent that the lesion is larger and more extensive than was suggested by the extent of calcifications on mammography or multifocal (Fig. 13.37). In such cases, each of the lesions is localized separately or the margins are bracketed with multiple wires under ultrasound guidance to better define its size. This maximizes the chance of complete excision during the first surgery, and minimizes the chances of residual tumor in the margins of the initial incision and the chances of local recurrence.

c) Third, sonographic exam during needle localization sometimes shows clearly invasive carcinoma that was not previously suspected (Fig. 13.38). While the diagnosis of invasive ductal carcinoma will likely be made histologically, it may be helpful for the pathologist to know in advance that there is sonographic evidence of invasion. This is especially

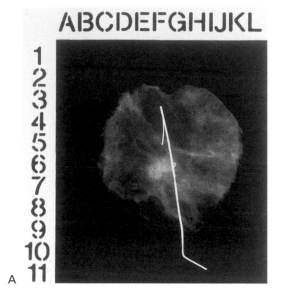

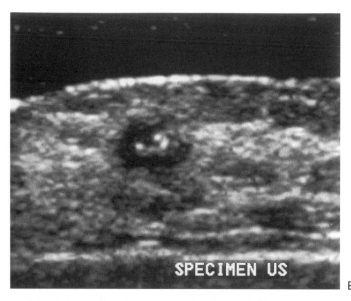

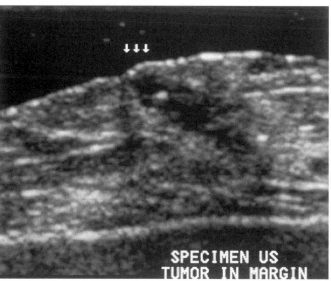

FIGURE 13.35. A: Specimen radiograph shows a few calcifications within a nodule that appears centered within the specimen on this single view. Radiographically, the margins appear clear. The needle localization was performed under ultrasound guidance. The diagnosis of ductal carcinoma in situ had previously undergone large-core vacuum-assisted needle biopsy approximately 10 weeks earlier. Note that the wire goes through the center of the mammotomy clip. **(B)** Sonography of the specimen shown in **(A)** shows the nodule and the calcifications that it contains. **(C)** Sonography of a different plane through the specimen shows involvement of a margin that was not detected on the routine one-view specimen radiograph. Orthogonal mammographic views of the specimen may have shown the positive margin. Based on sonography of the specimen, the positive margin was re-resected. Histology revealed a positive margin on the initial specimen, but clear margins on the re-resection specimen.

true if the pathologist uses a random sectioning method for evaluating excisional biopsy rather than the preferred serial section method. The 1% to 2% of patients reported to have pure DCIS metastatic to axillary lymph nodes almost certainly have had invasive malignancy that was missed by the pathologist (Fig. 13.13).

v) **Guiding percutaneous ductography for intraductal papillary lesions and guiding large-core vacuum-assisted biopsy of intraductal papillary lesions.** Preoperative localization of intraductal papillary lesions can be accomplished by ultrasound-guided galactography if standard galactography is not possible the day of surgery because secretions are not expressible, ductal cannulation has failed for technical reasons, or because there never was a nipple discharge (Fig. 13.39). A mixture of one-half methylene blue dye and one-half meg-

lumine iodinated contrast can be injected into the abnormal duct under ultrasound guidance to both stain the duct and to allow confirmation of the presence and location of the papilloma on mammograms taken after injection of contrast. When a very small intraductal papillary lesion occurs within an extensively arborizing ductal system (as shown by galactography), a combination of galactography (nipple cannulation or ultrasound-guided) and ultrasound-guided needle localization of papillary nodule can be performed. Ultrasound-guided percutaneous galactography has become much less important since the advent of ultrasound-guided mammotomy and large-core vacuum-assisted biopsy.

More than any other development, vacuum-assisted large-core needle biopsy has accelerated the role of ultrasound in evaluating nipple discharge. A definitive

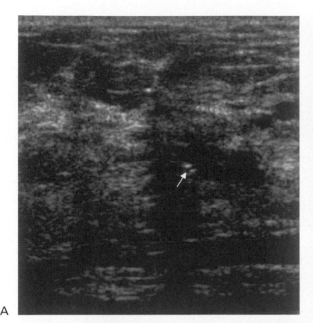
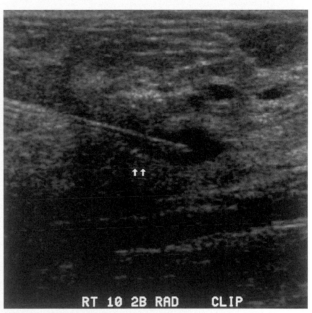

A

B

FIGURE 13.36. A: The post–vacuum-assisted seroma or hematoma makes an excellent target for needle localization. The mammotomy clip is visible on the posterior wall of the cavity *(arrow)*. Sonographic localization of the mammotomy cavity is preferred over mammographic localization of the mammotomy clip for two reasons. First, the sonographic localization is quicker and more precise. Second, any residual disease in the walls of the cavity is as likely to be on the opposite wall from the clip as on the same wall as the clip. If the cavity is 1 cm wide, a mammographic localization of ± 1 cm from the clip is accepted, and if the residual tumor lies on the opposite wall from the clip, the needle may be as far as 2 cm from the residual disease. However, if the center of the 1 cm cavity is localized under ultrasound guidance, the needle will never be more than 0.5 cm from the residual disease, regardless of the wall involved. **(B)** This image documents the localization needle passing into the center of the mammotomy cavity under ultrasound guidance. Note the mammotomy clip eccentrically located on the posterior wall of the cavity. In our experience, the average mammotomy cavity seroma or hematoma persists for 4 to 6 weeks. If there was a large post-biopsy hematoma, the cavity may persist longer. Most needle localizations performed more than 6 weeks after mammotomy will have to be targeted to the mammotomy clip under mammographic guidance.

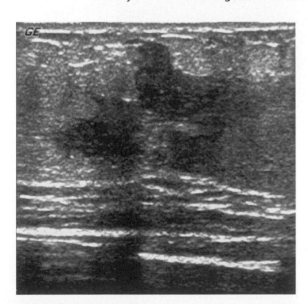

FIGURE 13.37. In some cases, the extent of the tumor than can be demonstrated sonographically is much greater than was suggested by the extent of mammographic calcifications. The few calcifications within this anterior lesion were visible mammographically. However, three additional foci of tumor were sonographically visible, one with calcifications (not shown in the plane of this image), and two additional noncalcified lesions. The histologic diagnosis was high nuclear grade ductal carcinoma in situ.

diagnosis is obtained in virtually all cases, and in 90% of cases, the offending nipple discharge for which the patient presents ccases permanently. A marking clip should be deployed in all cases so that the location can be found if the histology reveals DCIS or atypia. While mammotomy can be galactographically guided, it is far easier and more reliable to guide the biopsy using ultrasound. Thus, even if galactography is used to identify an intraductal papillary lesion, sonography is always performed prior to biopsy. For this reason, every patient with complaints of nipple discharge is now scheduled for both sonography and galactography. Sonography is performed first, with galactography to follow only if necessary. When sonography shows an intraductal papillary lesion to be the cause of nipple discharge, the galactogram is generally deferred, and the lesion is immediately subjected to ultrasound-guided mammotomy (Fig. 13.40). If sonography shows a definitive benign cause of nipple discharge (such as a communicating cyst), galactography may be deferred. However, if sonography does not show a definitive cause for nipple discharge, the galactogram is performed as scheduled because sonography may miss lesions that lie within ducts that are not dilated and

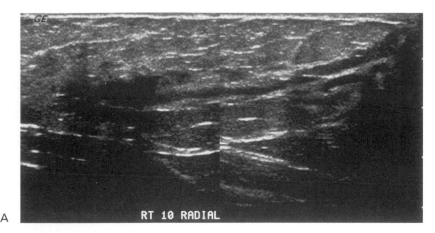

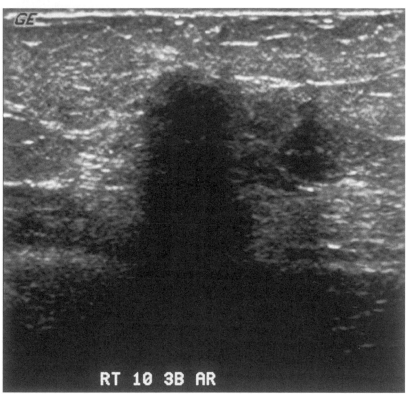

FIGURE 13.38. A: Sonography was performed to evaluate nipple discharge. Mammography showed BIRADS 4b calcifications in the 10-o'clock position in the right breast suspicious for intermediate nuclear grade ductal carcinoma in situ (DCIS). Sonography and galactography were scheduled with sonography performed first and showing a solid hypoechoic mass farther peripherally located than the usual large duct papilloma. An abnormally large duct leads from the lesion to the nipple. Ballottement caused no "color-swoosh," indicating that the echoes within the duct were likely DCIS, not merely blood or inspissated secretions. The findings are compatible with high nuclear grade DCIS. **(B)** Just peripheral to the lesion shown in **(A)** was an intensely shadowing mass that suggested the presence of too much desmoplasia for pure DCIS and the presence of invasive components of tumor not suspected on mammography. Galactography was deferred and the patient underwent ultrasound-guided large-core needle biopsy that showed invasive ductal and lobular carcinoma.

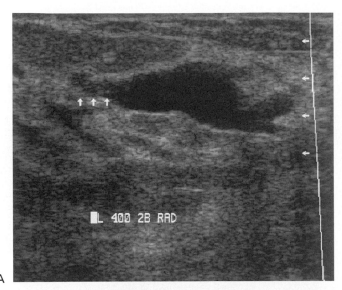
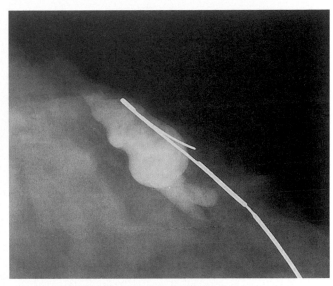

FIGURE 13.39. A: This patient presented with a mammographic nodule that sonography showed to be caused by a severely dilated mammary duct that was obstructed by an intraductal papillary lesion. In other planes, three additional intraductal papillary lesions were identified within the duct. Today, this lesion would undergo ultrasound-guided vacuum-assisted biopsy and a clip would be deployed. However, this patient presented before the advent of vacuum-assisted large-core needle biopsy. Ultrasound-guided galactography and needle localization were performed to enable excision. **(B)** Using a 50:50 mixture of blue dye and 60% iodinated contrast, the duct was punctured under ultrasound guidance, contrast and blue dye injected, and a wire deployed within the duct. Note the obstructing intraductal papillary lesion that was sonographically demonstrated *(arrow)*. Histology showed multiple benign intraductal papillomas.

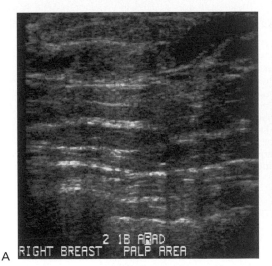
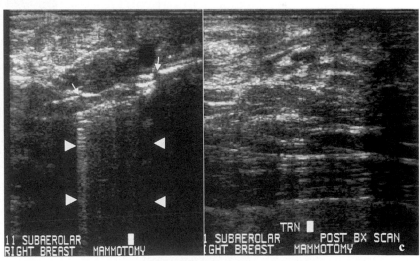

FIGURE 13.40. A: This large, intraductal papillary lesion caused the serous nipple discharge for which this patient presented. Ultrasound was the first diagnostic study performed after mammography. Because the ultrasound showed a definitive cause for nipple discharge, the galactogram was deferred and the patient was scheduled for ultrasound-guided vacuum-assisted biopsy. **(B)** The intraductal papillary lesion *(left)* during the vacuum-assisted biopsy. Note that the artifacts arising from the vacuum holes *(arrowheads)* in the needle aperture *(arrows)* are directly deep to the lesion. A clip was deployed at the end of the procedure. **(C)** No residual lesion *(right)* or duct ectasia immediately post-mammotomy. Histology revealed benign large duct papilloma. After the procedure, the nipple discharge cleared. At two years there is no sonographic evidence of recurrence and no clinical evidence of nipple discharge.

filled with secretions. However, even in cases where the lesion is initially missed by sonography and then diagnosed with galactography, second look ultrasound usually adequately shows the lesion to allow the mammotomy to be performed under ultrasound guidance.

vi) **Guiding aspiration and vacuum-assisted large-core needle biopsy or ultrasound-guided needle localization of intraductal and intracystic papillary lesions.** Sonography is the method of choice for showing intracystic and intraductal papillary lesions, including intracystic DCIS. When sonographic evaluation of a complex cyst reveals a worrisome papillary lesion, ultrasound-guided needle localization for excisional biopsy or ultrasound-guided core biopsy (usually after aspiration of fluid) can be performed. In such cases, aspiration of fluid for cytology is not sufficient, because of a high rate of false-negative cytology studies. If aspiration alone is performed, a significant majority of intracystic malignancies will be missed due to false-negative cytology. Additionally, if only aspiration is performed and the cytology is atypical or malignant, it may be difficult to find the residual solid component of the complex cyst at a later time if the fluid does not reaccumulate. When there is suspicion of intracystic malignancy and the election is made not to proceed straight to excisional biopsy, a combined ultrasound-guided aspiration/vacuum-assisted large-core needle biopsy is scheduled. In these cases, aspiration of fluid is performed to stabilize the papillary lesion for vacuum-assisted large-core needle biopsy, and is performed under continuous real-time guidance so that the sonographic appearance of the residual solid component is immediately apparent. Ultrasound-guided vacuum-assisted large-core needle biopsy is then immediately performed while the appearance of the residual solid component is fresh in our minds (Fig. 13.41). It should be anticipated that the lesion might be difficult to find for later excisional biopsy if removal is incomplete or if histology reveals malignancy or atypia. Therefore, a localizing mammotomy clip or an echogenic collagen plug is always deployed.

According to the literature, most malignant intracystic lesions are rather indolent lesions, usually papillary DCIS. However, this has not been our experience. We have seen the entire range of malignant histologies within intracystic papillary lesions, including aggressive lesions such as high grade invasive ductal, invasive lobular, medullary, and even metaplastic carcinomas. Thus, we do not feel that it should be assumed that intracystic lesions are indolent LNG DCIS lesions.

vii) **Guiding core needle biopsy of calcifications in the rare cases when stereotactic biopsy is not possible.** There are rare cases in which stereotactically guided large-core needle biopsy, mammotome biopsy, or needle localization of calcifications is not possible. This

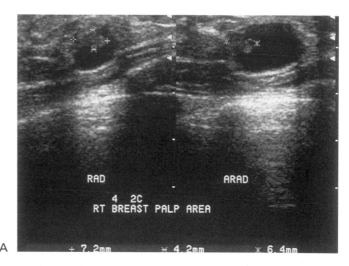

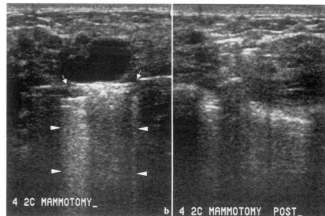

FIGURE 13.41. A: A complex cyst that contained a mildly suspicious (BIRADS 4a) mural nodule caused the palpable lump in this patient *(calipers).* **(B)** The mammotomy probe *(left)* deep to the lesion. Ring down artifacts arise from the vacuum holes *(arrowheads)* in the aperture *(arrows).* At the completion of the procedure, a mammotomy clip was deployed. **(C)** No residual lesion *(right).* The mammotomy clip is not visible in this image. Histology revealed low nuclear grade ductal carcinoma in situ involving the surface epithelium of an intracystic papillomas, and the patient subsequently underwent excisional biopsy, which revealed no residual malignant disease.

can occur when calcifications are too deep and close to the chest wall, and in patients who cannot lie prone. Ultrasound guidance can be used in these cases if the calcifications, nodule, or enlarged duct is identified in association with calcifications.

viii) **Evaluating axillary lymph nodes in patients with large, bulky, high nuclear grade DCIS lesions.** One to 2% of patients with DCIS have positive axillary lymph nodes. This implies that they have microscopic foci of invasion that were not diagnosed histologically. Positive nodes are most likely to occur in large, HNG DCIS lesions, where the lesion is so large that only portions of the tumor may be sampled for histologic evaluation. Therefore, in large lesions suspected of being DCIS, we evaluate axillary lymph nodes. If an abnormal axillary lymph node is found (Fig. 13.13), the primary lesion is reassessed for subtle signs of invasion, and both the abnormal appearing axillary lymph nodes and suspected areas of invasion undergo core biopsy with ultrasound guidance. If the axillary lymph node contains metastatic disease and/or the suspected area of invasion contains invasive carcinoma, the patient undergoes axillary dissection in addition to mastectomy. Additionally, any portion of the specimen that was not sectioned and histologically assessed undergoes histologic evaluation.

ix) **Evaluation of mammographic calcifications prior to biopsy.** The key to detection of most cases of DCIS is the presence of calcifications. Mammography is our best tool for detecting calcifications.

Is it possible that sonography could play a role in evaluating mammographic calcifications despite its lower sensitivity for them? To date it has not. The reason for this is simply that mammography is generally more sensitive than sonography for "microcalcifications." However, as the resolution of sonography improves, a larger percentage of mammographically visible calcifications are now becoming sonographically visible as well. Ten years ago, when we first began to explore this issue, sonography was only able to show calcifications in approximately half of the cases where calcifications were mammographically visible. However, our current data shows that we can identify calcifications in approximately 80% of cases where it is mammographically visible. With older equipment, we could rarely demonstrate calcifications smaller than 500 microns; but with newer higher frequency, broader bandwidth, higher dynamic range equipment, 1.5-dimensional array transducers, coded harmonics, and real-time compounding, we can now see calcifications as small as 200 microns (under ideal circumstances).

Calcifications that are sonographically visible are visible because of a combination of good spatial and good contrast resolution. The ultrasound beam at its optimal point of focus is approximately a millimeter wide for the best equipment currently available. However, that does not mean that calcifications smaller than the beam width are never demonstrable. It simply means that calcifications smaller than the beam width will be subject to volume averaging with surrounding tissues. If the calcification appears echogenic enough compared with surrounding tissues, it will still be visible despite volume averaging (however, calcifications that are smaller than the beam width will not cast acoustic shadows because the calcification must completely occlude the beam to cast a shadow). Any ultrasound developments that lead to either a narrower beam or better contrast resolution will improve our ability to see smaller calcifications. Our ability to see small calcifications is improved by 1.5-dimensional array transducers that produce a narrower beam over a greater range of depths that do standard 1-dimensional array transducers, especially in the near field. Coded harmonics and real-time compounding are recent developments that reduce artifacts, improve contrast resolution, and, therefore, also improve our ability to demonstrate calcifications (Figs. 13.42 and 13.43).

But equipment is not the only reason for variation in ability to demonstrate calcifications. The background tissue that surrounds the calcifications also affects their visibility. Since small calcifications will be subject to volume averaging with background tissues, calcifications whose bright echogenicity is volume averaged with hypoechoic surrounding tissues will be more readily demonstrated than those that are averaged with echogenic background tissues. HNG DCIS calcifications are better demonstrated sonographically than are LNG DCIS calcifications for several reasons. First, HNG calcifications tend to be larger and coarser. Second, HNG DCIS tends to more grossly distend ducts and lobules with isoechoic or hypoechoic tissue. Even when volume averaged, HNG DCIS calcifications tend to be visible

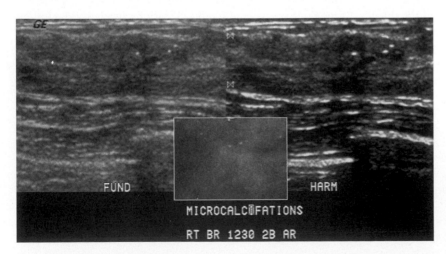

FIGURE 13.42. By decreasing artifact and improving spatial resolution, coded harmonics can make breast calcifications more apparent. The left image, obtained within fundamental imaging, shows these small punctate calcifications. However, because the contrast between the calcifications and surrounding tissues is less and there is greater volume averaging with fundamental imaging, the calcifications appear smaller and less bright than they do with coded harmonic imaging *(right image).*

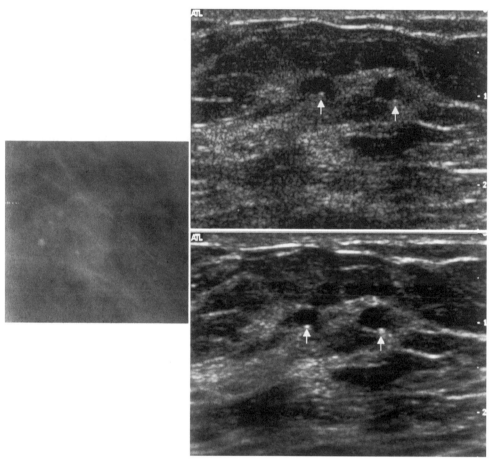

FIGURE 13.43. The upper image is obtained with conventional imaging. There is a single calculus in each of the two cysts. Because of temporal averaging and multiple angles of incidence, artifacts (particular speckle artifact) are decreased, and the calcifications appear brighter and better defined in the lower image obtained with real time compounding. Since both calcifications and speckle artifact are sonographically represented by little white dots, it should not be surprising that anything that suppresses the artifactual white dots of speckle will make the real white dots (the calcifications) more apparent. Note that the salt and pepper texture in the upper image has nearly been eradicated from the lower image, and the texture of the tissues appears much smoother with real time compounding.

because their echogenicity is being volume averaged with very "dark" tissues. LNG DCIS, on the other hand, has smaller calcifications, and is less likely to distend the ducts and lobules wherein the calcifications lie. The surrounding tissues with which LNG DCIS calcifications are volume averaged is more likely to be hyperechoic fibroglandular tissue that is so close in echogenicity to the calcifications that it obscures them.

While we are not quite in the realm of ultrasound microscopy yet, it is now possible to evaluate calcifications with great anatomic detail using commercially available equipment. We can now show the structures within which necrosis of malignancy leads to calcifications. We routinely see calcifications within tumor-laden ducts and cancerous lobules (Fig. 13.44).

Despite improvements in resolution, the sensitivity of sonography for calcifications is still lower than that of mam-

mography, so the argument could be made that sonography has no role in evaluation of calcifications. However, mammographic assessment of calcifications also has some limitations:

a) First, calcifications tend to reflect the DCIS components of disease rather than the invasive components. Therefore, stereotactically guided needle biopsy of calcifications is prone to "under-diagnose" the presence of invasion. The more extensive the calcification, the more likely the diagnosis of invasion is to be missed by stereotactically guided biopsy alone. In some cases, the presence of invasion is unsuspected until after lumpectomy. In other cases, it is detected on contrast-enhanced MRI and documented with "2nd look" ultrasound and ultrasound-guided biopsy. What we have learned from 2nd look ultrasound is that if sonography shows a solid mass

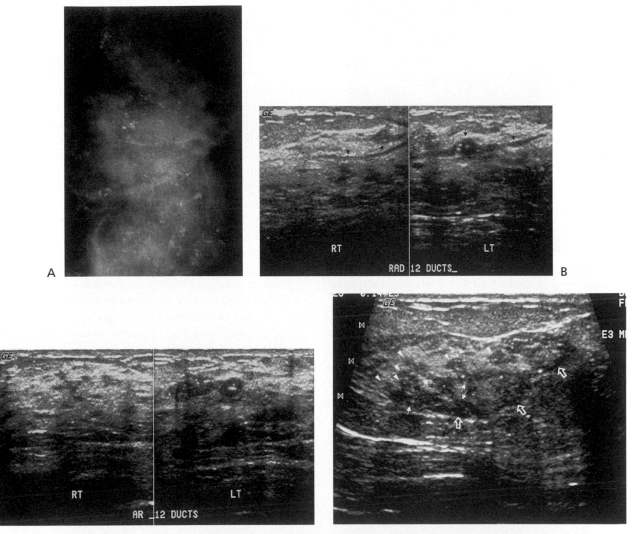

FIGURE 13.44. A: These calcifications are linear, branching, "snake skin" calcifications that are BIRADS 5 and indicate a high likelihood of high nuclear grade ductal carcinoma in situ (HNG DCIS). Because of the extent of the lesion, there is a high risk of at least microscopic invasion, but mammography does not show any direct evidence of invasion. **(B)** Sonography of the patient shown in **(A)** reveals the gross morphology of HNG DCIS. This split-screen image of the 12-o'clock locations in the right and left breast shows a long axis view of a normal duct in the right breast and a long axis view of a grossly enlarged duct distended with HNG DCIS on the left. Note the central calcifications in the abnormally enlarged duct on the left that indicate the presence of necrosis. Note that the degree of distention by DCIS of the left duct in the 12-o'clock position is not uniform. **(C)** Split-screen mirror images of the 12-o'clock areas of the right and left breasts obtained in the antiradial views shows normal and abnormal ducts in short axis. Note the size and number of normal ducts in the right breast. Note the grossly enlarged DCIS distended duct on the left that contains a dense luminal calcification indicating the presence of necrosis. Note that just medial to the grossly enlarged ducts is a cluster of less severely enlarged ducts. These appear more numerous than normal ducts in the contralateral mirror image location of the breast, suggesting that HNG DCIS forms new ducts as it grows. **(D)** This radial view shows that virtually all of the ducts and lobules within this lobe of the breast are involved with DCIS. A lobar duct courses from upper left to lower right *(hollow arrows)*. Several branch ducts are involved. There is extensive cancerization of lobules *(arrowheads)*. Punctate echoes representing calcifications are visible within the lobar duct, branch ducts, and cancerized lobules.

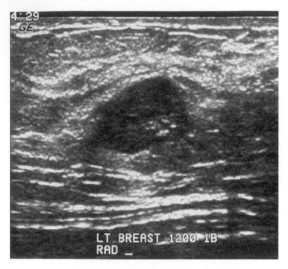

FIGURE 13.45. Sonography in the same patient that is shown in Figure 13.44 revealed a solid mass with a relative paucity of calcifications compared with the rest of the tumor. While calcifications may be seen within the invasive portion of carcinomas, they are most common in the ductal carcinoma in situ components. A solid nodule within an area of mammographic calcifications that has generally fewer calcifications than other parts of the lesion is likely to represent an invasive component of the lesion, and it should be biopsied with ultrasound guidance. Ultrasound-guided core biopsy of this nodule revealed high-grade invasive ductal carcinoma that was not suspected from mammography and would likely have been missed if only stereotactically guided biopsy of calcifications were performed.

within the area of calcifications that is absolutely or even relatively devoid of calcifications, the mass is likely to represent the invasive component of the tumor (Fig. 13.45). Ultrasound-guided biopsy of the solid nodule could confirm invasion that stereotactic biopsy might miss. Thus, one could make the argument that in order to better detect invasive components of tumor, a sonographic search of the calcification area for the presence of a BIRADS 4a or higher solid nodule is warranted prior to performing stereotactically guided biopsy of calcifications. In such cases, however, the ultrasound-guided biopsy would supplement the stereotactically guided biopsy, not replace it. Stereotactically guided biopsy of calcifications is still important in "mapping" the extent of DCIS components of disease.

b) Histologic evaluation of lumpectomy specimens is too frequently less than perfect. In many institutions, "random sectioning" rather than systematic serial sectioning of lumpectomy or mastectomy specimens is performed. In cases of extensive DCIS, random sectioning increases the likelihood that areas of invasion will be missed. Sonographic assessment of the calcification areas for a solid mass and ultrasound-guided biopsy of such solid nodules could help avoid this problem. Sonographic assessment of regional nodes and ultrasound-guided biopsy of grossly abnormal appearing nodes can also be helpful in documenting metastasis and avoiding the missed diagnosis of invasion (Fig. 13.13).

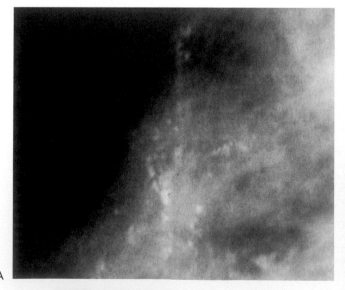
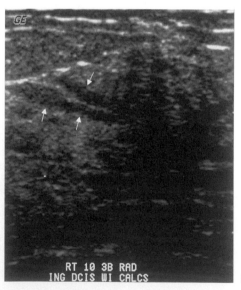

FIGURE 13.46. A: Mammography reveals BIRADS 5 intraductal calcifications highly suspicious for ductal carcinoma in situ (DCIS), most likely of high nuclear grade. **B:** Although this lesion was extensively calcified on mammograms, significant parts of the DCIS component of the lesion are not calcified. Note the branch pattern of enlarged ducts *(arrows)* that extends away from the tumor into the periphery of the breast and that contains no intraluminal calcifications. The extent of mammographic calcifications may underestimate the extent of disease, as it does in this case. Sonography may reveal noncalcified components of tumor that are not mammographically visible.

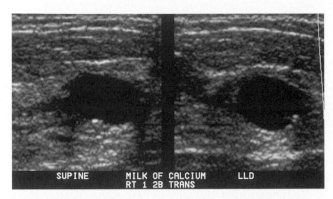

FIGURE 13.47. Sonography is capable of demonstrating milk-of-calcium as small stones within a cyst that can be made to move to the newly dependent part of the cyst when patient position is changed.

c) Not all DCIS components of the malignant lesion may be calcified. Sonography may reveal long duct extensions or branch patterns that do not contain calcifications. Sonographically guided biopsy of such components might more often lead to more accurate assessment of disease (Fig. 13.46).

d) Many mildly suspicious and nonspecific clustered calcifications represent FCC or BPD. The negative-to-positive biopsy rate for isolated calcifications is higher than that for ultrasound-guided biopsy of solid nodules. We have reduced the negative-to-positive biopsy ratio for solid nodules to 2:1. However, the negative to positive biopsy ratio for calcifications in most institutions remains 4 or 5:1. In some cases, sonography may show

milk of calcium – not milk, but tiny individual stones

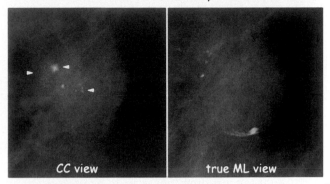

15 or 20 stones usually necessary for classical "teacup"

FIGURE 13.48. Milk-of-calcium is a previously described definitively benign (BIRADS 2) mammographic finding that can be used in sonography. On the craniocaudal view *(CC view)* taken with a vertical beam, the calcifications are punctate or granular, variable in size, and nonspecific *(arrowheads)*. On the true mediolateral view *(ML view)*, however, taken with a horizontal beam, the calculi layer in the dependent portion of the cyst. The appearance has been likened to milk in the bottom of a "teacup." Unfortunately, a dozen or more calculi are necessary to form a classical teacup. Fewer calculi result in a nonspecific punctate appearance to calcifications that lead to BIRADS 4 classification and biopsy.

mildly suspicious (BIRADS 4a) clustered calcifications on mammography to be definitively benign (BIRADS 2) sonographically. This is a fairly frequent occurrence for milk-of-calcium. Sonography shows milk-of-calcium to represent individual calculi within a cyst (Figure 13.47). While mammography can show more calcifications than

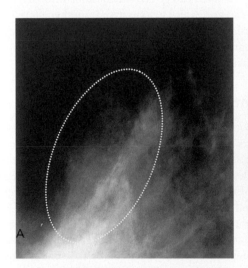
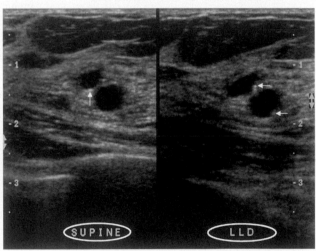

FIGURE 13.49. A: This was the only cluster of punctate calcifications present in either breast. It was new and had formed since the patient's last mammogram a year earlier. This is an upright mediolateral view and shows no milk-of-calcium "teacups." **(B)** The sonogram (obtained with real-time compounding) shows two small cysts, each with a single mobile calcification that moves to the left side of the cyst in the left lateral decubitus view. Sonography actually has the advantage over mammography in demonstrating milk-of-calcium because sonography requires only a single mobile calcification in each cyst for definitive diagnosis, while mammography requires many. Thus, many nonspecific calcifications on mammography can be shown to be milk-of-calcium by sonography.

sonography, a dozen or more calcifications must be present within a cyst to form a classical "teacup" appearance on horizontal beam mammography (Figure 13.48). Many, if not most breast cysts that contain milk-of-calcium contain too few calcifications to be documented as definitively benign "teacups" mammographically. Sonography, on the other hand, can easily demonstrate a single mobile calcification within a cyst (Figure 13.49). Thus, despite the overall advantage of mammography for demonstrating calcifications, sonography can often reveal a BIRADS 2 milk-of-calcium pattern when mammography is unable to do so, and ultrasound offers the possibility of avoiding biopsy in some cases where it would be required based on mammographic findings alone.

Sonographically guided needle biopsy staging of malignant breast disease prior to definitive surgery (either at the time of initial sonographic evaluation or in a "2nd look" role after staging contrast-enhanced MRI) is now well established and routine in our practice. It should be remembered, however, that the advantages of sonographic evaluation of certain benign calcifications are anecdotal at this time, and must be confirmed prospectively before sonographic information can be used in determining the need for biopsy.

SONOGRAPHY OF INVASIVE DUCTAL CARCINOMAS CONTAINING DUCTAL CARCINOMA IN SITU COMPONENTS

Effect of Ductal Carcinoma in Situ Components on Surface Characteristics and Lesion Shape

Approximately one-third of invasive NOS carcinomas are spiculated, while one-third of invasive NOS carcinomas appear circumscribed at gross pathologic examination, and an additional one-third have mixed spiculated and circumscribed appearance.

Most spiculated lesions do not undergo sonography for diagnosis, because the mammographic findings are BI-RADS 5, malignant. Such lesions usually undergo biopsy without additional imaging evaluation. The role of sonography in such patients is guiding needle biopsy or localization. Circumscribed carcinomas, on the other hand, are often mammographically nonspecific, and frequently require diagnostic sonography for further evaluation.

Mammographically circumscribed carcinomas may lack the "hard" suspicious sonographic findings that suggest the presence of invasive malignancy and that so readily allow their distinction from fibroadenomas. They may even be partially surrounded by a thin, echogenic pseudocapsule of compressed breast tissue similar to that seen around fibroadenomas. However, 85% of invasive ductal carcinomas have components of DCIS that may contribute to their

overall sonographic appearance. In such cases, the clues to the nature of the lesion may lie in surface characteristics and shapes that are "soft" suspicious sonographic findings suggesting the presence of intraductal (DCIS) components of tumor, not in the "hard" suspicious findings characteristic of spiculated lesions.

The invasive breast carcinomas that are mammographically circumscribed represent either high-grade invasive ductal carcinomas or special type tumors such as medullary, colloid (mucinous), or invasive papillary carcinomas. In our experience, the majority of such tumors are high-grade ductal carcinomas (that also tend to have relatively large HNG DCIS components), with only a minority of circumscribed lesions representing special type tumors. The DCIS components in mixed lesions may lie anywhere within the invasive tumor, but are most numerous in the periphery, and therefore, often affect the surface characteristics and shape of the lesion.

The HNG DCIS components within such lesions tend to grossly distend numerous peripheral ducts and lobules, leading to a microlobulated surface. Pagetoid spread of DCIS components toward the nipple that grossly distend large central ducts can give rise to the sonographic shape finding of duct extension. Retrograde growth of DCIS components within peripheral ducts and cancerization of lobules can give rise to the sonographic shape finding of branch pattern. In our experience, one or more of these three findings is present in most cases of so-called "circumscribed" invasive carcinomas. Thus, it is the DCIS components rather than the invasive components of such lesions that create the "soft" suspicious sonographic the appearance that appropriately allow us to categorize such lesions into BIRADS 4a or higher categories and help us avoid mischaracterizing malignant lesions as probably benign. These findings will be discussed and illustrated in the following section on extent of intraductal components.

Extent of Intraductal Component

As previously stated, approximately 85% of NOS breast carcinomas have a mixture of invasive and intraductal (DCIS) components. The percentage of DCIS components in mixed lesions varies greatly. When more than 50% of the lesion is DCIS, the lesion is considered to have extensive intraductal components (EIC).

The presence of extensive intraductal tumor (DCIS) within an invasive NOS lesion affects the prognosis in two ways, depending upon the type of treatment chosen. The first is that NOS tumors with an EIC are less likely to have lymph node and distant hematogenous metastases than are NOS tumors with lower percentages of intraductal components. Therefore, patients who have NOS tumors EIC *and who undergo mastectomy* have better long-term survival. On the other hand, patients who have NOS tumors with EIC *and who undergo lumpectomy or other breast-conserving surgery* have a higher risk of local recurrence. Thus, the presence of EIC improves survival prognosis if mastectomy is performed, but worsens local recurrence prognosis if breast conservation therapy is performed.

Most local recurrences result from inadequate resection of the primary tumor rather than new foci of tumor development. Because the DCIS components of mixed invasive and intraductal lesions tend to occur in the periphery of the lesion; because EIC tend to grow out from the periphery of the central invasive component into the surrounding ducts and lobules; and because these extensive intraductal components are generally nonpalpable even at the time of lumpectomy, they are often transected during lumpectomy, leaving residual intraductal components extending out from the walls of the lumpectomy cavity. Careful orientation of the lumpectomy specimen, inking, and histologic assessment of margins can detect residual disease in most, but not all, cases. However, positive margins require re-excision or mastectomy and extra surgical procedures. It would be better to either initially perform the appropriate surgery or to attempt induction chemotherapy prior to the definitive attempt to excise the lesion. Post-lumpectomy radiation therapy is designed to sterilize any residual disease that may exist after lumpectomy, but recent evidence suggests that radiation therapy does not completely kill residual DCIS components and prevent recurrence, but merely delays recurrence. Thus, appropriate excision of all components of disease remains the key to preventing local recurrence. However, since these components are nonpalpable, even during lumpectomy, the burden of presurgical diagnosis rests with the breast imager rather than the surgeon or pathologist, who can only diagnose residual disease after attempted lumpectomy. Appropriate presurgical diagnosis and mapping of intraductal components with targeted image-guided biopsy offers a better picture of the true extent of the disease.

Detection of EIC is probably best accomplished with contrast-enhanced MRI and a high resolution fat and water

suppressed sequence such as RODEO, but can also be done with ultrasound in many cases. Even in cases where staging contrast-enhanced RODEO sequence MRI is used to detect EIC, 2nd look ultrasound is usually necessary because MRI has so many false positives, and because MRI-guided biopsy is not readily available or economically feasible at this time. The extent of EIC must still be mapped out with ultrasound-guided vacuum-assisted large-core needle biopsy, and the lesion must then be bracketed with multiple wires to allow adequate excision. In some cases, MRI and 2nd look ultrasound may indicate that the lesion is too large for lumpectomy and the patient would be better served by either skin sparing mastectomy and reconstruction or a trial of induction chemotherapy.

Although MRI appears better for staging breast carcinoma and in demonstrating EIC than is ultrasound, (especially when the EIC is low nuclear grade) the breast sonographer who performs the initial diagnostic sonogram has the first opportunity to demonstrate EIC. In many cases of invasive carcinoma with EIC, sonography will be performed for evaluation of palpable or mammographic abnormalities long before the diagnosis of malignancy is histologically established. The "soft" suspicious sonographic findings that suggest the presence of EIC extending into the surrounding tissues away from the main tumor mass are duct extension and branch pattern. Microlobulation also increases the likelihood of EIC, but the intraductal components causing microlobulation do not necessarily extend as far into the surrounding tissues as do the DCIS components that create duct extensions and branch patterns.

Duct extension represents intraductal components of tumor growing into a central duct toward the nipple (Fig. 13.50). Since the lactiferous sinus portion of the main duct is often involved, the diameter of duct extensions can be quite large, up to 4 or 5 mm. Because the lactiferous sinus is so easily distensible, the width of the duct extension is unrelated to the nuclear grade of the tumor. Even LNG DCIS

duct extension – soft finding of DCIS –
single projection toward nipple

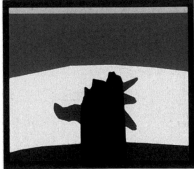 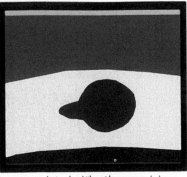

associated with other suspicious
findings

unassociated with other suspicious
findings

FIGURE 13.50. Duct extension usually consists of a single relatively large projection of intraductal tumor away from the tumor nodule toward the nipple. Because a duct extension often involves the highly distensible lactiferous sinus portion of the ductal system, it can be quite wide (up to 5 mm), and can extend all the way to the nipple. Duct extensions may be seen with nodules that have other "hard" sonographic findings that indicate the presence of invasive disease *(left image)*, in which case the duct extension represents a ductal carcinoma in situ (DCIS) component of the tumor and increases the likelihood of extensive intraductal components being present. The duct extension may be an isolated "soft" sonographic finding or may be associated with other soft findings *(right image)*. In most cases that lack hard findings, the lesion represents a benign large duct papilloma. However, 6% of such lesions contain DCIS and another 7% contain atypical ductal hyperplasia.

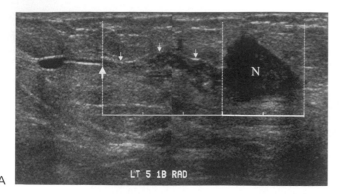
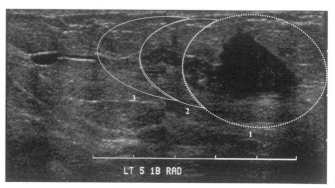

FIGURE 13.51. A: This duct extension *(arrows)* is very long, reaching 3 cm away from the main 2 cm nodule *(N)* toward the nipple. The combined tumor nodule and duct extension have a maximum diameter of 5 cm in this relatively small-breasted patient. **(B)** The duct extension is unlikely to be palpable by the surgeon at the time of lumpectomy, and therefore unlikely to be detected unless its existence is known prior to surgery. Thus, a wide excision with 1 cm margins *(oval #1)* will transect the duct extension. If the specimen is oriented and its margins inked and carefully inspected, the pathologist will likely detect the positive margin, and the surgeon will have to re-excise the positive margin, likely resulting in extension of the lumpectomy cavity 1 cm toward the nipple *(#2)*. However, the margin will still be positive. It is likely that the cosmesis will be unacceptable after an additional re-excision *(#3)*, and the patient will be advised that mastectomy is necessary. But three surgeries were necessary to arrive at the right treatment. Even worse, the positive margin might be missed, and 18 months or so later the patient will then have recurrent carcinoma along the course of the duct extension. A better approach would be to sonographically detect the duct extension, and perform ultrasound-guided core biopsy of the main nodule and ultrasound-guided mammotomy of the farthest extent of the duct extension to document the presence of extensive intraductal component 3 cm from the main nodule. Then the patient can be appropriately given one of three choices: mastectomy at the first rather than the third surgery, segmentectomy (using a multi-wire localization), or a trial of induction chemotherapy prior to attempted lumpectomy.

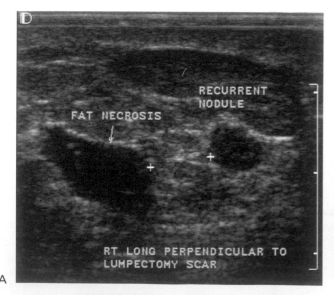
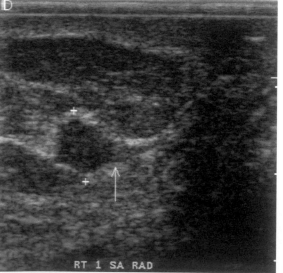

FIGURE 13.52. A: Missed ductal carcinoma in situ in duct extensions is a common cause for local recurrence. Approximately half of the local recurrences that we find sonographically occur along the course of the lobar duct from the lumpectomy cavity toward the nipple, as in this patient (nipple is toward right upper corner of image). **(B)** Radial image of the recurrent nodule shown in **(A)** shows it to lie within the duct. The recurrent nodule, which arose from a missed duct extension like its parent nodule, also has a duct extension growing toward the nipple *(arrow)*.

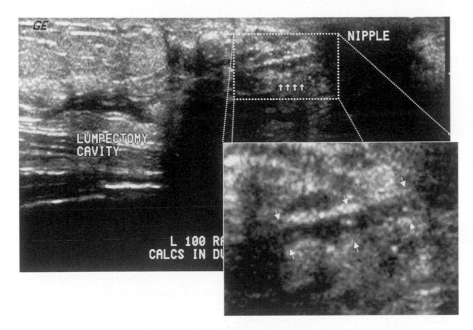

FIGURE 13.53. In this patient, the local recurrence is pure ductal carcinoma in situ and involves the subareolar portion of the lobar duct, which is distended with tumor and contains calcifications. Note peripherally how much farther the lumpectomy cavity lies. When sonographically evaluating post-lumpectomy patients for recurrence, it is important to assess the subareolar ducts that extend into the quadrant where the lumpectomy was performed as well as the immediate vicinity of the lumpectomy cavity.

can cause 4 or 5 mm wide duct extensions. The resistance to tumor grown within the central ducts is very low, so it is not unusual for tumor to grow down the main duct for several centimeters toward the nipple (Fig. 13.51). In our experience, transections of duct extensions toward the nipple from the lumpectomy cavity are one of the main causes of local recurrences that we see most commonly within the duct. This is true of both invasive and intraductal recurrences (Figs. 13.52 and 13.53). Duct extensions can even extend to and involve the nipple without causing obvious nipple retraction, and can contraindicate simple lumpectomy (Figs. 13.14 and 13.17). Occasionally, EIC may be manifest as calcifications extending toward the nipple in the absence of

gross duct distention (Fig. 13.18). Such calcified duct extensions are demonstrable by mammography, but most duct extensions shown by sonography do not contain calcifications, and therefore, are not mammographically demonstrable. Thus, the sonographic findings complement the mammographic findings in most cases. It is highly unlikely that long intraductal extensions of tumor will be palpable at the time of surgery, and thus, unlikely that they will be completely removed at the initial excision without the surgeon knowing of their existence prior to surgery. Our strategy is to perform ultrasound-guided core needle biopsy of the main tumor mass and ultrasound-guided vacuum-assisted large-core needle biopsy of the farthest extent of the duct ex-

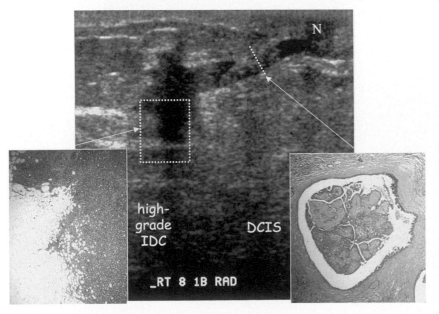

FIGURE 13.54. This high-grade invasive malignant lesion had a long duct extension that caused bloody nipple (N) discharge. The mass on the left is the invasive component of tumor. Note the taller than wide shape and angular margins that involve multiple Cooper's ligaments. The duct extension to the right side of the image represents the papillary ductal carcinoma in situ component of the disease. Areas of the duct extension had undergone hemorrhagic infarction, resulting in the bloody discharge. Areas of sclerosis and fibrosis represent older areas of infarction.

branch pattern – soft finding of DCIS multiple ducts (smaller) away
from nipple

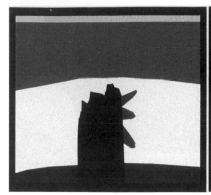
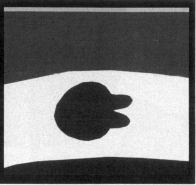

associated with other suspicious   unassociated with other suspicious
findings   findings

FIGURE 13.55. Branch pattern involves multiple small ducts that project peripherally off the main tumor mass away from the nipple. As is the case for duct extension, branch pattern can be associated with other "hard" findings (suggesting invasion), with other soft findings (favoring ductal carcinoma in situ [DCIS]), or may be an isolated finding. When associated with other hard findings *(left image)*, branch pattern suggests the presence of extensive intraductal components. When isolated or associated only with other soft findings, the presence of branch pattern usually indicates the presence of a large duct papilloma, but 6% of cases contain DCIS and another 7% contain atypical ductal hyperplasia.

tension in order to best document the extent of the tumor. At the time of surgical excision, multiple wires must be placed to outline the extent of the lesion (Fig. 13.54).

Branch pattern is another soft suspicious finding suggesting the presence of EIC. Branch pattern represents involvement of small ducts with DCIS that extend away from the main tumor nodule and nipple. Branch pattern can also be formed by cancerized lobules (Fig. 13.55). The peripheral ducts involved by branch pattern are small and relatively non-distensible compared with the central ducts involved by duct extension. Therefore, unlike duct extension, the diameters of branch patterns are correlated with the histologic grade of the tumor. High-grade invasive ductal carcinomas tend to have HNG DCIS components, and low-grade invasive ductal carcinomas tend to have LNG DCIS components. As discussed earlier, HNG DCIS tends to distend the ducts more and cause more periductal inflammatory and desmoplastic response than does LNG DCIS. Thus, large diameter branch patterns are associated with high-grade lesions, small branch patterns tend to be associated with high-grade lesions, and intermediate sized branch patterns tend to be associated with intermediate grade lesions (Fig. 13.56). Branch patterns are usually shorter than duct extensions, but in rare cases may extend far into the periphery. Like long duct extensions, long branch patterns can lead to local recurrences if not diagnosed and resected (Fig. 13.57). Branch patterns may readily extend into TDLUs, a pattern that indicates cancerized lobules (Fig. 13.44).

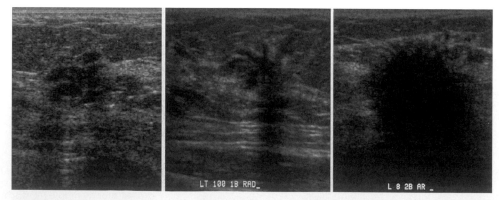

FIGURE 13.56. The width of the branch ducts in branch pattern correlates with the nuclear grade of the ductal carcinoma in situ (DCIS) components. Since the nuclear grade of the DCIS tends to correspond to the histologic grade of invasive components that are present, the width of the branches in branch pattern also correlates with the histologic grade of the invasive components of disease. Wide branches favor either high nuclear grade DCIS or DCIS or an underlying large duct papilloma (left image, histology revealed low nuclear grade DCIS forming in pre-existing papilloma). Medium width branches correlate with intermediate nuclear grade (ING) DCIS components (middle image, histology revealed intermediate grade invasive duct carcinoma with ING DCIS components). Thin branches suggest low nuclear grade (LNG) DCIS components (right image, histology revealed low grade invasive duct carcinoma with LNG DCIS components).

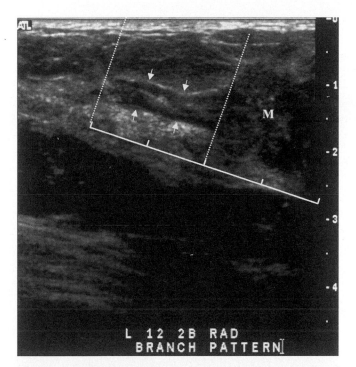

FIGURE 13.57. In most cases, branch pattern involvement of ducts by ductal carcinoma in situ (DCIS) components is much shorter than the involvement by duct extension. However, in a few cases, such as this one, branch pattern *(arrows)* may indicate the presence of DCIS components extending several centimeters away from the main lesion *(M)* into surrounding tissues. Such long branch patterns increase the risk of transection and positive margins during attempted lumpectomy.

The presence of heavy microlobulation is another soft suspicious sonographic finding that indicates an increased risk of EIC. Microlobulations can be caused by intraductal components of tumor and by cancerized lobules (Fig. 13.58). However, not all microlobulation represents intraductal components of tumor. Microlobulation can represent fingers of invasive tumor extending into surrounding tissues, intraductal components of tumor, or cancerous lobules. Microlobulations that are caused by fingers of invasive tumor tend to have angular margins and tend to be associated with a thick echogenic halo, while microlobulations resulting from intraductal components of tumor tend to be round and have a thin echogenic outer capsule (Fig. 13.59). Cancerized lobules tend to lack any sort of capsule, have a fluffy appearance, and are often connected to the main tumor or branch pattern by narrow waists that represent the extralobular terminal ducts (Fig. 13.60). As is the case for branch pattern, the size of microlobulation tends to correlate with the histologic grade of the lesion. High-grade invasive ductal carcinomas that have HNG DCIS components tend to have large microlobulations, low-grade invasive ductal carcinomas with LNG components tend to have small microlobulations, and intermediate grade lesions tend to have intermediate sized microlobulations (Fig. 13.61).

The relationship of sonographic findings to histologic grade of malignant solid nodules is complex, not simple. The grade of the lesion correlates not only with the size of branch pattern and microlobulations but also with sound

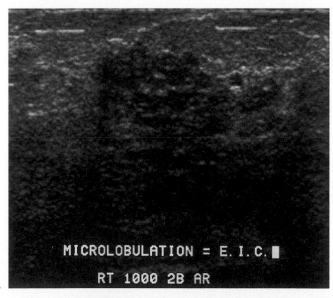

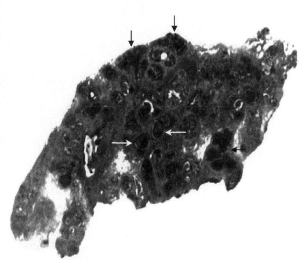

FIGURE 13.58. A: Microlobulations can be caused by ductal carcinoma in situ (DCIS) or invasive components of tumor. This nodule is composed of pure high nuclear grade DCIS and is heavily microlobulated not only on its surface, but internally. **(B)** The sub-gross low power histologic specimen of the nodule in **(A)** shows the microlobulations to be caused by ducts distended with tumor and comedonecrosis *(lighter homogeneous structures marked by white arrows)* and cancerous lobules *(darker, more heterogeneous structures marked by black arrows).*

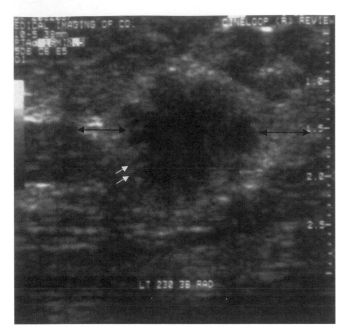

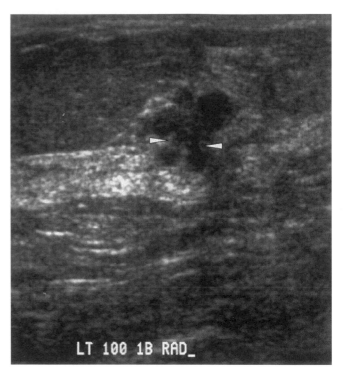

FIGURE 13.59. Internal microlobulations caused by invasive carcinoma are indistinguishable from those caused by ductal carcinoma in situ (DCIS). However, surface microlobulations caused by invasive carcinoma differ subtly from those caused by pure DCIS. The microlobulations caused by invasive carcinoma are frequently angular or pointed *(white arrows)* and associated with a thick, echogenic halo that represents spiculations too small to resolve individually. The thick echogenic halo is typically thickest along the lateral edges of the nodule *(black arrows)* because the laterally located spicules are oriented perpendicular to the beam and make stronger specular reflectors than do the spicules on the anterior and posterior surfaces of the nodule, where they are nearly parallel to the beam.

FIGURE 13.60. Microlobulations that are the result of cancerized lobules often extend away from the periphery of the nodule on narrow "stalks" that represent ductal carcinoma in situ within the extralobular terminal ducts *(arrowheads)*.

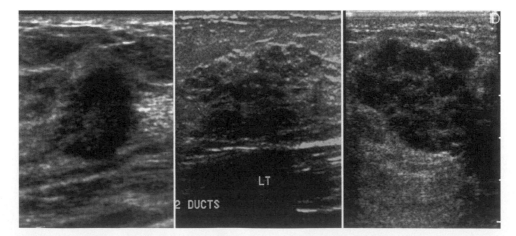

FIGURE 13.61. Like branch pattern, the size of microlobulations corresponds somewhat to the nuclear grade of the ductal carcinoma in situ components and/or the histologic grade of the invasive carcinoma that cause them. Low grade lesions tend to form small microlobulations *(left image)*, intermediate grade lesions tend to form intermediate sized microlobulations *(middle image)*, and high grade lesions tend to cause very large lobulations *(right image)*. Note that the high grade lesions also tend to be associated with enhanced through transmission of sound, while (in the absence of hemorrhage or cystic necrosis) low to intermediate grade lesions tend to have normal or decreased sound transmission.

transmission and the presence of spiculations or thick echogenic halo. Solid nodules associated with enhanced through transmission tend to be high grade, while those that cause acoustic shadowing tend to be low grade. Lesions that transmit sound similar to surrounding tissues may be low or intermediate grade. Lesions that are surrounded by a thick echogenic halo tend to be low or intermediate grade, while lesions that are circumscribed and encapsulated by a thin echogenic capsule are more likely to be high grade. However, a thin echogenic capsule that represents the intact duct wall always surrounds pure DCIS and DCIS components of invasive carcinomas, regardless of the nuclear grade.

It should be remembered that ultrasound generally can detect only intraductal components that grossly distend ducts and/or lobules in the periphery of the tumor. HNG DCIS components are the most likely to grossly distend the ducts to a degree that is sonographically detectable. On the other hand, LNG DCIS components of mixed tumors may not distend the surrounding ducts enough to be readily detectable by ultrasound or distinguished from normal ducts and lobules. Contrast-enhanced MRI with the RODEO sequence may have an advantage over ultrasound in demonstrating low nuclear grade EIC. Thus, a positive ultrasound is always more valuable than a negative ultrasound. If ultrasound shows findings suspicious for EIC, and these can be biopsied under ultrasound guidance, MRI may not be necessary. However, if ultrasound fails to show findings suggestive of EIC, MRI may still be warranted.

Ultrasound-guided core needle biopsy or mammotome biopsy, targeted not only at the primary tumor nodule but also at the suspected intraductal components of the lesion, may enable us to preoperatively confirm the presence of extensive intraductal components. For lesions whose combined invasive and intraductal components are too large for wide excision, skin sparing mastectomy and immediate reconstruction can be offered as a primary treatment option, avoiding the sequence of excision, re-excision, and then mastectomy, and most likely offering a better cosmetic result. Even in cases where the combined intraductal and invasive components are small enough to allow wide excision as an option, bracketing the margins and the ultrasound visible portion of the lesion with multiple localization wires may reduce the incidence of positive margins and the need for re-excision. Furthermore, sonographic evidence of EIC, especially if confirmed by ultrasound-guided core needle biopsy or mammotome biopsy, may indicate the need for postoperative radiation therapy and/or adjuvant chemotherapy. Finally, despite careful inking and histologic analysis of the margins, it is likely that the pathologist will miss some positive margins. Patients in whom positive margins are missed are more likely have local recurrences. Ultrasound-guided bracketing localization of intraductal components could potentially reduce the risk of "missed positive margins" and the rate of local recurrence.

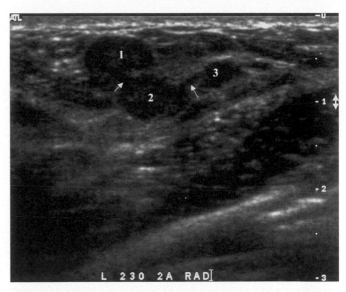

FIGURE 13.62. Careful serial section studies have shown that most cases of multifocal invasive ductal breast carcinoma really represent a single lesion that contains multiple separate foci of invasion connected by "bridges" of ductal carcinoma in situ *(arrows)*.

Multifocal or Multicentric Disease

The percentage of NOS tumors that are multifocal has been reported to be 25% to 50%. Multifocal disease may represent multiple synchronous foci of tumor formation, multiple foci of invasion connected by microscopic invasive disease, or multiple foci of invasion connected by gross DCIS components of disease (Fig. 13.62). Careful serial section studies suggest that most cases of multifocal carcinoma represent multiple foci of invasion in a single malignant lesion where the foci of invasion are connected by intraductal components of tumor (DCIS). Regardless of whether additional foci of invasive tumor are completely separate neoplasms or different areas of invasion within the same tumor, failure to remove all components will result in local treatment failure and increase the risk of metastatic disease and death (Fig. 13.63). Careful imaging evaluation with spot compression, magnification mammographic images, and ultrasound may be helpful in prospectively identifying additional foci of invasion and the intraductal connections between them, enabling the surgeon to perform the most appropriate primary therapy. The most common sites for satellite foci of invasive disease are at branch points of the ducts and in cancerized lobules (Fig. 13.64).

The exercise of examining the primary tumor nodule in radial and antiradial planes, specifically seeking intraductal components of tumor, improves the likelihood that we will detect and correctly diagnose multiple foci of invasion. This is true not only of cases where the ducts between the components are grossly distended with tumor but also in cases

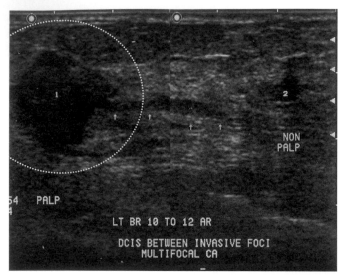

FIGURE 13.63. These two foci of invasive carcinoma lie several centimeters apart, but are connected by ductal carcinoma in situ (DCIS). The DCIS component of the larger lesion *(#1)* grossly distends the duct. The DCIS component of the smaller lesion *(#2)* may not be visible because the duct is tortuous and out of the plane of this image, it does not grossly distend that portion of the duct, or it has necrosed and regressed in that portion of the ductal system. The DCIS bridge is unlikely to be palpable at the time of lumpectomy, and it is likely to be transected by a wide excision *(white oval dotted line)* if the surgeon does not know the second focus of invasive tumor and DCIS bridge exist. As with the case for extensive intraductal components, the burden lies with the breast imager, and careful mapping of the lesion with selected multiple biopsies prior to attempted lumpectomy would be invaluable. We would perform core biopsy on the main nodule *(#1)* and vacuum-assisted biopsy on one additional focus of suspected tumor the farthest from the main nodule, facilitating selection of the best treatment option available to the patient.

where there are only microscopic connecting DCIS components if the normal ductal system is demonstrable. As is the case for EIC, multiple ultrasound-guided biopsies should be performed. The primary nodule and the addition focus farthest from the primary nodule are usually sufficient to document multiple foci of invasion. In most cases the patient

with multifocal disease will undergo mastectomy. However, if the foci are close together and lie within the same quadrant, a wide excision or segmentectomy may be performed. In cases where breast-conserving surgery is anticipated, placement of multiple wires under ultrasound guidance will be necessary.

SUMMARY

Ultrasound has less of a role to play in the diagnosis of pure DCIS than does mammography because mammography is a screening examination and sonography is a diagnostic procedure, and because mammography generally shows microcalcifications better than sonography. Nevertheless, in selected cases of DCIS, particularly those that present with palpable lumps and nonspecific mammographic opacities, ultrasound can be instrumental. Sonography is also useful for evaluating nipple discharge and intracystic lesions caused by DCIS. Most pure DCIS lesions contain only "soft" suspicious findings, such as duct extension, branch pattern, and calcifications, or the mixed finding of microlobulation. The presence of "hard" sonographic findings, such as spiculations, thick, echogenic halo, acoustic shadowing, and angular margins, suggests that there are invasive components to the lesion. Most pure DCIS lesions that are sonographically visible will be high nuclear grade lesions, because HNG DCIS more grossly distends ducts and lobules and/or incites periductal inflammatory and/or desmoplastic response that contribute to the sonographic conspicuity of the lesion. LNG DCIS may not enlarge ducts and lobules or incite enough periductal reaction to allow them to be sonographically distinguished from ducts and lobules affected by common benign processes such as FCC, benign proliferative epithelial disorders, or duct ectasia.

Ultrasound may also be of use in evaluating the DCIS components of mixed invasive and intraductal tumors

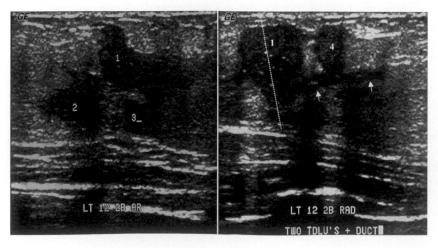

FIGURE 13.64. Satellite invasive lesions tend to occur at branch points in the ductal system and in cancerous lobules, as demonstrated in this case. The antiradial view *(left image)* shows three separate foci of tumor. However, because the image is obtained along the short axis of the ductal system, the relationship of the lesions to the ductal system is not apparent. In the long axis of the ductal system *(right image)* it is clear that each lesion represents a grossly enlarged cancerous lobule. Lobule #1 corresponds to the anterior lobule shown in the left image. Lobule #4 was out of the plane of the antiradial image. Note the calcifications in the tumor-distended duct that connects the cancerous lobules. The enhanced through transmission of sound correctly suggests that the lesion is high grade (the left image was obtained perpendicular to the right image through the plane shown by the dotted line).

where the presence of extensive intraductal component or multifocal disease can be suggested by sonographic findings. Finally, in some circumscribed invasive carcinomas, it is only the soft suspicious findings of the associated DCIS components that enable us to avoid falsely characterizing the lesion as probably benign.

While sonography is certainly much better for assessment of DCIS than we previously had believed, its role in DCIS is still being defined, meaning some caution is necessary. Although we are expanding the role ultrasound plays in DCIS and its future appears bright, it should be remembered that the standard of care is still based on mammographic findings. Mammography is still more sensitive than ultrasound for some cases of DCIS, especially cases of LNG DCIS. Thus, ultrasound will always be more valuable when positive or when able to guide intervention than when it is negative. This is especially true in cases with mammographically suspicious calcifications. Furthermore, while it seems likely that ultrasound will play a future role in determining whether mammographically suspicious calcifications require biopsy, its current role in assessing calcifications is not at all proved. At the present time, one should not cancel biopsy of mammographically suspicious findings because the ultrasound is "negative." On the other hand, if ultrasound shows a solid nodule within a bed of clustered calcifications that demonstrates one or more "hard" findings suspicious for invasion, one should definitely biopsy the solid nodule under ultrasound guidance as well as performing biopsy of the calcifications. The ultrasound-guided biopsy is likely to be the one that appropriately shows evidence of invasion, while biopsy of only the calcifications is more likely to result in preoperative under-diagnosis of invasion.

Similarly, the role of ultrasound in staging breast cancer is still evolving and is greatest when sonography is positive. When a solid nodule with BIRADS 4a or higher findings is found, whole breast sonography and assessment of axillary lymph nodes should be performed. Sonographically detected EIC, multifocal or multicentric disease, or sonographically abnormal axillary lymph nodes should be biopsied under ultrasound guidance as part of the preoperative staging procedure. This may preclude unnecessary staging MRI, sentinel node procedures, and will likely minimize positive margins, re-excisions, delayed mastectomies, and local recurrences. However, failure of ultrasound to demonstrate EIC or multifocal disease does not mean that staging MRI is not necessary. MRI may well be significantly more sensitive than sonography for staging breast cancer. However, MRI has many false positives, and 2nd look sonography will likely be necessary after MRI to "map" the lesion. Likewise, failure of sonography to demonstrate abnormal axillary lymph nodes simply means that there is no metastatic disease gross enough to be seen sonographically and does not mean that sentinel node procedure or axillary dissection is no longer necessary.

SUGGESTED READING

Origin of DCIS from the TDLU

Wellings SR, Jensen HM, Marcum RG. An atlas of subgross pathology of the human breast with special reference to possible precancerous lesions. *J Natl Cancer Inst* 1975;55:231–273.

Natural History of Untreated DCIS

Page DL, Dupont WD, Rogers LW, et al. Intraductal carcinoma of the breast: follow-up after biopsy only. *Cancer* 1982;49:751–758.

DCIS Is Not a Single Disease, but a Heterogeneous Group of Diseases

Evans AJ, Pinder S, Ellis IO, et al. Screening detected and symptomatic ductal carcinoma in situ: mammographic features with pathologic correlation. *Radiology* 1994;191:237–240.

Gump FE, Jicha DL, Ozello L. Ductal carcinoma in situ (DCIS): A revised concept. *Surgery* 1987;102:790–795.

Lennington WJ, Jensen RA, Dalton LW, et al. Ductal carcinoma in situ of the breast. Heterogeneity of individual lesions. *Cancer* 1994;73:118–124.

Millis RR, Thynne GSJ. In situ intraduct carcinoma of the breast: a long term follow-up study. *Br J Surg* 1975;62:957–962.

Silverstein MJ, Poller DN, Waisman JR, et al. Prognostic classification of breast ductal carcinoma in situ. *Lancet* 1995;345:1154–1157.

Mammography with DCIS

Bassett LW. Mammographic analysis of calcifications. *Radiol Clin North Am* 1990;30:93–105.

Dershaw DD, Abramson A, Kinne DW. Ductal carcinoma in situ: mammographic findings and clinical implications. *Radiology* 1989;170:411–415.

Ikeda DM, Andersson I. Ductal carcinoma in situ: Atypical mammographic appearances. *Radiology* 1989;172:661–666.

Kinkel K, Gilles R, Feger C, et al. Focal areas of increased opacity in ductal carcinoma in situ of the comedo type: mammographic-pathologic correlation. *Radiology* 1994;192:443–446.

Mitnik JS, Roses DF, Harris MN, et al. Circumscribed intraductal carcinoma of the breast. *Radiology* 1989;170:423–425.

Mammography Can Underestimate the Size of DCIS

Holland R, Hedriks JH, Verbeek AL, et al. Extent, distribution, and mammographic/histological correlations of breast ductal carcinoma in situ. *Lancet* 1990;335:519–522.

Comedo CA Ducts May be up to 2 to 3 mm in Size

Rogers LW. Carcinoma In Situ. In: Page DL, Anderson TJ, eds. *Diagnostic histopathology of the breast*, 1st ed. New York: Churchill Livingstone, 1993:159.

Sonographic Appearances of DCIS

Di Piro PJ, Meyer JE, Denison CM, et al. Image-guided core breast biopsy of ductal carcinoma in situ presenting as a noncalcified abnormality. *Eur J Radiol* 1999;30:231–236.

Durfee SM, Selland DL, Smith DN, et al. Sonographic evaluation of clinically palpable breast cancers invisible on mammography. *Breast J* 2000;6:247–251.

Gufler H, Guitrago-Tellz CH, Madjar H, et al. Ultrasound demonstration of mammographically detected calcifications. *Acta Radiol* 2000;41:217–221.

Hashimoto BE, Kramer DJ, Picozzi VJ. High detection rate of breast ductal carcinoma in situ calcifications on mammographically directed high-resolution sonography. *J Ultrasound Med* 2001;20: 501–508.

Moon WK, Im JG, Koh YH, et al. US of mammographically detected clustered calcifications. *Radiology* 2000;217:849–854.

Schoonjans JM, Brem RF. Sonographic appearance of ductal carcinoma in situ diagnosed with ultrasonographically guided large-core needle biopsy: correlation with mammographic and pathologic findings. *J Ultrasound Med* 2000;19:449–457.

Tochio H, Konishi Y, Hashimoto T, et al. Ultrasonographic features of noninvasive breast cancer. *Jap Jnl Med Ultrasonic* 1989;16(suppl II):543–544.

Tohno E, Cosgrove DO, Sloane JP. Malignant disease–primary carcinoma–ductal carcinoma in situ. In *Ultrasound Diagnosis of Breast Disease.* New York: Churchill Livingstone, 1994:178–179.

Intracystic Papillary Carcinoma

Carter D, Orr SL, Merino MJ. Intracystic papillary carcinoma of the breast. After mastectomy, radiotherapy or excisional biopsy alone. *Cancer* 1983;52:14–19.

Knelson MH, el Yousef SJ, Goldber RE, et al. Intracystic papillary carcinoma of the breast: mammographic, sonographic, and MR appearance with pathologic correlation. *J Comput Assist Tomogr* 1987,11:1074–1076.

Reuter K, D'Orsi CJ, Reale F. Intracystic carcinoma of the breast: the role of ultrasonography. *Radiology* 1984;153:233–234.

Rogers LW. Carcinoma in situ. In: Page DL, Anderson TJ, eds. *Diagnostic histopathology of the breast,* 1st ed. New York: Churchill Livingstone, 1993:186–187.

Soo MS, Williford ME, Walsh R, et al. Papillary carcinoma of the breast: Imaging Findings. *AJR Am J Roentgenol* 1995;164:321–326.

Tobin CE, Hendrix TM, Resnikoff LB, et al. Breast imaging case of the day. Multicentric intraductal papillary carcinoma. *Radiographics* 1996;16:720–722.

Sonography for Evaluation of Nipple Discharge

Hild F, Duda VF, Albert U, et al. Ductal oriented sonography improves the diagnosis of pathological nipple discharge of the female breast compared with galactography. *Eur J Cancer Prev* 1998;7(I): 57–62.

Local Recurrences are in the Region of the Primary Excision Site

Holland R, Hendriks JHCL, Verbeek ALM, et al. Clinical practice: extent, distribution, and mammographic/histologic correlations of breast ductal carcinoma in situ. *Lancet* 1990;319:519–522.

Lagios MD, Westdahl PR, Margolin FR, et al. Duct carcinoma in situ. Relationship of extent of noninvasive disease to the frequency of occult invasion, multicentricity, lymph node metastases, and short-term treatment failures. *Cancer* 1982;50:1309–1314.

Lagios MD. Biology of duct carcinoma in situ of limited extent. Prospective study of patients treated by tylectomy. *Lab Invest* 1986;54:34A.

Rahusen FD, Taets van Amerongen AH, van Diest PJ, et al. Ultrasound-guided lumpectomy of nonpalpable breast cancers: a feasibility study looking at the accuracy of obtained margins. *J Surg Oncol* 1999:72–76.

Extensive Intraductal Components

Connolly JL, Schnitt SJ. Miscellaneous features of carcinoma: extent of in situ disease. In: Page DL, Anderson TJ, eds. *Diagnostic histopathology of the breast,* 1st ed. New York: Churchill Livingstone, 1993:269–271.

Healey EA, Osteen RT, Schnitt SJ, et al. Can the clinical and mammographic findings at presentation predict the presence of an extensive intraductal component in early stage breast cancer? *Int J Radiat Oncol Biol Phys* 1989;17:1217–1221.

Holland R, Connolly JL, Gelman R, et al. The presence of an extensive intraductal component following a limited excision correlates with prominent residual disease in the remainder of the breast. *J Clin Oncol* 1990;8:113–118.

Lindley R, Bulman A, Parsons P, et al. Histologic features predictive of an increased risk of early local recurrence after treatment of breast cancer by local tumor excision and radical radiotherapy. *Surgery* 1989;105:13–20.

Satake H, Shimamoto K, Sawaki A, et al. Role of ultrasonography in the detection of intraductal spread of breast cancer: correlation with pathologic findings, mammography, and MR imaging. *Eur Radiol* 2000;10:1726–1732.

Schnitt SJ, Connolly JL, Harris JR, et al. Pathologic predictors of early local recurrence in stage I and stage II breast cancer treated by primary radiation therapy. *Cancer* 1984;53:1049–1057.

Schnitt SJ, Connolly JL, Silver B, et al. Updated results of the influence of pathologic features on treatment outcome in stage I and II breast cancer patients treated by primary radiation therapy. *Int J Radiat Oncol Biol Phys* 1985;suppl.I:104.

Schnitt SJ, Connolly JL, Khettry U, et al. Pathologic findings on re-excision of the primary site in breast cancer patients considered for treatment by primary radiation therapy. *Cancer* 1987;59:675–681.

Stomper PC, Connolly JL. Mammographic features predicting an extensive intraductal component in early stage infiltrating ductal carcinoma. *AJR Am J Roentgenol* 1992;158:269–272.

Tresserra F, Feu J, Grases PJ, et al. Assessment of breast cancer size: sonographic and pathologic correlation. *J Clin Ultrasound* 1999; 27:485–491.

Vicini FA, Eberlein TJ, Connolly JL, et al. The optimal extent of resection for patients with stages I or II breast cancer treated with conservative surgery and radiotherapy. *Ann Surg* 1991;214:200–204.

Multifocal Tumors

Berg WA, Gilbreath PL. Multicentric and multifocal cancer: whole-breast US in preoperative evaluation. *Radiology* 2000;214:59–66.

Fisher ER, Gregorio R, Redmond C, et al. Pathologic findings from the national surgical adjuvant breast project (protocol no. 4) I. Observations concerning the multicentricity of mammary cancer. *Cancer* 1975;35:247–254.

Lagios MD, Wesdahl PR, Rose MR. The concept and implications of multicentricity in breast carcinoma. *Pathol Annu* 1981;16:1123–1130.

Leopold KA, Recht A, Schnitt SJ, et al. Results of conservative surgery and radiation therapy for multiple synchronous cancers of one breast. *Int J Radiat Oncol Biol Phys* 1989;16:11–16.

Schwartz GF, Patchefsky AS. Non palpable in situ ductal carcinoma of the breast. Predictors of multicentricity and microinvasion and implications for treatment. *Arch Surg* 1989;124:29–32.

Ultrasound-Guided Percutaneous Galactography

Rissanen T, Typpo T, Tikkakoski T, et al. Ultrasound-guided percutaneous galactography. *J Clin Ultrasound* 1993;21:497–502.

Cancerization of Lobules

Azzopardi J. *Problems in breast pathology.* Philadelphia: WB Saunders, 1979:128–146, 266–273.

LN Mets from DCIS

Rosen PP, Braun DW Jr, Kinne DE. The clinical significance of pre-invasive breast carcinomas. *Cancer* 1980;46:919–925.

Smith RRL. Carcinoma in situ of the breast. *Cancer* 1977;40:1189–1193.

Paget's Disease of the Nipple

Rogers LW. Carcinoma in situ. In: Page DL, Anderson TJ, eds. *Diagnostic histopathology of the breast,* 1st ed. New York: Churchill Livingstone, 1993:184–186.

Mammotomy of Intraductal Papillary Lesions

Parker SH, Dennis MA, Stavros AT. Critical pathways in percutaneous breast intervention. *Radiographics* 1995;15:946–950.

Parker SH, Dennis MA, Stavros AT, et al. Ultrasound-guided mammotomy: a new breast biopsy technique. *JDMS* 1996;12:113–118.

Dennis MA, Parker S, Kaske TI, et al. Incidental treatment of nipple discharge caused by benign intraductal papilloma through diagnostic mammotome biopsy. *AJR Am J Roentgenol* 2000;174:1263–1268.

Sonographic Findings used to Assess Solid Breast Nodules

Stavros AT, Thickman D, Rapp CR, et al. Solid breast nodules: Use of Sonography to Distinguish Benign from Malignant Lesions. *Radiology* 1995;196:123–134.

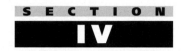

BIOPSY TECHNIQUES

14

MINIMALLY INVASIVE BIOPSY

STEVE H. PARKER

With increased screening mammography, ductal carcinoma in situ (DCIS) represents a growing percentage of breast cancers detected. For nonpalpable breast cancers, DCIS now represents up to 45% of all mammographically detected cancers (1–4). Wire-localized surgical biopsy of the breast has long been the most commonly accepted method of determining if a mammographic abnormality represents DCIS. Because surgical biopsy carries with it certain cost and morbidity drawbacks, physicians have investigated less invasive alternatives. As a result, wire-localized surgical biopsy of mammographic microcalcifications has begun to be supplanted by stereotactic-guided directional, vacuum-assisted biopsy (DVAB).

The transition from surgery to image-guided biopsy was initially attempted using fine-needle aspiration (FNA) and automated large-core biopsy (5–7). For the most part, however, surgeons and other pathologists have been reluctant to base definitive decision making on the results of FNA, especially in the setting of microcalcifications. This is understandable because FNA carries significant insufficient tissue and false-negative rates (5,6).

With the advent of automated core biopsy of the breast, a gradual shift from surgical breast biopsy to minimally invasive, percutaneous biopsy began. Because core biopsy of the breast resulted in a histologic (rather than a cytologic) diagnosis, a more definitive picture of the breast lesion could be painted (7,8). If the lesion turned out to be benign, such as a fibroadenoma, this diagnosis could be relied on and surgery avoided entirely. If the diagnosis turned out to be malignant, then a distinction between in situ and invasive carcinoma could frequently be made, allowing for the definitive therapeutic surgery to go forward with confidence. This process of core biopsy diagnosis prior to definitive surgery has been shown to dramatically decrease the number of surgeries performed in breast cancer patients (9,10). There is some evidence, however, that core biopsy of microcalcifications may be less reliable than core biopsy for solid lesions (8,11). This is consistent with the known, somewhat unpredictable presence of certain types of DCIS in and around calcifications (12). Thus, a missed diagnosis of DCIS may manifest as a result of the potential for sampling error inherent in the noncontiguous tissue acquisition of the core technique. Because of this, many radiologists and surgeons have recommended that microcalcifications undergo surgical excision and not core biopsy.

However, the introduction of DVAB instruments, such as the mammotome, has altered the negative perceptions of percutaneous biopsy of microcalcifications (13) (Fig. 14.1). Because the mammotome acquires tissue contiguously and can remove all the tissue in and around a cluster of calcifications, the theoretic possibility of sampling error is markedly lessened (Fig. 14.1). Clinical results have shown that there are far fewer partial agreements and underestimates (atypical ductal hyperplasia [ADH] and DCIS subsequently upgraded to DCIS and invasive carcinoma, respectively, at surgery) in the setting of microcalcifications when a mammotomy is performed instead of a core biopsy (14). Thus, there should now be little reason not to percutaneously biopsy microcalcifications and diagnose DCIS nonsurgically.

The question as to which specialties will emerge as the providers of minimally invasive breast biopsy is still unresolved. Radiologists have breast imaging and image-guided needle technique expertise, and have also developed and refined image-guided, minimally invasive breast biopsy. However, surgeons have traditionally handled complex clinical breast conditions and have been responsible for performing breast biopsy in the past. Obstetrical-gynecological physicians are also involved to some degree with breast care, and some have voiced a desire to enter the percutaneous breast biopsy arena. Regardless of what has previously existed, however, the surgeon who does very little breast work and has limited imaging skills is not likely to be the physician who will emerge as the accepted provider of minimally invasive breast biopsy. By the same token, the radiologist who spends the majority of time reading plain films and who has little training or experience in interventional radiology or ultrasound also is not likely to emerge as the preferred physician for breast biopsy. The reality is that image-guided breast biopsy should not be performed by physicians who do not have a dedicated focus on breast disease and who do not have the requisite training and experience in the new diagnostic techniques.

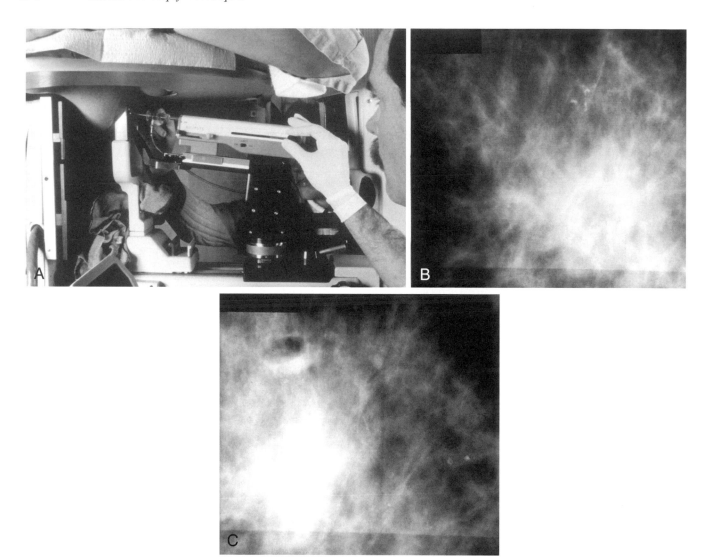

FIGURE 14.1. The Biopsys mammotome. **(A)** The mammotome configured for stereotactic biopsy. **(B)** Stereotactic view of a cluster of microcalcifications prior to mammotomy. **(C)** Opposite stereotactic view demonstrating an air-filled cavity in place of the calcifications.

GUIDANCE MODALITIES FOR PERCUTANEOUS BIOPSY OF DUCTAL CARCINOMA IN SITU

Several guidance modalities are available for percutaneous breast biopsy. The oldest (and previously most common) method of guiding needles into the breast was by palpation, although, in the age of mammography, few cases of DCIS manifest as palpable lesions. However, some physicians still use this method for guiding needles, especially fine needles. This guidance modality carries a major disadvantage—it relies on the sense of touch, which, when compared with the sense of sight, is considerably less powerful. The physician using an imaging modality rather than palpation to guide a biopsy has the significant advantage using the sense of sight in addition to, if necessary, the sense of touch.

Ultrasound generally is used to guide biopsies of breast masses rather than microcalcifications, and therefore is in-

frequently used in the diagnosis of DCIS (15). There are, however, some who subject all regions of calcifications to ultrasound in an attempt to define any possible associated infiltrating component. In addition, the calcifications associated with DCIS can occasionally be visualized sonographically, and ultrasound can then be used for biopsy guidance (Fig. 14.2). The calcifications associated with intermediate and high-grade DCIS tend to be more sonographically conspicuous, since they are generally larger. Also, there can be associated periductal inflammation manifested sonographically by a hypoechoic region surrounding the calcifications, thereby making them more conspicuous. Because calcifications are not easily seen with ultrasound, however, it is not usually the guidance modality of choice for minimally invasive diagnosis of DCIS.

If biopsy of an area of DCIS is performed with ultrasound, however, the ultrasound equipment used for needle guidance should be the same high-quality, state-of-the-art

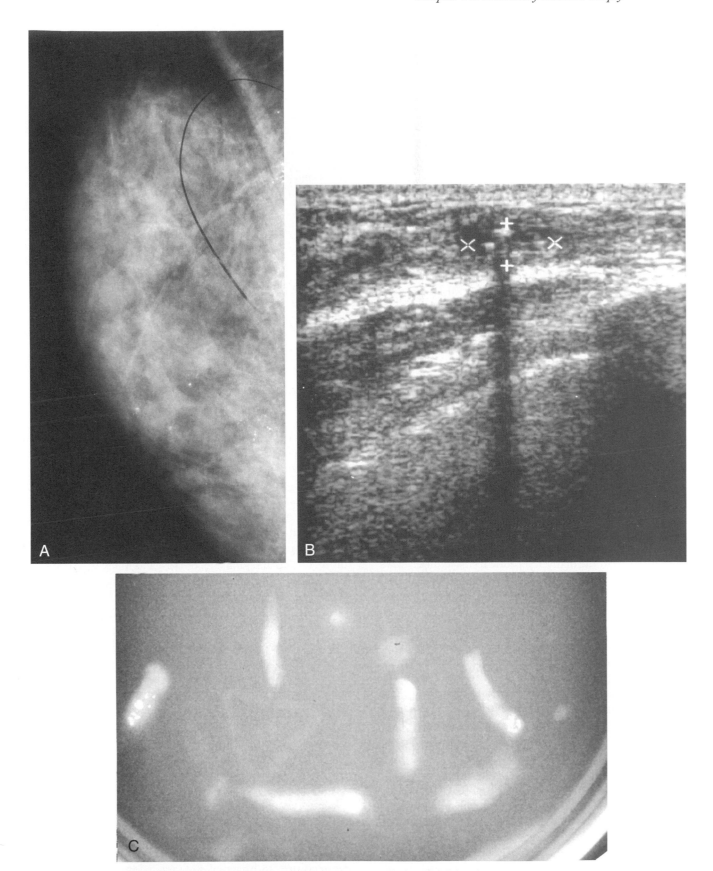

FIGURE 14.2. Ultrasound-guided biopsy of microcalcifications. **(A)** Cluster of microcalcifications in the axillary tail of the right breast. **(B)** Calcifications seen sonographically as small echogenicities, one of which exhibits posterior acoustic shadowing. **(C)** Specimen radiograph of the resultant core tissue.

equipment necessary for good diagnostic breast ultrasound. This is especially true to visualize and target any microcalcifications. The transducer should be a high-frequency (7.5 to 15.0 MHz), electronically focused linear array transducer with a fixed elevation plane focus of 2 cm or less. Additionally, the transducers should be broad bandwidth with a short pulse length. These characteristics will ensure the best axial and lateral spatial resolution, as well as the best contrast resolution (16). To be considered adequate, the equipment should easily visualize a 25-gauge needle within the breast.

Ultrasound-guided biopsies are generally faster than stereotactic guidance and use no ionizing radiation. For deep lesions in large, fatty, replaced breasts, however, digital stereotactic guidance is almost always preferred. The possibility of sonographically identifying deep calcifications in a large breast is remote. Ultrasound is best suited for smaller and average-size breasts, since the 7.5 to 15.0 MHz transducers required for the necessary resolution in the breast do not penetrate well beyond 3 to 4 cm. Although ultrasound is not usually employed for biopsy guidance in cases of possible DCIS, the physician must be adept at both diagnostic breast ultrasound and ultrasound-guided interventional procedures, including biopsy, to provide a global approach to the diagnosis of DCIS.

Because high-quality digital stereotactic mammography easily visualizes the calcifications that can be associated with DCIS, it should be the guidance modality of choice in most cases. Stereotactic mammography can be performed on upright, adapted standard mammography units ("add-on" units) or on dedicated, prone table units. Additionally, the stereotactic images can be obtained with conventional film-screen technique or with digital technique.

The add-on units have two advantages. They are much less expensive than the dedicated prone units, and they have the flexibility to be used to perform standard mammography when not being used for needle guidance. There are several disadvantages of the add-on units. The most bothersome problem is that patients have a tendency to move during the procedure. Any patient movement adversely affects the accuracy of the biopsy guidance. Additionally, the add-on units typically have less working room than the prone units. Finally, there is a greater tendency for the patient to have a vasovagal reaction, as the procedure generally takes place in the patient's view. Several manufacturers have attempted to address these problems by docking a biopsy table to the add-on unit on which the patient lies, or by using a flexible tube head.

The main advantage of the dedicated, prone table stereotactic unit is that it largely eliminates the problems associated with the add-on units enumerated above (17). Since the patient lies prone on the table, there is little or no chance for significant movement (Fig. 14.3). The patient does not see what is taking place beneath the table, so vasovagal reactions rarely occur. Additionally, there is considerably more working room under the table. The major disadvantage of

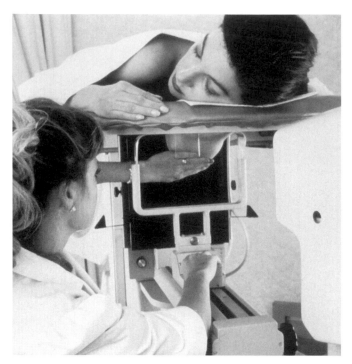

FIGURE 14.3. The Fischer Imaging prone stereotactic unit.

the dedicated prone unit is the cost. It generally costs about twice that of its add-on counterparts. Another disadvantage is that essentially its sole use is to guide needles. Thus, when no needle procedures are taking place, the equipment, and sometimes the room, stand idle. If the room is large enough, however, another standard mammography unit or a breast ultrasound unit (or both) can be placed in it.

Both manufacturers of dedicated prone stereotactic table units (Fischer Imaging and Lorad), and many of the add-on stereotactic units, can be furnished with digital imaging or film-screen capability. The advantages of film-screen stereotactic mammography are lower cost and full field-of-view. The cost of the film-screen units without digital capability is significantly less than the cost of the digital units, since the digital capability can almost double the cost of the stereotactic unit. Also, with film-screen, unlike the digital units, there is no restriction of the field-of-view. Thus, the entire breast can be visualized on the scout and stereotactic scout views. The disadvantages of film-screen include relatively poor contrast resolution, lengthy film development times, inability to postprocess and optimize the image, and generally higher radiation dose.

Most physicians believe that the advantages of digital stereotactic imaging outweigh its additional cost and clearly eliminate the disadvantages of the film-screen approach. The most salient advantage of digital imaging is the speed of image acquisition and display. Approximately 5 seconds after exposure, an image of the targeted area of the breast is displayed, compared with 5 minutes with the film-screen approach. With a percutaneous breast biopsy procedure,

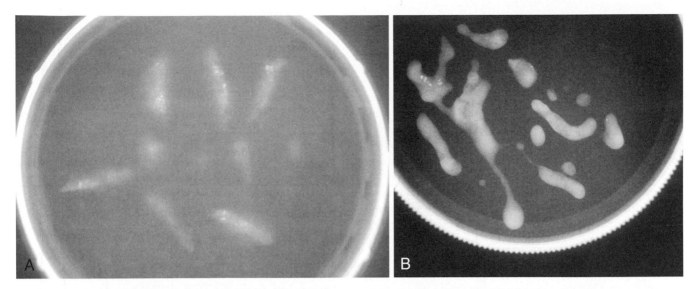

FIGURE 14.4. Specimen radiography. **(A)** Film-screen specimen radiograph. **(B)** Digital specimen radiograph demonstrating much better visualization of microcalcifications due to the increased contrast resolution (the same magnitude of improved calcification visualization is found with digital stereotactic mammography).

this represents a tremendous advantage because the multiple targeting readjustments and confirmation of targeting accuracy can be made with alacrity. Additionally, the digital technique provides greater contrast resolution compared with film-screen (Fig. 14.4). This is especially crucial in the percutaneous biopsy of possible DCIS lesions, because the microcalcifications are much more obvious than on film-screen, allowing for faster and more accurate targeting. The ability to postprocess the image also allows for better visualization of all lesions, including microcalcifications. The contrast and brightness can also be adjusted to better visualize the calcifications. Additionally, the lesion can be displayed at up to 8× magnification, the video can be reversed to display black on white instead of white on black, and edge enhancement algorithms can be used to better evaluate the nature and extent of the calcifications. All these image postprocessing maneuvers can improve microcalcification visualization and, therefore, the accuracy of DCIS diagnosis.

The "target on scout" software developed by Fred Burbank, M.D., in conjunction with Fischer Imaging allows the radiologist to target a lesion using the best of the two stereo scout views coupled with the straight (0°) scout view. Thus, lesion location is calculated using views obtained 15° apart rather than the traditional 30° apart. This is of great help when one of the two 15° scout views shows the lesion poorly or not at all, and can be especially crucial in cases of very faint, subtle calcifications that are associated with some types of DCIS. The straight scout view frequently shows this kind of calcification to best advantage. Additionally, the straight scout view performed with the needle in place in the breast allows the radiologist to see the position of the needle relative to the lesion in a more understandable, straightforward fashion. The view with the needle in place is especially

helpful for physicians in the early stages of learning the stereotactic biopsy technique, since it is possible to immediately discern if the needle is to the left or right of the targeted lesion (Fig. 14.5).

It is important to emphasize that the greatest enemy of a successful stereotactic biopsy is time. The more time that transpires during a biopsy, the greater the likelihood of patient movement, and, therefore, an unsuccessful biopsy. A prone, dedicated stereotactic table provides the longest possible window of time within which to do the stereotactic procedure. If one combines digital capability with a prone unit, one can perform the greatest amount of work within

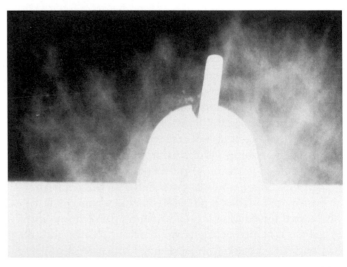

FIGURE 14.5. Target on scout technique shows scout view with mammotome probe in place (target calcifications are to the left of the probe shaft).

the longest period of time. Conversely, using a traditional add-on unit with film-screen capability, only a small amount of work restricted to a relatively short period of time can be accomplished. Thus, the ability to overcome any unanticipated adverse occurrences during a procedure is severely limited. On the other hand, with a dedicated prone unit that has digital imaging, it is possible to adjust to and overcome any multiple or sequential problems that may develop during the course of a stereotactic procedure and ultimately complete a successful procedure despite any adversities.

Because magnetic resonance imaging (MRI) is increasingly being used to evaluate the breast, and lesions have been identified that are not seen mammographically, there has been a desire to develop MRI-guided needle procedures of the breast (18). This may be especially useful for preoperatively determining the true extent of an area of DCIS or demonstrating DCIS in addition to an infiltrating carcinoma (19). Several approaches can be used. With MRI-compatible needles and appropriate guidance tools, a biopsy could conceivably take place within the MRI suite. With open configuration "interventional" magnets, the biopsy could take place with the patient in position for further images. Alternatively, the breast could be immobilized within a guidance device, and the biopsy could take place outside of the MRI suite according to coordinates generated by the MRI.

At this time, perhaps the best approach to a needle biopsy of an MRI-detected lesion is to use ultrasound subsequent to the breast MRI. An MRI-detectable marker can be placed on the skin overlying the lesion, and the region so-marked can then be carefully scanned with high-quality ultrasound. With DCIS, it is unlikely that a discrete lesion will be seen. However, a suspected region of DCIS identified by breast MRI can still be targeted for biopsy under ultrasound guidance, since the fibroglandular tissue and abnormal-appearing distended ductal structures can be identified sonographically in the area where the suspected DCIS resides. Because the specificity of breast MRI is low, ultrasound can add an additional "filter" to reduce the number of patients who are subjected to biopsy. Even with the ultrasound "filter," however, expanded ducts associated with benign proliferative fibrocystic change cannot be reliably distinguished from DCIS sonographically. Thus, when distended ducts are noted in the region of MRI enhancement, those ducts and the associated fibroglandular tissue are biopsied using ultrasound-guided mammotomy. The recently developed "hand-held" mammotome is well suited for this application. A post-biopsy marker is placed so that the region can be easily located for excision if DCIS is found. In addition, if the diagnosis is benign proliferative fibrocystic change, then the clip serves as a marker for subsequent breast MRI to prove that the biopsy did indeed canvas the appropriate tissue.

Although there is the possibility of using palpation, ultrasound, stereotactic mammography, and MRI as guidance

modalities for minimally invasive biopsy of DCIS, it seems most logical at present to concentrate on stereotactic mammography as the best means of targeting indeterminate or suspicious microcalcifications within the breast. Palpation alone should be considered a less accurate means of needle guidance, and MRI-guided capabilities are not yet refined and widely available. Ultrasound cannot usually visualize DCIS, but sometimes can be very useful. With appropriate use of stereotactic mammography, and occasionally ultrasound and MRI, virtually any mammographically-detected area of DCIS within the breast can be successfully and accurately targeted.

TISSUE ACQUISITION INSTRUMENTS

As noted earlier, fine-needle aspiration (FNA) has little place in the diagnosis of DCIS. FNA alone is incapable of distinguishing between in situ and invasive disease. Additionally, fine-needle aspiration biopsy (FNAB) has several other drawbacks. FNAB requires the skill of a highly trained breast cytopathologist if it is to have a chance of success. Cytopathologists are uncommon in the United States. There are many geographic locations, therefore, where the technique should not be used. Even with cytopathologic support, the biopsy does not provide histologic data, which are crucial for determining histologic grade and whether or not a cancer is invasive. False-negatives can be more difficult to distinguish from a truly benign lesion in an FNAB program compared with histologic biopsies. Because of the vagueness about the nature of many benign FNA biopsies, the referring physician and patient may be left uneasy about the conclusiveness of the biopsy. In this setting, the patient may go on to a surgical biopsy to confirm the benign nature of the lesion. Underscoring the failings of breast FNA are the early results of Radiology Oncology Group V (RDOG V), a National Cancer Institute–sponsored trial of percutaneous breast biopsy. In this trial, the FNA arm was discontinued after only 1 year because the results already had been shown to be statistically inferior to core biopsy.

Because of the drawbacks associated with FNAB, physicians began using core biopsy needles to improve the results of percutaneous breast biopsy (7,15,20–22). Manual "Tru-cut" core biopsy needles had been tried in the past and were found to be less adequate than FNAB in several studies (23,24). Therefore, the "modern" core biopsy era began with the introduction of automated core biopsy "guns." When these were combined with stereotactic mammographic or ultrasound guidance, the results were encouraging (25). These automated devices more consistently acquired sufficient tissue compared with the manual core or fine needles. Because the early studies demonstrated that the diagnostic quality of the cores improved with larger gauge needles, the 14-gauge automated core biopsy needle quickly became the standard. Early studies also demonstrated a significant difference between the "long-throw" (12 cm excursion) and the "short-throw" (less than 2 cm excursion) (26). The "short-throw" guns were noted to perform consistently worse, acquiring less tissue and poorer quality tissue than the long-throw guns.

It also became clear that two or three passes with the automated core biopsy needle did not always adequately sample an area to assure correct diagnosis. With further experience, it is now accepted by most radiologists that a minimum of five cores should be obtained in cases of nodules or densities, and a minimum of 10 cores should be obtained in cases of microcalcifications (27). The performance of specimen radiography of the cores helped to reinforce the need for more specimens in cases of microcalcifications. Since it has been shown that having calcifications within the cores improves the diagnostic yield of DCIS, an increased number of cores were found to be required to ensure that microcalcifications were indeed found consistently within the cores (27,28).

With automated core biopsy of the breast, documenting the accuracy of each procedure is important. This is done with stereotactic images that demonstrate the core needle in both "pre-fire" and "post-fire" positions (Fig. 14.6). These images should show the needle poised over the center of the lesion in the "pre-fire" position and coursing through the lesion in the "post-fire" position. Additionally, a post-biopsy stereo pair should be obtained to document a decrease in number of calcifications and/or small pockets of air throughout the calcifications, verifying the accuracy of the multiple core acquisitions. Finally, it is essential to perform a specimen radiograph of the resultant cores to verify that the cores do indeed contain calcifications (Fig. 14.4). With ultrasound-guided core biopsy, the needle is observed under continuous real-time visualization for assurance of targeting accuracy. For documentation purposes, however, ultrasound images of the needle in the pre- and post-fire positions are recorded. When the ultrasound biopsy is performed on a lesion containing calcifications, a specimen radiograph is also obtained. With automated core biopsy of the breast, one must achieve pinpoint targeting accuracy during the procedure, since the tissue acquisition process occurs in a "line-of-sight" fashion. Also, because of the frequently scant tissue acquired with core biopsy, it is not uncommon to harvest only a few or no calcifications, raising questions about the accuracy of the resultant diagnosis. Finally, because the core biopsy instrument must be inserted and removed for each individual core specimen, multiple insertions (sometimes 15 or more) are required to ensure sufficient tissue acquisition.

Because of these drawbacks and the potential for sampling error, stereotactic mammotome biopsy of calcifications is now preferred to stereotactic automated core biopsy (Fig. 14.1). The mammotome works on an entirely different principle than the automated biopsy guns. Instead of a "tru-cut"–style needle that collects tissue in a sample notch

and must be withdrawn after each pass, the mammotome uses vacuum, which helps pull tissue into and transport it back through the probe without having to withdraw each time. Not only does the mammotome acquire much greater amounts of tissue during each acquisition, but a given cluster of calcifications can be canvassed much more quickly and completely, since the device remains in the breast while the tissue containing the calcifications is harvested.

The mammotome probe consists of an outer, hollow sleeve with an aperture at its terminus (Fig. 14.7). Multiple small vacuum holes are positioned on the opposite side of this aperture. These holes are designed to actively pull adjacent breast tissue into the probe when the vacuum is activated. A hollow "cutter" with a sharpened end is positioned within the outer sleeve. After breast tissue is pulled into the probe, the cutter begins to rotate at high speed and is advanced through the tissue captured within the probe. A large breast specimen, nearly equal to the diameter of the entire probe and is usually much longer than the aperture, is subsequently captured in the cutter. The probe is rotated to position the sample bowl opening toward a different clock position (e.g., from 12-o'clock to one-thirty) in preparation for the next sample acquisition. The cutter is then withdrawn rearward within the outer sleeve of the probe, and the tissue specimen is carried back to a "knockout" pin that pushes the captured specimen out into a specimen chamber (Fig. 14.7). Suction is reapplied and the cutter re-advanced into the newly captured specimen from the 1:30 position. This process is continuously repeated as the probe is rotated entirely "around the clock." Contiguous tissue acquisition can be accomplished by acquiring tissue at 1.5-hour increments, thereby markedly reducing or eliminating the chance of sampling error. A side benefit of the mammotome vacuum is that it suctions most, if not all, of the blood that accumulates at the biopsy site, making subsequent stereotactic mammographic views much clearer for assessing adequacy of lesion targeting and/or removal.

The mammotome has been found to be especially useful for stereotactic biopsy of microcalcifications, and a much more accurate diagnosis of ADH and DCIS can be made compared with core biopsy. The ability to confidently acquire some of the calcifications in a given cluster of calcifications is extremely important to ensure a successful and accurate diagnosis. The mammotome makes the acquisition of most, if not all, of the calcifications in a given cluster effortless and speedy. This translates into fewer "partial agreements" or "underestimates" of disease (i.e., ADH upgraded to DCIS, and DCIS upgraded to invasive carcinoma at surgery). Thus, besides the theoretic decrease in false-negative diagnoses compared with core biopsy of calcifications, there is a definite, proven decrease in the number of "partial agreements" in the ADH and DCIS arena. With core biopsy, approximately 50% of the biopsies that result in the diagnosis of ADH are actually DCIS lesions, and approximately 20% of core biopsies that result in a diagnosis of

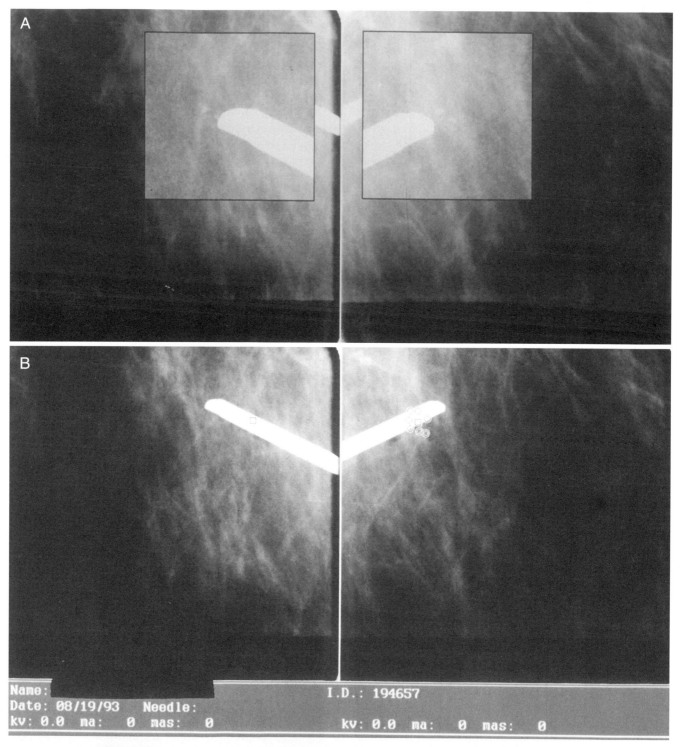

Name:
Date: 08/19/93   Needle:
kv: 0.0   ma: 0   mas: 0   I.D.: 194657
                                                kv: 0.0   ma: 0   mas: 0

FIGURE 14.6. Stereotactic core biopsy. **(A)** Pre-fire stereotactic views with magnified digital images. **(B)** Post-fire stereotactic views with conventional digital images.

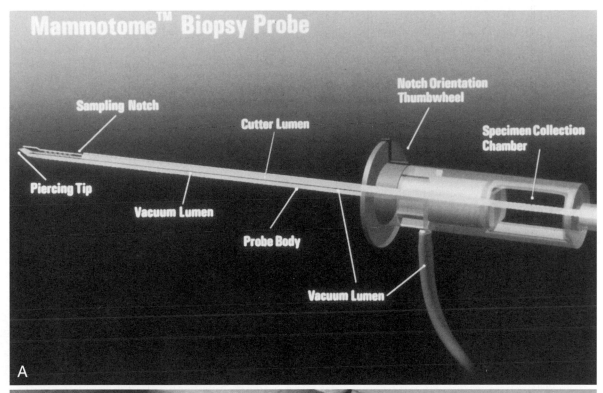

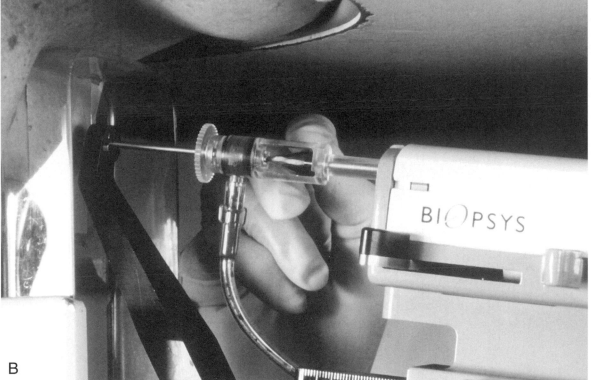

FIGURE 14.7. The mammotome structure. **(A)** The mammotome's components. **(B)** Tissue in specimen collection chamber.

DCIS are upgraded to invasive carcinoma at surgery (9,29,30). In contrast, with mammotomy these underestimates can be markedly reduced and even eliminated (14,31).

Some physicians have been concerned that when all of the calcifications have been removed during the biopsy, and the histologic diagnosis of the lesion is DCIS, it is difficult to relocalize the region for surgical lumpectomy. To address this problem, there are now a variety of marking devices that can be percutaneously placed at the biopsy site (Fig. 14.8). One such device is a catheter-delivered clip that is placed through the mammotome probe. Recently, another FDA-approved device, the SenoRx "GelMark," has become available for the same purpose. This device delivers multiple gelfoam pledgets through a catheter to fill the mammotome biopsy cavity. One of the pledgets contains a metallic marker that allows the biopsy site to be mammographically

visualized. The gelfoam pledgets also allow the biopsy site to be sonographically visualized, unlike the stand-alone biopsy clip. Whether using the catheter-delivered clip or the "Gel-Mark," the biopsy and post-biopsy marking or clipping can take place with a single probe insertion.

With the introduction of the mammotome, the percutaneous biopsy of microcalcifications representing DCIS lesions should become a more accepted practice. Highly suspicious calcifications, which are virtually certain to be DCIS based on the mammographic appearance alone, might still go straight to surgical excision rather than percutaneous biopsy. However, the surgeon must be willing to perform a therapeutic wide-excision lumpectomy as the initial surgery to justify this course of action. The surgeon must also be willing to accept that up to 10% of the time the diagnosis will be benign despite the highly suspicious mammographic findings. Thus, up to 10% of patients will have some degree

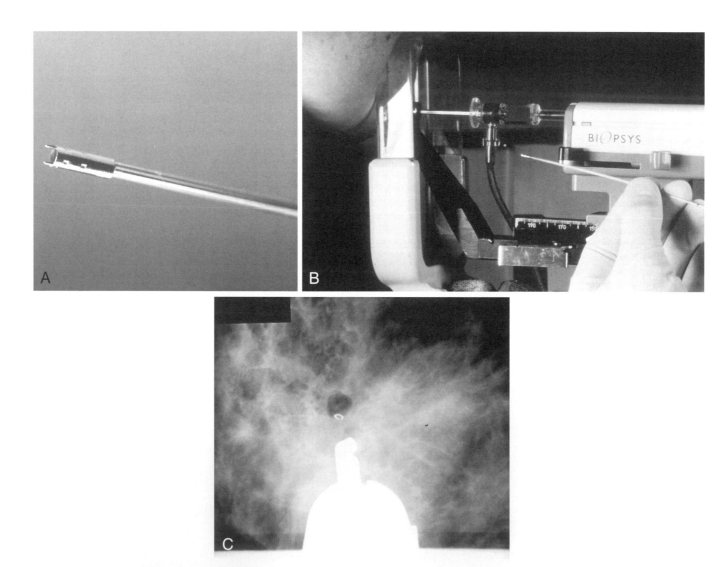

FIGURE 14.8. The MicroMark clip. **(A)** Clip in loaded position within delivery catheter. **(B)** Catheter is inserted into the forward lumen of the probe through the specimen collection chamber. **(C)** Clip in place in the anterior aspect of the mammotomy cavity.

of cosmetic deficit even though their lesion is found to be benign. Alternatively, a minimal surgical excision that subsequently necessitates a re-excision because of positive margins would not make for a more streamlined approach. In such instances, it would be better to perform the percutaneous biopsy prior to surgery. In any case, virtually all breast lesions that might represent DCIS can be percutaneously biopsied with confidence, reserving surgical excision for the therapy of breast cancer.

FUTURE

The rate of change in breast diagnosis and treatment will continue to accelerate. What is accepted today will become obsolete much more quickly than the approaches and procedures of the twentieth century. As automated core biopsy of the breast is replaced by "mammotomy," the percutaneous treatment of small cancers could quickly follow using an "excavation" technique with the mammotome. Using an 11-gauge mammotome, however, Liberman et al. (32) found residual malignancy in 73% of cases, even when the entire imaged lesion had been removed. Sequential analysis of the specimens obtained might provide more confident cancer margin evaluation. Minimally invasive "en bloc" resection may also prove to be therapeutic. The advanced breast biopsy instrument (ABBI, U.S. Surgical) device, which removes a 2 cm "plug" of breast tissue from the skin down to the lesion, has been and continues to be investigated. Initial reports, however, indicate that 64% to 100% of malignancies undergoing an ABBI procedure had positive margins (33). Radiofrequency (RF)-based minimally invasive excisional instruments are also under development for this purpose. This approach springs from a current device known as the "AnchorGuide," which utilizes multiple RF-energized wires that are extruded from a single RF needle to surround the calcifications representing the DCIS. An RF cutting wire can then be deployed around the anchoring wires to sever the excised tissue from the breast. Some form of in situ ablation may be forthcoming in addition to, or instead of, mammotomy. Investigators are currently considering cryotherapy, laser therapy, and in situ radiotherapy. Investigation of MRI-directed breast lesion laser therapy has recently begun (Steve Harms, M.D., personal communication, 2000). Whether the therapy is MRI guided or not, it seems that pre- and posttherapy breast MRI will be the most convincing means of determining the suitability for and the success of a minimally invasive therapeutic procedure.

SUMMARY

With the ability to perform good diagnostic mammography, breast ultrasound, and stereotactic or ultrasound-guided percutaneous biopsy, the percutaneous diagnosis of DCIS should proceed in a time-, cost-, and patient-effective manner. The definitive diagnosis of microcalcification lesions afforded by image-guided mammotomy, which entirely obviates surgery in benign states and streamlines the therapeutic surgery of DCIS, can now be routinely obtained. Preoperative knowledge of the extent and focality of the percutaneously diagnosed DCIS is now available through high-quality, high-resolution breast MRI. These techniques and procedures are best accomplished in a radiologic or multidisciplinary breast center. The future holds even more exciting challenges as percutaneous therapy of small DCIS lesions becomes a reality. Armed with the technology and techniques of the twenty-first century, truly we stand on the threshold of a new era.

REFERENCES

1. Morrow M, Schmidt R, Cregger B, et al. Preoperative evaluation of abnormal mammographic findings to avoid unnecessary breast biopsy. *Arch Surg* 1994;129:1091–1096.
2. Evans WP III, Starr AL, Bennos ES. Comparison of the relative incidence of impalpable invasive breast carcinoma and ductal carcinoma in situ in patients older and younger than 50 years of age. *Radiology* 1997;204:489.
3. Kopans DB, Moore RH, McCarthy K, et al. Positive predictive value of breast biopsy performed as a result of mammography: There is no abrupt change at age 50 years. *Radiology* 1996;200:357–360.
4. Sickles EA, Ominsky SH, Sollito RA, et al. Medical audit of rapid-throughput mammography screening practice: Methodology and results of 27,114 examinations. *Radiology* 1989;175:323–327.
5. Dowlatsahi K, Gent HJ, Schmidt R, et al. Non-palpable breast tumors: Diagnosis with stereotaxic localization and fine-needle aspiration. *Radiology* 1989;170:427–433.
6. Ciatto S, Del Turco MR, Bravetti P. Non-palpable breast lesions: Stereotaxic fine-needle aspiration cytology. *Radiology* 1989;173:57–59.
7. Parker SH, Lovin JD, Jobe WE, et al. Non-palpable breast lesions: Stereotactic automated large-core biopsies. *Radiology* 1991;180:403–407.
8. Parker SH, Burbank F, Jackman RJ. Percutaneous large-core breast biopsy: A multi-institutional study. *Radiology* 1994;193:359–364.
9. Jackman RF, Nowels KW, Shepard MJ, et al. Stereotaxic large-core needle biopsy of 450 nonpalpable breast lesions with surgical correlation in lesions with cancer or atypical hyperplasia. *Radiology* 1994;193:91–95.
10. Liberman L, Dershaw D, Rosen PP, et al. Stereotactic core biopsy of impalpable spiculated breast masses. *AJR Am J Roentgenol* 1995;165:551–554.
11. Berg WA. When is core breast biopsy or fine-needle aspiration not enough? *Radiology* 1996;198:313–315.
12. Holland R, Hendriks J, Verbeek A, et al. Extent, distribution, and mammographic/histological correlations of breast ductal carcinoma in situ. *Lancet* 1990;335:519–522.
13. Parker SH, Burbank F. State of the art. A practical approach to minimally invasive breast biopsy. *Radiology* 1996;200:11–20.
14. Burbank F. Stereotactic breast biopsy of ADH and DCIS lesions: Improved accuracy with directional, vacuum-assisted biopsy. *Radiology* 1997;202:843–847.

15. Parker SH, Jobe WE, Dennis MA, et al. US-guided automated large-core breast biopsy. *Radiology* 1993;187:507–511.
16. Stavros AT. Introduction to breast ultrasound. In: Parker SH, Jobe WE, eds. *Percutaneous breast biopsy.* New York: Raven Press, 1993:105–106.
17. Parker SH, Lovin JD, Jobe WE, et al. Stereotactic breast biopsies with a biopsy gun. *Radiology* 1990;176:741–747.
18. Fischer U, Vosshenrich R, Keating D, et al. MR-guided biopsy of suspect breast lesions with a simple stereotaxic add-on device for surface coils. *Radiology* 1994;192:272.
19. Soderstrom CE, Harms SE, Copit DS, et al. 3D RODEO breast MR imaging of lesions containing ductal carcinoma in situ. *Radiology* 1996;201:427.
20. Elvecrog E, Lechner MC, Nelson MT. Non-palpable breast lesions: Correlation of stereotaxic large-core needle biopsy and surgical biopsy results. *Radiology* 1993;188:453–455.
21. Myer JE. Value of large-core biopsy of occult breast lesions. *AJR Am J Roentgenol* 1992;158:991–992.
22. Mukkamala AR, Azher Q, Lawrence L, et al. Stereotaxic core needle biopsy of nonpalpable mammographic lesions. *Radiology* 1993;189(P):325.
23. Elston CW, Cotton RE, Davies CJ, et al. A comparison of the use of the "tru-cut" needle and fine-needle aspiration cytology in the pre-operative diagnosis of carcinoma of the breast. *Histopathology* 1978;2:239–254.
24. Shabot MM, Goldberg IM, Schick P, et al. Aspiration cytology is superior to tru-cut needle biopsy in establishing the diagnosis of clinically suspicious breast masses. *Ann Surg* 1982;196:122–126.
25. Parker SH, Jobe WE. Large-core breast biopsy offers reliable diagnosis. *Diagn Imag* 1990;12(10):90–97.
26. Hopper KD, Adendroth CS, Sturtz KW, et al. Automated biopsy devices: A blinded evaluation. *Radiology* 1993;187:653–660.
27. Liberman L, Dershaw DD, Rosen PP, et al. Stereotaxic 14-gauge breast biopsy: How many core biopsy specimens are needed? *Radiology* 1994;192:793–795.
28. Liberman L, Evans WP, Dershaw DD, et al. Radiography of microcalcifications in stereotaxic mammary core biopsy specimens. *Radiology* 1994;190:223–225.
29. Liberman L, Cohen MA, Dershaw DD, et al. Atypical ductal hyperplasia diagnosed at stereotaxic core biopsy of breast lesions: an indication for surgical biopsy. *AJR Am J Roentgenol* 1995;164:1111–1113.
30. Liberman L, Dershaw DD, Rosen PP, et al. Stereotaxic core biopsy of breast carcinoma: Accuracy at predicting invasion. *Radiology* 1995;194:379–381.
31. Liberman L. Clinical management issues in percutaneous core breast biopsy. *Radiol Clin North Am* 2000;38:791–807.
32. Liberman L, Dershaw DD, Rosen PP, et al. Percutaneous removal of malignant mammographic lesions at stereotactic vacuum-assisted biopsy. *Radiology* 1998;206:711–715.
33. Liberman L. Advanced breast biopsy instrumentation: Analysis of published experience. *AJR Am J Roentgenol* 1999;172:1413–1416.

15

BREAST BIOPSY AND ONCOPLASTIC SURGERY FOR THE PATIENT WITH DUCTAL CARCINOMA IN SITU: SURGICAL, PATHOLOGIC, AND RADIOLOGIC ISSUES

MELVIN J. SILVERSTEIN
SHELLEY NAKAMURA
EUGENE D. GIERSON
WEI-CHIANG HSIAO

LINDA LARSEN
CAROL WOO
YURI PARISKY
PULIN A. SHETH

RASHIDA SONI
WILLIAM J. COLBURN
ANDY SHERROD
PARVIS GAMAGAMI

In 1997, we published a chapter in the first edition of this text entitled: The Coordinated Biopsy Team: Surgical, Pathologic, and Radiologic Issues (1). The data and approaches presented in that chapter were based on patients seen through mid-1996 at the Van Nuys Breast Center. There have been significant changes during the last 6 years, and they are reflected in this chapter. Many of us here at the Harold E. and Henrietta C. Lee Breast Center at the University of Southern California/Norris Comprehensive Cancer Center have been fortunate to adopt some of the ideas and methods of the Van Nuys Breast Center (2) and to develop new tools as we proceeded into this millennium.

A coordinated biopsy team continues to be of great importance. It makes finding and completely excising ductal carcinoma in situ (DCIS) a much simpler task. That has not changed, but some of our approaches have.

With the development of high-quality screening mammography, it has become common to see an asymptomatic patient in whom routine mammography has revealed an area of microcalcifications. To make a diagnosis in the 1980s, this patient would have undergone wire-directed, open surgical breast biopsy (using a single wire) through a circumareolar or curvilinear incision. Because the approach at that time was for diagnosis only, and therefore not aggressive, if DCIS were found, there was a high probability that the margins would have been involved (less than 1 mm) and that a second operative procedure would have been required.

During the 1980s, approximately 70% to 75% of surgical biopsies for microcalcifications yielded benign diagnoses. In addition, surgeons did not fully appreciate the radial segmental distribution of most DCIS lesions or the importance of clear margins. During the 1980s, we irradiated all conservatively treated patients. We were not anxious to initially perform a wide segmental-type resection when the majority of lesions were benign, and we often accepted close or focally involved margins without suggesting re-excision. Our thought was that radiation therapy would deal with any residual cancer cells.

Our approach changed in the late 1980s. We had a greater appreciation of the extent and radial distribution of DCIS. We became more concerned with clear margins, and we lost our enthusiasm for radiation therapy for DCIS. The development of stereotactic core biopsy technology in the 1990s went hand in hand with our new thinking. It was now possible, using a specially designed table with the patient in the prone position, to make a preoperative diagnosis in most cases. This allowed preoperative consultation and planning in addition to only one trip to the operating room for definitive treatment. In this chapter, we will detail the evolution of our thought processes and our current management practices.

DIAGNOSTIC AND SURGICAL PRETREATMENT ISSUES

Radiologic Workup

The importance of high quality mammography and an experienced, dedicated breast radiologist cannot be overemphasized. From 1979 to 1982, the first 3 years of operation of the Van Nuys Breast Center (2), the center utilized a single mammography unit and films were sent across campus to the hospital's general radiologist for interpretation. During those 3 years, the Van Nuys group treated an average of only five patients with DCIS per year, and 84% of the lesions were palpable. In other words, they were diagnosed by clinical presentation rather than mammography. In late 1982, a full-time, experienced, dedicated mammographer joined the Van Nuys staff, and the older mammography unit was replaced with two state-of-the-art units and in-house processing. The average number of new patients with DCIS rapidly increased six-fold to 31 cases per year, 75% of which were nonpalpable and discovered mammographically. In 1987, the Van Nuys group added a third mammography unit, and the number of new cases from 1987 to 1993 increased to 37 per year, 83% of which were nonpalpable. In 1994, a fourth mammography unit was added, as well as a stereotactic unit. During the last 5 years of operation as a multidisciplinary breast center (1994 to 1998), they accrued 41 new patients with DCIS per year and 92% of their patients with DCIS presented with nonpalpable, clinically occult lesions (Fig. 15.1).

The Van Nuys Breast Center ceased operation as a multidisciplinary facility in mid-1998. From that time until the present, our efforts have been focused at the Harold E. and Henrietta C. Lee Breast Center at the Kenneth Norris, Jr. Comprehensive Cancer Center, Keck School of Medicine, University of Southern California (USC). During the first 30 months at this facility, we saw 152 new patients with DCIS (an average of 61 new DCIS cases per year). Only six (4%) had palpable masses or were symptomatic (nipple discharge). Ninety-three percent (142 patients) were discovered mammographically, while 3% (four patients) were diagnosed with DCIS as an incidental finding.

The most common mammographic finding was microcalcifications, frequently clustered and generally without an associated soft tissue abnormality. Overall, 83% (755/909)

of our patients with DCIS exhibited microcalcifications on preoperative mammography: 75% of patients with nuclear grade 1 lesions, 80% with grade 2 lesions, and 89% with grade 3 lesions. Eleven percent of patients had either a mass or an architectural distortion, and 6% had negative mammography. Since lower grade lesions are somewhat less likely to have mammographic calcifications (3), they are more difficult to find initially and more difficult to follow mammographically if treated conservatively.

Calcifications do not always map out the entire extent of a DCIS lesion, particularly in those cases without comedonecrosis. This is a major problem confronting surgeons today. Even though all the calcifications may be removed in a given case, the surgeon may be leaving some DCIS behind. In some cases, the majority of the calcifications are associated with benign changes. In other words, the DCIS lesion may be smaller, larger, or the same size as the calcifications that lead to its identification. The extent of calcifications tends to more closely approximate the size of high-grade DCIS than low-grade lesions (3–6).

When a mammographic abnormality (microcalcifications, a nonpalpable mass, a subtle architectural distortion, etc.) is found, further workup is indicated. This generally includes compression mammography, magnification views, and ultrasonography (6) (See Chapter 10, 11). We now ultrasound all patients with suspicious microcalcifications. In approximately 10% to 15% of patients, there is a mass that accompanies the microcalcifications that cannot been seen by mammography but that can be appreciated by ultrasound. When this occurs, we perform an ultrasound-guided, image-directed breast biopsy targeting the mass. The presence of a mass increases the possibility of invasive breast cancer.

Once a diagnosis of DCIS has been made, selected patients are evaluated by magnetic resonance imaging (MRI).

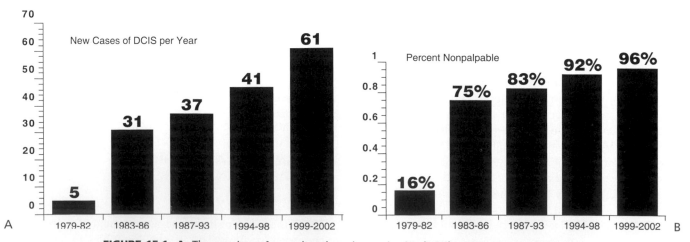

FIGURE 15.1. A: The number of new ductal carcinoma in situ (DCIS) cases per year at the Van Nuys Breast Center (1979 to 1998) and the Harold E. and Henrietta C. Lee Breast Center at the USC/Norris comprehensive Cancer Center, University of Southern California (1999 to 2002). **(B)** The percentage of nonpalpable DCIS cases by year seen at the Van Nuys Breast Center (1979 to 1998) and the Harold E. and Henrietta C. Lee Breast Center at the USC/Norris comprehensive Cancer Center, University of Southern California (1999 to 2002).

We have found MRI to be valuable in patients with very large DCIS lesions or in those who have calcifications in more than one quadrant and, therefore, possible multicentric disease (Chapter 12).

MRI is a promising technology with the potential to solve many breast cancer management problems (7). Currently, breast MRI is limited by lack of availability, inconsistent quality, and only moderate specificity. Although used at some institutions as an adjunct to mammography and ultrasound, breast MRI is not considered standard practice at this time. Breast MRI is currently indicated for patients with axillary metastasis with no known primary, inconclusive mammography after breast conservation or reconstruction, and for determining response to neoadjuvant chemotherapy. Breast MRI is helpful in pretreatment evaluation of local tumor extent and when evaluating a patient previously augmented with silicone- or saline-filled implants. The screening of high-risk patients is promising and should be re-evaluated pending the completion of several ongoing clinical trials.

Once the imaging workup is complete, the radiologist should render an opinion as to whether or not the lesion should be biopsied or followed. While mammographic follow-up in 3 to 6 months may be reasonable for many benign-appearing lesions, it can be an uncertain and anxiety-provoking option. If there is any question about the neoplastic nature of a lesion, we prefer that an accurate diagnosis, benign or malignant, be made in a timely fashion. Many low-grade DCIS lesions can remain unchanged in mammographic appearance for years. A delay of 3 to 6 months with a benign-appearing mammographic lesion, however, is quite reasonable. If by some chance a low-grade DCIS is missed, progression to invasion is not likely.

Biopsy

When biopsy is required, there are a number of ways that this can be achieved. During the last few years, percutaneous tissue acquisition techniques (also called "minimally invasive breast biopsy") have emerged as important diagnostic tools. These include (but are not limited to) fine-needle aspiration (FNA), large-core biopsy (18- to 14-gauge), vacuum-assisted core biopsy (14- to 8-gauge), and larger tissue acquisition systems. The Consensus Committee of the Image-Detected Breast Cancer Consensus Conference recently recommended that when breast biopsy is indicated percutaneous biopsy is preferred over open surgical procedures as the first biopsy procedure in most patients with image-detected abnormalities (7).

Fine needle aspiration (FNA) biopsy, while a good tool for solid lesions, is not a very good tool for DCIS, particularly for DCIS presenting as microcalcifications. While it is possible to use FNA for DCIS, FNA does not resolve the key question. By using mammography to localize the lesion, it is possible to obtain cancer cells with FNA, but since FNA cy-

tology deals with cellular morphology and not architectural detail, a cytopathologist cannot generally differentiate in situ from invasive carcinoma. Beyond that, many DCIS lesions are extremely difficult to diagnose even when the entire area of concern has been surgically removed using open biopsy and many histologic sections have been made. In the absence of a palpable lesion, FNA must be done under mammographic, stereotactic, or sonographic guidance, all of which require special radiographic skills and equipment.

Large-bore needle biopsy can be done with a variety of needles and is relatively easy if the lesion is palpable. If the lesion is nonpalpable, the biopsy can be directed by ultrasound or mammography. Initially, 18-gauge, 16-gauge, and then 14-gauge needles were used. These removed relatively small fragments of tissue and there was a fairly high upstaging rate (as much as 30% to 50%) when an open biopsy was performed after the needle biopsy (8–11): the smaller the core biopsy needle (18-gauge, for example), the higher the upstaging rate. This was remedied to some extent with the development of the vacuum-assisted tools. Initially, a 14-gauge mammotome was developed (Ethicon Endo-Surgery, Cincinnati, OH). This was followed by the 11-gauge and then the 8-gauge. The larger gauge vacuum-assisted tools take significantly larger pieces of tissue with an accuracy greater than 90% (11–13). Numerous other percutaneous tissue acquisition tools are currently under development.

While far better than FNA or needle core biopsy, vacuum-assisted breast biopsy continues to present some minor problems for DCIS. Since the biopsy specimen sample is relatively small, the possibility of invasion in an area of the lesion that was not sampled cannot be excluded. Decisions that require knowledge of whether or not invasion is present, such as axillary node dissection or sentinel node biopsy (in the case of invasive breast cancer), may need to be based on excision of the entire lesion rather than a minimally invasive breast biopsy. If multiple needle biopsies have been performed and the lesion is subsequently surgically removed, the area of the needle biopsies may be artificially disrupted, creating needle tracts and hematoma that can falsely mimic invasion and lymphatic involvement.

At the least aggressive end of the DCIS spectrum, the small biopsy samples occasionally make the distinction between atypical ductal hyperplasia (ADH) and ductal carcinoma in situ very difficult and sometimes impossible. Because of this, we generally recommend surgical biopsy when the percutaneous biopsy diagnosis is atypical ductal hyperplasia. At the other end of the spectrum, the diagnosis of microinvasion may be very difficult from a limited specimen.

In spite of these minor problems, percutaneous minimally invasive breast biopsy is extremely useful for preplanning the extent of resection in patients with DCIS. It is also valuable when there are multiple lesions in one or both breasts, and in patients who have been previously biopsied and do not want to undergo another open biopsy. It leaves a minimal scar. It is a relatively simple outpatient procedure and hematoma and infection complications are infrequent. In addition, subsequent mammograms show little architectural distortion following this type of biopsy.

A clip marking the biopsy site should be left in place if technically possible. It is not uncommon for a radiologist to remove the entire lesion if it is small. Wide local excision following percutaneous biopsy is difficult, and may be inaccurate if the radiologist has no marker around which to place the hooked wires. If there is a hematoma cavity, this may be localized using ultrasound.

Following any form of percutaneous breast biopsy (except FNA), we always wrap the patient with a 24 to 30 foot bias pressure dressing (Fig. 15.2) (Fisher Imaging, Inc., Denver, CO), using exactly the same technique that we use for open breast biopsy. With the combination of meticulous hemostasis and the bias pressure wrap, we have only had to drain six hematomas in more than 7,000 open biopsies. Even ecchymoses are unusual if this wrap is properly applied. By using the bias pressure wrap at the conclusion of stereotactic core biopsy, we have had no clinical hematomas and only an occasional ecchymosis.

Hematomas may compromise treatment when they occur after minimally invasive breast biopsy or open surgical biopsy (Fig. 15.3). If a significant hematoma occurs in the immediate postoperative period, we take those patients to the operating room within 24 hours and drain the hematoma. Because the surrounding tissue has not had sufficient time to respond, rapid intervention usually yields excellent cosmetic results that are virtually identical to what would have been achieved if there had been no hematoma.

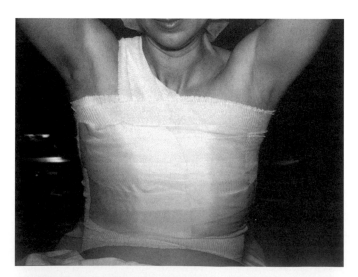

FIGURE 15.2. A cotton bias wrap (Fisher Imaging, Inc.) approximately 24 to 30 feet long has been used to apply pressure to the biopsy site. This patient is wide awake and cooperative after breast surgery using local anesthesia and intravenous sedation. The same bias wrap is used after mastectomy or axillary dissection done under general anesthesia. This wrap is left in place for 24 to 48 hours, and is used on all percutaneous needle biopsies (except fine needle aspirations), all open surgical biopsies, all axillary dissections, and all mastectomies.

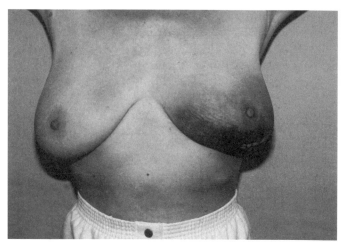

FIGURE 15.3. A 5-day postoperative 55-year-old patient from another facility. An 8-cm hematoma was evacuated in the operating room. As is generally the case, no significant bleeder was found. Drainage of the hematoma resulted in an excellent cosmetic result with no delay in her beginning radiation therapy.

Unfortunately, we often see patients from other facilities with well-established hematomas of 2 to 4 weeks duration (Fig. 15.4). These patients present a significant and difficult challenge, because the surrounding tissue becomes firm and inelastic. Draining the hematoma will leave an empty hole that fills with serum. If a drain is used, the overlying skin dents inward, yielding a poor cosmetic result. In these patients, the hematoma must either be allowed to resolve or it must be completely excised with a rim of surrounding tissue. If the patient has pure DCIS and the hematoma is not too large (5 cm or smaller), we may elect to allow the hematoma to resolve, although this may take many months. Some hematomas will drain spontaneously while they are being allowed to reabsorb. This represents a significant wound management problem for the patient.

The cosmetic results are poor when irradiating patients with a resolving hematoma. We are more likely to excise the hematoma and remodel the breast as well as possible for the patient with an invasive breast cancer that requires irradiation.

Percutaneous biopsy may spare as many as 80% of patients with histologically benign image-detected abnormalities from undergoing open surgical biopsy procedures. When a definitive diagnosis of cancer is made by minimally invasive breast biopsy, it permits optimal preoperative planning. This often results in definitive treatment with a single trip to the operating room and substantial cost savings for the overall course of patient management. For these reasons, percutaneous biopsy is preferred over an open needle-directed surgical procedure as the primary biopsy procedure in most patients with image-detected abnormalities.

When a diagnosis cannot be made by percutaneous breast biopsy, open surgical needle directed breast biopsy is generally indicated. A directed biopsy makes use of an aid,

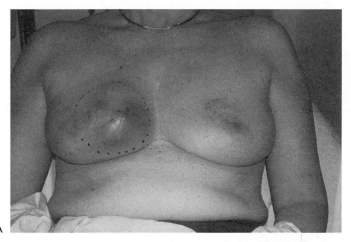

A

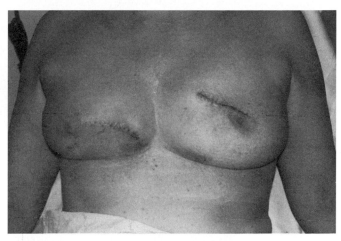

B

FIGURE 15.4. A 57-year-old patient who had undergone bilateral breast biopsies at another facility for suspicious microcalcifications. Curvilinear incisions rather than radial incisions were used. Ductal carcinoma in situ (DCIS) was found on both sides. The margins on the left side were involved. **(A)** She developed an 8 to 9 cm hematoma on the right side and was advised by her original surgeon to allow the hematoma to resolve and then follow with radiation therapy. **(B)** At the USC/Norris Cancer Center, the right hematoma was excised immediately through a radial incision and the breast was remodeled. No residual DCIS was found. The left DCIS was re-excised using a radial incision and flap advancement. A 5 mm invasive cancer and residual DCIS was found. With new 10 mm margins, no additional therapy was given on the right. On the left side, the new margins were 3 mm. She was treated with radiation therapy and tamoxifen. The photograph in **(B)** was taken 2 weeks after re-excision.

such as a hooked wire or a dye like methylene blue, to direct the surgeon to the nonpalpable mammographic abnormality. Because the wire is solid and can be palpated by the surgeon, it is more reliable than dye. Wire also aids the surgeon in attempting to achieve a clear margin. We have no problem with dye being used in conjunction with a wire, but dye has disadvantages by itself. Most important, the lesion may be difficult to find, which makes complete excision less likely. For DCIS, a single wire is better than dye without a wire, but may not be adequate in many cases. Multiple wires make complete excision much easier and more likely.

the widest possible margins (the limit, of course, being a mastectomy). From a cosmetic point of view, a much smaller amount of tissue should be removed, disturbing the breast as little as possible. Since more than 90% of currently diagnosed DCIS cases are both grossly nonpalpable and cannot be visualized, the surgeon essentially operates blindly. Multiple wires, to a major extent, solve this problem.

The first attempt to remove a cancerous lesion is critical. The first excision offers the best chance to remove the entire lesion in one piece and to achieve the best possible cosmetic result. We strongly recommend that an attempt be made by

TREATMENT ISSUES

Oncoplastic Surgery

Oncoplastic surgery combines sound oncologic surgical principles with plastic surgical techniques. Coordination of the two disciplines is encouraged, and may help to avoid poor cosmetic results after wide excision (Fig. 15.5). In addition, it may increase the number of women who can be treated with breast-conserving surgery rather than mastectomy by allowing surgeons to perform larger breast excisions with acceptable cosmetic results. While this textbook is devoted to DCIS, much of this information can be applied to patients with invasive breast cancer.

When excising a lesion that is probably DCIS, the surgeon faces two opposing goals: clear margins versus good cosmesis. From an oncologic point of view, the largest specimen possible should be removed in an attempt to achieve

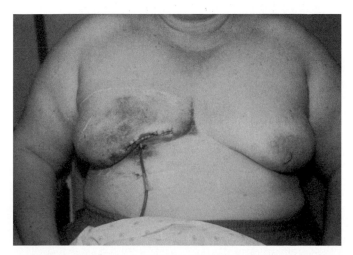

FIGURE 15.5. A 57-year-old patient from another hospital with a very poor cosmetic result from a non-oncoplastic excision.

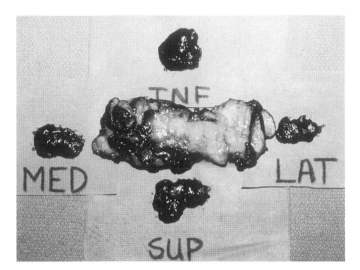

FIGURE 15.6. An excision specimen with four additional pieces that allegedly represent the new margins. The additional pieces are too small and do not reflect the true margins of the original specimen. A judgment on margin clearance based on these small additional pieces is likely to be wrong.

the surgeon to excise the entire lesion in a single piece of tissue. If the specimen is removed in multiple pieces rather than a single piece, there is little likelihood of accurately evaluating margins and size. Figure 15.6 shows an excision specimen with four additional pieces that allegedly represent the new margins. The additional pieces are too small and do not reflect the true margins of the original specimen. A judgment based on margin clearance on these small additional pieces is likely to be wrong. Figure 15.7 is a better attempt at complete margin re-excision, but even these larger pieces fail to completely re-excise the biopsy cavity.

Once the diagnosis of DCIS has been made by percutaneous biopsy and after the patient has been fully counseled and has elected breast conservation, a complete excision using an oncoplastic approach is attempted. We currently use two (Fig. 15.8) to four (Fig. 15.9) wires to bracket all DCIS lesions (14,15). The wires are placed approximately 10 mm from the edges of the lesion. We never remove a possible DCIS using a single wire, since it may result in incomplete removal of the abnormality, calcifications at the edge of the specimen (Fig. 15.10), positive histologic margins, and the need to re-excise the biopsy cavity. The bracketing wire technique does not guarantee complete removal during the initial biopsy, but it makes it more likely. Incomplete excisions are more likely to result when the mammographic abnormality does not correspond to the entire extent of the lesion (16). This is more likely to occur in low-grade rather than high-grade lesions (4,5). The failure to perform specimen radiography in every wire-directed case may also lead to incomplete excision, since immediate feedback from the radiologist as to the adequacy of the excision is lacking.

Segmentectomy Using a Radial Incision

The whole-organ studies of Holland and Faverly (3–5) have clearly demonstrated the radial nature of the disease. This has also been confirmed by more recent studies (17). Due to the radial distribution of most DCIS, we try to plan our incision accordingly; most of our incisions are radial, like the spokes of a wheel.

Figure 15.11 shows a patient with a curvilinear lateral incision made in the 3-o'clock position of the left breast at another facility. The medial margin extending toward the nipple was positive. After mammography, she was re-excised using a radial incision and four guide wires. The entire lateral segment down to and including the pectoralis major fascia was removed. The surrounding tissue was then undermined with electrocautery or the harmonic scalpel (Ethicon Endo-Surgery, Inc., Cincinnati, OH). After the tissue was undermined, it was advanced with deep sutures, and all layers were then closed.

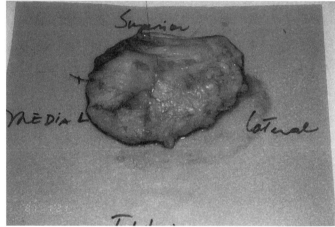

A

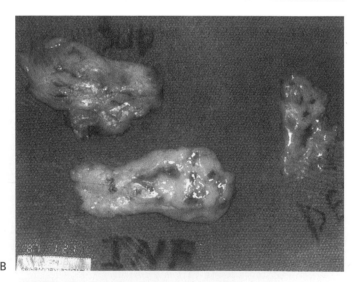

B

FIGURE 15.7. A better attempt at complete margin re-excision than Figure 15.6, but even these larger pieces fail to completely re-excise the biopsy cavity. **(A)** is the original excision. **(B)** is the additional tissue removed.

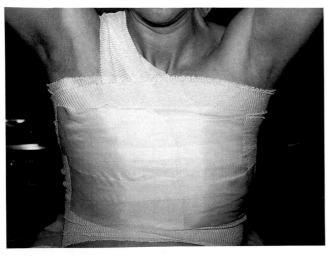

COLOR FIGURE 15.2. A cotton bias wrap (Fisher Imaging, Inc.) approximately 24 to 30 feet long has been used to apply pressure to the biopsy site. This patient is wide awake and cooperative after breast surgery using local anesthesia and intravenous sedation. The same bias wrap is used after mastectomy or axillary dissection done under general anesthesia. This wrap is left in place for 24 to 48 hours, and is used on all percutaneous needle biopsies (except fine needle aspirations), all open surgical biopsies, all axillary dissections, and all mastectomies.

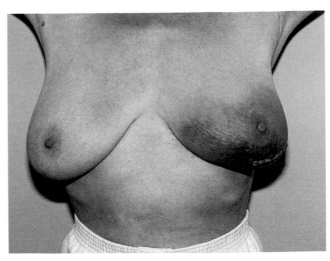

COLOR FIGURE 15.3. A 5-day postoperative 55-year-old patient from another facility. An 8-cm hematoma was evacuated in the operating room. As is generally the case, no significant bleeder was found. Drainage of the hematoma resulted in an excellent cosmetic result with no delay in her beginning radiation therapy.

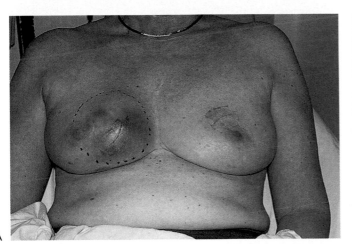

A

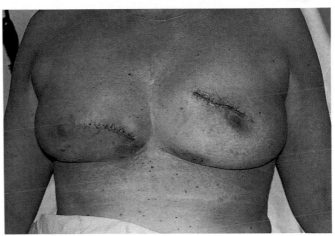

B

COLOR FIGURE 15.4. A 57-year-old patient who had undergone bilateral breast biopsies at another facility for suspicious microcalcifications. Curvilinear incisions rather than radial incisions were used. Ductal carcinoma in situ (DCIS) was found on both sides. The margins on the left side were involved. **(A)** She developed an 8 to 9 cm hematoma on the right side and was advised to allow the hematoma to resolve and then followed with radiation therapy. **(B)** At the USC/Norris Cancer Center, the right hematoma was excised through a radial incision and the breast was remodeled. No residual DCIS was found. The left DCIS was re-excised using a radial incision and flap advancement. A 5 mm invasive cancer and residual DCIS was found. With new 10 mm margins, no additional therapy was given on the right. On the left side, the new margins were 3 mm. She was treated with radiation therapy and tamoxifen. The photograph in **(B)** was taken 2 weeks after re-excision.

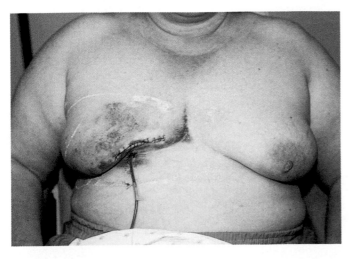

COLOR FIGURE 15.5. A 57-year-old patient from another hospital with a very poor cosmetic result from a non-oncoplastic excision.

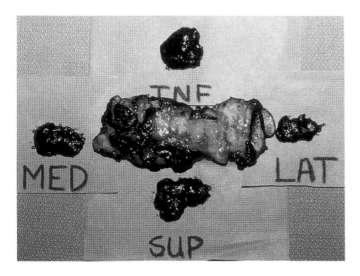

COLOR FIGURE 15.6. An excision specimen with four additional pieces that allegedly represent the new margins. The additional pieces are too small and do not reflect the true margins of the original specimen. A judgment on margin clearance based on these small additional pieces is likely to be wrong.

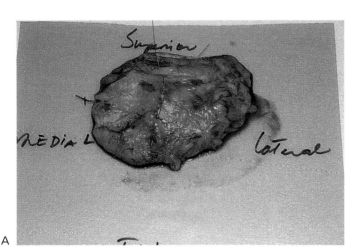

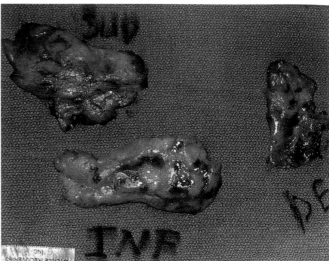

COLOR FIGURE 15.7. A better attempt at complete margin re-excision than Figure 15.6, but even these larger pieces fail to completely re-excise the biopsy cavity. **(A)** is the original excision. **(B)** is the additional tissue removed.

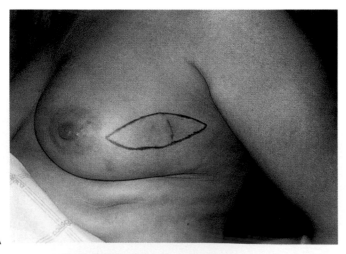

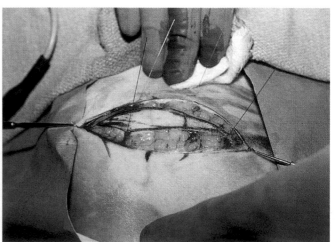

COLOR FIGURE 15.11. A 45-year-old patient in whom a curvilinear lateral incision has been made in the 3-o'clock position of the left breast at another facility. **(A)** The medial margin, extending toward the nipple was positive. After mammography, the lesion was re-excised using a radial incision and four guide wires. **(A, B)** The entire lateral segment down to and including the pectoralis major fascia was removed. *(continued)*

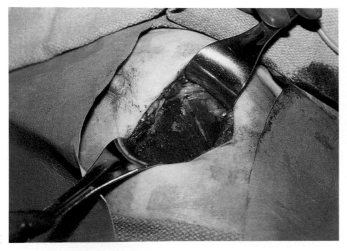
C

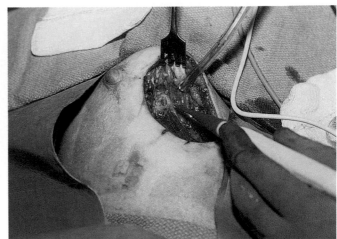
D

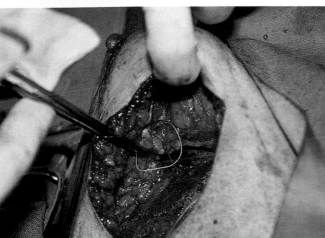
E

COLOR FIGURE 15.11. *(Continued)*. **(C)** The surrounding tissue is then undermined with the electrocautery or the harmonic scalpel (Ethicon Endo-Surgery, Inc., Cincinnati, OH). **(D)** After the tissue has been undermined, it is advanced with deep sutures **(E)**.

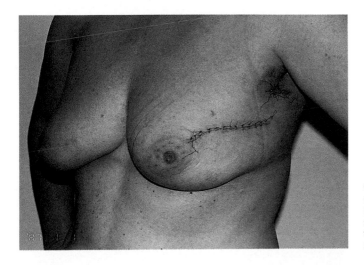

COLOR FIGURE 15.12. A 38-year-old patient 5 days post-left-lateral-to-upper-outer-quadrant segmental resection for ductal carcinoma in situ. The drain was removed on postoperative day 1. The sutures were removed immediately after this photograph was taken. The left breast is slightly smaller than the right, but the overall cosmetic result is excellent.

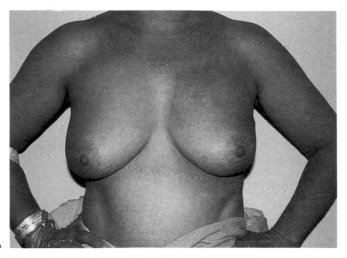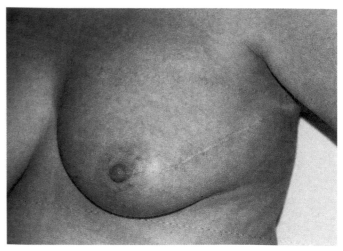

COLOR FIGURE 15.13. A: A 44-year-old patient 6 months after left lateral segmental resection for ductal carcinoma in situ. No radiotherapy was given. The left breast is slightly smaller than the right. **(B)** Oblique view of the patient in **(A)**. The scar is well healed.

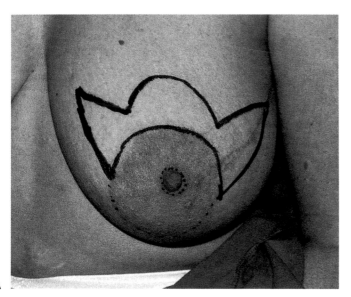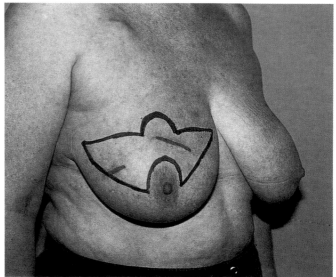

COLOR FIGURE 15.14. Typical batwing incision plans. These incisions can be used in any patient with a medium to large sized breast. The wings of the incision can be designed to allow removal of lesions anywhere from the 8-o'clock to the 4-o'clock position (clockwise).

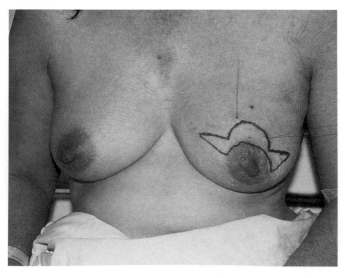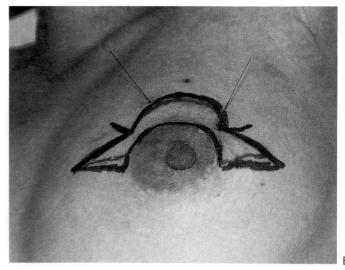

COLOR FIGURE 15.15. A 51-year-old patient with a 55 mm ductal carcinoma in situ. **(A)** Frontal view with batwing treatment plan drawn and two hooked wires are in place bracketing the lesion. **(B)** Close-up frontal view. Patient is lying down. *(continued)*

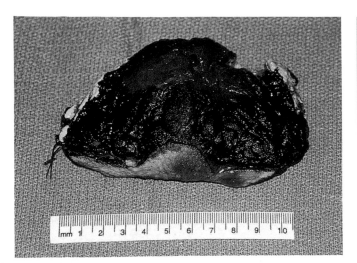

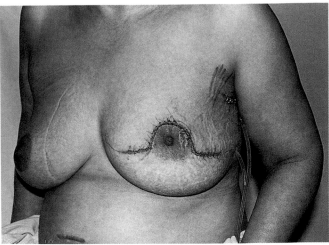

C

D

COLOR FIGURE 15.15. *(Continued).* **(C)** 12 cm batwing-shaped specimen has been excised and color coded prior to sectioning. The skin has some blue discoloration from sentinel lymph node biopsy that was performed in this case because of the large size of the lesion. **(D)** The patient 2 days postoperative after her bias pressure wrap has been removed. There is no ecchymosis or hematoma. There is some blue discoloration of the skin from sentinel lymph node biopsy. The breast shape and symmetry is excellent. The drain is in place and was removed immediately after taking this photograph. The patient was then re-wrapped with a bias pressure dressing for another 24 hours.

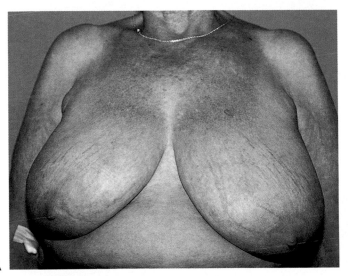

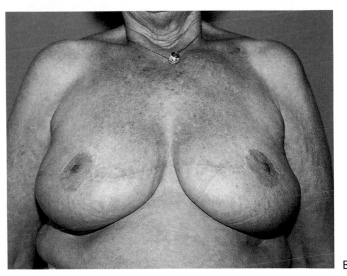

A

B

COLOR FIGURE 15.16. A: A 69-year-old patient with a 20 mm ductal carcinoma in situ in the right breast, 12-o'clock position, above the nipple areolar complex. **(B)** She underwent bilateral batwing segmental resections. More than 500 grams of tissue was removed from both sides. On the right side, all margins were clear by 15 mm or more. No disease was found on the left. No additional treatment was given (no radiotherapy or tamoxifen). There has been no recurrence of disease more than 7 years after the original surgery.

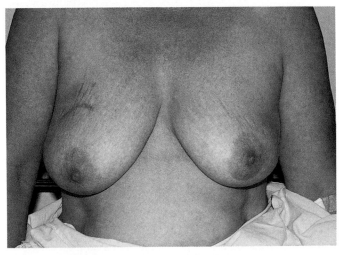

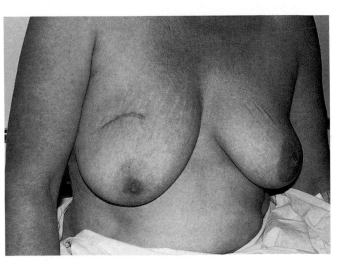

A

B

COLOR FIGURE 15.17. A 53-year-old patient with large upper-outer-to-upper-central ductal carcinoma in situ (DCIS). **(A)** This patient underwent multiple previous excision attempts elsewhere through a transverse upper central incision for a large DCIS. The margins were persistently positive inferiorly, toward the nipple. **(B)** Oblique view. *(continued)*

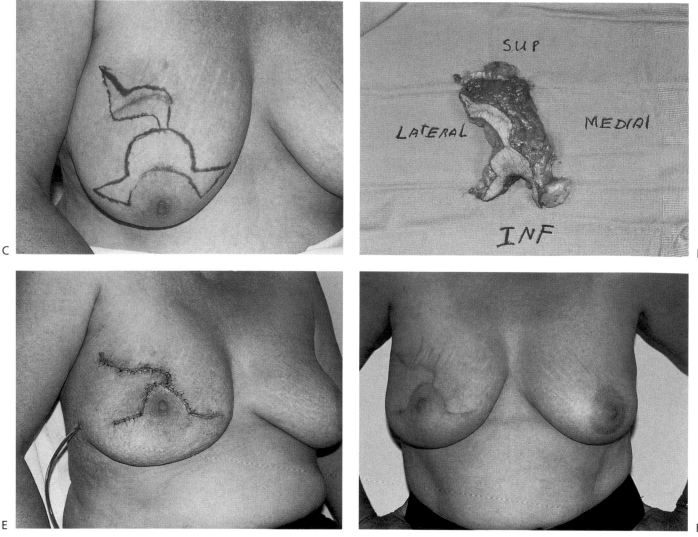

COLOR FIGURE 15.17. *(Continued).* **(C)** Incision plan: batwing with re-excision of previous biopsy site; elevate and reduce the right breast, which is fortunately a bit larger than the left. The incision will convert the upper transverse incision to a radial resection. **(D)** The excision specimen before color coding. It weighed 142 grams. **(E)** 2 days postoperative. There is no hematoma or ecchymosis. The symmetry is good. The shape is excellent. The drain was removed immediately after taking this picture. **(F)** 1 month postoperative.

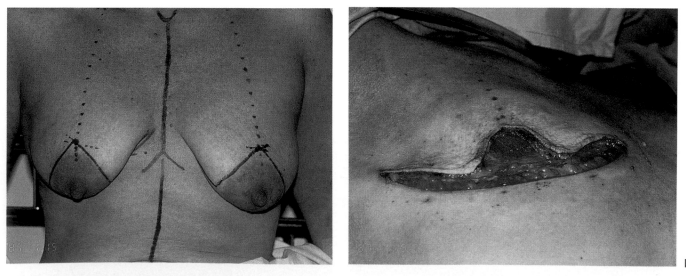

COLOR FIGURE 15.18. A 44-year-old patient with a 70 mm right-sided ductal carcinoma in situ. Due to the large size of her lesion and the relatively small size of her breast, she was not thought to be a candidate for breast conservation. **(A)** Preoperative treatment plan. A right mastectomy with sentinel node biopsy will be performed through a reduction excision. The right nipple-areola complex will be removed. A left mastopexy will be performed through a standard reduction mammoplasty incision. **(B)** The right mastectomy has been performed through a reduction mammoplasty incision. The nipple-areolar complex has been removed. *(continued)*

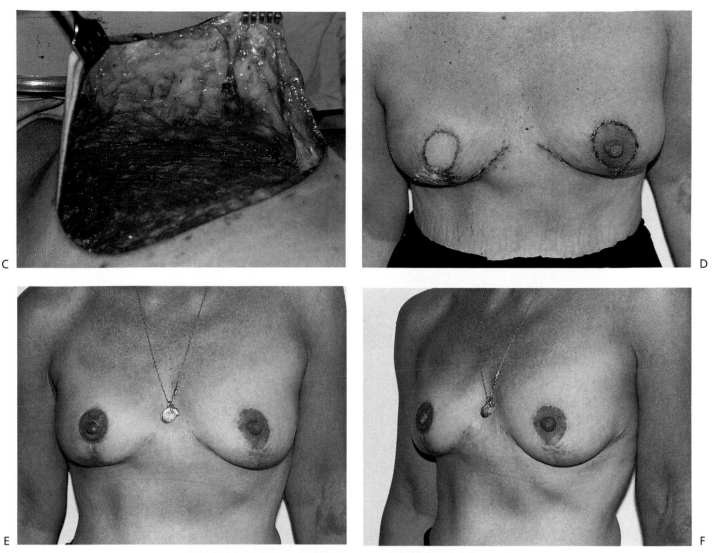

COLOR FIGURE 15.18. *(Continued).* **(C)** Isosulfan blue, which has turned green, was used to find the sentinel node and can be seen in lymphatics on the superior flap. The skin flaps are thin and viable. The pectoralis major muscle fascia has been removed with the mastectomy specimen. **(D)** 1 month postoperative. The right immediate reconstruction was performed with a pedical TRAM flap. **(E)** 6 months postoperative. The right nipple areola has been reconstructed with a local flap and tattooing. **(F)** Oblique view after reconstruction.

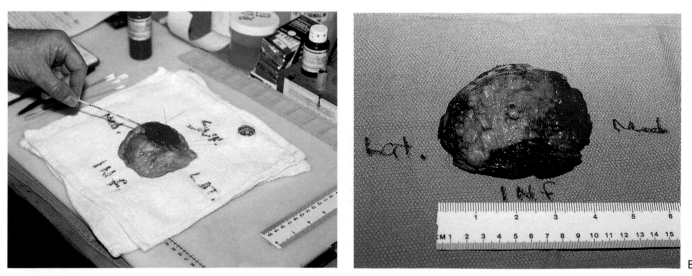

COLOR FIGURE 15.19. Inking the specimen. **(A)** The pathologist has been given an oriented specimen. The specimen radiograph has been taken and the pathologist has begun the color coding with red ink for the superior surface. **(B)** A completely color coded specimen with a different color ink marking each surface.

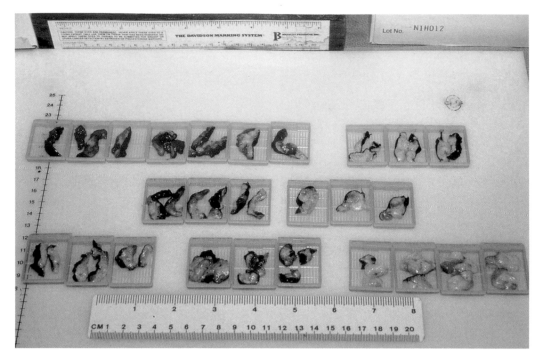

COLOR FIGURE 15.20. The specimen has been color coded, serially sectioned, and sequentially submitted.

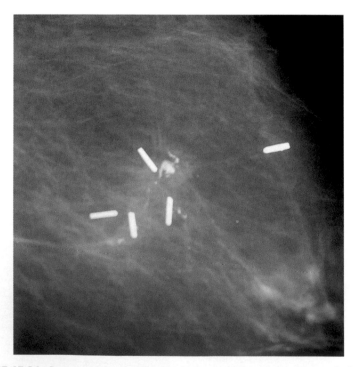

COLOR FIGURE 15.21. Postoperative mediolateral mammogram. Metal clips mark the biopsy cavity.

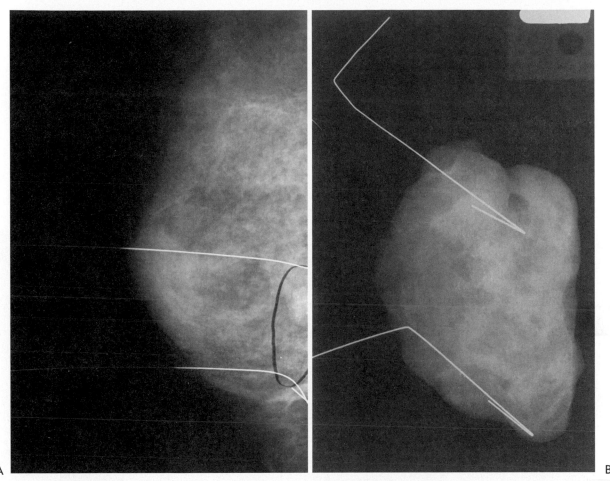

A B

FIGURE 15.8. A: Mediolateral mammogram taken after insertion of two bracketing wires around an area of microcalcifications in the extreme posterior aspect of the right breast. **(B)** Magnification specimen radiograph of two wire–directed breast biopsy showing a cluster of microcalcifications with mammographically clear margins (same patient as Figure 15.5 A).

We drain most segmental resections for 24 to 48 hours and completely close the wound in layers, constantly checking and reappraising the cosmetic result. In contrast to the old axiom that "the seroma is your friend," we feel exactly the opposite. We prefer the wound to heal with as little seroma and blood as possible. Regardless of how the wound is closed, there will always be a small amount of fluid in the biopsy cavity, but we prefer to minimize it.

This type of segmental resection may change the size and shape of the breast, but good cosmetic results are generally achieved (Figs. 15.12 and 15.13).

Segmentectomy Using a Reduction Mammoplasty Incision

In a fully counseled woman with a larger breast that might benefit from a reduction mammoplasty or a mastopexy, and whose DCIS is in position in the breast that allows complete removal through a reduction or a mastopexy incision, we use an appropriately designed re-

duction incision. For lesions in the lower hemisphere of the breast (the 4-o'clock to 8-o'clock position, going clockwise), a standard reduction incision is used. For lateral, superior, or medial lesions (the 8-o'clock to 4-o'clock position, going clockwise), we often use a "batwing" incision (Fig. 15.14). Both of these approaches allow the lesion to be generously removed (specimens are typically 200 grams or more) while preserving the contour of the breast. In both, the nipple areolar complex is elevated from its original position (Fig. 15.15). We do not generally adjust the contralateral breast at the same time; we prefer to know the final pathology and margin status, in particular, before altering the appearance of the opposite breast. However, after thorough discussion, in some cases and if it is possible, the patient may decide she is willing to accept the risks and prefers a single operation (Fig. 15.16).

If permanent microscopic sections reveal involved margins and the residual breast is amenable to re-excision, we often wait as long as 3 months for the inflammatory response and induration to subside before re-excising a DCIS

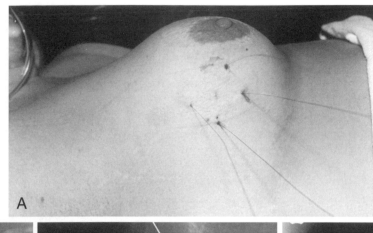

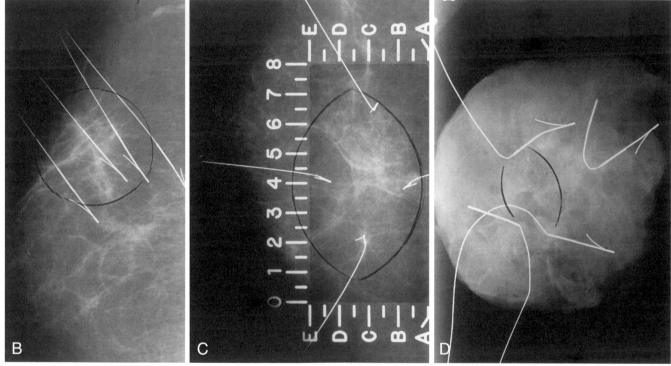

FIGURE 15.9. A: Preoperative photograph of a patient with four wires in place. **(B)** Mediolateral mammogram taken after insertion of four bracketing wires around an area of architectural distortion and microcalcifications. **(C)** Craniocaudal mammogram taken after insertion of four bracketing wires around an area of architectural distortion and microcalcifications [same patient as **(B)**]. **(D)** Magnification specimen radiograph of four wire–directed breast biopsy showing a cluster of microcalcifications and the architectural distortion excised with mammographically clear margins.

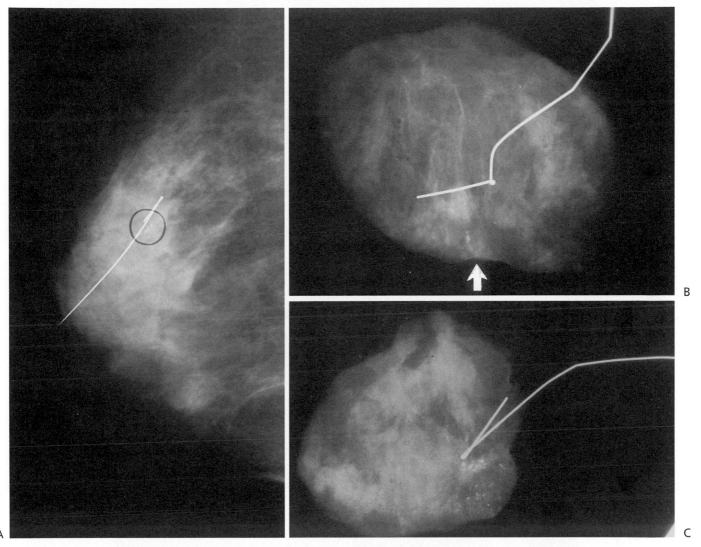

FIGURE 15.10. A: Mediolateral mammogram taken after insertion of a single bracketing wire. The wire placement is perfect in that it is extremely close to the microcalcifications and goes 1 cm beyond them. **(B)** Magnification specimen radiograph of a single wire–directed breast biopsy showing a cluster of microcalcifications at the edge of the biopsy specimen *(arrow)* in spite of perfect wire placement [same patient as **(A)**]. **(C)** Specimen radiograph of another patient with a perfectly placed single wire in which the microcalcifications extend to the edge of the specimen and have been incompletely removed.

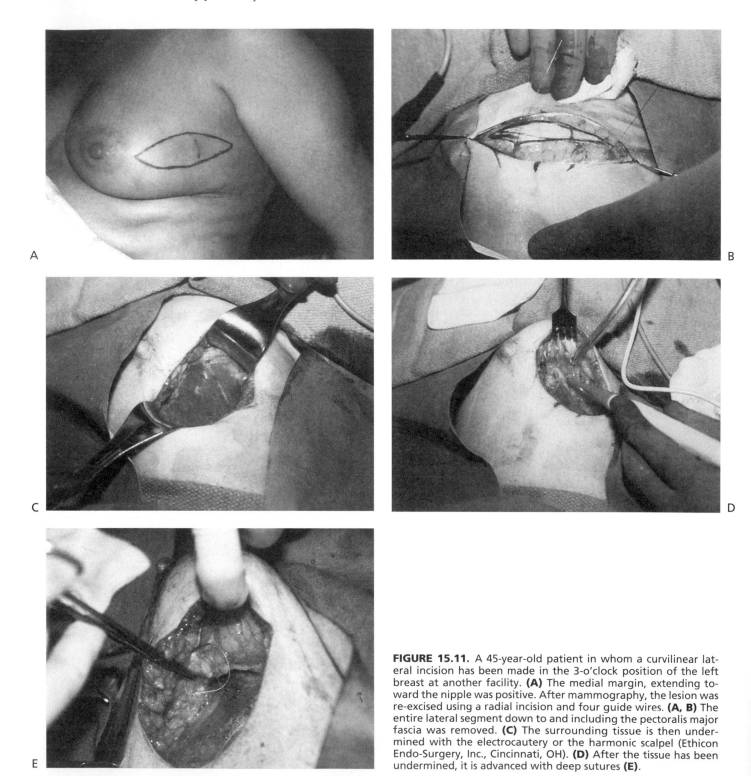

FIGURE 15.11. A 45-year-old patient in whom a curvilinear lateral incision has been made in the 3-o'clock position of the left breast at another facility. **(A)** The medial margin, extending toward the nipple was positive. After mammography, the lesion was re-excised using a radial incision and four guide wires. **(A, B)** The entire lateral segment down to and including the pectoralis major fascia was removed. **(C)** The surrounding tissue is then undermined with the electrocautery or the harmonic scalpel (Ethicon Endo-Surgery, Inc., Cincinnati, OH). **(D)** After the tissue has been undermined, it is advanced with deep sutures **(E)**.

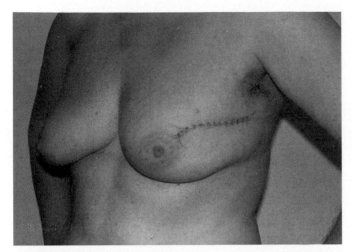

FIGURE 15.12. A 38-year-old patient 5 days post-left-lateral-to-upper-outer-quadrant segmental resection for ductal carcinoma in situ. The drain was removed on postoperative day 1. The sutures were removed immediately after this photograph was taken. The left breast is slightly smaller than the right, but the overall cosmetic result is excellent.

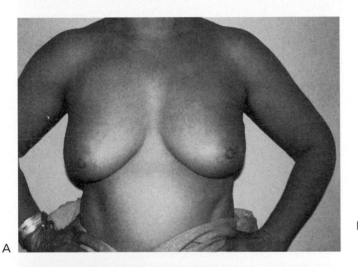

A

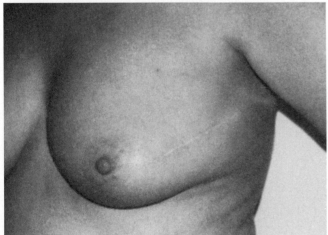

B

FIGURE 15.13. A: A 44-year-old patient 6 months after left lateral segmental resection for ductal carcinoma in situ. No radiotherapy was given. The left breast is slightly smaller than the right. **(B)** Oblique view of the patient in **(A)**. The scar is well healed.

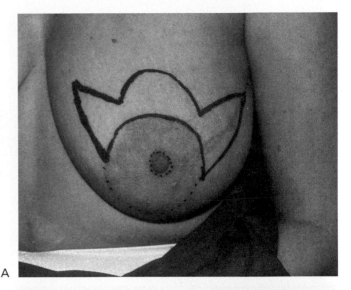

A

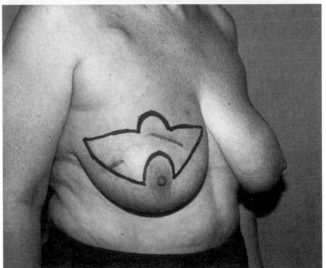

B

FIGURE 15.14. Typical batwing incision plans. These incisions can be used in any patient with a medium to large sized breast. The wings of the incision can be designed to allow removal of lesions anywhere from the 2-o'clock to the 4-o'clock position (clockwise) and from the 8-o'clock to the 10-o'clock position.

lesion. As mentioned earlier, there is little chance that a DCIS lesion will progress in 3 months, and the cosmetic results from re-excision are generally better after a sufficient period of wound healing and resolution. Figure 15.17 shows a 53-year-old patient with a large upper-outer-to-upper central DCIS. After numerous excisions through an upper central incision, margins remained positive. We allowed the wound to heal for three additional months and re-excised it using a modified batwing combined with re-excision of the old scar. This approach converted her resection to a radial segmentectomy with excellent cosmetic results.

In patients with lesions that are mammographically too large to yield clear margins and acceptable cosmetic result, we prefer to go directly to skin-sparing mastectomy and au-

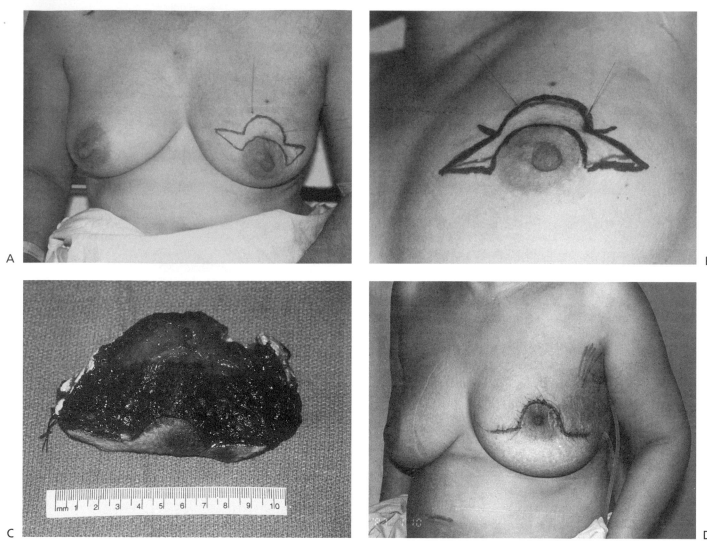

A   B

C   D

FIGURE 15.15. A 51-year-old patient with a 55 mm ductal carcinoma in situ. **(A)** Frontal view with batwing treatment plan drawn and two hooked wires are in place bracketing the lesion. **(B)** Close-up frontal view. Patient is lying down. **(C)** 12 cm batwing-shaped specimen has been excised and color coded prior to sectioning. The skin has some blue discoloration from sentinel lymph node biopsy that was performed in this case because of the large size of the lesion. **(D)** The patient 2 days postoperative after her bias pressure wrap has been removed. There is no ecchymosis or hematoma. There is some blue discoloration of the skin from sentinel lymph node biopsy. The breast shape and symmetry are excellent. The drain is in place and was removed immediately after taking this photograph. The patient was then re-wrapped with a bias pressure dressing for another 24 hours.

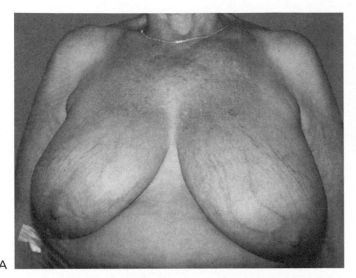
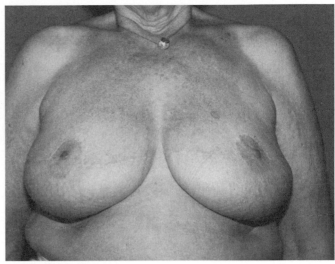

A B

FIGURE 15.16. A: A 69-year-old patient with a 20 mm ductal carcinoma in situ in the right breast, 12-o'clock position, above the nipple areolar complex. **(B)** She underwent bilateral batwing segmental resections. More than 500 grams of tissue was removed from both sides. On the right side, all margins were clear by 15 mm or more. No disease was found on the left. No additional treatment was given (no radiotherapy or tamoxifen). There has been no recurrence of disease more than 7 years after the original surgery.

tologous reconstruction, generally with a transverse rectus abdominus myocutaneous (TRAM) flap. After performing only a percutaneous minimally invasive breast biopsy in these patients, we are seldom faced with a skin incision in the wrong place or a biopsy scar that needs re-excision. Figure 15.18 shows a patient with a large right sided lesion who underwent a right mastectomy using a standard reduction incision and a simultaneous contralateral left mastopexy. During a mastectomy, we have no hesitation adjusting the contralateral breast since little else can be done on the ipsilateral side.

Handling of the Biopsy Specimen/Tissue Processing

Needle localization, intraoperative specimen radiography, and correlation with the preoperative mammogram should be performed in every nonpalpable case (7). Margins should be inked or dyed (Fig. 15.19), and specimens should be serially sectioned at 2 to 3 mm intervals (Fig. 15.20). The tissue sections should be arranged and processed sequentially. We generally fix the specimen in a combined alcohol formalin mixture (commercial Pen-Fix) for variable lengths of time depending on fat content. Fattier specimens may be fixed over night before sectioning, while more fibrous specimens may be sectioned and submitted for processing after only 4 to 6 hours. Ideally the entire specimen is submitted, which was our practice through mid-1998. Currently, for very large pieces of tissue, the economic climate is such that it is often unfeasible to submit the entire specimen in every case. We now submit the entire specimen when it will not exceed 30 to 40 cassettes. Beyond this threshold, additional sections as

defined grossly or by specimen radiography may be submitted according to a working schematic that maintains orientation. Following initial histopathologic review, additional sections are submitted if needed to determine the overall dimensions and finalize accurate margins of the disease process.

Pathologic reporting should include a determination of nuclear grade, an assessment of the presence or absence of comedo-type necrosis, the measured size or extent of the lesion, the margin status with measurement of the closest margin, a description of all architectural subtypes with their relative amounts of each, and the presence or absence of microinvasion.

Tumor size should be determined by direct measurement or, for smaller lesions, ocular micrometry from stained slides. For larger lesions, a combination of direct measurement and estimation based on the distribution of the lesion in a sequential series of slides should be used. The proximity of DCIS to an inked margin should be determined by direct measurement or ocular micrometry. The closest single distance between any involved duct containing DCIS and an inked margin should be reported.

The Coordinated Biopsy Team

Removal of nonpalpable lesions is best performed with an integrated and coordinated team consisting of a surgeon, a radiologist, and a pathologist. To obtain the most reliable results, the radiologist who places the wires must be experienced, as must the surgeon who removes the lesion, and the pathologist who processes the tissue.

At The Van Nuys Breast Center, we were fortunate to have been able to develop an optimal system for wire-

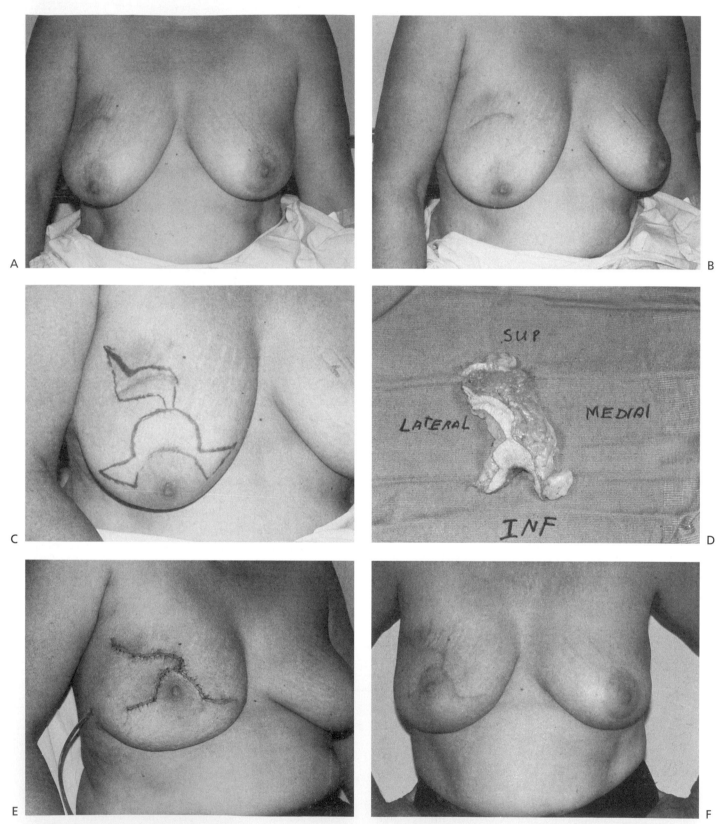

FIGURE 15.17. A 53-year-old patient with large upper-outer-to-upper-central ductal carcinoma in situ (DCIS). **(A)** This patient underwent multiple previous excision attempts elsewhere through a transverse upper central incision for a large DCIS. The margins were persistently positive inferiorly, toward the nipple. **(B)** Oblique view. **(C)** Incision plan: batwing with re-excision of previous biopsy site; elevate and reduce the right breast, which is fortunately a bit larger than the left. The incision will convert the upper transverse incision to a radial resection. **(D)** The excision specimen before color coding. It weighed 142 grams. **(E)** 2 days postoperative. There is no hematoma or ecchymosis. The symmetry is good. The shape is excellent. The drain was removed immediately after taking this picture. **(F)** 1 month postoperative.

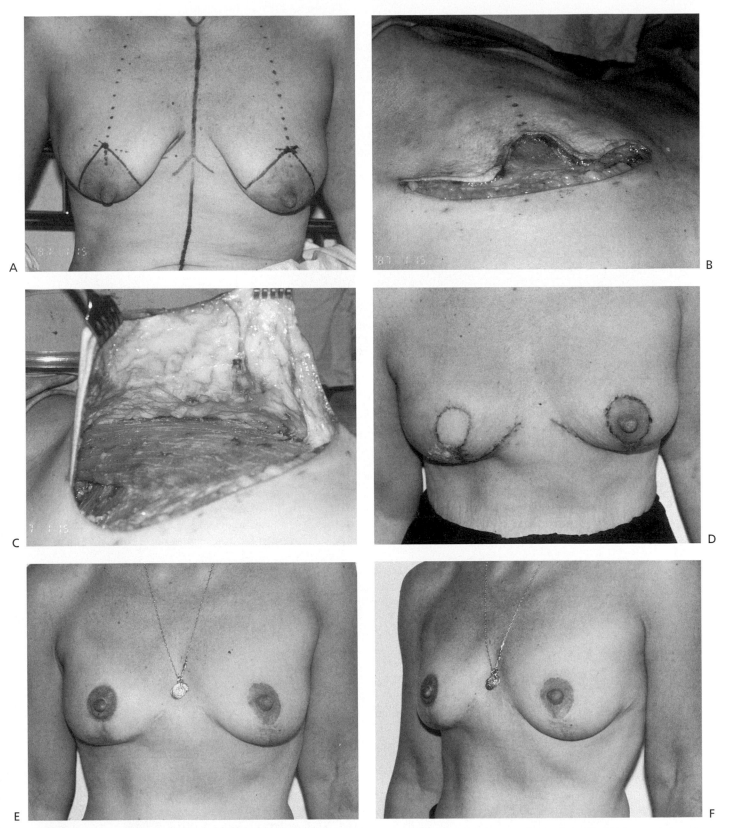

FIGURE 15.18. A 44-year-old patient with a 70 mm right-sided ductal carcinoma in situ. Due to the large size of her lesion and the relatively small size of her breast, she was not thought to be a candidate for breast conservation. **(A)** Preoperative treatment plan. A right mastectomy with sentinel node biopsy will be performed through a reduction excision. The right nipple-areola complex will be removed. A left mastopexy will be performed through a standard reduction mammoplasty incision. **(B)** The right mastectomy has been performed through a reduction mammoplasty incision. The nipple-areolar complex has been removed. **(C)** Isosulfan blue, which has turned green, was used to find the sentinel node and can be seen in lymphatics on the superior flap. The skin flaps are thin and viable. The pectoralis major muscle fascia has been removed with the mastectomy specimen. **(D)** 1 month postoperative. The right immediate reconstruction was performed with a pedical TRAM flap. **(E)** 6 months postoperative. The right nipple areola has been reconstructed with a local flap and tattooing. **(F)** Oblique view after reconstruction.

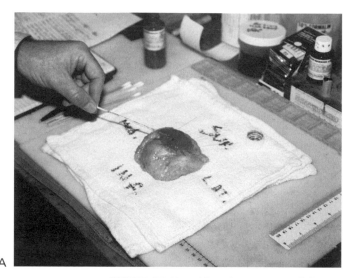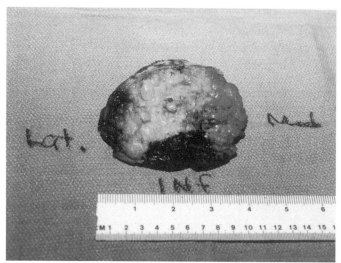

FIGURE 15.19. Inking the specimen. **(A)** The pathologist has been given an oriented specimen. The specimen radiograph has been taken and the pathologist has begun the color coding with red ink for the superior surface. **(B)** A completely color coded specimen with a different color ink marking each surface.

directed breast biopsy. A pathologist was always present in the operating room to receive the specimen and to be three-dimensionally oriented to the specimen's exact position in the patient. The pathologist then took the specimen to the radiology department, only 100 feet away and on the same floor, where specimen radiology was carried out under the direction of the radiologist who placed the wires and in the presence of the pathologist who maintained proper orientation of the tissue as it made its way from department to department.

We believe it is a mistake for the pathologist to perform the specimen radiology in the pathology department and interpret the film, particularly if the mammographic abnormality is a subtle mass or an architectural distortion. The pathologist should not be responsible for determining whether or not the surgeon has properly removed a subtle abnormality that was initially identified by the radiologist. We realize that specimen radiography is commonly performed by the pathologist in many facilities in the United States. It is often far quicker and more convenient this way

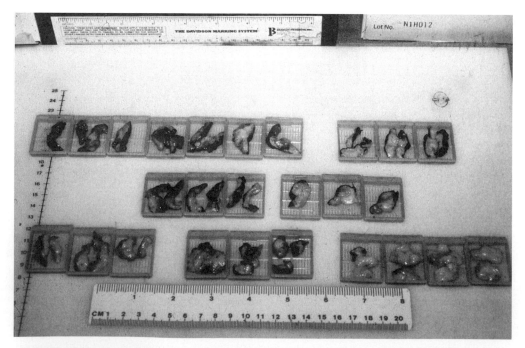

FIGURE 15.20. The entire specimen has been color coded, serially sectioned, and sequentially submitted.

and, for many cases, probably completely adequate. However, ideally, the radiologist who initially identified the lesion should place the wires, read the specimen radiograph, and inform the surgeon and the pathologist that the proper area has been removed and that the margins appear adequate by specimen radiography. There is a greater risk of error when multiple radiologists and/or pathologists are involved who pass the case to and from one another.

Once the radiologist confirms that the proper area has been removed, the pathologist returns to the pathology laboratory to ink or dye the specimen. We use a different color for each marginal surface (Fig. 15.19). If one of these different colored margins is involved on final histopathologic evaluation, we know which color-coordinated surface of the biopsy needs to be re-excised.

We generally fix the specimen and then serially section and submit the entire specimen sequentially for histologic evaluation (Fig. 15.20) with a slide legend denoting histologic margins and other areas of pathologic interest. No tissue should be discarded. Frozen sections should not be performed on nonpalpable lesions for either diagnosis or margin assessment because of the loss of tissue due to the frozen section process. In addition, because much of the specimen is fat, which does not freeze well, frozen sections are technically difficult to perform, often inaccurate, and may be extremely difficult to interpret. Most importantly, however, definitive treatment should not be decided upon until permanent sections have been thoroughly evaluated. Hormone receptors, DNA analysis, HER2/neu, etc., can be determined on paraffin fixed tissue if invasive cancer is found. Currently, these markers have no clinical role in the DCIS treatment-selection process (7). Cytologic touch preps to evaluate margins may be appropriate in some cases.

Once the surgeon has been told that the proper area has been removed, the biopsy cavity should be marked with metallic clips (Fig. 15.21). This will identify the area of the biopsy if radiation therapy is elected or if there is a subsequent local recurrence. Clips will focus the radiologists attention during the years of follow-up, and they can be used for wire placement guidance should re-excision be necessary.

The surgeon should perform a cosmetic closure. When a large amount of tissue has been removed, flap advancement is often required. This is done by undermining the surrounding breast tissue at the level of the pectoralis fascia and advancing it with deep sutures (Fig. 15.11). As previously mentioned, the patient is wrapped with a 24 to 30 foot bias pressure dressing (Fig. 15.2) over fluff gauze at the conclusion of the procedure.

The Management of Large, Histologically Unproven Lesions

If the lesion is large (greater than 40 mm) and the diagnosis unproven, we suggest stereotactic vacuum-assisted

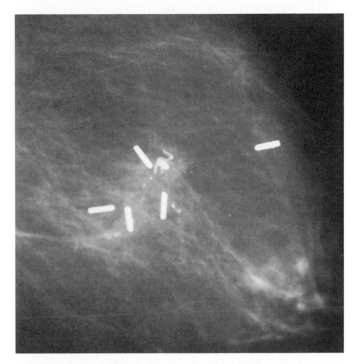

FIGURE 15.21. Postoperative mediolateral mammogram. Metal clips mark the biopsy cavity.

biopsy as a first step to prove that malignancy is present. If the patient is motivated for breast conservation, a multiple wire directed excision can be planned. This gives the patient the best chance at clear margins and good cosmesis. The best option for completely removing a large lesion is with a large initial resection, and the best chance at good cosmesis is with a small initial excision. It is the surgeon's job to optimize these two opposing goals. A large quadrant resection should not be performed unless there is histologic proof of malignancy. An extremely suspicious mammogram without histologic proof of malignancy is insufficient. We will not perform a quadrant resection without microscopic proof of cancer. This type of resection may lead to varying degrees of breast deformity, and the patient will be quite unhappy should the diagnosis prove to be benign.

As lesions get larger, the likelihood of invasion increases (18). Therefore, we routinely perform a sentinel node biopsy on all patients with DCIS large enough to warrant a mastectomy. In addition, if the patient is undergoing an upper outer quadrant excision for a large DCIS, we perform sentinel node biopsy through the same incision. If the lesion is not in the upper outer quadrant, we do not do a sentinel node biopsy because it requires a separate incision, which we believe is not warranted for patients with DCIS.

If a large lesion appears to involve more than one quadrant on mammography, we generally biopsy two areas separated by at least 50 mm. If both biopsies reveal DCIS, we discourage the patients from having breast conservation.

Histologic Excision Margins

Earlier in this chapter, we mentioned how tissues should be processed and the importance of marking all margins. When this has been done properly and the pathologist reports the margins to be free of disease, what does that mean? Does it really mean that the entire lesion has been excised? First, we must define what is meant by clear margins. An initial problem is that a consensus on what constitutes a clear margin is lacking. Different researchers use different criteria. Our group initially used 1 mm in all directions, but we will show that 1 mm is inadequate.

Solin et al. (19) have used 2 mm. The National Surgical Adjuvant Breast Project (NSABP) (20) requires that the tumor not be transected; only a few adipose cells or collagen between the tumor and the inked margin are needed to call the margin clear. Holland and associates (21) require normal breast structures between the tumor and the inked margin. The Nottingham group (22) has required 10 mm in all directions. The work of Faverly et al. (4) suggests that 10 mm would be an excellent choice for clear margins. Using serial subgross technique, they showed that only 8% of DCIS lesions have gaps (skip lesions) greater than 10 mm. More recently, Chan et al. (23) have shown the importance of clear margins.

We have looked at the importance of margins in our patients treated with breast conservation. Figure 15.22 compares the actuarial local recurrence-free rates when 1 mm or more is used as the definition of a clear margin. Conservatively treated tumors with a margin of 1 mm or more had a 17% local recurrence rate at 10 years. Those with less than 1 mm experienced a 47% local recurrence rate at 10 years. When the margin is 10 mm, there is a dramatic decrease in the local recurrence rate. Conservatively treated tumors with a margin of 10 mm or more had only a 5% local recurrence rate at 10 years. Those with less than 10 mm had a 30% local recurrence rate at 10 years (Fig. 15.23). As mentioned

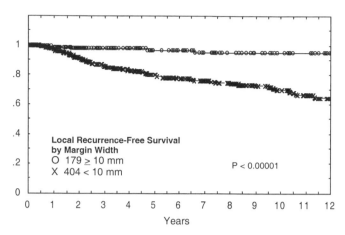

FIGURE 15.23. Probability of local disease-free survival comparing margins greater than 10 mm with margins less than 10 mm for 583 breast conservation patients.

above, the three-dimensional work of Faverly and associates (4) suggests that skip areas are generally less then 10 mm in length and that 10 mm margins may be the gold standard. Our results and the low rate of local recurrence initially reported by the Nottingham group (6%) support this conclusion (22) (Chapter 27).

However, 10 mm margins in every direction may be difficult to achieve in some cases while obtaining good cosmesis. In the operating room, the surgeon is faced with a difficult problem: a lesion that generally can neither be seen nor felt. The best chance for a complete excision with widely clear margins comes with the placement of multiple hooked-wires around a lesion whose extent is well delineated by microcalcifications. If the lesion extends significantly beyond the calcifications, complete excision is far less likely and will only occur if the surgeon is not only competent but lucky. If the lesion is not marked by microcalcifications, it is even more difficult to completely excise.

OUR CURRENT MANAGEMENT OVERVIEW

We currently manage patients with suspicious nonpalpable mammographic lesions in the following manner. Our first step is to get a minimally invasive percutaneous biopsy, generally with an 11-gauge vacuum assisted tool, if technically possible. If the diagnosis of DCIS is made, the patient is thoroughly counseled about the nature of the disease, paying particular attention to the size and distribution of her disease as determined mammographically. We always perform ultrasound on suspicious findings, including microcalcifications. In selected patients, we obtain MRI.

If the patient is a good candidate for breast conservation (an area of DCIS that can be completely removed with clear margins without dramatically deforming the breast), and she is anxious to preserve her breast, we generally perform a 4-wire directed segmental resection using either a radial in-

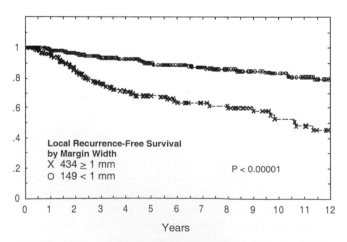

FIGURE 15.22. Probability of local disease-free survival comparing margins greater than 1 mm with margins less than 1 mm for 583 breast conservation patients.

cision to take advantage of the radial distribution of DCIS, a batwing reduction, or a standard reduction incision. An adequate amount of overlying skin is always removed. The entire segment is resected down to and including the pectoralis major muscle fascia. This guarantees that the anterior and posterior margins will be clear. If widely clear margins, 10 mm or more in the other four directions (superior, inferior, medial, and lateral) are obtained, postoperative radiation therapy is not recommended, regardless of nuclear grade, comedonecrosis, tumor size, or age (24,25) (Chapters 45, 47). If the margins are 1 to 9 mm, re-excision or radiation therapy may be added. For patients with margins less than 1 mm, we re-excise or convert to a mastectomy, generally with immediate reconstruction.

Once satisfied with the removal of the primary lesion, an oncoplastic closure is performed by undermining the surrounding tissue for a distance of 4 to 5 cm in every direction and then advancing it with deep sutures. We drain most lesions for 24 to 48 hours and completely close the wound in layers, constantly checking and reappraising the cosmetic result. We prefer the wound to heal with as little seroma and blood as possible.

In patients whose lesions are mammographically too large to yield clear margins and an acceptable cosmetic result, we go directly to skin-sparing mastectomy and reconstruction, generally with a TRAM flap. Having performed only a percutaneous minimally invasive breast biopsy in these patients, we are seldom faced with a skin incision in the wrong place or a biopsy scar that needs re-excision.

Some DCIS lesions are much larger than they mammographically appear, and may be extremely difficult to completely excise. These patients are probably better served with skin-sparing mastectomy and autologous reconstruction. We do not spare the nipple. On occasion, we have spared the areola.

Patients with DCIS treated with breast conservation should be closely followed. Currently, at the Lee Breast Center within the USC/Norris Comprehensive Cancer Center, they are physically examined every six months indefinitely. Mammography is performed every six months on the ipsilateral breast and yearly on the contralateral breast.

SUMMARY

Most DCIS detected today will be nonpalpable and detected by mammography with microcalcifications as the most common finding. It is not uncommon for DCIS to be larger than expected by mammography, to involve more than a quadrant of the breast, and to be unicentric and radial in its distribution.

Preoperative evaluation should include film-screen mammography with magnification and ultrasonography. If technically possible, a percutaneous image-guided biopsy should be performed. Following the establishment of the diagnosis,

the patient can be apprised of all alternative procedures, including their risks and advantages. If the patient is motivated for breast conservation, the surgeon and radiologist should carefully plan the procedure using multiple wires to map out the extent of the lesion. The first attempt at excision is the best chance to get a complete excision with a good cosmetic result. Once the multiple-wire-directed excisional biopsy has been done, two factors can be evaluated: the cosmetic result and the histopathology.

If the cosmetic result is acceptable and the margins are clear, the patient can proceed with breast conservation. If the initial margins are involved, consideration can be given to a re-excision procedure versus mastectomy with immediate reconstruction. The patient should be apprised of the fact that re-excision may yield a poor cosmetic result and margins may continue to be involved. For most patients, re-excision can be delayed for 2 to 3 months to allow for adequate wound healing. This, in turn, may yield a better cosmetic result at the time of re-excision.

After the establishment of the diagnosis, the patient may not be a good candidate for breast conservation due to the large size of the lesion relative to the size of her breast, multicentricity, etc. If this is the case, skin-sparing mastectomy with immediate reconstruction should be discussed, and if the patient is a candidate for and interested in it, plastic surgical consultation should follow.

REFERENCES

1. Silverstein MJ, Gamagami P, Colburn WJ. Coordinated biopsy team: Surgical, pathologic, and radiologic issues. In: *Ductal Carcinoma In Situ of the Breast,* 1st ed. Silverstein MJ. Baltimore: Williams & Wilkins, 1997:333–342.
2. Silverstein MJ. The Van Nuys Breast Center: The First Free-Standing Multidisciplinary Breast Center. *Surg Oncol Clin N Am* 2000;9(2):159–175.
3. Holland R, Hendriks JHCL. Microcalcifications associated with ductal carcinoma in situ: mammographic-pathologic correlation. *Semin Diagn Pathol* 1994;11(3):181–192.
4. Faverly DRG, Burgers L, Bult P, et al. Three-dimensional imaging of mammary ductal carcinoma is situ: Clinical implications. *Semin Diagn Pathol* 1995;11(3):193–198.
5. Holland R, Hendriks JHCL, Verbeek ALM, et al. Extent, distribution, and mammographic/histological correlations of breast ductal carcinoma in situ. *Lancet* 1990;335:519–522.
6. Tabar L, Dean PB. Basic principles of mammographic diagnosis. *Diagn Imag Clin Med* 1985;54:146–157.
7. Consensus Committee. Consensus Conference on Image-Detected Breast Cancer. *J Am Coll Surg* 2001;193:297–302.
8. Dershaw DD, Morris EA, Liberman L, et al. Nondiagnostic stereotactic core breast biopsy: Results of re-biopsy. *Radiology* 1996;198:323–325.
9. Jackman RJ, Nowels KW, Shepard MJ, et al. Stereotactic large core needle biopsy of 450 nonpalpable breast lesions with surgical correlation in lesions with cancer or atypical hyperplasia. *Radiology* 1994;193:91–95.
10. Liberman L, Cohen MA, Dershaw DD, et al. Atypical ductal hyperplasia diagnosed at stereotactic biopsy of breast lesions: An indication for surgical biopsy. *AJR Am J Roentgenol* 1995;164:1111–1113.

11. Liberman L. Clinical management issues in percutaneous core breast biopsy. *Radiol Clin North Am* 2000;38(4):791–807.

12. Burbank F. Stereotactic breast biopsy: Comparison of 14- and 11-gauge mammotome probe performance and complication rates. *Am Surg* 1997;63:988–995.

13. Burbank F. Stereotactic breast biopsy of atypical ductal hyperplasia and ductal carcinoma in situ lesions: Improved accuracy with directional, vacuum-assisted biopsy instrument. *Radiology* 1997; 202:843–847.

14. Silverstein MJ, Gamagami P, Colburn WJ, et al. Nonpalpable breast lesions: Diagnosis with slightly overpenetrated screen-film mammography and hook wire–directed breast biopsy in 1014 cases. *Radiology* 1989;171:633–638.

15. Silverstein MJ, Gamagami P, Rosser RJ, et al. Hooked-Wire-Directed Breast Biopsy and Overpenetrated Mammography. *Cancer* 1987;59:715–722.

16. Noguchi S, Aihara T, Koyama H, et al. Discrimination between multicentric and multifocal carcinomas of breast through clonal analysis. *Cancer* 1994;74:872–877.

17. Thompson JZ, Evans AJ, Pinder SE, et al. Growth pattern of ductal carcinoma in situ (DCIS): A retrospective analysis based on mammographic findings. *Br J Cancer* 2001;85:225–227.

18. Lagios MD, Westdahl PR, Margolin FR, et al. Duct Carcinoma in situ: Relationship of extent of noninvasive disease to the frequency of occult invasion, multicentricity, lymph node metastases, and short-term treatment failures. *Cancer* 1982;50:1309–1314.

19. Solin LJ, Yet I-T, Kurtz J, et al. Ductal carcinoma in situ (intraductal carcinoma) of the breast treated with breast-conserving surgery and definitive irradiation. Correlation of pathologic parameters with outcome of treatment. *Cancer* 1993;71:2532–2542.

20. Fisher ER, Sass R, Fisher B, et al. Pathologic findings from the National surgical Adjuvant Breast Project (Protocol No. 6) I. Intraductal carcinoma (DCIS). *Cancer* 1986;57:197–208.

21. Holland R, Veling SHJ, Mravunac M, et al. Histologic multifocality of Tis, T1-2 Breast carcinomas. Implications for clinical trials of breast conserving surgery. *Cancer* 1985;56:979–990.

22. Sibbering DM, Blamey RW. Nottingham Experience. In: Silverstein MJ, ed. *Ductal Carcinoma In Situ of the Breast,* 1st ed. Baltimore: Williams & Wilkins, 1997:367–372.

23. Chan KC, Knox WF, Sinha G, et al. Extent of incision margin width required in breast conserving surgery for ductal carcinoma in situ. *Cancer* 2001;91:9–16.

24. Silverstein MJ, Lagios MD, Craig PH, et al. A prognostic index for ductal carcinoma in situ of the breast. *Cancer* 1996;77:2267–2274.

25. Silverstein MJ, Lagios MD, Groshen S, et al. The influence of margin width on local control in patients with ductal carcinoma in situ (DCIS) of the breast. *N Engl J Med* 1999;340:1455–1461.

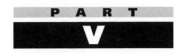

PART V

PATHOLOGY

16

PRACTICAL PATHOLOGY OF DUCTAL CARCINOMA IN SITU: HOW TO DERIVE OPTIMAL DATA FROM THE PATHOLOGIC EXAMINATION

MICHAEL D. LAGIOS

Successful breast conservation therapy for ductal carcinoma in situ (DCIS), with or without irradiation, is highly dependent on a thorough pathologic evaluation of the disease, its grade and extent, and, in particular, the status of the margins and the exclusion of invasion. Inadequate recognition and evaluation of these pathologic factors can lead to both over- and undertreatment of the patient. Such practice is characteristic of several published randomized trials with unacceptably high local recurrence rates, metastatic events, and cause-specific deaths within relatively short follow-up intervals, most of which reflects the lack of recognition and treatment of invasive disease.

This chapter reviews recognized prognostic factors for DCIS and describes the essential pathologic techniques needed to define them in a particular patient. Recommended pathologic techniques derive from the authors' experience with ductal carcinoma in situ over the past 25 years. Several cost analyses are offered to contrast the costs of recommended pathology procedures with the costs of medical treatments currently recommended by others.

In the past 20 years, there has been a tenfold or greater increase in the frequency of DCIS and a similar increase in breast conservation for this disease. At present, two-thirds of the newly diagnosed cases of DCIS, the majority of small size, are treated by some form of breast conservation in the United States (1,2). Prospective studies performed during this interval have revealed a number of pathologic features that have statistical significance for local control in programs of breast-conservation therapy (BCT) (3–8), and these have been recognized by an international consensus on the pathology of DCIS (9) and are reviewed in detail in this chapter.

Unlike the standard pathologic examination for invasive disease, in which representative samples are generally sufficient to establish reliable margins and size for purposes of therapy, DCIS is a diagnosis of exclusion. Resections for DCIS cannot exclude invasive disease, microscopic margin involvement, or determine size (extent) by conventional tis-

sue sampling designed for palpable lesions. Occult invasive carcinomas within such a resection, often of T1mic or T1a size, are easily missed when half or less of the tissue is sampled. Margins that may be involved by microscopic DCIS not associated with microcalcifications and surrounded by fatty breast tissue are not palpable, visible, or imageable. For DCIS, reliable analyses of outcome of BCT require complete tissue processing (CTP), not sampling. Prospective studies that are based on conventional tissue sampling, e.g., National Surgical Adjuvant Breast Project (NSABP) protocols B-17 and B-24 and European Organization for Research and Treatment of Cancer (EORTC) 10853, are characterized by very high local recurrence rates with or without irradiation, small but telling frequencies of distant metastases as first events, and a large number of cause-specific deaths within short follow-up periods (10–13). In B-17, with 8 years of follow-up, local recurrence rates for the ipsilateral breast were 12% with and 27% without irradiation and an additional 1.5% exhibited local regional or distant metastases as first events (without a preceding local in-breast recurrence), and a comparable number died of the disease. In contrast, data from the Van Nuys Breast Center, Van Nuys, CA, for DCIS of comparable size (<10 mm) at 8 years of follow-up were 9.6% and 12.2% with no metastatic first events (6,7), and none was evident in our initial study with a 10-year local recurrence rate of 16% in patients treated by BCT without irradiation (14). Solin et al. (15) noted only one metastatic first event in a 15-year follow-up of 270 patients in a collaborative study of DCIS treated with BCT with irradiation.

COMPLETE SEQUENTIAL TISSUE PROCESSING

Both the early work at the Children's Hospital of San Francisco by my colleagues (3,4,16) on DCIS treated with BCT without irradiation and the much larger prospective database from the Van Nuys Breast Center (5–7), which included nonrandomized patients treated both with and without irradiation, were based on complete sequential tissue processing (CST), which provided the greatest likelihood of excluding minimal invasive disease, microscopic margin involvement, and confirming size. Analyses of DCIS by CST have permitted the identification of subsets of patients with DCIS with a local control rate at 8 years varying from 97% for those with margins greater than 10 mm or a negative re-excision (7) or 99% for Van Nuys Prognostic Index (VNPI) scores of 3 or 4 (6).

Arguments against CST have cited the additional costs and time required to process a large resection for DCIS. This argument has merit only if one were to process all mammographically directed diagnostic needle localized biopsies, the majority for microcalcification, as if they contained DCIS. On average, only 20% to 33% of such resections in the recent past would be expected to contain any type of carcinoma. However, at present, large resections for mammographically detected DCIS are increasingly being based on a preoperative diagnosis achieved by stereotactic biopsy. Stereotactic technology can reliably identify at least DCIS in most cases in which microcalcification marks the in situ carcinoma, particularly with vacuum-assisted technology. CST is then used only for the 25% to 30% of resections for which the stereotactic core biopsy has already documented DCIS or atypical ductal hyperplasia. Seventy percent to 75% of patients with mammographic findings that previously would have gone on to open biopsy are spared both the morbidity and expense of an open procedure. Another way to look at the relative costs of CST for DCIS is to compare two well-documented approaches: one based on methodical tissue processing with mammographic pathologic correlation and the other on conventional tissue sampling with adjunct radiation therapy and tamoxifen based on the results of NSABP B-17 and B-24 in which the resection was only sampled and margins defined as nontransection.

Silverstein et al. (6,7) showed that the expected mean 8-year local recurrence rate is 0.7% for DCIS with VNPI

TABLE 16.1. COMPARATIVE LOCAL (IN-BREAST) RECURRENCES: VAN NUYS PROGNOSTIC INDEX SCORE OF 3 OR 4, >10-MM MARGIN, <10-MM SIZE, NATIONAL SURGICAL ADJUVANT BREAST PROJECT B-24 ADJUVANT RADIATION THERAPY, ANDTAMOXIFEN

	N	R	%
VNPI score 3–4	131	1	0.75*
>10-mm margin	93	2	2.1
<10-mm size	163	20	12.2
NSABP B-24	899	63	11.0†

* Mean of 96 months of follow-up.
† Projected 96-month outcome.
VNPI, Van Nuys Prognostic Index; NSABP, National Surgical Adjuvant Breast Project.

TABLE 16.2. HOW EXPENSIVE IS COMPLETE TISSUE PROCESSING FOR DUCTAL CARCINOMA IN SITU?

- Assume mean 20 blocks in addition to conventional 10 sample blocks, 30 total for complete tissue processing per patient
- $6.00 per block × 30 × 100 patients = $18,000
- Assume 30 min of pathologist time to review 30 slides @ $120/hr × 100 = $6,000
- Total cost per 100 patients = $24,000

scores 3 or 4 and 3% for all DCIS with margins of 10 mm or more or a negative re-excision (Table 16.1). Compared with B-17, in which the irradiated arm had a 12% local recurrence rate and a 1.5% distant or locoregional failure rate at 8 years, careful surgery and meticulous pathology can provide a much higher level of local control and survival, but with larger costs in pathology.

Let us assume that the standard resection for DCIS of 30 to 45 g requires 30 blocks (cassettes) for CTP. Conventional pathology practice, as exemplified by NSABP B-17, B-24 and the recently published EORTC 10853 trial, would sample the same resection on average in ten blocks for those with clear margins, 12 overall (11), or a median of 17 (17). A single block processed as a slide for examination at present costs approximately $6.00. For 100 patients, the total costs of slide preparation would be $18,000 (Table 16.2). Providing a generous allotment of time (30 minutes) and compensation for the pathologist to review these 30 slides at $120.00 per hour per 100 patients is $6,000.00. Total pathology costs for CTP and professional examination per 100 patients is $24,000. This figure is slightly inflated because it assigns the costs of the conventional ten-block sampling and pathology examination to the CTP costs.

How expensive are the adjuvant therapies recommended by the NSABP (B-17, B-24) to provide optimal local control in their practice? Let us assume only health maintenance organization reimbursement for radiation therapy: whole breast without node bearing areas at 80% of Medicare reimbursement (i.e., approximately $7,000) (Table 16.3). For 100 patients, this is $700,000. Tamoxifen mandated for 5 years at $5.00 per day per 100 patients is $912,500. Total adjuvant therapy costs $1,612,500 per 100 patients.

Bracketed wire resections for DCIS planned after an initial diagnostic core biopsy results in a 60% success rate in achieving 10-mm margins (M. J. Silverstein, personal com-

TABLE 16.3. HOW EXPENSIVE IS RADIATION THERAPY/TAMOXIFEN THERAPY FOR DUCTAL CARCINOMA IN SITU?

- Assume 80% Medicare reimbursement rate for whole breast
- Radiation therapy exclusive of node-bearing areas
- $7,000 per patient × 100 = $700,000
- Tamoxifen @ $5.00/d × 5 yr × 100 = $912,500
- Total adjuvant therapy costs per 100 patients = $1,612,500

TABLE 16.4. PENNYWISE, POUND FOOLISH COST BENEFIT ANALYSIS PER 100 PATIENTS FOR RADIATION/TAMOXIFEN THERAPY VS. COMPLETE TISSUE PROCESSING

- Assume 10% patients spared RTX/tamoxifen by confirmed adequate resection with CTP
- 10% RTX/tamoxifen cost = $161,250 − costs CTP/100 = $24,000 = potential cost savings = $137,250
- Cost savings = 5.7 × costs of CTP if only 10% spared adjuvant treatment

RTX, radiation therapy; CTP, complete tissue processing.

munication, 2001). An additional 20% can be provided adequate margins with a subsequent attempt at re-excision. However, to not favor this thesis, I will assume that CTP can only establish 10-mm margins or negative re-excisions in 10% of patients with DCIS who elect BCT (rather than the 60% to 80% who in reality can be provided adequate margins). How do these costs compare?

Let us assume that the 10% of these patients with DCIS and adequate margins do not require adjuvant therapies (Table 16.4). The savings are $161,250, (10% of $1,612,500) minus the costs of CTP for all 100 patients ($24,000). The cost savings per 100 patients using CTP and assuming a benefit of only 10% for the entire group is $137,250, a figure nearly six times the cost of CTP alone. If 60% of the patients were benefited, the cost savings would be $919,375.

The problem at present is that reimbursement is allocated not for the disease but for the specific specialists who bill. Pathologists under the existing reimbursement schedule are not sufficiently compensated to break even processing resections for DCIS in their entirety, but that is an artificial administrative restraint that sets equal rates of compensation for a shave excision of a seborrheic keratosis (one slide per 1 minute) and a vacuum-assisted stereotactic biopsy with six to eight levels (six to 16 slides per 15 to 25 minutes).

The cost analysis is based on 80% Medicare reimbursement in the San Francisco Bay area in October 2000. Pathology reimbursement at $120 per hour exists only in the imagination. The cost of slide preparation at $6.00 per slide is the current actual cost for outside proprietary laboratories.

MAMMOGRAPHIC PATHOLOGIC CORRELATION

An essential first step in pathologic evaluation of the 90% of DCIS resections predicated on mammographic, nonpalpable findings is mammographic correlation (Fig. 16.1). The pathologist must know what the mammographic target is and by correlation with preoperative imaging and specimen radiography determine to what extent the pathology specimen has sampled the mammographic tar-

get and to what extent it is associated, for example, with microcalcification. Regardless of the fact that mammographers will be rendering an intraoperative decision on whether the mammographic target has been sampled, the final and definitive correlation awaits pathologic examination. It is the role of the pathologist not only to identify the pathologic process by conventional microscopic examination, but, in addition, to indicate whether microcalcification or a mass identified mammographically represents DCIS or a mixture of benign and neoplastic processes and whether the mammographic target is incidental to the DCIS, marks it only in part, or has a close association with it. Such evaluation is part of the recommendations of the Consensus Conference on DCIS (9) and a subsequent international consensus conference on image-detected breast cancer (18). These determinations can have a large impact on treatment recommendations. For example, a pathologic evaluation that indicates that microcalcifications represent DCIS, but fails to note that only a minute portion of the process is associated with microcalcification, can result in additional surgery that will not likely result in an adequate excision.

Pathology reports on mammographically directed biopsies and resections for DCIS frequently fail to indicate the nature of the mammographic target and the extent of its association. Some such reports to this day fail to indicate that the biopsy or resection was mammographically directed at all. Because most DCIS is now detected by occult mammographic microcalcification, this type of correlation is a requirement for any adequate pathologic examination for that disease. The pathologist must review at least the specimen x-ray before examining and blocking the tissue.

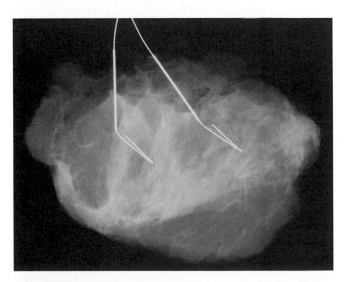

FIGURE 16.1. Specimen radiograph of the intact specimen oriented by sutures is available to the pathologist at the time of gross examination. He or she can visually examine the specimen x-ray to obtain some orientation to the mammographic target. Note the microcalcifications below the right-hand wire tip. These represent recurrent ductal carcinoma in situ.

ORIENTATION OF THE SPECIMEN

Orientation of the specimen permits directed intraoperative re-excisions for specific margins if they are found to be close on specimen radiographic or gross examination. Orientation can be preserved by radiopaque sutures or metallic clips used in a standardized protocol, but these markers must be placed into the specimen while it is still at least partially in situ, not after it is free of the biopsy cavity. The orientation of a soft, irregular piece of fat cannot be reliably recalled after it is excised even by those who otherwise walk on water.

In our practice, the pathologist receives the oriented specimen directly in the operating room and carries both the specimen and the localizing films to the radiology department where he or she assists in preparing the specimen for x-ray. A 12 o'clock suture (long) and an anterior suture (short) permit a specimen x-ray in which the orientation is preserved in the film. The sutures also facilitate fixation (see below) and can more readily be removed than metallic staples. Two views of the specimen are normally attempted, one in which it is laid flat with the deep surface down on the film and a second with rotation. The specimen is normally placed in a plastic disposable bag with a zip lock, and this facilitates attempts at rotating it to obtain a 90-degree orthogonal view, although that is rarely achieved completely. It is important to realize that the weight of the plastic compression plate is sufficient to flatten any irregularities of the surface of the specimen, and certainly it is not necessary to compress the specimen by screwing the wing nuts down. That type of compression only results in the fat of the specimen being fractured, which can create false cleavage planes in the tissue into which ink can run.

INTRAOPERATIVE EVALUATION

Based on an intraoperative specimen x-ray, the surgeon is informed whether he or she has obtained the target and provided estimates of the size of the margin based on radiography. If the margin is determined to be close, a directed intraoperative re-excision for a specific margin is performed. In the absence of a close mammographic or gross margin, there is no attempt to routinely re-excise the margins. Such shave re-excisions of the biopsy cavity wall, in my experience, are unlikely to achieve an adequate re-excision when it is necessary, rarely encompass the entirety of the cavity surface, and are difficult to analyze unless carefully marked intraoperatively. Guidi et al. (19) showed a 39% false-positive rate for re-excision shaved margins. Frozen sections do not provide a reliable estimate of margin status for DCIS intraoperatively. Fatty resections cannot be cut at standard cryostat temperatures, and, given the microscopic nature of DCIS in most circumstances,

choosing a margin to freeze is an entirely random exercise. Imprint cytologic evaluation of margins that can work for invasive cancers involving a margin is not a practical technique for microscopic disease involving ducts that may measure less than 0.1 mm in diameter transected at a fatty surface.

INKING OF MARGINS
Artifactual Margins and Inking Surfaces

Selective inking of margins is a standard recommendation for resected breast cancers and the recommendation of the Consensus Conference (9) on DCIS. Inking should be performed so that an easily identifiable surface marked with a specific colored ink can be recognized in the subsequent histologic section as a margin.

The margins of the resection can be compromised, however, even before inking by improper, rough handling of the specimen. Most breast resections contain considerable amounts of fat, which is as fragile as aspic. Simply placing a resection specimen on a dry towel as it is handed off in the operating suite can compromise the true margin, some of which will adhere to the fabric. This can result in the loss of several millimeters of tissue and reduce the remaining margin width, increasing the VNPI score. Telfa or any other nonadherent material such as discarded plastic wrap from an instrument tray is better than dry, sterile toweling.

Most such resections for mammographically identified DCIS should make their way to the radiology department where they can be subject to further battery. Commonly, the radiology technician will compress the fragile specimen in a Dubin device in the process of obtaining a specimen x-ray. Unfortunately, the compression plate is often too vigorously screwed down, thus fracturing the tissue and creating false tissue planes that, when inked, can make interpretation of the actual margin difficult. The weight of the compression plate alone is sufficient to flatten the surface of the specimen and to obtain excellent specimen radiographs without mechanical compression

In our practice, the entire deep surface of the specimen is first inked black, and then the specimen is turned over so that its anterior or superficial aspect is available. The 12 o'clock and anterior sutures are identified and an imaginary line is drawn between 12 o'clock and the anterior suture and extended to the 6 o'clock pole of the resection. The medial half of this superficial surface demarcated by this imaginary line is then inked in red, the lateral half in green. We have found that ink can be applied more uniformly and more quickly if the ink is applied in a rolling motion with a swab rather than being daubed (Fig. 16.2). The specimen is then immersed in Bouin's solution for 30 seconds and immediately suspended in fixative (Fig. 16.3).

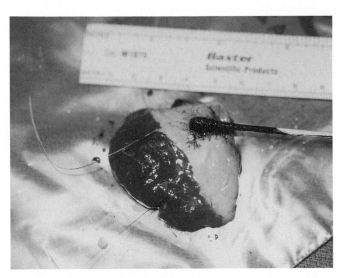

FIGURE 16.2. Inking a specimen with the swab technique. The anterior surface is exposed, and the medial half demarcated by the 12 and 6 o'clock sutures has been inked in red. Note that ink does not run all over the surface.

FIXATION

In our practice, inked specimens are not immediately sectioned (fresh) but rather fixed in their entirety. We prefer 10% alcoholic formalin (i.e., one part saturated formaldehyde solution in nine parts absolute ethanol). The alcoholic formalin more rapidly hardens the tissue so that it can be blocked on the same day except for the largest resections.

The specimen is suspended in 20 times its volume of alcoholic formalin fixative by the 12 o'clock suture; thus, orientation is better preserved even in the fixed specimen, and

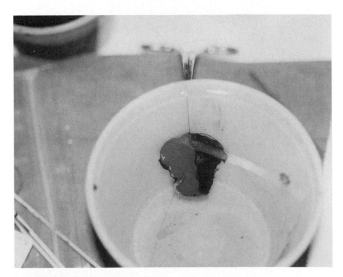

FIGURE 16.3. The inked specimen is immersed for 30 seconds in Bouin's solution to fix the ink to the specimen. The specimen is now suspended in 20-fold its volume in alcohol formalin. Note suspension by 12 o'clock suture, which allows the specimen to fix in an oriented fashion.

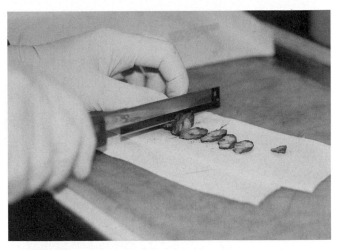

FIGURE 16.4. Three to four hours later, the fixed specimen is sectioned transversely from 12 to 6 o'clock using inked surfaces and sutures as guides. A large disposable blade allows uniform 2.5-mm thick segments to be cut.

the fixation time is reduced. After 2 to 4 hours, depending on the size of the resection, the specimen is removed from the fixative, and transverse sections are prepared from 12 to 6 o'clock at 2.5-mm intervals (Fig. 16.4). Each of these segments demonstrates the black deep surface and superficial surfaces marked red and green. These segments are arranged on a paper sheet cut to correspond to the size of standard mammogram film. The segments are arranged in sequence (Fig. 16.5), and the entirely sectioned specimen is x-rayed again if the mammographic target was microcalcification. The entire specimen is processed in sequence. The pathology report documents into which lettered cassette each segment was processed (e.g., segment 1A, 2B, 3C, D, 4E, F, 5G, H, I). Microcalcifications corresponding to the mammographic target are identified in segments 4 to 6 and 8. With this record and the sequentially and totally embedded resection, the extent of DCIS can be determined by calculation and all margins evaluated at least at 2.5-mm intervals, and occult microinvasion can be largely eliminated (Fig. 16.6).

The intact fixed specimen is cut with a large disposable blade (Accublade) rather than a scalpel blade. Segments prepared in this manner are of more uniform thickness and can be more easily handled. They also permit a more uniform specimen radiographic appearance when the specimen is x-rayed again than do those segments that are prepared from unfixed tissue.

PROGNOSTIC FACTORS

Three prognostic factors have been shown to be important in local control of DCIS after attempts at BCT. These are the extent of disease in the breast (and its corollary the residuum after an attempt at excision), the status of margins

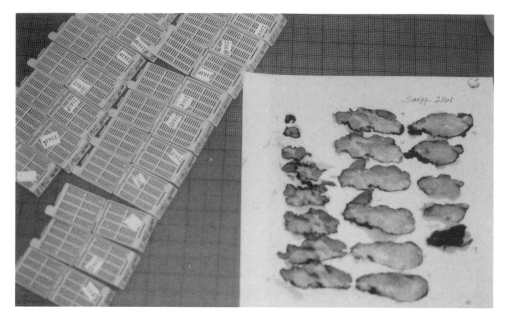

FIGURE 16.5. The bracketed wire resection specimen is fixed and then sectioned at 2.5-mm intervals, and the sections arranged in sequence for a second specimen x-ray. Nineteen cassettes are required to process this specimen in sequence.

(also reflecting residual disease in the breast), and the grade of the DCIS. The most significant of these, uncorrected for margins, is grade (5,14). High nuclear grade (3) and necrosis together define a group of DCIS at much higher risk of local recurrence and invasive transformation. The grade of a DCIS is largely independent of the conventional classifica-

tion. For example, high nuclear grade lesions can exhibit any architectural pattern, and low nuclear grade lesions likewise (3,20). There is a growing consensus that classifications based on nuclear grade and necrosis can stratify the majority of patients with DCIS at risk of short-term local recurrence and invasive transformation (3,5,8,21) after BCT

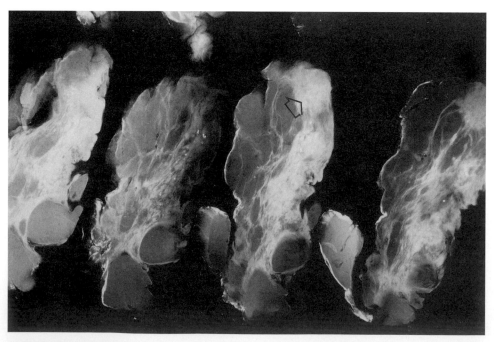

FIGURE 16.6. The second specimen x-ray helps to orient the pathologist to the extent of microcalcification and which margins (by reference to the adjacent inked gross sections that are examined side by side) might be close or involved. The two right-hand slices contained a surprise not apparent in the preoperative mammogram and only subtly appreciated in the intact specimen x-ray (Fig. 16.1), an 8-mm invasive duct carcinoma (*arrow*).

with or without irradiation. Most of these short-term recurrences are associated with DCIS exhibiting nuclear grade 3 morphology and significant coagulative necrosis. Most, but not all, such lesions would be conventionally classified as comedo DCIS. Studies using conventional classification schemes have shown that the most of short-term failures relate to comedo-type DCIS (22). It should be recalled that comedo DCIS is not synonymous with high nuclear grade. Some lesions exhibiting comedonecrosis and a solid growth pattern are composed of intermediate (nuclear grade 2) and in a few cases low-grade nuclei (nuclear grade 1), both of which would be defined as intermediate grade in the Van Nuys Classification.

Very little information is available regarding the potential of low-grade (i.e., noncomedo type) DCIS after biopsy or breast conservation therapy. It is clear that, in the short term (5 to 10 years), few local recurrences or invasive transformations occur, but Page et al. (23), in a recent update of the only study of low-grade DCIS with adequate follow-up (24), noted a substantial delayed recurrence rate, i.e., approximately 37% at 30 years of follow-up. Although the sample is small, it is significant that recurrences were in the same quadrant and in some cases in the site of the prior biopsy, a biology identical to that of higher grade DCIS and a risk that does not diminish after menopause. This biology should be contrasted with that of marker lesions (e.g., atypical ductal hyperplasia, atypical lobular hyperplasia, and lobular carcinoma in situ), which generally do not predict the side of involvement and in which relative risk diminishes postmenopausally (25–27).

GRADE AND CLASSIFICATION

There are several published classifications of DCIS that use nuclear grade and necrosis as the major distinguishing features of specific subtypes. The separations achieved by these classifications are different and in part may have an impact on interpretation of outcome results. DCIS characterized by grade 3 nuclear morphology and necrosis is uniformly classified as high grade (3,5,8,21). The EORTC classification (20), although not using conventional nuclear grade or necrosis as major discriminates, would also regard this as high-grade or, in their terminology, poorly differentiated DCIS. Fisher et al. (11), in an initial analysis of B-17 pathology, noted that DCIS with grade 3 nuclei (poor nuclei) and DCIS that exhibited larger areas of necrosis (more than one-third of ducts involved) had a higher local recurrence rate but reported these results separately, not analyzing the risk associated with two features in concert. Despite the differences in classification, it would appear that high-grade DCIS could be recognized uniformly; all investigators have shown that high-grade subtypes so defined have the highest risk of local recurrence and invasive transformation.

The separate classifications are less consistent with regard to the remainder of the heterogeneous noncomedo group:

DCIS with grade 3 nuclei but without necrosis, an infrequent association, is classified as high grade by Silverstein et al. (5) but as noncomedo (a lower grade) by Solin et al. (8). Lagios et al. (3) and Silverstein et al. (5) use nuclear grade to separate the remaining DCIS groups; however, Lagios et al. classify low-grade DCIS as grade 1 nuclei without necrosis and intermediate-grade DCIS as grade 2 with or without necrosis. Silverstein et al. separate DCIS with nuclear grades 1 and 2 based on necrosis. Group 2 (low grade) may exhibit grade 1 or 2 nuclei but no necrosis, whereas DCIS with grade 1 or 2 nuclei but with any necrosis is classified as intermediate (group 3). Solin et al. (8) regard all DCIS without grade 3 nuclei as noncomedo. Despite these differences in classification, all investigators have shown a substantially diminished local recurrence rate for DCIS not characterized by grade 3 nuclei and necrosis. Moreover, in those studies in which DCIS are divided into three groups instead of the dichotomous comedo/noncomedo, there is a recognizable intermediate group (intermediate grade, group 2, intermediately differentiated) that exhibits a morphology and risk between low- and high-grade DCIS.

In an analysis of the influence of histologic grading on local recurrence, Solin et al. (8) noted recurrence rates of 20% for high-grade DCIS compared with 5% for low-grade lesions at 87 months of follow-up. These results are not dissimilar from our study in which recurrence rates were projected as 28% for similarly defined high-grade DCIS and 6% for lower grade DCIS at 120 months of follow-up. At 124 months of actual follow-up, local recurrence rates are 33% and 2.3%, respectively, for these two groups.

Silverstein et al. (5) confirmed the significance of nuclear grade and necrosis on local recurrence–free survival after BCT for DCIS. With an 8-year actuarial follow-up, group 1 DCIS (low or intermediate nuclear grade without necrosis) had a 2% recurrence rate, group 2 DCIS (low or intermediate nuclear grade with necrosis) had a 6% recurrence rate, and group 3 DCIS (any nuclear grade 3 regardless of necrosis) had a 16% recurrence rate. Collins et al. (28) corroborated the Van Nuys grading scheme with a 62-month follow-up with figures for low, intermediate, and high grade for local recurrence rates of 0%, 8%, and 25%, respectively. Pertinent to the discussion of the role of radiation therapy was the inability of the study to demonstrate any significant difference in local control with or without irradiation for the two lower grade groups (groups 1 and 2). Only for high-grade DCIS (group 3) did radiation therapy provide a benefit for local control.

Several papers compare the utility of various existing DCIS classifications, in terms of identifying subgroups with different outcomes and their reproducibility. Badve et al. (29) compared recurrence-free survival rates among DCIS subgroups defined by five different classification schemes. Only those schemes based on nuclear grade were able to distinguish subgroups with different risks of recurrence; the conventional architectural classification was unable to do so. The Van Nuys Classification, based on nuclear grade and necrosis, achieved the highest *p* value (0.001) among those tested. Douglas-Jones et al. (30) and Bethwaite et al. (31) found the Van Nuys Classification to have the highest level of interobserver agreement among those tested. Sneige et al. (32) compared interobserver reproducibility of the Lagios nuclear grading system for DCIS in a setting of six pathologists with previous training. Complete agreement among the six observers was achieved in 35% and five of the six observers agreed in 36% of 125 cases. Leong et al. (33) have shown that nuclear grade alone or in combination with necrosis showed that the best correlation between an DCIS and concurrent invasive ductal carcinoma, and nuclear grade was clearly associated with specific suites of biomarkers and most clearly was associated with the proliferative index as determined by MIB-1.

The most recent update of the pathology of B-17 (34) is exceptional among analyses of the impact of nuclear grade on the outcome of DCIS in finding no correlation. A previous pathology analysis of B-17 (11) had shown that poor nuclear grade (i.e., grade 3, high grade), margin status, and extent of necrosis were significant predictors of local recurrence. Now only an extent of comedonecrosis in more than one-third of the involved ducts is a significant predictor, not grade III nuclei, although these two features were analyzed separately and not combined as they are in most classifications. Nonetheless, poor nuclear grade continues to be a risk marker in a sister study of the NSABP, B-24, associated with local recurrence rates in that study (12).

Fisher et al. (34) attempted to apply the Van Nuys (pathology) Classification (5) to their data but, because of their definition of necrosis (absent/slight versus moderate/marked), were not able to identify subsets equivalent to the Van Nuys low-grade (group 1) DCIS (without necrosis) or to the intermediate (group 2) DCIS (good nuclear grade with any degree of necrosis).

Bijker et al. (17), in a pathology analysis of the EORTC 10853 randomized trial of irradiation versus lumpectomy for DCIS, noted that nuclear grade, histologic type (20), and, for a subset of analyzable patients, the Van Nuys Classification (5) all showed significant correlation with outcome in the nonirradiated arm, but the association was less pronounced in the irradiated arm. These features were not significant predictors for local recurrence in a multivariate analysis that combined both arms; however, poorly differentiated DCIS (group 3, high grade) subtypes were significantly associated with local recurrences (in situ and invasive combined), distant metastases, and death from disease within the 5.4-year current follow-up and at comparable rates regardless of radiation therapy. These findings can be explained in part by the inability of the EORTC trial to con-

trol for either the adequacy of the resection or the thoroughness of the pathologic examination.

Most studies of DCIS treated by BCT, with or without irradiation, have shown the highest rates of local recurrence among those patients with high-grade DCIS because this subset has the shortest mean interval to recurrence when margins are inadequate, i.e., when residual disease is likely to have been left in the breast (3,6,8,22). Metastatic events and death from disease in both EORTC 10853 and B-17 most likely reflect undetected invasive disease at the onset.

EXTENT OF DISEASE

Clinical concern with the evaluation of size or extent of the area of the breast occupied by DCIS was an early focus during the development of BCT for this disease. Using a serial subgross sectioning technique correlated with specimen radiography, developed by Egan et al. (35), a clear association was shown between the likelihood of invasive growth and the extent of disease (16). The technique of Egan et al. permitted a correlative radiographic and pathologic mapping of areas of involvement by DCIS. These were extensively sampled from mastectomy material. The initial concern was whether occult invasion might exist in the breast separate from an adequately excised focus of DCIS. This was shown not to be the case. Treatment planning for areas of DCIS of 25 mm or less, which were completely excised by the standards of the day, were not associated with occult areas of invasion in those cases that subsequently progressed to mastectomy. Silverstein et al. (36) demonstrated a similar correlation between the extent of disease and the likelihood of invasion, as did Patchefsky et al. (37). What was not clearly described at the time was that the invasive focus always occurred within the area occupied by DCIS and that the area occupied by DCIS had a segmental distribution, as clearly noted subsequently (38,39). Using the same serial subgross technique but applying it to radial segments of the breast, which more closely approximates the true anatomy of the ductal system, Holland and colleagues (38) were able to more clearly define the relationships of DCIS to mammographic microcalcification and to the remaining breast. They identified different distribution patterns among DCIS of different subtypes. High-grade DCIS (poorly differentiated) was more closely defined by the extent of mammographic microcalcifications, and, therefore, its extent could be estimated with more certainty preoperatively. It was also associated with fewer discontinuities or "skip areas" in its distribution, and, therefore, attempts at surgical excision were more likely to be successful. In contrast, DCIS of lower grades (intermediate and well differentiated) were poorly associated with microcalcification and often exhibited a discontinuous distribution. However, Faverly et al. (39) note that 85% of low-grade (well-differentiated) DCIS would be excised with a 10-mm margin. Despite the greater likelihood of residual disease, lower grades of DCIS have a much lower frequency of local recurrence after attempts at BCT, at least in the first 10 years of follow-up.

Determination of the size or extent of DCIS requires a sequential method of CTP with correlated mammography. This was the recommendation of the DCIS Consensus Conference (9) and the Image Guided Breast Cancer Consensus Conference (18) and was the method used at Children's Hospital (3,4,16) and the Van Nuys Breast Center (5–7,40) as well as the method used for the primary resection at Jefferson University (22). Without this type of methodology, the extent of DCIS, the margin status, or the absence of invasive foci cannot be reliably established.

The two published randomized trials of DCIS (10–13, 17,34) had to rely on size as documented in the pathology reports submitted by the contributing laboratories. Bijker et al. (17) noted that only 25% of the cases entered in the EORTC 10853 had size recorded in the microscopic section or conclusion of the report. Of these 25%, 91% were recorded as less than 2 cm, and 68% as less than 1 cm, but no reliable size or extent was available for 75% of entered patients. Fisher et al. (34) attempted to define the size retrospectively for B-17, but 80% were mammographically detected without a specific size recorded. Retrospectively attempting to determine size by measuring the greatest extent in a slide, when neither all the slides nor all the cases were available for review, and by following a nonsequential method of pathologic sampling, which had been the major method of examination employed, is a bootless enterprise.

Vicini et al. (41) used the number of the slides, each representing a corresponding block and tissue sample, as an alternative to sizing DCIS by the use of sequential tissue processing with mammographic correlation as advocated here. They showed that this number is significant in multivariate analysis for outcome in their own database. Given a standard method of tissue sampling, or sequential processing, and a standard block of tissue, there will be an association between the number of slides and the extent of DCIS and outcome. Although this method may be easier to accomplish, it does not lend itself to reproducibility between laboratories. Depending on the thoroughness of the tissue sampling in various laboratories, the same extent of DCIS might be documented in as few as three or as many as 15 blocks (Fig. 16.4).

The United Kingdom/Australia New Zealand DCIS trial mandated pathologic evaluation of size and correlation with specimen radiography, but the specifics of their methods await a subsequent pathology analysis, which is in preparation (42) (Chapter 44).

MARGIN STATUS

Assessment of resection margins has been a major focus in BCT in the United States with the increased use of that surgical procedure in the mid-1970s. The most common method of margin assessment is based on the use of India ink or some other permanent dye and selective sampling. This method works well for invasive carcinomas, for most of which a likely area of involved margins can be estimated by palpation and can be confirmed with few appropriate sections. The method is impracticable in DCIS, in which the lesion is generally nonpalpable and grossly invisible and may not be uniformly associated with microcalcification. In these circumstances, margins must be completely examined rather than sampled. This frequently increases substantially the number of tissue samples or blocks prepared; however, neither margin involvement nor occult microinvasion can be excluded without CTP. Even so, this only samples the tissue at 2- to 3-mm intervals, and, therefore, margin involvement can still be missed with CTP. The likelihood of finding a positive margin, however, can be markedly increased by CTP in comparison with sampling 30% to 50% of the resection. Differences in the kind of tissue processing used can contribute significantly to outcome results for BCT in DCIS (43).

The definitions of an adequate margin initially used by several investigators (3,16, 40) were too narrow to accommodate most cases of DCIS, which exhibited a discontinuous distribution. A standard acceptable margin at the time was 1 mm (3,40), although the NSABP used anything short of transection of an involved duct as adequate. The work of Holland et al. (38) and Silverstein (50) subsequently documented that a 1-mm margin was inadequate. Silverstein et al., in analyzing the results of initial attempts at excision biopsy, noted that 45% of DCIS, which were thought to be adequately excised, had residual disease either at re-excision or mastectomy and that the size of the free margin was directly related to local recurrence–free survival rate, all other factors being equal (7). Even using a definition of an adequate margin of 1 mm, however achieves a better local recurrence–free survival rate than did the NSABP B-17 criterion of nontransection, e.g., 16% local recurrence at a mean of 124 months of follow-up (14) versus 22% local recurrence rate at a mean of 43 months of follow-up (10) (Fig. 16.5).

Margins are one of the three features that are significant predictors in multivariate analyses for local recurrence in DCIS. In the VNPI (6), margins were weighted as less than 1 mm (score 3), 1 to 9.9 mm (score 2), and 10 mm or more or negative re-excision (score 1). The VNPI was an initial attempt to develop a clinicopathologic scoring system to assess the risk of local recurrence among patients with DCIS treated with BCT. Analysis of the database clearly showed that there were large differences between DCIS of different nuclear grade and subtypes. However, after its publication, the data were reanalyzed to evaluate the individual contribution of each predictor separately. When DCIS is analyzed by margin status equivalent to 10 mm or more or a negative re-excision, the differences between various subtypes defined by nuclear grade or nuclear grade and necrosis become inconsequential. Local recurrence–free survival rates for high-grade DCIS (nuclear grade 3 with or without necrosis) with 10 mm or more margins projected to 10 years of actuarial follow-up are 92%, and for intermediate- and low-grade DCIS, they are virtually 100% (7,44).

It is clear from this reanalysis that nuclear grade, subtype, and size only are only pertinent for local recurrence when there is a high risk of residual disease. Given that an estimated 92% of all local recurrences reflect residual (unresected) disease, it is the biology of the residual disease that defines most short-term local recurrences in DCIS.

Because of the importance of an adequate resection in achieving an outstanding local recurrence–free survival and in eliminating the need for radiation therapy, defining the margin status for a patient with DCIS should be of paramount importance in pathology practice. Until practice standards change substantially, and they are beginning to, margins will continue to be poorly defined in cases of DCIS. Consequently, DCIS subtyping by nuclear grade and necrosis will continue to be important in estimating the risk of local recurrence for many patients.

In the EORTC 10853 randomized trial (17), margins are significant for local control, and, more particularly, patients with involved/uncertain or unspecified margins treated by radiation were not significantly benefitted relative to patients with free margins without radiation treatment (recurrence rates: involved/uncertain, 19.7% with irradiation versus free margins without irradiation, 14.6%). Data on margins were compiled from the pathology reports of the contributing institutions; 49% were reported as free without specification, whereas another 5% were free with a measured margin width.

Vicini et al. (41) noted that both the margins and the number of terminal duct lobular units (TDLUs) exhibiting cancerization of lobules within 5 mm of the margin were significant for local control in a multivariate analysis of 146 patients, all of whom were treated by radiation therapy. In the Van Nuys database, DCIS and cancerization of lobules are considered equivalent, and the smallest margin width is measured to establish the margin status. Goldstein et al. (45), in an earlier report of the same data, noted that margins were not significant for outcome. However, all the margin definitions employed (margin widths: >2 mm, <2 mm, and focally and more extensively transected) would have been considered suboptimal in the Van Nuys database, which uses less than 1 mm as a cutoff. In all likelihood, an additional 1 mm of margin width would be expected to add

little to local control in a program of breast conservation without irradiation, but these differences would be reduced further by irradiation. Moreover, although margin status as defined was not significant, the number (five or more) of ducts with DCIS or foci of cancerization of lobules within 4.2 mm of the margin was significant for 5-year actuarial local recurrence rates.

In the 8-year update of the pathology analysis of B-17 (34), margin status was classified as free versus uncertain/involved and was not significant for ipsilateral recurrence. Indeed, there was very little difference between free and uncertain/involved margins in either treatment arm. However, this should not be surprising given the definition of a free margin as nontransection. The differences between a free and an involved margin with that definition can amount to less than 0.1 mm. The differences in margin status in B-17 (11) were originally noted to be significant for local control, particularly in the nonirradiated arm. Part of the loss of significance for margins at this later analysis may represent the impact of patients with free margins but less than 1 mm in width who continue to experience recurrence because of residual disease, as has been shown by the work of Holland et al. (38) and Silverstein (50).

The published data from the United Kingdom DCIS trial (42) (Chapter 44) does not include the authors' definition of a free margin, but all patients entered were required to have complete local excision, confirmation of the excision by specimen radiography, and microscopically free margins. Radiation therapy had a significant impact on ipsilateral recurrence ($p < 0.01$), both in situ and invasive (hazard ratios: 0.4 to 0.41), with a total ipsilateral recurrence rate of 8.4% at a median 3-years of follow-up. This recurrence rate is far lower than comparable rates reported by the NSABP B-17 and the EORTC 10853 and likely reflect the impact of meticulous surgical technique, the use of correlative specimen radiography, and a histologically defined margin.

VAN NUYS PROGNOSTIC INDEX

Weighting the prognostic factors of grade, extent, and margin width has been accomplished in the VNPI (6), which provides summary scores varying from 3 to 9 for DCIS. In this system, tumor grading is weighed: 1 for low-grade (group 1) lesions defined as nuclear grades 1 and 2 without necrosis; 2 for intermediate-grade (group 2) lesions defined as nuclear grade 1 or 2 with necrosis; and 3 for high-grade (group 3) lesions, defined as nuclear grade 3. Size is weighed 1, 2, and 3 as 15 mm or less, 16 to 40 mm, and 40 mm or more, respectively. Margin width is weighted: 1 for margins 10 mm or more or with a negative re-excision, 2 for margins between 1 and 9.9 mm, and 3 for margins less than 1 mm. Adding these individual scores produces prognostic groups with summary scores of 3 and 4, 5 to 7, and 8 and 9. Local recurrence rates are lowest for VNPI scores of 3 and 4 (<1%) and highest for scores 8 and 9 (60%). Radiation therapy provides no benefit for VNPI scores of 3 or 4, a 13% benefit for scores 5, 6, or 7, and a large benefit for VNPI scores 8 and 9. However, despite the large difference in local recurrence rate in the VNPI 8 and 9 group, dependent on irradiation, both irradiated and nonirradiated patients have such high recurrence rates that radiation therapy is not a practical therapeutic option. Additionally, if one analyzes VNPI scores of 5 to 7 by the grade of DCIS, it is clear that most of the suboptimal local recurrence–free survival in that subset reflects patients with high-grade (nuclear grade 3) DCIS. The increase in local recurrence rates for intermediate-grade DCIS with margins of 1 to 9.9 mm is more modest, i.e., a local recurrence–free survival rate of 93% at 8 years, and there is virtually no benefit from radiation therapy at 8 years. Analysis of the data based on margins, however, shows that the differences between different grades of DCIS all resected with a 10-mm margin or greater are not statistically significant. An adequate margin eliminates the clinical differences in outcome and the benefit of irradiation for all subgroups (7,44). Collins et al. (28) have recently corroborated the utility of the VNPI among 96 patients treated only by excision with a median 62-months of follow-up. Margins defined as negative, close, or positive had the greatest impact on 5-year local recurrence rates: 8%, 25%, and 100%, respectively. The Van Nuys Prognostic Index is updated in Chapter 45 to include age.

MULTICENTRICITY AND MULTIFOCALITY

The literature on the multicentricity and multifocality of DCIS remains confusing because of the different definitions, methods of tissue processing, and sampling techniques used and differences in the perspective of the investigators. Two groups of investigators, both of whom used the serial subgross technique of examination of Egan et al. (35) exemplify this problem. The focus of Lagios et al. (46) was on the question of residual disease after segmental mastectomy (lumpectomy), a new and radical direction for American surgeons at the time. They defined as multicentric any focus lying beyond 5 cm of the border of the resection. In most cases, this defined involvement in another quadrant. Holland et al. (38) and Faverly et al. (39), although clearly concerned about the success of a surgical resection, were focused more on the distribution of the disease. Multicentric, by very definition, required a 4-cm zone of uninvolved breast tissue between the primary and any potential multicentric site. Discontinuous foci of DCIS within 4 cm were defined as multifocal. Holland et al. noted that only 5% of DCIS were multicentric using this definition. To what extent these data reflect the large size of

DCIS in their patient population remains unknown. However, Faverly et al. (38) reported that 63% of the DCIS studied at mastectomy had an extent greater than 5 cm (50 mm), whereas Lagios et al. (3), in a similar mastectomy series, noted that 52% were 25 mm or less and 25% were 50 mm or more. Lagios et al. (16) had previously shown that neither multicentricity nor occult invasion was a feature of the smaller, mammographically detected lesions less than 25 mm. Truly multicentric carcinomas, as defined by Holland et al. (38), are infrequent but in my experience minimally represent 5% of invasive carcinomas.

MICROINVASION

Microinvasion, as used in our laboratory, refers to foci of invasive cancer with maximum diameters of 1 mm or less. This is now officially recognized in the TMN system as T1mic. Larger areas of invasive growth are termed minimal invasive carcinoma. These comprise the original minimal invasive group as defined by Gallagher (51), those 1 to 5 mm in maximum diameter (T1a) and the more loosely defined minimal invasive carcinomas that may measure as much as 10 mm in maximum diameter (T1b).

A diagnosis of microinvasion requires all the features of invasive growth, i.e., extension of the lesion beyond the confines of a ductolobular unit, the development of a desmoplastic stroma, and an appropriate histology.

Unfortunately, microinvasion can be mimicked by artifact, duct sclerosis, and entrapment, for example, and represents one of the most commonly revised diagnoses on review. In speaking with a number of pathologists, I have noted that there is a common philosophy that indicates that it is better to call an equivocal focus of microinvasion than to define the process as DCIS and comment on the equivocal areas. Our own standard in this laboratory requires that evidence of invasion be present and that equivocal foci of microinvasion not be defined as invasive disease.

Common processes that have led to a misdiagnosis of microinvasion include crush and electrocautery artifact at the edge of a biopsy specimen, colonization of areas of sclerosing adenosis by DCIS, ductal sclerosis with entrapment of neoplastic epithelium within the area of the pre-existing duct or ductolobular unit, cancerization of lobules with an associated very striking lymphocytic host reaction, and larger ducts showing desquamation of ductal epithelium misinterpreted as vascular invasion. Included with such processes is the implantation of neoplastic epithelium along needle tracts after both fine-needle aspiration and stereotactic core biopsy procedures.

Technical problems related to tissue handling, processing, and sectioning contribute significantly to misinterpretation of microinvasion. Several simple and inexpensive procedures

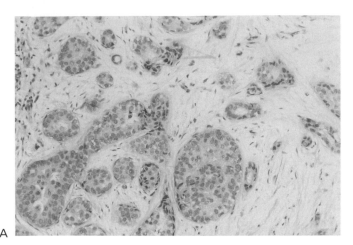
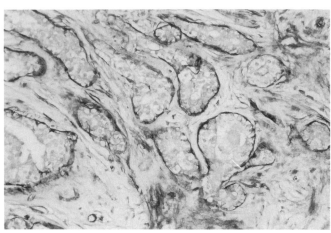

FIGURE 16.7. A core biopsy of a palpable mass was interpreted as intermediate-grade invasive ductal carcinoma. **A:** Careful scrutiny reveals compressed myoepithelial nuclei at the periphery of these sharply demarcated cell groups, many of which show a refractile, hyaline basement membrane. **B:** Subsequent smooth muscle actin immunohistochemistry demonstrates a confluent band of myoepithelial processes appearing as a dark border outlining the ductal walls of this area of adenosis and excluding an invasive diagnosis. No invasive carcinoma was demonstrated at mastectomy.

can reduce this error rate. First, surgeons should be cautioned to avoid higher electrocautery voltages when excising diagnostic biopsy material. "Frying" tissue not only can preclude a diagnosis but will make margin evaluation and receptor and other immunohistochemistries impossible.

Second, adequate fixation time will avoid many sins. For diagnostic problems in well-fixed tissue, several superficial levels of the block can often clarify the process. The addition of markers for the epithelial-stromal junction, specifically the use of labeled smooth muscle actin antisera, which identifies myoepithelial elements, and, to a lesser extent, type IV collagen antisera, can define many equivocal structures, dis-

torted and compressed, as intraductal and thereby exclude invasion (Fig. 16.7).

A diagnosis of microinvasion has serious implications for the likely treatment that the patient may receive. Patients with DCIS are not candidates for adjuvant chemotherapy or radiation therapy after mastectomy, and certainly most of the currently detected cases are not candidates for axillary dissection.

Being aware of the possible pitfalls in interpreting artifact and other benign distorting processes such as microinvasion may permit the pathologist to avoid misdiagnosis. Additionally, appropriate use of levels and occasionally special

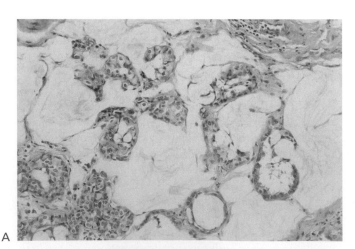
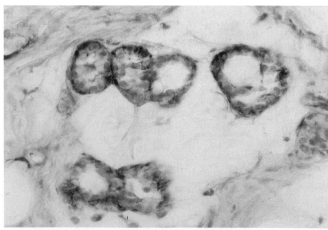

FIGURE 16.8. A patient sought a second opinion regarding the need for adjuvant therapy for this T1b, node-negative invasive mucinous carcinoma. **A:** Microscopic review demonstrated that cancer cell groups were not floating in the mucin but were tenuously anchored by collagen fibers, not a feature of mucinous carcinoma. **B:** Subsequent smooth muscle actin immunohistochemistry demonstrates characteristic darkly stained myoepithelial elements at the periphery of the cell groups defining an intact ductal wall. The diagnosis was revised to low-grade ductal carcinoma in situ with mucocele formation, and the question of adjuvant therapy became moot.

stains or immunoperoxidase preparations may permit clarification of an equivocal focus (Fig. 16.8).

CANCERIZATION OF LOBULES

Cancerization of lobules refers to DCIS involving small TDLUs with minimal architectural distortion, a process

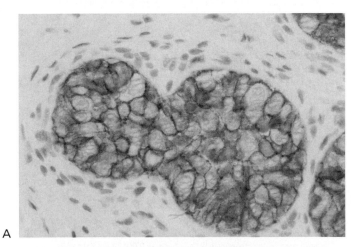

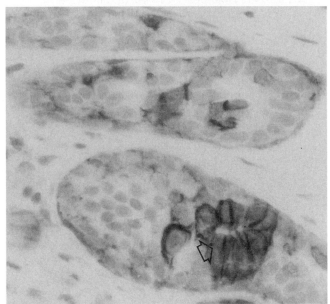

FIGURE 16.9. Two cases of solid intraductal moderately pleomorphic proliferations extensively involving the breast in patients with T1c invasive ductal carcinoma had generated a differential diagnosis of cancerization of lobules [i.e., ductal carcinoma in situ (DCIS) involving a lobular structure] versus lobular carcinoma in situ. Cancerization of lobules carries the same weight as extensive intraductal carcinoma and would have jeopardized breast conservation, whereas lobular carcinoma in situ would not. **A:** E-cadherin immunohistochemistry demonstrates membrane-limited, uniform reaction product characteristic of a ductal lesion and, given the differential diagnosis, defining cancerization of a lobule, i.e., DCIS. **B:** In contrast, only residual luminal ductal cells show membrane staining in this solid proliferation (*arrow*). Absence of E-cadherin staining is characteristic of lobular neoplasia.

that can be overlooked or in some cases misinterpreted as lobular neoplasia because of the frequent tendency to exhibit a solid growth pattern without architectural acinar features when TDLUs are minimally involved with DCIS. The term cancerization reflects an erroneous conception of the growth of DCIS from larger ducts in which it originated in retrograde fashion into TDLUs. Wellings et al. (47) demonstrated that DCIS and lobular neoplasia originate within the TDLU or lobule, not in larger extralobular ducts, but the term cancerization persists as an anachronism.

Cancerization of lobules has always been thought to have the same significance as DCIS with regard to local recurrence–free survival. Goldstein et al. (45) corroborated this interpretation by demonstrating the significance of cancerization of lobules to predict local recurrence when it lay within 5 mm of a margin.

Separating cancerization of lobules from lobular neoplasia can be difficult, and misinterpretation can drastically alter recommendations for therapy: lobular neoplasia has no impact on local control, whereas cancerization of lobules has the same significance as DCIS. This separation is facilitated by the use of E-cadherin immunohistochemistry (Fig. 16.9). Acs et al. (48) which reveals a strong membrane associated E-cadherin marker in all ductal epithelium including DCIS and cancerization of lobules but fails to show any comparable membrane reaction product in 95% of lobular lesions. In those few lobular lesions that have some evidence of E-cadherin, reaction product is distributed in a focal and meager fashion (49). In a group of lesions for which there was no pathologic consensus, diagnosis as either lobular or ductal, Goldstein et al. (49) were able to demonstrate that most were lobular based on E-cadherin immunohistochemistry. For the problematic lesion that cannot be distinguished by morphologic criteria alone, E-cadherin immunohistochemistry appears to offer an independent analytic tool.

REFERENCES

1. Ernster VL, Barclay J, Kerlikowske K, et al. Incidence of and treatment for ductal carcinoma in situ of the breast. *JAMA* 1996; 275:913–918.
2. Winchester DP, Mench HR, Osteen RT, et al. Treatment trends for ductal carcinoma in situ of the breast. *Ann Surg Oncol* 1995;2: 207–213.
3. Lagios MD, Margolin FR, Westdahl PR, et al. Mammographically detected duct carcinoma in situ: frequency of local recurrence following tylectomy and prognostic effect of nuclear grade on local recurrence. *Cancer* 1989;63:618–624.
4. Lagios MD. Duct carcinoma in situ: pathology and treatment. *Surg Clin North Am* 1990;4:853–871.
5. Silverstein MJ, Poller DN, Waisman JR, et al. Prognostic classification of breast ductal carcinoma in situ. *Lancet* 1995;345: 1154–1157.
6. Silverstein MJ, Lagios MD, Craig PH, et al. A prognostic index for ductal carcinoma of the breast in situ. *Cancer* 1996;77: 2267–2274.

7. Silverstein MJ, Lagios MD, Groshen S, et al. The influence of margin width on local control of ductal carcinoma in situ of the breast. *N Engl J Med* 1999;340:1455–1461.

8. Solin LJ, Yeh IT, Kurtz J, et al. Ductal carcinoma in situ (intra-ductal carcinoma) of the breast treated with breast-conserving surgery and definitive irradiation: correlation of pathologic parameters with outcome of treatment. *Cancer* 1993;71:2532–2542.

9. The Consensus Conference Committee. Consensus conference on the classification of ductal carcinoma in situ. *Cancer* 1997;80:1798–1802.

10. Fisher B, Costantino J, Redmond C, et al. Lumpectomy compared with lumpectomy and radiation therapy for the treatment of intraductal breast cancer. *N Engl J Med* 1993;328:1581–1586.

11. Fisher ER, Costantino J, Fisher B, et al. Pathologic findings from the National Surgical Adjuvant Breast Project (NSABP) Protocol B-17: intraductal carcinoma (ductal carcinoma in situ). *Cancer* 1995;75:1310–1319.

12. Fisher B, Dignam J, Wolmark N, et al. Lumpectomy and radiation therapy for the treatment of Intraductal breast cancer: findings from National Surgical Adjuvant Breast and Bowel Project B-17. *J Clin Oncol* 1998;16:441–452.

13. Julien JP, Bijker N, Fentiman IS. Radiotherapy in breast-conserving treatment for ductal carcinoma in situ: first results of the EORTC randomized phase III trial 10853. *Lancet* 2000;355:528–533.

14. Lagios MD. Duct carcinoma in situ: controversies in diagnosis, biology and treatment. *Breast J* 1995;1:68–78.

15. Solin LJ, Kurtz J, Fourquet A, et al. Fifteen-year results of breast conserving surgery and definitive breast irradiation for the treatment of ductal carcinoma in situ of the breast. *J Clin Oncol* 1996;14:754–763.

16. Lagios MD, Westdahl PR, Margolin FR, et al. Duct carcinoma in situ: relationship of extent of noninvasive disease to the frequency of occult invasion, multicentricity, lymph node metastases, and short-term treatment failures. *Cancer* 1982;50:1309–1314.

17. Bijker N, Peterse JL, Duchateau L, et al. Risk factors for recurrence and metastasis after breast-conserving therapy for ductal carcinoma in situ: analysis of European Organization for Research and Treatment of Cancer Trial 10853. *J Clin Oncol* 2001;19:2263–2271.

18. International Consensus Conference Committee. Image-detected breast cancer: state of the art diagnosis and treatment. *J Amer Coll Surg* 2001;193:247–302.

19. Guidi AJ, Connolly JL, Harris JR, et al. The relationship between shaved margin and inked margin status in breast excision specimens. *Cancer* 1997;79:1568–1573.

20. Holland R, Peterse JL, Millis RR, et al. Ductal carcinoma in situ: a proposal for new classification. *Semin Diagn Pathol* 1994;11:167–180.

21. Sneige N, McNesse MD, Atkinson EN, et al. Ductal carcinoma in situ treated with lumpectomy and irradiation: histo-pathological analysis of 49 specimens with emphasis on risk factors and long-term results. *Hum Pathol* 1995;126:642–649.

22. Schwartz GF, Finkel GC, Garcia JG, et al. Subclinical ductal carcinoma in situ of the breast. Treatment by local excision and surveillance alone. *Cancer* 1992;70:2468–2474.

23. Page DL, Dupont WD, Rogers LW, et al. Continued local recurrence of carcinoma 15–25 years after diagnosis of low grade ductal carcinoma of the breast treated only by biopsy. *Cancer* 1995;76:1197–1200.

24. Page DL, Dupont WD, Rogers LW, et al. Intraductal carcinoma of the breast: followup after biopsy only. *Cancer* 1982;49:751–758.

25. Page DL, Dupont WD, Rogers LW, et al. Atypical hyperplastic lesions of the female breast: a long follow-up study. *Cancer* 1985;55:2698–2708.

26. Dupont WD, Page DL. Risk factors for breast cancer in women with proliferative breast disease. *N Engl J Med* 1985;312:146–151.

27. London SJ, Connolly JL, Schnitt SJ, et al. A prospective study of benign breast disease and risk of breast cancer. *JAMA* 1992;267:941–944.

28. Collins L, Lester S, Cooper A, et al. Ductal carcinoma in situ (DCIS) treated with excision alone: predictors of local recurrence. US–Canadian Acad Pathol Annual Meeting, 1997. (abstract 80).

29. Badve S, Ahern RP, Ward AM, et al. Prediction of local recurrence of ductal carcinoma of the breast using five histological classifications: a comparative study with long follow-up. *Hum Pathol* 1998;29:915–923.

30. Douglas-Jones AG, Gupta SK, Attanoos RL, et al. A critical appraisal of six modern classifications of ductal carcinoma in situ of the breast: correlation with grade of associated invasive disease. *Histopathology* 1996;29:397–409.

31. Bethwaite P, Smithe N, Delahunt B, et al. Reproducibility of new classification schemes for the pathology of ductal carcinoma in situ of the breast. *J Clin Pathol* 1998;51:450–454.

32. Sneige N, Lagios MD, Schwarting R, et al. Interobserver reproducibility of the Lagios nuclear grading system for ductal carcinoma in situ. *Hum Pathol* 1998;30:257–262.

33. Leong AS, Sormunen RT, Vinyuvat S, et al. Biologic markers in ductal carcinoma in situ and concurrent infiltrating carcinoma. A comparison of eight contemporary grading systems. *Am J Clin Pathol* 2001;115:709–718.

34. Fisher B, Dignam J, Tan-Chu E, et al. Pathologic findings from the National Surgical Adjuvant Breast Project (NSABP) eight-year update of Protocol B-17. *Cancer* 1999;86:429–438.

35. Egan RL, Ellis JR, Powell RW. Team approach to the study of disease of the breast. *Cancer* 1971;71:847–854.

36. Silverstein MJ, Waisman JR, Gierson ED, et al. Radiation therapy for intraductal carcinoma. Is it an equal alternative? *Arch Surg* 1991;126:424–428.

37. Patchefsky AS, Schwartz GF, Finkelstein SD, et al. Heterogeneity of intraductal carcinoma of the breast. *Cancer* 1995;75:1219–1221.

38. Holland R, Veling SHJ, Marvunac M, et al. Histologic multiplicity of T1s, T1-2 breast carcinomas. Implications for clinical trials of breast conserving surgery. *Cancer* 1985;56:979–990.

39. Faverly D, Burgers L, Bult P, et al. Three dimensional imaging of mammary ductal carcinoma in situ: clinical implications. *Semin Diagn Pathol* 1994;11:193–198.

40. Silverstein MJ, Waisman JR, Gamagami P, et al. Intraductal carcinoma of the breast (208) cases. Clinical factors influencing treatment choice. *Cancer* 1990;55:102–108.

41. Vicini FA, Kestin LL, Goldstein NS, et al. Relationship between excision volume, margin status, and tumor size with the development of local recurrence in patients with ductal carcinoma in situ treated by breast-conserving therapy. *J Surg Oncol* 2001;76:245–254.

42. George W, Houghton J, Cuzick J, et al. Radiotherapy and tamoxifen following complete local excision (CLE) in the management of ductal carcinoma in situ (DCIS): preliminary results from the UK DCIS trial. *Proc Am Soc Clin Oncol* 2000;19:70A.

43. Page DL, Lagios MD. Pathologic analysis of the National Surgical Adjuvant Breast Project (NSABP) B-17 trial. *Cancer* 1995;75:1219–1221.

44. Lagios MD, Silverstein MJ. Ductal carcinoma in situ. The success of breast conservation therapy: a shared experience of two single institutional non-randomized prospective studies. *Surg Oncol Clin North Am* 1997;6:385–392.

45. Goldstein NS, Kestin L, Vicini F. Intraductal carcinoma of the breast. Pathologic features associated with local recurrence in patients treated with breast-conserving therapy. *Am J Surg Pathol* 2000;24:1058–1067.

46. Lagios MD. Multicentricity of breast carcinoma demonstrated by routine correlated serial subgross and radiographic examination. *Cancer* 1977;40:1726–1734.
47. Wellings SR, Jensen HM, Marcum RG. An atlas of subgross pathology of human breast with special reference to possible precancerous lesions. *J Natl Cancer Inst* 1975;55: 231–273.
48. Acs G, Lawton TJ, Rebbeck TR, et al. Differential expression of E-Cadherin in lobular and ductal neoplasms of the breast and its biologic and diagnostic implications. *Am J Clin Pathol* 2001;115: 85–98.
49. Goldstein NS, Bassi D. Watts JC, et al. E-cadherin reactivity of 95 noninvasive ductal and lobular lesions of the breast. *Am J Clin Pathol* 2001;115:534–542.
50. Silverstein MJ. Can intraductal breast carcinoma be excised completely by local excision? *Cancer* 1994;73:2985–2989.
51. Gallagher MS, Martin JE. An orientation to the concept of minimal breast cancer. *Cancer* 1971;53:681–684.

17

THE VAN NUYS DUCTAL CARCINOMA IN SITU CLASSIFICATION: AN UPDATE

DAVID N. POLLER
MELVIN J. SILVERSTEIN

This updated chapter describes a simple reproducible histologic classification system that categorizes ductal carcinoma in situ (DCIS) by risk of local recurrence and details the results of long-term follow-up in a large series of patients with DCIS, confirming the prognostic value of the Van Nuys DCIS Classification. Newly published studies confirming the reproducibility and pathologic prognostic value of the Van Nuys DCIS Classification are presented and discussed.

DCIS is not a single disease but rather a spectrum of disease. This concept is based on histologic and architectural differences, molecular and cytogenetic findings (1,2), and clinical evidence showing a higher rate of local recurrence in DCIS with high nuclear grade (3–7) or necrosis (4,6–9). Current evidence suggests that DCIS is in most cases a unicentric high-risk factor for the subsequent development of invasive breast carcinoma (10). Because DCIS is a spectrum of diseases, various pathologic classifications have been proposed (11–17), although none has found universal acceptance.

Pathologic subclassification of DCIS can be used to predict prognosis after breast conservation. A simple, reproducible histologic classification system that categorizes DCIS by risk of local recurrence would be extremely helpful. However, the contribution to outcome by three important variables generally not considered part of the histologic subtype (age, lesion size, and margin width) suggests that pathologic subtype cannot be relied on in isolation (18,19) (see Chapter 45). Unfortunately, many published studies of DCIS rarely include reliable size and margin data. Larger DCIS lesions tend to demonstrate a higher pathologic grade (18) and in some studies have been shown to be more likely to have involved margins (18). This has a profound influence on rates of local control of disease after breast conservation.

COMEDO VERSUS NONCOMEDO DUCTAL CARCINOMA IN SITU: AN OVERSIMPLIFICATION

Studies have shown that nuclear grade and comedonecrosis (6,8,13,20,21) are important factors in predicting the risk of local recurrence after breast conservation. Pathologists have attempted to classify DCIS by using nuclear grade or combinations of nuclear grade with other features (1,11,13,14, 17,21–24) such as differentiation and cytoarchitectural differentiation (12), architecture (25), the presence or absence of comedonecrosis (1), or various combinations of factors. Although these classifications can be used by most pathologists, there is some discordance among pathologists in the subclassification of DCIS (11,26–30), and the classifications do not always generate prognostically different subgroups. It is important, therefore, to use pathologic features that are of prognostic importance and show reproducibility among pathologists.

Historically, architecture was thought to be the most important distinguishing feature of DCIS. Traditionally, most pathologists have divided DCIS into five or six architectural subtypes (papillary, micropapillary, cribriform, solid, clinging, and comedo), often grouping the first five together as noncomedo and comparing them with comedo (31). Necrosis in DCIS is frequently associated with high nuclear grade (13,14,23–25,31). Comedonecrosis and/or high nuclear grade are associated with a higher proliferation fraction in DCIS (32–41) and HER2/neu (c-erbB-2) gene amplification or protein overexpression (37–39,41–49) and, by inference, are more likely to show aggressive clinical behavior. DCIS without necrosis tends to be the opposite. These systems do not take into account rarer subtypes of DCIS such as clear cell, endocrine, cystic hypersecretory, apocrine, and encysted papillary DCIS (1). Thus, division by architecture, comedo versus noncomedo, is an oversimplification and not applicable in all cases because it does not always reflect the biology of the underlying disease. Although the findings in comedo/noncomedo DCIS are typically as stated above, any architectural subtype may present with any nuclear grade with or without comedonecrosis. It is not uncommon for high nuclear grade noncomedo lesions to express markers similar to high-grade comedo lesions. Such lesions may require more aggressive treatment. Furthermore, mixtures of various architectural subtypes within a single biopsy speci-

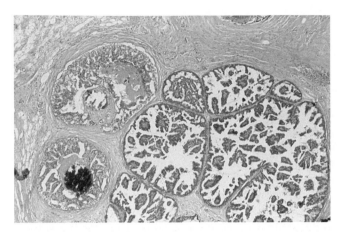

FIGURE 17.1. Right side of the field reveals a low-grade micropapillary ductal carcinoma in situ (DCIS) without obvious necrosis seen on low power on the right, although high-power microscopic examination is required to confirm that fewer than five pyknotic nuclei are present to exclude the presence of necrosis here. The left side of the field shows two foci of intermediate-grade cribriform DCIS with obvious necrosis/microcalcifications (magnification 20×).

men are common. In the Van Nuys series, 72% of all lesions had significant amounts of two or more architectural subtypes (Fig. 17.1).

A WORKING DEFINITION OF NECROSIS

In the previous edition, we stated that "there is no uniform agreement among pathologists of exactly how much comedo DCIS must to be present before considering a lesion to be comedo DCIS." In our original publication of the Van Nuys DCIS Classification (21), we considered a lesion comedo if it was predominantly comedo, i.e., most of the lesion was made up of the comedo subtype. Generally that meant that at least 50% of the lesion demonstrated comedo architecture. However, a lesion consisting of 40% comedo, 30% cribriform, and 30% micropapillary would be considered predominantly comedo. Moriya and Silverberg (50,51) required 70% of the lesion to be comedo before calling it a comedo lesion. The Nottingham group (15) used comedonecrosis to divide DCIS in three groups based on morphology and cellular necrosis. Tumors in which 75% of the lesion showed central lumina containing necrotic debris surrounded by large pleomorphic viable cells in solid masses were classified as pure comedo subtype. Tumors that showed a smaller amount (less than 75% but at least 5%) of necrotic neoplastic cells of ductal origin within duct lumina and did not otherwise have a pure comedo pattern were classified as DCIS with necrosis or non–pure comedo. Tumors that showed no evidence of necrosis in any of the tissue examined were classified as DCIS without necrosis (15). Using this classification, S-phase fraction and c-erbB-2 protein expression were shown to be associated with the amount of

necrosis and outcome as measured by local recurrence. We are now advocating a simplified working definition of necrosis for the Van Nuys DCIS Classification as described by Douglas-Jones et al. (27). Their definition for necrosis is "eosinophilic cellular debris containing five or more pyknotic nuclei. Calcification is regarded as a surrogate of necrosis if it is accompanied by 5 or more pyknotic nuclei." This definition of necrosis has been shown by Douglas-Jones and colleagues to have high interobserver reproducibility (27). This definition would include all cases of DCIS in the discussion above regarded as comedo DCIS but also includes any other architectural subtype of DCIS that fulfills these minimum criteria for necrosis. As stated in the previous edition, "the distinction between comedo and non-comedo DCIS is flawed since virtually any architectural subtype may present with any nuclear grade, with or without necrosis. Architecture, without a strict set of universally agreed upon criteria (which currently do not exist), is a poor way to classify DCIS."

EVOLUTION OF THE VAN NUYS DUCTAL CARCINOMA IN SITU CLASSIFICATION

Nuclear grade is a better prognostic indicator than architecture and has emerged, along with lesion size and margin width (18), as an important histopathologic factor for identifying aggressive behavior (1,13,14,20,52). In late 1994, in an analysis of our own series, limiting the analysis to patients with DCIS treated with excision plus radiation therapy, we found that nuclear grade was the only significant factor, by multivariate analysis, that predicted for local recurrence of both DCIS and invasive breast cancer (52).

This result led us in early 1995 to a more detailed analysis in which we used all patients who had received breast-preservation treatment in our series (excision only and excision plus radiation therapy) (53). At that time, we analyzed 16 prognostic factors and found that nuclear grade, tumor size, margin width, and comedonecrosis were all significant predictors of local recurrence by univariate analysis. Based on this, we devised a new pathologic DCIS classification, the Van Nuys DCIS Classification (21). We used two statistically important predictors of local recurrence: the presence or absence of high nuclear grade and comedonecrosis. Both factors are thought to be indicators of tumor biology. Since its publication, the utility of the Van Nuys Classification has been independently validated (3,11,26,27,29,30,54). Most of these studies show that this DCIS classification, employing a combination of high grade, compared with intermediate/low nuclear grade, and the presence or absence of necrosis, shows good interobserver reproducibility and that the Van Nuys Classification is predictive of clinical outcome after breast conservation (3,11,26,27,29).

Sloane et al. (29) examined 33 cases of DCIS among a working group of 23 European pathologists who categorized them using five recently published classifications: that of the European Pathologists Working Group (12); one based entirely on nuclear grade with categories of high, intermediate, and low as currently in use in the United Kingdom National Health Service and European Commission–funded breast screening programs; the same classification as in previously with only two categories, i.e., high nuclear grade and other; the Van Nuys Classification (21), and a two-category classification based entirely on the presence or absence of comedonecrosis. Of the three systems with three categories, the Van Nuys Classification gave the highest overall kappa statistic of 0.42. Others gave similar values of 0.37 and 0.35, showing that assessing cell polarization in addition to nuclear grade neither improves nor worsens consistency. In all three tricategory systems, the middle category was associated with the lowest kappa value. Of the two systems with two categories, that based on nuclear grade gave the highest overall kappa value of 0.46 and that based on comedonecrosis the lowest of 0.34. The most robust histologic features in this study of interobserver reproducibility were high- and low-grade nuclei and necrosis as long as the latter did not involve the recognition of a comedo growth pattern. The authors commented of this study that these kappa values probably represent the maximum achievable, at least by reasonable numbers of pathologists in everyday practice.

A second study (11) examined the in situ component of 180 cases of screen-detected infiltrating ductal carcinoma of the breast using six published classifications, including the Van Nuys Classification. All cases were evaluated independently by two experienced observers to assess interobserver variation. Interobserver disagreements were most common in the assessment of architecture and least common in the assessment of necrosis. For cytonuclear grade, most disagreements (62.2%) involved the distinction between low and intermediate as against 33.9% disagreements for intermediate versus high. The Van Nuys Classification was commended by the authors for its well-defined criteria (with no requirement for percentage estimations) and its applicability to small numbers of ducts as well as its proven prognostic importance.

In the third study, a case-control study of 141 patients with long-term follow-up, the ability of five morphologic DCIS classifications to predict recurrence after local excision was compared (3). No significant correlation between recurrence and a traditional classification based on architecture was found, nor with necrosis when a scheme based principally on architectural features was employed. A significant correlation between histology and recurrence was observed using the Van Nuys Classification. A correlation was also found between recurrence and differentiation as defined by nuclear features and cell polarization in a classification formulated by Holland et al. (12), but this failed to reach statistical significance at the 5% level. A stronger and statistically significant correlation was found with nuclear

grade using the classification currently employed by the United Kingdom National Health Service and European Commission–funded breast screening programs. Whether the tumor recurred as in situ or invasive carcinoma was unrelated to histologic classification, as was the time course over which it occurred. It was commented that the findings strongly supported the use of nuclear grade to identify cases of DCIS at high risk of recurrence after local excision but that further work was necessary to determine whether nuclear grade or necrosis was more appropriate to subdivide the non–high-grade cases.

The fourth study, an interobserver reproducibility study (26), was performed to compare the interobserver variation in the pathologic classification of DCIS of the breast using two recently proposed classification schemes, that of Holland et al. (12) and the Van Nuys DCIS Classification (21). Eleven pathologists classified a set of 25 cases of DCIS chosen to reflect a range of lesions, using a traditional architectural classification together with the modified cytonuclear grading scheme of Holland et al. and the Van Nuys Classification scheme. Participating pathologists received a standard tutorial, written information, and illustrative photomicrographs before their assessment of the cases. The interobserver agreement was poorest when using the architectural scheme (kappa = 0.44), largely owing to variations in classifying lesions with a mixed component of patterns (kappa = 0.13). Agreement was better using the modified cytonuclear grading scheme (kappa = 0.57), with most consistency achieved using the Van Nuys scheme (kappa = 0.66). Most discordant results using the latter scheme were owing to inconsistency in assessing the presence or absence of luminal necrosis. The authors concluded that both of the new classification schemes assessed in this study were an improvement over the traditional architectural classification system for DCIS and resulted in more reproducible pathologic assignment of cases. In their opinion, the Van Nuys Classification scheme was easy to apply, even to small areas of DCIS, resulting in acceptable interobserver agreement between reporting pathologists.

The fifth study (27) examined inter- and intraobserver agreement in the assessment of cytologic grade and intraductal necrosis in pure DCIS of the breast. Sixty unselected cases with illustrated, previously defined diagnostic criteria were circulated to 19 practicing pathologists. There was overall moderate agreement for cytonuclear grade in three categories with 71% agreement, weighted kappa = 0.36; intraduct necrosis in three categories (absent, present, extensive) showing 76% agreement, weighted kappa = 0.57; and the Van Nuys Classification showing 73% agreement, weighted kappa = 0.48. There was 69.6% interobserver agreement for cytonuclear grade assessment, weighted kappa = 0.52, and 68.3% agreement for intraductal necrosis, weighted kappa = 0.48. These results were interpreted as suggesting that individual variation rather than precision of the pathologic criteria contributed to the lack of agreement. The authors concluded that moderate interpathologist agreement could be achieved by nonspecialist pathologists with better agreement on necrosis than nuclear grade. There was evidence of consistent individual bias toward over- or underscoring cytonuclear grade, which could be corrected with adequate and prompt feedback.

The sixth study by Wells et al. (30) assessed the diagnostic agreement and reproducibility of the Holland et al. (12), modified Lagios (16), and Van Nuys classifications (21). Seven nonexpert pathologists and three experts evaluated 40 slides of DCIS according to the three classifications. Twenty slides were reinterpreted by each nonexpert pathologist. Diagnostic accuracy (nonexperts compared with experts) and reproducibility were evaluated using kappa statistics. This study was flawed in that study tickbox questionnaire used by the participants had three nuclear grade categories for the Van Nuys Classification rather than two; high grade and non-high grade. This error lead to incorrect conclusions being made regarding the reproducibility of the Van Nuys Classification (55).

The seventh study by Warnberg et al. (54) evaluated the correlation with prognosis for two classification systems of DCIS. Using the Holland et al. system (12) and the Van Nuys system, 195 cases were reclassified by two pathologists (21). The relapse-free survival by histopathologic subgroup and by nuclear grade only was estimated for 149 women treated with breast-conserving surgery. There were 32 ipsilateral recurrences, 19 in situ and 13 invasive. There was no difference in relapse-free survival between the three groups in the Van Nuys Classification, with overall agreement between the two observers in 79% and 64% of the cases, according to the Holland et al. and Van Nuys systems, respectively. The authors identified one group of 13 patients with well-differentiated DCIS with no ipsilateral recurrences using the Holland et al. system (12) and found that the Holland et al. system showed greater interobserver agreement. The significance of this apparent greater interobserver agreement for the Holland et al. classification (12) must be questioned in the light of the qualifying statement in the article that indicates that only one clinically experienced pathologist participated in the study and that the degree of interobserver agreement should "be regarded as a test of whether these systems are easy to learn."

UPDATE OF THE VAN NUYS CLASSIFICATION

Patients and Methods

The Van Nuys Classification defines three groups of patients with DCIS by using the presence of high nuclear grade (nuclear grade 3) to select the most aggressive group (group 3). The remaining non–high-grade lesions (nuclear grades 1 or 2) are then separated by the presence (group 2) or absence (group 1) of necrosis (Fig. 17.2). Nuclear grade

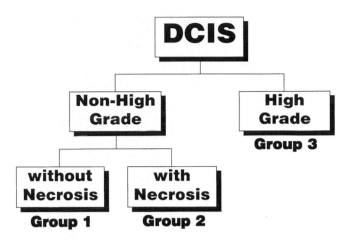

FIGURE 17.2. Van Nuys Classification of ductal carcinoma in situ (DCIS). Patients with DCIS are separated into high nuclear grade and non-high nuclear grade. Non-high nuclear grade cases are then separated by the presence or absence of necrosis. Lesions in group 3 (high nuclear grade) may or may not show necrosis. (From Silverstein MJ, Poller DN, Waisman JR, et al. Prognostic classification of breast ductal carcinoma in situ. *Lancet* 1995;345:1154–1157, with permission.)

(13,22) and necrosis are scored as follows (21). Low-grade nuclei (grade 1) are defined as nuclei one to 1.5 red blood cells in diameter with diffuse chromatin and inapparent nucleoli. Intermediate-grade nuclei (grade 2) are defined as nuclei one to two red blood cells in diameter with coarse chromatin and infrequent nucleoli. High-grade nuclei (grade 3) are defined as nuclei with a diameter greater than two red blood cells with vesicular chromatin and one or more nucleoli. The definition of necrosis is now modified slightly. Necrosis is now considered to be present for any architectural pattern of DCIS in which central lumina contain necrotic neoplastic cells of ductal origin with the minimum criterion of the presence eosinophilic cellular debris within ductal spaces containing at least five or more pyknotic nuclei. Calcification is regarded as a surrogate of necrosis if it is accompanied by five or more pyknotic nuclei. This definition is from Douglas-Jones et al. (27). No quantitative requirement is made for a specific amount of high nuclear grade DCIS or necrosis. Occasional desquamated or individually necrotic cells are ignored and are not scored as necrosis.

Group 1 DCIS consists of non–high-grade DCIS without necrosis (Fig. 17.3). Group 2 consisted of non–high-grade DCIS with necrosis (Fig. 17.4). Group 3 consisted of all high-grade DCIS with or without necrosis (Fig. 17.5). The classification was initially applied to a series of 425 consecutive patients with histologically confirmed DCIS treated at the Van Nuys Breast Center, Van Nuys, CA, between 1979 and 1994 and published in *The Lancet* (21) in 1995. In 1998, one of us (M.J.S.) moved to the University of Southern California (USC). The same prospective pathologic data collection system was introduced there, and patients accrued by M.J.S. at USC are included in the

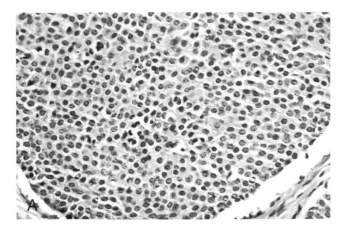

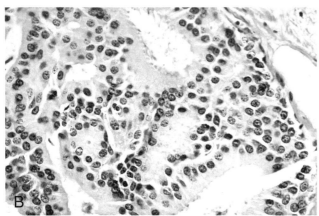

FIGURE 17.3. Group 1 ductal carcinoma in situ (non-high grade without necrosis). **A:** Low nuclear grade (grade 1) without necrosis (group 1) (magnification 250×. **B:** Intermediate nuclear grade (grade 2) without necrosis (group 1) (magnification ×250).

database, which has been renamed the Van Nuys/USC database. Through December 2000, the Van Nuys/USC series grew to 909 patients.

A total of 326 patients were treated by mastectomy and, therefore, did not have the ipsilateral breast at risk after treatment; 583 patients were treated with breast preservation (346 by excision alone and 237 by excision and radiation therapy). Because the likelihood of local recurrence is low for patients treated with mastectomy, their inclusion would artificially improve the local recurrence data. Therefore, only the 583 patients who were treated with breast preservation (with 109 local recurrences) are used in the Kaplan-Meier calculations of local recurrence.

Treatment was not randomized. Patients with large lesions (≥4 cm), true multicentricity, or involved margins not amenable to re-excision were advised to undergo mastectomy (usually with immediate breast reconstruction). Patients with smaller lesions (≤4 cm) and microscopically clear surgical margins were generally treated with excision alone or excision plus radiation therapy. However, some patients with larger lesions elected breast preservation, whereas others with lesions smaller than 4 cm elected mastectomy.

Until 1988, all patients with DCIS who elected breast conservation were advised to add breast irradiation to their treatment. Most patients accepted this recommendation; a few refused and were treated with careful clinical follow-up without irradiation. Beginning in 1989, the physicians at the Van Nuys Breast Center were no longer convinced with

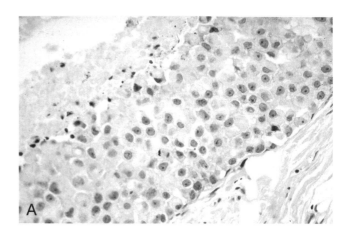

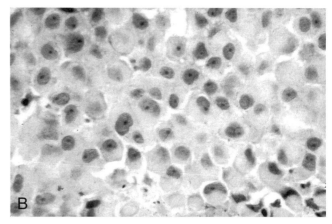

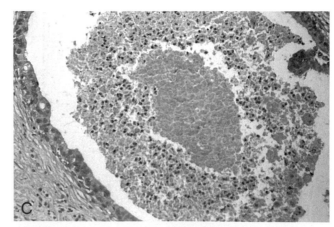

FIGURE 17.4. Group 2 ductal carcinoma in situ (non-high grade with necrosis). **A:** Intermediate-grade nuclei (grade 2) with necrosis seen in the upper right hand corner (group 2) (magnification ×250). **B:** High-power view of **A**. Note minimally pleomorphic nuclei with nucleolar development and rare mitotic figures (group 2) (magnification ×400). **C:** Low-grade lesion with marked central necrosis (group 2) (magnification ×100)

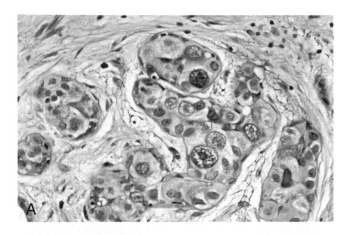

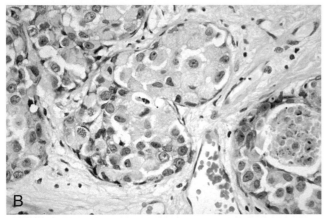

FIGURE 17.5. A: High-grade (group 3) ductal carcinoma in situ (DCIS) without necrosis involving a small lobule (magnification ×400). **B:** High-grade (group 3) DCIS with necrosis (duct on right) involving a small lobule (magnification ×250).

the overall value of radiation therapy for DCIS, and all patients who had breast conservation with clear biopsy margins (defined at that time as ≥1 mm) were offered the option of careful clinical follow-up without radiation therapy. Most patients accepted this option; a few refused and were treated with breast irradiation. Outside patients with DCIS referred to our radiation oncologists for radiation therapy

continued to be treated with radiation therapy in accordance with the wishes of their referring physicians.

Eighty-nine percent of patients treated with excision plus radiation therapy had nonpalpable lesions compared with 94% of excision only patients (p = NS). The mean tumor diameter was 18 mm for patients treated with excision and radiation therapy and 15 mm for patients treated with excision only ($p < 0.01$). In addition to the fact that treatment selection was not randomized, the difference in tumor size supports the conclusion that the Breast Center's patients treated with radiation therapy and patients treated with excision alone should not be directly compared.

Level 1 and 2 axillary dissections were done routinely until 1988; thereafter, a lower axillary sampling was performed in some patents treated with mastectomy. Beginning in 1995, a sentinel lymph node biopsy was performed on patients who underwent mastectomy. Whole-breast external beam irradiation (40 to 50 Gy) was performed on a 4 or 6 MeV linear accelerator. Some patients received a boost of 10 to 20 Gy to the tumor bed by an iridium 192 implant or linear accelerator (Chapter 37). Disease-free survival rates for each group were estimated by the Kaplan-Meier method. The statistical significance between survival curves was determined by the log-rank test.

Results: Analysis by Treatment

One hundred eleven patients experienced local failure: two patients treated with mastectomy (both invasive recurrences) and 109 patients treated with breast preservation (47 invasive recurrences, 62 DCIS) (Table 17.1). Ninety-eight of the 109 (90%) patients treated with breast preservation recurred at or near the primary lesion, suggesting that the most likely cause for local failure was inadequate initial resection (in other words, disease was left behind). Eight patients developed metastatic breast cancer in addition to their local recurrence. No patient developed distant disease without a local recurrence. Five patients have died of breast cancer. Fifty additional patients have died of other causes without recurrence of their breast cancer.

TABLE 17.1. TYPES OF RECURRENCES BY TREATMENT: 909 PATIENTS WITH DUCTAL CARCINOMA IN SITU

	Mastectomy	Excision Plus Irradiation	Excision Only	Total
Local only	1	42	60	103
Local plus distant	1	6	1	8
Distant only	0	0	0	0
Total	2	48	61	111
Invasive	2	22	25	49
DCIS only	0	26	36	62
Total	2	48	61	111

DCIS, ductal carcinoma in situ.

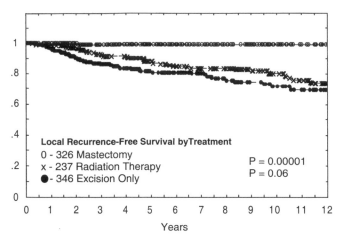

FIGURE 17.6. Local recurrence–free survival by treatment for 909 nonrandomized patients. The difference between mastectomy and either form of breast preservation is highly significant. The difference between excision only and excision with radiation therapy trends toward significant. If a statistic weighted more toward the earlier years of the study is used, then patients who were treated with radiation therapy have a statistically significant benefit despite the fact that the patients are not randomized and the patients treated with radiation therapy had larger lesions.

Figure 17.6 shows the local recurrence–free survival for the three forms of treatment. Mastectomy is clearly superior to both forms of breast preservation ($p = 0.00001$) in terms of local recurrence. In terms of the truly important end point, breast cancer–specific survival, there was no significant difference regardless of treatment (Fig. 17.7).

Despite the differences between patients who received radiation therapy and those who did not (the patients treated with excision only had smaller lesions and have been followed for a shorter period), there was a trend toward a significant difference in favor of those who received radiation therapy. When analyzed by the log-rank test, the p value was 0.06, as shown in Figure 17.6, but when analyzed by a statistic that puts more weight on the earlier part of the curve (Gehan's Wilcoxon), the value was significant ($p = 0.008$). This trend supports the conclusions of the prospective randomized trials that have shown that radiation therapy reduces local recurrence rate.

Two patients treated with mastectomy developed a local recurrence of invasive disease. One patient developed a solitary bone metastasis but has remained healthy without additional recurrence for more than 16 years. There have been no breast cancer deaths in the mastectomy group.

Sixty-one patients treated with excision alone developed local recurrence (25 invasive, 36 DCIS). One patient developed metastatic disease and died of breast cancer.

Forty-eight patients who received postexcisional radiation therapy developed local recurrences (22 invasive, 26 DCIS). Six developed metastatic disease, four of whom have died of breast cancer. There is no statistical difference in

breast cancer–specific mortality among the three treatment options (Fig. 17.7) ($p = NS$).

Three hundred five level 1 and 2 axillary node dissections (average number of nodes removed $= 18$) and 58 node samplings (six or fewer nodes) have been done. In two patients, both treated with mastectomy, positive nodes were found (0.6%). A single positive node was found in one patient and two positive nodes in the second. Thorough sectioning of the breast did not reveal the invasive focus in either case. Neither patient has developed metastatic disease. Routine axillary node dissection is clearly not indicated for patients with DCIS (56).

Beginning in 1995, sentinel node biopsies have been performed on patients with DCIS who underwent mastectomy. Through 2000, 66 additional patients underwent this procedure, five (6%) had one positive node by immunohistochemistry. All were negative by hematoxylin-eosin staining. None of these patients has developed metastatic disease. None has been treated as stage II disease.

Analysis Using the Van Nuys Classification

Patient and tumor characteristics for all three Van Nuys Classification groups are shown in Table 17.2. Size, nuclear grade, and HER2/neu overexpression were statistically different for all groups. The differences from group to group for p53 were not significant. If groups 1 and 2 are combined and compared with group 3, estrogen receptor and progesterone receptor are statistically different.

Forty-seven of 109 (43%) of recurrences in patients treated with breast preservation were invasive: six of 14 (43%) in group 1, 11 of 26 (42%) in group 2, and 30 of 69 (43%) in group 3.

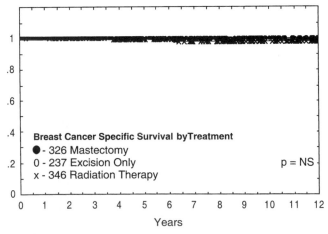

FIGURE 17.7. Breast cancer–specific mortality by treatment for 909 nonrandomized patients. There were no deaths in the mastectomy group. There were four deaths among patients treated with radiation therapy and one death among patients treated with excision alone. The differences are not statistically significant.

TABLE 17.2. TUMOR CHARACTERISTICS BY VAN NUYS CLASSIFICATION: 909 PATIENTS WITH DUCTAL CARCINOMA IN SITU

	Van Nuys Group 1 Non–High-Grade DCIS without Necrosis	Van Nuys Group 2 Non–High-Grade DCIS with Necrosis	Van Nuys Group 3 High-Grade DCIS
No. of patients (n = 909)	254	273	382
Average follow-up (mo)	92	88	73
Average size (mm) (n = 909)	18	25	32
Average nuclear grade (n = 922)	1.48	1.92	3.00
Average DNA (n = 76)	1.27	1.20	1.55
Average S phase (n = 56)	4.67	5.71	7.60
% ER positive (n = 149)	89%	76%	49%
% PR positive (n = 144)	89%	60%	53%
% HER2/neu positive (n = 204)	11%	31%	56%
% p53 positive (n = 157)	8%	13%	20%
Local recurrences (BCT only) (n = 109)	14/176 (8%)	26/166 (16%)	69/241 (29%)
Invasive local recurrences (BCT only) (n = 47)	6/14 (43%)	11/26 (42%)	30/69 (43%)
12-yr LRFS (BCT only) (n = 583)	87%	74%	55%
Deaths	0	2	3

DCIS, ductal carcinoma in situ; BCT, breast conservation therapy; LRFS, local recurrence–free survival; ER, estrogen receptor; PR, progesterone receptor.

There were two local invasive recurrences in patients treated with mastectomy. Initially, both lesions were large (a 45-mm group 2 lesion and a 100-mm group 3 lesion). The group 2 lesion was a local recurrence in the skin flap of a skin-sparing mastectomy. The other was a skin flap recurrence after standard mastectomy and implant reconstruction. The latter patient developed a solitary bone metastasis 2 years after her invasive recurrence and is currently alive and well without evidence of disease 16 years after the recurrence. The average follow-up for all patients is 83 months.

Figure 17.8 shows the local recurrence free–survival for all 583 patients treated with breast preservation analyzed by Van Nuys Classification group. Figures 17.9, 17.10, and 17.11 show each breast preservation subgroup (Van Nuys Classification groups 1, 2, and 3) divided into those patients who were treated with excision alone versus those treated with excision plus radiation therapy. There is no difference in the local recurrence rate by treatment for patients with group 1 or 2 lesions. There is, however, a statistically significant benefit for group 3 patients who received radiation therapy.

As mentioned above, there have been five deaths: none in group 1, two in group 2, and three in group 3. Three of four patients treated with radiation therapy developed inflammatory type recurrences with dermal lymphatic involvement. There is no statistical difference in breast cancer–specific survival among the three classification groups.

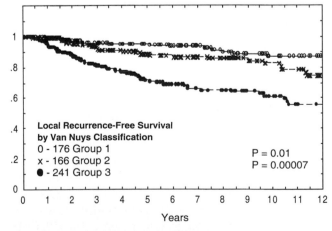

FIGURE 17.8. Local recurrence–free survival by Van Nuys Classification group for 583 patients treated with breast conservation. Local recurrence–free survival is statistically different for each group ($p \leq 0.01$).

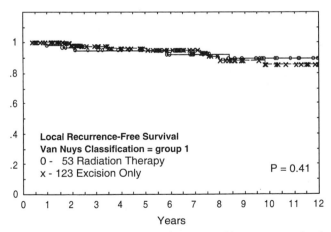

FIGURE 17.9. Local recurrence–free survival by treatment (excision plus radiation therapy versus excision alone) for 176 Van Nuys Classification group 1 patients (non–high-grade ductal carcinoma in situ without necrosis) (p = NS).

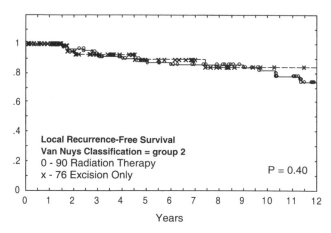

FIGURE 17.10. Local recurrence–free survival by treatment (excision plus radiation therapy versus excision alone) for 166 Van Nuys Classification group 2 patients (non–high-grade ductal carcinoma in situ with necrosis) (*p* = NS).

DISCUSSION

There is accumulating evidence that DCIS is a heterogeneous disease, part of a spectrum ranging at one end from typical hyperplasia to atypical intraductal hyperplasia to high nuclear grade DCIS with comedonecrosis at the opposite end (1). The evidence for this statement is derived from both morphologic and cytogenetic studies. The cytogenetics and molecular biology of DCIS have been discussed elsewhere in this book (see Chapters 5 and 8), but suffice it to say that there is much evidence now for accumulation of chromosomal deletions in the transition from usual type hyperplasia to atypical intraductal hyperplasia and through the morphologic spectrum of DCIS to invasive carcinoma (2). The spectrum of disease concept for DCIS is borne out by the fact that, after breast-conservation treatment, DCIS without necrosis shows a lower rate of local recurrence than DCIS with necrosis (13–15,20), as does low nuclear grade

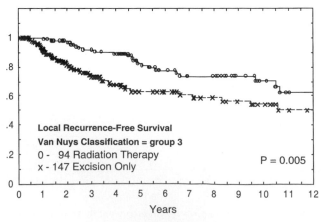

FIGURE 17.11. Local recurrence–free survival by treatment (excision plus radiation versus excision only) for 241 Van Nuys Classification group 3 patients (high-grade ductal carcinoma in situ) (*p* = 0.005).

DCIS when compared with high nuclear grade DCIS (1,13,14). Because DCIS is a heterogeneous disease, some lesions may require no treatment other than excisional biopsy. Other lesions may require complete excision with clear margins of 10-mm width (19), others require the addition of radiation therapy after complete excision, and yet others may be best treated by mastectomy. Several classifications of DCIS have been devised in an attempt to sort this heterogeneous group of lesions into usable subcategories that define patient outcome.

The Van Nuys Classification was developed as the next step of an earlier joint Nottingham proposal for a DCIS classification (15), which used one main feature, the presence or absence of comedonecrosis, but did not use nuclear grade. To qualify for the worst prognostic group in the Nottingham Classification, called pure comedo, 75% of the lesion had to be comedo DCIS. In Van Nuys, interobserver difficulties arose in assessing an accurate percentage of necrosis within a given tumor. In addition, because nuclear grade was not used, high-grade lesions such as large-cell, solid DCIS without necrosis were classified as DCIS without necrosis (15), the best prognostic group in the Nottingham Classification. There are 31 high-grade lesions without necrosis in this series, six of which have recurred (19%). Using the Nottingham Classification, these 31 cases fall into the most favorable prognostic group (DCIS without necrosis); in the Van Nuys Classification, they are in the least favorable group (high-grade DCIS, group 3) (21).

The Van Nuys Classification was devised by statistical modeling based on outcomes (local recurrences) of patients treated in Van Nuys. Based on the results of previous statistical analyses, it was thought to be extremely important to select all high nuclear grade lesions first, placing them into the worst prognostic group, before separating the cases by the presence or absence of comedonecrosis.

The suggestion has been made that there is an association between the differentiation of DCIS and the histologic grade of coexistent invasive cancer when DCIS is found in association with invasive carcinoma (50,57). This finding could imply that nuclear grade, an essential component of the Van Nuys Classification system for DCIS, might be an important factor in predicting progression of in situ breast carcinomas to invasive disease.

Although there is discordance among pathologists in recognizing subtypes of DCIS, particularly at the lower grade end of the DCIS spectrum (58,59), there is good agreement among pathologists concerning the presence or absence of comedonecrosis in DCIS (27). There is also evidence that comedonecrosis and/or high nuclear grade in DCIS is associated with c-erbB-2 (HER2/neu) gene amplification or c-erbB-2 protein overexpression (37–39,41–49) and with p53 protein expression or p53 gene mutation (33,37,39,41,43, 46,60–70), both of which are thought to be markers of adverse prognosis in invasive breast cancer. In addition, DCIS with comedonecrosis and/or high nuclear grade is more likely to lack estrogen receptor α (1,39,44,49,60,71–76) or progesterone receptor expression (39,44,49,60,61). Thus far, studies of estrogen receptor β in DCIS are too limited to make inferences with respect to estrogen receptor β and nuclear grade or necrosis in DCIS.

A DCIS pathology report should contain an assessment of nuclear grade, the presence or absence of necrosis, a description of architecture and growth pattern, the size of the lesion, the presence or absence of associated microcalcifications, and a measurement of the proximity to the nearest plane of excision (margin width) after correlation of the pathologic findings with the specimen radiograph (77). Unfortunately, there are no clear and universally agreed-on criteria for some of these categories. Hence, when DCIS cases are evaluated by a number of pathologists, there is some discordance (58,59,78).

The Van Nuys Classification alleviates some of the discordance, and most studies show that it is easy to apply (3,11,26,27,29), has prognostic significance (3), has high interobserver reproducibility (11,26,27,29), and is based on two prognostic features that are both biologically important and easy to recognize (3,11,26,27,29). Once the diagnosis of DCIS is made, the high-grade lesions are selected and assigned to group 3. The remaining lesions are then separated by necrosis. The presence or absence of comedonecrosis can be accurately judged by most pathologists as can high nuclear grade (27). No other decisions need be made to use this classification. Because we make no quantitative requirements regarding the amount of high-grade DCIS or necrosis, the classification is easy to apply.

We have chosen high nuclear grade as the most important factor in our classification because there is general agreement that patients with nuclear grade 3 lesions are likely to do worse than patients with low-grade lesions (13). We have chosen comedonecrosis because it is easy to recognize and its presence also suggests a poor prognosis (15,20,25). The presence of comedonecrosis may reflect a rapid growth phase that outstrips current blood supply or increased tumor apoptosis (79,80).

The most difficult part of most classifications is nuclear grading (78), particularly the identification of intermediate-grade lesions, which may reflect heterogeneity of nuclear grade within individual lesions. The subtleties of the intermediate-grade lesion are not relevant to our classification because only high nuclear grade (grade 3) needs to be recognized. The cells must be large and pleomorphic, lack architectural differentiation and polarity, and have prominent nucleoli and coarse clumped chromatin; generally, mitoses should be present.

The proposed classification is useful because it divides DCIS into three distinct groups with markedly different risks of local recurrence after breast-conservation therapy. However, classification alone is not adequate for selecting appropriate treatment. Three other factors (tumor size, margin width, and age) and perhaps others are of importance when determining appropriate treatment. The combination of tumors size, margin width, pathologic classification, and

age has been integrated into a modified Van Nuys Prognostic Index (18) and are further discussed in Chapter 45.

The low rates of local recurrence in patients with group 1 DCIS may be owing to the fact that these lesions do not have microcalcifications. When they recur, if they do not develop microcalcifications, their detection is likely to be difficult. It will be extremely important to follow all group 1 patients for a prolonged period because the diagnosis of recurrence is likely to be more difficult in these patients and detection will likely be delayed.

Because all conservatively treated patients are included in Figure 17.8, the recurrence rates at 12 years will probably be no worse than those estimated here: 13% for group 1, 26% for group 2, and 45% for group 3. If wider margins are obtained or radiation therapy is used, recurrence rates will decrease.

Pathologic classification is a valuable tool, but without the integration of other important factors such as margin width, tumor size, and age, it will only be of marginal value in the treatment selection process. A very large group 1 lesion may require mastectomy because its size makes complete excision, with an acceptable cosmetic result, almost impossible, whereas a small, high-grade group 3 lesion, well marked by mammographic microcalcifications, may be completely excised easily with near perfect cosmesis and can easily be treated with breast preservation. Pathologic classifications that do not take into account significant prognostic factors relating to local recurrence cannot be used as the sole guideline for treatment decision making.

SUMMARY

The details of a prognostic classification for DCIS are presented. Three groups of patients with DCIS are defined based on the presence or absence of high nuclear grade and comedonecrosis: group 1, non–high-grade DCIS without necrosis; group 2, non–high-grade DCIS with necrosis; group 3, high-grade DCIS with or without necrosis. There were 109 local recurrences in 583 patients treated with breast preservation: 8% (14 of 176) in group 1, 16% (26 of 166) in group 2, and 29% (69 of 241) in group 3. The 12-year actuarial local recurrence-free survival was 87%, 74%, and 55%, respectively (all $p < 0.01$). The Van Nuys Classification is in accord with current molecular and clinical evidence, defining three distinctly different and easily recognizable groups, each one of which has a different likelihood of local recurrence if treated with breast conservation. However, pathologic classification, regardless of which one is used, is not adequate by itself for determining appropriate treatment for patients with DCIS.

REFERENCES

1. Poller DN, Ellis IO. Ductal carcinoma in situ (DCIS) of the breast. In: Kirkham N, Lemoine N, eds. *Progress in pathology*, 2nd ed. London: Churchill-Livingstone, 1995.

2. O'Connell P, Pekkel V, Fuqua S, et al. Analysis of loss of heterozygosity in 399 premalignant breast lesions at 15 genetic loci. *J Natl Cancer Inst* 1998;90:697–703.

3. Badve S, A'Hern RP, Ward AM, et al. Prediction of local recurrence of ductal carcinoma in situ of the breast using five histological classifications: a comparative study with long follow-up. *Hum Pathol* 1998;29:915–923.

4. Boyages J, Delaney G, Taylor R. Predictors of local recurrence after treatment of ductal carcinoma in situ: a meta-analysis. *Cancer* 1999;85:616–628.

5. Lagios MD, Silverstein MJ. Ductal carcinoma in situ. The success of breast conservation therapy: a shared experience of two single institutional nonrandomized prospective studies. *Surg Oncol Clin North Am* 1997;6:385–392.

6. Ringberg A, Idvall I, Ferno M, et al. Ipsilateral local recurrence in relation to therapy and morphological characteristics in patients with ductal carcinoma in situ of the breast. *Eur J Surg Oncol* 2000;26:444–451.

7. Van Zee KJ, Liberman L, Samli B, et al. Long term follow-up of women with ductal carcinoma in situ treated with breast-conserving surgery: the effect of age. *Cancer* 1999;86:1757–1767.

8. Fisher E, Dignam J, Tan-Chiu E, et al. Pathologic findings from the National Surgical Adjuvant Breast Project (NSABP) eight-year update of Protocol B-17: intraductal carcinoma. *Cancer* 1999;86:429–438.

9. Sneige N, McNeese MD, Atkinson EN, et al. Ductal carcinoma in situ treated with lumpectomy and irradiation: histopathological analysis of 49 specimens with emphasis on risk factors and long term results. *Hum Pathol* 1995;26:642–649.

10. Faverly DR, Burgers L, Bult P, et al. Three dimensional imaging of mammary ductal carcinoma in situ: clinical implications. *Semin Diagn Pathol* 1994;11:193–198.

11. Douglas-Jones AG, Gupta SK, Attanoos RL, et al. A critical appraisal of six modern classifications of ductal carcinoma in situ of the breast (DCIS): correlation with grade of associated invasive carcinoma. *Histopathology* 1996;29:397–409.

12. Holland R, Peterse J, Millis R, et al. Ductal carcinoma in situ: a proposal for a new classification. *Semin Diagn Pathol* 1994;11:167–180.

13. Lagios MD. Duct carcinoma in situ. Pathology and treatment. *Surg Clin North Am* 1990;70:853–871.

14. Ottesen GL, Graversen HP, Blichert-Toft M, et al. Ductal carcinoma in situ of the female breast. Short-term results of a prospective nationwide study. The Danish Breast Cancer Cooperative Group. *Am J Surg Pathol* 1992;16:1183–1196.

15. Poller DN, Silverstein M, Galea M, et al. Ductal carcinoma in situ of the breast: A proposal for a new simplified histological classification. Association between cellular proliferation and c-erbB-2 expression. *Mod Pathol* 1994;7:257–262.

16. Scott MA, Lagios MD, Axelsson K, et al. Ductal carcinoma in situ of the breast: reproducibility of histological subtype analysis. *Hum Pathol* 1997;28:967–973.

17. Tavassoli FA. Ductal carcinoma in situ: introduction of the concept of ductal intraepithelial neoplasia. *Mod Pathol* 1998;11:140–154.

18. Silverstein MJ, Lagios MD, Craig PH, et al. A prognostic index for ductal carcinoma in situ of the breast. *Cancer* 1996;77:2267–2274.

19. Silverstein MJ, Lagios MD, Groshen S, et al. The influence of margin width on local control of ductal carcinoma in situ of the breast. *N Engl J Med* 1999;340:1455–1461.

20. Schwartz GF, Finkel GC, Garcia JC, et al. Subclinical ductal carcinoma in situ of the breast. Treatment by local excision and surveillance alone. *Cancer* 1992;70:2468–2474.

21. Silverstein MJ, Poller DN, Waisman JR, et al. Prognostic classification of breast ductal carcinoma-in-situ. *Lancet* 1995;345:1154–1157.

22. Lagios MD, Margolin FR, Westdahl PR, et al. Mammographically detected duct carcinoma in situ. Frequency of local recurrence following tylectomy and prognostic effect of nuclear grade on local recurrence. *Cancer* 1989;63:618–624.

23. Rosen P, Oberman H. Intraepithelial (preinvasive or in situ) carcinoma. In: Rosen P, Oberman H, eds. *Atlas of tumor pathology—tumors of the mammary gland*. Washington, DC: Armed Forces Institute of Pathology, 1993:119–156.

24. Lennington WJ, Jensen RA, Dalton LW, et al. Ductal carcinoma in situ of the breast. Heterogeneity of individual lesions. *Cancer* 1994;73:118–124.

25. Bellamy COC, McDonald C, Salter DM, et al. Noninvasive ductal carcinoma of the breast. The relevance of histologic categorization. *Hum Pathol* 1993;24:16–23.

26. Bethwaite P, Smith N, Delahunt B, et al. Reproducibility of new classification schemes for the pathology of ductal carcinoma in situ of the breast. *J Clin Pathol* 1998;51:450–454.

27. Douglas-Jones AG, Morgan JM, Appleton MA, et al. Consistency in the observation of features used to classify duct carcinoma in situ (DCIS) of the breast. *J Clin Pathol* 2000;53:596–602.

28. Sloane JP, Amendoeira I, Apostolikas N, et al. Consistency achieved by 23 European pathologists from 12 countries in diagnosing breast disease and reporting prognostic features of carcinomas. European Commission Working Group on Breast Screening Pathology. *Virchows Arch* 1999;434:3–10.

29. Sloane JP, Amendoeira I, Apostolikas N, et al. Consistency achieved by 23 European pathologists in categorizing ductal carcinoma in situ of the breast using five classifications. European Commission Working Group on Breast Screening Pathology. *Hum Pathol* 1998;29:1056–1062.

30. Wells WA, Carney PA, Eliassen MS, et al. Pathologists' agreement with experts and reproducibility of breast ductal carcinoma-in-situ classification schemes. *Am J Surg Pathol* 2000;24:651–659.

31. Page DL, Rogers LW. Carcinoma in situ (CIS). In: Page DL, Anderson TJ, eds. *Diagnostic histopathology of the breast*. Edinburgh: Churchill-Livingstone, 1987:157–192.

32. Barnard N, Hall P, Lemoine N, et al. Proliferative index in breast carcinoma determined in situ by Ki67 immunostaining and its relationship to clinical and pathological variables. *J Pathol* 1987;152:287–295.

33. Bobrow LG, Happerfield LC, Gregory WM, et al. Ductal carcinoma in situ: assessment of necrosis and nuclear morphology and their association with biological markers. *J Pathol* 1995;176:333–341.

34. Brower ST, Ahmed S, Tartter PI, et al. Prognostic variables in invasive breast cancer: contribution of comedo versus noncomedo in situ component. *Ann Surg Oncol* 1995;2:440–444.

35. Christov K, Chew K, Ljung B, et al. Cell proliferation in hyperplastic and in situ carcinoma lesions of the breast estimated by in vivo labeling with bromodeoxyuridine. *J Cell Biochem Suppl* 1994;19:165–172.

36. Locker AP, Horrocks C, Gilmour AS, et al. Flow cytometric and histological analysis of ductal carcinoma in situ of the breast. *Br J Surg* 1990;77:564–567.

37. Moreno A, Lloveras B, Figueras A, et al. Ductal carcinoma in situ of the breast: correlation between histologic classifications and biologic markers. *Mod Pathol* 1997;10:1088–1092.

38. Poller DN, Galea M, Pearson D, et al. Nuclear and flow cytometric characteristics associated with overexpression of the c-erbB-2 oncoprotein in breast carcinoma. *Breast Cancer Res Treat* 1991;20:3–10.

39. Zafrani B, Leroyer A, Fourquet A, et al. Mammographically-detected ductal in situ carcinoma of the breast analyzed with a new classification. A study of 127 cases: correlation with estrogen and

progesterone receptors, p53 and c-erbB-2 proteins, and proliferative activity. *Semin Diagn Pathol* 1994;11:208–214.

40. Meyer J. Cell kinetics of histologic variants of in situ breast carcinoma. *Breast Cancer Res Treat* 1986;18:11–17.

41. Albonico G, Querzoli P, Ferretti S, et al. Biological profile of in situ breast cancer investigated by immunohistochemical technique. *Cancer Detect Prev* 1998;22:313–318.

42. Allred DC, Clark GM, Molina R, et al. Overexpression of HER-2/neu and its relationship with other prognostic factors change during the progression of in situ to invasive breast cancer. *Hum Pathol* 1992;23:974–979.

43. Dublin EA, Millis RR, Smith P, et al. Minimal breast cancer: evaluation of histology and biological marker expression. *Br J Cancer* 1999;80:1608–1616.

44. Leal CB, Schmitt FC, Bento MJ, et al. Ductal carcinoma in situ of the breast. Histologic categorization and its relationship to ploidy and immunohistochemical expression of hormone receptors, p53, and c-erbB-2 protein. *Cancer* 1995;75:2123–2131.

45. Lodato RF, Maguire HC Jr, Greene MI, et al. Immunohistochemical evaluation of c-erbB-2 oncogene expression in ductal carcinoma in situ and atypical ductal hyperplasia of the breast. *Mod Pathol* 1990;3:449–454.

46. Perin T, Canzonieri V, Massarut S, et al. Immunohistochemical evaluation of multiple biological markers in ductal carcinoma in situ of the breast. *Eur J Cancer* 1996;32A:1148–1155.

47. Ramachandra S, Machin L, Ashley S, et al. Immunohistochemical distribution of c-erbB-2 in in situ breast carcinoma-a detailed morphological analysis. *J Pathol* 1990;161:7–14.

48. Somerville JE, Clarke LA, Biggart JD. c-erbB-2 overexpression and histological type of in situ and invasive breast carcinoma. *J Clin Pathol* 1992;45:16–20.

49. Wilbur DC, Barrows GH. Estrogen and progesterone receptor and c-erbB-2 oncoprotein analysis in pure in situ breast carcinoma: an immunohistochemical study. *Mod Pathol* 1993;6:114–120.

50. Moriya T, Silverberg SG. Intraductal carcinoma (ductal carcinoma in situ) of the breast. A comparison of pure noninvasive tumors with those including different proportions of infiltrating carcinoma. *Cancer* 1994;74:2972–2978.

51. Moriya T, Silverberg S. Intraductal carcinoma (ductal carcinoma in situ) of the breast: Analysis of pathologic findings of 85 pure intraductal carcinomas. *Int J Surg Pathol* 1995;3:83–92.

52. Silverstein MJ, Barth A, Poller DN, et al. Ten-year results comparing mastectomy to excision and radiation therapy for ductal carcinoma in situ of the breast. *Eur J Cancer* 1995;31A:1425–1427.

53. Silverstein M, Barth A, Waisman J, et al. Predicting local recurrence in patients with intraductal breast carcinoma (DCIS). *Proc Am Soc Clin Oncol* 1995;14:117.

54. Warnberg F, Nordgren H, Bergh J, et al. Ductal carcinoma in situ of the breast from a population-defined cohort: an evaluation of new histopathological classification systems. *Eur J Cancer* 1999;35:714–720.

55. Poller DN. Use of the Van Nuys DCIS Classification. *Am J Surg Pathol* 2001;25:543–545.

56. Silverstein MJ, Gierson ED, Waisman JR, et al. Axillary lymph node dissection for T1a breast carcinoma. Is it indicated? *Cancer* 1994;73:664–667.

57. Lampejo O, Barnes D, Smith P, et al. Evaluation of infiltrating ductal carcinomas with a DCIS component: correlation of the histologic type of the in situ component with grade of the infiltrating component. *Semin Diagn Pathol* 1994;11:215–222.

58. Rosai J. Borderline epithelial lesions of the breast. *Am J Surg Pathol* 1991;15:209–221.

59. Schnitt SJ, Connolly JL, Tavassoli FA, et al. Interobserver reproducibility in the diagnosis of ductal proliferative breast lesions using standardized criteria. *Am J Surg Pathol* 1992;16:1133–1143.

60. Allred DC, O'Connell P, Fuqua SA, et al. Immunohistochemical studies of early breast cancer evolution. *Breast Cancer Res Treat* 1994;32:13–18.

61. Bobrow LG, Happerfield LC, Gregory WM, et al. The classification of ductal carcinoma in situ and its association with biological markers. *Semin Diagn Pathol* 1994;11:199–207.

62. Chitemerere M, Andersen TI, Holm R, et al. TP53 alterations in atypical ductal hyperplasia and ductal carcinoma in situ of the breast. *Breast Cancer Res Treat* 1996;41:103–109.

63. Done SJ, Arneson NC, Ozcelik H, et al. p53 mutations in mammary ductal carcinoma in situ but not in epithelial hyperplasias. *Cancer Res* 1998;58:785–789.

64. Douglas-Jones AG, Navabi H, Morgan JM, et al. Immunoreactive p53 and metallothionein expression in duct carcinoma in situ of the breast. No correlation. *Virchows Arch* 1997;430:373–379.

65. Kanthan R, Xiang J, Magliocco AM. p53, ErbB2, and TAG-72 expression in the spectrum of ductal carcinoma in situ of the breast classified by the Van Nuys system. *Arch Pathol Lab Med* 2000;124:234–239.

66. Lukas J, Niu N, Press MF. p53 mutations and expression in breast carcinoma in situ. *Am J Pathol* 2000;156:183–191.

67. Munn KE, Walker RA, Menasce L, et al. Mutation of the TP53 gene and allelic imbalance at chromosome 17p13 in ductal carcinoma in situ. *Br J Cancer* 1996;74:1578–1585.

68. O'Malley FP, Vnencak-Jones CL, Dupont WD, et al. p53 mutations are confined to the comedo type ductal carcinoma in situ of the breast. Immunohistochemical and sequencing data. *Lab Invest* 1994;71:67–72.

69. Poller DN, Roberts EC, Bell JA, et al. p53 protein expression in mammary ductal carcinoma in situ: relationship to immunohistochemical expression of estrogen receptor and c-erbB-2 protein. *Hum Pathol* 1993;24:463–468.

70. Rajan PB, Scott DJ, Perry RH, Griffith CD. p53 protein expression in ductal carcinoma in situ (DCIS) of the breast. *Breast Cancer Res Treat* 1997;42:283–290.

71. Pallis L, Wilking N, Cedermark B, et al. Receptors for estrogen and progesterone in breast carcinoma in situ. *Anticancer Res* 1992;12:2113–2115.

72. Poller DN, Snead DR, Roberts EC, et al. Oestrogen receptor expression in ductal carcinoma in situ of the breast: relationship to flow cytometric analysis of DNA and expression of the c-erbB-2 oncoprotein. *Br J Cancer* 1993;68:156–161.

73. Bur M, Zimarowski M, Schnitt S, et al. Estrogen receptor immunohistochemistry in carcinoma in situ of the breast. *Cancer* 1992;69:1174–1181.

74. Giri DD, Dundas SA, Nottingham JF, et al. Oestrogen receptors in benign epithelial lesions and intraduct carcinomas of the breast: an immunohistological study. *Histopathology* 1989;15:575–584.

75. Barnes R, Masood S. Potential value of hormone receptor assay in carcinoma in situ of the breast. *Am J Clin Pathol* 1990;94:533–537.

76. Malafa M, Chaudhuri B, Thomford NR, et al. Estrogen receptors in ductal carcinoma in situ of breast. *Am Surg* 1990;56:436–439.

77. Schwartz GF, Solin LJ, Olivotto IA, et al. Consensus Conference on the Treatment of In Situ Ductal Carcinoma of the Breast, April 22–25, 1999. *Cancer* 2000;88:946–954.

78. Elston C, Sloane J, Amendoeira I, et al. Causes of inconsistency in diagnosing and classifying intraductal proliferations of the breast. *Eur J Cancer* 2000;36:1769–1772.

79. Gandhi A, Holland PA, Knox WF, et al. Evidence of significant apoptosis in poorly differentiated ductal carcinoma in situ of the breast. *Br J Cancer* 1998;78:788–794.

80. Bodis S, Siziopikou KP, Schnitt SJ, et al. Extensive apoptosis in ductal carcinoma in situ of the breast. *Cancer* 1996;77:1831–1835.

ANGIOGENESIS IN DUCTAL CARCINOMA IN SITU OF THE BREAST

STUART J. SCHNITT

Angiogenesis is a critical factor in both local growth and metastasis of solid tumors including breast cancers. The seminal studies of Folkman and colleagues in the 1960s clearly demonstrated that the formation of new blood vessels is necessary for solid tumors to enlarge beyond a few millimeters in size (1–3). More recently, many, but not all, studies of patients with invasive breast cancer have indicated that there is a significant association between the number of blood vessels in the tumor stroma, a reflection of the extent of angiogenesis, and the likelihood of developing metastatic disease and death from breast cancer (4–6).

Although angiogenesis appears to be critically important in invasive breast cancer, an understanding of the role of angiogenesis in the early stages of breast cancer development and progression is arguably even more crucial. Studies in both experimental animals and humans have indicated that at least some preinvasive breast lesions, including examples of ductal carcinoma in situ (DCIS), are capable of inducing neovascularization. The results of these studies suggest, therefore, that angiogenesis is an early event in the development of breast cancer. These observations have important biologic and clinical implications.

In this chapter, the subject of angiogenesis in preinvasive breast lesions is reviewed, with particular emphasis on angiogenesis in DCIS.

EXPERIMENTAL STUDIES

During the past 20 years, several studies in experimental systems have attempted to assess the angiogenic potential of preinvasive breast lesions. Gimbrone and Gullino (7,8), using an *in vivo* assay for neovascularization involving the intraocular transplantation of mammary tissues onto rabbit irises, reported that normal, hyperplastic, and neoplastic murine breast tissues, in ascending order of frequency, were capable of inducing angiogenesis. Furthermore, they demonstrated that among the hyperplastic lesions, those with the highest frequency of angiogenesis also had the

highest rate of neoplastic transformation. Using the same technique, Brem and Gullino (9) reported that neovascularization was also induced by murine mammary papillomatous lesions. Brem et al. (10) subsequently reported similar findings with tissues transplanted from human breast lesions and cited a neovascularization induction rate of 20% to 30% with tissues from benign hyperplasias. Fragments with in situ carcinoma and invasive carcinoma yielded neovascularization induction rates of 66% and 65%, respectively. The authors suggested that the assay was of potential use in predicting which benign biopsies were angiogenic and possibly at higher risk of neoplastic transformation. Ziche and Gullino (11) subsequently used the *in vivo* rabbit ocular transplant assay to demonstrate that various multiply passed cell lines (including a human mammary epithelial cell line) developed the ability to induce neovascularization before becoming tumorigenic.

The results of these studies provide strong experimental evidence that at least some preinvasive breast lesions are capable of inducing angiogenesis and that the ability to induce angiogenesis is an early event in the development of breast cancer.

HUMAN STUDIES

Studies of angiogenesis in DCIS in humans have largely focused on the evaluation of the extent and/or pattern of microvessels seen in association with DCIS and on the evaluation of angiogenic factors in DCIS.

Vascularity in Ductal Carcinoma in Situ

Several investigators have studied angiogenesis in preinvasive breast lesions in humans, with particular emphasis on DCIS. Ottinetti and Sapino (12) used tissue sections immunostained for factor VIII–related antigen to highlight microvessels and found that the mean vessel size was increased in DCIS and benign hyperplastic lesions compared with normal breast tissue but that the density of microvessels was not statistically different in the three groups. However, only ten cases of DCIS were evaluated, and therefore an analysis of microvessel density (MVD) among DCIS subtypes could not be performed. Similarly, Porter et al. (13), also using sections immunostained for factor VIII, reported that the mean vessel size was increased in neoplastic (in situ and invasive) and hyperplastic breast lesions compared with normal breast but found no significant differences in MVD among the four groups. However, only five cases of DCIS were included in this study. In contrast, using hematoxylin and eosin–stained sections and sections immunostained for laminin, Samejima and Yamazaki (14) reported that the stroma associated with DCIS was significantly more vascular than the stroma of invasive cancer and that both invasive and in situ cancers were significantly more vascular than benign lesions and normal breast parenchyma. Weidner et al. (15,16) noted a "ring of neovascularization" surrounding DCIS in five of 22 invasive breast cancers (23%) with a component of DCIS and considered this to represent a response to angiogenic factors elaborated by the adjacent DCIS.

In the first detailed study of angiogenesis in DCIS, Guidi et al. (17) evaluated 55 cases of DCIS unassociated with invasive cancer using sections immunostained for factor VIII. These investigators noted two major patterns of microvessels in association with DCIS: a diffuse stromal pattern and a cuff or rim of microvessels immediately adjacent to the basement membrane of involved ducts. In all cases in that study, a variable number of microvessels was present diffusely in the stroma surrounding the lesion. The MVD associated with these DCIS lesions was assessed using both a semiquantitative scale (1+ to 3+) and quantitative vessel counts. Semiquantitatively, the majority of cases (53%) had an overall MVD score of 2+; 22% of cases were 1+ and 25% were 3+ (representing lesions with the highest MVD) (Fig. 18.1). Quantitatively, a continuum of microvessel counts was observed, ranging from 17 to 80 vessels per 100× field, with a mean of 42.9 ± 16.6 vessels per 100× field. There was a significant relationship between the semiquantitative assessment of MVD and the quantitative microvessel counts. Lesions with 1+, 2+, and 3+ MVD scores had mean microvessel counts of 25.8 ± 7.1, 40.5 ± 10.5, and 60.9 ± 15.1 vessels per 100× field, respectively ($p < 0.05$ for all comparisons).

In 54 of the 55 cases, there was sufficient benign breast tissue on the same slide as the DCIS to permit comparison of DCIS-associated MVD with that of the uninvolved breast tissue. In 38 cases (70%), including 14 of 14 cases with 3+ MVD, 21 of 28 cases with 2+ MVD, and three of 12 cases with 1+ MVD, microvessels were clearly more prominent in association with the DCIS than with the benign breast tissue.

These investigators also related the stromal MVD in DCIS to the histologic features of the lesions, the expression of the protein product of the HER2/*neu* (c-erbB-2) oncogene, and the proliferation index of these lesions as determined by immunostaining with a monoclonal antibody

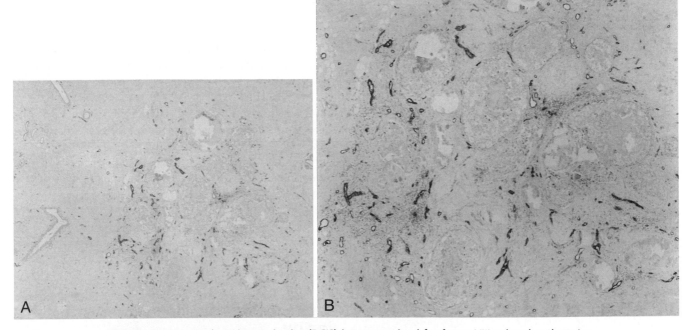

FIGURE 18.1. Ductal carcinoma in situ (DCIS) immunostained for factor VIII–related antigen to highlight microvessels. **A:** Microvessels are clearly more numerous in association with the DCIS than in the stroma of the adjacent benign breast tissue, which is present on the left side of this figure. **B:** Higher power view demonstrating microvessels in stroma surrounding DCIS.

known as Ki-S1 (18). The presence of 3+ MVD was significantly associated with comedo subtype ($p = 0.004$), predominant nuclear grade 3 ($p = 0.05$), marked stromal desmoplasia ($p = 0.05$), and HER2/neu protein expression ($p = 0.03$). In addition, a high Ki-S1 proliferation index was associated with 3+ MVD ($p = 0.05$). HER2/*neu* oncogene expression and a high Ki-S1 proliferation index were both more frequent in comedo than in noncomedo lesions ($p = 0.03$ and $p = 0.05$, respectively). The association between MVD score and stromal desmoplasia was independent of comedo subtype because no significant association between desmoplasia and tumor subtype was observed. Tumors with the combination of comedo histology and marked stromal desmoplasia had a 3+ MVD score in 83% of cases compared with 18% of all other lesions.

The second major pattern of microvessels observed by Guidi et al. (17) was the presence of a prominent cuff of microvessels in immediate apposition to the basement membrane of involved spaces, identical to the ring of neovascularization described by Weidner et al. (15,16) in DCIS associated with invasive breast cancer. This phenomenon was identified in 21 of the 55 cases (38%) (Fig. 18.2). Although the cuffing pattern of microvessels was more commonly seen in lesions with prominent MVD (8% of 1+, 41% of 2+, and 57% of 3+ MVD cases; $p = 0.03$), six DCIS lesions (11%) showed 3+ MVD but no vascular cuffing around involved spaces. No significant association was observed between quantitative microvessel counts and the cuffing pattern. There was also no significant association between the cuffing pattern and any of the histologic features (including histologic subtype), HER2/*neu* expression, or the Ki-S1 proliferation index. The cuffing pattern, characterized by either a complete or partial periductal ring of vessels, was also observed in 32 of 40 cases (80%) of DCIS studied by Bose et al. (19). This incidence is higher than the 38% incidence noted by Guidi et al. (17), and this difference may be related to differences in criteria used for determining the presence of the cuffing pattern. Nonetheless, like Guidi et al. (17), Bose et al. (19) also failed to note a significant correlation between the presence of a periductal cuff of microvessels and histologic subtype of DCIS, although a complete periductal ring was more common in lesions of the comedo type than in noncomedo lesions.

Engels et al. (20) evaluated patterns of vascularity in 75 formalin-fixed, paraffin-embedded specimens of cases of DCIS, also using immunostaining for factor VIII–related antigen. These investigators observed the same two vascular patterns first noted by Guidi et al.: a diffuse increase in stromal vascularity and a dense rim of microvessels adjacent to ductal basement membranes. Overall, 57% of the DCIS cases in this study showed diffuse vascularity and 62% showed the periductal rim pattern. The presence of these two patterns was highly correlated, with both patterns present in 47% of the cases. In addition, both patterns were most often seen in association with high-grade DCIS.

Lee et al. (21) also confirmed these two patterns of microvessels in association with DCIS. In a study of 41 formalin-fixed, paraffin-embedded specimens of cases of DCIS, these investigators assessed the relationships among patterns of vascularity, inflammation, and histologic features of DCIS. In that study, the extent of perivascular inflammatory cell clusters was significantly associated with the stromal pattern of vascularity, whereas the intensity of diffuse inflammation was associated with the periductal rim pattern. As noted by Guidi et al. (17), these authors also found that the diffuse pattern of stromal vascularity, but not the perivascular rim pattern, was significantly associated with HER2/*neu* expression in the DCIS cells. In another study, Bhoola et al. (22) evaluated MVD in 74 formalin-fixed, paraffin-embedded cases of DCIS using factor VIII–related antigen immunostains and computer-assisted image analysis. In contrast to the studies cited above, these investigators found no relationship between the extent of vascularization and the histologic features of DCIS when microvessels were quantified in this manner.

Most recently, Teo et al. (23) studied a series of DCIS cases using several different antiendothelial cell antibodies. They found that the immunophenotype of the vessels seen in association with DCIS differed from that seen in vessels surrounding normal breast lobules. In particular, DCIS lesions showed a greater density of CD34- and CD31-positive vessels and a lower density of factor VIII–related antigen-positive vessels than normal lobules. These observations suggest that studying the vascular phenotype may be as important as evaluating the number and pattern of microvessels in gaining a more complete understanding of the angiogenesis associated with DCIS.

Angiogenic Factors in Ductal Carcinoma in Situ

Several studies of angiogenic factors in DCIS have provided further evidence that DCIS lesions are capable of inducing

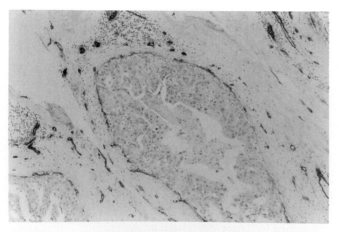

FIGURE 18.2. Ductal carcinoma in situ (DCIS) immunostained for factor VIII–related antigen to highlight microvessels. A cuff of microvessels is present around this involved space.

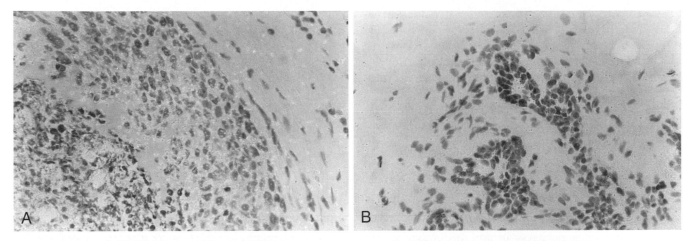

FIGURE 18.3. In situ hybridization for vascular permeability factor/vascular endothelial growth factor (VPF/VEGF) mRNA. **A:** The cells in this comedo DCIS lesion show intense labeling (indicated by the numerous grains) that is accentuated adjacent to the area of central necrosis. **B:** In contrast, normal duct and lobular epithelial cells show only weak labeling for VPF/VEGF mRNA.

angiogenesis. Brown et al. (24) studied the expression of the potent angiogenic substance vascular permeability factor (VPF), also known as vascular endothelial growth factor (VEGF) (25), in a series of breast lesions. The tumor cells in all four examples of DCIS studied strongly expressed VPF/VEGF mRNA as determined by in situ hybridization performed on frozen sections. The epithelial cells immediately adjacent to areas of necrosis showed the most intense labeling (Fig. 18.3). Furthermore, the endothelial cells of small stromal blood vessels near these DCIS lesions showed strong labeling for the mRNA of two VPF/VEGF receptors, flt-1 and kdr. In some areas, VPF/VEGF receptor mRNA expression in endothelial cells was present in a periductal cuffing pattern (Fig. 18.4), identical to the cuffing pattern of vessels identified around involved ducts on sections immunostained for factor VIII.

In a subsequent study, Guidi et al. (26) used mRNA in situ hybridization to evaluate VPF/VEGF expression in formalin-fixed, paraffin-embedded sections of 46 specimens from DCIS cases. Expression of this angiogenic factor by the DCIS cells was greater than that seen in the adjacent benign breast tissue in 96% of the evaluable cases. In addition, the extent of VPF/VEGF expression was significantly associated with the degree of angiogenesis in these lesions as determined from sections immunostained for factor VIII–related antigen. Finally, these investigators also noted that high-grade DCIS lesions more commonly showed high levels of expression of VPF/VEGF mRNA than lower grade lesions.

Other studies have assessed the potential role of the angiogenic factor thymidine phosphorylase (also know as platelet-derived endothelial cell growth factor) in the angiogenesis associated with DCIS. Engels et al. (27) documented increased expression of this substance in tumor cells, stromal cells, and endothelial cells in a series of DCIS cases and found that high levels of thymidine phosphorylase expres-

sion as determined by immunohistochemistry were significantly associated with the periductal rim pattern of vascularity. Lee et al. (28) also studied the relationship between thymidine phosphorylase expression and vascularity in DCIS. Using an immunohistochemical stain for thymidine phosphorylase, these investigators found expression of this angiogenic factor in both tumor cells and perivascular inflammatory cells (particularly macrophages) in cases of DCIS. These authors also found a significant association between thymidine phosphorylase expression and vascularity in DCIS. However, in contrast with Engels et al. (27), Lee et al. (28) noted that thymidine phosphorylase expression was associated with the stromal pattern of vascularity but not with the periductal rim pattern.

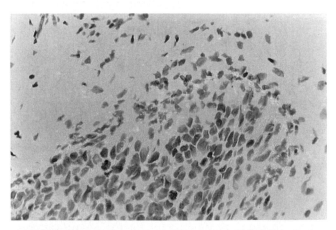

FIGURE 18.4. In situ hybridization for mRNA of the vascular permeability factor/vascular endothelial growth factor receptor kdr. There is intense labeling of endothelial cells in a cuffing pattern around the periphery of this involved duct. This is similar to the cuffing pattern of microvessels seen in some examples of ductal carcinoma in situ immunostained for factor VIII (compare with Fig. 18.2).

In summary, the results of these studies in human tissues clearly indicate that (i) some DCIS lesions are associated with increased stromal vessels in a diffuse and/or cuffing pattern around involved spaces, (ii) DCIS cells produce angiogenic factors including the potent angiogenic factor VPF/VEGF, and (iii) microvessels near the DCIS show strong expression for two VPF/VEGF receptors. Taken together, these data provide compelling evidence that at least some cases of DCIS have angiogenic capability.

CLINICAL IMPLICATIONS

The observation that some preinvasive breast lesions are capable of inducing angiogenesis in the surrounding stroma has several important clinical implications. It is possible, for example, that angiogenesis may be a marker for DCIS lesions with an increased risk for progression to invasive carcinoma or a marker for lesions with a greater potential to metastasize rapidly once stromal invasion has occurred. The finding of loss of expression of the antimetastasis gene *nm23* in comedo-type DCIS lesions (29), which are the DCIS lesions most often associated with prominently increased stromal microvessels in a diffuse pattern, lends support for this contention. However, the relationship between angiogenesis in DCIS and the likelihood of tumor progression can only be assessed in studies in which MVD in DCIS is related to clinical outcome in cohorts of patients treated with breast-conserving therapy.

It is also possible that angiogenesis associated with benign hyperplastic lesions may be a marker for an increased risk of breast cancer development. In a pilot study, Guinebretiere et al. (30) suggested that the risk of breast cancer increases with the density and concentration of microvessels in benign breast biopsy specimens. In that study, patients whose benign breast biopsy specimens had the highest number of microvessels had a sevenfold risk of developing breast cancer compared with those with fewer stromal microvessels in their benign biopsy specimens. Furthermore, this risk appeared to be independent of the presence of atypical hyperplasia. Although these results are based on a small number of patients and must be considered preliminary, they suggest a potentially valuable means for identifying patients with benign breast biopsy specimens who have a higher risk of developing breast cancer, and this approach merits further study.

The presence of angiogenesis in preinvasive breast lesions also raises the possibility that imaging modalities based on lesional vascularity, such as contrast-enhanced magnetic resonance imaging, may be useful for the identification of preinvasive lesions in which the angiogenic phenotype is present (31–33).

Finally, the identification of preinvasive lesions with angiogenic capability may identify a subset of patients in whom antiangiogenic therapy might be of value in the prevention of the development of invasive breast cancer, either alone or in combination with other chemopreventive agents. Results from the ongoing clinical trials assessing the value of antiangiogenic therapy in patients with invasive breast cancer (5,34–36) may shed light on this important issue.

SUMMARY

The results of the experimental and human studies reviewed here provide convincing evidence that some preinvasive breast lesions, including many examples of DCIS, are capable of inducing angiogenesis in the surrounding stroma. These findings indicate that angiogenesis is an early event in the development of breast cancer that may precede stromal invasion. A more thorough understanding of the role of various angiogenic and antiangiogenic factors in preinvasive breast lesions will provide further insight into this important biologic phenomenon, and this could, in turn, result in new diagnostic, prognostic, and therapeutic approaches to these lesions.

REFERENCES

1. Folkman J. What is the evidence that tumors are angiogenesis dependent? *J Natl Cancer Inst* 1990;82:4–6.
2. Blood CH, Zetter BR. Tumor interactions with the vasculature: angiogenesis and tumor metastasis. *Biochim Biophys Acta* 1990; 1032:89–118.
3. Folkman J. The role of angiogenesis in tumor growth. *Semin Cancer Biol* 1992;3:65–71.
4. Weidner N. Intratumor microvessel density as a prognostic factor in cancer. *Am J Pathol* 1995;147:9–19.
5. Gasparini G, Harris AL. Clinical implications of the determination fo tumor angiogenesis in breast carcinoma: much more than a new prognostic tool. *J Clin Oncol* 1995;13:765–782.
6. Weidner N. Angiogenesis as a predictor of clinical outcome in cancer patients. *Hum Pathol* 2000;31:403–405.
7. Gimbrone MA, Gullino PM. Neovascularization induced by intraocular xenografts of normal, preneoplastic, and neoplastic mouse mammary tissues. *J Natl Cancer Inst* 1976;56:305–318.
8. Gimbrone MA, Gullino PM. Angiogenic capacity of preneoplastic lesions of the murine mammary gland as a marker of neoplastic transformation. *Cancer Res* 1976;36:2611–2620.
9. Brem SS, Gullino PM. Angiogenesis. A marker for neoplastic transformation of mammary papillary hyperplasia. *Science* 1977; 195:880–882.
10. Brem SS, Jensen HM, Gullino PM. Angiogenesis as a marker of neoplastic lesions of the human breast. *Cancer* 1978;41:239–244.
11. Ziche M, Gullino PM. Angiogenesis and neoplastic progression in vitro. *J Natl Cancer Inst* 1982;69:483–487.
12. Ottinetti A, Sapino A. morphometric evaluation of microvessels surrounding hyperplastic and neoplastic mammary lesions. *Breast Cancer Res Treat* 1988;11:241–248.
13. Porter PL, Patton KF, Self SA, et al. A quantitative study of blood vessels size and density in normal and neoplastic breast tissue. *Lab Invest* 1993;68:18A (abst).
14. Samejima N, Yamazaki K. A study on the vascular proliferation in tissues around the tumor in breast cancer. *Jpn J Surg* 1988;18: 235–242.

15. Weidner N, Semple JP, Welch WR, et al. Tumor angiogenesis and metastasis — Correlation in invasive breast carcinoma. *N Engl J Med* 1991;324:1–8.
16. Weidner N. The relationship of tumor angiogenesis and metastasis with emphasis on invasive breast carcinoma. *Adv Pathol Lab Med* 1992;5:101–121.
17. Guidi AJ, Fischer L, Harris JR, et al. Microvessel density and distribution in ductal carcinoma in situ of the breast. *J Natl Cancer Inst* 1994;86:614–619.
18. Kreipe H, Heidebrecht HJ, Hansen S, et al. A new proliferation-associated nuclear antigen detectable in paraffin-embedded tissues by the monoclonal antibody Ki-S1. *Am J Pathol* 1993;142: 3–9.
19. Bose S, Lesser ML, Norton L, et al. Immunophenotype of intra-ductal carcinoma. *Arch Pathol Lab Med* 1996;120:81–85.
20. Engels K, Fox SB, Whitehouse RM, et al. Distinct angiogenic patterns are associated with high-grade in situ ductal carcinomas of the breast. *J Pathol* 1997;181:207–212.
21. Lee AH, Happerfield LC, Bobrow LG, et al. Angiogenesis and inflammation in ductal carcinoma in situ of the breast. *J Pathol* 1997;181:200–206.
22. Bhoola S, DeRose PB, Cohen C. Ductal carcinoma in situ of the breast: frequency of biomarkers according to histologic subtype. *Appl Immunohistochem Mol Morphol* 1999;7:108–115.
23. Teo NB, Shoker BS, Shaaban A, et al. Angiogenesis in ductal carcinoma in situ of the breast is related to the presence of invasive carcinoma and risk of recurrence. *Lab Invest* 2001;81: 38A (abst).
24. Brown LF, Berse B, Jackman RW, et al. Expression of vascular permeability factor (vascular endothelial growth factor) and its receptors in breast cancer. *Hum Pathol* 1995;26:86–91.
25. Dvorak HF, Brown LF, Detmar M, et al. Vascular permeability factor/vascular endothelial growth factor, endothelial growth factor, microvascular permeability, and angiogenesis. *Am J Pathol* 1995;146:1029–1039.
26. Guidi AJ, Schnitt SJ, Fischer L, et al. Vascular permeability factor (vascular endothelial growth factor) expression and angiogenesis in patients with ductal carcinoma in situ of the breast. *Cancer* 1997;80:1945–1953.
27. Engels K, Fox SB, Whitehouse M, et al. Up-regulation of thymidine phosphorylase expression is associated with a discrete pattern of angiogenesis in ductal carcinomas in situ of the breast. *J Pathol* 1997;182:414–420.
28. Lee AH, Dublin EA, Bobrow LG. Angiogenesis and expression of thymidine phosphorylase by inflammatory and carcinoma cells in ductal carcinoma in situ of the breast. *J Pathol* 1999;187:285–290.
29. Royds JA, Stephenson TJ, Rees RC, et al. Nm23 protein expression in ductal in situ and invasive human breast carcinoma. *J Natl Cancer Inst* 1993;85:727–731.
30. Guinebretiere JM, Monique GL, Gavoille A, et al. Angiogenesis and risk of breast cancer in women with fibrocystic disease. *J Natl Cancer Inst* 1994;86:635–636.
31. Adler DD, Wahl RL. New methods for imaging the breast: techniques, findings, and potential. *AJR Am J Roentgenol* 1995;164: 19–30.
32. Gilles R, Zafrani B, Guinebretiere J-M, et al. Ductal carcinoma in situ: MR imaging-histopathologic correlation. *Radiology* 1995; 196:415–419.
33. Williams MB, Pisano ED, Schnall MD, et al. Future directions in imaging of breast diseases. *Radiology* 1998;206:297–300.
34. Talks KL, Harris AL. Current status of antiangiogenic factors. *Br J Haematol* 2000;109:477–489.
35. Kerbel RS. Tumor angiogenesis: past, present and the near future. *Carcinogenesis* 2000;21:505–515.
36. Rosen L. Antiangiogenic strategies and agents in clinical trials. *Oncologist* 2000;5[Suppl 1]:20–27.

THE LOCAL DISTRIBUTION OF DUCTAL CARCINOMA IN SITU OF THE BREAST: WHOLE-ORGAN STUDIES

ROLAND HOLLAND
DANIEL R. G. FAVERLY

WHAT CAN WE LEARN FROM WHOLE-ORGAN STUDIES OF THE BREAST?

Currently, for the management of selected cases of ductal carcinoma in situ (DCIS) breast-conserving treatment has been accepted as an alternative to mastectomy despite reported rates of local recurrence varying from 20% to 30% after excision alone and approximately 10% if local radiotherapy is included (1,2). Approximately half of all recurrences are invasive, some of which may lead to death. By careful selection of patients, based on the extent and distribution of the tumor in the breast, the risk of local recurrence after breast-conserving treatment can be minimized. Whole-organ studies allow us to explore the pattern of spread and extent of DCIS, thereby contributing to an optimal patient selection for breast-conserving treatment.

When resecting a DCIS, in most cases, the surgeon can only rely on the extent of the mammographic microcalcifications associated with the tumor because grossly the lesion is generally neither palpable nor visible. The mammographic extent of these microcalcifications often differs from the real histopathologic extent of the tumor. The whole-organ technique is a useful approach that allows us to gain insight in the mammographic-pathologic size correlation of DCIS. Furthermore, it allows us to assess the relationship between margin width and amount of residual tumor by simulating incrementally increasing margin widths around the index tumor in mastectomy specimens.

Various studies concluded that residual foci of DCIS are the most likely sources of local recurrence after breast-conserving treatment in some types of invasive carcinomas, in particular those with an extensive intraductal component spreading through the ductal network beyond the invasive mass (3,4). Whole-organ studies facilitated the exploration of both the extent and pattern of spread of this DCIS component, thereby contributing to a rational choice of treatment.

WHOLE-ORGAN TECHNIQUE

The correlated radiologic-histologic whole-organ technique for studying breast lesions was first described by Egan (5)

and is used by relatively few investigators because it is a rather time-consuming, laborious approach (6–8). To use this method, whole-organ sections of the chilled breast are taken every 5 mm, and each one is radiographed. Tissue blocks for paraffin sections are obtained from radiologically suspicious lesions (i.e., those with microcalcifications or architectural distortions) and from areas showing grossly suspicious changes. In any whole-breast specimen from our series, an average of 25 tissue blocks was taken from the quadrant containing the index lesion, as well as random samples from other quadrants, the nipple, and the central area beneath the nipple-areolar complex. Both the precise site of the blocks sampled and the microscopically verified type and extension of each lesion were indicated on the specimen x-ray. All these data were transferred to a two-dimensional topographic breast chart for further evaluation (Fig. 19.1). A diagnostic biopsy specimen, taken before the mastectomy, was handled similarly with the use of specimen x-rays after a careful orientation of the specimen.

This correlated radiographic-histologic whole-organ technique allows a detailed reconstruction of the site, extent, and distribution of the tumor foci in the breast, and, more specifically, the assessment of potential tumor multifocality or multicentricity. Additionally, it can estimate the mammographic extent of the microcalcifications and the histopathologic extent of the tumor, resolving any difference between the mammographic and histologic size of DCIS. All these data have paramount importance with respect to an optimal choice of treatment and for designing treatment protocols, especially for a breast-conserving approach to DCIS.

MULTICENTRICITY/MULTIFOCALITY

The terms multicentricity and multifocality are often used interchangeably in the literature, causing great confusion if study results are to be compared. We adopted the definition of Fisher et al. (9) for multicentric distribution: a tumor involvement in two or more remote areas separated by uninvolved glandular tissue (3 to 4 cm in our studies), in contrast to a unicentric tumor with a single area of involvement. A unicentric tumor, however, is often multifocal, spreading over a large field with many small, microscopic tumor foci around the index tumor and may reach a total size of as large as 5 to 10 cm across. These foci are directly related to the index tumor in contrast to a multicentric tumor distribution in which the fields of tumor are unrelated to each other.

Several investigators (10–13) have assessed the distribution of DCIS within the breast with an incidence ranging from 0% to 80% for multifocality and multicentricity. This wide range may be explained mainly by the diversity of the pathologic procedures applied and the lack of uniformity in the definitions. For example, in one study with a reported multifocality of 75%, any additional DCIS foci found after an excision biopsy were regarded as evidence of multifocality (14); in another (15), multicentricity was defined as the occurrence of DCIS foci in quadrants other than that of the original site of the biopsy with a reported incidence of 78%. None of these studies considered potential connections between the index and residual tumor or assessed the distance between them.

In our studies, we applied the correlated radiologic-pathologic technique in combination with subgross sectioning and extensive sampling in a series of 119 mastectomies harboring DCIS [82 from a previous series (16) and 37 cases from a recent series (17)] and concluded that typically DCIS does not have a multicentric distribution. In these series, there appeared to be a single multicentric process with two separate areas of DCIS unrelated to each other. Usually the tumor foci were evenly distributed within a particular region, corresponding most likely to a breast segment, without intervening areas of uninvolved breast tissue. In practical terms, this implies that two apparently separate areas of malignant mammographic microcalcifications usually do not represent separate fields of DCIS but rather a large tumor in which the two mammographically identified fields are connected by DCIS, which is mammographically invisible owing to the lack of detectable-size microcalcifications. The entire field should, therefore, be considered involved and treated by the surgeon accordingly. The concept that DCIS is not a multicentric process is supported by clinical data showing that local tumor recurrence after breast-conserving treatment of DCIS typically appears in the vicinity of the biopsy site (18–20).

DCIS is regarded as a genuine multifocal process owing to its histologic appearance in the two-dimensional plane section showing multiple separate tumor foci on the cross section of the tumorously involved ductal network. However, if intraductal tumor growth on three-dimensional studies appears to be continuous rather than discontinuous, these tumor spots may not necessarily represent separate foci. The issue of whether DCIS grows continuously or discontinuously has two important implications: first, the reliability of pathologic margin assessment of surgical specimens and second, the understanding of the natural history of DCIS (continuous growth suggests a one-spot and discontinuous growth a multiple-spot tumor origin).

We studied the growth pattern of DCIS by combining the correlated radiographic-histologic whole-organ method with a three-dimensional technique (21). The paraffin-embedded tissue blocks containing the histologically identified areas of DCIS were deparaffinized and prepared for stereomicroscopy. First, we identified the apparently separate DCIS foci in the conventional hematoxylin and eosin slide and then explored potential ductal connections between these foci in the 2- to 3-mm thick sections of the original paraffin block, whereupon the thick section was re-embedded and an additional series of hematoxylin and eosin slides were made to determine whether the connecting duct contained tumor. If a discontinuous growth was observed, the greatest distance between the tumor foci was measured and recorded.

In this study, a consecutive series of 60 patients was treated for DCIS by mastectomy (22). The three-dimensional analysis reflected the heterogeneous histologic nature of DCIS and showed the various growth patterns ranging from massively filled galactophoric tubes of the poorly differentiated type (Fig. 19.2A, B, solid pattern) to the delicate coralliform-like structures of the well-differentiated type (Fig. 19.2C, D, micropapillary/clinging pattern). The study established that DCIS may grow continuously by extending through the glandular tree (Fig. 19.2A, B, E, F) but that it may also have a discontinuous (genuine multifocal) distribution with nonaffected interposed ductal segments (Fig. 19.2C, D). In this series, continuous and discontinuous growth patterns were found with equal frequency (Table 19.1). However, whereas poorly differentiated DCIS showed a predominantly continuous growth (90% of the cases), the well-differentiated DCIS, in contrast, presented a discontinuous (multifocal) distribution in most of the cases (70%). The intermediately differentiated DCIS did not show any particular pattern; both continuous and discontinuous growth was observed.

We measured the length of the uninvolved breast tissue (gap) interposed between the tumor foci (Table 19.2). Of the 30 cases with discontinuous growth, 19 (63%) had gaps smaller than 5 mm and 25 (83%) had gaps smaller than 10 mm. Of all studied DCIS tumors, irrespective of histologic type, 8% (five of 60) showed a discontinuous growth with gaps wider than 10 mm.

These results have a direct implication on the reliability of the margin assessment of surgical specimens. In cases of poorly differentiated DCIS, margin assessment should, theoretically, be more reliable than in well-differentiated DCIS. In a multifocal process with discontinuous growth, the surgical margin may lie between the tumor foci, giving the false impression of a free margin. However, the likelihood of such an error is theoretically low because the tumor foci are fairly evenly distributed and the gaps between the foci are usually narrow. Nevertheless, these findings may

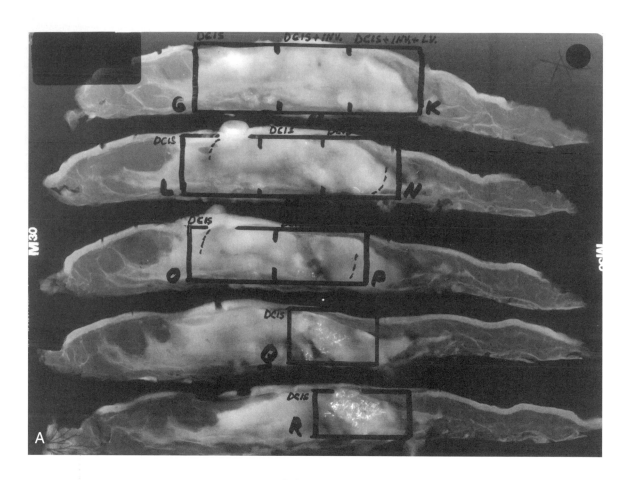

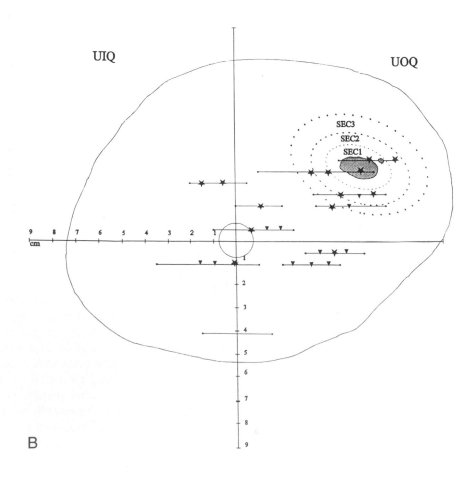

TABLE 19.1. HISTOLOGIC CLASSIFICATION OF DUCTAL CARCINOMA IN SITU: RELATIONSHIP TO GROWTH PATTERN

DCIS Type	Total (%)	Multifocal (%)	Continuous (%)
Well-differentiated	27 (45)	19 (70)	8 (30)
Intermediately differentiated	9 (15)	5 (56)	4 (44)
Poorly differentiated	19 (32)	2 (10)	17 (90)
Mixed	5 (8)	4 (80)	1 (20)
Total no. of cases	60	30	30

DCIS, ductal carcinoma in situ.
From Faverly RG, Burgers L, Bult P, Holland R. Three-dimensional imaging of mammary ductal carcinoma in situ: clinical implications. *Semin Diagn Pathol* 1994;11:193–198, with permission.

provide an explanation for reported cases with apparently free margins and, despite that, with short-time local recurrences.

EXTENT AND MAMMOGRAPHIC-PATHOLOGIC CORRELATION

Although DCIS is typically not a multicentric process, it is frequently extensive. Therefore, complete surgical excision is often not feasible. This is supported by the results of clinical studies showing a significant recurrence rate in the vicinity of the biopsy site in patients treated by lumpectomy alone without postoperative radiotherapy. In a series of 115

DCIS cases, Lagios et al. (23), reported 52% to have a tumor size of 25 mm or smaller. Seventy-nine patients with mammographically detected DCIS with an average tumor size of 7 mm were treated by excision alone. The resection margins were carefully assessed for completeness and considered negative. However, as many as 19% of the patients with poorly differentiated DCIS recurred in an average follow-up period of 26 months, casting doubt on the adequacy of the resections and the original size assessment of the tumors. In the series of Silverstein et al. (24), only 18% of the 208 lesions were smaller than 2 cm. In approximately half of the patients who were selected for breast-conserving treatment, the margins of the initial biopsy were involved. This suggests that the extent of the lesions was greater than orig-

TABLE 19.2. LARGEST DISTANCE OF UNINVOLVED BREAST TISSUE BETWEEN TUMOR FOCI: RELATIONSHIP TO DUCTAL CARCINOMA IN SITU TYPE

Size of Largest Gap	Frequency (%)	Well-Differentiated	Intermediately Differentiated	Poorly Differentiated	Mixed
No gap	30 (50)	8	4	17	1
<5 mm	19 (32)	12	3	1	3
5–10 mm	6 (10)	3	1	1	1
>10 mm	5 (8)	4[a]	1	0	0
Total	60	27	9	19	5

[a] One well-differentiated ductal carcinoma in situ had a 40-mm gap of uninvolved parenchyma between two tumor areas and was defined as multicentric.
From Faverly RG, Burgers L, Bult P, Holland R. Three-dimensional imaging of mammary ductal carcinoma in situ: clinical implications. *Semin Diagn Pathol* 1994;11:193–198, with permission.

FIGURE 19.1. The whole-organ technique. **A:** One of the specimen x-rays of a series of five of a total of 26 breast slices of a mastectomy specimen (4 to 5 mm thick) harboring a large process of poorly differentiated ductal carcinoma in situ (DCIS) with typical mammographic microcalcifications. Both the precise site of the blocks sampled for histologic examination and the microscopically verified type and extension of each lesion are indicated on the specimen x-ray. All such data are then transferred to a two-dimensional topographic breast chart for further evaluation. **B:** Topographic chart of a mastectomy specimen harboring an invasive carcinoma with an extensive DCIS component. The axes are centered on the nipple. The outer limits of the specimen are indicated by thin lines. ✱, DCIS foci; ▼, atypical ductal hyperplasia foci; |—|, fields sampled for histology; gray zones, invasive carcinoma; dotted lines, the edges of the three segmental resections with margins of 1, 2, and 3 cm around the invasive tumor. The whole-organ technique allows a detailed reconstruction of the site, the extent and distribution of the tumor foci in the breast and, more specifically, the assessment of potential tumor multifocality and multicentricity.

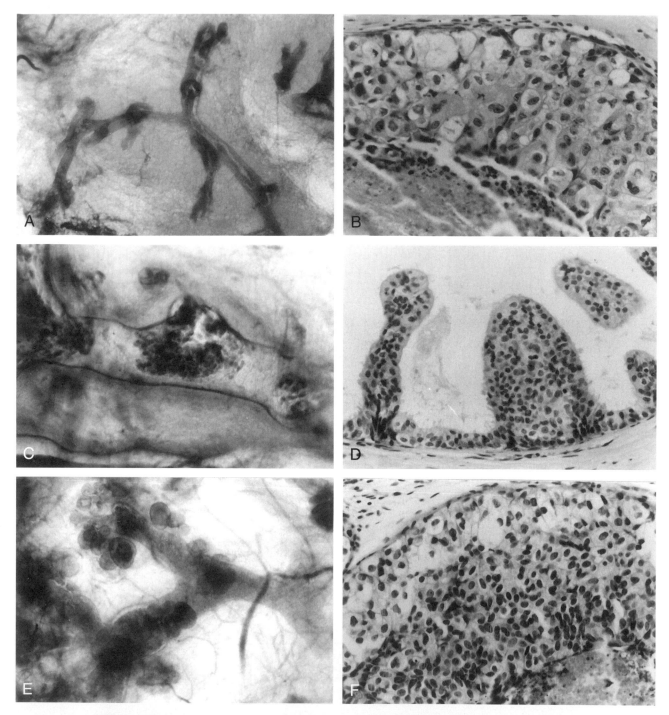

FIGURE 19.2. Subgross **(A)** and histologic **(B)** views of a poorly differentiated ductal carcinoma in situ (DCIS). The ductal tree is continuously involved by the tumor that is composed of cells with markedly pleomorphic nuclei. There is extensive central necrosis present (**A**, Mayer's hematoxylin, magnification ×7; **B**, hematoxylin and eosin, magnification ×500). **C, D:** This example of well-differentiated micropapillary/clinging DCIS shows an unequivocal multifocal growth pattern. After re-embedding and serial sectioning, the connecting segment of the duct between the DCIS foci appeared normal and is lined with a single layer of flattened luminal cells (**C**, Mayer's hematoxylin, magnification ×20; **D**, hematoxylin and eosin, magnification ×500). **E, F:** This case illustrates the continuous growth pattern in a well-differentiated DCIS. Note the round, oval-shaped monotonous nuclei characteristic of good cytonuclear differentiation in association with some central necrosis (**E**, Mayer's hematoxylin, magnification ×12; **F**, hematoxylin and eosin, magnification ×500). (From Faverly RG, Burgers L, Bult P, Holland R. Three-dimensional imaging of mammary ductal carcinoma in situ: clinical implications. *Semin Diagn Pathol* 1994;11:193–198, with permission.)

inally assessed. Fisher et al. (1,20) reported on 391 women treated by lumpectomy alone for very small DCIS tumors. As many as 64 (16.4%) developed an ipsilateral breast recurrence with an average follow-up of 43 months. All these studies contradict the often-heard statement that with the large-scale use of mammography, the currently detected DCIS lesions are all small tumors.

In our recent consecutive series of 59 DCIS cases, 51 of which were detected by mammography, 42% were 2 cm or smaller and thus 58% were larger. Only 17% were 1 cm or less (17) (Table 19.3).

Because most DCIS are nonpalpable, the mammographic estimate is the sole guide for resection. Therefore, data on the mammographic pathologic correlation of the tumor size are essential for guiding the extent of surgery. The mammographic extent of a DCIS was defined as the greatest distance between the most peripherally located clusters of suspicious microcalcifications, and the histologic extent as the greatest distance between the most peripherally located, histologically verified DCIS foci. Histologic evaluation supported by correlation with the x-ray of the sliced specimen allows a pre-

TABLE 19.3. SELECTED DATA ON 59 DCIS CASES ASSESSED BY FOUR MAMMOGRAPHIC VIEWS (1986–1993)

Detected by mammography (%)	
Yes	51 (86)
No	8 (14)

Mammographic Microcalcifications	
Present	51 (86)
Absent	8 (14)

Mammographic Size of Area Containing Microcalcifications	
≤10 mm	10 (20)
11–20 mm	17 (33)
21–30 mm	8 (16)
30 mm	16 (31)

Histologic Size of DCIS	
≤10 mm	10 (17)
11–20 mm	15 (25)
21–30 mm	7 (12)
30 mm	27 (46)

Surgical Treatment	
Simple mastectomy	37 (63)
Biopsy with reexcision	10 (17)
Biopsy only	12 (20)

(Reproduced by permission from Holland R, Hendriks JHCL. Microcalcifications associated with ductal carcinoma in situ: mammographic-pathologic correlation. Semin Diagn Pathol 1994;11:190.)

TABLE 19.4. DIFFERENCE BETWEEN HISTOLOGIC AND MAMMOGRAPHIC SIZE IN 35 OF 59 CASES WITH MAMMOGRAPHIC SIZE ≤30 MM

Type of DCIS	Number of Cases	Difference in Size (%) Histologic Size > Than Mammographic Size	
		≤20 mm	>20 mm
Poorly differentiated	14	11 (79)	3 (21)
Well-differentiated	14	12 (86)	2 (14)
Intermediately differentiated	7	6 (86)	1 (14)

(Reproduced by permission from Holland R, Hendriks JHCL. Microcalcifications associated with ductal carcinoma in situ: mammographic-pathologic correlation. Semin Diagn Pathol 1994;11:191.)

cise and reproducible assessment of the extent of any DCIS present. Our whole-organ studies showed that mammography, based on the significant microcalcifications, generally underestimates the histologic or real size of DCIS by an average of 1 to 2 cm. In the series of 35 DCIS cases with mammographic sizes as large as 3 cm, the size difference was less than 2 cm in more than 80% of the cases (17) (Table 19.4). Based on these data, the relationship between incrementally increased margin sizes and the chance of resecting the entire tumor can be calculated. If this series of 35 DCIS cases had been resected with a 1-cm margin around the mammographic lesion, 34% would have had incomplete excision. With a 2- or 3-cm margin, this percentage decreases to 17% and 11%, respectively (Table 19.5). These data indicate that in any DCIS tumor, at least a 2-cm margin should be resected around the field of the mammographic calcifications to limit the amount of residual tumor to a minimum.

Recently, Silverstein et al. (25,26) showed that margin width is most likely the strongest predictor of local recurrence and that breast irradiation has little additional effect if the lesion is completely excised with margin widths exceeding 10 mm. Using conventional two-view mammography, the mammographic assessment of size in cases of well-differentiated DCIS turned out to be less accurate (16). This can be explained by the poor visualization and perception of the fine-granular microcalcifications that are usually associated with this type of DCIS. In contrast, the linear, branch-

TABLE 19.5. TOTAL TUMOR CLEARANCE BY MARGIN WIDTH: 35 CASES WITH MAMMOGRAPHIC SIZE ≤3 CM

Margin Beyond Mammographic Tumor	Total Tumor Clearance (%)
1 cm	23/35 (66%)
2 cm	29/35 (83%)
3 cm	31/35 (89%)

ing, and coarse-granular microcalcifications of the poorly differentiated type are easier to recognize on the mammogram. By using magnification views in addition to the standard views, however, equal accuracy in size assessment can be achieved in both DCIS types. Therefore, magnification views should always be included for the assessment of suspicious microcalcifications.

EXTENSIVE INTRADUCTAL COMPONENT

A related issue is the invasive tumor with an extensive intraductal component (EIC). An original study from the Joint Center for Radiation Therapy in Boston reported an increased risk of local recurrence if this particular tumor characteristic was present (27). Various other studies confirmed this finding with recurrence rates of some 20% for EIC-positive patients compared with 5% to 10% for EIC-negative patients (28–30).

Several histopathologic definitions have been formulated for EIC, most of which cannot be applied reproducibly. In practical terms, EIC-positive tumors are invasive cancers with predominant DCIS foci near the index tumor extending to several centimeters beyond the edge of the tumor. It was hypothesized that the origin of the recurrence of EIC-positive tumors might be a large burden of residual DCIS left behind in the remainder of the breast after a limited excision and that such a tumor burden might not be fully eradicated by the conventional dose of radiation therapy.

In a collaborative study with the Joint Center for Radiation Therapy group, we assessed the extent of DCIS by applying the whole-organ technique in 214 patients with an invasive ductal carcinoma measuring 5 cm or less and treated by mastectomy (4). Overall, 14% of the tumors had prominent DCIS (defined as showing six or more microscopic low-power fields of intraductal carcinoma). In 12% of the cases, such a burden of DCIS was present beyond 2 cm from the edge of the invasive tumor and even beyond 4 cm in 5%. These results proved the existence of a subgroup accounting for some 15% of invasive ductal cancers that were associated with a large presence of intraductal cancer. These tumors are very likely less suitable for breast-conserving treatment and should be treated by more extensive surgery including mastectomy. More than half of these EIC-positive tumors can be recognized preoperatively by mammography showing the DCIS-associated microcalcifications. For an accurate assessment of the extent of the process, magnification views are mandatory.

SUMMARY

For decades, the usual approach to breast cancer has been to obtain histologic confirmation of cancer by means of a diagnostic biopsy followed by a mastectomy. Apart from the index tumor, other fields of the breast received little attention. Two events completely changed this attitude: the introduction of mammography and the introduction of breast-conserving treatment as an alternative to mastectomy. Mammography was the first modality to provide images of the whole breast and detect nonpalpable lesions such as microcalcifications and small densities. It became important to explore the pathologic background of these images to facilitate the mammographic differentiation of benign and malignant processes. The whole-organ technique proved to be a very useful method for the correlation of the various mammographic changes with histopathology.

The breast-conserving approach established that breast cancers often are not limited processes but are usually associated with multiple foci of subclinical tumor spreading around the index lesion and treatment, by surgery or radiation therapy, or both, should involve the entire diseased field. The whole-organ mammographic-pathologic mapping technique proved to be a noble method to study the pattern of subclinical tumor distribution associated with the various types of breast cancers, thereby assessing potential tumor multicentricity and multifocality. Whole-organ studies demonstrated that:

1. The distribution of cancer in the breast (in both invasive and noninvasive disease) is seldom multicentric but is often multifocal.
2. Multifocality of tumors usually implies multiple foci of DCIS rather than multiple foci of invasive tumor.
3. A large amount of residual DCIS is usually the source of local recurrence.
4. DCIS is often an extensive process, even if mammographically detected. Complete removal usually necessitates a wide excision with at least a 2-cm margin around the mammographic field of microcalcifications, of which the outer 1 cm should be microscopically tumor free.
5. The growth pattern of DCIS can be both continuous (usually the poorly differentiated type), suggesting a one-spot origin, or discontinuous (usually the well-differentiated type), suggesting a genuine multifocal origin.

The clinical implications of these findings are largely determined by the histologic type of DCIS, either with a high- or low-grade malignant potential. There is now general agreement among investigators that it is useful to divide DCIS into high-, intermediate-, and low-grade subtypes (31,32). This subclassification is mainly based on cytonuclear features such as nuclear pleomorphism and size, architectural differentiation, and the presence of necrosis. Recently, we proposed the terms poorly differentiated for high-grade and well differentiated for low-grade DCIS (31).

One might argue that patients with high-grade DCIS and patients with low-grade DCIS should be treated differently in terms of the use of radiation therapy and the extent of surgery. Involved margins and residual tumor should theoretically be associated with different levels of risk for local recurrence in general, and for the ability to progress to an invasive process in particular, in cases of high-grade, poorly differentiated and low-grade, well-differentiated DCIS. Silverstein et al. (32) reported on the 8-year, disease-free survival of 133 patients treated with excision and radiation therapy. The recurrence rates were 0%, 10%, and 34% for DCIS with nuclear grades 1, 2, and 3, respectively. Comparing, in a subsequent evaluation of the data (33), the disease-free survival between the treatment groups of excision alone and excision plus radiotherapy, a significant difference was only seen in group 3, i.e., the group of poorly differentiated DCIS. As a consequence, whereas negative margins seem to be an essential requirement and radiation therapy should be routinely given in cases of poorly differentiated DCIS, a subset of well-differentiated tumors with ample microscopically negative negative margins may be managed without irradiation. More clinical data are needed to establish the minimal safe management for the low-grade, well-differentiated type of DCIS.

A meticulous pathologic margin assessment is an essential part of any breast-conserving protocol. This should include the inking of the specimen, the use of specimen mammography before and after the sectioning of the specimen, and the generous sampling of the area of microcalcifications and margins. Pathologists should be trained to assess the expected amount of residual DCIS in the remainder of the breast as either none to minimal, moderate, or massive, using the quantitative involvement of the biopsy margins as a guideline. Whole-organ studies reveal that this is feasible in more than 80% of the cases if there is close cooperation among the radiologist, surgeon, and pathologist.

REFERENCES

1. Fisher B, Dignam J, Wolmark N, et al. Lumpectomy and radiation therapy for the treatment of intraductal breast cancer: findings from National Surgical Adjuvant Breast and Bowel Project B-17. *J Clin Oncol* 1998;16:441–452.
2. Julien JP, Bijker N, Fentiman IS, et al. Radiotherapy in breast-conserving treatment for ductal carcinoma in situ: first results of the EORTC randomised phase III trial 10853. *Lancet* 2000;355:528–533.
3. Vicini F, Recht A, Abner A, et al. Recurrence in the breast following conservative surgery and radiation therapy for early-stage breast cancer [monograph]. *J Natl Cancer Inst* 1992;11:33–39.
4. Holland R, Connolly J, Gelman R, et al. The presence of an extensive intraductal component (EIC) following a limited excision correlates with prominent residual disease in the remainder of the breast. *J Clin Oncol* 1990;8:113–118.
5. Egan RL. Multicentric breast carcinomas: clinical-radiographic pathologic whole organ studies and 10-year survival. *Cancer* 1982;49:1123–1130.
6. Lagios MD, Westdahl PR, Rose MR. The concept and implications of multicentricity in breast carcinoma. *Pathol Annu* 1981;16:83–102.
7. Holland R, Veling SH, Mravunac M, et al. Histologic multifocality of Tis, T1-2 breast carcinomas. *Cancer* 1985;56:979–990.
8. Morimoto T, Okazaki K, Komaki K, et al. Cancerous residue in breast conserving surgery. *J Surg Oncol* 1993;52:71–76.
9. Fisher ER, Leeming R, Anderson S, et al. Conservative management of intraductal carcinoma (DCIS) of the breast. *J Surg Oncol* 1991;47:139–147.
10. Patchefsky AS, Schwartz GF, Finkelstein SD, et al. Heterogeneity of intraductal carcinoma of the breast. *Cancer* 1989;63:731–741.
11. Ashikari R, Hajdu SI, Robbins GF. Intraductal carcinoma of the breast. *Cancer* 1971;28:1182–1187.
12. Alpers CE, Wellings SR. The prevalence of carcinoma in situ in normal and cancer-associated breasts. *Hum Pathol* 1985;16:796–807.
13. Posner MC, Wolmark N. Noninvasive breast carcinoma. *Breast Cancer Res Treat* 1992;21:155–164.
14. Ringberg A, Palmer B, Linell F, et al. Bilateral and multifocal breast carcinoma. A clinical and autopsy study with special emphasis on carcinoma in situ. *Eur J Surg Oncol* 1991;17:20–29.
15. Simpson T, Thirlby RC, Dail DH. Surgical treatment of ductal carcinoma in situ of the breast. 10- to 20-year follow-up. *Arch Surg* 1992;127:468–472.
16. Holland R, Hendriks JHCL, Verbeek ALM, et al. Extent, distribution and mammographic/histological correlations of breast ductal carcinoma in situ. *Lancet* 1990;335:519–522.
17. Holland R, Hendriks JHCL. Microcalcifications associated with ductal carcinoma in situ: mammographic-pathologic correlation. *Semin Diagn Pathol* 1994;11:181–192.
18. Schwartz GF, Finkel GC, Garcia JC, et al. Subclinical ductal carcinoma in situ of the breast: treatment by local excision and surveillance alone. *Cancer* 1992;70:2468–2474.
19. Solin LJ, Yeh IT, Kurtz JM, et al. Ductal carcinoma in situ (intraductal carcinoma) of the breast treated with breast conserving surgery and definitive irradiation. *Cancer* 1993;1:2532–2542.
20. Fisher B, Costantino J, Redmond C, et al. Lumpectomy compared with lumpectomy and radiation therapy for the treatment of intraductal breast cancer. *N Engl J Med* 1993;328:1581–1586.
21. Faverly DRG, Holland R, Burgers L. An original stereomicroscopic analysis of the mammary glandular tree. *Virchows Arch* 1992;421:115–119.
22. Faverly DRG, Burgers L, Bult P, et al. Three-dimensional imaging of mammary ductal carcinoma in situ: clinical implications. *Semin Diagn Pathol* 1994;11:193–198.
23. Lagios MD, Margolin FR, Westdahl PR, et al. Mammographically detected duct carcinoma in situ: frequency of local recurrence following tylectomy and prognostic effect of nuclear grade on local recurrence. *Cancer* 1989;63:618–624.
24. Silverstein MJ, Waisman JR, Gamagami P, et al. Intraductal carcinoma of the breast (208 cases): clinical factors influencing treatment choice. *Cancer* 1990;66:102–108.
25. Silverstein MJ, Lagios MD, Groshen S, et al. The influence of margin width on local control of ductal carcinoma in situ of the breast. *N Engl J Med* 1999;340:1455–1461.
26. Silverstein MJ. Current status of the Van Nuys Prognostic Index for patients with ductal carcinoma in situ of the breast. *Semin Breast Dis* 2000;3:220–228.
27. Boyages J, Recht A, Connolly J, et al. Early breast cancer: predictors of breast recurrence for patients treated with conservative surgery and radiation therapy. *Radiother Oncol* 1990;19:29–41.
28. Jacquemier J, Kurtz JM, Amalric R, et al. An assessment of extensive intraductal component as a risk factor for local recurrence after breast-conserving therapy. *Br J Cancer* 1990;61:873–876.
29. Veronesi U, Luini A, Galimberti V, et al. Conservation approaches for the management of stage I/II carcinoma of the breast. Milan Cancer Institute trials. *World J Surg* 1994;18:70–75.

30. Borger JH, Kemperman HWPM, Hart AAM, et al. Risk factors in breast-conservation therapy. *J Clin Oncol* 1994;12:653–660.

31. Holland R, Peterse JL, Millis RR, et al. Ductal carcinoma in situ: a proposal for a new classification. *Semin Diagn Pathol* 1994;11: 167–180.

32. Silverstein MJ, Barth A, Poller ED, et al. Ten-year results com-paring mastectomy to excision and radiation therapy for ductal carcinoma in situ of the breast. *Eur J Cancer* 1995;31A:1425–1427.

33. Silverstein MJ, Poller DN, Waisman JC, et al. Prognostic classi-fication of breast ductal carcinoma-in-situ. *Lancet* 1995;345: 1154–1157.

LARGE-SECTION (MACROSECTION) HISTOLOGIC SLIDES

MARIA P. FOSCHINI
TIBOR TOT
VINCENZO EUSEBI

Large-section (macrosection) histologic slides were first used for examining breast parenchyma at the beginning of the twentieth century. This method was termed "a whole cleared mount" and led to remarkable data about the normal anatomy and neoplastic transformation of the mouse mammary tree (1). Macrosections were used to examine the relationship between neoplastic lesions and the surrounding tissue in the human breast for the first time by Ingleby and Holly in 1939 (2). Subsequently the method was modified, improved, and, to some extent, simplified (3–11).

Macrosections allow the pathologist to quickly screen the complete surgical specimen and identify barely visible lesions. If the tissue is cleared and examined further with a stereomicroscope, a three-dimensional view of the mammary gland can be seen (11). Studies based on such subgross analysis have led to important insights into modern breast pathology such as the correlation between mammographic and pathologic tumor extent (5,10,12–16) and the structural distribution of ductal carcinoma in situ (DCIS) (16). Nevertheless, the use of macrosections has never become popular in studying breast specimens, despite the many advantages of this method that have led to its common use for studying brain and prostate specimens.

During the past two decades, the introduction of breast screening programs has led to an increasing number of specimens containing DCIS and minute invasive carcinomas. New problems in breast pathology have arisen as a result, especially because of the increased use of breast-conserving therapy. Knowledge of the exact extent of each lesion, its size, the presence of multifocality, the detection of foci of microinvasion, and correct assessment of the status of resection margins are all vital data need to make treatment decisions. In addition, the diffusion of and improved quality of mammography have increased the need to obtain precise correlation between mammographic and pathologic findings.

We think that the use of macrosections meets all these needs. Recent papers have suggested that large sections yield important information, for both research and routine diagnostic purposes (17).

TECHNIQUE

Breast macrosections can be created for two purposes: to obtain large histologic sections allowing high-power microscopic examination and for three-dimensional tissue reconstruction using a low-power stereomicroscope. In both cases, correct orientation and careful slicing of the specimen are critical to obtain a precise correlation with radiologic findings and to assess resection margins. The method described here has been in use in our departments in Bologna and Falun for 6 and 15 years, respectively, and is essentially similar to that described by Jackson et al. (17).

The specimen is received fresh, oriented with metallic wires and/or marking sutures that indicate the margin nearest to the nipple and at least two other margins (usually the right and superior). Radiography of the surgical specimens is performed, taking care to orient the radiograph in the same manner as the gross specimen (Fig. 20.1). The surgical margins of the specimen may be marked with black ink.

For histologic examination, sections are taken with an appropriate surgical blade (or large knife) in areas thought to be abnormal on radiography or macroscopic visual examination. The section must include the lesion or the area of microcalcifications in the plane of its largest diameter. Each section is between 0.3 and 0.5 cm thick. Mastectomy specimens are usually sectioned perpendicular to the skin, extending to the deep margin of resection. Quadrantectomy specimens are sliced horizontally (parallel to the cutting table) or, alternatively, radially; care is taken to orient the section so it extends from the margin closer to the central portion of the breast toward the periphery.

Sections are fixed flat overnight in 10% buffered formalin and then embedded in paraffin as specified below, taking care to maintain the orientation during the embedding pro-

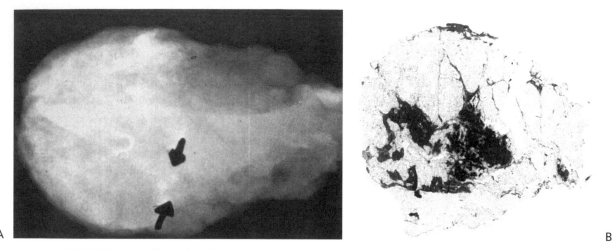

FIGURE 20.1. Radiography of the surgical specimen obtained with a Faxitron **(A)** shows a cluster of microcalcification (*arrows*). The corresponding macrosection shows extensive ductal carcinoma in situ **(B)**.

cedure and using a cellulose acetate white membrane filter. Specimens are processed in a tissue vacuum infiltrator processor. On the first day, the specimen is bathed first in 70% alcohol (three 30-minute baths), followed by 95% alcohol (two 1-hour baths), followed by absolute alcohol (three 1-hour baths). On the second day, xylene (two 3-hour baths) is followed by melted paraffin (left overnight). On the third day, the tissue is put in molten paraffin for 4 hours and then cooled and embedded in paraffin. Sections 5 μm thick are obtained using a dedicated microtome, mounted on large slides, and then routinely stained with hematoxylin and eosin.

The section is then examined microscopically and compared with the mammogram to identify the site of the lesion. The size of the lesion, if neoplastic, is then measured with an ocular micrometer in accordance with European guidelines (18). The distance from the nearest margin is also recorded.

For quadrantectomies, one or two additional macrosections are submitted that are contiguous with those taken because of the presence of mammographic abnormalities. These additional sections are also embedded, but hematoxylin and eosin slides are obtained from them only if a malignancy is found. Blocks are taken from these additional slices in positions that correspond with the location of the neoplastic lesion, perpendicular to the previous macrosections, both from the superior and inferior margins. In this manner, virtually all margins around the lesion are examined.

The total time of the full procedure, including processing the additional sections, is 4 days. Immunohistochemistry and special stains can be obtained in the same manner as for specimens processed in other ways.

When the goal is to perform three-dimensional reconstructions, the large paraffin blocks must be remelted. A slice of the embedded tissue, no thicker than 1 mm, is pro-

duced using a sharp knife. The sample is immersed in several xylol baths for at least 24 hours to remove the remaining paraffin. The specimen is rehydrated in three baths of absolute alcohol, each lasting at least 1 hour each, followed by 2 hours in 70% alcohol, and a final bath overnight in water. The slice is then stained in Harris hematoxylin for 7 minutes, washed in tap water, differentiated in acidic alcohol for approximately 10 minutes, and washed again. After a thorough washing, the slice is dehydrated through a series of 70% alcohol, absolute alcohol, alcohol and xylol, and xylol, and finally cleared in methylsalicylate.

RESULTS OF STUDIES USING MACROSECTIONS

Subgross Breast Anatomy

Stereomicroscopic studies described the changes of the mammary tree occurring during breast development from childhood through puberty to sexual maturation (6,7,9) and the benign modifications occurring as adulthood progresses (Fig. 20.2) (19,20). Studies of adult breasts demonstrated two basic patterns of normal breast parenchyma. The first is rich in lobular structures and has been termed the "adenotic" pattern. The second one is characterized by only rare lobules and ductules and has been termed the "atrophic" pattern (9,21).

Three-Dimensional Reconstruction of the Spread of Ductal Carcinoma in Situ

Early three-dimensional studies of cancerous breasts demonstrated that foci of invasive carcinomas were often associated with in situ carcinoma or atypical hyperplasia (5). Observations that the first neoplastic changes occur in the terminal duct lobular unit led to the hypothesis that most

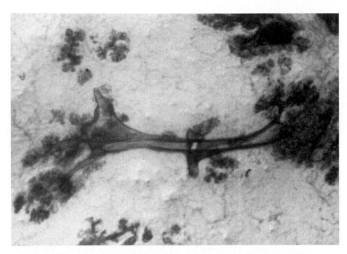

FIGURE 20.2. Stereomicroscopic view of nonneoplastic mammary tree shows several lobules departing from a duct with related terminal duct lobular units.

breast cancers, both the lobular and ductal types, originate in the terminal duct lobular unit (Fig. 20.3) (22).

The incidence of multicentricity of DCIS and invasive ductal carcinoma in studies using conventional specimen sampling (using small blocks) varies from 13% to 65% (23,24). Multicentricity is more common in patients with a family history of breast cancer (25). Nevertheless, Mai et al. (26) recently found that invasive duct carcinomas, DCIS, and atypical ductal hyperplasia are usually found in the same breast segment. Specifically, in 90% of 30 cases studied, these neoplastic lesions were confined to a single glandular tree (or lobe).

These data are consistent with those of Faverly et al. (16) who found that DCIS can grow in two patterns: continuous and discontinuous. Poorly differentiated DCIS were characterized by a continuous growth pattern (extending along the same duct without visible gaps) in 90% of cases (27).

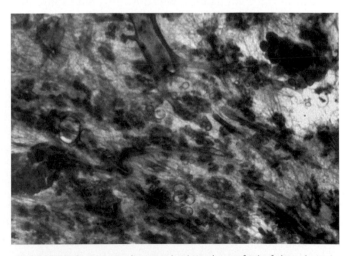

FIGURE 20.3. Stereomicroscopic view shows foci of ductal carcinoma in situ growing in distended terminal duct lobular units.

The cells of well-differentiated DCIS also proliferate along the same duct but in a discontinuous pattern, leaving segments of uninvolved duct between segments of tumor.

This conclusion was also reached by Ohtake et al. (28) in a computerized three-dimensional reconstruction of the breast tree. They evaluated 20 quadrantectomies performed for primary invasive breast carcinomas and found that in 80% of the cases, DCIS was limited to only one glandular tree (or lobe) that was close to the invasive tumor.

Thus, these data point toward DCIS originating within a single lobe. Nevertheless, cases are seen in routine practice in which there are two or more neoplastic foci far apart from one another or even in different quadrants. The possibility that such cases demonstrate multiple, independently arising cancers cannot be excluded. However, the possible existence (not yet conclusively demonstrated) of anastomosing channels between different lobes must be taken in consideration (28). Finally, a single ductal breast tree might extend from one quadrant into neighboring quadrants. In these cases, the neoplastic growth would thus still be confined to a single lobe but would give a false impression of multifocality. This issue needs further study. We believe that only three-dimensional analysis and the use of macrosections can solve this problem.

Correlation Between Mammography and Large-Section Histology

Knowledge of subgross mammary anatomy is important in the interpretation of radiographic findings. The use of mammographic screening in asymptomatic women has greatly expanded our knowledge of the range of radiographic patterns seen in the normal breast parenchyma. A relationship between the presence of certain mammographic parenchymal patterns and an increased risk for developing breast cancer has been demonstrated. This was recently reviewed by Tot et al. (15), who distinguished five mammographic parenchymal patterns and characterized their radiographic features, histologic finding on macrosections, and three-dimensional subgross anatomic features. Mammographic pattern I, typically found in younger women, was characterized by abundant terminal duct lobular units, supported by fibrous and adipose tissue. Mammographic patterns II and III were typically observed in older women and were characterized by atrophy of terminal duct lobular units and ducts and the predominance of adipose tissue. In mammographic pattern III, dilated retroareolar ducts and fibrosis were also seen. Progression from pattern I to II occurred during the usual involution of the breast tissue after menopause, but in patients using hormonal replacement therapy partial reversion to pattern I was also seen. Mammographic pattern IV was present in approximately 12% of women 40 to 74 years of age and did not change over time. This pattern was characterized by nodular densities measuring 3 to 6 mm in greatest dimension, which histologically corresponded mainly to sclerosing adenosis, microcysts, and fibroadenomatous change. Mammographic pattern V was present in approximately 6% of the women and corresponded to the presence of extensive fibrous modification of the interlobular stroma, which obscured the diagnostic details on mammography (except for microcalcifications).

Early histologic-mammographic correlation studies were mainly devoted to invasive carcinomas and described tumor margins, the type of infiltration, and modifications of the mammary tissue adjacent to carcinomas (29,30). More recently, emphasis has been placed on the detection of DCIS through the study of microcalcifications (31,32). Microcalcifications associated with poorly differentiated (comedo-type) DCIS typically appear linear on mammography, often with branching coarse granules (31). On histology, these correspond to granular calcifications deposited on the nuclear DNA of necrotic cells (33). In contrast, microcalcifications associated with well-differentiated DCIS present on a mammogram as multiple clusters of minute calcifications. On histology, they correspond to lamellar bodies and calcium deposits associated with mucins (33).

Using macrosections, it is possible to compare the spatial extent of microcalcifications, as seen in tissue, to that seen on a mammogram. It soon became apparent that mammography underestimated the size of neoplastic lesions. Holland et al. (32) found that in 85% of their cases, the area of calcifications on a mammogram was smaller than the corresponding lesion seen in the macrosection (Fig. 20.4).

Resection Margins

Correct assessment of resection margins has become an urgent and important problem because of the popularity of less radical surgical techniques (34,35). Data on the patterns of growth and distribution of invasive and in situ carcinomas indicate that the distance between the neoplastic cell population and resection margin should not be less than 10 mm if all tumor cells are to be resected (16,36). Patients with margins less than 10 mm in width should be treated with radiotherapy (36), especially in cases with poorly differentiated DCIS.

To adequately map resection margins, numerous small conventional histologic blocks are required, thus making a thorough routine examination of quadrantectomy specimens an expensive and time-consuming procedure. Macrosections can be helpful for this task. As previously noted, macrosections can be cut and oriented according to the mammographic findings in the individual case. This allows easy detection of the extent of tumor spread into the adjacent parenchyma and of the exact distance between the tumor and the margins. In addition, as the orientation is maintained during the embedding process, it is possible to establish which surgical margins are involved. Macrosections, also helpful in revealing multiple foci of carcinoma, can show minute neoplastic foci near the resection margin,

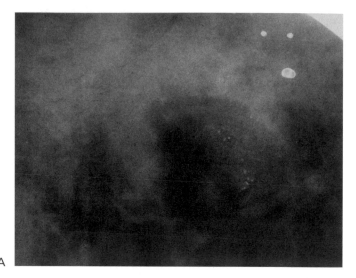

A

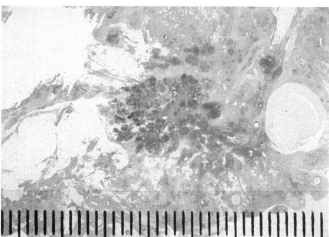

B

FIGURE 20.4. Microcalcifications seen on mammography **(A)**. The macrosection shows that the corresponding neoplastic lesion extends beyond the area of calcifications **(B)**.

which eliminates the bias resulting from directing most attention to the main lesion revealed by mammography, and minor foci are undetected. Admittedly, one can assess margin status only in the plane of sectioning of a macrosection. This problem, however, is overcome by obtaining parallel macrosections and additional orthogonal blocks as described previously. In this manner, virtually all margins around the tumor can be examined; the total number of blocks needed is far less than the number required if the entire quadrant were embedded using conventional small blocks. For nodules smaller than a quadrant, usually only two or three macrosections are needed for a thorough histologic examination (Figs. 20.5 and 20.6).

Assessment of the Size of the Neoplastic Lesion

This issue was emphasized by Jackson et al. (17) who compared two series, one studied with conventional histology

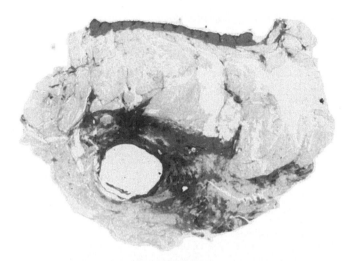

FIGURE 20.5. Quadrantectomy specimen removed after a mammotome biopsy. In the macrosection, the hole created by the mammotome biopsy is surrounded by additional neoplastic lesion that extends to the deep surgical margin.

and the other with macrosections. With macrosections, the size of the invasive carcinoma could be determined for all cases (Fig. 20.7). In contrast, size could be measured for only 63% of the 99 cases studied with conventional small blocks. They also found that macrosections were more accurate in detecting and measuring the size of the DCIS. DCIS was found more frequently in association with invasive carcinomas on specimens assessed by macrosection (80%) than in cases processed using small blocks (63%). In addition, it was easier to determine the size of the foci of the DCIS, those found in macrosections being larger. In mea-

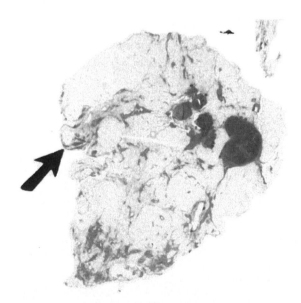

FIGURE 20.6. Macrosection from a quadrantectomy specimen performed for infiltrating ductal carcinoma. On the margin opposite to the lesion (*arrow*), a small area of ductal carcinoma in situ is present.

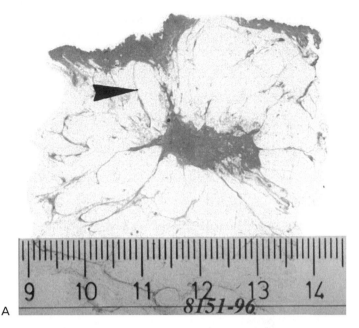

A

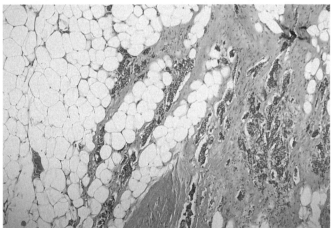

B

FIGURE 20.7. Infiltrating ductal carcinoma. **A:** Macrosection provides a reliable tool to measure the size of the neoplastic area. The thin peripheral extension of the tumor (*arrow*) was not seen by naked-eye examination. **B:** Minute foci of neoplastic cells extend into the fat tissue (magnification ×40).

suring the neoplastic area, in accordance with European guidelines (18), we measure the widest diameter of an invasive carcinoma in a single plane. If the invasive tumor is surrounded by DCIS, we provide a second measurement that includes the whole neoplastic area.

CONCLUSIONS

The usefulness of macrosections and subgross analysis of breast tissue both for research and routine clinical purposes has been amply demonstrated. Current understanding of breast pathology and mammographic-histologic correlation is based on studies using macrosections. In addition, the use of macrosections in routine clinical practice confidently allows the assessment of the size and distribution of the neoplastic lesion and the margin status, which are critical factors in determining patient suitability for breast-conserving therapy.

Increased workload and financial cost are often given as reasons for not performing whole-organ studies in daily practice. However, complete preparation of macrosections using our procedure requires only 4 days, which is only slightly longer than the time needed for conventional blocks. The diagnostic advantages and accuracy of macrosections are so great that we believe that it is worth waiting an extra day for the diagnosis. The cost of macrosections is identical to, if not lower than, the cost of processing the multiple conventional blocks required to yield the same information. Thus, we believe that macrosections should be much more widely used than they are at present.

REFERENCES

1. Dalton AJ. Histogenesis of the mammary gland of the mouse. In Moulton FR., ed. *A symposium on mammary tumors in mice.* Washington, DC: American Association for the Advancement of Science, 1949:39–46.
2. Ingleby H, Holly C. A method for the preparation of serial slices of the breast. *Bull Int Assoc Med Museum* 1939;19:93–96.
3. Parks AG. The microanatomy of the breast. *Ann R Coll Surg Engl* 1959;24:235–231.
4. Marcum RG, Wellings SR. Subgross pathology of the human breast: method and initial observations. *J Natl Cancer Inst* 1969;42:115–121.
5. Gallager HS, Martin JE. Early phases in the development of breast cancer. *Cancer* 1969;24:1170–1178.
6. Tanaka Y, Oota K. A stereomicroscopic study of the mastopathic human breast. I. Three dimensional structures of abnormal duct evolution and their histologic entity. *Virchows Arch* 1970;349:195–214.
7. Tanaka Y, Oota K. A stereomicroscopic study of the mastopathic human breast. II. Peripheral type of duct evolution and its relation to cystic disease. *Virchows Arch* 1970;349:215–228.
8. Migliori E. Un metodo di studio submacroscopico della mammella umana intera. *Tumori* 1975;61:357–363.
9. Sarnelli R, Orlandi F, Migliori E, et al. Morfologia submicroscopica della mammella: reperti semeiologici, nomenclatura e possibilita di applicazione del metodo. *Pathologica* 1980;72:139–87.
10. Egan RL. Multicentric breast carcinomas: clinical-radiographic-pathologic whole organ studies and 10-year survival. *Cancer* 1982;49:1123–1130.
11. Faverly D, Holland R, Burgers L. An original stereomicroscopic analysis of the mammary glandular tree. *Virchows Arch* 1992;421:115–119.
12. Jensen HM, Rice JR, Wellings SR. Preneoplastic lesions in the human breast. *Science* 1976;191:295–297.
13. Gallager HS, Martin JE. The study of mammary carcinoma by mammography and whole organ sectioning. *Cancer* 1969;23:855–873.
14. Fisher ER, Posada H, Ramos H. Evaluation of mammography based upon correlation of specimen mammograms and histopathologic findings. *Am J Clin Pathol* 1974;62:60–72.
15. Tot T, Tabar L, Dean PB. The pressing need for better histologic-mammographic correlation of the many variations in normal breast anatomy. *Virchows Arch* 2000;437:338–344.
16. Faverly DRG, Burgers L, Bult P, et al. Three dimensional imaging of mammary ductal carcinoma in situ: clinical implications. *Semin Diagn Pathol* 1994;11:193–198.
17. Jackson PA, Merchant W, McCormick CJ, et al. A comparison of large block macrosectioning and conventional techniques in breast pathology. *Virchows Arch* 1994;425;243–248.
18. Bussolati G. Linee guida relative alla citopatologia mammaria in corso di programmi di screening mammografico. *Pathologica* 1999;91:203–208.
19. Wellings SR, Alpers CE. Subgross pathologic features and incidence of radial scars in the breast. *Hum Pathol* 1984;15:475–479.
20. Wellings SR, Alpers CE. Apocrine cystic metaplasia: subgross pathology and prevalence in cancer-associated versus random autopsy breasts. *Hum Pathol* 1987;381–386.
21. Sarnelli R, Squartini F. Cancerous versus noncancerous breasts. A comparative morphological analysis of the entire glandular tree of the breast. *Virchows Arch* 1989;414:257–262.
22. Wellings SR, Jensen HM. On the origin and progression of ductal carcinoma in the human breast. *J Natl Cancer Inst* 1973;50:1111–1118.
23. Fisher ER, Gregorio R, Redmond C, et al. Pathologic findings from the national surgical adjuvant breast project (protocol no. 4). 1) Observations concerning the multicentricity of mammary cancer. *Cancer* 1975;35:247–254.
24. Rosen PP, Fracchia AA, Urban JA. Residual mammary carcinoma following simulated partial mastectomy. *Cancer* 1975;35;739–747.
25. Lagios MD. Multicentricity of breast carcinoma demonstrated by routine correlated serial subgross and radiographic examination. *Cancer* 1977;40:1726–1734.
26. Mai KT, Yazdi HM, Burns BF, et al. Pattern of distribution of intraductal and infiltrating ductal carcinoma: a three-dimensional study using serial coronal giant sections of the breast. *Hum Pathol* 2000;31:464–474.
27. Holland R, Peterse JL, Millis RR, et al. Ductal carcinoma in situ: a proposal for a new classification. *Semin Diagn Pathol* 1994;11:167–180.
28. Ohtake T, Abe R, Kimijima I, et al. Intraductal extension of primary invasive breast carcinoma treated by breast conservative surgery. *Cancer* 1995;76:32–45.
29. Qualheim RE, Gall EA. Breast carcinoma with multiple sites of origin. *Cancer* 1957;10:460–468.
30. Tellem M, Prive L, Meranze DR. Four-quadrant study of breasts removed for carcinoma. *Cancer* 1962;15:10–17.
31. Holland R, Hendriks JHCL. Microcalcifications associated with ductal carcinoma in situ: mammographic-pathologic correlation. *Semin Diagn Pathol* 1994;11:181–192
32. Holland R, Hendriks JHCL, Verbeek ALM, et al. Extent, distribution and mammographic/histological correlations of breast ductal carcinoma in situ. *Lancet* 1990;335:519–522.
33. Foschini MP, Fornelli A, Peterse JL, et al. Microcalcifications in ductal carcinoma in situ of the breast. *Hum Pathol* 1996;27:178–183.
34. Silverstein MJ, Gierson ED, Colburn WJ, et al. Can intraductal breast carcinoma be excised completely by local excision? Clinical and pathologic predictors. *Cancer* 1994;73:2985–2989.
35. Silverstein MJ, Lagios MD, Groshen S, et al. The influence of margin width on local control of ductal carcinoma in situ of the breast. *N Engl J Med* 1999;340:1455–1461.
36. Silverstein MJ, Lagios MD. Use of predictors of recurrence to plan therapy for DCIS of the breast. *Oncology (Huntingt)* 1997;11:393–415.

21

PREDICTING LOCAL RECURRENCE IN PATIENTS WITH DUCTAL CARCINOMA IN SITU

RICHARD SPOSTO
MELINDA S. EPSTEIN
MELVIN J. SILVERSTEIN

Although large, randomized trials of patients with ductal carcinoma in situ (DCIS) have shown that radiation therapy reduces the local recurrence rate of both noninvasive and invasive cancer (1–4), there continues to be controversy as to whether one can identify subgroups of patients for whom conservative surgery alone is sufficient therapy (1,5–11). Clearly, it is essential that the physician and patient carefully evaluate the comparative risks and benefits of different treatment choices (12,13), but the extent to which this can be done depends on a thorough understanding of the predictors of local recurrence in DCIS. Over the past 10 years, there has developed a greater understanding of the important patient and tumor characteristics that determine local recurrence risk in DCIS. The use of postoperative radiation therapy, nuclear grade, presence of necrosis, pathologic tumor size, patient age, and width of the resection margin have all been associated with different risks of local recurrence (14–21). The purpose of this chapter is not to address the issue of optimal treatment for DCIS but rather to investigate in detail, based on a large series of carefully evaluated patients with DCIS, which features of the patient, the tumor, and the surgical outcome are most relevant in assessing the risk of local recurrence in patients with DCIS.

PATIENTS AND METHODS

The study cohort comprised 909 independent diagnoses of pathologically confirmed DCIS diagnosed from 1971 through 2000. No patients with invasive or microinvasive breast cancer were included. Treatment was not randomized. The cohort represents an update of the patient cohort used in previous reports (7,19,22), as well as an extension of this cohort to include patients treated by one of us (M.J.S.) since 1998 at the University of Southern California Norris Comprehensive Cancer Center.

Treatment

Treatment was not determined as part of a randomized study. Rather, patients were advised of treatment options depending on the characteristics of their disease and the current state of knowledge about the treatment of DCIS. (Refer to Chapter 17 for the details about treatment selection.)

Tumor Pathology, Tumor Size, and Resection Margins

Pathologic evaluation included determination of the histologic subtype, nuclear grade, presence or absence of comedonecrosis, maximal diameter of the lesion, and margin width, as previously described (7). Tissue was processed completely and sequentially. Nuclear grade and necrosis were scored by previously described methods (23) (see Chapter 17).

The size of small lesions was determined by direct measurement or ocular micrometry of specimens stained on slides. The size of large lesions was determined by a combination of direct measurement and estimation using three-dimensional reconstruction within a sequential series of slides. For example, a lesion that measured 5 mm on a single slide but that extended across 10 sequential sections was estimated to be 25 mm in size because the average size of each block was 2.5 mm. For the purposes of statistical analysis, tumor size was categorized as 15 mm or less, 16 to 40 mm, and more than 40 mm.

Margin width was determined by direct measurement or ocular micrometry. The smallest single distance between the edge of the tumor and an inked line delineating the margin of normal tissue was reported. Margins in patients who underwent repeated excision and in whom no additional DCIS was found were reported as being at least 10 mm in width. For the purposes of statistical analysis, margin width was categorized as less than 1 mm, 1 to 9 mm, and 10 mm or more.

STATISTICAL CONSIDERATIONS

The primary end point for statistical analysis was recurrence-free survival (RFS), which is the minimum time from diagnosis to noninvasive or invasive recurrence. Patients who died of causes apparently unrelated to breast cancer are not counted as events. RFS is essentially synonymous with local RFS because only one patient relapsed distant from the original tumor before local relapse, and this patient was diagnosed with a local relapse within 6 months. Follow-up through the end of 2000 was used in the analysis.

Plots and estimates of RFS percentages were computed using the product-limit estimate. Univariate differences between treatment and prognostic groups were tested using the log-rank test. Multivariate analysis was based on Cox regression analysis. Confidence intervals for relative failure rates were based on the partial likelihood estimates and standard errors obtained from the Cox model. Tests of significance in the Cox model were based on the partial likelihood ratio χ^2 test (24).

RESULTS

Characteristics of the patients and their tumors are summarized in Tables 21.1 and 21.2. Most patients were diagnosed and treated in the past two decades, with more than half treated after 1990. Median age was 51 years, with 10% of patients younger than 40 years of age and 9% older than 70 years of age at diagnosis.

Eighty-six percent of patients had tumors that were not palpable on physical examination, and 49% had tumors with the largest dimension 15 mm or less. There was a significant association between palpability and tumor size: 9.5% of tumors measuring 15 mm or less were palpable compared with 18% of tumors larger than 15 mm ($p < 0.001$, χ^2 test).

TABLE 21.1. PATIENT AND GROSS TUMOR CHARACTERISTICS

	All Patients		Conservative Rx Only	
	No.	%	No.	%
No. of breasts with DCIS				
1	845	93	552	95
2	64	7	31	5
Year of diagnosis				
1971–1980	36	4		4
1981–1990	382	42		41
1991–2000	491	54		55
Age at diagnosis (yr)				
20–29	9	1	3	1
30–39	78	9	42	7
40–49	310	34	190	32
50–59	263	29	179	31
60–69	160	18	111	19
70–79	76	8	49	8
80–89	13	1	9	2
Tumor size by pathology (mm)				
≤15	443	49	369	63
16–40	276	30	167	29
>40	190	21	47	8
Tumor resection margin (mm)				
≥10	179	31	179	31
1–9	255	44	255	44
<1	149	25	149	25
NA (mastectomy)	326	—		
Treatment				
Mastectomy	326	36		
Radiation therapy	237	26	237	41
None	346	38	346	59

Rx, treatment; DCIS, ductal carcinoma in situ; NA, not applicable.

TABLE 21.2. MICROSCOPIC TUMOR CHARACTERISTICS

	All Patients		Conservative Rx Only	
	No.	%	No.	%
Nuclear grade				
I	154	17	116	20
II	373	41	226	39
III	382	42	241	41
Necrosis				
Present	625	69	383	66
Absent	284	31	200	34
Estrogen receptor positive				
Yes	98	66	68	72
No	51	34	26	28
Unknown	760	—	489	—
Progesterone receptor positive				
Yes	90	63	67	72
No	54	37	26	28
Unknown	765	—	490	—
HER2/neu receptor positive				
Yes	73	56	37	32
No	131	44	80	68
Unknown	705	—	466	—

Rx, treatment.

Three hundred twenty-six patients (36%) were treated with mastectomy, 237 (26%) with breast-conserving surgery and radiation therapy, and 346 (38%) with conservative surgery alone. Of the 583 patients treated with conservative surgery, 31% has wide resection margins ($\geq$10 mm) and 25% had close margins (<1 mm). Not unexpectedly, there is a significant association between the width of the resection margin and tumor size, with a wide excision ($\geq$10 mm) achieved in 34% of patients with tumors measuring 15 mm or less, 28% of tumors measuring 16 to 40 mm, and 13% of tumors measuring more than 40 mm ($p < 0.001$). Patients with a wider resection margin also less commonly received radiation therapy as part of their treatment; 25% of patients with wide excision were treated with radiation therapy compared with 43% with intermediate resection margin and 56% with close margin ($p < 0.0001$).

Nuclear grade was highly associated with the presence of necrosis in the tumor specimen. 16% of grade 1 tumors, 67% of grade 2 tumors, and 92% of grade 3 tumors displayed some necrosis ($p < 0.0001$).

In the comparatively small number of tumors for which estrogen receptor (ER), progesterone receptor (PR), or HER2/neu receptor status was available, there was an apparent association with nuclear grade: 86% of grade 1, 80% of grade 2, and 49% of grade 2 tumors were ER positive ($p < 0.0005$); 71% of grade 1, 70% of grade 2, and 53% of grade 3 tumors were PR positive ($p < 0.10$); 26% of grade 1, 23% of grade 2, and 56% of grade 3 tumors were

HER2/neu positive ($p < 0.0001$). Furthermore, ER and PR were positively associated with each other ($p < 0.0001$), and each was negatively associated with HER2/neu status ($p = 0.0005$ and $p < 0.0001$, respectively).

RECURRENCES

There was a total of 111 recurrences: two in patients treated with mastectomy, 48 in patients treated with excision plus radiation therapy, and 61 in patients treated with excision alone. Forty-nine of the 111 recurrences (44%) were invasive.

UNIVARIATE ANALYSIS OF SELECTED PROGNOSTIC FACTORS

The initial focus of the analysis of RFS was on selected patient and tumor characteristics that had previously been reported to be associated with DCIS recurrence. These factors were age, tumor size, tumor resection margin, treatment, nuclear grade, the presence of comedonecrosis, ER and PR positivity, and HER2/neu receptor positivity. These analyses were restricted to patients that had been treated with conservative surgery with or without radiation therapy. Tables 21.3 and 21.4 and Figures 21.1 through 21.7 summarize these results.

TABLE 21.3. UNIVARIATE ANALYSIS OF LOCAL RECURRENCE BY PATIENT AND GROSS TUMOR CHARACTERISTICS

Characteristic	No. of Patients	8-yr RFS (Est. ± SE) (%)	12-yr RFS (Est. ± SE) (%)	p Value
Age at diagnosis (yr)				
<40	45	64 ± 8	55 ± 9	<0.0002[a,b]
40–60	385	78 ± 3	69 ± 4	
>60	153	89 ± 3	84 ÷ 5	
Tumor size by pathology (mm)				
≤15	369	88 ± 2	79 ± 3	<0.0001[a,b]
16–40	167	68 ± 4	62 ± 5	
>40	47	50 ± 10	21 ± 16	
Tumor resection margin (mm)				
Mastectomy	326	99 ± 1	99 ± 1	<0.0001[b]
≥10	179	95 ± 2	95 ± 2	<0.0001[a,b]
1–9	255	81 ± 3	73 ± 4	
<1	149	62 ± 5	46 ± 6	
Treatment				
Mastectomy	326	99 ± 1	99 ± 1	<0.0001
Radiation therapy	237	83 ± 3	73 ± 4	0.13[a]
None	346	76 ± 3	69 ± 4	

[a] Mastectomy cases excluded.
[b] Log-rank test for trend.
RFS, recurrence-free survival; Est., estimate; SE, standard error.

TABLE 21.4. UNIVARIATE ANALYSIS OF LOCAL RECURRENCE BY MICROSCOPIC TUMOR CHARACTERISTICS

Characteristic	No. of Patients	8-yr RFS (Est. ± SE) (%)	12-yr RFS (Est. ± SE) (%)	p Value
Nuclear grade				
I	116	91 ± 3	87 ± 4	<0.0001[b]
II	226	87 ± 3	77 ± 4	
III	241	65 ± 4	55 ± 5	
Necrosis				
Present	383	75 ± 3	64 ± 4	0.0001[a]
Absent	200	88 ± 3	84 ± 4	
Estrogen receptor positive				
Yes	68	64 ± 8	c	0.32[a]
No	26	47 ± 11	c	
Progesterone receptor positive				
Yes	67	62 ± 9	c	0.14[a]
No	26	51 ± 11	c	
HER2/neu receptor positive				
Yes	37	65 ± 9	c	0.012[a]
No	80	79 ± 5	c	

[a] Mastectomy cases excluded.
[b] Log-rank test for trend.
[c] Data too sparse for estimation.
RFS, recurrence-free survival; Est., estimate; SE, standard error.

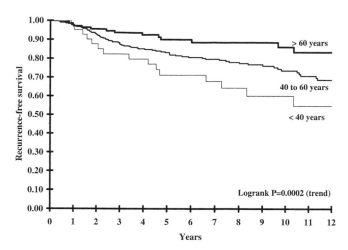

FIGURE 21.1. Age at diagnosis (conservatively treated patients only).

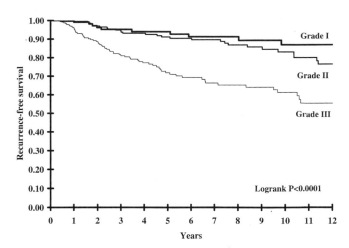

FIGURE 21.3. Nuclear grade (conservatively treated patients only).

Age at Diagnosis

Patients younger than 40 years of age and those 40 to 60 years of age had a significantly higher recurrence rate than older women (older than 60 years) ($p = 0.0002$, logrank test for trend, Fig. 21.1). Of the women in the oldest age category, 89% were free of recurrence at 8 years compared with only 64% of women in the youngest age category.

Tumor Characteristics

Tumor size was significantly associated with RFS. Eight-year RFS was 88% in women with tumors less than 15 mm in maximum dimension compared with 68% and 50% in women with intermediate- (16 to 40 mm) and large- (greater than 40 mm) size tumors ($p < 0.0001$, log-rank test for trend; Fig. 21.2). Higher nuclear grade and the presence of necrosis in the tumor specimen were both signifi-

cantly associated with a worse outcome. Of patients with grade 1 tumors, 91% were relapse free at 8 years compared with 87% and 65% of patients with grade 2 and 3 tumors, respectively ($p < 0.0001$; Fig. 21.3). Of patients with tumors with comedonecrosis, 75% were relapse free compared with 88% of patients with tumors that did not display necrosis ($p < 0.0001$; Fig. 21.4).

ER, PR, and HER2/neu receptor expression data were available for fewer than 25% of the tumors. Neither ER nor PR status was significantly associated with RFS ($p = 0.32$ and $p = 0.14$). Although this nonsignificance might be attributed to the small sample size available, the difference in 8-year RFS between receptor-positive and -negative tumors also was not extremely large: 64% versus 47% for ER status and 62% versus 51% for PR status. HER2/neu status was nominally significantly associated with outcome ($p = 0.012$), with 65% of patients with HER2/neu-positive tumors relapse free at 8 years compared with 79% of patients with HER2/neu-negative tumors.

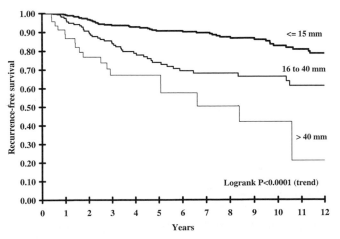

FIGURE 21.2. Pathologic tumor size (conservatively treated patients only).

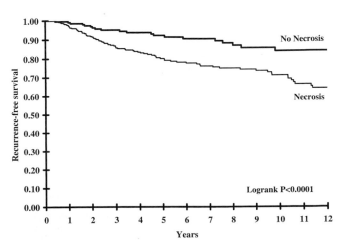

FIGURE 21.4. Any necrosis in the tumor specimen (conservatively treated patients only).

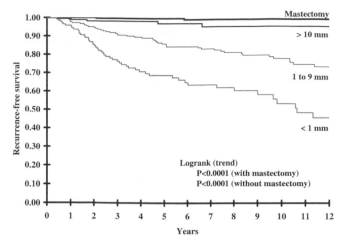

FIGURE 21.5. Resection margin (all patients).

Treatment Factors

Patients whose initial treatment was mastectomy had a significantly lower recurrence rate ($p < 0.0001$; Fig. 21.5), with only 1% of these patients having a recurrence within 8 years of treatment. Among patients treated conservatively, the width of the resection margin was significantly associated with outcome. Of the women with wide margins, 95% were recurrence free at 8 years compared with 81% with intermediate margins and 62% with close margins ($p < 0.0001$) (Fig. 21.5). Patients treated with radiation therapy had an 83% 8-year RFS compared with 76% for patients treated without radiation therapy (Fig. 21.6; $p = 0.13$). It is important to note that these univariate analyses of treatment factors are confounded by the association between tumor size, resection margin, and radiation therapy administration. A more accurate picture of their joint effects is obtained in the multivariate analysis below.

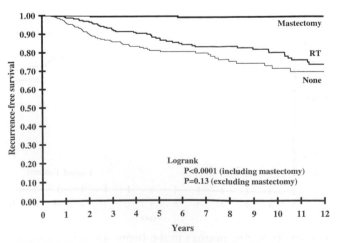

FIGURE 21.6. Treatment at diagnosis (all patients).

MULTIVARIATE ANALYSIS OF UNIVARIATELY SIGNIFICANT FACTORS

Many of the prognostic factors in this population that were significant in the univariate analyses above are correlated (e.g., tumor size and resection margin, tumor necrosis, and nuclear grade). A Cox multivariate analysis was performed to identify which of these factors were independent predictors of RFS. The factors that were included in this analysis were nuclear grade, age at diagnosis, tumor size, margin width, necrosis, and treatment. As in the univariate analyses, patients who had undergone a mastectomy were excluded from the analysis. The rate of recurrence in the mastectomy group is exceedingly small, and its inclusion would not qualitatively affect the relative failure rate estimates or the conclusions from the analysis.

The results of the multivariate analysis are displayed graphically in Figure 21.7. This figure shows the relative failure rate and 95% confidence interval for all the factors included in the model. Also shown is the p value for significance of the factor in the model. Nuclear grade, age at diagnosis, tumor size, resection margin, and treatment remain strongly significant prognostic factors in the model. The presence of necrosis, although highly significant in the univariate analysis, was not significant in the multivariate analysis, although the relative failure rate of 1.6 was still considerably larger than 1 for this factor.

This model predicts that patients with grade 3 tumors have a 2.2-fold higher recurrence rate than patients with grade 1 tumors, with grade 2 tumors associated with a 1.2-fold higher recurrence rate.

Patients at intermediate and young ages have a 2.3- and 3.2-fold higher recurrence rate, respectively, than do the oldest patients. Similarly, patients with intermediate- and large-size tumors have a 2.2- and 3.3-fold higher recurrence rate than do patients with small tumors.

Tumor resection margin is by far the most significant and important factor associated with recurrence rate. Patients with intermediate and close margins have a 6.4- and 12.1-fold higher risk of recurrence than do patients with resection margin of at least 10 mm.

Finally, patients who received radiation therapy had a risk of failure of 0.45, less than half of that for patients who did not receive radiation therapy, after controlling for the other factors in the model. This relative risk reduction is similar to that reported by the National Surgical Adjuvant Breast Project (5,9) (Chapter 42) and the European Organization for Research and Treatment of Cancer (3,4).

TYPE OF RECURRENCE

An open question in the treatment of DCIS is whether radiation therapy is not only more effective in preventing any disease recurrence, but whether it is particularly effective in

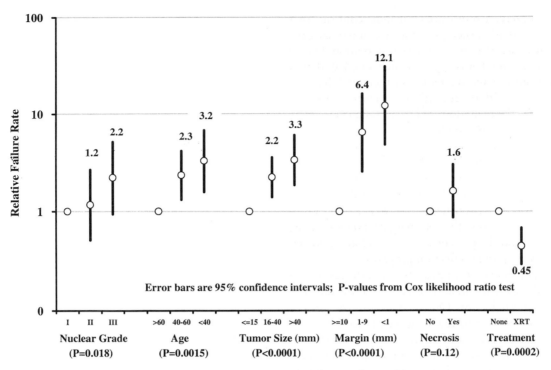

FIGURE 21.7. Cox multivariate analysis of factors affecting ductal carcinoma in situ recurrence-free survival (conservatively treated patients only).

preventing invasive cancer recurrences. Figure 21.8 shows the cumulative incidence of invasive recurrence by treatment. Figure 21.9 shows the cumulative incidence of noninvasive recurrence by treatment. It is evident from this analysis that, at least in this cohort, there is very little evidence of a differential effect of radiation therapy in preventing invasive recurrence. The 8-year cumulative incidence of invasive recurrence is 1 ± 1% for mastectomy, 7 ± 2% for radiation therapy, and 10 ± 2% for excision alone. For noninvasive recurrence, the 8-year rates are 0.63 ± 0.44%, 9 ± 2%, and 14 ± 3%, respectively.

CONCLUSIONS

The analysis of this prospectively pathologically evaluated cohort of patients treated for DCIS demonstrates that there are several factors in addition to treatment that are important determinants of the likelihood of local recurrence. Clearly, from the point of view of preventing local recurrence, mastectomy is the most effective treatment regardless of other features of the patient or tumor. Only 1% of the patients in this cohort treated with mastectomy experienced a recurrence of disease. In the group of patients treated with

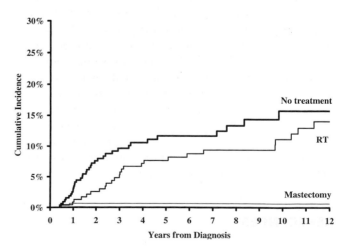

FIGURE 21.8. Cumulative incidence of invasive recurrence by treatment.

FIGURE 21.9. Cumulative incidence of noninvasive recurrence by treatment.

conservative surgery, a multivariate analysis confirms that the addition of radiation therapy is effective in reducing the local recurrence rate. Patients who receive radiation therapy have a recurrence rate that is approximately one-half that of patients who did not receive radiation therapy. This estimate agrees closely with the reduction in recurrence risk obtain from the two large randomized trials designed to study this question (1,3,4,9) (Chapter 42).

In addition to radiation therapy, however, it is clear that other factors are also important determinants of prognosis. The most prominent of these is clearly the width of the resection margin that is achieved by the conservative surgery. Patients with wide resection margins have a 12-fold lower failure rate than patients with close margins. Nuclear grade, age, tumor size, and the presence of necrosis have a smaller but nonetheless important effect on prognosis.

It is important here to distinguish between the relative reduction in risk owing to radiation therapy and the practical importance of this reduction. Our analyses confirm the benefit of radiation therapy in reducing recurrence rate. Furthermore, there is no evidence from our analysis that this approximately 50% reduction in failure rate does not apply equally to any identifiable subgroup of patients in the cohort, e.g., a group of patients with a wide resection margin and low nuclear grade who receive radiation therapy will likely have half the failure rate when compared with a similar cohort without radiation. This is consistent with the notion that radiation therapy is effective in eliminating cancer in the fraction of patients who have postsurgical residual disease despite apparently pathologically clear and wide margins. It is also true, however, that a patient who achieves a wide (>10 mm) resection margin that is documented by careful pathologic examination of the resected tissue will have a much smaller chance of having viable postsurgical residual disease than one with a clear but close margin. This is reflected in the 12-fold lower risk of failure in patients with wide resection margins compared with those with close margins. From our data, a 55-year-old patient with a 10-mm tumor of nuclear grade 2 whose tumor is resected with a margin greater than 10 mm margin has only approximately a 3% chance of local recurrence by 8 years even without radiation therapy. The key question is not whether radiation therapy will cut this risk in half, which we must assume that it will, but whether the reduction from a 3% to 1.5% chance of local failure is worth the morbidity associated with radiation therapy, especially when one considers the very high rate of successful retreatment with additional surgery and radiation therapy in the small number of patients who do experience a recurrence.

REFERENCES

1. Fisher ER, Costantino J, Fisher B, et al. Pathologic findings from the National Surgical Adjuvant Breast Project (NSABP) Protocol B-17. Intraductal carcinoma (ductal carcinoma in situ). The National Surgical Adjuvant Breast and Bowel Project Collaborating Investigators. *Cancer* 1995;75:1310-1–319.

2. Fisher B, Dignam J, Wolmark N, et al. Tamoxifen in treatment of intraductal breast cancer: National Surgical Adjuvant Breast and Bowel Project B-24 randomised controlled trial. *Lancet* 1999;353:1993–2000.

3. Bijker N, Peterse JL, Duchateau L, et al. Risk factors for recurrence and metastasis after breast-conserving therapy for ductal carcinoma-in-situ: analysis of European Organization for Research and Treatment of Cancer Trial 10853. *J Clin Oncol* 2001; 19:2263–2271.

4. Julien JP, Bijker N, Fentiman IS, et al. Radiotherapy in breast-conserving treatment for ductal carcinoma in situ: first results of the EORTC randomised phase III trial 10853. EORTC Breast Cancer Cooperative Group and EORTC Radiotherapy Group. *Lancet* 2000;355:528–533.

5. Fisher B, Costantino J, Redmond C, et al. Lumpectomy compared with lumpectomy and radiation therapy for the treatment of intraductal breast cancer. *N Engl J Med* 1993;328:1581–1586.

6. Silverstein MJ, Lagios MD. Benefits of irradiation for DCIS: a Pyrrhic victory [published erratum appears in *Lancet* 2000;355:1190]. *Lancet* 2000;355:510–511.

7. Silverstein MJ, Lagios MD, Groshen S, et al. The influence of margin width on local control of ductal carcinoma in situ of the breast. *N Engl J Med* 1999;340:1455–1461.

8. Fisher ER, Dignam J, Tan-Chiu E, et al. Pathologic findings from the National Surgical Adjuvant Breast Project (NSABP) eight-year update of Protocol B-17: intraductal carcinoma. *Cancer* 1999;86:429–438.

9. Fisher B, Dignam J, Wolmark N, et al. Lumpectomy and radiation therapy for the treatment of intraductal breast cancer: findings from National Surgical Adjuvant Breast and Bowel Project B-17. *J Clin Oncol* 1998;16:441–452.

10. Silverstein MJ, Lagios MD, Martino S, et al. Outcome after invasive local recurrence in patients with ductal carcinoma in situ of the breast. *J Clin Oncol* 1998;16:1367–1373.

11. Gottlieb N. San Antonio Breast Cancer Symposium explores DCIS "battleground." *J Natl Cancer Inst* 2000;92:295–297.

12. Hwang ES, Esserman LJ. Management of ductal carcinoma in situ. *Surg Clin North Am* 1999;79:1007–1030.

13. Winchester DP, Jeske JM, Goldschmidt RA. The diagnosis and management of ductal carcinoma in-situ of the breast. *CA Cancer J Clin* 2000;50:184–200.

14. Pinder SE, Evans AJ, Ellis IO. Ductal carcinoma in situ of the human breast: clinico-pathological aspects. *Ann Ital Chir* 1999;70:343–347.

15. Hetelekidis S, Collins L, Silver B, et al. Predictors of local recurrence following excision alone for ductal carcinoma in situ. *Cancer* 1999;85:427–431.

16. Holland PA, Gandhi A, Knox WF, et al. The importance of complete excision in the prevention of local recurrence of ductal carcinoma in situ. *Br J Cancer* 1998;77:110–114.

17. Lagios MD. Heterogeneity of duct carcinoma in situ (DCIS): relationship of grade and subtype analysis to local recurrence and risk of invasive transformation. *Cancer Lett* 1995;90:97–102.

18. Silverstein MJ, Poller DN, Waisman JR, et al. Prognostic classification of breast ductal carcinoma-in-situ. *Lancet* 1995;345:1154–1157.

19. Silverstein MJ, Lagios MD, Craig PH, et al. A prognostic index for ductal carcinoma in situ of the breast. *Cancer* 1996;77:2267–2274.

20. Van Zee KJ, Liberman L, Samli B, et al. Long term follow-up of women with ductal carcinoma in situ treated with breast-conserving surgery: the effect of age. *Cancer* 1999;86:1757–1767.

21. Vicini FA, Goldstein NS, Kestin LL. Pathologic and technical considerations in the treatment of ductal carcinoma in situ of the breast with lumpectomy and radiation therapy. *Ann Oncol* 1999;10:883–890.

22. Silverstein MJ, Barth A, Poller DN, et al. Ten-year results comparing mastectomy to excision and radiation therapy for ductal carcinoma in situ of the breast. *Eur J Cancer* 1995;31A:1425–1427.

23. Lagios MD. Duct carcinoma in situ. Pathology and treatment. *Surg Clin North Am* 1990;70:853–871.

24. Kalbfleisch J, Prentice R. *The statistical analysis of failure time data.* New York: John Wiley & Sons, 1980.

22

THE DIAGNOSTIC REPRODUCIBILITY OF DUCTAL CARCINOMA IN SITU

WENDY A. WELLS

"An ideal histological classification of DCIS should be clinically useful and correlate with the local recurrence rate of DCIS and with the development of invasive carcinoma. The classification needs to provide unequivocal definitions of the terms used, be applicable to all histological appearances and manifestations of DCIS, be simple and quick to apply, be applicable to small numbers of ducts and, ideally, should show no inter or intra-observer error" (1).

Ductal carcinoma in situ (DCIS) of the breast is a heterogencous lesion with variable biologic behavior, which currently accounts for more than 20% of mammographically detected breast lesions (2,3). In combination with tumor size and margin status (4), mammographic correlation (5), and other selected biologic markers (6–13), the histologic appearances help predict the clinical behavior of DCIS lesions.

Multiple classifications of DCIS have been proposed since 1993 (6,11,14–18) (see Chapters 17 and 63). Most de-emphasize the importance of architectural pattern but retain a three-tier system of final tumor grade (low, intermediate, and high) and include criteria such as nuclear grade, necrosis, and cellular polarization. Rarely have these various classifications been evaluated for diagnostic reproducibility at the time of publication (16), and subsequent studies to assess criteria of reproducibility have invariably involved pathologists with an expertise in breast pathology rather than nonspecialist pathologists (19).

The constant publication of new or modified classifications for DCIS presents a dilemma to many practicing pathologists who must digest variable changes in criteria definitions and convey these changes in a meaningful and consistent way to their clinical colleagues. It also presents problems for researchers who are seeking to study treatment effectiveness based on prognostic factors. If the diagnostic criteria are not reproducible, then disease outcome studies based on these criteria will be virtually meaningless.

This chapter compares and contrasts the published reproducibility studies for the histologic criteria of DCIS by reviewing their methods, statistical analyses, and conclusions. It is hoped that an evaluation of these studies will determine which consistently reproducible histologic criteria should form the basis of a DCIS classification.

METHODS

Study Sets

The method most commonly used to assess diagnostic reproducibility in surgical pathology is to ask the participating pathologists to evaluate representative slides from multiple cases according to the classification(s) or criteria being tested.

Origin of the Study Set

A set of study slides is either compiled from cases originating at the study institution or representative slides are submitted from the institutions of the participating pathologists. If the study set is from one institution, the complexity of the cases may be biased toward that institution (usually an academic center), but there will be a uniformity of tissue processing, cutting, and staining. If the participating pathologists from varying institutions provide the cases, the study set complexity may be more representative of community-based practice. The representative slides submitted from multiple laboratories may already be stained, and the study participants may be asked to comment on the quality of each slide, as part of the study, to ascertain whether the slide quality affected their interpretation. Some reproducibility studies request that representative tissue blocks or unstained slides from participating laboratories be sent to the study institution to ensure uniform staining and/or cutting.

Compilation and Distribution of the Study Set(s)

If the study is assessing diagnostic reproducibility in the everyday practice of pathologist groups, then the slides selected should be consecutive cases, over a defined period of time or selected according to the normal distribution of cases for that group of practices (20). If the study focuses on distinguishing between very specific diagnostic areas (such as ductal hyperplasia without atypia versus atypical ductal hyperplasia versus low-grade DCIS), then a preselected group of slides will make up the study set. In this case, discrepancies in diagnostic agreement must be weighed against the incidence of these entities occurring in normal practice and the impact that this poor reproducibility may have on subsequent under- or overtreatment (21). Any slide identifiers that may introduce bias into the interpretation must be removed or covered and a study code applied to each slide. Then, the study coordinator either must rotate the same set of study slides separately to all the participants or assemble multiple identical study sets. In the latter case, each group of slides must be checked to ensure that identical diagnostic material is present on each slide recut.

Evaluation of the Study Set(s)

Some studies mark specific regions of the slides in the study set to draw the attention of the participant to that area (22). In many studies, the participants are asked to evaluate the histologic criteria of more than one classification scheme on the same study slide set (1,22–25). In these cases, there may be bias owing to the requirement to interpret slightly different criteria close together. Rater fatigue should also not be underestimated. A solution is to ask the participants to assess the study set for the first classification, then fax the completed pathology reporting form to the study coordinator. Upon receipt of this fax, the appropriate reporting form for the next classification can be sent, after a reasonable period has elapsed (23).

Reporting Sheets

To facilitate data collection, a standardized reporting form is often devised for use by all the study participants. The histologic criteria being tested are summarized in list form and the participants are required to check the presence, absence, or grade of each criterion. Such a reporting form may limit the diagnostic interpretations of the participants because its format, by definition, discourages wordy comments and its layout may differ from the more familiar reporting templates routinely used by the participants. The coordinator compiling the reporting form may also introduce interpretation bias when details of the criteria to be tested are summarized or condensed from the original publications.

Some classifications use an algorithm to link some criteria into final grades or groups. In the Van Nuys Classification (18), a high nuclear grade (with or without necrosis) is defined as group 3. Of the remaining nonhigh nuclear grades (low and intermediate), those with necrosis are defined as group 2 and those without necrosis are defined as group 1. Most reproducibility studies do not address who (the project coordinators or the participants) derive these final groups and whether mistakes were made, in retrospect, using the al-

gorithm. For example, in one study that assessed reproducibility of the Van Nuys Classification, the participants derived the final group for each case (23). The reporting form in this study provided definitions of three nuclear grades and necrosis identical to those given in the original publication of the Van Nuys Classification (18). The participants then used their designations of nuclear grade and necrosis to derive a final DCIS group, according to the published algorithm. In this study, the mistakes made by the participants in deriving this final group have been attributed to a poorly designed reporting form (26). Critics of the study's reporting form believed that if the participants had been given only two options for nuclear grade (high and nonhigh), rather than three options (high, intermediate, and low), then fewer mistakes would have been made in the derivation of the final algorithm for each case. However, the histologic criteria for three nuclear grades were distinctly described in the original classification paper (18) rather than just defining the morphologic criteria for a high nuclear grade and then stating that all other nuclear features should be called nonhigh. The nonspecialist pathologists in this study were interpreting the published literature of this classification as they must do in their daily practice, and any interpretation difficulties should be reported and evaluated in the statistical analysis.

Prestudy Sets/Training Sessions

All reproducibility studies vary in the amount of information that is provided to the participants before, during, and after a reproducibility study. Some studies simply provide copies of the original publications detailing the criteria to be tested. Others also provide a summary of the criteria and/or teaching sets of the diagnostic entities being tested and/or formal tutorials emphasizing the relevant criteria. Because community-based pathologists are less likely to be part of group discussions of controversial criteria, the introduction of such study sets/training sessions into a reproducibility study does not reflect either the everyday practice of most pathologists or their ability to interpret new histologic criteria as they are published. If these published details are not precise and simple, then reproducibility will be invariably poor. It has been postulated that continuous, sufficient feedback between pathologists, when diagnosing controversial criteria, improves both inter- and intraobserver reproducibility (1). This is best achieved when pathologists meet regularly in small groups (such as interdepartmental conferences) rather than infrequently participating in large, quality assurance slide circulation programs in which the feedback of peer opinion may be delayed weeks or months.

The Gold Standard Diagnosis

When a group of pathologists take part in a diagnostic reproducibility study, their interpretations must be compared with a gold standard diagnosis, be it the retrospective, consensus diagnoses of all the participants or of one of the investigators. In surgical pathology, there is a tradition of seeking a second opinion from experts in the appropriate field in cases of poor diagnostic reproducibility. In breast pathology, common areas where confirmatory expert opinions are sought include the distinction between atypical ductal hyperplasia or low-grade DCIS, the presence or absence of microinvasive carcinoma, and the differentiation between a radial scar and a tubular carcinoma. A group of pathologists may come to a consensus diagnosis, but that diagnosis may not necessarily be the same as that rendered by the expert who originally defined the criteria being interpreted.

To date, one study has assessed the diagnostic accuracy and reproducibility of three DCIS classifications by comparing the results of nonspecialist pathologists with those of three breast pathology experts, each a proponent of one of the three evaluated classifications (23). In this study, the three experts were considered to provide the gold standard diagnosis. The final DCIS grade and nuclear grade (low, intermediate, or high) were assessed most accurately using the Holland Classification (15). An intermediate DCIS grade was assessed most accurately using the Holland Classification (15) and the Modified Lagios Classification (16). A high nuclear grade was assessed most accurately using the Van Nuys Classification (18). The Van Nuys interpretation of necrosis (present or absent) was the definition of necrosis reported most accurately (18). Overall, in this study of American pathologists, the final DCIS grade was reported best using the Holland Classification (15). Nuclear grade (cytodifferentiation), according to the Holland Classification, and the presence or absence of necrosis, according to the Van Nuys Classification, were the criteria diagnosed most accurately and reproducibly.

Specialists Versus Nonspecialist Participants

Most of the reproducibility studies involve pathologists with a specialist interest in breast pathology (22,24,25). These studies do not necessarily reflect how community-based, nonspecialist pathologists may interpret the histologic criteria detailed in the various DCIS classification publications. Two studies directly compare the performance of specialists and nonspecialists, one comparing the results of the nonspecialists with those of three international experts (as described above) (23) and the other comparing the performance of the nonspecialists and specialists compared with the consensus of these observers (1). The latter study determined that there was no difference in diagnostic agreement between these two groups.

Statistical Analysis for Agreement

Interrater Reproducibility

This compares the ability of different observers (raters) to classify topics into one of several groups and is well described by Altman (27). A simple approach for measuring agreement would be to see how many agreements were made by two pathologists (A and B) in categorizing 60 cases of DCIS into one of three nuclear grades (low, intermediate, or high). The following example is adapted from that described by Altman (27) (Table 22.1).

The number of exact agreements between the two pathologists is 37 (8 + 20 + 9). If both pathologists had agreed on every diagnostic category, the total number of agreements would have been 60. For these two pathologists, the overall agreement is 37/60 = 0.62 (62%). However, this method of assessing agreement does not take into consideration where in the table there is agreement or that some of the agreement may have been by chance. A more meaningful measure of agreement would be to consider the agreement in excess of that which may occur by chance.

Pathologist A evaluates a case as high nuclear grade 15 times (6 + 9). Pathologist B evaluates a case as high nuclear grade 19 times (10 + 9), but both pathologists only agree on this diagnosis in nine cases. Of the possible 60 options in the frequency table, the expected frequency of the two pathologists making the same diagnosis of a high nuclear grade by chance is $(15 \times 19)/60$. The expected frequency of the two pathologists making the same diagnosis of an intermediate nuclear grade by chance is $(35 \times 28)/60$.

TABLE 22.1. NUCLEAR GRADE ASSESSMENTS MADE BY TWO PATHOLOGISTS IN 60 CASES OF DCIS

Pathologist A	Pathologist B			
	Low Nuclear Grade	Intermediate Nuclear Grade	High Nuclear Grade	Total
Low nuclear grade	**8**	2	0	10
Intermediate nuclear grade	5	**20**	10	35
High nuclear grade	0	6	**9**	15
Total	13	28	19	60

The number of agreements expected by chance for each diagnostic category are:

Low nuclear grade: (10*13)/60 =   2.17
Intermediate nuclear grade: (35*28)/60 = 16.33
High nuclear grade: (15*19)/60 =   4.75
Total: 23.25

The total number of agreements expected by chance is 23.25, which, as a proportion of the total, is 23.25/60 = 0.39.

Because 1.00 represents maximum agreement, then the agreement in excess of that which may occur by chance by these two pathologists is 1.00 − 0.39.

Thus, the pathologists' diagnostic agreement, after accounting for chance (0.62 − 0.39) as a proportion of theoretical maximum agreement, in excess of chance (1.00 − 0.39), will be

$$(0.62 - 0.39)/(1.00 - 0.39)$$
$$0.23/0.61$$
$$0.38$$

This measure of agreement is kappa, which has a maximum value of 1.00 when there is perfect agreement and a value of 0 when there is no agreement better than by chance. The kappa statistic is commonly used in reproducibility studies involving multiple participants and the assessment of multiple criteria. However, the kappa value and corresponding strength of agreement are not intuitive. In the medical literature, the interpretation of kappa values between 0 and 1 is often attributed to Landis and Koch (28) (Table 22.2).

Intrarater Reproducibility

This is also assessed by the kappa statistic. Two recently published reproducibility studies looked at both interrater (between group) and intrarater (within group) reproducibility and showed similar results. In both studies, some participants were required to re-evaluate randomly selected slides from the original study, and the separate assessments were compared. In the study by Wells et al. (23), the intrarater reproducibility was better than interrater reproducibility, suggesting that each nonspecialist pathologist had established their own fixed definitions of the criteria, even if these did

TABLE 22.2. THE INTERPRETATION OF KAPPA STATISTICS

Value of Kappa	Strength of Agreement
<0.20	Poor
0.21–0.40	Fair
0.41–0.60	Moderate
0.61–0.80	Good
0.81–1.00	Excellent

not correlate well with the published criteria. In the study by Douglas-Jones et al. (1), intrarater agreement was considered moderate. This study also analyzed consistency of performance of individual observers by comparing the degree to which their interpretations differed from the consensus. The study showed a consistent individual bias toward either over- or underscoring of the nuclear grade.

Weighted Kappas

The kappa statistic treats all disagreements equally. Sometimes, it may be preferable to weight a disagreement according to the magnitude of that disagreement. In the previously described example, the optimal treatment algorithm and subsequent clinical outcome may be affected by diagnosing a DCIS lesion as low nuclear grade rather than high. The weighted kappa is calculated by giving weights to the frequencies in each cell of the table depending on how far that cell is away from the diagonal that indicates full agreement. Weighted kappa values are usually higher than their unweighted counterparts because the disagreements are more likely to be by just one category (intermediate nuclear grade versus high nuclear grade) rather than several (low nuclear grade versus high nuclear grade).

The kappa statistic is dependent on the number of participating observers and diagnostic categories being evaluated. This must be taken into consideration when kappa statistics from different studies are compared.

Limitations of Reproducibility Studies

Ideally, reproducibility studies should recapitulate the usual working conditions of the pathologist community. The comparison of multiple reproducibility studies (detailed below) shows that the following criteria differ from study to study and thus must be regarded as limitations in the interpretation and comparison of the results in such studies.

- The potential for tissue sampling, processing, and staining variability interfering with the interpretation of the slide study sets.
- The performance comparisons of pathologists with and without specialist interests in breast pathology.
- The bias introduced by the presence or absence of prestudy training tutorials or criteria summaries.
- The influence of marking specific areas on the slide to draw the attention of the participating pathologist to that region.
- The artificial environment of a study set assessment without the usual constraints of time and work pressure.
- The influence that a uniform reporting form may have on final diagnostic interpretations because its format discourages wordy comments and may differ from the reporting templates routinely used by the participants.

- The incorrect use of algorithms by the participants to characterize a final grade, as in the Van Nuys Classification (see above).
- A variation in the number of participants and the number of diagnostic categories being assessed in each study, limiting the direct comparison of kappa statistic evaluations.

INTERNATIONAL VARIATIONS IN DUCTAL CARCINOMA IN SITU CLASSIFICATION SCHEMES

In the United States, no one DCIS classification scheme is used. Most community-based pathologists list multiple criteria in their breast surgical pathology reports, such as nuclear grade, necrosis (presence, absence, type) and pattern(s) but do not extrapolate those criteria into a specific classification system. However, because many surgeons in the United States use the Van Nuys Prognostic Index (4) as a basis for developing their treatment algorithms, the nuclear grade and presence or absence of necrosis can be used (together with tumor size and margin status) to evaluate that Prognostic Index. Pathologists in the United States do not report cellular polarization despite the recommendation to do so when the Consensus Committee's report was published (14).

In Europe, the DCIS classification recommended by the European Pathologists Working Group (EPWG), based on the Holland Classification, is widely used, although several studies have shown comparable reproducibility when the criterion of polarization is dropped (22,24,25). Unlike in Europe, reproducibility studies involving large groups of breast pathologist specialists in the United States have not been attempted, despite the fact that nonspecialist pathologists there remain unclear as to which several proposed classifications they should pursue. Interestingly, one reproducibility study from the United States comparing multiple classifications (23) showed that the classification advocated by the EPWG provided the best overall diagnostic accuracy and agreement among the U.S. pathologists. The level of agreement among U.S. pathologists for the EPWG classification (kappa = 0.46) was higher than that observed among 23 European pathologists who have a special interest in breast pathology for the same classification system (kappa = 0.37) (25). It was also noted that the European study recorded best overall agreement for the Van Nuys Classification (kappa = 0.42), a classification used more often in the United States. This finding may represent the increased concentration and attention required to review the set of slides according to an unfamiliar classification system but begs the question why pathologists throughout the world cannot agree on one classification scheme (Table 22.3).

CONCLUSIONS

Review of the current reproducibility studies for DCIS classifications suggest that evaluations of nuclear grade and necrosis should be included in a reproducible DCIS classification:

Nuclear grade. Nearly all these studies indicate that a two-tier system (high grade versus nonhigh grade) for nuclear grade correlates with the best diagnostic reproducibility. Some of the studies use the definitions for nuclear grade given in the Van Nuys scheme and others show the best reproducibility for a high nuclear grade (compared with low and intermediate grades), according to the nuclear criteria described in the EPWG (Holland) scheme. If a high nuclear grade is the only category that is repeatedly reproducible, then only the specific cytologic characteristics for this nuclear grade (be they according to the EPWG, Van Nuys, or a combination of both classifications) should be defined. Descriptions for any other grades should be excluded.

Necrosis. All but one of the studies discussed conclude that necrosis is most reproducibly reported when divided into a two-tier scheme (present or absent). Because this categorization was first defined in the Van Nuys scheme, then it seems logical that this definition for necrosis be used.

Review of the current reproducibility studies for DCIS classifications suggests that the following criteria are best not included in a reproducible DCIS classification.

Polarization (architectural differentiation). In studies comparing the Holland Classification as originally published and the classification adopted by the EPWG Breast Screening Program and the U.K. Breast Screening Program based on the cytodifferentiation criteria of the Holland Classification but without polarization (25,29), the reproducibility was found to be comparable. The presence or absence of an evaluation of polarization does not appear to worsen or improve overall DCIS grade assessment or reproducibility.

Architectural pattern(s). Poor reproducibility of architectural patterns is well documented because of the heterogeneity of DCIS lesions and the multiple number of patterns recognized (22,25,31).

Special-type DCIS pattern(s). The rare special-type DCIS patterns (such as micropapillary and apocrine) are independently classified in two published DCIS classification schemes (15,16) but are incorporated into others (18). There is evidence that a pure micropapillary pattern is more commonly associated with extensive disease (6,32,33). However, the poor diagnostic reproducibility of these special type lesions (6,23,34) calls into question whether reliable predictions of their clinical behavior can be made.

SUMMARY

The relevance and reproducibility of one published set of diagnostic criteria for classifying DCIS compared with an-

TABLE 22.3. A COMPARISON OF REPRODUCIBILITY STUDIES TO DATE

A critical appraisal of six modern classifications of DCIS of the breast: correlation with grade of associated invasive carcinoma (24)

Participants	Two specialists, both European
Materials	All from the study institution (academic center), specific areas on slide not marked, criteria for each classification summarized on separate cards as reference during the slide reviews
Prestudy tutoring	None
Statistical analysis	Number of disagreements as a percentage of the total
Aim	Categorization of DCIS into six possible groups:
	Architecture classification: traditional classification based on architecture (6)
	Holland Classification: EPWG classification based on cytodifferentiation (low, intermediate, and high nuclear grades) and polarization (15)
	Cytonuclear grade classification: defines nuclear cytologic features of malignant cells (low, intermediate, and high) using the same criteria as for invasive carcinoma (29)
	Extent of necrosis classification: extensive necrosis, DCIS with necrosis, and DCIS without necrosis (13)
	Van Nuys Classification: high nuclear grade, nonhigh grade with necrosis, nonhigh grade without necrosis (18)
	Nottingham Classification: pure comedo, nonpure comedo, or absent necrosis (11)
Results	The fewest disagreements were observed with the extent of necrosis classification (17.7%), followed by the Van Nuys (21.1%), the Nottingham (22.2%), the cytonuclear grade (29.4%), the Holland (30.5%), and the architecture classifications (34.4%).
	For the cytonuclear grade classification, most disagreements were seen distinguishing between low and intermediate grades (62.2%) compared with between intermediate and high grades (33.9%).
Conclusion	The Van Nuys Classification is commended for its acceptable interobserver agreement, precisely defined, simple rules, application to a small number of ducts and its significant clinical correlates.

Reproducibility of new classification schemes for the pathology of DCIS of breast (22)

Participants	All specialists, all New Zealand pathologists
Materials	Submitted from two affiliated centers, sections cut and stained centrally, specific areas of tumor (average of 9 mm^2) marked
Prestudy tutoring	45-min tutorial on the diagnostic criteria of the classifications, written information, and a set of illustrative photomicrographs
Statistical analysis	Kappa statistic (interrater)
Aim	Categorization of DCIS into three possible groups:
	Traditional classification based on architecture (30)
	ECWGBSP and U.K. Breast Screening Program scheme based on cytodifferentiation, identical to the EPWG but without polarization (29)
	Van Nuys Classification: high nuclear grade, nonhigh grade with necrosis, nonhigh grade without necrosis (18)
Results	Highest interrater kappa for Van Nuys (0.66).
	Interrater kappa for the ECWGBSP and U.K. Breast Screening Program of 0.57 with the most consistent assignment for the poorly differentiated (high-grade) category.
	Lowest kappa for the traditional classification (0.44 for one architectural pattern and 0.13 for mixed patterns).
Conclusions	The use of the Van Nuys Classification is recommended, but a better definition of necrosis for cases in the nonhigh nuclear grade group is needed.

Consistency achieved by 23 European pathologists in categorizing DCIS of the breast using five classifications (25)

Participants	All specialists, all European
Materials	Submitted from 20 participants as blocks, sections cut and stained centrally, specific areas on slide not marked, copies of published articles for each classification sent to participants
Prestudy tutoring	None
Statistical analysis	Kappa statistic (interrater), weighted for three-way classifications
Aim	Categorized DCIS into five possible groups:
	EPWG classification based on cytodifferentiation (low, intermediate, and high nuclear grades) and polarization (15)
	ECWGBSP and U.K. Breast Screening Program scheme based on cytodifferentiation, identical to the EPWG, but without polarization (29)
	Adapted ECWGBSP and U.K. Breast Screening Program, two nuclear categories (high, as defined by EPWG, and other) but no polarization
	Van Nuys, high nuclear grade, nonhigh nuclear grade with necrosis, nonhigh nuclear grade without necrosis (18)
	Pure comedo, nonpure comedo necrosis, or absent (11)

(continues)

TABLE 22.3. *CONTINUED*

Results	Highest interrater kappa for Van Nuys (0.42).
	Comparable kappa for EPWG with and without assessing polarization (0.37 and 0.35).
	Lowest kappa for the intermediate nuclear grades.
	Good reproducibility for presence or absence of necrosis as long as a comedo pattern did not need to be recognized.
Conclusions	The best reproducibility was found for a two-tier nuclear grade system (high and low) with necrosis (as long as a comedo pattern did not have to be recognized).
	Pathologists' agreement with experts and reproducibility of Breast DCIS classification schemes (23)
Participants	Nonspecialist pathologists (7) from the U.S. and expert pathologists (3) from the U.S. and Europe
Materials	All from the study institution (academic center), specific areas on slide not marked, copies of published articles for each classification sent to participants, slide recirculation to assess intrarater agreement
Prestudy tutoring	None
Statistical analysis	Kappa statistic (inter- and intrarater)
	Assessed both diagnostic reproducibility (among the nonexperts) and diagnostic accuracy (nonexperts compared with experts)
Aim	Categorized DCIS into three possible groups:
	EPWG classification based on cytodifferentiation (low, intermediate, and high nuclear grades) and polarization (15)
	Van Nuys, high nuclear grade, nonhigh grade with necrosis, nonhigh grade without necrosis (18)
	Modified Lagios, three-tier nuclear grade (low, intermediate, and high) and necrosis (extensive, focal, absent) scheme (16)
Results	Best diagnostic reproducibility overall, using EPWG (kappa = 0.49).
	Best accuracy for final DCIS and nuclear grade according to EPWG (kappas of 0.53 and 0.49, respectively).
	Best accuracy for intermediate nuclear grade using EPWG and Modified Lagios but for high nuclear grade using Van Nuys.
	Most accurate interpretation of necrosis using Van Nuys (present or absent) rather than the Modified Lagios (extensive, focal, absent) (kappas of 0.59 and 0.45, respectively) but comparable reproducibility.
	Consistently high intrarater reproducibility compared with interrater reproducibility.
Conclusion	Final DCIS grade and nuclear grade according to EPWG and presence or absence of necrosis according to Van Nuys are the most reproducible criteria.
	Consistency in the observation of features used to classify DCIS of the breast (1)
Participants	Specialists and nonspecialists, all European
Materials	Submitted by the participants as unstained sections and stained centrally, specific areas on slide not marked
Prestudy tutoring	Criteria outlined and photomicrographs sent to the participants
Statistical analysis	Kappa statistic (inter- and intrarater)
Aim	Categorized DCIS into four possible groups:
	DCIS heterogeneity
	ECWGBSP and U.K. Breast Screening Program scheme based on cytodifferentiation, identical to that of the EPWG, but without polarization (29)
	Necrosis (absent, focal/punctate, or extensive) according to the Consensus classification (14)
	Derivation of the Van Nuys score (by the project coordinator) using the designated nuclear grades and amount of necrosis
Results	Agreement for cytologic grade in three categories (kappa = 0.47).
	Agreement for necrosis in three categories (kappa = 0.57).
	Agreement for Van Nuys scheme (kappa = 0.48).
	Similar diagnostic agreement for specialists and nonspecialists.
	Moderate intrarater agreement for nuclear grade and necrosis.
Conclusions	Better agreement for a three-tier scheme of necrosis than a three-tier scheme of nuclear grade.
	Comparable agreement for nonspecialists as specialists.

DCIS, ductal carcinoma in situ; EPWG, European Pathologists Working Group; ECWGBSP, European Commission Working Group on Breast Screening Pathology.

other published set remain a serious issue. To ensure optimal treatment for a patient with DCIS, the histologic criteria must be diagnostically reproducible among pathologists with and without expertise in breast pathology interpretation before studies attempting to predict tumor recurrence rates can be meaningful (35). The superior reproducibility of nuclear grade and necrosis, compared with other proposed criteria in DCIS classifications, has now been established. Cooperation of pathologist's worldwide is needed to establish one internationally accepted set of simple and clear definitions, with few subcategories, all tested for reproducibility among pathologists with and without expertise in breast pathology interpretation. This may be facilitated by slide study sets, photomicrographs, or digitized images on the Internet in addition to the information provided in the standard publication format. However, it may be that the importance of reproducible histologic criteria in predicting tumor progression and behavior is surpassed by the accurate and standardized pathologic assessment of excised margin status and lesion size in conjunction with the radiologic and clinical factors.

REFERENCES

1. Douglas-Jones A, Morgan JM, Appleton MAC, et al. Consistency in the observation of features used to classify duct carcinoma in situ (DCIS) of the breast. *J Clin Pathol* 2000;53:596– 602.
2. Choi W, Parker B, Pierce J, et al. Regional differences in the incidence and treatment of carcinoma in situ of the breast. *Cancer Epidemiol Biomarkers Prev* 1996;4:317–320.
3. Ernster V, Barclay J, Kerlikowske K, et al. Incidence of and treatment for ductal carcinoma in situ of the breast. *JAMA* 1996;12:913–918.
4. Silverstein MJ, Lagios MD, Craig PH, et al. A prognostic index for ductal carcinoma-in-situ. *Cancer* 1996;77:2267–2274.
5. Holland R, Hendriks J. Microcalcifications associated with ductal carcinoma in situ: mammographic-pathologic correlation. *Semin Diagn Pathol* 1994;11:181–192.
6. Bellamy C, McDonald C, Salter D, et al. Non-invasive ductal carcinoma of the breast. The relevance of histologic categorization. *Hum Pathol* 1993;24:16–23.
7. Bobrow L, Happerfield L, Gregory WM, et al. The classification of ductal carcinoma in situ and its association with biological markers. *Semin Diagn Pathol* 1994;11:199–207.
8. Bur M, Zimarowski M, Schnitt S, et al. Estrogen receptor immunohisto-chemistry in carcinoma in situ of the breast. *Cancer* 1992;69:1174–1181.
9. Killeen J, Namiki H. DNA analysis of ductal carcinoma in situ of the breast. A comparison with histological features. *Cancer* 1991;68:2602–2607.
10. Meyer J. Cell kinetics of histologic variants of in situ breast carcinoma. *Breast Cancer Res Treat* 1986;7:171–180.
11. Poller D, Silverstein M, Galea M, et al. Ductal carcinoma in situ of the breast: a proposal for a new simplified histological classification association between cellular proliferation and c-erbB-2 protein expression. *Mod Pathol* 1994;7:257–262.
12. Zafrani B, Leroyer A, Fourquet A, et al. Mammographically-detected ductal in situ carcinoma of the breast analyzed with a new classification. A study of 127 cases: correlation with estrogen and progesterone receptors, p53 and c-erb-B2 proteins and proliferative activity. *Semin Diagn Pathol* 1994;11:208–214.
13. Douglas-Jones AG, Schmid KW, Bier B, et al. Expression in duct carcinoma in situ of the breast. *Hum Pathol* 1995;26:217–222.
14. Consensus Statement; Consensus Conference on the Classification of Ductal Carcinoma in Situ. Cancer 1997;80:1798–1802.
15. Holland R, Peterse J, Millis R, et al. Ductal carcinoma in situ: a proposal for a new classification. *Semin Diagn Pathol* 1994;11:167–180.
16. Scott MA, Lagios MD, Axelsson K, et al. Ductal carcinoma in situ of the breast: reproducibility of histological subtype analysis. *Hum Pathol* 1997;28:967–973.
17. Tavassoli FA, Man Y. Morphofunctional features of intraductal hyperplasia, atypical intraductal hyperplasia, and various grades of intraductal carcinoma. *Breast J* 1995;1:155–162.
18. Silverstein M, Poller D, Waisman J, et al. Prognostic classification of breast ductal carcinoma-in-situ. *Lancet* 1995;345:1154– 1157.
19. Sneige N, Lagios M, Schwarting R, et al. Interobserver reproducibility of the Lagios nuclear grading system for ductal carcinoma in situ. *Hum Pathol* 1999;30:257–262.
20. Wells WA, Carney PA, Eliassen MS, et al. Statewide study of diagnostic agreement in breast pathology. *J Natl Cancer Inst* 1998;90:142–145.
21. Schnitt S, Connolly J, Tavassoli F, et al. Interobserver reproducibility in the diagnosis of ductal proliferative breast lesions using standardized criteria. *Am J Surg Pathol* 1992;16:1131–1143.
22. Bethwaite P, Smith N, Delahunt B, et al. Reproducibility of new classification schemes for the pathology of ductal carcinoma in situ of the breast. *J Clin Pathol* 1998;51:450–454.
23. Wells WA, Carney PA, Eliassen MS, et al. Pathologists' agreement with experts and reproducibility of breast ductal carcinoma in situ classification schemes. *Am J Surg Pathol* 2000;24:651– 659.
24. Douglas-Jones AG, Gupta SK, Attanoos RL, et al. A critical appraisal of six modern classifications of ductal carcinoma in situ of the breast (DCIS): correlation with grade and associated invasive carcinoma. *Histopathology* 1996;29:397–409.
25. Sloane JP, Amendocira I, Apostolikas N, et al. Consistency achieved by 23 European pathologists in categorizing ductal carcinoma in situ of the breast using five classifications. *Hum Pathol* 1998;29:1056–1062.
26. Wells WA, Carney PA, Eliassen MS, et al. Pathologists' agreement with experts and reproducibility of breast ductal carcinoma in situ classification schemes (response to letter to the editor). *Am J Surg Pathol* 2001;25(4):543–545.
27. Altman D. *Practical statistics for medical research*. London, Glasgow, New York, Tokyo, Melbourne, Madras: Chapman and Hall, 1991.
28. Landis JR, Koch GG. The measurement of observer agreement for categorical data. *Biometrics* 1977;33:159–174.
29. National Coordinating Group for Breast Screening Pathology. Pathology reporting in breast cancer screening. In: 2nd ed. Sheffield: NHSBSP Publications, 1995:23–27.
30. Rogers L. Carcinoma-in-situ. In: Page D, T A, eds. *Diagnostic histopathology of the breast*. Edinburgh: Churchill-Livingstone, 1987:157–192.
31. Sloane J, Ellman R, Anderson T, et al. U.K. National Coordinating Group for Breast Screening Pathology. *Eur J Cancer* 1994;30A:1414–1419.
32. Patchefsky A, Schwartz G, Finkelstein SD. Heterogeneity of intraductal carcinoma of the breast. *Cancer* 1989;63:731–741.
33. Lennington W, Jensen R, Dalton LW, et al. Ductal carcinoma in situ of the breast. Heterogeneity of individual lesions. *Cancer* 1994;73:118–124.
34. O'Malley FP, Page DL, Nelson EH, et al. Ductal carcinoma in situ of breast with apocrine cytology: definition of a borderline category. *Hum Pathol* 1994;25:164–168.
35. Badve S, A'hern RP, Ward AM, et al. Prediction of local recurrence of ductal carcinoma in situ of the breast using five histological classifications: a comparative study with long follow-up. *Hum Pathol* 1998;29:915–923.

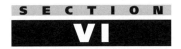

TREATMENT OF DUCTAL
CARCINOMA IN SITU

23

SURGICAL OVERVIEW OF THE TREATMENT OF DUCTAL CARCINOMA IN SITU

MONICA MORROW
ERIKA BRINKMANN

The appropriate local therapy for ductal carcinoma in situ (DCIS) is controversial, and total mastectomy, excision and radiation therapy, and excision alone have all been advocated as management strategies. This wide variety of treatment options results from uncertainty about the natural history of DCIS, with those who regard the disease as an obligate precursor of malignancy advocating traditional cancer treatments and those who believe that not all DCIS will progress to invasive carcinoma favoring a policy of excision and observation in selected cases. Evaluation of the results of different local therapies is complicated by changes in the presentation of DCIS over time and differences in the extent of the mammographic and pathologic evaluation of DCIS. Additionally, most studies are retrospective and involve small numbers of nonuniformly treated patients followed for limited periods. These problems make comparisons between patients treated in different ways difficult. This chapter reviews the data on the local therapy of DCIS and describes our approach to patient assessment and treatment.

MASTECTOMY

Mastectomy is a curative treatment for approximately 98% of patients with DCIS, whether gross or nonpalpable, and a therapy for which all patients are eligible (1–8). As illustrated in Table 23.1, most of the data on the efficacy of mastectomy come from patients with clinically evident DCIS. Despite the fact that clinically evident DCIS might be more biologically aggressive than its mammographic counterpart, recurrences after mastectomy are rare. Recurrent carcinoma after a mastectomy for DCIS may be owing to two mechanisms. First, undetected invasive carcinoma may be present at the time of the mastectomy. This is particularly true in older reports in which histologic sampling of the mastectomy specimen was often limited when compared with current standards. Gillis et al. (9) reported that 28% of 50 lesions diagnosed as DCIS were found to contain invasion when additional sections were taken. In a similar study, Brown et al. (10) found that 15% of 52 cases diagnosed as DCIS contained invasive carcinoma. More recently, the central pathology review for the National Surgical Adjuvant Breast Project (NSABP) DCIS protocol B-17 identified only five of 818 randomized cases in which unrecognized invasive carcinoma was present, suggesting that this is a less frequent problem today (11).

The size of the surgical biopsy specimen that is taken will also influence the likelihood of identifying invasive carcinoma in patients initially diagnosed with DCIS. Rosen et al. (12) identified invasive carcinoma in only three of 53 (6%) mastectomy specimens after an excisional biopsy demonstrating intraductal carcinoma. In contrast, approximately 10% to 20% of patients diagnosed by core biopsy as having DCIS are found to have invasive carcinoma (13). The likelihood of invasive carcinoma being present increases as the size of the intraductal carcinoma increases (14,15), and occult invasion is also seen more frequently in cases of high-grade (comedo) DCIS (14). These findings also suggest that a small proportion of patients with DCIS who undergo breast-conserving therapy will be understaged owing to the failure to identify occult foci of invasive carcinoma, and more accurate staging may be responsible for some of the differences in recurrence and survival seen in patients undergoing mastectomy and those treated with breast conservation. The ability to identify clinically occult foci of invasive carcinoma is one of the advantages of the treatment of DCIS by mastectomy.

In general, patients with DCIS found to have invasive carcinoma in mastectomy specimens were excluded from the series reported in Table 23.1. However, the data discussed earlier indicate that unrecognized or unsampled invasive carcinoma in patients with DCIS has the potential to explain the 1% to 2% failure rate seen after mastectomy.

TABLE 23.1. RESULTS OF TREATMENT OF DCIS WITH SIMPLE MASTECTOMY

Study	Years	Follow-Up	No. of Patients	% Nonpalpable	No.
Sunshine et al. (1)	1960–1972	10 yr	74	0	4
Von Rueden & Wilson (2)	1960–1981	?	45	9	0
Ashikari et al. (3)	1965–1975	11 yr	92	0	0
Schuh et al. (4)	1965–1984	5.5 yr	51	33	1
Kinne et al. (5)	1970–1976	11.5 yr	101	59	1
Arnesson et al. (38)	1978–1984	77 mo	28	100	0
Ward et al. (7)	1979–1983	10 yr	123	20	1
Silverstein (Chapter 29)	1979–2000	81 mo	326	76	2

An additional explanation for recurrent carcinoma after a mastectomy for DCIS is incomplete removal of the breast tissue. Residual breast tissue has the potential to develop carcinoma, either invasive or intraductal, which would be manifest as recurrence. The failure of recurrence rates after mastectomy to increase with longer follow-up intervals suggests that most cases of recurrence are owing to undiagnosed invasive carcinoma rather than the malignant transformation of residual breast tissue.

Until recently, mastectomy was the most common treatment for DCIS in the United States. Analysis of DCIS treatment data collected by the National Cancer Institute's Surveillance, Epidemiology and End Results Program between 1983 and 1992 revealed a significant decline in the proportion of DCIS cases treated by mastectomy in the United States (from 71% to 43.8%) and an increase in those treated by lumpectomy (from 25.6% to 53.3%) (16). Treatment patterns for DCIS varied widely by geographic region. In 1992, 57.7% of cases of DCIS in New Mexico but only 28.8% of cases in Connecticut were treated with mastectomy.

BREAST-CONSERVING THERAPY

Various factors have stimulated interest in the treatment of DCIS with less than total mastectomy. These include the large increase in the number of clinically occult cases of DCIS being identified by screening mammography, uncertainty regarding the natural history of mammographically detected DCIS, and the acceptance of breast-conserving therapy for the treatment of invasive carcinoma.

BREAST CONSERVATION WITH EXCISION AND RADIATION THERAPY

The acceptance of breast-conserving therapy as a treatment for invasive carcinoma has led to the use of excision and radiation therapy to treat DCIS. No randomized trial has directly compared the treatment of DCIS by mastectomy with treatment by excision and radiation therapy, and such a trial is unlikely to be done. The assumption that because these two treatments have been repeatedly shown to result in equal survival for patients with invasive carcinoma, the same will be true for patients with DCIS, is flawed because of the fundamental difference between invasive carcinoma and DCIS. In patients with invasive carcinoma, the risk of metastatic disease is present at the time of diagnosis and in most cases is not altered by local recurrence in the breast. In DCIS, the risk of metastases at the time of diagnosis is negligible, and an invasive local recurrence carries with it the risk of increased breast cancer mortality. The appropriateness of excision and radiation therapy as a treatment for DCIS should be determined by the incidence of invasive recurrence in the breast and the results of salvage therapy.

Several authors have reported their experiences with excision and radiation therapy for the treatment of DCIS, and these reports are summarized in Table 23.2 (17–23). Solin et al. (23) reported the results of 268 women with 270 breasts treated with excision and radiation therapy and followed for a median of 10.3 years. Gross excision of the tumor was carried out in all cases, but margin status was unknown in 120 cases and only 15% of patients underwent re-excision. The median whole-breast dose of radiation was 50 Gy, and 65% of patients received a boost to the primary tumor site. Forty-five local failures were observed, and the 15-year actuarial rate of local failure was 19%. The median time to local failure was 5.2 years, but 14% of the recurrences were seen after 10 years of follow-up. Half of the local recurrences were invasive carcinoma and the 15-year cause-specific survival rate was 96%. However, a separate analysis of 42 patients who recurred demonstrated a 5-year actuarial cause-specific survival rate of 85% for this subgroup of patients (24). This study is noteworthy for the large number of patients and the long duration of follow-up. Although many of the surgical excisions would not be considered adequate by today's standards, the 15-year cause-specific mortality rate for the entire group was low, supporting the idea that excision and radiation therapy are safe treatment.

Solin et al. (25) performed a separate analysis of 110 patients with clinically occult, mammographically detected tumors. The 10-year actuarial rate of local recurrence in this

TABLE 23.2. RESULTS OF TREATMENT OF DUCTAL CARCINOMA IN SITU BY EXCISION AND IRRADIATION

Study	No. of Patients	Follow-Up (mo)	% Recurrence	% Invasive
McCormick et al. (17)	54	36[a]	18	30
Silverstein (Chapter 29)	237	106[a]	12/20 (5-/10-yr actuarial)	46
Silverstein et al. (43)	213	81[a]	17	51
Ray et al. (19)	56	67[a]	9	20
Hiramatsu et al. (20)	76	74[b]	9	57
Fisher et al. (B-06) (21)	27	83[a]	7	50
Stotter et al. (22)	42	92[b]	9	100
Solin et al. (23)	268	130[b]	19 (15-yr actuarial)	53
Fisher et al. (B-17) (46)	411	90[a]	11	36
Julien et al. (EORTC) (49)	502	51[b]	11	45

[a] Mean.
[b] Median.
EORTC, European Organization for Research and Treatment of Cancer.

series was 14%, and the median interval to recurrence was 5 years. These figures do not differ significantly from those seen in their larger series, which included patients with both clinically evident and mammographically detected DCIS.

BREAST CONSERVATION WITH EXCISION ALONE

Natural History of Ductal Carcinoma in Situ

Data from the Surveillance Epidemiology and End Results Program demonstrate that although age-adjusted DCIS incidence rates increased 3.9% annually from 1973 to 1983, there was a 17.5% annual rate of increase between 1983 and 1992 (26). This dramatic increase in the incidence (or perhaps detection) of DCIS corresponds to an increased use of screening mammography and has raised questions about the biologic potential of mammographic DCIS to progress to invasive carcinoma because a corresponding increase in the incidence of invasive carcinoma has not been observed. To address this question, Gapstur et al. (27) compared risk factors for DCIS and invasive breast cancer in a cohort of 37,105 women followed for 9 years in which 1,240 incident breast cancers occurred. No differences in risk factors or the magnitude of risk conveyed by these factors were observed between invasive carcinoma and DCIS. This suggests that both entities are part of the same biologic process.

A major limitation in the attempt to define treatment options for the patient with DCIS is our lack of knowledge of the natural history of the disease. However, autopsy data and information from patients with DCIS who were misdiagnosed as having benign disease provide some information about the biologic potential of DCIS. Autopsy studies of women without breast cancer show significant variation in the incidence of unsuspected DCIS. Bartow et al. (28) identified only one case of DCIS in a series of 519 autopsies,

which included 229 white women, 156 Hispanic women, and 134 American Indian women. Alpers and Wellings (29) noted DCIS in 6% of 185 breasts from random autopsies, and Nielson et al. (30) reported a 14% incidence of DCIS at autopsy. A much higher incidence of DCIS was noted in the contralateral breast of women with breast cancer (29,30). These data suggest that not all DCIS will progress to invasive carcinoma within a woman's lifetime. Further support for this idea comes from studies of women initially diagnosed as having benign breast disease and found on subsequent pathology review to have DCIS. These studies antedate the use of modern mammography, and no attempt was made to assess margin status, so the completeness of excision remains uncertain. Page et al. (31,32) identified 25 such cases in a review of 11,760 breast biopsies. After 15 years of follow-up, seven women had developed invasive carcinoma at a mean of 6.1 years from the time of biopsy. This incidence of carcinoma represents a relative risk of 11 compared with age-matched controls. A subsequent report of this study with the follow-up period extended to a median of 24 years demonstrated that the relative risk of cancer development remained constant and was 9 at 30 years (32). In a similar study, Betsill et al. (33) described 25 women with untreated DCIS, with complete follow-up available for only ten of the women. At an average follow-up of 21.6 years, seven patients had developed invasive carcinoma. In both reports, all the carcinomas were in the same breast in which the biopsy showed DCIS and usually in the same quadrant. A much lower relative risk of carcinoma development was noted by Eusebi et al. (34). They reported 80 cases of DCIS, only two of which were high grade, which were followed for a mean of 17.5 years. Eleven patients developed invasive carcinoma, and five had recurrent DCIS for a total recurrence rate of 20%. The relative risk of invasive carcinoma was twice that of the general population. In all these studies, most cases were low-grade, noncomedo lesions, representing one extreme of the histologic spectrum of DCIS. However, the results of these clinical studies support the findings of the autopsy reports that not all DCIS will progress to invasive carcinoma.

Results of Treatment with Excision Alone

Several investigators examined the use of excision alone as a treatment for DCIS (6,11,21,35–40). Most of these studies suggest that patients with large, high-grade DCIS lesions are poor candidates for treatment with excision alone. In most studies of treatment with excision alone, patients have been highly selected, usually based on small lesion size and low histologic grade or absence of comedonecrosis. Schwartz et al. (41) identified only 70 patients between 1978 and 1990 for whom excision alone was appropriate, whereas Silverstein et al. (8) found that approximately one-third of 333 patients in their series underwent excision alone. Solin et al. (25) retrospectively applied criteria for treatment with excision alone to a group of 110 patients with mammographically detected DCIS treated with excision and radiation therapy and found only 21 suitable patients.

Recurrence rates after excision alone range from 13% to 43% and are highly dependent on the patient selection criteria employed, method used to calculate the recurrence rate, and length of follow-up (Table 23.3). In general, higher rates of local failure are observed in studies that include clinically evident DCIS and those with longer follow-up periods. Gallagher et al. (39) reported 17 patients treated with excision alone, with a 38% recurrence rate at a median follow-up of 60 months. However, one-half of the patients followed for more than 9 years (n = 8) developed local failure. Fisher et al. (21) reported 21 patients with DCIS treated with local excision alone as part of NSABP protocol B-06. These patients were originally diagnosed as having invasive cancer and later were reclassified as having DCIS, and

all but one had palpable tumors. At a mean follow-up of 83 months, a 43% breast recurrence rate was noted, similar to that reported by Gallagher et al. (39).

More recent studies (18,36,42) using more highly selected patients have reported lower rates of local failure. In general, the patients in these studies were selected based on small tumor size and/or low histologic grade.

Lagios (42) (see also Chapter 25) reported 79 patients with DCIS 25 mm or smaller (mean size: 7 mm) who were treated with excision alone. At a median follow-up of 130 months, 16 patients (20%) had a recurrence in the breast, two of whom, however, had a recurrence after 17 years of follow-up, suggesting the possibility that these were new cancers rather than recurrences. Most of the recurrences in the series of Lagios occurred in patients with high-grade DCIS. The 15-year actuarial recurrence rate for patients with nuclear grade 1 or 2 lesions was 8%, whereas it was 35% for patients with nuclear grade 3 DCIS. In a similar study, Schwartz et al. (36,41) (Chapter 26) observed a recurrence rate of 14% in 191 women with 194 DCIS lesions. The patients were followed up for a median of 53 months after excision alone. Sixteen percent of these patients had DCIS detected as an incidental finding, and none of these patients had a recurrence.

More recently, Silverstein et al. (43) suggested that all DCIS lesions were appropriate for treatment with excision alone, provided that a margin of normal breast tissue of 1 cm or more was obtained in all directions. This was based on a retrospective study of 469 patients who had been treated with breast-conserving surgery with or without postoperative radiation therapy. At 8 years of follow-up, no difference in the incidence of local recurrence between patients treated with excision alone and those treated with excision and radiation therapy was seen if a margin width was greater than 1 cm. However, lesions treated with excision alone

TABLE 23.3. RESULTS OF TREATMENT OF DUCTAL CARCINOMA IN SITU BY EXCISION ALONE

Study	No. of Patients	Follow-Up (mo)	% Recurrence	% Invasion
Carpenter et al. (35)	28	38[a]	18	20
Schwartz (Chapter 26)	256	76[a]	24/41 (5-/10-yr actuarial)	37
Baird et al. (37)	30	43[a]	13	25
Silverstein (Chapter 29)	346	70[a]	19/28 (5-/10-yr actuarial)	41
Silverstein et al. (43)	256	81[a]	15	42
Arnesson (89)	169	80[b]	16/22 (5-/10-yr actuarial)	36
Fisher et al. (B-06) (21)	21	83[a]	43	55
Gallagher et al. (39)	13	100[b]	38	60
Millis & Thynne (40)	9	120[a]	22	100
Lagios (Chapter 25)	79	130[b]	18 (15-yr actuarial)	56
Fisher et al. (B-17) (46)	403	90[a]	26	51
Julien et al. (EORTC) (49)	500	51[b]	17	48

[a] Mean.
[b] Median.
EORTC, European Organization for Research and Treatment of Cancer.

were significantly smaller than those treated with radiation therapy. Perhaps more important, treatment with excision alone was more frequent in the later years of the study, raising the possibility that improvements in mammography and pathologic evaluation may be responsible for some of the outcomes. This is well illustrated in the study of Hiramatsu et al. (44), in which local failure rates of patients treated with excision and radiation therapy from 1976 to 1985 and 1986 to 1990 were compared. The incidence of local failure decreased from 12% to 2% at 6.5 years, although the dose of radiation did not change. This strongly suggests that findings from retrospective studies in which patients are accrued over long periods cannot be regarded as definitive but should serve as the basis of prospective studies.

Breast recurrences after the treatment of DCIS with excision alone are evenly divided between invasive carcinoma and recurrent DCIS in most reports (Table 23.3). A notable exception is the report of Schwartz et al. (36), in which only 24% of breast recurrences were invasive carcinoma in their initial report (41). This has increased and in Chapter 26, Schwartz reports an invasive recurrence rate of 37% of 256 cases. This is now similar to other investigators.

The likelihood of invasive recurrence is the critical determinant of outcome in DCIS because recurrent intraductal carcinoma carries no risk of breast cancer mortality. Whether the high incidence of noninvasive recurrence in the study of Schwartz et al. was owing to aggressive mammographic surveillance or the successful identification of a subset of patients with DCIS of low malignant potential is uncertain. It has been suggested that invasive recurrences only occur in cases of high-grade DCIS (45). Further confirmation of this observation would provide a compelling argument for the treatment of low-grade DCIS with excision alone.

Randomized Trials of Breast Conservation

Data from three prospective, randomized trials are available to address the issue of the benefit of radiation therapy in the treatment of DCIS. As previously mentioned, NSABP protocol B-06 was designed to evaluate the local therapy of invasive carcinoma (21). Seventy-eight patients with DCIS alone were identified on review of pathologic material. At a mean follow-up of 83 months, no local failures were observed in the 28 patients treated with mastectomy compared with a 7% (two of 27) local failure rate in the patients treated with radiation therapy and a 43% (nine of 21) failure rate in patients treated with lumpectomy alone.

The NSABP also reported the results of B-17, a trial specifically designed to evaluate the role of radiation therapy in DCIS (11,46). In this study, 818 patients were randomized to excision alone or excision plus 5,000 cGy radiation to the breast. Histologically negative margins, defined as tumor-filled ducts not touching inked surfaces, were required, and only 9% of the irradiated patients received a boost dose

to the tumor bed. Eighty percent of the patients in the study had mammographically detected tumors. At a mean follow-up of 90 months, there was a 59% reduction in the annual incidence of ipsilateral breast cancer recurrence in the radiation therapy group. Although the incidence of both invasive and intraductal breast recurrence was reduced with radiation therapy, the main benefit was in reducing invasive recurrences: although the rate of noninvasive cancer was reduced by 47%, the rate of invasive cancer was decreased by 71%. At 8 years of follow-up, the recurrence rate of DCIS was reduced from 13.4% to 8.2% ($p = 0.007$) with the addition of radiation therapy and the incidence of invasive breast recurrence was reduced from 13.4% to 3.9% ($p < 0.0001$). However, there was no significant difference in the overall survival rate between the groups at 8 years, with a 94% survival rate in the lumpectomy group and a 95% survival rate in the lumpectomy plus radiation group. A subsequent pathologic analysis of 623 of the patients enrolled in the study assessed the relationship between pathologic variables and breast cancer recurrence at 8-years of follow-up in an effort to identify subgroups of women who did not benefit from radiation therapy and, conversely, women who were at increased risk of breast cancer recurrence (47). Overall, the frequency of local failure rate was reduced from 31% to 13% ($p = 0.0001$) with radiation therapy. The only pathologic feature shown to be an independent risk factor for breast cancer recurrence was moderate to marked comedonecrosis. A subgroup of patients who did not benefit from radiation therapy could not be identified in this study. For the most favorable subgroup, those with absent or slight comedonecrosis and negative margins, the absolute benefit of radiation therapy was a 7% reduction in recurrence at 8 years. Based on these findings, the authors concluded that the use of radiation therapy is appropriate for all patients with intraductal carcinoma, although the magnitude of benefit will vary with the absolute risk of recurrence.

The results of the NSABP study have been criticized as being inadequate to address the issue of whether some patients with DCIS do not require radiation therapy (48) owing to failure to evaluate specimens with the detailed pathologic and mammographic techniques in use today to determine the size of a lesion and the completeness of resection. Although this is true, this randomized study clearly demonstrates that when DCIS is evaluated using standard mammographic and pathologic techniques available in any hospital, the use of radiation therapy will reduce the risk of a breast recurrence.

The third and most recent prospective, randomized study to address the benefit of radiation therapy was the European Organization for Research and Treatment of Cancer trial 10853 (49). In this study, 1,010 women with DCIS of 5 cm or less were treated with excision to negative margins and randomized to no further treatment or to whole-breast irradiation (50 Gy over 5 weeks). The 4-year, relapse-free survival rate was 84% in the group treated with excision alone and 91% in the group treated with excision plus radiation therapy ($p = 0.005$). Risk reduction for recurrent DCIS was 35%, and for recurrent invasive tumor, it was 40%. The results of this trial confirm the findings of NS-ABP B-17 that there is a benefit from radiation therapy in DCIS but fail to support a differential effect on invasive recurrence.

MANAGEMENT OF THE AXILLA

Regardless of whether mastectomy or breast conservation is chosen as a local therapy, axillary dissection is not indicated. The risk of axillary metastases is less than 4% in most series and in recent studies of mammographically detected DCIS approaches zero (Table 23.4) (2,3,18,23,50,51). There is little rationale for performing axillary dissection in patients undergoing breast-conserving surgery. The risk of occult invasion and associated axillary metastases is highest in patients with gross DCIS and those with large and high-grade lesions (14). These patients frequently require mastectomy for complete lesion removal. Complete removal of the axillary tail of the breast often results in the removal of some of the low axillary nodes, providing reassurance that they are not involved with tumor. Because the incidence of nodal metastases is low even with microinvasive carcinoma, we do not perform a formal axillary dissection for any patients with DCIS.

Recently, lymphatic mapping and sentinel lymph node biopsy have been advocated by some centers for either all patients with DCIS (52–57) or selected cases in which microinvasion is more likely to be present. In a study by Pendas et al. (53), 87 patients diagnosed with DCIS underwent sentinel lymph node biopsy, with lymph nodes evaluated by serial sectioning, hematoxylin and eosin staining, and cytokeratin immunohistochemical staining. Five of 87 patients (6%) had metastatic disease present in the sentinel lymph nodes. Three of the patients with positive sentinel lymph nodes were positive by cytokeratin immunohistochemical staining alone. Klauber-DeMore et al. (52) performed sentinel lymph node biopsy on 76 patients with DCIS and examined the lymph nodes by serial sectioning, hematoxylin and eosin staining, and cytokeratin immunohistochemical staining. Nine of the 76 patients (12%) had sentinel lymph nodes positive for metastases. These data would suggest that a higher rate of occult invasive disease with axillary metastases is present in cases diagnosed as DCIS than was previously realized. However, findings of axillary metastases in as many as 12% of patients with DCIS are not compatible with the known risks of breast cancer death at 10 years after breast conservation (2% to 3%) and mastectomy (1% to 2%) for the treatment of DCIS (58).

Studies have demonstrated that the diagnosis of DCIS by core needle biopsy underestimates the presence of invasive disease in 20% to 29% of cases (59,60). We developed selection criteria for lymphatic mapping and sentinel lymph node biopsy for cases of DCIS diagnosed by core needle biopsy. DCIS in which invasion is found tends to have predictable histologic features, with high nuclear grade, comedonecrosis, and often to occur in a background of altered, desmoplastic stroma or lymphocytic infiltration (61). In addition, larger, palpable DCIS lesions are likely to contain foci of invasion. For this reason, we perform sentinel lymph node biopsy for large, high-grade DCIS lesions that require mastectomy to encompass the entire lesion and in cases of gross DCIS.

TAMOXIFEN

The NSABP P-1 chemoprevention trial demonstrated that tamoxifen reduced the risk of development of invasive breast cancer by 49% and of noninvasive breast cancer by 50% in women at increased risk of the disease (62). Based on this evidence, it seemed likely that tamoxifen would reduce the risk of invasive breast cancer and recurrent DCIS in patients diagnosed with DCIS.

NSABP B-24 was a randomized, controlled trial to determine whether lumpectomy, radiation therapy, and tamoxifen were of greater benefit than lumpectomy and radiation therapy alone for the treatment of DCIS (63). In this study, 1,804 patients with DCIS treated with breast-conserving surgery and radiation therapy were randomized to receive either tamoxifen (20 mg daily) or placebo for 5 years.

TABLE 23.4. AXILLARY NODE METASTASES IN DUCTAL CARCINOMA IN SITU

Study	Year	No. of Patients	% Metastases
Ashikari et al. (3)	1971	113	0.9
Baker (BCDDP) (51)	1979	212	1.0
Von Reuden & Wilson (2)	1984	32	0
Solin et al. (23)	1995	86	0
Winchester et al. (NCDB) (50)	1995	10,946	3.7
Silverstein (Chapter 29)	2002	427	0.5

BCDDP, Breast Cancer Diagnosis and Demonstration Project; NCDB, National Cancer Data Base.

Margins were positive for DCIS in 16% of enrolled patients. After a median follow-up of 74 months, patients who had taken tamoxifen had a lower incidence of total breast cancer events at 5 years than their counterparts (8.2% versus 13.4%, $p = 0.0009$). Breast cancer events were defined as ipsilateral disease, contralateral disease, or metastases. A reduced rate of ipsilateral breast cancer in the tamoxifen group was apparent only for invasive tumors, with a 44% reduction over the placebo group. This benefit was evident in the subgroups of women with positive margins and those with comedonecrosis. The cumulative incidence of all contralateral breast tumors occurring at 5 years (as first events) was 2.0% in the tamoxifen group and 3.4% in the placebo group.

Congruent with the NSABP P-1 results, tamoxifen reduces the risk of breast cancer events in women with DCIS. The magnitude of benefit is relatively small and is greater in women treated with breast-conserving surgery than in those treated with mastectomy. In considering the use of tamoxifen in individual patients with DCIS, its benefits must be carefully weighed against its risks, particularly in postmenopausal women at risk of thromboembolic events and endometrial cancer.

PROGNOSTIC CLASSIFICATIONS FOR DUCTAL CARCINOMA IN SITU

The available data clearly indicate that the term DCIS encompasses a heterogeneous group of lesions that vary in their presentation, histologic characteristics, and, most important, the potential to progress to invasive carcinoma. The ideal classification system for DCIS would separate those lesions that will become invasive carcinoma from those destined to remain as DCIS because recurrent or persistent DCIS poses no threat to the patient. DCIS lesions have been shown to vary in the expression of hormone receptors (64), the c-erbB-2 oncogene (64–66), the bcl-2 gene (67), and markers of proliferation (64–66). However, clinical studies to indicate that any of these features correlate with the risk of development of invasive carcinoma are lacking.

In the absence of a marker predictive of the risk of progression to invasive carcinoma, markers that predict the risk of recurrence after local therapy have been proposed. Histologic subtype and grade of DCIS have been the most widely studied predictive factors for recurrence. The use of histologic subtyping is complicated by the fact that many DCIS lesions, particularly those that are large, display more than one pattern (58). In one series of 100 consecutive cases, 30% of noncomedo lesions showed a mixed histologic pattern and 42% of comedo lesions also contained areas of noncomedo DCIS (68). Despite these limitations, histologic subtype alone or in combination with nuclear grade appears to be predictive of the risk of local failure after treatment with excision and radiation therapy or excision alone.

Schwartz et al. (41) observed that 32% of patients with comedo DCIS experienced local recurrence after treatment with excision alone compared with only 3% of those with noncomedo histology. Similar findings were reported by Lagios et al. (69) in a study in which a 35% local failure rate was seen in patients with high-grade DCIS compared with 8% for patients with low- or intermediate-grade DCIS.

In patients treated with excision and radiation therapy, high nuclear grade and comedo histology are predictive of early local recurrence, but the predictive power of these factors is lost in studies with long-term follow-up. Silverstein et al. (70) observed an 11% rate of local failure in patients with comedo DCIS compared with a 2% failure rate in noncomedo DCIS in 96 patients at a median follow-up of 45 months. However, when the median follow-up period was extended to 62 months, no difference in the rate of local failure based on histologic subtype was observed (18).

Similar findings were noted by Solin et al. (71) in their multi-institutional study of 172 patients. In an early report of this study, the 5-year rate of local recurrence was 12% for patients with the combination of nuclear grade 3 and comedo histology compared with 3% for patients lacking this combination of histologic features, a highly significant difference. When the median follow-up time was extended to 10.3 years, the failure rate in the comedo plus nuclear grade 3 subgroup was 18% compared with 15% in the other group, an insignificant difference (23). These findings suggest that the importance of high nuclear grade and the comedo subgroup in predicting local recurrence may be overemphasized in studies with short durations of follow-up.

The extent of the surgical resection or status of the inked margins also appears to be predictive of the risk of breast recurrence. Although uncertain or involved margins were not a significant predictor of local failure for patients treated with excision alone or excision and radiation therapy in NSABP B-17 at 8 years of follow-up (46), this may reflect the definition of a negative margin (tumor cells not touching the ink) used in this study. Because DCIS is known to grow discontinuously in the duct (72) and postexcision mammography to document complete removal of calcifications was not routinely employed, it is quite possible that patients with positive and negative margins were not reliably separated in this study. Multiple nonrandomized studies suggest that margin status is important in predicting recurrence. McCormick et al. (17) reported close or involved margins in 30% of patients experiencing local failure, whereas only 4% of patients in whom local control was maintained had close or involved margins. Solin et al. (25) also found margin status to be a predictor of local failure with a crude local recurrence rate of 7% for patients with negative margins, 14% for patients with unknown margins, and 29% in patients with close or positive margins in their series of 110 patients with mammographically detected DCIS. Hiramatsu et al. (20) examined the relationship between total volume of excision and local recurrence and found that the 10-year actuarial rate of local recurrence for patients with a total excision volume of less than 60 cm was 25% compared with 0% in those with 60 cm or more excised ($p = 0.04$) (3).

An increasing number of studies suggests that patient age may influence outcome in DCIS. Solin et al. (25) observed a 25% rate of local failure in patients treated with excision and radiation therapy aged 50 or younger compared with 2% in patients older than 50, despite the fact that nuclear grade, tumor size, and margin status did not differ between groups. The median time to local failure was also shorter in the younger patients (4.9 versus 8.7 years). Vicini et al. (73) reviewed 146 patients diagnosed with DCIS and treated with breast conservation followed by radiation therapy from 1980 to 1993. The rate of local failure at 10 years was 26.1% in patients younger than 45 years of age versus 8.6% in older women. The difference in invasive recurrence was especially noteworthy, with younger patients having a 19.9% incidence of invasive recurrence at 10 years, whereas women 45 years of age and older had only a 3.2% rate of invasive recurrence. In multivariate analysis of factors associated with invasive failure, only nuclear grade and patient age were independent predictors. Van Zee et al. (74,75) also observed higher rates of local failure after treatment with excision and radiation therapy or excision alone in women younger than age 40 than in their older counterparts. However, the addition of breast irradiation to excision did reduce the rate of local failure in all age groups. Goldstein et al. (76) examined the pathologic features of DCIS in three different age groups (ages younger than 45 years, 45 to 59 years, and older than 60 years) to explain why young patient age at diagnosis is a risk factor for recurrence. Younger patients more frequently had higher nuclear grade DCIS (grade 3: 69%, 60%, and 39%, respectively; $p = 0.003$) and comedonecrosis (72%, 62%, and 44%, respectively; $p = 0.01$). Younger patients also had smaller initial biopsy specimens (maximum dimensions: 4.3 cm, 5.2 cm, and 5.7 cm, respectively; $p = 0.004$) and more frequent close or positive margins (89%, 61%, and 64%, respectively; $p = 0.03$). Thus, younger patients with DCIS may have increased recurrence risk owing to higher grade DCIS with central necrosis and smaller initial excision volumes. The results of these retrospective studies were confirmed in the NSABP B-24 trial. Local recurrence rates after treatment with excision and radiation therapy were 3.3% in women younger than 49 years of age compared with 1.3% in women age 50 years and older (63). A possible explanation of these results may be the presence of higher circulating levels of estrogen in the younger patients because estrogen has known promotional effects on breast cancer cell lines.

Other studies have suggested that a family history of breast cancer may affect the risk of local failure after excision and radiation therapy. McCormick et al. (17) reported that 40% of patients failing locally had a family history of a first-degree relative with breast cancer versus 11.4% of patients in whom local control was maintained. Similarly, Hiramatsu et al. (20) observed a 37% failure rate in patients with a family history of breast cancer compared with 9% in those without a family history. Szelei-Stevens et al. (77) evaluated the combined influence of family history of breast cancer and young age on outcome by treatment method. One hundred twenty-eight patients with DCIS were treated with mastectomy, lumpectomy alone, or lumpectomy and radiation therapy, with a median follow-up of 8.7 years. Patients with a positive family history had a 10.3% local recurrence rate versus a 2.3% in patients with a negative family history. Of women 50 years of age and younger, the local recurrence rate was 9.1% compared with 2.4% for women older than 50 years of age. Women with a positive family history and younger than 50 years of age had a local recurrence rate of 20%. Importantly, all women who had a recurrence had undergone lumpectomy alone.

TREATMENT SELECTION

Although all patients with DCIS are candidates for mastectomy, many can also be treated with breast preservation with or without radiation therapy. The evaluation of a patient's suitability for breast preservation begins with an assessment of the extent of the DCIS lesion. Magnification mammography is essential for this evaluation. Holland et al. (78,79) noted that conventional two-view mammography (craniocaudal and mediolateral oblique views only) underestimates the extent of well-differentiated DCIS by 2 cm in 47% of cases. The use of magnification views reduces this discrepancy to only approximately 14% of cases. An accurate determination of lesion size allows preoperative selection of those patients who are appropriate candidates for breast preservation and minimizes the number of surgical procedures that are needed to achieve an adequate negative margin. Morrow et al. (80) reported the results of magnification mammography in 263 patients, including 51 with DCIS, who were clinical candidates for breast conservation. Breast preservation was successfully carried out in 97% of patients found to have localized tumors by magnification mammography compared with only 38% of patients with extensive multifocal or multicentric disease identified by mammography. Kearney and Morrow (81) reported 173 patients evaluated with magnification mammography, in whom a diagnostic excision to negative margins was attempted. Negative margins were obtained in 161 patients (93%) with a single surgical procedure. These data indicate that the extent of DCIS can be identified preoperatively in most patients, avoiding attempts at breast preservation in those with extensive disease.

Needle localization should be used to guide the excision of all nonpalpable lesions. Placement of the biopsy guide within 1 cm of the target allows removal of the lesion with a limited amount of normal breast tissue and is an achievable goal (82). Bracketing wires may be useful in patients with extensive calcifications who are candidates for breast-conserving surgery, but we do not find them necessary for routine cases. Placement of the surgical incision over the area of pathology rather than at the entry point of the wire improves exposure and often allows the use of a smaller incision. Electrocautery should be avoided until after the specimen is removed because cautery may distort or destroy small lesions, making an accurate pathologic diagnosis difficult or impossible. Specimen mammography is essential to confirm the excision of calcifications. In cases in which calcifications are extensive or approach the edge of the surgical specimen, postexcision mammograms are useful to confirm the removal of all suspicious calcifications. Gluck et al. (83) did postexcision mammograms with spot compression views on 43 women who required re-excision for positive or unknown margins after a diagnosis of breast carcinoma. Twenty-eight patients had DCIS, and the positive predictive value for residual calcifications as an indicator of residual tumor was 0.67, which increased to 0.9 when more than five calcifications were present. Waddell et al. (84) reported similar findings in a retrospective review of 67 patients treated for DCIS between 1995 and 1998 who underwent postexcision mammography. Residual microcalcifications were identified in 16 patients (24%). Twelve patients underwent wide re-excision and two patients underwent mastectomy. Residual DCIS was identified in nine of 14 patients (64%). These studies confirm that postexcision mammography can be a valuable adjunct to specimen radiography and pathologic analysis to ensure that adequate excision of DCIS has been achieved.

Although core biopsy is the diagnostic procedure of choice for indeterminate calcifications (Breast Imaging Reporting and Data System 4) and for highly suspicious calcifications (Breast Imaging Reporting and Data System 5) suitable for treatment with a breast-conserving approach, we have prospectively demonstrated that a diagnosis with core biopsy does not offer any advantages over needle localization and excision with regard to achieving negative margins with a single excision (85).

A detailed pathologic evaluation is also needed and should include orientation and inking of the specimen and a measurement of both specimen and tumor sizes. The difficulties with size measurement in DCIS have been discussed. Reporting the number of blocks in which DCIS is present and the lesion size is often useful. The correlation of microcalcifications with DCIS (i.e., DCIS present only in areas of calcification or in calcification and adjacent breast tissue) and the presence of calcification in benign disease should be noted. If margins are negative, the proximity of the lesion to the margin should be stated, and when margins are involved, the extent of the involvement should be noted. The demonstration that DCIS, particularly low- to intermediate-grade lesions, grows in a discontinuous fashion (86) indicates that a significant amount of residual tumor

may be present at the biopsy site even when the margin is negative. Thus, margin status and postexcision mammography are complementary means of assessing the adequacy of resection.

Contraindications to breast preservation with excision and radiation therapy are similar to those defined for invasive carcinoma (87). These include a history of therapeutic irradiation of the breast, evidence of multicentric tumor, and diffuse indeterminate or malignant-appearing microcalcifications that would preclude follow-up. A large tumor-to-breast ratio is a relative contraindication.

Although high-grade or comedo DCIS has a higher rate of short-term recurrence than low-grade DCIS, the presence of high-grade histology alone is not a contraindication to breast-conservation treatment because most of these patients will not experience local failure. Contraindications to breast preservation with excision alone are less well defined. However, recurrence rates for gross DCIS, high-grade or comedo lesions, and large areas of DCIS (>20 mm) treated with excision alone are high, and these findings are considered contraindications in most centers. The inability to salvage a patient treated with excision alone with further excision and radiation therapy (for example, owing to small breast size) is a relative contraindication to treatment with excision alone. Although the ability to treat local recurrence with further breast preservation with re-excision and radiation therapy is one of the advantages of initial treatment with excision alone, only 44% of patients in the NSABP B-17 underwent such therapy after recurrence (11). A similar low rate of secondary breast preservation has been reported in randomized trials of patients with invasive carcinoma treated with excision alone (88).

After determining a patient's suitability for breast preservation, treatment options should be discussed in detail. The risk of recurrent DCIS and invasive breast cancer, the treatment implications of a recurrence, and the risk of breast cancer death should all be considered. The risk of breast cancer death 10 years after a mastectomy is 1% to 2%. It is likely that the major force of breast cancer mortality will be evident in the first 10 years after treatment, given that death is presumably owing to occult microinvasive disease present at the time of diagnosis. The risk of death after excision and radiation therapy at 10 years is approximately 3%, little different than that seen after mastectomy. However, because the time to local recurrence is often prolonged, it is likely that additional breast cancer-associated mortality will occur after 10 years, and comparisons of breast cancer mortality rates 30 years after treatment may show greater differences than those discussed here. The importance to patients of these small differences will vary and patient age will certainly influence treatment selection. Conversely, improvements in patient selection in recent years are likely to result in fewer breast recurrences than reported in currently available studies with 10- and 15-year follow-up periods. The addition of tamoxifen to local therapy offers the opportunity for additional risk reduction. Today, a spectrum of treatments ranging from excision alone to excision plus radiation therapy; excision, radiotherapy, and tamoxifen; and mastectomy is available for women with DCIS. The chance of breast cancer death is small with each approach, and individual attitudes toward risk and benefit will play a major role in treatment selection.

REFERENCES

1. Sunshine JA, Moseley HS, Fletcher WS, et al. Breast carcinoma in situ. A retrospective review of 112 cases with a minimum 10-year follow-up. *Am J Surg* 1985;150:44–51.
2. Von Rueden DG, Wilson RE. Intraductal carcinoma of the breast. *Surg Gynecol Obstet* 1984;158:105–111.
3. Ashikari R, Huvos AG, Snyder RE. Prospective study of non-infiltrating carcinoma of the breast. *Cancer* 1977;39:435–457.
4. Schuh ME, Nemoto T, Penetrante RB, et al. Intraductal carcinoma. Analysis of presentation, pathologic findings and outcome of disease. *Arch Surg* 1986;121:1303–1307.
5. Kinne DW, Petrek JA, Osborne MP, et al. Breast carcinoma in situ. *Arch Surg* 1984;124:33–36.
6. Silverstein MJ, Barth A, Poller DN, et al. Ten-year results comparing mastectomy to excision and radiation therapy for ductal carcinoma in situ of the breast. *Eur J Cancer* 1995;31:1425–1427.
7. Ward BA, McKhann CF, Ravikumar TS. Ten-year follow-up of breast carcinoma in situ in Connecticut. *Arch Surg* 1992;127:1392–1395.
8. Silverstein MJ, Poller DN, Waisman JR, et al. Prognostic classification of breast ductal carcinoma in situ. *Lancet* 1995;345:1154–1157.
9. Gillis DA, Dockerty MB, Clagett OT. Preinvasive intraductal carcinoma of the breast. *Surg Gynecol Obstet* 1960;110:555–562.
10. Brown PW, Silverman J, Owens E, et al. Intraductal "non-infiltrating" carcinoma of the breast. *Arch Surg* 1976;111:1063–1067.
11. Fisher B, Costantino J, Redmond C, et al. Lumpectomy compared with lumpectomy and radiation therapy for the treatment of intraductal breast cancer. *N Engl J Med* 1993;328:1581–1586.
12. Rosen PP, Senie R, Schottenfeld D, et al. Noninvasive breast carcinoma. Frequency of unsuspected invasion and implications for treatment. *Ann Surg* 1979;189:377–382.
13. Morrow M. When can stereotactic core biopsy replace excisional biopsy? A clinical perspective. *Breast Cancer Res Treat* 1995;36:1–9.
14. Lagios MD, Westdahl PR, Margolin FR, et al. Duct carcinoma in situ. Relationship of noninvasive disease to the frequency of occult invasion, multicentricity, lymph node metastases, and short-term treatment failures. *Cancer* 1982;50: 1309–1314.
15. Patchefsky AS, Schwartz GF, Finklestein SD, et al. Heterogeneity of intraductal carcinoma of the breast. *Cancer* 1989;63:731–741.
16. Ernster VL, Barclay J, Kerlikowske K, et al. Incidence of and treatment for ductal carcinoma in situ of the breast. *JAMA* 1996;275:913–918.
17. McCormick B, Rosen PP, Kinne D, et al. Duct carcinoma in situ of the breast: an analysis of local control after conservation surgery and radiotherapy. *Int J Radiat Oncol Biol Phys* 1991;21:289–292.
18. Silverstein MJ, Cohlan BF, Gierson ED, et al. Duct carcinoma in situ: 227 cases without microinvasion. *Eur J Cancer* 1992;28:630–634.
19. Ray GR, Adelson J, Hayhurst E, et al. Ductal carcinoma in situ of the breast: results of treatment by conservative surgery and definitive irradiation. *Int J Radiat Oncol Biol Phys* 1993;28:105–111.
20. Hiramatsu H, Bornstein BA, Recht A, et al. Local recurrence after conservative surgery and radiation therapy for ductal carcinoma in situ. Possible importance of family history. *Can J Sci Am* 1995;1:55–61.
21. Fisher ER, Leeming R, Anderson S, et al. Conservative management of intraductal carcinoma (DCIS) of the breast. *J Surg Oncol* 1991;47:139–147.
22. Stotter AT, McNeese M, Oswald MJ, et al. The role of limited surgery with irradiation in primary treatment of ductal in situ breast cancer. *Int J Radiat Oncol Biol Phys* 1990;18:283–287.
23. Solin LJ, Kurtz J, Fourquet A, et al. Fifteen-year results of breast-conserving surgery and definitive breast irradiation for the treatment of ductal carcinoma in situ of the breast. *J Clin Oncol* 1996; 14:754–763.
24. Solin LJ, Fourquet A, McCormick B, et al. Salvage treatment for local recurrence following breast conserving surgery and definitive irradiation for ductal carcinoma in situ (intraductal carcinoma) of the breast. *Int J Radiat Oncol Biol Phys* 1994;309:3–9.
25. Solin LJ, McCormick B, Recht A, et al. Mammographically detected, clinically occult ductal carcinoma in situ (intraductal carcinoma) treated with breast conserving surgery and definitive irradiation. *Can J Sci Am* 1996;2:158–165.
26. Ernster VL, Barclay J, Kerlikowske K, et al. Incidence of and treatment for ductal carcinoma in situ of the breast. *JAMA* 1996;275:913–918.
27. Gapstur SM, Morrow M, Sellers TA. Hormone replacement therapy and risk of breast cancer with a favorable histology: results of the Iowa Women's Health Study. *JAMA* 1999;281:2091–2097.
28. Bartow SA, Pathak DR, Black WC, et al. Prevalence of benign, atypical and malignant breast lesions in populations at different risk for breast cancer. A forensic autopsy study. *Cancer* 1994;60:2751–2760.
29. Alpers CE, Wellings SR. The prevalence of carcinoma in situ in normal and cancer associated breasts. *Hum Pathol* 1985;16:796–807.
30. Nielsen M, Jensen J, Andersen J. Precancerous and cancerous breast lesions during lifetime and at autopsy. A study of 83 women. *Cancer* 1984;54:612–615.
31. Page DL, Dupont WD, Rogers LW, et al. Intraductal carcinoma of the breast: follow-up after biopsy only. *Cancer* 1982;49:751–758.
32. Page DL, Dupont WD, Rogers LW, et al. Continued local recurrence of carcinoma 15–25 years after a diagnosis of low grade ductal carcinoma in situ of the breast treated only by biopsy. *Cancer* 1995;76:1197–1200.
33. Betsill WL, Rosen PP, Lieberman PH, et al. Intraductal carcinoma. Long-term follow-up after treatment by biopsy alone. *JAMA* 1978;239:1863–1867.
34. Eusebi V, Feudale E, Foschini M, et al. Long-term follow-up of in situ carcinoma of the breast. *Semin Diagn Pathol* 1994;1:223–235.
35. Carpenter R, Boulter PS, Cooke T, et al. Management of screen detected ductal carcinoma in situ of the female breast. *Br J Surg* 1981;76:564–567.
36. Schwartz GF, Schwarting R, Cornfield DB, et al. Sub-clinical duct carcinoma in situ of the breast (DCIS): treatment by local excision and surveillance alone. *Proc Am Soc Clin Oncol* 1996;15:101.
37. Baird RM, Worth A, Hislop G. Recurrence after lumpectomy for comedo-type intraductal carcinoma of the breast. *Am J Surg* 1990;159:479–481.

38. Arnesson LG, Smeds S, Fagerberg G, et al. Follow-up of two treatment modalities for ductal carcinoma in situ of the breast. *Br J Surg* 1989;76:672–675.
39. Gallagher WJ, Koerner FC, Wood WC. Treatment of intraductal carcinoma with limited surgery: long-term follow-up. *J Clin Oncol* 1989;7:376–380.
40. Millis RR, Thynne GSJ. In situ intraductal carcinoma of the breast: a long-term follow-up study. *Br J Surg* 1975;62:957–962.
41. Schwartz GF, Finkel GC, Garcia JC, et al. Subclinical ductal carcinoma in situ of the breast. Treatment by local excision and surveillance alone. *Cancer* 1992;70:2468–2474.
42. Lagios MD. Evaluation of surrogate endpoint biomarkers for ductal carcinoma in situ. *J Cell Biochem* 1994;19[Suppl]:186–188.
43. Silverstein MJ, Lagios MD, Groshen S, et al. The influence of margin width on local control of ductal carcinoma in situ of the breast. *N Engl J Med* 1999;340:1455–1461.
44. Hiramatsu H, Bornstein BA, Recht A, et al. Local recurrence after conservative surgery and radiation therapy for ductal carcinoma in situ. *Cancer J Sci Am* 1995;1:55–61.
45. Bellamy COC, McDonald C, Salter DM, et al. Noninvasive ductal carcinoma of the breast. The relevance of histologic categorization. *Hum Pathol* 1993;24:16–23.
46. Fisher B, Dignam J, Wolmark N, et al. Lumpectomy and radiation therapy for the treatment of intraductal breast cancer: findings from National Surgical Adjuvant Breast and Bowel Project B-17. *J Clin Oncol* 1998;16:441–452.
47. Fisher ER, Dignam J, Tan-Chiu E, et al. Pathologic findings from the National Surgical Adjuvant Breast Project (NSABP) eight-year update of protocol B-17: intraductal carcinoma. *Cancer* 1999;86:429–438.
48. Page DL, Lagios MD. Pathologic analysis of the National Surgical Adjuvant Breast Project (NSABP) B-17 Trial. Unanswered questions remain unanswered concerning current concepts of ductal carcinoma in situ. *Cancer* 1995;75:1219–1221.
49. Julien JP, Bijker N, Fentiman IS, et al. Radiotherapy in breast-conserving treatment for ductal carcinoma in situ: first results of the EORTC randomised phase III trial 10853. EORTC Breast Cancer Cooperative Group and EORTC Radiotherapy Group. *Lancet* 2000;355:528–533.
50. Winchester DP, Menck HR, Osteen RT, et al. Treatment trends for ductal carcinoma in situ of the breast. *Ann Surg Oncol* 1995;2:297–213.
51. Baker L. Breast cancer detection demonstration project. Five-year summary report. *Cancer* 1982;32:194–225.
52. Klauber-DeMore N, Tan LK, Liberman L, et al. Sentinel lymph node biopsy: is it indicated in patients with high-risk ductal carcinoma-in-situ and ductal carcinoma-in-situ with microinvasion? *Ann Surg Oncol* 2000;7:636–642.
53. Pendas S, Dauway E, Giuliano R, et al. Sentinel node biopsy in ductal carcinoma in situ patients. *Ann Surg Oncol* 2000;7:15–20.
54. Cox CE, Bass SS, Ku NN, et al. Sentinel lymphadenectomy: a safe answer to less axillary surgery? *Recent Results Cancer Res* 1998;152:170–179.
55. Dupont EL, Ku NN, McCann C, et al. Ductal carcinoma in situ of the breast. *Cancer Control* 1999;6:264–271.
56. Bembenek, A, Reuhl T, Markwardt J, et al. Sentinel lymph node dissection in breast cancer. *Swiss Surg* 1999;5:217–221.
57. Hohenberger P, Reuhl T, Markwardt J, et al. Sentinel node detection in breast carcinoma. *Chirurg* 1998;69:708–716.
58. Morrow M, Schnitt SJ, Harris JR. Ductal carcinoma in situ and microinvasive carcinoma. In: Harris JR, Lippman ME, Morrow M, et al., eds. *Diseases of the breast*, 2nd ed. Philadelphia: Lippincott Williams & Wilkins, 2000:383–401.
59. Lee CH, Carter D, Philpotts LE, et al. Ductal carcinoma in situ diagnosed with stereotactic core needle biopsy: can invasion be predicted? *Radiology* 2000;217:466–470.
60. Liberman L, Dershaw DD, Rosen PP, et al. Stereotaxic core biopsy of breast carcinoma: accuracy of predicting invasion. *Radiology* 1995;194:379–381.
61. Silver SA, Tavassoli FA. Mammary ductal carcinoma in situ with microinvasion. *Cancer* 1998;82:2382–2390.
62. Fisher B, Costantino JP, Wickerham DL, et al. Tamoxifen for prevention of breast cancer: report of the National Surgical Adjuvant Breast and Bowel Project P-1 Study. *J Natl Cancer Inst* 1998;90:1371–1388.
63. Fisher B, Dignam J, Wolmark N, et al. Tamoxifen in treatment of intraductal breast cancer: National Surgical Adjuvant Breast and Bowel Project B-24 randomised controlled trial. *Lancet* 1999;353:1993–2000.
64. Zafrani B, Leroyer A, Fourquet A, et al. Mammographically detected ductal carcinoma in situ carcinoma of the breast analyzed with a new classification. A study of 127 cases: correlation with estrogen and progesterone receptors, p53 and c-erbB-2 proteins and proliferative activity. *Semin Diagn Pathol* 1994;11:208–214.
65. Evans AJ, Pinder SE, Ellis DE, et al. Correlations between the mammographic features of ductal carcinoma in situ (DCIS) and c-erbB-2 oncogene expression. *Clin Radiol* 1994;49:559–562.
66. Guidi AJ, Fischer L, Harris JR, et al. Microvessel density and distribution in ductal carcinoma in situ of the breast. *J Natl Cancer Inst* 1994;86:614–619.
67. Siziopikou KP, Prioleau JE, Harris JR, et al. Bcl-2 expression in the spectrum of preinvasive breast lesions. *Cancer* 1996;77:499–506.
68. Lennington WJ, Jensen RA, Dalton LW, et al. Ductal carcinoma in situ of the breast: heterogeneity of individual lesions. *Cancer* 1994;73:118–124.
69. Lagios MD, Margolin FR, Westdahl PR, et al. Mammographically detected duct carcinoma in situ: frequency of local recurrence following tylectomy and prognostic effect of nuclear grade on local recurrence. *Cancer* 1989;68:618–624.
70. Silverstein MJ, Waisman JR, Gamagami P, et al. Intraductal carcinoma of the breast (208 cases): clinical factors influencing treatment choice. *Cancer* 1990;66:102–108.
71. Solin LJ, Yeh IT, Kurtz J, et al. Ductal carcinoma in situ (intraductal carcinoma) of the breast treated with breast conserving surgery and definitive irradiation. Correlation of pathologic parameters with outcome of treatment. *Cancer* 1993;71:2532–2542.
72. Morrow M. Understanding ductal carcinoma in situ: a step in the right direction. *Cancer* 1999;86:357–377.
73. Vicini FA, Kestin LL, Goldstein NS, et al. Impact of young age on outcome in patients with ductal carcinoma-in-situ treated with breast-conserving therapy. *J Clin Oncol* 2000;18:296–306.
74. Van Zee KT, Liberman L, McCormick B, et al. Long-term follow-up of DCIS treated with breast conservation: effect of age and radiation. Presented at the 49th Cancer Symposium of the Society of Surgical Oncology. Atlanta, GA, March 22, 1995.
75. Van Zee KJ, Liberman L, Samli B, et al. Long term follow-up of women with ductal carcinoma in situ treated with breast-conserving surgery: the effect of age. *Cancer* 1999;86:1757–1767.
76. Goldstein NS, Vicini FA, Kestin LL, et al. Differences in the pathologic features of ductal carcinoma in situ of the breast based on patient age. *Cancer* 2000;88:2553–2560.
77. Szelei-Stevens KA, Kuske RR, Yantsos VA, et al. The influence of young age and positive family history of breast cancer on the prognosis of ductal carcinoma in situ treated by excision with or

without radiation therapy or by mastectomy. *Int J Radiat Oncol Biol Phys* 2000;48:943–949.

78. Holland R, Hendriks JHCL, Verbeek ALM, et al. Extent, distribution, and mammographic histological correlations of breast ductal carcinoma in situ. *Lancet* 1990;335:519–522.

79. Holland R, Hendriks JHCL. Microcalcifications associated with ductal carcinoma in situ: mammographic-pathologic correlation. *Semin Diagn Pathol* 1994;11:181–192.

80. Morrow M, Schmidt R, Hassett C. Patient selection for breast conservation therapy with magnification mammography. *Surgery* 1995;118:621–626.

81. Kearney TJ, Morrow M. Effect of re-excision on the success of breast-conserving surgery. *Ann Surg Oncol* 1995;2:303–307.

82. Gallagher WJ, Cardenosa G, Rubens JR, et al. Minimal-volume excision of non-palpable breast lesions. *Am J Radiol* 1989;153:957–961.

83. Gluck BS, Dershaw DD, Liberman L, et al. Microcalcifications on postoperative mammograms as an indicator of adequacy of tumor excision. *Radiology* 1993;188:469–471.

84. Waddell BE, Stomper PC, DeFazio JL, et al. Post-excision mammography is indicated after resection of ductal carcinoma-in-situ of the breast. *Ann Surg Oncol* 2000;7:665–668.

85. Morrow M, Venta LA, Stinson T, et al. A prospective comparison of stereotactic core biopsy and surgical excision as diagnostic procedures for breast cancer patients. *Ann Surg* 2001; 233:537–541.

86. Faverly D, Burgers L, Bult P, et al. Three-dimensional imaging of ductal carcinoma in situ: clinical implications. *Semin Diagn Pathol* 1994;11:193–198.

87. Winchester D, Cox J. Standards for breast conservation treatment. *CA Cancer J Clin* 1992;42:134–162.

88. Morrow M, Harris JR, Schnitt SJ. Local control following breast conserving surgery for invasive cancer: results of clinical trials. *J Natl Cancer Inst* 1995;87:1669–1673.

24

OVERVIEW OF CONSERVATIVE SURGERY AND RADIATION THERAPY DUCTAL CARCINOMA IN SITU

BARBARA FOWBLE

Breast-conservation therapy for ductal carcinoma in situ (DCIS) resulted as an extension of the conservative approach for early-stage invasive cancer.

The initial reports of conservative surgery and radiation therapy for DCIS reflected our then limited understanding of the natural history and biologic significance of the disease. DCIS was viewed as a single clinical entity and was often treated in a manner similar to that of an invasive cancer. In the multi-institution study reported by Solin et al. (1), 32% of patients with DCIS had an axillary dissection, 37% had irradiation of the regional nodes, and 4% received adjuvant chemotherapy or hormonal therapy. The clinical and pathologic heterogeneity of DCIS was not appreciated. Patients who presented with physical findings (palpable mass, bloody nipple discharge) were not distinguished from those whose cancer was detected solely by mammography or as an incidental finding (Table 24.1). Detailed mammographic and pathologic correlation was not performed. The pathologic assessment was often incomplete with little or no information regarding the histologic subtype (2–6). Margins of resection were unknown in the majority of patients in the earlier series. Despite these limitations, the published results from single institutions and the multi-institutional study initiated by Solin et al. (1) provided important information regarding the role of conservative surgery and radiation therapy in the treatment of DCIS. This chapter reviews the results of conservative surgery and radiation therapy for DCIS reported from retrospective series and prospective randomized trials.

RATIONALE FOR CONSERVATIVE SURGERY AND RADIATION THERAPY OF DUCTAL CARCINOMA IN SITU

The rationale for conservative surgery and radiation therapy in the treatment of DCIS is based on its demonstrated effectiveness in the treatment of early-stage invasive cancer and its ability to decrease the incidence of ipsilateral breast tumor recurrence after wide excision alone (7–9). The rationale for treatment directed to the entire breast is related to the reported incidence of multicentricity and occult invasive cancer observed in mastectomy specimens from patients with DCIS.

The reported incidence of multicentricity ranges from 0% to 47% when random sectioning of the breast is performed (10–16). A 1% to 32% incidence of multicentricity (17–20) has been reported in series in which a more detailed pathologic analysis using the serial subgross and correlated mammography technique was employed. Some of these differences can also be attributed to variations in the definition of multicentricity that has included foci of DCIS in quadrants separate from the primary or foci of DCIS at distances greater than 4 to 5 cm from the primary. The incidence of multicentricity has been correlated with the method of detection, tumor extent, and histologic subtype of DCIS and ranges from 19% to 38% for DCIS detected solely by mammography (10,14,21,22) to 25% for DCIS presenting as a palpable mass (10). Multicentricity has not been reported in DCIS detected as an incidental finding at the time of biopsy for a benign lesion (14,22). Multicentricity has been observed in 52% of cases of DCIS larger than 2.5 cm compared with 14% for those 2.5 cm or smaller (20). Multicentricity has been reported in 71% (23) and 86% (14,24) of micropapillary DCIS compared with 10% to 30% for the comedo, solid, cribriform, and papillary histology (10,14,23,24).

With the increased use of breast-conservation therapy for DCIS, there has been a renewed interest in assessing more precisely the pathologic extent and distribution of DCIS within the breast. Studies (18,25,26) using the subgross pathologic and mammographic technique or three-dimensional stereoscopic examination have reported that true multicentricity, i.e., separate and independent foci of DCIS, occurs in only 1% to 2% of the cases studied. In most cases, DCIS spreads in a contiguous manner and most often in a

TABLE 24.1. CHARACTERISTICS OF DUCTAL CARCINOMA IN SITU IN RETROSPECTIVE SERIES AND RANDOMIZED TRIALS OF CONSERVATIVE SURGERY AND RADIATION THERAPY

Study	% Detected on Mammography	% Negative Margins	% Low Grade or Noncomedo	Median Follow-Up (yr)
Retrospective series				
McCormick et al. (5)	67	30	—	3
Warneke et al. (68)	80	43	71	3
Kuske et al. (4)	65	23	42	4
Ray et al. (69)	71	23	47	5
Fowble et al. (45)	100	62	36	5.3
White et al. (63)	88	77	54	5.7
Van Zee et al. (70)	62	23	54	6.2
Solin et al. (43)	47	24	50	6.2
Hiramatsu et al. (6)	71	45	—	6.2
Cataliotti et al. (71)	57	—	60	6.6
Amichetti et al. (56)	28	—	55	6.8
Kestin et al. (33)	100	67	77	7
Vicini et al. (48)	89	68	79	7.2
Beron et al. (50)	89	89	59	7.5
Fourquet et al. (52)	63	—	62	9
Collaborative group (1,34,38,40,72)				
All patients	42	35	41	10.3
Mammo only	100	53	—	9.4
Mirza et al. (73)	65	52	—	11
Randomized trials				
NSABP B-17 (7,51)	83	63	50	8.5
NSABP B-24 (41)	84	75	50	6.2
EORTC (8,47)	73	79	72	5.4

NSABP, National Surgical Adjuvant Breast Project; EORTC, European Organization for Research and Treatment of Cancer.

central direction toward the nipple (26). Comedo histology and age younger than 40 years have been associated with more extensive disease in some series (26). Faverly et al. (18), in an analysis of 60 mastectomy specimens containing DCIS ranging in size from 2 to 14 cm, reported that 48% of the cases demonstrated multifocality, i.e., two or more foci separated by an apparently uninvolved portion of duct system of 4 cm or smaller. In 82% of the multifocal cases, the distances between foci were less than 5 mm. Multifocality was more common with intermediate- (45%) and low-grade (30%) lesions. Multifocality has also been observed in patients undergoing re-excision after an initial excision for DCIS with negative margins. Fisher et al. (27) reported that 24% of patients in the National Surgical Adjuvant Breast Project (NSABP) B-17 trial who underwent excision with negative margins (defined as no tumor at the inked margin) had residual DCIS at the time of re-excision. The finding of residual DCIS appears to be related to the width of the initial tumor-free margin. Silverstein et al. (28) reported that 43% of 53 patients with DCIS who underwent re-excision after excision with margins of 1 mm or more had residual DCIS. Goldstein et al. (29) and Ratanawichitrasin et al. (30) found residual DCIS in 45% and 31% of patients, re-

spectively, whose initial margins were 2 mm or less. In a series of 102 cases from the Fox Chase Cancer Center (Philadelphia, PA) with initial margins of 2 mm or less, residual DCIS was found in 28%. For initial margins greater than 2 mm, Ratanawichitrasin et al. (30) reported residual DCIS in 17%, and at the Fox Chase Cancer Center, we found residual DCIS in six of 70 patients (9%). Residual DCIS at the time of re-excision or mastectomy after an initial excision has also been correlated with higher nuclear grade, increasing tumor size, and increasing number of slides with DCIS (28–30).

Therefore, although multicentricity is rare, DCIS can produce contiguous involvement of the ductal system that may extend over relatively large distances. The normal breast contains 16 to 24 different (four to six per quadrant) ductal-lobular structures with a corresponding number of collecting ducts at the nipple. The ductal anastomoses connecting different systems are most prominent in the region of the nipple corresponding to the propensity for DCIS to exhibit a central pattern of extension (26).

Despite these pathologic studies, the ability to assess accurately the extent and distribution of DCIS remains a problem in clinical practice. For patients presenting with a mass on physical examination or mammography, the clinical and pathologic size of the DCIS can be assessed by measuring the size of the mass. For patients presenting with mammographic calcifications only, assessment of the size and extent of DCIS is more difficult. With conventional two-view mammography, the radiographic extent of these calcifications underestimates the pathologic extent of DCIS in 80% to 85% of patients (25). Holland et al. (17) reported that the pathologic extent was greater than the mammographic calcifications by more than 2 cm for 47% of the noncomedo DCIS compared with only 16% of the comedo DCIS. With the addition of magnification views, this discrepancy was decreased for the noncomedo lesions (14% >2 cm) but not for the comedo lesions (21% >2 cm) (25). Several methods have been employed to determine the pathologic extent of DCIS in these patients. The most accurate method requires serial and sequential sectioning of the entire specimen. Size is then calculated by determining the number of blocks with DCIS and their relationship to one another assuming a 2.5- to 3-mm distance between blocks. This method is used in the Van Nuys Prognostic Index (31). The NSABP measures the pathologic site of DCIS as the largest area on a given slide (32). Others have assessed size by the number of blocks containing DCIS versus the total number of blocks examined (33). Knowledge of the size and extent of DCIS is important for the clinician in determining appropriate treatment. Underestimation of the extent of DCIS may result in suboptimal treatment.

The incidence of occult invasive cancer at the time of diagnosis of DCIS ranges from 2% to 21% (10,13,15,20). Occult invasion is more common with increasing tumor size greater than 5 cm (16,20) and comedo histology (10,24,34) and has not been reported in DCIS detected incidentally (14,22). Moriya and Silverberg (35) reported solid growth pattern and high nuclear grade as the most important histopathologic features associated with invasive cancer in the presence of DCIS.

Based on the foregoing discussion, treatment directed to the entire breast (i.e., radiation therapy or mastectomy) for DCIS would seem most appropriate for patients in whom a wide excision is least likely to remove all foci of tumor (i.e., those with an increased risk of multicentricity or multifocality) or in whom there is a risk of occult invasive cancer. Patients in the former category include low nuclear grade or noncomedo DCIS and, in the latter, high nuclear grade or comedo DCIS.

RESULTS OF RETROSPECTIVE SERIES OF CONSERVATIVE SURGERY AND RADIATION THERAPY FOR DUCTAL CARCINOMA IN SITU

The first published report of the results of conservative surgery and radiation therapy for DCIS was from the University of Pennsylvania (36). The initial 14 patients in this study and six others were combined with 20 patients treated at the Joint Center for Radiation Therapy in Boston for a second report (37). Sixty-eight percent of the patients had a palpable mass, and of the 20 patients in whom tumor size was available, 14 had tumors 2 cm or smaller. The 5-year actuarial breast recurrence rate was 10% and the 5-year actuarial survival rate was 100%. Table 24.2 presents the results from numerous retrospective series. With median follow-up periods varying from 3 to 11 years, the crude breast recurrence rate ranges from 0% to 18%. The characteristics of the patients treated are presented in Table 24.1. Approximately two-thirds of these patients had mammographically detected DCIS; 50% were low nuclear grade or noncomedo and less than 50% had negative margins of resection. The variations in the incidence of breast recurrence in these series reflect differences in patient selection, mammographic and pathologic assessment, and differences in the follow-up period.

In an effort to obtain long-term results of conservative surgery and radiation therapy for DCIS, nine institutions initially and subsequently 10 in the United States and Europe collaborated to establish a database. The details of this database and an update of the results are presented in Chapter 33. For this discussion, the database is referred to as the collaborative group. The 15-year actuarial risk of a breast recurrence in the 268 patients reported by the collaborative group was 19% (1,38). The median follow-up for these patients was 10.3 years. The National Federation of Cancer Centers in France also collected data on 387 patients with DCIS treated from 1970 to 1981 with mastectomy (268 patients), excision alone (74 patients), or excision and radiation therapy (45 patients). The median follow-up was 7 years. The 10-year breast recurrence rate for the 45 patients treated with excision and radiation therapy was 12% (39).

RESULTS OF CONSERVATIVE SURGERY AND RADIATION THERAPY FOR MAMMOGRAPHICALLY DETECTED DUCTAL CARCINOMA IN SITU

Many of the series reporting the results of conservative surgery and radiation therapy for DCIS have included patients whose disease was detected as a physical finding (palpable mass, bloody nipple discharge). It is difficult to compare the results of these series with those of observation series of mammographically detected DCIS. Table 24.3 presents the results of series of conservative surgery and radiation therapy for mammographically detected DCIS. The 5-year actuarial ipsilateral breast tumor recurrence (IBTR) rate ranges from 0% to 12% with 10-year rates of 8% to 23%. The initial collaborative group study reported a 10-year actuarial IBTR rate of 14% for all patients and 8% for those with negative margins (40). In an expanded series of

TABLE 24.2. RESULTS OF CONSERVATIVE SURGERY AND RADIATION THERAPY FOR DUCTAL CARCINOMA IN SITU: RETROSPECTIVE SERIES

Study	No. of Patients	% Ipsilateral Breast Tumor Recurrence	Median Follow-Up (yr)
McCormick et al. (5)	54	18	3
Warneke et al. (68)	21	0	3
Haffty et al. (3)	60	7	3.6
Kuske et al. (4)	70	4	4
Bullock et al. (74)	43	7	5
Kurtz et al. (75)	47	4	5
Ray et al. (69)	56	9	5
Ciatto et al. (76)	37	5	5.5
Solin et al. (43)	51	10	5.7
White et al. (63)	53	6	5.7
Hiramatsu et al. (6)	76	9	6.2
Van Zee et al. (70)	65	10	6.2
Cataliotti et al. (71)	83	7	6.6
Amichetti et al. (56)	139	9	6.8
Fourquet et al. (French cancer centers) (39)	45	12	7.0
Fisher et al. (77,78)	27	7	7.1
Vicini et al. (48)	146	12	7.2
Beron et al. (50)	185	16	7.5
Fourquet et al. (52)	153	16	9
Solin et al. (collaborative group) (1)	268	17	10.3
Delouche et al. (79)	18	5	11
Mirza et al. (73)	87	13	11

422 patients, the 10-year actuarial IBTR rate was 11% (38). For patients with negative margins, the rate was 9%. The results of conservative surgery and radiation therapy from the prospective randomized trials of DCIS are also presented in Table 24.3. The majority of patients in these trials had mammographically detected DCIS (Table 24.1). The 5-year IBTR rate ranges from 9% to 13% with 8-year rates of 12% and 16% (7,8,41).

TABLE 24.3. RESULTS OF CONSERVATIVE SURGERY AND RADIATION THERAPY FOR MAMMOGRAPHICALLY DETECTED DUCTAL CARCINOMA IN SITU

Study	No. of Patients	Actuarial Ipsilateral Breast Tumor Recurrence %		Median Follow-Up (yr)
Retrospective series		5 yr	10 yr	
Kuske et al. (4)	44	7	—	4
Fowble et al. (45)	110	1	15	5.3
Hiramatsu et al. (6)	54	2	23	6.2
Sneige et al. (53)	31	0	8	7.2
Kestin et al. (60)	151	8	9	7.3
Beron et al. (50)	185[a]	12	20	7.5
Solin et al. (collaborative group) (38)	418	6	11	9.4
Prospective randomized trials		5 yr	8 yr	
Fisher et al. NSABP B-17 (7)	411[a]	9	12	(7.5)[b]
Fisher et al. NSABP B-24 (41)	902[a]	13	—	6.2
EORTC 10853 (8,47)	502[a]	12	16	4.2

[a] Majority mammographically detected.
[b] Mean.
NSABP, National Surgical Adjuvant Breast Project; EORTC, European Organization for Research and Treatment of Cancer.

PROGNOSTIC FACTORS FOR IPSILATERAL BREAST TUMOR RECURRENCE (IBTR)

Several factors have been analyzed for their ability to predict for a breast recurrence in patients undergoing conservative surgery and radiation therapy for DCIS. These include clinical factors such as age, method of detection, the presence of a bloody nipple discharge, and a positive family history. Pathologic factors have included the histologic subtype based on architectural pattern, nuclear grade, the presence or absence of necrosis, and margins of resection. Treatment-related factors include re-excision and total radiation dose. An analysis of these factors is presented in Tables 24.4 through 24.8.

Clinical factors associated with IBTR rates are presented in Tables 24.4 and 24.5. An increased IBTR rate has been associated with the method of detection as a physical finding when compared with mammographic detection only. In the NSABP B-24 trial in which all patients received radiation therapy, the method of detection was a significant predictor for IBTR. Two series reported an increased breast recurrence rate in patients who presented with a bloody nipple

discharge (42,43). However, in the collaborative group study, the 10-year actuarial IBTR rate was 20% for the 25 patients with a bloody nipple discharge compared with 15% for 245 patients who did not have this finding (1). The influence of a positive family history on IBTR rates has been variable with some series suggesting an increased risk of recurrence (5,6) and others (44–46) finding no such correlation. The influence of age on IBTR rates is presented in Table 24.5. This subject is discussed in detail in Chapter 36. Most of the series confirm an increased risk of IBTR rate in younger women variously defined as age younger than 40, 45, or 50 years. In the NSABP B-24 trial (41), age younger than 50 years was a significant predictor of IBTR. In the European Organization for Research and Treatment of Cancer (EORTC) randomized trial 10853, the IBTR rate was 23% for the 22 women 40 years of age or younger who received radiation therapy compared with 12% for the 415 women older than 40 years of age (47). Wider surgical resections may diminish the risk of an IBTR in these women (48). In the study by Vicini et al. (48), younger women had more dispersed areas of DCIS but a similar total number of slides with DCIS. Fisher and Fisher (49) suggest that not all re-

TABLE 24.4. CLINICAL FACTORS ASSESSED FOR THEIR IMPACT ON IPSILATERAL BREAST TUMOR RECURRENCE AFTER CONSERVATIVE SURGERY AND RADIATION THERAPY

Method of Detection	% Ipsilateral Breast Tumor Recurrence		Interval Reported (yr)
	Physical Examination	Mammography Only	
White et al. (63)	20 (6)	5 (46)	5 act.
Bijker et al. (EORTC 10853) (47)	17 (115)	11 (322)	5.4 med.
Hughes et al. (80)	20 (5)	14 (22)	5.3 med.
Fisher et al. (NSABP B-24) (41)	14 (144)	9 (755)	6.2 med.
Fisher et al. (NSABP B-06) (78)	7 (27)	—	7 mean
Fisher et al. (NSABP B-17) (7)	17 (81)	10 (330)	7.5 mean
Sneige et al. (53)	22 (18)	3 (31)	7.2 med.
Hiramatsu et al. (6)	14 (22)	23 (54)	10 act.
Vicini et al. (48)	29 (16)	10 (132)	10 act.
Solin et al. (collaborative group) (1)	18 (96)	13 (113)	10 act.

Family History	Negative	Positive	Interval Reported (yr)
McCormick et al. (5)	13 (45)	44 (9)	3 med.
Fowble et al. (45)	0 (72)	5 (34)	5 act.
Szelei-Stevens et al. (44)	0 (25)	0 (10)	6 med.
Hiramatsu et al. (6)	9 (58)	37 (17)	10 act.
Harris et al. (46)	16 (91)	8 (55)	10 act.

(), number of patients; act., actuarial; med., median; EORTC, European Organization for Research and Treatment of Cancer; NSABP, National Surgical Adjuvant Breast Project.

TABLE 24.5. RESULTS OF CONSERVATIVE SURGERY AND RADIATION THERAPY FOR DUCTAL CARCINOMA IN SITU RELATED TO PATIENT AGE

Study	Definition Young (yrs)	IBTR% Young	IBTR% Old	Interval Reported (yr)
Retrospective series				
Solin et al. (collaborative group) (1)	<40	30 (32)	7 (267)	10 act.
Solin et al. (38) (mammography only)	<40	31 (31)	6–13 (391)	10 act.
Cutuli et al. (81)	<40	27 (NS)	15 (NS)	8 act.
Van Zee et al. (70)	<40	33 (6)	8 (49)	6 act.
Fowble et al. (45)	≤40	25 (8)	0 (102)	5 act.
Fourquet et al. (52)	≤40	30 (24)	14 (129)	10 act.
Harris et al. (46)	<40	8 (12)	10 (131)	7.1 med.
Park et al. (82)	<50	6 (66)	0 (109)	5 min.
Vicini et al. (48)	<45	26 (31)	9 (117)	10 act.
Hiramatsu et al. (6)	≤50	12 (39)	17 (37)	10 act.
Szelei-Stevens et al. (44)	≤50	0 (NS)	0 (NS)	6 med.
Randomized trials				
Fisher et al. NSABP B-17 (7)	<50	15 (137)	9 (274)	8
Fisher et al. NSABP B-24 (41)	<50	16 (300)	7 (599)	5
Bijker et al. EORTC 10853 (47)	≤40	23 (22)	12 (415)	5.4 med.

(), number of patients; NS, not stated; act., actuarial; med., median; min., minimum; NSABP, National Surgical Adjuvant Breast Project; EORTC, European Organization for Research and Treatment of Cancer.

currences of DCIS can be attributed to residual disease, and some may arise *de novo* in a field of premalignant change destined to malignant transformation over time. This phenomenon may account in part for the increased risk of IBTR observed in younger women.

Tables 24.6 through 24.8 present pathologic factors assessed for their impact on ipsilateral breast tumor recurrence rates in patients with DCIS treated with conservative surgery and radiation therapy. As previously discussed assessment of the size and extent of DCIS is difficult in patients whose sole presentation is that of mammographic calcifications. In addition, few series have correlated the size and extent of DCIS with clinical outcome. The absence of this information reflects the failure to document the mammographic size (mass or calcifications) or the reliance on gross examination of the pathologic specimen even when mammographic calcifications were the only finding on presentation. Table 24.6 presents IBTR rates related to clinical and pathologic tumor size. There appears to be little correlation with outcome and size as determined by mammographic measurements or the area on a given slide in patients receiving radiation therapy. However, in the NSABP B-17, the IBTR rate was 27% for patients with scattered calcifications compared with 9% for clustered calcifications 1 cm or smaller and 16% for clustered calcifications larger than 1 cm (7). Size determined by the three-dimensional reconstruction as advocated by the Van Nuys Prognostic Index and the total number of slides with DCIS have been correlated with IBTR rates (33,50).

For the most part, there is little correlation with the architectural pattern and IBTR rates when using the categories of comedo versus noncomedo (Table 24.7). In the collaborative group study, the 10-year actuarial IBTR rate was 17% for the 77 patients with comedo histology compared with 15% for the 114 patients with noncomedo histology. The patients with noncomedo DCIS had a longer median interval to failure (6.5 versus 3.1 years) and therefore series with shorter follow-up may report an increased IBTR rate in the comedo lesions. The influence of nuclear grade on IBTR rates in patients receiving radiation therapy has been variable. In the NSABP B-17 trial, there were no significant differences in IBTR rates in patients receiving radiation therapy when comparing nuclear grade good with nuclear grade poor tumors (51). However, high nuclear grade has been associated with an increased risk of IBTR in some retrospective series (48,50,52). In the collaborative group study (1), the 10-year actuarial IBTR rate was 13% for nuclear grade 1 tumors, 16% for nuclear grade 2, and 21% for nuclear grade 3. There is limited information regarding the impact of necrosis on IBTR rates. In the NSABP B-24 trial in which all patients received radiation therapy, comedonecrosis was a significant predictor of IBTR (41). However, in the NSABP B-17, the IBTR rate was 13% for DCIS with none or focal areas of necrosis compared with 14% for moderately marked necrosis in the patients who received radiation therapy. The collaborative group (1) reported no correlation with IBTR rates and the presence of moderately marked necrosis in contrast to two

TABLE 24.6. RESULTS OF CONSERVATIVE SURGERY AND RADIATION THERAPY OF DUCTAL CARCINOMA IN SITU RELATED TO TUMOR SIZE

Size	% Ipsilateral Breast Tumor Recurrence Tumor Size (cm)			Interval Reported (yr)
	<1–1.5	>1–1.5	>4	
Clinical				
Solin et al. (1) (collaborative group)[a]	12 (162)	15 (44)	—	10 act.
Solin et al. (38) (mammography only)[a]	12 (197)	12 (37)	—	10 act.
Fisher et al. (NSABP B-17) (7)	10 (209)	12 (112)	—	7.5 mean
Pathologic				
3-D reconstruction				
Beron et al. (50)	7 (108)	29 (65)	55 (11)	8 act.
Area on a slide				
Fisher et al. NSABP B-17 (51)	5 (62)	11 (81)	—	8.5 mean
Fowble et al. (45)	0 (43)	0 (10)		5 act.
Bijker et al. EORTC 10853 (47)	11 (79)	7 (29)		5.4 med.
No. of slides	<6	≥6		
Kestin et al. (33)	7 (91)	18 (41)		10 act.

[a] ≤2 cm versus 2.1–5 cm.
act., actuarial; NSABP, National Surgical Adjuvant Breast Project; 3-D, three dimensional; EORTC, European Organization for Research and Treatment of Cancer; med., median.

other retrospective series and the EORTC 10853 randomized trial (47,52,53).

The influence of resection margin status on IBTR rates is presented in Table 24.8. In the NSABP B-17 trial, margin status was not significantly correlated with IBTR. However, a negative margin was defined as no tumor at the inked margin and patients with unknown margins were included with those with positive margins. In the NSABP B-24 trial, margin status was a significant predictor of IBTR (41). The lack of significance of margin status in the NSABP B-17 trial and its statistical significance in the NSABP B-24 may be owing to the numbers of patients in the trials. In both trials, positive margins had a higher IBTR rate, although in the NSABP B-17 trial, the absolute difference was 4%, and in the B-24, it was 7% (Table 24.8). However, the number of patients analyzed in the B-17 trial for margin status who received radiation therapy was 320 compared with 899 in the B-24 for radiation therapy alone and 899 for radiation therapy and tamoxifen (47). The EORTC 10853 trial reported a 16% IBTR rate in patients with close (≤1 mm) or positive margins who received radiation therapy compared with 12% for those with margins greater than 1 mm and 7% for those with a negative re-excision (47). For the retrospective series, all but one (6) demonstrated a higher recurrence rate in patients with close (<1 to 2 mm) or positive margins. The width of the negative margin that best minimizes the risk of IBTR after radiation therapy is controversial, with some series advocating 2 mm (40,45,48,54) and others 1 cm

(55). It is unlikely that one margin width will be applicable to all patients. As previously noted, wider margins may be needed in younger women and in those lesions with a greater propensity for multifocality, i.e., larger tumor size, micropapillary histology, or nuclear grade 3 tumors.

The identification of clinical or pathologic factors that best predict an increased risk of IBTR in patients receiving radiation therapy remains controversial. Table 24.9 presents a summary of some of the retrospective series as well as the NSABP B-24 prospective randomized trial. The series vary with the method of detection of DCIS, with some focusing only on mammographically detected lesions, and with the thoroughness of the pathologic evaluation. Age and resection margin status are fairly consistently identified as factors correlating with IBTR rates. Both of these factors were significant in the NSABP B-24 trial in which all patients received radiation therapy. However, neither of these was significant in the NSABP B-17 trial in which patients were randomized to observation or radiation therapy. In both trials, women 49 years of age or younger and those with positive margins had an increased risk of IBTR. The finding of statistical significance in the B-24 trial could be attributed to larger patient numbers. The size and extent of DCIS when assessed were often clinical or as the area on a given slide (1,40,41,45,54,56) and account for the fact that extent of DCIS does not appear to predict IBTR in patients receiving radiation therapy. However, Kestin et al. (33) assessed the extent of DCIS by the number of slides with DCIS and

TABLE 24.7. PATHOLOGIC FACTORS ASSESSED FOR THEIR IMPACT ON IPSILATERAL BREAST TUMOR RECURRENCE AFTER CONSERVATIVE SURGERY AND RADIATION THERAPY FOR DUCTAL CARCINOMA IN SITU

Histologic Subtype	% Ipsilateral Breast Tumor Recurrence		Follow-Up (yr)
	Comedo	Noncomedo	
Kuske et al. (4)	12 (25)	0 (NS)	4 med.
Solin et al. (43)	7 (14)	4 (26)	5 act.
Fowble et al. (45)	0 (37)	0 (32)	5 act.
Hughes et al. (80)	13 (8)	22 (9)	5.3 med.
Bijker et al. (EORTC 10853) (47)	15 (165)	11 (228)	5.4 med.
White et al. (63)	6 (18)	6 (34)	5.7 med.
Cataliotti et al. (71)	9 (33)	6 (50)	6.6 mean
Bornstein et al. (42)	22 (27)	20 (10)	6.8 med.
Sneige et al. (53)	11 (18)	10 (31)	7.2 med.
Beron et al. (50)	35 (75)	26 (110)	10 act.
Vicini et al. (48)	13 (33)	12 (115)	10 act.
Solin et al. (collaborative group) (1)	17 (77)	15 (114)	10 act.

Nuclear Grade	1	2	3	Follow-Up (yr)
Solin et al. (43)	0 (8)	6 (17)	7 (15)	5 act.
Hughes et al. (80)	0 (6)	25 (4)	28 (7)	5.3 med.
Bijker et al. (EORTC 10853) (47)	4 (156)	14 (125)	18 (112)	5.4 med.
Cataliotti et al. (71)	5 (44)		8 (25)	6.6 mean
Bornstein et al. (3)	100 (1)	19 (16)	20 (20)	6.8 med.
Sneige et al. (53)	0 (7)	6 (17)	4 (16)	7.2 med.
Beron et al. (50)	7 (27)	13 (92)	24 (66)	7.5 med.
Fisher et al. (NSABP B-17) (51)	12 (160)		15 (160)	8.5 med.
Fourquet et al. (52)	10 (32)		20 (113)	10 act.
Vicini et al. (48)	10 (106)		19 (42)	10 act.
Solin et al. (collaborative group) (1)	13 (34)	16 (76)	21 (81)	10 act.

Necrosis	None	Focal	Moderate/ Marked	Follow-Up (yr)
Bijker et al. (EORTC 10853) (47)	4 (112)		16 (135)	5.4 med.
Fisher et al. (NSABP B-24) (41)		7 (446)	13 (433)	6.2 med.
Sneige et al. (53)	0 (19)	17 (30)		7.2 med.
Fisher et al. (NSABP B-17) (51)		13 (178)	14 (142)	8.5 mean
Fourquet et al. (52)	9 (61)		24 (84)	10 act.
Solin et al. (collaborative group) (1)	20 (31)	16 (96)	13 (64)	10 act.

(), number of patients; med., median; act., actuarial; EORTC, European Organization for Research and Treatment of Cancer; NSABP, National Surgical Adjuvant Breast Project.

Beron et al. (50) used the serial and sequential sectioning method. Both of these series found a correlation with size and extent of DCIS and IBTR rates. Necrosis was identified as a significant predictor of IBTR in the NSABP B-24 trial, the EORTC 10853 trial, and the series reported by Sneige et al. (53) and others (41,47). Architectural pattern has been a significant factor in two series (4,50).

Silverstein et al. (57,58) (see Chapter 45) proposed the Van Nuys Prognostic Index as a means of classifying DCIS and assessing outcome. The index includes tumor size, margin width, and morphology which uses a combination of nuclear grade and comedonecrosis. There are three categories for each of the factors, and each is assigned a score of 1, 2, or 3 as follows: size less than 15 mm, 16 to 40

TABLE 24.8. IPSILATERAL BREAST TUMOR RECURRENCE RATES RELATED TO RESECTION MARGIN STATUS DUCTAL CARCINOMA IN SITU TREATED WITH CONSERVATIVE SURGERY AND RADIATION THERAPY

Study	Definition Negative	BTR%			Interval Reported (yr)
		Negative	Close	Positive	
Retrospective series					
Cutuli et al. (81)	NS	10 (NS)		30 (NS)	8 act.
Chan et al. (83)	>1 mm	0 (12)	33 (6)		3.9 mean
Hiramatsu et al. (6)	>1 mm	11 (34)	9 (11)	0 (11)	10 act.
Beron et al. (8)	>1 mm	12 (124)	25 (61)		7.5 med.
Weng et al. (54)	>2 mm	4 (23)		31 (13)	8.5 med.
Solin et al.	>2 mm	7 (42)	29 (17)		9.3 med.
(collaborative group) (38,40)		9 (222)		24 (40)	10 act.
Vicini et al. (48)	>2 mm	9 (99)	16 (49)		10 act.
Ray et al. (69)	>2 mm	8 (13)		38 (8)	5 med.
Fowble et al. (45)	>2 mm	0 (68)		8 (20)	5 act.
Randomized trials					
Fisher et al. (NSABP B-17) (51)	1 cell	13 (267)		17 (53)	8.5 mean
Fisher et al. (NSABP B-24) (41)	1 cell	8 (675)		15 (224)	6.2 med.
Bijker et al. (EORTC 10853) (47)	>1 mm	8 (98)	16 (32)		5.4 med.

NS, not stated; (), number of patients; act., actuarial; med., median; NSABP, National Surgical Adjuvant Breast Project; EORTC, European Organization for Research and Treatment of Cancer.

mm, and larger than 41 mm; margins 10 mm or more, 1 to 9 mm, and less than 1 mm; and pathology low- or intermediate-grade without necrosis, low- or intermediate-grade with necrosis, and high-grade with or without necrosis. Scores for each factor are totaled to yield a final score of 3 to 9. For patients receiving radiation therapy with scores of 3 to 4, the disease-free survival rate was 100%; for scores of 5, 6, or 7, it was 85%, and for scores of 8 and 9; it was 36%. In a univariate analysis limited to the patients receiving radiation therapy, size, margin status, histology, nuclear grade, and necrosis significantly predicted IBTR (59). In multivariate analysis, only the nuclear grade was significant. Kestin et al. (60) found that the Van Nuys Prognostic Index was not a significant predictor for IBTR in patients receiving radiation therapy. However, these authors did not routinely employ the serial and sequential method of sectioning the entire specimen and a margin of 2 mm or less was scored as 3.

Boyages et al. (61) reported a meta-analysis of predictors for IBTR in patients with DCIS treated with breast-conservation therapy. The analysts included 18 retrospective studies and the NSABP B-17 trial. Factors analyzed included architectural pattern, necrosis, nuclear grade, and tumor size. For patients receiving radiation therapy, all these factors were associated with an increased IBTR rate; however, the absolute increase ranged from 3.4% to 8.4%.

Treatment-related factors that have been assessed for their impact on IBTR rates after radiation therapy include the volume of resection, the use of re-excision, total radiation dose, and tamoxifen. Larger excision volumes (6,48,62) have resulted in significantly decreased recurrence rates, especially in young women (48). Similarly, re-excisions have resulted in lower IBTR rates in some series (6,63) but not others (48). There has been no correlation with the total radiation dose and IBTR rates (1,42,43,56) in the range of 5,000 to 6,600 cGy. One of the most important factors predicting an increased risk of IBTR is the presence of residual malignant-appearing calcifications on a mammogram before radiation therapy. Seven patients have been reported in whom all malignant-appearing calcifications were not removed before radiation therapy, and all have recurred in the treated breast (5,53,54). Vicini et al. (48) reported a 14% 10-year actuarial IBTR rate in women who did not have a preradiation mammogram compared with 4% for those who did. The American College of Radiology, the American College of Surgeons, the College of American Pathologists, and the Society of Surgical Oncology published standards for the diagnosis and treatment of DCIS in 1998 (64). These standards state that a "postoperative mammogram is essential to ensure that microcalcifications have been removed in patients having breast-conservation treatment with or without irradiation." If no residual calcifications are demonstrated on the standard views, magnification views are indicated.

TABLE 24.9. FACTORS CORRELATING WITH IPSILATERAL BREAST TUMOR RECURRENCE AFTER CONSERVATIVE SURGERY AND RADIATION THERAPY FOR DUCTAL CARCINOMA IN SITU

Study	Method of Detection	Pathologic Factor(s) Evaluated	Significant Factor(s)
Collaborative group (3,38)	Mammography only	Margins only	Age, margins
	All	Yes	None
Fowble et al. (45)	Mammography only	Yes	Age
Kestin et al. (33)	All	Yes	Age, no. of slides of DCIS, extent of DCIS at margin, absence of calcifications in DCIS
Sneige et al. (53)	All	Yes	Margins, residual calcifications, necrosis, periductal fibrosis
McCormick et al. (5)	All	Margins only	Margins, FH, residual calcifications
Hiramatsu et al. (6)	All	Margins only	Extent of surgery, FH
Catalotti et al. (71)	All	Yes	None
Beron et al. (50)	All	Yes	Architectural pattern, size, margins
Amichetti et al. (56)	All	Except margins	Size borderline
Kuske et al. (4)	All	Except margins	Architectural pattern, menopausal status
Weng et al. (54)	All	Yes	Margins
Fourquet et al. (52)	All	Except margins	Age, necrosis, absence of calcifications
Fisher et al. (NSABP B-24) (41)	All	Yes	Age, margins, comedonecrosis method of detection
Bijker et al. (EORTC 10853) (47)	All	Yes	Age, method of detection, grade, necrosis, architectural pattern, margins

DCIS, ductal carcinoma in situ; FH, family history.

The role of tamoxifen in the treatment of DCIS in patients receiving radiation therapy has been evaluated by two prospective randomized trials (9,41). In the United Kingdom trial, 1,694 women with mammographically detected DCIS were randomized to radiation therapy with or without tamoxifen or observation with or without tamoxifen. With a median follow-up of 3 years, there was no statistically significant benefit in terms of IBTR or contralateral breast cancer with tamoxifen (9). The NSABP B-24 trial randomized 1,804 women with DCIS to radiation therapy with or without tamoxifen. In contrast to the NSABP B-17 trial, eligibility for the B-24 trial included women with mammographic evidence of scattered calcifications or more than one focus of malignant-appearing calcifications or masses and positive resection margins. The 5-year cumulative incidence of an IBTR was 13.4% in the patients receiving radiation therapy only and 8.2% in the patients who re-

ceived radiation therapy and tamoxifen ($p = 0.0009$) (41). The 5-year cumulative incidence of an ipsilateral invasive cancer was decreased from 4.2% to 2.1% ($p = 0.03$) with tamoxifen. The 5-year cumulative incidence of an ipsilateral noninvasive recurrence was 5.1% without tamoxifen and 3.9% with tamoxifen ($p = 0.43$). The absolute benefit of tamoxifen in decreasing IBTR rates was greatest for women 49 years of age and younger (16% no tamoxifen versus 10% tamoxifen), those with positive or unknown margins (15% no tamoxifen versus 9% tamoxifen), comedonecrosis (13% no tamoxifen versus 9% tamoxifen), and mammographically detected DCIS (9% no tamoxifen versus 5% tamoxifen). Although tamoxifen decreased the risk of a contralateral breast cancer (3.4% no tamoxifen versus 2% tamoxifen), statistical significance was noted only for a decrease in contralateral noninvasive cancers (1.1% versus 0.2%, $p = 0.02$).

PATTERNS OF BREAST RECURRENCE AFTER CONSERVATIVE SURGERY AND RADIATION THERAPY FOR DUCTAL CARCINOMA IN SITU AND RESULTS OF SALVAGE MASTECTOMY

Patterns of breast recurrence in patients with DCIS treated with conservative surgery and radiation therapy are presented in Tables 24.10 and 24.11. Most recurrences occur in the vicinity of the original primary tumor, and approximately 50% are invasive cancers. In the NSABP B-17 trial, the 8-year cumulative incidence of an invasive recurrence in patients treated with conservative surgery and radiation therapy was 3.9%, whereas the 8-year cumulative incidence of a noninvasive recurrence was 8.2% (7).

Table 24.11 presents the incidence of ipsilateral invasive breast cancer after conservative surgery and radiation therapy for DCIS from retrospective series and prospective randomized trials. With varying follow-up periods, the incidence ranges from 0% to 9%. There is limited information regarding factors that predict an invasive IBTR. Vicini et al. (48) reported a higher incidence of invasive recurrences in young women (younger than 45 years). Silverstein et al. (59)

reported that the most significant predictor of an invasive recurrence after conservative surgery and radiation therapy was nuclear grade. Two retrospective series and the collaborative group study have correlated invasive recurrences with noncomedo histology (5,53,65). In the NSABP B-24 trial, comedonecrosis was associated with more noninvasive recurrences (41). In the EORTC 10853, there was no correlation with the risk of an invasive recurrence and histologic type classified as well, intermediate, or poorly differentiated (47). However, distant metastases were more frequent in patients whose invasive recurrence followed an initial diagnosis of poorly differentiated DCIS. Invasive recurrence rates were correlated with architectural pattern and were 2% for the clinging/micropapillary pattern compared with 11% for cribriform DCIS and 9% for solid or comedo DCIS. Distant metastases were also more common with solid or comedo DCIS. The interval to an invasive recurrence has been reported to be longer than a noninvasive recurrence (1,27), the same (66), or shorter (6).

Surgical salvage of an IBTR, either invasive or noninvasive, has been mastectomy in the majority of patients. In some selected patients, further attempts at breast conservation have been employed. Table 24.12 presents the results

TABLE 24.10. PATTERNS OF IPSILATERAL BREAST TUMOR RECURRENCE IN PATIENTS WITH DUCTAL CARCINOMA IN SITU TREATED WITH CONSERVATIVE SURGERY AND RADIATION THERAPY

Study	No. of Patients	Location Recurrence Vicinity Primary (%)	Pathology Recurrence Invasive (%)
Retrospective series			
Bullock et al. (74)	3	—	33
Howard et al. (84)	3	100	67
Kuske et al. (4)	3	—	100
Kurtz et al. (75)	3	67	100
Fowble et al. (45)	3	33	100
Haffty et al. (3)	4	—	25
Ray et al. (69)	5	80	20
Solin et al. (43)	5	60	40
Hiramatsu et al. (6)	7	85	57
McCormick et al. (5)	8	60	37
Mirza et al. (73)	11	—	55
Kestin et al. (60)	13	69	77
Fourquet et al. (52)	24	56	72
Silverstein et al. (67)	36	—	50
Solin et al. (collaborative group) (65)	42	71	55
Solin et al. (collaborative group) (66) (mammography detected)	42	69	52
Randomized trials			
Fisher et al. (NSABP B-17) (7)	47	84	36
Julien et al. (EORTC 10853) (8)	53	—	45
Fisher et al. (NSABP B-24) (41)	87	—	46

NSABP, National Surgical Adjuvant Breast Project; EORTC, European Organization for Research and Treatment of Cancer.

TABLE 24.11. IPSILATERAL INVASIVE BREAST TUMOR RECURRENCE AFTER CONSERVATIVE SURGERY AND RADIATION THERAPY IN MAMMOGRAPHICALLY DETECTED DUCTAL CARCINOMA IN SITU

Study	No. of Patients	Ipsilateral Invasive Breast Tumor Recurrence (%)	Median Follow-Up (yr)
Retrospective series			
Solin et al. (collaborative group) (66)	422	5	9.3
Beron et al. (50)	185	9	7.5
Sneige et al. (53)	31	0	7.2
Hiramatsu et al. (6)	54	2	6.2
Vicini et al. (85)	105	7	6.1
Fowble et al. (45)	110	3	5.3
Randomized trials			
Fisher et al. (NSABP B-17) (7)	411	4	(7.5)[a]
Fisher et al. (NSABP B-24) (41)	902	4	6.2
Julien et al. (EORTC 10853) (8)	502	5	4.2

[a] Mean.
NSABP, National Surgical Adjuvant Breast Project; EORTC, European Organization for Research and Treatment of Cancer.

of salvage therapy for an IBTR after conservative surgery and radiation therapy for DCIS. Salvage of a noninvasive recurrence has ranged from 93% to 100%. Approximately 80% of invasive recurrences are salvaged. The results of salvage treatment for an IBTR in patients treated with conservative surgery and radiation therapy by the collaborative group institutions have been reported by Solin et al. (65,66). The first report included patients whose DCIS was detected by clinical findings and/or mammography (65). The second report included only those patients whose DCIS was initially detected mammographically (66). In the first report, 42 of the 44 patients who developed a recurrence un-

TABLE 24.12. RESULTS OF SALVAGE TREATMENT IN PATIENTS WITH DUCTAL CARCINOMA IN SITU INITIALLY TREATED WITH CONSERVATIVE SURGERY AND RADIATION THERAPY

Study	Total No. of Patients	Salvage Recurrence		% DOD
		Noninvasive	Invasive	
Retrospective series				
Howard et al. (84)	3	2/2	1/1	0
Kuske et al. (4)	3	—	3/3	0
Kurtz et al. (75)	3	—	2/3	33
Fowble et al. (45)	3	—	2/3	0
Haffty et al. (3)	4	3/3	1/1	0
Ray et al. (69)	5	4/4	1/1	0
Solin et al. (43)	5	3/3	2/2	0
Hiramatsu et al. (6)	7	3/3	3/4	14
McCormick et al. (5)	8	5/5	3/3	0
Mirza et al. (73)	11	4/4	5/6	9
Kestin et al. (60)	13	3/3	9/10	8
Fourquet et al. (52)	24	6/6	14/18	0
Silverstein et al. (67)	36	18/18	14/18	11
Solin et al. (collaborative group) (65)	42	19/19	19/23	10
Solin et al. (collaborative group) (66) (mammography detected)	42	18/18	19/23	8
Randomized trials				
Fisher et al. (NSABP B-17) (7)	47	28/30	15/17	4
Julien et al. (EORTC 10853) (8)	53	—	—	8

NSABP, National Surgical Adjuvant Breast Project; EORTC, European Organization for Research and Treatment of Cancer; DOD, dead of disease.

derwent salvage mastectomy, and 81% of those received no additional treatment. Fifty-five percent of the recurrences were invasive. The median interval to recurrence was 5.1 years. The 5-year cause-specific survival rate after recurrence was 84% with an overall survival rate of 78%. None of the patients with a noninvasive recurrence developed distant metastases compared with 22% of those with an invasive recurrence. In the second report, 37 of the 42 recurrences were treated with salvage mastectomy. Sixty-nine percent of the patients had no adjuvant therapy. Fifty-five percent of the recurrences were invasive. The median interval to a recurrence was 4.8 years. After treatment, 5-year overall and cause-specific survival rates were 93%. Distant metastases developed in 17% of the patients with invasive recurrences and in none of the patients with noninvasive recurrences. Silverstein et al. (67) reported outcome of salvage therapy for 36 patients with an IBTR after conservative surgery and radiation therapy. Fifty percent of the recurrences were invasive. The median interval to an invasive recurrence was 5.5 years, 2.8 years for a noninvasive recurrence, and 4.7 years for all recurrences. None of patients with a noninvasive recurrence developed distant metastases compared with 28% of those with an invasive recurrence. In the NSABP B-17 trial (7), 47 women developed an isolated ipsilateral breast tumor recurrence after radiation therapy, of which 36% were invasive cancers. Distant metastases developed in 7% of the noninvasive recurrences and 6% of the invasive recurrences. Twenty-seven percent of noninvasive recurrences that were treated with excision without a mastectomy developed a second recurrence in the treated breast. There were no chest wall recurrences in the patients treated with mastectomy.

These studies support the excellent salvage of noninvasive recurrence with mastectomy. The prognosis of an invasive recurrence appears to be similar to that of a *de novo* invasive cancer.

SURVIVAL AFTER CONSERVATIVE SURGERY AND RADIATION THERAPY FOR DUCTAL CARCINOMA IN SITU

Mortality related to DCIS is owing to the presence of an occult invasive breast cancer or the subsequent development of an invasive cancer that may arise *de novo* or from the progression of residual DCIS to an invasive cancer. Breast cancer mortality after conservative surgery and radiation therapy for DCIS should be low because 50% of the recurrences are noninvasive, and virtually all these as well as 80% of the invasive recurrences are salvaged. Table 24.13 presents overall and cause-specific survival rates from retrospective series and prospective randomized trials. Breast cancer mortality rates ranges from 0% to 5%. These studies suggest that long-term survival for conservative surgery and radiation therapy in the treatment of DCIS is excellent and comparable with that achieved with mastectomy (39,59).

TABLE 24.13. SURVIVAL IN PATIENTS WITH DUCTAL CARCINOMA IN SITU AFTER CONSERVATIVE SURGERY AND RADIATION THERAPY

Retrospective Series	No. of Patients	Cause-Specific (Overall) Survival (%)	
		10 Yr	15 Yr
Solin et al. (collaborative group) (1,40)	268	97 (94)	96 (87)
Mammography detected	110	96 (93)	
Mirza et al. (73)	87	97	97
Hiramatsu et al. (6)	76	96	
Bullock et al. (74)	43	100	
Beron et al. (50)	185	97	
Fowble et al. (45)	110	100	
Kestin et al. (60)	146	99 (97)	
Amichetti et al. (56)	139	100 (93)	
Fourquet et al. (52)	153	98 (98)	

Randomized Trials		4 Yr	5 Yr	8 Yr
Fisher et al. (NSABP B-17) (7)	411	(99)	(98)	(96)
Fisher et al. (NSABP B-24) (41)	902		(97)	
Julien et al. EORTC 10853) (8)	502	(99)		

NSABP, National Surgical Adjuvant Breast Project; EORTC, European Organization for Research and Treatment of Cancer.

The incidence of contralateral breast cancer in patients treated with radiation therapy for DCIS is presented in Table 24.14. The incidence ranges from 2% to 10% depending on the length of follow-up. The NSABP B-17 trial reported no significant increase in contralateral breast cancer in women who received radiation therapy (7). However, the EORTC trial (8) reported a significant increase in contralateral breast cancer with radiation therapy at 4 years (3% versus 1%, $p = 0.01$). However, it is unlikely that the early appearance of these contralateral breast cancers could be attributed to radiation therapy. By 12 years, there were more contralateral breast cancers in the observation patients.

SUMMARY

Numerous retrospective studies and three prospective randomized trials have established the role of conservative surgery and radiation therapy in the treatment of DCIS. Despite the limitations of some of the early efforts, an appreciation for the heterogeneity of DCIS both in terms of clinical presentation, mammographic findings, pathologic features, extent of disease in the breast, and, more recently, biologic markers has emerged. We have discovered the importance of the mammographic and pathologic correlation,

TABLE 24.14. CONTRALATERAL BREAST CANCER IN PATIENTS WITH DUCTAL CARCINOMA IN SITU TREATED WITH CONSERVATIVE SURGERY AND RADIATION THERAPY

Study	Incidence of Contralateral Breast Cancer (%)	Interval Reported (yr)
Retrospective series		
Solin et al. (collaborative group) (1)	6	10.3 med.
Mammography detected (38)	6	9.3 med.
Kestin et al. (60)	9	10 act.
Fourquet et al. (52)	7	10 act.
Mirza et al. (73)	10	11 med.
Solin et al. (43)	4	5.7 med.
Fowble et al. (45)	2	5.3 med.
Randomized trials		
Fisher et al. (NSABP B-17) (7)	6	7.5 mean
Fisher et al. (NSABP B-24) (41)	3	6.2 med.
Julien et al. (EORTC 10853) (8)	4	4.2 med.

med., median; act., actuarial; NSABP, National Surgical Adjuvant Breast Project; EORTC, European Organization for Research and Treatment of Cancer.

surgical technique, and margins of resection in minimizing the risk of a breast recurrence in patients treated with conservative surgery and radiation therapy. The identification of factors associated with a significant risk of breast recurrence in these patients will help to define the group of patients for whom breast-conservation therapy is not appropriate. The current challenge is to identify a group of patients with DCIS in whom radiation may be omitted.

REFERENCES

1. Solin LJ, Kurtz J, Fourquet A, et al. Fifteen year results of breast conserving surgery and definitive breast irradiation for the treatment of ductal carcinoma in situ (intraductal carcinoma of the breast). *J Clin Oncol* 1996;14:754–763.
2. Stotter AT, McNeese M, Oswald MJ, et al. The role of limited surgery with irradiation in primary treatment of ductal in situ breast cancer. *Int J Radiat Oncol Biol Phys* 1990;18:283.
3. Haffty BG, Peschel RE, Papdopoulis D, et al. Radiation therapy for ductal carcinoma in situ of the breast. *Conn Med* 1990;54:482–484.
4. Kuske RR, Bean JM, Garcia DM, et al. Breast conservation therapy for intraductal carcinoma of the breast. *Int J Radiat Oncol Biol Phys* 1993;26:391–396.
5. McCormick B, Rosen PP, Kinne D, et al. Duct carcinoma in situ of the breast: an analysis of local control after conservative surgery and radiotherapy. *Int J Radiat Oncol Biol Phys* 1991;21:289–292.
6. Hiramatsu H, Bornstein BA, Recht A, et al. Local recurrence after conservative surgery and radiation therapy for ductal carci-

noma in situ. Possible importance of family history. *Cancer J Sci Am* 1995;1:55–61.
7. Fisher B, Dignam J, Wolmark N, et al. Lumpectomy and radiation therapy for the treatment of intraductal breast cancer: Findings from National Surgical Adjuvant Breast and Bowel Project B-17. *J Clin Oncol* 1998;16:441–452.
8. Julien J-P, Bijker N, Fentiman IS, et al. on Behalf of the EORTC Breast Cancer Cooperative Group and EORTC Radiotherapy Group. Radiotherapy in breast-conserving treatment for ductal carcinoma in situ: first results of EORTC randomised phase III trial 10853. *Lancet* 2000;355:528–533.
9. George WD, Houghton J, Cuzick J, et al. Radiotherapy and tamoxifen following complete local excision in the management of ductal carcinoma in situ (DCIS): preliminary results from the UK DCIS trial. *Proc Am Soc Clin Oncol* 2000;19:70(abst).
10. Fentiman IS, Fagg N, Millis RR, et al. In situ ductal carcinoma of the breast: implications of disease pattern and treatment. *Eur J Surg Oncol* 1986;12:261–266.
11. Fisher ER, Sass R, Fisher B, et al. Pathologic findings from the National Surgical Adjuvant Breast Project (Protocol 6). II. Relation of local breast recurrence to multicentricity. *Cancer* 1986;57:1717–1724.
12. Brown PW, Silverman J, Owens E, et al. Intraductal "non-infiltrating" carcinoma of the breast. *Arch Surg* 1976;111:1063–1067.
13. Schuh ME, Nemoto T, Penetrante RB, et al. Intraductal carcinoma. Analysis of presentation, pathologic findings and outcome of disease. *Arch Surg* 1986;121:1303–1307.
14. Schwartz GF, Patchefsky AS, Finklestein SD, et al. Nonpalpable in situ ductal carcinoma of the breast. Predictors of multicentricity and microinvasion and implications for treatment. *Arch Surg* 1989;124:29.
15. Rosen PP, Senie R, Schottenfeld D, et al. Non-invasive breast carcinoma: frequency of unsuspected invasion and implications for treatment. *Ann Surg* 1979;189:377.
16. Silverstein MJ, Waisman JR, Gamagami P, et al. Intraductal carcinoma of the breast (208 cases). Clinical factors influencing treatment choice. *Cancer* 1990;66:102–108.
17. Holland R, Hendriks JHCL, Verbeek ALM, et al. Extent, distribution and mammographic/histologic correlations of breast ductal carcinoma in situ. *Lancet* 1990;335:519–522.
18. Faverly DRG, Burgers L, Bult P, et al. Three dimensional imaging of mammary ductal carcinoma in situ: clinical implications. *Semin Diagn Pathol* 1994;11:193–198.
19. Ohuchi N, Furuta A, Mori S. Management of ductal carcinoma in situ with nipple discharge. Intraductal spreading of carcinoma is an unfavorable pathologic factor for breast-conserving surgery. *Cancer* 1994;74:1294–1302.
20. Lagios MD, Westdahl PR, Margolin FR, et al. Duct carcinoma in situ: relationship of extent of noninvasive disease to the frequency of occult invasion, multicentricity, lymph node metastases and short term treatment failures. *Cancer* 1982;50:1309–1314.
21. Wobbes TH, Tinnemans JGM, van der Sluis RF. Residual tumor after biopsy for non-palpable ductal carcinoma in situ of the breast. *Br J Surg* 1989;76:185.
22. Gump FE, Jicha DL, Ozello L. Ductal carcinoma in situ (DCIS): a revised concept. *Surg* 1987;102:790–795.
23. Bellamy COC, McDonald C, Salter DM, et al. Noninvasive ductal carcinoma of the breast. The relevance of histologic categorization. *Hum Pathol* 1993;24:16–23.
24. Patchefsky AS, Schwartz GF, Finkelstein SD, et al. Heterogeneity of intraductal carcinoma of the breast. *Cancer* 1989;63:731–741.
25. Holland R, Hendricks JHCL. Microcalcifications associated with ductal carcinoma in situ: mammographic-pathologic correlation. *Semin Diagn Pathol* 1994;11:181–192.

26. Ohtake T, Abe R, Kimijima I, et al. Intraductal extension of primary invasive breast carcinoma treated by breast-conservative surgery. Computer graphic three-dimensional reconstruction of the mammary duct-lobular systems. *Cancer* 1995;76:32–42.

27. Fisher ER, Costantino J, Palekar AS, et al. Pathologic findings from the National Surgical Adjuvant Breast Project (NSABP) protocol B-17. Intraductal carcinoma (ductal carcinoma in situ) [Letter]. *Cancer* 1995;76:2385–2387.

28. Silverstein MJ, Gierson ED, Colburn WJ, et al. Can intraductal breast carcinoma be excised completely by local excision? Clinical and pathologic predictors. *Cancer* 1994;73:2985–2989.

29. Goldstein NS, Kestin LL, Vicini FA. Pathologic features of initial biopsy specimens associated with residual intraductal carcinoma on re-excision in patients with ductal carcinoma in situ of the breast referred for breast conserving therapy. *Am J Surg Pathol* 1999;23:1340–1348.

30. Ratanawichitrasin A, Rybicki LA, Steiger E, et al. In predicting the likelihood of residual disease in women treated for ductal carcinoma in situ. *J Am Coll Surg* 1999;188:17–21.

31. Lagios MD, Silverstein M. Ductal carcinoma in situ. The success of breast conservation therapy. A shared experience of two single institutional non-randomized prospective studies. *Surg Oncol Clin North Am* 1997;6:385–392.

32. Fisher ER. National Surgical Adjuvant Breast Project (NSABP) Experience: pathology. In: Silverstein MJ, ed. *Ductal carcinoma in situ of the breast.* Baltimore: Williams & Wilkins, 1997:259–269.

33. Kestin LL, Goldstein NS, Lacerna MD, et al. Factors associated with local recurrence of mammographically detected ductal carcinoma in situ in patients given breast-conserving therapy. *Cancer* 2000;88:596–607.

34. Hardman PDJ, Worth A, Lee U. The risk of occult invasive breast cancer after excisional biopsy showing in-situ ductal carcinoma of comedo pattern. *Can J Surg* 1989;32:56–60.

35. Moriya T, Silverberg SG. Intraductal carcinoma (ductal carcinoma in situ) of the breast. A comparison of pure noninvasive tumors with those including different proportions of infiltrating carcinoma. *Cancer* 1994;74:2972–2978.

36. Findlay PA, Goodman R. Radiation therapy for treatment of intraductal carcinoma of the breast. *Am J Clin Oncol* 1983;6:281.

37. Recht A, Danoff BF, Solin LJ, et al. Intraductal carcinoma of the breast: results of treatment with excisional biopsy and irradiation. *J Clin Oncol* 1985;3:1339–1343.

38. Solin LJ, Fourquet A, Vicini FA, et al. Mammographically detected ductal carcinoma in situ of the breast treated with breast-conserving surgery and definitive breast irradiation: Long-term outcome and prognostic significance of patient age and margin status. *Int J Radiat Oncol Biol Phys* 2001;50:991–1002.

39. Fourquet A, Zafrani B, Campana F. Breast conserving treatment of ductal carcinoma in situ. *Semin Radiat Oncol* 1992;2:116–124.

40. Solin LJ, McCormick B, Recht A, et al. Mammographically detected clinically occult ductal carcinoma in situ (intraductal carcinoma) treated with breast-conserving surgery and definitive breast irradiation. *Cancer J Sci Am* 1996;2:158–165.

41. Fisher B, Dignam J, Wolmark N, et al. Tamoxifen in treatment of intraductal breast cancer: National Surgical Adjuvant Breast and Bowel Project B-24 randomized controlled trial. *Lancet* 1999;353:1993–2000.

42. Bornstein BA, Recht A, Connolly JL, et al. Results of treating ductal carcinoma in situ of the breast with conservative surgery and radiation therapy. *Cancer* 1991;67:7–13.

43. Solin LJ, Fowble BL, Schultz DJ, et al. Definitive irradiation for intraductal carcinoma of the breast. *Int J Radiat Oncol Biol Phys* 1990;19:843–850.

44. Szelei-Stevens KA, Kuske RR, Yantsos VA, et al. The influence of young age and positive family history of breast cancer on the prognosis of ductal carcinoma in situ treated by excision with or without radiation therapy or by mastectomy. *Int J Radiat Oncol Biol Phys* 2000;48:943–949.

45. Fowble B, Hanlon AL, Fein DA, et al. Results of conservative surgery and radiation for mammographically detected ductal carcinoma in situ (DCIS). *Int J Radiat Oncol Biol Phys* 1997;38:949–957.

46. Harris EER, Schultz DJ, Peters CA, et al. Relationship of family history and outcome after breast conservation therapy in women with ductal carcinoma in situ of the breast. *Int J Radiat Oncol Biol Phys* 2000;48:933–942.

47. Bijker N, Peterse JL, Duchateau L, et al. Risk factors for recurrence and metastasis after breast-conserving therapy for ductal carcinoma in situ: Analysis of European Organization for Research and Treatment of Clinical Trial 10853. *J Clin Oncol* 2001;19:2263–2271.

48. Vicini FA, Kestin LL, Goldstein NS, et al. Impact of young age on outcome in patients with ductal carcinoma in situ treated with breast-conserving therapy. *J Clin Oncol* 2000;18:296–306.

49. Fisher ER, Fisher B. Relation of a recurrent intraductal carcinoma (ductal carcinoma *in situ*) to the primary tumor. *J Natl Cancer Inst* 2000;92:288–289.

50. Beron P, Lewinsky BS, Silverstein MJ. Breast conserving therapy for ductal carcinoma in-situ. The Van Nuys experience with excision plus radiation therapy. In: Silverstein MJ, ed. *Ductal carcinoma in situ of the breast.* Baltimore: Williams & Wilkins, 1997:405.

51. Fisher ER, Dignam J, Tan-Chiu E, et al. for the National Surgical Adjuvant Breast and Bowel Project (NSABP). Eight-year update of protocol B-17. *Cancer* 1999;86:429–439.

52. Fourquet A, Zafrani B, Campana F, et al. Institut Curie Experience. In: Silverstein MJ, ed. *Ductal carcinoma in situ of the breast.* Baltimore: Williams & Wilkins, 1997:391–397.

53. Sneige N, McNeese MD, Atkinson EN, et al. Ductal carcinoma in situ treated with lumpectomy and irradiation: histopathologic analysis of 49 specimens with emphasis on risk factors and long term results. *Hum Pathol* 1995;26:642–649.

54. Weng EY, Juillard GJF, Parker RG, et al. Outcomes and factors impacting local recurrence of ductal carcinoma in situ. *Cancer* 2000;88:1643–1649.

55. Silverstein MJ, Lagios MD, Groseh S, et al. The influence of margin width on local control of ductal carcinoma in situ of the breast. *N Engl J Med* 1999;340:1455–1461.

56. Amichetti M, Caffo O, Richetti A, et al. Ten-year results of treatment of ductal carcinoma in situ (DCIS) of the breast with conservative surgery and radiotherapy. *Eur J Cancer* 1997;33:1559–1565.

57. Silverstein MJ, Poller DN, Waisman JR, et al. Prognostic classification of breast ductal carcinoma-in-situ. *Lancet* 1995;345:1154–1157.

58. Silverstein MJ, Lagios MD, Craig PH, et al. A prognostic index for ductal carcinoma in situ of the breast. *Cancer* 1996;77:2267–2274.

59. Silverstein MJ, Barth A, Poller DN, et al. Ten year results comparing mastectomy to excision and radiation therapy for ductal carcinoma in situ of the breast. *Eur J Cancer* 1995;31:1425–1427.

60. Kestin LL, Goldstein NS, Martinez AA, et al. Mammographically detected ductal carcinoma in situ treated with conservative surgery with or without radiation therapy. Patterns of failure and 10-year results. *Ann Surg* 2000;231:235–245.

61. Boyages J, Delaney G, Taylor R. Predictors of local recurrence after treatment of ductal carcinoma in situ. *Cancer* 1999;85:616–628.

62. Hwang E-S, Samli B, Tran KN, et al. Volume of resection in patients treated with breast conservation for ductal carcinoma in situ. *Ann Surg Oncol* 1998;5:757–763.

63. White J, Levine A, Gustafson G, et al. Outcome and prognostic factors for local recurrence in mammographically detected ductal carcinoma in-situ of the breast treated with conservative surgery and radiation therapy. *Int J Radiat Oncol Biol Phys* 1995;31:791–797.

64. Winchester DP, Strom EA. Standards for diagnosis and management of ductal carcinoma in situ (DCIS) of the breast. *CA Cancer J Clin* 1998;48:108–128.

65. Solin LJ, Fourquet A, McCormick B, et al. Salvage treatment for local recurrence following breast-conserving surgery and definitive irradiation for ductal carcinoma in situ (intraductal carcinoma) of the breast. *Int J Radiat Oncol Biol Phys* 1994;30:3–9.

66. Solin LJ, Fourquet A, Vicini F, et al. Salvage treatment for local recurrence after breast-conserving surgery and radiation as initial treatment for mammographically detected ductal carcinoma in situ of the breast. *Cancer* 2001;91:1090–97.

67. Silverstein MJ, Lagios MD, Martino S, et al. Outcome after invasive local recurrence in patients with ductal carcinoma in situ of the breast. *J Clin Oncol* 1998;16:1367–1373.

68. Warneke J, Grossklaus D, Davis J, et al. Influence of local treatment on the recurrence rate of ductal carcinoma in situ. *J Am Coll Surg* 1995;180:683–688.

69. Ray GR, Adelson J, Hayhurst E, et al. Ductal carcinoma in situ of the breast: results of treatment by conservative surgery and definitive irradiation. *Int J Radiat Oncol Biol Phys* 1993;28:105–111.

70. Van Zee KJ, Liberman L, Samli B, et al. Long term follow-up of women with ductal carcinoma in situ treated with breast-conserving surgery. The effect of age. *Cancer* 1999;86:1757–1767.

71. Cataliotti L, Distante V, Pacini P, et al. Florence experience. In: Silverstein MJ, ed. *Ductal carcinoma in situ of the breast.* Baltimore: Williams & Wilkins, 1997:449–54.

72. Solin LJ, Recht A, Fourquet A, et al. Ten-year results of breast-conserving surgery and definitive irradiation for intraductal carcinoma (ductal carcinoma in situ) of the breast. *Cancer* 1990;68:2337–2344.

73. Mirza NQ, Vlastos G, Meric F, et al. Ductal carcinoma in situ: long-term results of breast-conserving therapy. *Ann Surg Oncol* 2000;7:656–64.

74. Bullock CG, Magnant C, Ayoob M, et al. The utility of conservative surgery and radiation therapy in ductal carcinoma-in-situ. *Int J Radiat Oncol Biol Phys* 1993;27:268(abst).

75. Kurtz JM, Jacquemier J, Torhorst J, et al. Conservation therapy for breast cancers other than infiltrating ductal carcinoma. *Cancer* 1989;63:1630–1635.

76. Ciatto S, Grazzini G, Iossa A, et al. In situ ductal carcinoma of the breast—analysis of clinical presentation and outcome in 156 consecutive cases. *Eur J Surg Oncol* 1990;16:220–224.

77. Fisher ER, Sass R, Fisher B, et al. Pathologic findings from the National Surgical Adjuvant Breast Project (protocol 6). I. Intraductal carcinoma (DCIS). *Cancer* 1986;57:197–208.

78. Fisher ER, Leiming R, Anderson S, et al. Conservative management of intraductal carcinoma (DCIS) of the breast. *J Surg Oncol* 1991;47:139–147.

79. Delouche G, Bachelot F, Premont M, et al. Conservation treatment of early breast cancer: long term results of complications. *Int J Radiat Oncol Biol Phys* 1987;13:29–34.

80. Hughes KW, Lee AKC, McLellan R, et al. Breast-conserving therapy for patients with ductal carcinoma in situ. *Breast Dis* 1996;9:255–268.

81. Cutuli B, on behalf of the Breast Cancer Group of the French Cancer Centers. Pathologic findings from the National Surgical Adjuvant Breast Project (NSABP) eight-year update of protocol B-17. *Cancer* 2000;88:1976–1977.

82. Park CC, Recht A, Gelman R, et al. The impact of young age on outcome after breast-conserving surgery and radiation therapy for carcinoma in situ of the breast (DCIS). *Int J Radiat Oncol Biol Phys* 2000;48:293–294.

83. Chan KC, Knox WF, Sinha G, et al. Extent of excision margin width required in breast conserving surgery for ductal carcinoma in situ. *Cancer* 2001;91:9–16.

84. Howard PW, Locker AP, Dowle CS, et al. In situ carcinoma of the breast. *Eur J Surg Oncol* 1989;15:328–332.

85. Vicini FA, Lacerna MD, Goldstein NS, et al. Ductal carcinoma in situ detected in the mammographic era: an analysis of clinical, pathologic, and treatment-related factors affecting outcome with breast-conserving therapy. *Int J Radiat Oncol Biol Phys* 1997;39:627–635.

25

THE LAGIOS EXPERIENCE

MICHAEL D. LAGIOS

Ductal carcinoma in situ (DCIS) of the breast is currently a growing clinical problem and a focus of both great controversy and intense basic research. DCIS is a potential neoplastic process that straddles the boundary between a nonmotile cellular proliferation to one capable of metastatic growth. It is a model system for the elucidation of the molecular biology of invasion.

A PERSONAL HISTORY

Twenty-five years ago I completed my Army service and entered private practice in San Francisco, CA, joining a pathology group at a community hospital that serviced some of the wealthiest areas of the city. Our patients had no financial limitations on their access to treatment and received a quality of care that could not be duplicated in today's medical economic environment. Despite their resources, patients with breast cancer presented with tumors averaging 30 mm in maximum diameter, and nearly all were treated with modified radical mastectomy. Fifty percent were found to have nodal metastases, and 40% had a recurrence or died of the disease within 8 years of treatment. DCIS was a rare anomaly in this setting, with one or two cases seen per year; so few that, on average, one pathologist in our group would have experienced a single case every 2 years.

Xeromammography, the first of the new generation of mammographic technologies, was introduced in our hospital in 1973. Although medicine is often reluctant to accept new technology, the advent of xeromammography promptly followed the now historic success of the mammographic screening trial of the Health Insurance Plan of New York (1). Many patients began to be referred by their primary care physicians and, to some extent, by surgeons for mammographic screening. The American Cancer Society began publicizing and supporting this new early detection tool for breast cancer, and an increasing interest in breast cancer began to be reflected in medical publications, both lay and scientific. Within 18 months of the inception of xeromammographic screening, the average size of invasive breast cancers at our hospital decreased from 30 to 18 mm; the proportion of patients with negative nodes increased, and, dramatically, the frequency of in situ duct carcinomas increased threefold to approximately 15% of all new breast cancers detected (2). However, despite the smaller size of both invasive and in situ cancers, most patients continued to be treated with mastectomy.

In June 1975, I attempted to use the serial subgross technique of Egan et al. (3) to evaluate mastectomy material. Initially, the mastectomy specimen was sectioned freehand, slicing the entire frozen breast into segments approximately 5 to 6 mm thick with a large carving knife. The slices were then arranged in sequence and the entire series were x-rayed. Within a few months, however, a colleague who had developed tennis elbow by this effort and who as a Yale undergraduate had dated a young woman who later married the heir of the Hobart Manufacturing firm, managed to secure a donation of a Hobart rotary meat slicer designed for delicatessen use. This markedly simplified the sectioning of mastectomy specimens, increased the number of sections, and became standard for our pathology department in late 1975 (4).

Our modification of the serial subgross technique of Egan et al. permitted sectioning of an entire mastectomy specimen in 2.5-mm intervals. Every slice was reviewed in sequence, both visually and radiographically. The distribution of clinical (palpable) invasive cancers and small, occult separate invasive and in situ subclinical cancers could be mapped out. Most important, this technique allowed us to delineate the distribution of particular lesions, specifically DCIS. We could now test the prevailing logic that DCIS was multicentric, commonly associated with invasion, and on occasion associated with lymph node metastases.

It soon became evident that there were two main populations of patients with DCIS: one with extensive disease largely detected by conventional physical examination and a second group with generally small, focal lesions detected only by mammographic microcalcifications. The more extensive disease averaged 60 mm in size, and nearly 50% harbored occult areas of invasion as detected by the serial subgross technique. Two percent of patients with extensive disease exhibited small axillary metastases. Fifteen percent of patients with extensive disease developed a postmastectomy recurrence or died of their disease within 7 years of follow-up. Such patients seemed to validate the historical treatment of total mastectomy, generally with lymph node dissection, for DCIS.

In contrast, the small focal lesions that were adequately excised by the standards of the time were not associated with occult areas of invasion in the mastectomy specimen; 86% were judged to be unifocal using the contemporary definition of multicentricity. None was associated with axillary metastases and none died of disease. No residual DCIS of any kind was the prevalent finding at mastectomy for most patients with small focal lesions that had been previously excised.

At this point, I began to question the necessity of modified radical mastectomy for DCIS of small size, and in collaboration with Phillip Westdahl, a courageous and inquisitive surgeon, then in his mid-60s, we proposed that some patients with DCIS whose lesions were small and adequately excised might be offered an option of follow-up alone. A small number of patients chose what was seen at that time (1975 to 1976) as a risky, experimental endeavor. During the mid-1970s, we worked in an informational vacuum regarding mammographically detected DCIS. There would be no published literature on this subject for another 7 years, and the first modern publication of radiation therapy for DCIS would not appear until 1983 (5,6).

I believed that small foci of DCIS that were adequately excised might have a risk comparable with that of lobular carcinoma in situ, which at the time was an interesting if not controversial model for noninvasive breast cancer (7–10). The biologic distinction between lobular carcinoma in situ as a marker lesion and DCIS as a variable obligate precursor to invasive growth still lay in the future.

We had no understanding of the most appropriate selection criteria at the onset, except that the lesion would have to be small and adequately incised. Selection criteria were developed on a trial-and-error basis. We learned that margins had to be marked and pathologically clear, all tissue had to be processed, and mammographic correlation was essential preoperative, intraoperative with specimen radiograms, and postoperative. We learned that microcalcifications, although not a reliable marker of disease extent, were a requisite for accepting a case for lumpectomy, for without them, there was no way to estimate the size of the lesion or the adequacy of the excision. We limited candidates for lumpectomy to those whose lesions were 25 mm or less based on the results of our subgross mastectomy series that had shown that there were no cases of DCIS 25 mm or smaller in diameter that exhibited occult invasion elsewhere in the breast (11).

Although our excision-only treatment for mammographically detected DCIS had been mentioned in 1977 (4), we first published in detail on the subject in 1982 (11), establishing selection criteria based on our "large" series of a mere 20 patients! These studies evolved in an environment in which a then young radiologist, Frederick Margolin, became dedicated to developing a successful screening and early detection program.

At the suggestion of two colleagues, P. P. Rosen and D. L. Page, we reviewed and classified all our DCIS cases in 1987. Perhaps being swayed by the prognostic significance of nuclear characteristics in the evaluation of invasive carcinomas, I chose to look at nuclear grade and necrosis as significant features in a new classification. The initial published classification, based on 79 patients, had four categories that were designated by architectural features but characterized by nuclear grade and necrosis. Two were high grade but differed only by architecture (12). These were collapsed subsequently into a single high-grade group (13). This latter three-tiered classification achieved a remarkable separation among the small number of cases available for evaluation. All but one of the local recurrences occurred in the high-grade subset and the single remaining recurrence in the intermediate-grade subset. There were no recurrences in the low-grade subset at the time of publication in 1989.

The significance of high nuclear grade and necrosis for local recurrence was corroborated by Solin et al. (14), in a two-tiered system (comedo versus noncomedo) in which nuclear grade 3 morphology and comedonecrosis resulted in a 20% local recurrence rate at 86 months, as opposed to a 5% local recurrence rate for all other noncomedo subtypes combined. Further corroboration of the importance of nuclear grade on local recurrence–free survival was provided by the works of Bellamy et al. (15), Ottesen et al. (16), and Silverstein et al. (17) and given the approximation of comedo with high nuclear grade subtypes by the work of Schwartz et al. (18).

Some features of my initial classification were limited by the small number of cases that I had available. Although necrosis was noted to occur in high- and intermediate-grade DCIS, none of the low-grade lesions exhibited necrosis. Larger series by Silverstein et al. (17) and Holland et al. (19) would later make clear that necrosis can occur in association with any nuclear grade, although clearly it is far more common in high-grade DCIS. Additionally, high nuclear grade lesions that exhibit no necrosis are occasionally encountered, but none was tabulated in my initial series.

The effect of size on local recurrence rate was evident in my small group of 79 patients when the group was divided into those with lesions smaller and larger than 12.5 mm, despite the fact that by design, no candidate for breast-conservation therapy with a lesion larger than 25 mm was accepted. Silverstein et al. (17,20), who initially employed radiation therapy in their program of breast-conservation therapy, accepted some larger lesions, with a substantial number larger than 25 mm and 6% larger than 40 mm in extent. In their study, there was a significant difference in local recurrence–free survival between patients with DCIS 15 mm or less, 16 to 40 mm, or 41 mm or greater in size; however, the differences between the size groups are smaller if the analysis is limited to those in the best margin category, i.e., 10 mm or more of free margin. The problem with the comparison is that surgical resection with good margins (>10 mm) in a patient with DCIS with a lesion 41 mm or larger is difficult to accomplish.

The definition of an adequate margin varies in the published studies of DCIS. Intrinsically, we want to have larger margins, but in the early period of the study, the operative procedure for a suspect group of microcalcifications was most commonly a diagnostic biopsy, and it was not designed as an excision biopsy for a known carcinoma. In California, in particular, concerns about cosmesis limited the tissue volume resected and as a result many clear margins were quite limited. Some were 1 mm or less. It is now clear that margins that are this limited are inadequate for local control. High-grade DCIS in the study of Silverstein et al. (17,20) dramatically illustrates this: For high-grade DCIS with margins of 10 mm or greater, local recurrence–free survival was 92% at 86 months but dropped to 40% when margins were 1 mm or less for the high-grade subset.

Developing a program in which margins are carefully evaluated is not easy. It requires a rigorous protocol of tissue processing and mammographic correlation and, in particular, for multi-institutional trials, a willingness to attempt an adequate excision. This point is exemplified by National Surgical Adjuvant Breast Project protocol B-17 (Chapter 42) in which margins of 1 mm or less were accepted as free. In fact, anything short of actual transection of the involved duct was classified as a free margin. Accepting this definition for a margin to be considered free has a lot to do with the 21% local recurrence rate in the nonirradiated treatment arm at a mean follow-up of 43 months.

FOLLOW-UP OF THE ORIGINAL 79 PATIENTS OF LAGIOS ET AL.

Follow-up of the original 79 patients reported in 1989 now averages 135 months (Table 25.1) with an overall actuarial local recurrence rate of 22% at 15 years (Fig. 25.1), 58% of which were invasive events. Despite this, there were no

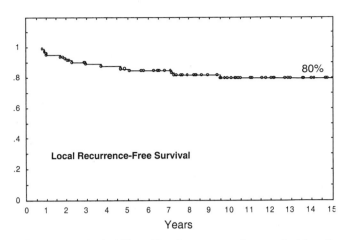

FIGURE 25.1. Probability of local recurrence-free survival for all 79 patients treated with excision alone.

cause- (breast cancer) specific deaths or patients who developed distant metastases. Two patients with high-grade (nuclear grade 3 and necrosis) DCIS developed invasive recurrences with axillary metastases. The first with a single micrometastasis was reported previously (13). More recently, a second patient had a recurrence with bilateral invasive breast carcinomas and axillary metastases after 18 years of follow-up. Follow-up time beyond a patient's date of death or recurrence was censored in this calculation. However, the most recently accessioned case among the 79 was included 14 years ago (1987).

Recurrences were predominantly seen among the high-grade DCIS (nuclear grade 3) subset (Table 25.2). This subset accounts for 82% of all recurrences at 135 months. Ultimately, two recurrences in patients with low-grade (nuclear grade 1) DCIS were detected mammographically. Both were low-grade in situ recurrences in patients whose original margins were less than 1 mm at the initial excision and

TABLE 25.1. PATIENT DEMOGRAPHICS

No. of patients	79
Average follow-up	135 mo
Average age	55 yr
Average tumor size	7.8 mm
Average nuclear grade	2.04
Recurrences	17 (22%)
Invasive recurrences	10 (13%)
Invasive recurrences/all recurrences	10/17
Breast cancer deaths	0
Other deaths	11 (14%)

TABLE 25.2. PATHOLOGIC SUBSETS

	No. Pts	Recurrences (%)
Necrosis		
Present	42	14 (33%)
Absent	37	3 (8%)
Size (mm)		
≤15	71	13 (18%)
≥16	8	4 (50%)
Margins (mm)		
≥10	15	2 (13%)
1–9	61	12 (20%)
≤1	3	3 (100%)
Grade		
1	33	2 (6%)
2	10	1 (10%)
3	36	14 (39%)

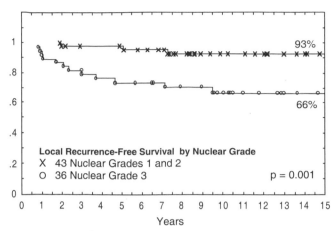

FIGURE 25.2. Probability of local recurrence–free survival by nuclear grade (nuclear grades 1 and 2 versus nuclear grade 3) for 79 patients treated with excision alone. The difference between the two curves is statistical significant ($p = 0.001$).

whose disease, in retrospect, clearly demonstrated a multifocal pattern of involvement in the breast.

The most dramatic information obtained from this retrospective review is the impact that margin width makes on outcome (Table 25.2), with local recurrences varying from 13% for the widest margin subset to 100% for the narrowest margin subset, a 7.7-fold difference.

A Kaplan-Meier actuarial projection of all 79 patients with DCIS to 15 years revealed a 39% recurrence rate for the nuclear grade 3 (high-grade) subset versus only 7% for the combined subsets of nuclear grades 1 and 2 (Fig. 25.2). This experience should be contrasted with the 15-year follow-up recently reported by Solin et al. (21) in which recurrences among the high-grade DCIS subset (nuclear grade 3 and necrosis) treated with lumpectomy and radiation therapy experienced a recurrence rate nearly matched by the comparison group (18% versus 15%). The current follow-up of this small initial group of 79 patients treated with breast conservation, a database independent of the far larger Van Nuys/University of Southern California compilation, dramatically confirms the prognostic value of grade, margins, and size codified in the Van Nuys Prognostic Index (20) (Table 25.2).

CONCLUSION

Looking back at the past quarter century, I see an accelerating transition from the initial timid steps toward breast-conservation therapy for DCIS, which were met with much skepticism and some derision, even in San Francisco, to a juncture at which we have identified reproducible and reliable prognostic features from which an individual patient's risk can be estimated in quantitative terms. We cannot as yet accurately predict which patients even in the high-grade subset are most likely to experience a recurrence.

Just a few years ago, great interest in obtaining archival paraffin blocks to identify oncogenes in patients with DCIS who subsequently had a recurrence peaked only to pass with the failure to be able to use such markers to identify the subset most likely to have a recurrence. However, it may be that markers such as HER-2/neu that identify 75% to 85% of the large cell type DCIS, those with the greatest predilection for subsequent invasive growth, can be manipulated to abort the cascade of molecular events that presage invasion. Tamoxifen and other selective estrogen receptor modulators (SERMS) have achieved a remarkably wide usage as chemopreventative agents in patients at risk and in those with DCIS in the United States despite the minute size and inconsistent appearance of a benefit in randomized trials. A recent consensus conference concluded that the role of tamoxifen in the management of DCIS was uncertain (22). True chemoprevention, at least in terms of invasive transformation, has not yet been achieved with available interventional agents. Let us hope that it may be achieved and brute surgery banished to that dark reliquary that buries a host of ancient therapies, confining them like blackblood in the tomb of Atreus.

REFERENCES

1. Shapiro S, Strax P, Vanet W. Periodic breast cancer screening in reducing mortality from breast cancer. *JAMA* 1971;215:1777–1785.
2. Margolin FR, Lagios MD. Development of mammography and breast services in a community hospital. *Radiol Clin North Am* 1987;25:973–982.
3. Egan RL, Ellis JR, Powell RW. Team approach to the study of disease of the breast. *Cancer* 1969;71:847–854.
4. Lagios MD. Multicentricity of breast carcinoma demonstrated by routine correlated serial subgross and radiographic examination. *Cancer* 1977;40:1726–1734.
5. Findlay P, Goodman R. Radiation therapy for treatment of intraductal carcinoma of the breast. *Am J Clin Oncol* 1983;6:281–285.
6. Montague ED, et al. Conservative treatment of non-invasive and small-volume invasive breast cancer. In: *Breast carcinoma: current diagnosis and treatment*. Philadelphia: Mosby,1986;429–432.
7. Wheeler JE, Enterline HT, Roseman JM, et al. Lobular carcinoma in situ of the breast. Long term follow-up. *Cancer* 1974;34:554–563.
8. Giordano JM, Klopp CT. Lobular carcinoma in situ: incidence and treatment. *Cancer* 1973;31:105–109.
9. Rosen PP, Lieberman PH, Braun DW Jr, et al. Lobular carcinoma in situ of the breast. Detailed analysis of 99 patients with average follow-up of 24 years. *Am J Surg Pathol* 1978;2:225–251.
10. Haagensen CD, Lane N, Lattes R, et al. Lobular neoplasia (so-called lobular carcinoma in situ) of the breast. *Cancer* 1978;42:737–769.
11. Lagios MD, Westdahl PR, Margolin FR, et al. Duct carcinoma in situ: relationship of extent of noninvasive disease to the frequency of occult invasion, multicentricity, lymph node metastases, and short-term treatment failures. *Cancer* 1982;50:1309–1314.
12. Lagios MD, Margolin FR, Westdahl PR, et al. Mammographically detected duct carcinoma in situ. Frequency of local recurrences following tylectomy and prognostic effect of nuclear grade on local recurrence. *Cancer* 1989;63:619–624.

13. Lagios MD. Duct carcinoma in situ: pathology and treatment. *Surg Clin North Am* 1990;70:853–871.

14. Solin LJ, Yeh IT, Kurtz J, et al. Ductal carcinoma in situ (intraductal carcinoma) of the breast treated with breast-conserving surgery and definitive irradiation: correlation pathologic parameters with outcome of treatment. *Cancer* 1993;71:2532–2542.

15. Bellamy COC, McDonald D. Salter DM, et al. Non-invasive ductal carcinoma of the breast. The relevance of histologic categorization. *Hum Pathol* 1993;24:16–23.

16. Ottesen GL, Graversen HP, Bilcher-Toft M, et al. Ductal carcinoma in situ of the female breast. Short-term results of a prospective nationwide study. *Am J Surg Pathol* 1992;16:1183–1196

17. Silverstein MJ, Poller DN, Waisman JR, et al. Prognostic classification of breast ductal carcinoma in situ. *Lancet* 1995;345:1154–1157.

18. Schwartz GF, Finkel GC, Garcia JG, et al. Subclinical ductal carcinoma in situ of the breast. Treatment by local excision and surveillance alone. *Cancer* 1992;70:2468–2474.

19. Holland R, Peterse JL, Millis RR, et al. Ductal carcinoma in situ: a proposal for new classification. *Semin Diagn Pathol* 1994;11:167–180.

20. Silverstein MJ, Lagios MD, Craig PH, et al. A prognostic index for ductal carcinoma in situ of the breast. *Cancer* 1996;77:2267–2274.

21. Solin LJ, Kurtz J, Fourquet A, et al. Fifteen-year results of breast-conserving surgery and definitive breast irradiation for the treatment of ductal carcinoma in situ of the breast. *J Clin Oncol* 1996;14:754–763.

22. International Breast Cancer Consensus Conference. Image-detected breast cancer: state of the art diagnosis and treatment. *J Am Coll Surg* 2001;193:297–302.

26

TREATMENT OF SUBCLINICAL DUCTAL CARCINOMA IN SITU OF THE BREAST BY LOCAL EXCISION AND SURVEILLANCE: AN UPDATED PERSONAL EXPERIENCE

GORDON FRANCIS SCHWARTZ

How much easier it would make the practice of medicine if we could easily summarize a few observations, type them into a computer, and sit back and await precise instructions for care, based on an analysis of these observations, however complicated we make the algorithm. Perhaps fortunately for those of us who still take pride in our clinical skills, that time has not yet arrived. Certainly, the entity that we designate by a hodgepodge of names, including ductal carcinoma in situ (DCIS), intraductal, noninvasive, noninfiltrating ductal carcinoma, and in situ ductal carcinoma, might benefit from such a system because both diagnosis and treatment of this particular breast lesion provoke assertive albeit conflicting opinions from renowned clinicians and pathologists. Currently, there may be no more controversial diagnosis in the breast cancer spectrum. Admittedly, the options of therapy are few—the treatment of the breast (and infrequently the axilla), but the differences among these treatments are formidable to the patients who must make these decisions and live with them. This dilemma about the treatment of DCIS became a matter of public debate in March 1996, by the publication of geographically related disparities in treatment for this disease (1). Although treatment has generally shifted from mastectomy toward breast conservation, the increased detection of DCIS has led, at least until recently, to an actual increase in the number of mastectomies performed for this disease.

The diagnosis of DCIS has become increasingly commonplace within the past few years because mammography for screening asymptomatic women (at least for women older than 50 years of age and, in our own opinion, for those between 40 and 50 as well) has been embraced as a major advance in the discovery of earlier malignancies and because notable improvements in mammographic technique, such as magnification films, have detected even smaller, subtle changes within the breast. In the past several years, our own data indicate that as many as one-fourth of nonpalpable breast cancers (those detected by mammography) will prove to be DCIS. As implied by the name, DCIS seems to arise within ducts of the breast that become greatly dilated as the process evolves. In the usual scenario, when necrosis occurs within the lumina of the ducts, the precipitation of radiographically opaque inorganic material, usually containing calcium, leads to the mammographic discovery of these areas of intraductal disease as areas of clustered "calcifications" on a mammogram. It had been assumed that, if the process continues without interference, the involved ducts grow in number and volume until finally discovered by the patient or physician as a palpable mass. At some time in this process, the formerly intraductal, cytologically malignant but biologically noninvasive, cells, penetrate through the basement membrane of the ducts, and the disease becomes invasive, with all the implications of any invasive carcinoma.

Within the past generation, the inevitable progression of DCIS to invasive carcinoma has been challenged (2). Whether there are circumstances such that the identification of DCIS at some early stage in its natural history will obviate the obligatory treatment of the entire breast, with minimal risk to the patient of developing a subsequent, life-threatening cancer, has become a topic of great debate. If, as now accepted, DCIS is not always accompanied by invasion and/or does not necessarily progress to this stage, to prescribe lesser treatment for DCIS than for invasive carcinoma implies an obligation to recognize the time at which the identification and excision of DCIS at this one site might be treatment enough. This premise, however, also implies that the eradication of DCIS at one location ensures that the site detected is no greater in significance than what might be a concurrent, as yet undetected, but more important (invasive), finding at another location within the same breast.

Controversy about DCIS begins with its definition. Initially, Haagensen (3) and others were careful to separate the term intraductal from the term noninfiltrating. The terms were not then considered synonyms. Those cases of intraductal carcinoma described by Haagensen were palpable lesions, and many (29%) were accompanied by metastasis to axillary lymph nodes (4). Although many similar tumors may fail to exhibit areas of invasion when examined under light microscopy, it is probably preferable to comment that invasion may not have been seen "in the sections studied." As the mammographic detection of smaller masses, then only as areas of nonpalpable calcifications, became more common as radiographic techniques improved, these distinctions became blurred, and over time the terms noninvasive, intraductal, noninfiltrating, and DCIS have become interchangeable. As currently used, they define the absence of invasive carcinoma. The separation of clinical from subclinical DCIS to permit a more careful comparison of equivalent diseases was first suggested by Gump et al. (5), and their distinction also has great implications for treatment. At least to us, DCIS presenting as a palpable mass, nipple erosion (Paget's carcinoma), or nipple discharge is not the same as DCIS presenting as an area of calcifications on a screening mammogram or discovered as an incidental finding in a specimen of breast tissue removed for another reason.

In any discussion about treatment, therefore, it is first appropriate to define the disease. Inasmuch as staging systems for breast cancer have not yet addressed this issue and all DCIS is considered stage 0, Tis, the subdivision of DCIS into categories for consideration is somewhat arbitrary (6). It is easier to discuss clinical DCIS (that producing a palpable mass of more than 1 cm), nipple erosion, or nipple discharge from the treatment viewpoint than subclinical DCIS, detected by mammography or as an incidental finding. If there are patients in whom DCIS is not inexorably followed by invasive cancer, as current data indicate, we do not consider women with clinical DCIS currently among that group. Currently, we believe that, except for highly selected patients, until data are available that refute this recommendation, patients with clinically detected DCIS should continue to undergo treatment that includes the entire breast, i.e., irradiation or mastectomy, and in selected patients, the axilla, at least sentinel lymph node biopsy (SLNB). Exceptions to this dictum might be made for those patients with small, palpable but biologically/histologically favorable types of DCIS.

Therefore, using this definition, the term palpable DCIS is almost an oxymoron. As a palpable mass, a carcinoma may be largely intraductal, but it should not be considered noninvasive. As already noted, the appropriate designation should probably be no invasion documented in the sections studied. Except for these specially selected patients, these allegedly intraductal but palpable lesions are often accompanied by microinvasion, even when not seen, and the appropriate treatment addresses the entire breast and, arguably, the axilla as well.

Some of these predominantly intraductal but palpable lesions may achieve considerable size (i.e., more than 5 cm in diameter) and may be accompanied by clinically involved axillary nodes. They are characterized by their firmness, fairly well delimited margins, and an abundance of malignant-appearing calcifications on mammography. Patients with these large lesions are usually not candidates for radiation therapy because of the difficulty of excising all the calcifications that permeate the ducts contiguous to and even at great distance from the mass itself. The palpable masses called DCIS that radiotherapists currently covet remain small ones, amenable to wide local excision with clear surgical margins.

Paget's carcinoma, presenting as nipple erosion, is a form of breast carcinoma that grows initially within the milk sinuses of the nipple and extends within the ducts beneath the nipple in an apparently intraductal, but not necessarily in situ, manner. The development of the disease may be multicentric within the breast, and patients with Paget's disease infrequently have axillary node metastasis, unless a mass accompanies the nipple and areolar findings. Tempting as it may be to consider less aggressive surgical procedures, mastectomy with axillary dissection has remained the treatment of choice except in unusual situations. The mammograms in Paget's disease may be helpful in defining the retroareolar spread of disease. Although not well described in the literature, it has been our observation that calcifications in a branching distribution in the retroareolar area may help to outline the intraductal spread of Paget's disease, proving its widespread character and the need for mastectomy (7).

Although it is not necessarily true that the absence of retroareolar calcifications proves a more limited distribution of disease, when the calcifications are seen to be distributed in this pattern, the failure of any procedure that does not treat the entire breast can be appreciated. Nevertheless, my colleagues and I have treated several women with Paget's carcinoma with radiation therapy only, not even excising the nipple and areolar complex, but this choice is tenable only when the biopsy of the nipple indicates what we believe is the relatively confined distribution of disease (7). These several patients have also been quite vocal and unequivocal in their desire to retain their breast. Despite this limited success with what should be considered a quasiexperimental approach, Paget's carcinoma should be considered as clinical DCIS, at the least. Untreated, Paget's carcinoma is inevitably, albeit slowly, progressive.

Patients presenting with spontaneous nipple discharge owing to intraductal carcinoma are tempting candidates for treatment with something less than mastectomy. Because the mammograms in these patients rarely show evidence of mass or calcifications, and the usual morphology of the malignant cells is less rather than more aggressive, why not consider these patients within the group to be followed up with surveillance alone? That had been our initial query as we began to search for patients with DCIS that might be candidates for local excision alone. However, after the first two patients so treated had a recurrence relatively quickly and we then reviewed the mastectomy specimens from other patients with the same presenting symptoms, we became more convinced that nipple discharge as the first sign of DCIS implies an uncertain intraductal, usually multicentric, distribution peripherally. At least in the traditional sense, it is impossible to perform a lumpectomy in these patients that conclusively circumscribes the macroscopic disease. Irradiation as an alternative to mastectomy is not usually suitable because, if one believes that the macroscopic extent of the disease must be excised before irradiation, the nipple and areola must be, by definition, part of the tissue removed. Additionally, if one also believes in additional irradiation to the site of the primary lesion, there is no specific site to boost.

Treatment of the axilla in patients with clinical DCIS detected as nipple discharge is more controversial than the same consideration in patients with intraductal carcinoma detected as Paget's disease or a palpable mass. If frank invasion is present, treatment includes the same attention to the axilla as for any other invasive cancer. When invasion is questioned, even if termed focal or microinvasive, a SLNB is an acceptable consideration, with further dissection if the axilla is positive.

It is difficult to justify treatment of the axilla when the microscopic sections fail to detect any invasion. However, most of these particular patients are currently treated with mastectomy, and a truly total mastectomy includes the removal of the axillary prolongation (tail of Spence) of the breast. Thus, some of the lowermost axillary lymph nodes, those in what would be called by anatomists the external mammary group and even a few in the central or scapular group of the level I nodes, which are impossible to separate from the axillary tail tissue, may be included within the specimen. Some surgeons have advocated performing a SLNB in all patients undergoing mastectomy for DCIS because this procedure is less morbid than a formal axillary dissection. However, ease of use and lack of complications should not be an excuse for performing SLNB. When microinvasion is found, this is an appropriate consideration as part of mastectomy but not for pure DCIS. Guidelines for SLNB in DCIS with microinvasion are the same as those for SLNB in frankly invasive carcinoma.

Whether radiation therapy is an alternative to mastectomy for both invasive carcinoma and DCIS is another contentious point in the contemporary literature. Recurrence in the same breast that occurs after irradiation usually implies mastectomy, but this should not be a greater threat to life for these patients (with DCIS) than for the women who have undergone breast conservation for invasive cancers and who then have a local recurrence. In our own experience with more than 1,000 patients with invasive stage 1 and 2 invasive breast cancers treated with radiation therapy, the same 10-year outcome was documented for those without local recurrence and those who had a recurrence in the breast only, without concurrent systemic disease (8). It would be logical to presume that women with DCIS would do at least as well, if not better. Data published by radiation oncologists thus far seem to concur with this assumption (9,10).

The current controversy, therefore, with respect to DCIS, concerns the patients who have subclinical disease, i.e., that which is detected by mammography within areas of clustered calcifications or as an incidental finding when biopsy is performed for another reason, whether palpable or not (11). In the latter cases, the detection of DCIS is truly serendipitous. Although it is generally accepted that many patients with DCIS, if untreated, do not subsequently develop invasive carcinoma of the same breast, the ability to distinguish which women will be spared has eluded us. The reports that discuss the implied natural history of this disease in patients untreated because the diagnosis was initially overlooked fail to demonstrate that even a simple majority of these patients progressed to invasive carcinoma (2). Nevertheless, until relatively recently, mastectomy had been the treatment of choice for this disease, and currently, the generally accepted choice is either mastectomy or radiation therapy, depending on the availability and influence of radiation therapists on local tradition (1,9,10,12,13). In our own practice, needle-guided biopsy for mammographically detected lesions was initiated in 1974, and, until 1978, mastectomy was the customary "reward" for those patients who were diligent enough to have their cancers (DCIS) detected in such an early stage. As the exponential increase in patients with subclinical DCIS was noted in response to technical improvements in mammography and the greater acceptance of screening mammography by the medical profession and the public alike, questions relating to the extent of disease within the breast, the possibility of occult invasion, and the likelihood of axillary metastasis began to be addressed.

In 1975, Lagios et al. began to offer selected patients with DCIS the option of local excision only (13). Their studies of these women have been the most elegant and their follow-up has been the longest. Thus far, 12.6% of their patients have developed local recurrence, either further DCIS or invasive duct carcinoma, after a median follow-up of 68 months. Independently influenced by similar observations and in response to patients' greater participation in their own health care, in 1978, we began to offer highly selected patients the same option, local excision alone, with the caveat that perhaps as many as 30% to 40% (our initial estimates) of patients so treated would develop a subsequent invasive carcinoma of the same breast. Having championed the surveillance option for patients with lobular carcinoma in situ (LCIS) (or lobular neoplasia) from the inception, extrapolation from LCIS to DCIS was understandable if not accurate. The observations of Haagensen et al. (14) on LCIS afforded a firmer commitment to the surveillance option for LCIS. At the time that this study was initiated, however, there was little information available about patients with

DCIS treated with local excision alone. Since that time, other reports have been published, but they have almost invariably addressed DCIS generically, without separating those cases that we consider subclinical from the others. Thus, it has been difficult and almost impossible to glean meaningful information about the treatment of subclinical DCIS from the extant literature.

In 1992, my colleagues and I reported our own initial experience with 72 cases of subclinical DCIS in 70 patients treated with local excision and surveillance alone (15). The mean and median follow-up periods of these 72 breasts were 49 months and 47 months, respectively, with the longest follow-up being 168 months. Of this group, all were detected as calcifications on a screening mammogram or as an incidental finding in a biopsy performed for another reason (60 and 12, respectively). Eleven patients (15.3%) had a recurrence, either further DCIS (8) or invasive duct carcinoma (3), the recurrence being detected from 8 to 85 months after the initial diagnosis.

Our rate of recurrence was comparable with that reported by Lagios et al. (13); we differed only in the likelihood of invasion. They noted that half of the recurrences in their series were invasive. As most DCIS investigators report their experience and those of others, most accept this number (i.e., approximately one-half) as the proportion of invasive recurrences to expect after local excision alone. Our data continue to support a lower percentage of invasive second events (15).

Comparing treatment of DCIS with lumpectomy only and lumpectomy and radiation therapy, the National Surgical Adjuvant Breast Project reported the results of their protocol B-17 in 1993 and again in 1998 (16,17). In the earlier study, in which patients were treated with lumpectomy alone, there was a 5-year actuarial local recurrence rate of 21%; for lumpectomy and radiation therapy, the failure rate was 10%. In the later study, after 8 years of follow-up, with a mean of 90 months, the local failure rate was 25.8% and 11.4%, respectively, for the lumpectomy alone and the lumpectomy and radiation therapy groups. Based on the initial and subsequent follow-up studies, the National Surgical Adjuvant Breast Project continues to recommend radiation therapy for all women with DCIS when breast preservation is employed.

In 2000, similar results, i.e., fewer second events in the ipsilateral breast, were reported by the European Organization for Research and Treatment of Cancer Breast Cancer Cooperative Group and European Organization for Research and Treatment of Cancer Radiotherapy Group when radiation therapy was employed after local excision for DCIS compared with local excision alone (91% versus 84%, respectively, after 4 years) (18). Approximately one-half of the second events were invasive after excision plus radiation therapy or excision alone. There were 100 patients followed up for a median of 4.25 years after treatment (19). Similar criteria for inclusion were used in this study as in the National Surgical Adjuvant Breast Project study.

These represent two large studies that confirm that radiotherapy after the diagnosis of DCIS reduces the likelihood of a second event in that breast.

Despite valid criticisms raised about both of these studies, those of us who still recommend local excision only for selected patients with DCIS do so because these widely read and accepted reports failed to contain any subset analysis, based on morphologic or biologic parameters that might identify subgroups of the population with DCIS who might fare as well with local excision alone. In some respects, these reports, carrying the weight of prospective clinical trials by two respected groups of investigators, are a giant leap backward in the study of DCIS. My colleagues and I and others have strongly emphasized the importance of multiple factors, such as size, margin status, nuclear grade, necrosis, steroid hormone receptors, growth rate, immunohistochemical markers, that may determine the likelihood of recurrence after breast conservation (9,13,15,20–23). Various combinations of these factors may predict more precisely which patients can be treated with breast conservation alone, which require radiation, and which might be treated best with mastectomy (21,22). Irrespective of which data one accepts as more valid, no existing data challenge the observations that most women with DCIS treated with local excision alone do not have a second event in that breast and that, even if they do, the likelihood that they will succumb to breast cancer is very small. If women are denied the opportunity to be treated with local excision and surveillance alone, we will never learn who will not benefit from the additional radiation therapy.

Therefore, encouraged by our initial success, we have continued to offer selected patients with DCIS the opportunity to be treated with local excision and surveillance alone. As of September 30, 2001, we have treated 352 women with local excision and surveillance alone. This is one of the largest series of women treated in this manner by a single surgeon in a single practice. Of this number, 256 breasts in 249 women have been followed up for more than 1 year. The cutoff for our follow-up calculations is December 31, 2000, and it is this group for which the following data apply. Patients accrued since January 1, 2001, have not been considered for survival and follow-up data.

The mean and median follow-up periods of this group of 256 breasts are 75.6 and 66.5 months, respectively, with the longest follow-up being 247 months. In this entire group of breasts, there have been 71 second events (27.7%), either DCIS or invasive cancer. Of this group with second events, 45 of 71 (63.4%) were DCIS only, and the remaining 26 cases (36.6%) were invasive recurrences (Table 26.1). No distinction was made between microinvasive and frankly invasive cancer. These observations suggest, however, that only a small proportion of these carefully selected women with subclinical DCIS will develop a potentially life-threatening (i.e., invasive) cancer. The number of occurrences of subsequent invasive cancers in these cases continues to be

TABLE 26.1. LOCAL RECURRENCE AFTER EXCISION ALONE

Total no. of breasts treated by local excision and surveillance: 256
Total no. of second events observed: 71 (27.7%)[a]
DCIS cases only as second event: 45 (63.4%)[b] (17.6%)[c]
Invasion as second event (including microinvasion): 26 (36.6%)[b] (10.2%)[c]

[a] Percentage of entire group of 256.
[b] Percentage of second events.
[c] Percentage of entire group of 256.
DCIS, ductal carcinoma in situ.

less than described by most investigators. The usually quoted figure is approximately one-half DCIS and one-half invasive recurrence. Our figure is approximately two-thirds DCIS and one-third invasive, either microinvasion or frankly invasive cancer (Figs. 26.1, 26.2, and 26.3).

Additionally, as we have continued follow up of these patients who have incurred a second event, there has been only one subsequent death from breast cancer. This occurred in a woman who was 65 years old at the time of her initial diagnosis of DCIS. This was a minute focus of DCIS in an area of atypical ductal hyperplasia. The re-excision specimen showed additional minute foci of DCIS with widely clear margins. She was lost to follow-up, but we learned that 2 years later she developed bilateral (node-negative) invasive carcinoma for which she underwent bilateral mastectomy. On the side of the prior DCIS, she developed DCIS with two microscopic foci of invasion. This second event was not in the same quadrant as the earlier DCIS. On the contralateral side, the invasive cancer was 1.3 cm in diameter. She subsequently died of metastatic breast cancer. It is likely that the contralateral disease had been present but undetected at the time of the DCIS diagnosis and that the contralateral cancer was the lethal one. Although she must be tallied as a death owing to breast cancer, the circumstances are certainly questionable as to the relationship to her having been initially treated for DCIS with local excision and surveillance alone.

The Kaplan-Meier curves created from our data are not quite as optimistic as we had hoped they might be, with the long-term projections of second events being as high as 50% in the 20 years after diagnosis. However, the number of patients who have had more than 8 years of follow-up is quite small, so that making projections based on their follow-up is risky. Even if the data are projected correctly, the long-term projections of an invasive second event remain low.

Another interesting observation in this group of women is the time from initial diagnosis until the second event. Forty of the 71 (56%) had a second event within 36 months of the initial diagnosis. Of these 40, 60% of the DCIS second events and 50% of the invasive second events occurred within this 3-year interval (Figs. 26.4,

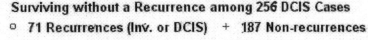
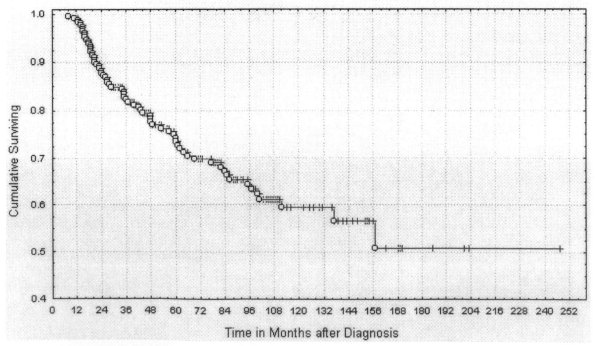

FIGURE 26.1. Surviving without a recurrence among 256 ductal carcinoma in situ (DCIS) cases: 71 recurrences (invasive or DCIS) + 187 nonrecurrences.

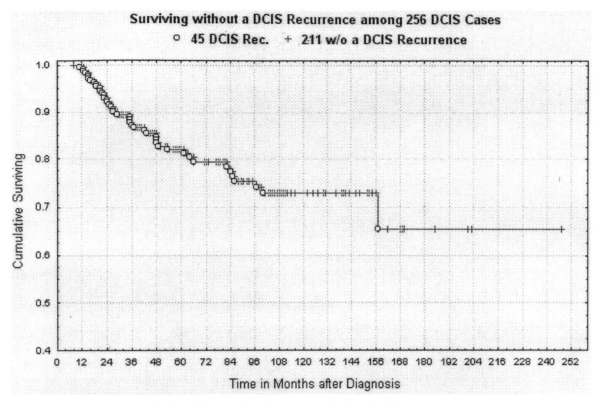

FIGURE 26.2. Surviving without a ductal carcinoma in situ (DCIS) recurrence among 256 DCIS cases: 45 DCIS recurrences + 211 with no DCIS recurrence.

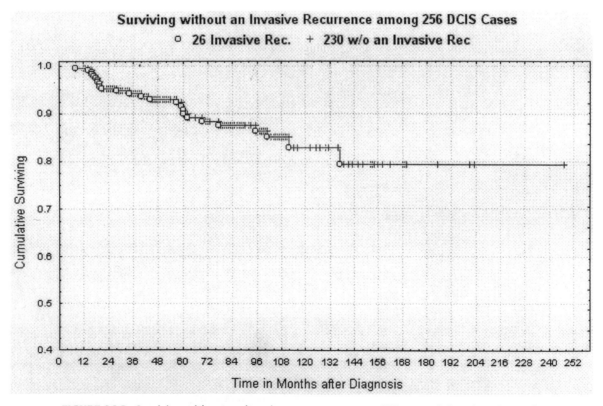

FIGURE 26.3. Surviving without an invasive recurrence among 256 cases of ductal carcinoma in situ: 26 with invasive recurrence + 230 without invasive recurrence.

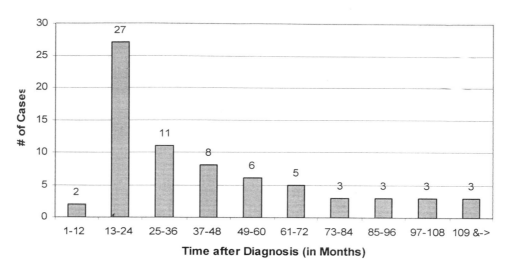

FIGURE 26.4. Seventy-one recurrences in a group of 256 DCIS breasts (DCIS and inv. recurrences).

26.5, and 26.6). Speculating about the growth rates of these and other cancers, it is tempting to suggest that these patients did not have a recurrence, but a persistence of incompletely excised DCIS in the same area of the breast. The second event occurred in the index quadrant, at or near the same site as the initial finding in all but two of our patients. If these observations stand and can be confirmed, they provide clues to the natural history of this disease. Moreover, if the breast is not treated with more than a wide local excision at the site, that breast remains at the

same risk of developing a new, unrelated cancer as the other breast. We should never expect recurrence to be zero. These observations also make us reluctant to use the term recurrence for the second events that occur in the same breast. Within this initial 3-year time period after the initial diagnosis, and perhaps even longer, whatever happens in that same breast is almost certainly persistence rather than recurrence of the disease initially detected. Because the calcifications that prompted the biopsy occur only after some degree of intraductal necrosis, we know that, de-

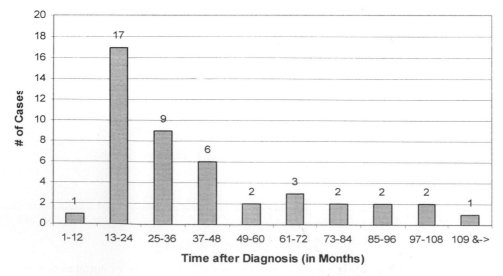

FIGURE 26.5. Forty-five DCIS recurrences in a group of 256 DCIS breasts.

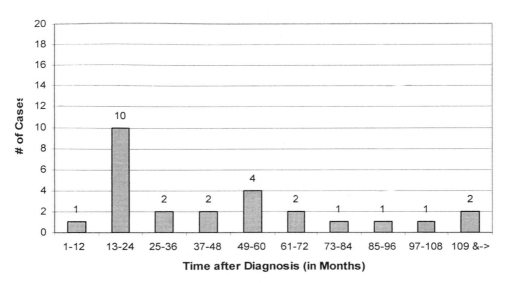

FIGURE 26.6. Twenty-six invasive recurrences in a group of 256 DCIS breasts.

spite a successful local excision, there may be additional microscopic disease elsewhere in the same breast. For those women in whom this additional disease is or becomes clinically significant, progression through the natural history of DCIS will produce more calcifications and lead to subsequent detection similar to the first episode.

If our observations about second events are considered further, only approximately 10% of these women with DCIS developed invasive cancer after local excision alone. Even if this number is higher, should we be treating 100% of this group of women with radiation therapy (or mastectomy) if only this small proportion will develop a theoretically life-threatening cancer subsequently? Additionally, because an ipsilateral second event after radiation therapy usually implies the need for mastectomy, does the use of radiation therapy at the time of the initial diagnosis preclude an additional attempt at treatment with further local excision alone (18)? Of our patients who have experienced their second event as DCIS alone, several have chosen to continue surveillance alone, without radiation or mastectomy. This includes one woman with bilateral DCIS with bilateral recurrence.

Age at diagnosis continues to be another contentious issue with respect to the likelihood of ipsilateral second events (24–26). We divided our group of 256 breasts into younger and older subsets, using age 50 as the divisor (Figs. 26.7, 24.8, and 26.9). We have not observed a statistically significant difference between these two groups with respect to second events, either further DCIS or invasive cancer. Whether further discrimination, using decile-divided age groups will show a difference is a difficult statistical manipulation because the number of women with DCIS diagnosed in their 20s or 30s is small. (Only 15 patients in this

series were younger than age 40). In our group of 256 breasts with DCIS, a plurality of cases occurred in the two age deciles between 40 and 60.

If those publications that conclude that there is a greater risk of a second event if the initial diagnosis was made at a younger age included more women with nuclear grade 3 DCIS, it might be expected that they would incur a greater likelihood of a second event. In a subset of 127 of our 256 breasts with nuclear grade determined precisely according to the classification conference of 1997 (27), using age 50 as the divisor into two groups, the younger group showed a slightly higher average nuclear grade, but this did not reach statistical significance ($p = 0.19$) Perhaps publications that suggest a higher likelihood of recurrence in younger women are seeing more patients with higher nuclear grade, and their observations may be based on nuclear grade rather than age alone. It is certainly for these young women for whom the magical algorithm is most important. Mastectomy is a paradoxical and ironic reward for diligence and early detection. Parenthetically, we have not yet observed a second event occur in a woman younger than 50 with nuclear grade 1 DCIS.

Documenting these observations about the nature of recurrence is crucial. If careful surveillance detects a second event while it is yet noninvasive, patients may be more enthusiastic about this alternative to mastectomy or irradiation because of the implication that recurrence (as DCIS only) does not endanger the patient. If a sizable segment of the group treated with excision and surveillance, however, does develop invasive carcinoma subsequently, there will be a small fraction of this group who will undoubtedly die of this disease, and for those women, however few, the price of surveillance was too high.

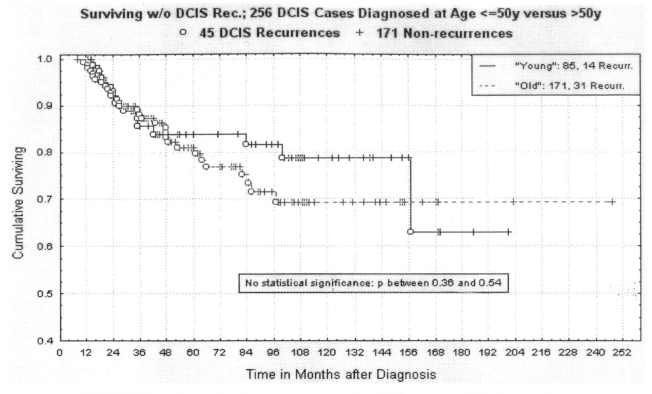

FIGURE 26.7. Surviving without ductal carcinoma in situ (DCIS) recurrence: 256 DCIS cases diagnosed at age 50 years and younger versus at 51 years of age and older, 45 DCIS recurrences + 171 nonrecurrences.

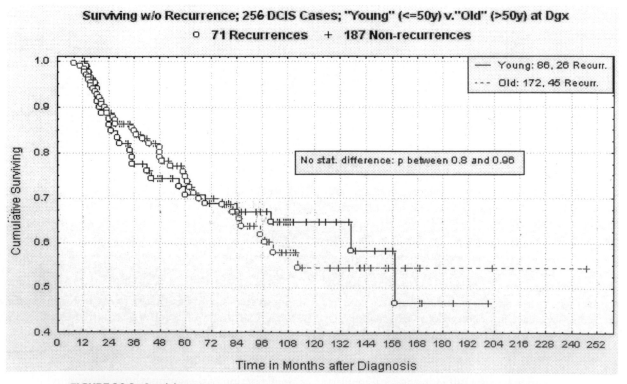

FIGURE 26.8. Surviving without recurrence: 256 cases of ductal carcinoma in situ, young (50 years of age or younger) versus old (51 years of age and older) at diagnosis, 71 recurrences + 187 nonrecurrences.

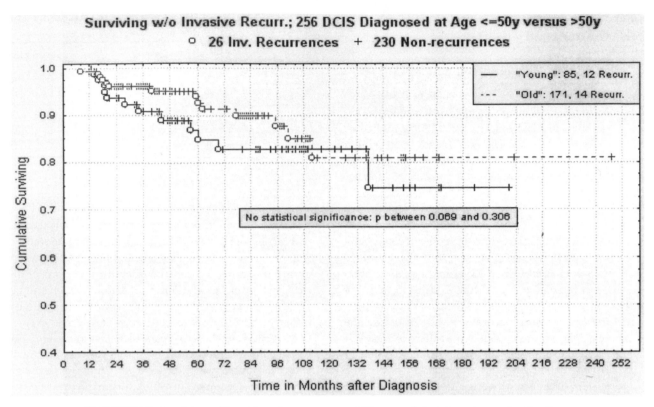

FIGURE 26.9. Surviving without invasive recurrence: 256 cases of ductal carcinoma in situ diagnosed at age 50 years and younger versus 51 years and older, 26 invasive recurrences + 230 non-recurrences.

Therefore, the challenge to those of us who would advocate local excision and surveillance as an option for those women whose subclinical DCIS is detected by screening mammography is to define precisely the ultimate risk of developing invasive cancer, not further DCIS, and not only the likelihood that this unfortunate event might occur but also within what period of time. We must try to develop biologic markers that predict who is at greatest risk; currently, size, margins, and morphology (comedo/necrosis) are the criteria often cited to suggest that some patients with DCIS are more likely than others to develop recurrence. Most investigators divide DCIS into several separate subsets based on morphologic criteria. These usually include comedo, cribriform, solid, papillary, and micropapillary types, and each has distinctive microscopic features. Attempts to correlate cytometric and histologic characteristics of these several varieties of DCIS have been undertaken, and the comedo type is considered the most biologically aggressive (10,15,20–22,28,29).

Our own comparisons of the findings within biopsies and those within subsequent mastectomy specimens (when we used to treat all patients with DCIS this way) have helped to define the risks of multicentricity and microinvasion associated with these various subsets of subclinical DCIS (28,29). For example, the incidental finding of DCIS in a specimen of tissue removed for another reason has not

been associated with either microinvasion or multicentricity, and no patient with incidental DCIS treated with excision and surveillance has yet developed a recurrence (15). When we reviewed our mastectomy specimens, we also noted the tendency for the comedo type of DCIS to be more likely accompanied by microinvasion and/or multicentricity. Similarly, although there was no maximum or minimum number of involved ducts that guaranteed the presence or absence of multicentricity or microinvasion, there was a trend, as might be expected, that the greater the volume of DCIS, the more likely was there to be accompanying microinvasion and/or multicentricity (28,29).

This analysis of microinvasion and multicentricity in mastectomy specimens has not yet been related to clinical observations of recurrence in our own group of patients treated with excision and surveillance. One would expect a greater incidence of recurrence in the patients with the comedo type of DCIS than the other histologic categories if recurrence were related directly to these cytologic and cytodynamic traits. In our own patients with subclinical DCIS treated with excision and surveillance alone, this was initially true in the first group of 72 patients. The greater likelihood of recurrence in patients with the comedo type of DCIS has not been statistically significant as we have accumulated more information through December 1999. The trend, however, still remains in that direction. Notwithstanding this observation, most patients with DCIS of the comedo type have not (yet) recurred.

The morphology and nuclear grade of the malignant cells and the degree of intraductal necrosis are the features associated with comedocarcinoma that are generally thought to predict local recurrence. We and others believe that the current division of DCIS into the five subsets named is not precise enough. Because the majority of DCIS is detected within clustered calcifications and intraductal, cellular necrosis leading to calcification is the hallmark of detection of these lesions, it is not surprising that comedocarcinoma is the most common single histologic type of DCIS encountered. It is the presence of intraductal necrosis that necessitates use of the term comedo as a modifier. Perhaps the implication of intraductal necrosis needs to be reconsidered. All the lesions that were formerly defined as the comedo type of DCIS may need to be reclassified, based on other attributes both biologic (e.g., nuclear grade) and morphologic. For example, in 128 cases of DCIS for which we determined the nuclear grade according to the recommendations of the 1997 consensus conference, there is a slightly significant difference in the likelihood of a second event ($p = 0.051$) between nuclear grade 1 and nuclear grades 2 and 3. There was no difference between nuclear grades 2 and 3 (27).

The first such attempt at categorizing subsets of DCIS to devise treatment algorithms is that proposed by Silverstein et al. (21,22), the Van Nuys Prognostic Index. Despite several valid criticisms (26), this represents the first time that investigators tried to fit an algorithm to individual patient circumstances to justify differences in treatment recommendations. Whether this index can be consistently and reproducibly used elsewhere by surgeons, pathologists, and radiation oncologists in less dedicated practices remains a dilemma.

We have been able to validate the Van Nuys Prognostic Index in our own practice to a limited degree. Learning early in our own experience that those patients whose Van Nuys score would be considered 8 or 9 have a high likelihood of developing a second event because of large size, inability to clear margins adequately, and biologic aggressiveness, and almost all of them have been treated with mastectomy. We have been able to calculate the Van Nuys score for 152 breasts, and as the score increases from 3 (the lowest possible score) to 7, the likelihood of a second event also increases (Table 26.2). Because we have accrued a large group of patients, all of whom have undergone local excision by the same surgeon, are followed up with surveillance alone without supplemental radiation therapy, and whose slides and paraffin blocks have been studied by the same pathologists, criticisms about reproducibility may be mitigated. We have added the immunohistochemical determinations of hormone receptors, nuclear antigen Ki-67, and gene products p53, C-erbB2, and p21 to our database. Whatever additional contributions these markers may offer to the DCIS

TABLE 26.2. VAN NUYS INDEX DETAILED IN 152 BREASTS

Score	No.	%	Second Events
8	1	00.7	01 = 100%
7	4	03	01 = 25%
6	20	13	11 = 55%
5	32	21	16 = 50%
4	49	32	07 = 14%
3	46	31	04 = 09%

treatment algorithm is currently only speculative. However, we do have preliminary data concerning the effects of these markers on the likelihood of a second event after local excision only. The values of estrogen and progesterone receptors do not thus far predict a second event. Ki-67 values higher than 10% seem to be modest predictors of a second event. For the oncogene p53, values higher than 2% positivity for mutated p53 are modest predictors of a second event, and for c-erbB2 (Her-2-neu), again there was a small increase in the likelihood of a second event between a negative value and each positive value, i.e., 1+, 2+, and 3+ in the group of 92 DCIS specimens in which this marker was measured. The difference in rate of recurrence was significant at $p = 0.05\%$ in each of the subgroups, negative versus 1+, 1+ versus 2+, and 2+ versus 3+, and negative versus any positive value (Fig. 26.10).

One highly significant difference ($p = 0.007$) was noted when the two markers p53 and c-erbB2 were combined. With p53 less than 5% and c-erbB2 less than 2+ versus p53 greater than 5% and c-erbB2 2+ or greater, a second event was more likely to occur within 2 years of initial diagnosis (Fig. 26.11). These conclusions, however, are based on only 85 breasts in which these two markers were both determined, not the entire group. Because the number of second events was only 19, despite the statistical significance noted, one must be careful when extrapolating from this small number of patients and second events.

These rudimentary observations, however, further validate the need to accrue more patients into trials of surveillance alone and measurement of these various prognostic markers. By doing so, the algorithm that would define how patients best fit into each treatment option might be not so distant.

For the time being, a pragmatic approach should be adopted to allow the accrual of patients into clinical trials that use local excision only with careful, lifetime surveillance as an alternative to mastectomy or radiation therapy for highly selected patients with subclinical DCIS. Our own approach is quite similar to that advocated by Lagios et al. (13). At the time of needle-guided biopsy, because no treatment plans depend on them, frozen sections of excised tissue are not performed. All the fresh tissue is examined by the surgical pathologist.

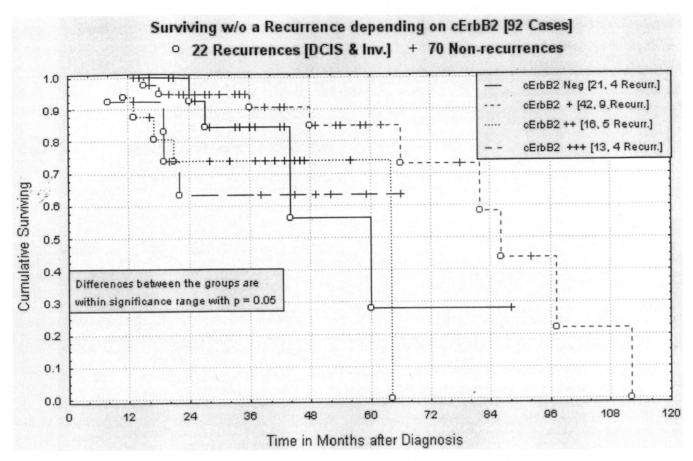

FIGURE 26.10. Surviving without a recurrence depending on c-ErbB2 (92 cases): 22 recurrences (ductal carcinoma in situ and invasive carcinoma) + 70 nonrecurrences.

We do differ with Lagios et al. in our perception of the importance of inking surgical margins. The careful excision of a small area of calcifications is more difficult than a breast biopsy performed for a palpable lesion, especially if the surgeon wishes to spare a small breast from a significant cosmetic deformity. Not infrequently it may require a second specimen to ensure that the mammographic abnormality has been removed. Because most needle-guided biopsies still prove to be for benign disease (our current benign-to-malignant ratio is 3%:2% to 41% of needle-guided biopsies proving to be for malignant disease), the pathologist's enthusiasm for the appropriately defined specimen must be tempered by the surgeon's and the patient's concern about the overall outcome. Moreover, these specimens are not smooth marbles that lend themselves to being coated by India ink in a uniform way. The excised tissue contains nooks and crannies related to varying proportions of fat, stromal elements and glandular breast tissue that may be encountered. Rather than sacrifice a large volume of normal tissue to ensure that margins are clear, because margins are irrelevant in benign disease, re-excision of the primary site with separate dissection of the margins and base of the wound and the application of metallic clips to these sites is our preferred alternative. This is especially appropriate for the

many patients with DCIS who have been referred for treatment recommendations after initial biopsy and diagnosis elsewhere. Re-excision of the primary site and dissection of wound margins and base are more precise than inking the margins of the specimen because the specimen is almost never uniform in its consistency or shape. This technique of securing clear margins was accepted as an alternative to inking by the consensus conference committees on the classification and treatment of DCIS in 1997 and 1999 (27,30).

Additionally, the application of metallic clips to wound margins and base offers precise localization of this site on subsequent mammograms. Because the second event is most commonly detected as new calcifications at the same site as the primary lesion, using these clips to demarcate this area on subsequent mammograms facilitates the radiologist's detection of a new problem. We have used this technique of clipping wound margins and base for almost 15 years to prepare patients for radiation therapy after local excision (and axillary dissection) for invasive carcinomas. Both radiation therapists and radiologists have found it most helpful to determine the site of the previous lesion accurately in this way. When the specimen is sent to the pathologist, grossly apparent areas of abnormality may be examined by frozen section, and if malignancy is confirmed, a portion of

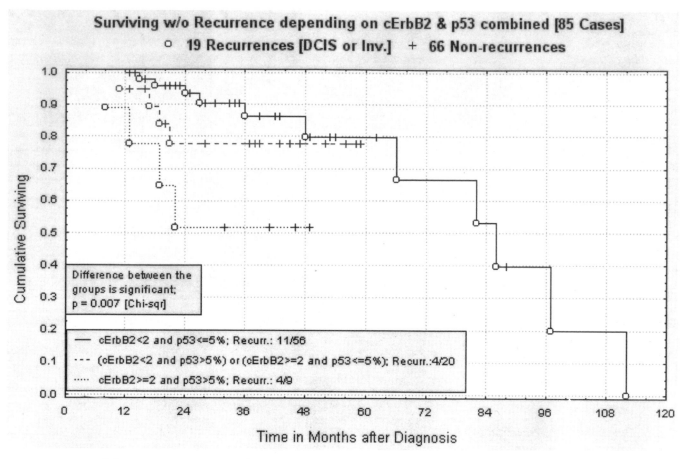

FIGURE 26.11. Surviving without recurrence depending on cErb-B2 and p53 combined (85 cases): 19 recurrences (ductal carcinoma in situ or invasive carcinoma) + 65 nonrecurrences.

the specimen may be saved for receptor and immuno-histopathologic studies. It is more important, however, to determine invasion, if present, than these other studies because treatment decisions, at least currently, are more likely to be related to the presence of invasion than to the quantification of, for example, receptors. Moreover, these studies may be performed subsequently, even more accurately, on formalin-fixed tissue from the paraffin blocks by immunohistochemical assay.

The earlier detection of mammographic abnormalities has even led to greater technical difficulties for the surgeon and surgical pathologists. More often than not, there are no grossly apparent abnormalities in the breast tissue even though the calcifications are known to be within the specimen. We rely on the radiologist to confirm the presence of the calcifications within the excised tissue by specimen radiography, and often a clip is placed at the exact site within the specimen, as small as it may be. Both the specimen and specimen radiograph are sent to the surgical pathologists so they can be alerted to the exact site of the area of greatest concern, even within an already small specimen.

With respect to other clinical decisions about the choice of patients with DCIS for treatment with local excision and surveillance, we agree with Lagios et al. and Silverstein et al.

that the lesion must be subclinical and found on the basis of mammographic calcifications or as an incidental finding. However, many of these small areas of DCIS are not easily defined by a single dimension, i.e., diameter. Some are rectangular or irregular as DCIS propagates along the course of intramammary ducts. Perhaps a preferable measurement should be the total area of DCIS, the greatest length times the greatest width, as measured on the mediolateral or craniocaudal mammographic projection. If this concept were adopted, then an area of approximately 6 cm^2 of calcifications would be considered the relative upper limit of the area to be treated. The breast should be large enough to allow the removal of a greater volume of tissue without creating a major cosmetic defect. The specimen radiograph should confirm the excision of the area in question, or a postoperative mammogram is indicated to substantiate this important criterion.

Another major reason to regard excision and surveillance as an option for many of these patients is the difficulty in diagnosis. Although DCIS and atypical ductal hyperplasia are not difficult to distinguish from each other in most cases, the line separating borderline lesions is fuzzy rather than precise, and skilled pathologists often interpret the same slides differently (31). If the pathologist's report does not address these subtleties and merely implies benign or malignant, without a modifier, there may be major differences in treatment recommendations. It is, therefore, important to resist an immediate decision when subclinical DCIS is found and to review and re-review the entire specimen. Borderline lesions such as atypical ductal hyperplasia should not be radiated. Such lesions are appropriately treated with surveillance alone, even if there is disagreement between knowledgeable pathologists about the exact diagnosis.

That the patient must recognize the limits of our current knowledge about this disease is implicit in the mutual agreement between patient and physician to choose surveillance as an option. A clear understanding of the biology and natural history of the disease that we call subclinical DCIS still eludes us. As clinicians, we have been involved in the care of too many women with often lethal breast cancers, so that reluctance to abandon traditional treatment in favor of lesser options is understandable. Our respect for breast cancer is too great. Overkill has always been assumed to be a more sound philosophy than "underkill" when dealing with malignancy. If we could be convinced that some diseases that we currently call malignant, such as DCIS, are not inevitably followed by invasive, life-threatening cancers and that even if a recurrence does develop, there is a second opportunity for successful interference, perhaps there would be greater enthusiasm for less rather than more treatment. Unless we can, however, enroll our patients in protocols that follow rather than always treat this disease, we will never know which, if any, women with DCIS can be followed without facing the specter of subsequent invasive breast cancer.

REFERENCES

1. Ernster VL, Barclay J, Kerlikowske K, et al. Incidence of and treatment for ductal carcinoma in situ of the breast. *JAMA* 1996;275:913–918.
2. Betsill WL Jr, Rosen PP, Lieberman PH, et al. Intraductal carcinoma: long-term follow-up after treatment by biopsy alone. *JAMA* 1978;239:1963–1967.
3. Haagensen CD. *Diseases of the breast*, 3rd ed. Philadelphia: WB Saunders, 1986:782.
4. Haagensen CD. *Diseases of the breast*, 3rd ed. Philadelphia: WB Saunders, 1986:788.
5. Gump FE, Jicha DL, Ozello L. Ductal carcinoma in situ (DCIS): a revised concept. *Surgery* 1987;102:790–795.
6. Fleming ID, Cooper JS, Henson DE, et al. *AJCC cancer staging manual*, 5th ed. Philadelphia: Lippincott Williams & Wilkins, 1997.
7. Schwartz GF, Carter WB, Finkel GC. Paget's carcinoma of the breast. *Surg Oncol Clin North Am* 1993;2: 93–106.
8. Schwartz GF, Kim R, Topham AK. Local recurrence following breast conservation for stage I and II invasive carcinoma: ten year follow-up. Presented at the 49th Cancer Symposium of the Society of Surgical Oncology, Atlanta, GA, March 21–24, 1996.
9. Solin LJ, Recht A, Fourquet A, et al. Ten-year results of breast-conserving surgery and definitive irradiation for intraductal carcinoma (ductal carcinoma in situ) of the breast. *Cancer* 1991;68:2337–2344.
10. Solin LJ, Kurtz J, Fourquet A, et al. Fifteen-year results of breast-conserving surgery and definitive breast irradiation for the treatment of ductal carcinoma in situ of the breast. *J Clin Oncol* 1996;14:754–763.
11. Pierce SM, Schnitt SJ, Harris JR. What to do about mammographically detected ductal carcinoma-in-situ? *Cancer* 1992;70:2576–2578.
12. Silverstein MJ, Cohlan, BF, Gierson ED, et al. Duct carcinoma in situ: 227 cases without invasion. *Eur J Cancer* 1992;28:630–634.
13. Lagios MD, Westdahl PR, Margolin FR, et al. Duct carcinoma in situ: relationship of extent of noninvasive disease to the frequency of occult invasion, multicentricity, lymph node metastasis and short-term treatment failures. *Cancer* 1982;59:1309–1314.
14. Haagensen CD, Lane N, Lattes R, et al. Lobular neoplasia (so-called lobular carcinoma in situ) of the breast. *Cancer* 1978;42: 737–769.
15. Schwartz GF, Finkel GC, Garcia JC, et al. Subclinical ductal carcinoma in situ of the breast: treatment by local excision and surveillance alone. *Cancer* 1992;70:2468–2474.
16. Fisher B, Constantino J, Redmond C, et al. Lumpectomy compared with lumpectomy and radiation therapy for the treatment of intraductal breast cancer. *N Engl J Med* 1993;328:1581–1586.
17. Fisher ER, Dignan J, Tan-Chiu E, et al. Pathologic findings from the National Surgical Adjuvant Breast Project (NSABP) eight-year update of protocol B-17. *Cancer* 1999;86:429–438.
18. Silverstein MJ, Lagios MD. Benefits of irradiation for DCIS: a Pyrrhic victory. *Lancet* 2000;355:510–511.
19. Julien JP, Bijker N, Fentiman IS, et al. Radiotherapy in breast-conserving treatment for ductal carcinoma in situ: first results of the EORTC randomized phase III trial 10853. EORTC Breast Cancer Cooperative Group and EORTC Radiotherapy Group. *Lancet* 2000;355:528–533.
20. Lagios MD. Duct carcinoma in situ: pathology and treatment. *Surg Clin North Am* 1990;70:853–871.
21. Silverstein MJ, Poller DN, Waisman JR, et al. Prognostic classification of breast ductal carcinoma-in-situ. *Lancet* 1995;345:1154–1157.
22. Silverstein MJ, Lagios MD, Craig PH, et al. A prognostic index for ductal carcinoma in situ of the breast. *Cancer* 1996;77:2267–2274.
23. Schwartz GF, Schwarting R, Cornfield DB, et al. Sub-clinical duct carcinoma in situ of the breast (DCIS): treatment by local excision and surveillance alone. *Proc Am Soc Clin Oncol* 1996;15: 101.
24. Van Zee KJ, Petrek JA, Liberman L, et al. Long-term follow-up of DCIS treated with breast conservation: the effect of age and radiation. *Cancer* 1999;86:1757–1767.
25. Solin LJ, Fourquet A, Vicini F, et al. Mammographically detected ductal carcinoma in situ of the breast treated with breast-conserving surgery and definitive irradiation: long-term outcome and prognostic significance of patient age and margin status. *Int J Radiat Oncol Biol Phys* 2001;50:991–1002.
26. Schnitt SJ, Harris JR, Smith BL. Developing a prognostic index for ductal carcinoma in situ of the breast: are we there yet? *Cancer* 1996;77:2189–2192.
27. Consensus Conference Committee. Consensus Conference on the Classification of Ductal Carcinoma in Situ, April 25–28, 1997. *Cancer* 1997;80:1798–1802.
28. Schwartz GF, Patchefsky AS, Finkelstein SD, et al. Nonpalpable in situ ductal carcinoma of the breast. *Arch Surg* 1989;124:29–32.
29. Patchefsky AS, Schwartz GF, Finkelstein SD, et al. Heterogeneity of intraductal carcinoma of the breast. *Cancer* 1989;63:731–741.
30. Schwartz GF, Solin LJ, Olivotto IA, et al. and the Consensus Conference Committee. Consensus Conference on the Treatment of In Situ Ductal Carcinoma of the Breast. *Cancer* 2000;88:946–954.
31. Rosai J. Borderline epithelial lesions of the breast. *Am J Pathol* 1991;15:209–221.

27

DUCTAL CARCINOMA IN SITU: EXPERIENCE AT NOTTINGHAM CITY HOSPITAL 1973 THROUGH 2000

ROGER W. BLAMEY   R. DOUGLAS MACMILLAN   RAJAM S. RAMPAUL
ANDREW J. EVANS   POPPY VALASSIADOU   D. MARK SIBBERING
YASMIN WAHEDNA   JACKIE READ   SARAH E. PINDER

The Breast Cancer Unit at Nottingham City Hospital was established in 1973. The work of the unit has increased steadily over the years so that now symptomatic referrals are received from a population of approximately 1 million women; cases are also diagnosed from population-based mammographic screening for women of ages 50 to 64, which has been carried out since 1988. The unit screens 72,000 women by invitation every 3 years.

Nottingham City Hospital lies within the Trent Health Region in the English Midlands, the region has a population of 4.7 million. The direction and audit of National Health Service Screening are carried out on a regional basis. Women requiring breast surgery are treated within 11 breast units in the Trent region that are staffed by specialists in breast cancer in all disciplines. All cases of breast cancer in the Trent region are under the care of one of the 21 breast surgeons working in the breast units.

This chapter covers the experience in Nottingham or the Trent region as a whole, in four aspects of DCIS:

Diagnostic. Most cases of ductal carcinoma in situ (DCIS) now have preoperative tissue diagnosis. Several cases thought to be DCIS only from preoperative diagnostic triple assessment are found on histology of the surgical specimen to contain invasive carcinoma (not simply microinvasion). This section examines the current sensitivity of the preoperative diagnosis of DCIS and the number of cases in which the presence of unsuspected invasive disease is found postoperatively.

Survival. Deaths from breast cancer or regional node metastases are seen in a few cases without prior local recurrence or contralateral cancer. These represent the rate of metastatic spread from an invasive focus not discovered in the pathologic specimen. Deaths from breast cancer after DCIS are more frequent in women who develop a local recurrence as their first event. These represent cancers in which inadequate local control leads to death. This section examines survival in all cases of DCIS diagnosed at Nottingham City Hospital between 1973 and 1998.

Screening. National Health Service mammographic population screening by invitation to all women of ages 50 to 64 every 3 years was introduced in 1988. This section examines the Trent region experience of the cases of DCIS detected in the first 6 years of the mammographic screening program, between 1988 and 1994.

Treatment with wide local excision without radiation therapy. Faced with an increase in case numbers of a hitherto relatively uncommon problem, treatment policy was reassessed at Nottingham City Hospital in 1988. Mastectomy was advised for patients with DCIS 40 mm or greater in diameter. Patients with DCIS less than 40 mm were offered breast-conserving surgery with a widely clear margin depth and without the addition of radiation therapy. This section examines the recurrence rate of the latter procedure and the factors leading to local recurrence.

ASPECTS OF THE DIAGNOSIS OF DUCTAL CARCINOMA IN SITU

DCIS may present as Paget's disease of the nipple, nipple discharge, or a breast lump. Because population screening was introduced in 1988 in the United Kingdom, most cases are now diagnosed by screening and have no clinical signs. The commonest mammographic finding is microcalcification.

Two hundred sixty-nine cases of pure DCIS were diagnosed at screening between 1988 and 2001, 87% of which showed microcalcification. In recent years, the mean size of screening-detected lesions has decreased from 34 mm to 25 mm because of more aggressive investigation of small clusters of calcification. Of screening-detected DCIS, 69% of cases are high grade, 18% intermediate grade, and 13% low grade.

The introduction of core biopsy in 1994 and digital stereotaxis in 1997 have aided the preoperative diagnosis of DCIS, but the diagnosis remains more difficult than in cases of invasive disease. The absolute sensitivity in DCIS for core biopsy is 80%. The introduction of the mammotome at Nottingham City Hospital has not appreciably increased the preoperative diagnosis of DCIS, but the mammotome is more accurate in diagnosing invasive foci within areas of DCIS.

Another preoperative diagnostic aspect is whether the lesion is wholly DCIS or contains invasive carcinoma. For this study, we looked at 140 women seen in our diagnostic clinics in whom core biopsy had shown only DCIS; 47 presented symptomatically and 93 were discovered at screening.

On clinical examination, 25 women had clinical lesions indicating probable invasive carcinomas and 17 of the symptomatic women had normal mammograms. In 96 women at preoperative triple assessment, all modalities (clinical examination, imaging by x-ray mammography and ultrasonography and histopathology of needle core biopsy) indicated no abnormality or that only DCIS appeared to be present (e.g., no tether nor palpable lump, calcification on x-ray with no mass lesion seen, histopathology of needle core showing DCIS only). The final postoperative histology of these cases showed significant invasive carcinoma (excluding microinvasion strictly defined as no focus of invasive carcinoma greater than 1 mm in extent) in 46 of the 96 cases (48%).

Invasive cancer is therefore present in approximately 50% of cases thought preoperatively to be only DCIS. This indicates the need for a thorough examination of the operative specimen by the histopathologist. Although axillary clearance should not be performed in DCIS to avoid side effects with a very low chance of positive nodes being found (see next two sections), it does seem prudent to obtain prognostic information by low axillary node sampling at operation because it otherwise means that the 50% found to have invasive carcinoma need node sampling at a second operation. Patients with low-grade DCIS on core biopsy rarely have occult invasion, and axillary sampling in this subgroup is not necessary (1).

Clusters of calcification with more than 40 flecks that show high-grade DCIS on core biopsy have a 48% chance of being invasive carcinoma, and further preoperative biopsies should be undertaken.

SURVIVAL AFTER DUCTAL CARCINOMA IN SITU

At Nottingham City Hospital from 1973 to 1998, 331 patients were diagnosed and treated for DCIS; the age range was 25 to 74 years with a median of 55. Seventy-four were diagnosed between 1973 and 1987 compared with 1,519 invasive cancers (DCIS then being 4.6% of all cancers) and 257 between 1988 and 1998 compared with 2,165 invasive cancers (10.7% of all cancers now being DCIS). This rise in the percentage of cases of DCIS was brought about by the introduction of mammographic screening in 1988; before that date the presentations were mostly symptomatic. Of the cases diagnosed at Nottingham since 1988, 116 presented with symptoms, 125 were detected at screening, and 17 were referred from other units.

The operations performed were breast-conserving surgery in 111 cases, simple (total) mastectomy in 151, and subcutaneous mastectomy with preservation of all skin including the nipple and insertion of a silicone prosthesis in 67.

Seven of these women died of breast cancer (2%). One died without proven local or regional recurrence or contralateral breast cancer. Two patients (one died of breast cancer and one is still alive) developed regional lymph node recurrence without prior local recurrence. This means that these latter three patients must have had small invasive tumors despite only DCIS being found on postoperative pathologic assessment. Four women died after a local recurrence, giving a death rate from breast cancer of 13% in those 28 with a local recurrence compared with less than 1% in those without. Because 22 of the 28 local recurrences were invasive, this is not surprising. Even though the percentage of local recurrences containing invasive carcinoma is higher in this series than the usually reported 50% (see section on ductal carcinoma detected in the first 6 years of the National Health Service Screening Program in the Trent region), this emphasizes the importance of local control and careful postoperative surveillance for early detection of local recurrence.

Local recurrence developed in 28 cases. No local recurrences occurred after simple mastectomy. In five cases, local recurrence occurred in the retained nipple after subcutaneous mastectomy. Because of this, a policy was instituted in 1988 of marking the cut surface under the nipple on the operative specimen; if DCIS of the nipple ducts is seen on histology, the nipple and areola area are now treated with radiation therapy. We have seen no further nipple recurrences since this policy was introduced. There were 23 local recurrences in the 117 women treated with breast-conserving surgery by lumpectomy (early in the series) or wide local excision or cone excision for Paget's disease.

The disease-specific survival rate at 5, 10, and 15 years for simple mastectomy was 97.5%, and for treatment with breast conservation, the rates were 100%, 97.5%, and 86.7% at 5, 10, and 15 years, respectively.

DUCTAL CARCINOMA IN SITU DETECTED IN THE FIRST 6 YEARS OF THE NATIONAL HEALTH SERVICE BREAST SCREENING PROGRAM IN THE TRENT REGION (1988 THROUGH 1993)

This retrospective study looked at the results of multicenter treatment of DCIS detected in one UK screening region during the first 6 years of the National Health Service Breast Screening Program.

Between January 1988 and December 1993, 392,030 women were screened at the 11 screening units within the region; 301 cases of DCIS or DCIS with microinvasion were diagnosed and case notes were retrieved for 297 of these. Most cases (n = 253) were detected at the prevalent screens. For recurrence analysis, all cases were censored at 80 months of follow-up.

In 44 cases, diagnostic excisional biopsy was the only surgical procedure performed. In the remaining 257 cases, a therapeutic procedure was carried out once the diagnosis of DCIS had been achieved (either preoperatively or by open surgical biopsy). Of the 257 patients, 140 were treated initially with wide local excision; 17 of these (12%) required conversion to mastectomy and 10 re-excision at the margins to achieve clear excision margins. Overall, the final operation was wide local excision in 123 patients and mastectomy in 134; 154 (51%) patients received no adjuvant therapies, 139 were treated with tamoxifen, and 24 were treated with radiation therapy.

The grade of lesion was recorded in only 47% of cases, and where known, 81% were designated high grade. Microinvasion (definition, p. 323) was recorded as definitely present in 30 cases (10%). Margins were reported as clear in 264 (88%) of cases. An axillary procedure was performed in 91 cases, with a median number of four nodes sampled; no positive nodes were detected.

Over the minimum 80-month follow-up period, 28 cases of local recurrence were recorded; of these, 15 were invasive. There were significant differences in the rates of local recurrence by operation type, with excisional biopsies having a 20% recurrence rate compared with 12% after wide local excision and 1% after mastectomy. Spread to lymph nodes was found in four cases at surgery for local recurrence. The median time to recurrence was 30.5 months (range, 5 to 80). Three new cases of primary disease in the contralateral breast were recorded.

Nineteen patients died, with death owing to breast cancer in six cases (2%). Distant metastases are present in one further patient and one patient had a regional recurrence. The median time to death owing to breast cancer was 47 months. The overall recurrence-free survival rate was 91% at 5 years.

Until the 1980s, the usual surgical management of DCIS was with mastectomy, with very low rates of local recurrence and survival rates approaching 100%. Local recurrence after surgical treatment of DCIS is best avoided because approximately one-half of the recurrences are invasive, and in this series, local recurrence was associated with significant lymph node spread. In these cases, because lymph node spread was not seen in any case at the primary operation, the prognosis had changed from close to a 100% survival rate to threatened mortality. This emphasizes the importance of careful postoperative follow-up of DCIS treated with wide local excision with mammography and clinical examination to detect any local recurrence early.

The overall local recurrence rate in this study was relatively high (9% at 5 years). Most of the local recurrences occurred in the groups treated with biopsy alone or wide local excision and very few in those treated with mastectomy.

In all respects, the experience within the whole region mirrors that in Nottingham. Local recurrence is uncommon after mastectomy but too high for comfort after wide local excision. In no case has an axillary node been found to be involved at surgery for the primary tumor. The overall survival rate is 98% but is poorer after local recurrence.

TREATMENT WITH WIDE LOCAL EXCISION WITHOUT INTACT BREAST IRRADIATION

Trials (2) studying the addition of intact breast radiation therapy (IBRT) to wide local excision have shown that IBRT reduces the risk of local recurrence (refs RWB). However, these may also be interpreted as showing that most of the women treated without IBRT escape local recurrence; this suggests that either surgical technique or the biologic characteristics of the tumors must be responsible for local recurrence.

Most of the cases detected at breast cancer screening are small so that patients tend to seek breast-conserving surgery for what they understand to be essentially a precancerous lesion.

High-grade DCIS may increase the chance of local recurrence, but more than 70% of the total of the Nottingham cases are assessed as high grade in the primary specimen, making grade an unsatisfactory criterion for selection of cases for wide local excision. The importance of clear margins in the avoidance of local recurrence in DCIS has been demonstrated (3), as has the width of the margin of clear tissue around the tumor (4).

Since 1988, women with DCIS less than 40 mm in diameter (usually assessed on mammography) were offered the option of wide local excision. The protocol demanded a histologically clear margin width of at least 10 mm. A specimen x-ray was taken so that the surgeon could re-excise close margins at the first operation. The technique was previously described (5). A cylinder of breast tissue between skin and muscle was taken and no skin was excised; the remaining breast tissue was apposed to fill the gap, with a good cosmetic result in more than 70% of cases (6). The operative specimens were carefully oriented with sutures marking the margins at surgery and the whole surface of the specimen was inked. Careful histologic assessment of the circumferential margins of the operative specimen was carried out. Because the surgeon went up to the skin and down to the muscle, these surfaces were not sampled. Cases with circumferential margins less than 10 mm were either advised to undergo mastectomy (if there appeared to be extensive in situ change at the margin or if multiple margins were involved) or re-excision of the involved margin.

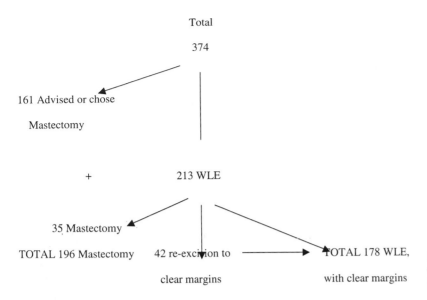

Total

374

161 Advised or chose

Mastectomy

+   213 WLE

35 Mastectomy

TOTAL 196 Mastectomy   42 re-excision to ⟶ TOTAL 178 WLE,

clear margins   with clear margins

FIGURE 27.1. Surgical treatment of cases of ductal carcinoma in situ diagnosed at Nottingham City Hospital between January 1988 and December 2000.

The patients did not receive IBRT or tamoxifen. Patients were seen regularly in the follow-up clinic and underwent mammography of the treated breast every year.

From 1988 to 2000, 374 cases of DCIS were diagnosed; 161 were either advised on grounds of tumor size or chose to undergo mastectomy as their first operation; 213 who had opted for wide local excision received this as their first therapeutic operation (73 of these had a previous diagnostic operation). Of the 213 patients who underwent wide local excision (Fig. 27.1), 77 required further surgery because of involved margins, defined as tumor at or within 10 mm of the margin of the specimen; 35 were treated with simple or subcutaneous mastectomy and 42 had re-excision of the involved margin. This left 178 women who had been treated with wide local excision with circumferential margins finally clear to a depth of 10 mm and without IBRT. The further analysis relates to these 178.

Local recurrence is defined as any recurrence in the treated breast, without attempting to make histologic differentiation between recurrence and new tumor. All but one local recurrence occurred in the same site as the previous excision; there were four contralateral primary tumors. On these bases, at least one and possibly four of the apparent recurrences was a new tumor.

At a median of 38 months (range, 6 to 150), there have been 21 local recurrences. The actuarial rate of local recurrence is 22% at 10 years (Fig. 27.2). The length of follow-up is important because the rate of local recurrence does not alter over the first 10 years. Twelve of the recurrences were in situ and nine were invasive (one of whom died of metastatic spread). An earlier report (5) on the first 50 cases in this series was encouraging, and this report is less so. This recurrence rate is in contrast to the rate of 5% at 84 months reported by Silverstein et al. (4) for cases of DCIS excised with a 10-mm margin. However, de Mascarel et al. (7) re-

ported a high recurrence rate for even low-grade tumors with a 10-mm margin width without IBRT.

With a recurrence rate of more than 2% per year, even though the curve appears to be exponential and the rate may decrease substantially (Fig. 27.2) after 10 years of follow-up, the relative risk reduction gained by IBRT appears worthwhile, and for the present, IBRT should be advised.

However, the fact remains that most women with widely clear margins treated without IBRT do not develop a local recurrence. Subgroup analyses in this series have shown factors that may be promising for further study.

Local recurrence was related to the pathologic size of DCIS, with local recurrence in three of seven cases larger than 30 mm in diameter.

Age at diagnosis appears important, with those younger than 50 years of age faring considerably worse (Fig. 27.3). This is akin to the situation in invasive carcinoma (8) but might also be related to most cases of DCIS in patients older than 50 being detected at screening and therefore smaller.

Another factor that may prove important in the prediction of local recurrence is the need for a second therapeutic operation to achieve clear margins (Fig. 27.4). This has also been reported from the European trial of therapy for DCIS (9). This might be owing to there being more extensive disease than appreciated on histology in this situation or to poor surgical identification of the margin to be excised at the second operation (possibly by inaccurate marking of the margins at the first operation).

CONCLUSION

Most cases of DCIS are diagnosed preoperatively by needle core biopsy carried out with ultrasonography or stereotactic

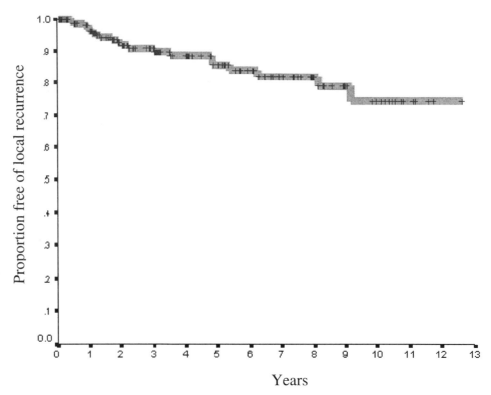

FIGURE 27.2. Local recurrence: all patients treated with wide local excision and without intact breast irradiation at Nottingham City Hospital from 1988 to 2000 (n = 178).

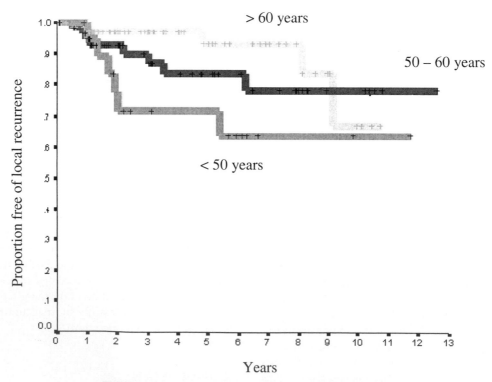

FIGURE 27.3. Local recurrence by age at time of surgery.

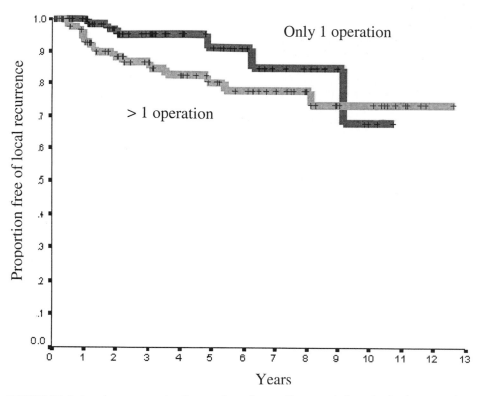

FIGURE 27.4. Local recurrence by the number of operations needed to obtain clear margins.

x-ray mammographic guidance. Fifty percent of cases that appear from triple assessment to be in situ only in fact have a significant invasive component. We therefore advise sampling of the low axilla (by four-node or sentinel techniques) in all such cases, with the possible exception of cases assessed by needle biopsy as low grade (1).

When pathologic examination of the surgical specimen has revealed DCIS only and no invasive tumor, the prognosis is excellent. However, in the minority of those treated with wide local excision who have a local recurrence (approximately one-half of which are invasive), more than 10% subsequently die of breast cancer, emphasizing the importance of completeness of excision and the early detection of local recurrence; there should be careful follow-up surveillance after wide local excision by regular clinical examinations and mammography.

Local recurrence is rare after mastectomy or subcutaneous mastectomy (with the precaution of examining the nipple ducts carefully and adding nipple irradiation where indicated) but is more common after wide local excision. IBRT reduces local recurrence and, although many patients without IBRT do not develop a local recurrence, we have failed to keep the rate low enough with our policy of substantial margins of clear breast tissue around the tumor. We therefore at present recommend IBRT for all cases treated with wide local excision.

DCIS is frequently extensive. It seems unlikely that in situ carcinoma can invade the breast more easily than in-

vasive carcinoma. One possibility is that the risk of breast tissue subsequently showing DCIS arises from a mutation during adolescent breast development, a time during which there are many cell divisions. If the mutation occurs early in breast development, the whole of the lobe undergoes a change to DCIS, the histologic expression of which may occur years later, with the radiologic and clinical manifestations following that. If the mutation occurs later in breast development, then only a group of lobules or a single lobule undergoes the change, producing a small lesion. This has the implication that completeness of histologic excision may sometimes leave tissue that will only later express DCIS histologically, which may account for recurrences seen when margins had appeared widely clear. This hypothesis gains support from the finding of Lakhani et al. (10) that the histologically normal tissue around breast cancers shows a loss of heterozygosity and from reports of the rate of local recurrence actually increasing with years of follow-up in low-grade tumors (11).

REFERENCES

1. Bagnall MJC, Evans AJ, Wilson ARM, et al. Predicting invasion in mammographically detected microcalcification. *Clin Radiol* 2001;56:828–832.
2. Fisher B, Dignam J, Wolmark N, et al. Lumpectomy and radiation therapy for the treatment of intraductal breast cancer: find-

ings from National Surgical Adjuvant Breast and Bowel Project B-17. *J Clin Oncol* 1998;16:441–452.

3. Boyages J, Delaney G, Taylor R. Predictors of local recurrence after treatment of ductal carcinoma in situ: a meta-analysis. *Cancer* 1999;85:616–628.

4. Silverstein MJ, Lagios MD, Groshen S, et al. The influence of margin width on local control of ductal carcinoma in situ of the breast. *N Engl J Med* 1999;340:1455–1461.

5. Sibbering DM, Blamey RW. Nottingham experience. In: Silverstein MJ, ed. *Ductal carcinoma in situ of the breast.* Baltimore: Williams & Wilkins, 1997:367–372.

6. Al-Ghazal SK, Blamey RW, Stewart J, et al. The cosmetic outcome in early breast cancer treated with breast conservation. *Eur J Surg Oncol* 1999;25:566–570.

7. de Mascarel I, Bonichon F, MacGrogan G, et al. Application of the Van Nuys Prognostic Index in a retrospective series of 367 ductal carcinomas in situ of the breast examined by series macroscopic sectioning: practical considerations. *Breast Cancer Res Treat* 2000;61:151–159.

8. Locker AP, Ellis IO, Morgan DAL, et al. Factors influencing local recurrence after excision and radiotherapy for primary breast cancer. *Br J Surg* 1989;76:890–894.

9. Bijker N, Peterse JL, Duchateau L, et al. Risk factors for recurrence and metastasis after breast conserving therapy for ductal carcinoma-in-situ: analysis of European Organization for Research and Treatment of Cancer Trial 10853. *J Clin Oncol* 2001; 19:2263–2271.

10. Lakhani SR, Chaggar, R, Davies, S, et al. Genetic alterations in 'normal' luminal and myoepithelial cells of the breast. *J Pathol* 1999;189:496–503.

11. Page DL, Dupont WD, Rogers LW, et al. Continued local recurrence of carcinoma 15–25 years after a diagnosis of low grade ductal carcinoma in situ of the breast treated only by biopsy. *Cancer* 1995;76:1197–1200.

DUCTAL CARCINOMA IN SITU: THE MEMORIAL SLOAN-KETTERING CANCER CENTER EXPERIENCE

KIMBERLY J. VAN ZEE
PATRICK I. BORGEN

Through the years, ductal carcinoma in situ (DCIS) has accounted for an increasing proportion of breast cancers. Before the use of screening mammography, DCIS accounted for only 1% to 2% of all breast carcinomas. With great improvements in mammographic technique and the widespread use of screening mammography, DCIS now represents up to 30% to 40% of mammographically detected breast malignancies (1). At Memorial Sloan-Kettering Cancer Center (MSKCC), we treat over 2,500 breast malignancies each year, with DCIS accounting for about 20% of all breast cancers treated by the surgical service.

Coincident with the rise in incidence of DCIS has been the detection of smaller and smaller lesions. Although in the past, most patients with DCIS presented with a palpable mass, most are now identified by a small area of microcalcification on a screening mammogram. Thus, in many ways, the DCIS seen today is a different entity from that seen decades ago.

The optimal management of DCIS remains a major challenge. Although the traditional treatment was mastectomy, the adoption of breast-conserving surgery for DCIS was inevitable after prospective, randomized studies demonstrated that breast conservation and mastectomy yield similar survival outcomes for selected patients with invasive breast cancer (2–7). It must be remembered, however, that DCIS is not simply early invasive breast cancer. Unlike invasive breast carcinoma, DCIS has a nearly 100% cure rate with mastectomy (8). Also, with breast conservation, DCIS appears to have a higher local-relapse rate than similarly treated invasive breast cancer. In studies of breast conservation for DCIS with long-term follow-up, local recurrences continue to be observed even at 10 to 15 years (9,10). In addition, it has been repeatedly found that among local recurrences after breast conservation for DCIS, approximately 50% contain invasive carcinoma (9,11–16). Thus, mastectomy remains the gold standard against which all other proposed treatment strategies must

be judged. Yet, in contrast to invasive carcinoma, there has been no prospective or randomized study comparing total mastectomy with conservative surgery for DCIS.

DIAGNOSIS

Mammography

The importance of state-of-the-art, high-resolution mammographic technique and experienced mammographers cannot be overstated. When reviewing the mammograms from an outside institution, if they are not of an acceptable quality, one must have a low threshold for repeating the mammogram. Repeat mammograms should be performed if an area in the breast is unclear or the films are of less than optimal quality. This may involve simply a two-view standard mammography, or it may entail several additional views and magnification views.

Galactography

Nipple discharge is the third most common presentation of DCIS, after findings of either a mammographic abnormality or a palpable mass. In the patient who presents with a normal mammogram, no palpable masses, and spontaneous unilateral nipple discharge from a single duct, we often recommend a galactogram to further elucidate the problem.

The secreting duct is cannulated with a 30- to 31-gauge blunt-ended sialogram cannula, and water-soluble contrast medium (iothalamate meglumine 60%) is injected using hand pressure (17). Injection is stopped when there is reversal of flow at the nipple or when the patient experiences fullness or discomfort. Usually only 0.2 to 3 mL of contrast are needed. Craniocaudal and 90-degree lateral magnification mammograms are then obtained to confirm the opacification of the appropriate duct. Abnormal galactograms are those with filling defects within the duct, wall irregularity, abrupt luminal changes, or cutoff of the column of contrast material.

We have shown that, in addition to imaging the abnormality, localizing the lesion with preoperative galactography assists in ultimate identification of the causative etiology. In a study of women undergoing preoperative galactography, all (16 of 16) had specific pathology identified, whereas only 20 of 30 (67%) women undergoing major duct excision alone had a lesion found that would explain the nipple discharge (17). It should be noted that in both groups, the same proportion of women were found to have carcinoma (2/16 and 4/30).

Magnetic Resonance Imaging

As more experience has been gained with magnetic resonance imaging (MRI) of the breast, breast imagers are appreciating that DCIS sometimes can be visualized even in the absence of physical or mammographic findings.

At MSKCC, examinations are performed on a 1.5-T magnet using a dedicated breast coil (18). Sagittal fat-suppressed T2-weighted images are obtained as well as sagittal fat-suppressed T1-weighted images before and after gadolinium diethylenetriamine pentaacetic acid administration. Subtraction images are then generated. Findings suggestive of DCIS on postgadolinium images are areas of enhancement that are linear and nodular or clumped.

Evaluation with MRI is currently considered in several situations. In patients with nipple discharge in whom a galactogram is unsuccessful, MRI may be helpful in localizing the causative lesion and in predicting the presence of malignancy. In women with biopsy-proven DCIS or highly suspicious mammograms, MRI can sometimes better assess the full extent of DCIS that is underrepresented mammographically. Likewise, in women with positive margins after attempted wide excision, MRI can be helpful in the assessment of residual disease. We have found that in women at high risk of breast cancer by virtue of a personal history of breast cancer, lobular carcinoma in situ, or atypical ductal hyperplasia (ADH), or because of a strong family history of breast cancer, screening with MRI has an acceptable false-positive rate and can occasionally detect DCIS that is nonpalpable and mammographically occult.

Diagnostic Biopsy

In most cases, DCIS is now detected by mammography as a nonpalpable area of microcalcifications. To confirm the diagnosis of DCIS, a histologic examination must be performed. This can be done by mammographically guided, needle-localized excisional biopsy or stereotactic needle core biopsy (19). In the case of a palpable lesion, nipple discharge, or an abnormality seen only by MRI, other surgical biopsy techniques are used.

Excisional Biopsy

The technical aspects of this biopsy are critical. Ideally, the goal is to obtain widely clear margins while sparing as much breast tissue as possible. In the case of a palpable lesion, the incision is made in the skin overlying the palpable lesion, in the direction of Langer's lines. If the lesion is very high or low in the breast, the incision may be made somewhat more centrally than the lesion. The surgeon must at all times consider the possibility that a mastectomy will later be required. Careful placement of the biopsy incision can facilitate a cosmetic result after mastectomy with or without reconstruction.

The specimen should be removed en bloc, and then oriented. We use short and long sutures to mark the superior and lateral margins, respectively. In the case of a palpable lesion, frozen-section analysis is highly reliable in predicting the presence of carcinoma.

Excisional Biopsy with Preoperative Mammographic Localization

In the case of a mammographically detected lesion, one option for diagnosis is a mammographically guided, needle localization biopsy. At our institution, a thin-hooked wire with a 2-cm reinforced portion is used. Multiple bracketing wires are commonly employed at MSKCC to assist the surgeon in excising a relatively large area of calcifications. This technique uses multiple mammographically guided wires to delineate the boundaries of the calcifications, thereby increasing the likelihood that the surgeon will completely excise all calcifications and obtain negative margins (20).

In the operating room, the surgeon should make a careful assessment of the location of the lesion with respect to the course of the wire(s) from the skin to the lesion and the relationship of the lesion to the tip of the wire(s). The wire(s) may be entering the skin at a location distant from the lesion itself. In most cases, the wire(s) enter the breast at a point more peripheral than the lesion. The mammograms obtained after placement of the localizing wire(s) should be studied before making the incision. Again, thought must be given to incision placement and the possibility of a mastectomy sometime in the future. We do not necessarily attempt to excise core biopsy or localization wire tracts.

The specimen is removed en bloc and oriented. A specimen radiograph is always obtained for a mammographically localized masses. This increases the likelihood that the mammographic lesion of interest has been included in the specimen. We have found it useful to orient the specimen with clips, which are visualized on the specimen radiograph and can sometimes alert the surgeon to the presence of calcifications extending to or near a particular margin. Orthogonal specimen radiographs can be very helpful in evaluating proximity of the calcifications to the margins. Observation of an apparent close margin then allows excision of an additional margin during the same procedure. Frozen-section examination should not typically be performed at the time of mammographically directed biopsy of microcalcifications because the ability to identify the appropriate area to sample is quite limited. In addition, analysis of the permanent sections may be compromised, especially with regard to microinvasion. The specimen is sent to pathology with a specific request to ink the margins. A post-biopsy mammogram is usually obtained, both to confirm that the entire lesion has been removed and to document the new "baseline" appearance of the breast that has undergone biopsy.

Excisional Biopsy with Preoperative Magnetic Resonance Imaging Localization

Excisional biopsy with MRI-guided placement of a localizing wire is now possible. This recently developed technology allows localization of lesions that are nonpalpable and mammographically occult but visible on MRI. In spite of this, we have found that a mammogram performed after the MRI-guided wire placement is still helpful in guiding the surgeon during the excision. The surgical procedure is similar to that used for excisional biopsy with preoperative mammographic localization, except that a specimen radiograph usually does not demonstrate the lesion.

Major Duct Excision with Preoperative Galactogram

In the patient who presents with persistent spontaneous unilateral nipple discharge from a single duct, major duct excision is performed to obtain tissue for diagnosis. We have found that the yield of this procedure is increased by the use of galactography (17). We sometimes perform a diagnostic galactogram initially, with a repeat galactogram done immediately before surgery. This preoperative galactogram is obtained with a combination of contrast medium and methylene blue dye to enable the surgeon to clearly visualize the duct in question. Using this technique in a small number of patients, we have found that the proportion of patients in whom a causative lesion was identified increased from 67% to 100% (17).

Stereotactic Core Biopsy

In the past decade, stereotactic core biopsy has become widely available. The majority of DCIS lesions are detected by microcalcifications or a mass lesion on mammography. When a lesion is detected mammographically, material may be obtained for histologic diagnosis via stereotactic core biopsy, and there are many instances in which a stereotactic biopsy greatly facilitates the diagnosis and treatment of DCIS (21). In women of advanced age or with comorbid conditions where the mammographic lesion is found to be benign, a surgical procedure may be avoided. In women with multifocal disease by mammography, core biopsies showing DCIS in widely separated areas in the breast will facilitate the decision to go directly to mastectomy for treatment (22). In the previously conserved breast, particularly after radiation, a core biopsy may provide a less invasive method to evaluate mammographic findings that are indeterminate (23).

There are, however, limitations to the use of stereotactic biopsy in patients with DCIS. In cases in which 14-gauge stereotactic biopsy reveals DCIS, 20% will have invasive carcinoma found at the time of surgery (24,25). The finding of invasion at the time of surgery may require that the patient return for axillary node dissection as a separate procedure. Second, in noncomedo and comedo DCIS treated surgically at our institution, a 14-gauge stereotactic core biopsy done before surgery found only ADH in 60% and 30% of cases, respectively (26). Of all 14-gauge stereotactic core biopsies that show ADH, 50% will have carcinoma (intraductal or invasive) at open surgical biopsy (27). These limitations should be kept in mind when planning the diagnosis and treatment of an individual patient. Underestimation of disease has decreased with the adoption of the 11-gauge, directional, vacuum-assisted breast biopsy device, because of the larger volume of tissue sampled. With this device, only 10% of cases yielding ADH at stereotactic biopsy revealed DCIS at surgical biopsy, and only 5% of lesions that yielded DCIS at stereotactic biopsy revealed infiltrating carcinoma at open biopsy (28).

In cases of microcalcifications that are highly suspicious for DCIS and appear to be amenable to excision and breast conservation, one may go directly to surgical biopsy. In these cases, surgery will inevitably be performed, either for definitive treatment or for diagnosis if the findings are benign by stereotactic core biopsy. For these highly suspicious calcifications, 14-gauge stereotactic biopsy reduces the number of procedures necessary in less than 50% of cases (19). Conversely, stereotactic core biopsy obviates a surgical procedure in 42% of women and does result in a modest cost savings. Also, obtaining a definitive diagnosis preoperatively can assist the surgeon in planning an adequate excision and may increase the chance that negative margins are achieved in one surgical procedure.

PATHOLOGY

It is important that the biopsy specimen be carefully processed and that histologic examination of the material be performed by a pathologist with experience in breast disease. In a specimen showing DCIS, a description including nuclear grade, architectural subtype (micropapillary, papillary, cribriform, solid, comedo), and distribution (i.e., single tumor focus, dispersed, focal with peripheral extension) is useful in characterizing the lesion for the clinician. Assigning a size to DCIS is often difficult owing to its ductal distribution and resultant dispersed appearance on histologic sectioning, but an attempt to do so is very helpful in making treatment plans. At MSKCC, the specimen is serially sectioned at 2- to 3-mm intervals from one end to the other. Tissue sections are then submitted in sequence. This is helpful in reconstructing the total extent of DCIS in the specimen.

The evaluation of margins is of utmost importance. All margins should be inked before sectioning the specimen. At MSKCC, a different color of ink is used for each margin to facilitate identification and orientation of close or positive margins. The presence of involved or questionable margins is probably the most important risk factor for recurrence (29–31).

As with mammograms, all pathologic material from outside institutions should be reviewed. The challenge of distinguishing DCIS from severely atypical hyperplasia is well documented. When, in a survey by Rosai (32), five experienced breast pathologists were asked to independently evaluate ten proliferative ductal lesions, diagnoses ranged from benign hyperplasia to DCIS in three cases, and in only two cases did four of the five pathologists agree. In cases of borderline pathology (i.e., ADH versus DCIS), pathologic review by a pathologist with a special interest in breast disease is desirable.

DEFINITIVE TREATMENT

The treatment of patients with DCIS is one of the most controversial topics in surgery today. As outlined in the introduction, although prospective trials defining the optimal management of DCIS have not been performed and despite the realization that the two diseases have substantial differences, treatment algorithms for invasive breast cancer have been widely adopted. Despite the fact that we are a tertiary referral center for cancer patients and tend to see a more advanced stage of disease at diagnosis than is generally seen in the community, approximately 60% of women with DCIS have breast-conserving surgery. This underscores our commitment to breast conservation.

Mastectomy

Mastectomy provides a standard with which other proposed therapeutic modalities should be compared. Among patients who have undergone mastectomy for DCIS, the disease-specific mortality rate should be 1% or less. In a series of 101 patients with DCIS treated with mastectomy at MSKCC, only one death had resulted from breast cancer at a median follow-up of 11.5 years (33).

Although we believe that mastectomy should be mentioned to all patients with DCIS as one of their treatment options, it is strongly recommended to those in whom negative margins are not obtainable, disease is grossly multicentric, or in whom the lesion is large enough that adequate resection will cause a poor cosmetic result.

For intraductal carcinoma, however, it is difficult to accept a surgical treatment that is more aggressive and disfiguring than that necessary for invasive carcinoma. One approach to mastectomy that addresses this problem is the use of a skin-sparing incision. In selected patients, an incision that includes only the nipple-areolar complex may be utilized to perform the mastectomy. In others, a "tennis racquet" incision, which includes the circumareolar incision with a lateral extension, is appropriate. If a tissue expander is to be used, a very small ellipse including the nipple-areolar complex with small triangles of skin medially and laterally allows a small, linear scar. Although more difficult and time-consuming, excellent cosmesis may be achieved with this skin-sparing approach (34). If the skin flaps are dissected in the same plane as in the traditional approach, the recurrence rates should be equivalent. Retrospective series suggest that long-term recurrence rates are equivalent to conventional mastectomy for invasive carcinoma (35).

In performing a mastectomy for DCIS, the same care must be taken as is taken with invasive disease. Residual breast tissue puts a woman at risk of residual intraductal carcinoma that may progress to invasion. In addition, failure to remove as much breast tissue as possible creates the potential for the subsequent development of additional breast cancer. Flaps are raised in the superficial fascial plane, leaving only a thin layer of subcutaneous adipose tissue on the dermis. When the anatomically correct plane is defined, blood loss is minimal and flaps are of uniform thickness.

Historically, in the case of extensive DCIS requiring a mastectomy, a low level I axillary node dissection was often performed at the time of the mastectomy. This was done out of concern that areas of invasion would be found in the specimen. We and others (36,37) evaluated the role of lymphatic mapping and sentinel lymph node biopsy in this situation. We examined patients in whom there had been concern that an invasive component would be identified in the specimen obtained at definitive surgery (extensive DCIS requiring mastectomy, extensive comedocarcinoma, presence of a mammographic or palpable mass, the presence of lymphovascular invasion in the absence of identifiable stromal invasion, suspicion of microinvasion), but in whom only DCIS was found. These patients comprised only a small proportion of our total DCIS patients, about 20%. In these patients, with "high-risk" DCIS, we found nine of 76 (12%) had positive sentinel nodes (38) Of these nine patients, two (22%) had macrometastases. Presumably, these axillary nodal metastases originated in invasive carcinoma that was unidentifiable in the breast. In view of these data, we consider evaluating the axilla with sentinel lymph node biopsy if a mastectomy is being performed for DCIS or if there is concern that invasion may be present. Because historically women with DCIS have a survival rate of 99%, questions arise regarding the clinical significance of micrometastases in these women. At MSKCC, we are creating a registry for women with DCIS and nodal metastases so that we can evaluate the prognostic importance of micrometastases in these patients over time.

After mastectomy, most women are candidates for immediate reconstruction. One method is the immediate placement of a subpectoral tissue expander that is later exchanged for a subpectoral saline implant. Other methods include the transfer of autogenous tissue from another area of the body (e.g., rectus abdominis or latissimus dorsi muscle).

Breast Conservation

As mentioned previously, there are no prospective, randomized studies that compare the results of breast conservation with those of mastectomy for DCIS. Two randomized studies have examined treatment options for DCIS, the National Surgical Adjuvant Breast and Bowel Project B-17 trial (15) and the European Organization for Research and Treatment of Cancer 10853 trial (16). In the National Surgical Adjuvant Breast and Bowel Project B-17 trial, with 7.5 years of follow-up, 26.8% of patients developed local recurrence after excision alone compared with 12.1% after excision and radiation therapy (15). In the European Organization for Research and Treatment of Cancer 10853 trial with 4.25 years of follow-up, 16.6% of patients had local recurrence after excision alone compared with 10.6% after excision and radiation therapy (16).

In reported retrospective series with at least 60 months of follow-up, local recurrence rates range from 12% to 63% for excision alone (14,15, 38–44) and from 6% to 21% for excision followed by adjuvant breast irradiation (9,10,14,15, 43–52). In a series of 150 patients treated at MSKCC from 1978 through 1990, we found 6-year actuarial recurrence rates of 20.7% and 9.6% among patients treated with excision alone and excision followed by radiation therapy, respectively (43). To date, with a median follow-up of more than 6 years, the overall disease-specific survival rate in this group is 100%.

After a biopsy that reveals DCIS, a re-excision is often necessary. This is done in the case of grossly or microscopically positive margins or if the margins are negative but close (within one high-power field, 40×). Because we know that even negative margins do not preclude residual disease, widely clear margins are desirable. A re-excision with minimal or no residual disease generally is a good indicator of complete resection.

Factors that we consider important in making treatment recommendations to a woman with DCIS include the size of the lesion, histologic subtype, presence of necrosis, nuclear grade, and margin status. Patients with small, noncomedo, low-grade lesions with widely clear margins are considered to be candidates for wide excision alone. Lesions that are somewhat larger or are of comedo subtype or high

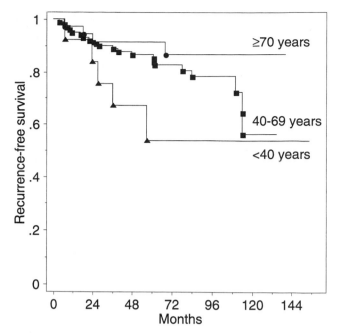

FIGURE 28.1. Local recurrence–free survival among women with ductal carcinoma in situ treated at Memorial Sloan-Kettering Cancer Center with breast conservation, by age. (From Van Zee KJ, Liberman L, Samli B, et al. Long term follow-up of women with ductal carcinoma in situ treated with breast-conserving surgery. *Cancer* 1999;86:1757–1767, with permission.)

nuclear grade are best treated by both wide excision and radiation therapy. At MSKCC, most patients with DCIS who undergo breast-conserving surgery are referred to a radiation oncologist for adjuvant radiation therapy.

Recent experience at our institution suggests that an additional factor that should be considered is age. We reviewed the records of 150 women with DCIS treated with breast conservation at our institution through 1990 (43). Among these women, there was a significantly lower risk of local recurrence with increasing age (Fig. 28.1), both in women who received adjuvant radiation and those who did not (Table 28.1).

For invasive breast carcinoma treated with breast conservation, others have reported a lower local recurrence rate in older women (45,53–59). Veronesi et al. (57) theorized that this may be due to the fact that with age, "the complex structure of the mammary gland disappears and the breast is

TABLE 28.1. THE MEMORIAL SLOAN-KETTERING CANCER CENTER EXPERIENCE WITH DUCTAL CARCINOMA IN SITU TREATED BY BREAST CONSERVATION: 6-YEAR ACTUARIAL RECURRENCE RATES BY AGE

	<40 Yr	40–69 Yr	≥70 Yr
Wide excision alone	59.2%	19.1%	14.4%
Wide excision and breast irradiation	33.3%	8.5%	0.0%

reduced to a fatty organ with scattered islands of fibroepithelial tissue, without connections between them." If these findings for invasive breast cancer are indeed attributable to a less interconnected ductal system in older women, the discrepancy in local relapse rates seen in invasive carcinoma should be even more pronounced with intraductal disease. Vicini et al. (52) recently confirmed our findings in a series of similar size. Thus, it appears that for DCIS, local recurrences are less likely in the older patient, and that this is another factor that should be considered when treating a woman with DCIS (43).

Most important, we believe that a treatment plan must be individualized. Relevant options and the current state of knowledge regarding them must be discussed with the patient in order for her to participate in the decision-making process. Only then can the best treatment plan be devised.

TAMOXIFEN

Tamoxifen has been used for decades in the treatment of women with invasive breast cancer. The NSABP P-1 trial, published in 1998, showed that the risk of breast cancer development in high-risk women could be reduced by tamoxifen administration (60). Then, in 1999, NSABP B-24 showed that among women with DCIS undergoing breast-conserving surgery followed by radiation, there was a reduction in ipsilateral (and contralateral) breast cancer among those taking tamoxifen compared with those taking placebo (ipsilateral rate 8.2% vs. 13.4%) (61). Therefore, a discussion of tamoxifen is often undertaken with women with DCIS, and an increasing number of these patients are referred for further discussions with a medical oncologist.

RECURRENCES

Diagnosis

Women who undergo breast-conserving treatment for DCIS should be carefully monitored for recurrences and for new primaries in the ipsilateral or contralateral breast. In any woman undergoing breast conservation for DCIS that presented as microcalcifications, a postoperative mammogram should be obtained as soon as the postoperative discomfort allows and certainly before initiation of radiation therapy. This postoperative mammogram ensures the complete resection of all microcalcifications. In addition, a mammogram should be obtained 6 months after surgery. This provides a new baseline mammogram of the ipsilateral breast and a basis for comparison of future mammograms. At 1 year post-surgery, bilateral annual mammography may be resumed.

As a patient undergoes follow-up screening mammography, the radiologist should be alert to signs of recurrent disease. The most common mammographic manifestation of local recurrence after breast-conserving treatment for DCIS

is recurrent calcifications in the same quadrant as the original DCIS (62).

In the patient in whom a recurrence is suspected on mammography, stereotactic core biopsy is often desirable. Needle localization surgical biopsy may also be performed but may have higher morbidity in the irradiated breast. Fine needle aspiration, core biopsy, or open surgical biopsy may be used for a suspicious palpable lesion.

Treatment

In women in whom a recurrence is detected after wide excision alone, we may consider reconservation. A wide excision is performed, and if widely negative margins are achieved, the patient may be offered breast conservation, but this time followed by breast irradiation.

Women who develop recurrences of DCIS after treatment with wide excision and radiation therapy are not candidates for breast conservation. In addition, they may not be good candidates for reconstruction with an implant because of the loss of elasticity of the skin with radiation. They may, however, be candidates for breast reconstruction using autogenous tissue transfer.

CONCLUSION

DCIS represents not a single disease entity but rather a spectrum of disease ranging from clinically insignificant, incidentally discovered lesions to aggressive, widespread disease with the potential for invasion and eventual metastasis. The physician endeavoring to treat carcinoma of the breast must identify where along this continuum the patient lies to match the treatment with the severity of the disease. We believe that there is no single treatment plan that is appropriate for all patients; rather, a treatment plan must be individualized for each woman. Relevant options and the current state of knowledge regarding these options must be discussed with the patient for her to fully understand the situation and choose the best options for her.

It is likely that in the future, identification of subsets of patients best managed by each treatment option will be greatly facilitated by the characterization of genetic lesions in DCIS. We are currently actively involved in characterizing molecular lesions in microdissected specimens from patients with DCIS (63). A move from a descriptive to a functional understanding of the disease may allow the much more precise design of each individual's treatment plan in the future.

REFERENCES

1. Ernster VL, Barclay J, Kerlikowske K, et al. Incidence of and treatment for ductal carcinoma in situ of the breast. *JAMA* 1996; 275:913–918.

2. Fisher B, Redmond C, Poisson R, et al. Eight-year results of a randomized clinical trial comparing total mastectomy and lumpectomy with or without irradiation in the treatment of breast cancer. *N Engl J Med* 1989;320:822–828.

3. Sarrazin D, Le MG, Arriagada R, et al. Ten-year results of a randomized trial comparing a conservative treatment to mastectomy in early breast cancer. *Radiother Oncol* 1989;14:177–184.

4. Veronesi U, Banfi A, Salvadori B, et al. Breast conservation is the treatment of choice in small breast cancer: long-term results of a randomized trial. *Eur J Cancer* 1990;26:668–670.

5. Blichert-Toft M, Rose C, Andersen JA, et al. Danish randomized trial comparing breast conservation therapy with mastectomy: six years of life-table analysis. *J Natl Cancer Inst Monogr* 1992;11:19–25.

6. van Dongen JA, Bartelink H, Fentiman IS, et al. Randomized clinical trial to assess the value of breast-conserving therapy in stage I and II breast cancer, EORTC 10801 trial. *J Natl Cancer Inst Monogr* 1992;11:15–18.

7. Jacobson JA, Danforth DN, Cowan KH, et al. Ten-year results of a comparison of conservation with mastectomy in the treatment of stage I and II breast cancer. *N Engl J Med* 1995;332:907–911.

8. Ashikari R, Huvos AG, Snyder RE. Prospective study of non-infiltrating carcinoma of the breast. *Cancer* 1977;39:435–439.

9. Solin LJ, Kurtz J, Fourquet A, et al. Fifteen-year results of breast-conserving surgery and definitive breast irradiation for the treatment of ductal carcinoma in situ of the breast. *J Clin Oncol* 1996;16:754–763.

10. Mirza NQ, Vlastos G, Meric F, et al. Ductal carcinoma-in-situ: long-term results of breast-conserving therapy. *Ann Surg Oncol* 2000;7:656–664.

11. Fisher ER, Leeming R, Anderson S, et al. Conservative management of intraductal carcinoma (DCIS) of the breast. *J Surg Oncol* 1991;47:139–147.

12. Solin LJ, Recht A, Fourquet A, et al. Ten-year results of breast-conserving surgery and definitive irradiation for intraductal carcinoma (ductal carcinoma in situ) of the breast. *Cancer* 1991;68:2337–2344.

13. Fisher B, Costantino J, Redmond C, et al. Lumpectomy compared with lumpectomy and radiation therapy for the treatment of intraductal breast cancer. *N Engl J Med* 1993;328:1581–1586.

14. Silverstein MJ, Lagios MD, Craig PH, et al. A prognostic index for ductal carcinoma in situ of the breast. *Cancer* 1996;77:2267–2274.

15. Fisher B, Dignam J, Wolmark N, et al. Lumpectomy and radiation therapy for the treatment of intraductal breast cancer: findings from National Surgical Adjuvant Breast and Bowel Project B-17. *J Clin Oncol* 1998;16:441–452.

16. Julien J-P, Bijker N, Fentiman IS, et al. Radiotherapy in breast-conserving treatment for ductal carcinoma in situ: first results of the EORTC randomised phase III trial 10853. *Lancet* 2000;355:528–533.

17. Van Zee KJ, Ortega-Perez G, Emery M, et al. Preoperative galactography increases the diagnostic yield of major duct excision for nipple discharge. *Cancer* 1998;82.

18. Olson J, Morris E, Van Zee K, et al. Magnetic resonance imaging facilitates breast conservation for occult breast cancer. *Ann Surg Oncol* 2000;7:411–415.

19. Liberman L, LaTrenta LR, Van Zee KJ, et al. Stereotactic core biopsy of calcifications highly suggestive of malignancy. *Radiology* 1997;203:673–677.

20. Liberman L, Kaplan J, Van Zee KJ, et al. Bracketing wires for preoperative breast needle localization *AJR Am J Roentgenol* 2001;177:565–572.

21. Liberman L, LaTrenta LR, Dershaw DD, et al. Impact of core biopsy on the surgical management of impalpable breast cancer. *AJR Am J Roentgenol* 1997;168:495–499.

22. Liberman L, Dershaw DD, Rosen PP, et al. Core needle biopsy of synchronous ipsilateral breast lesions: impact on treatment. *AJR Am J Roentgenol* 1996;166:1429–1432.

23. Liberman L, Dershaw DD, Durfee S, et al. Recurrent carcinoma after breast conservation: diagnosis with stereotaxic core biopsy. *Radiology* 1995;197:735–738.

24. Liberman L, Dershaw DD, Rosen PP, et al. Stereotaxic core biopsy of breast carcinoma: accuracy at predicting invasion. *Radiology* 1995;194:379–381.

25. Jackman RJ, Nowels KW, Shepard MJ, et al. Stereotaxic large-core needle biopsy of 450 nonpalpable breast lesions with surgical correlation in lesions with cancer or atypical hyperplasia. *Radiology* 1994;193:91–95.

26. Liberman L, Dershaw DD, Glassman JR, et al. Analysis of cancers not diagnosed at stereotactic core breast biopsy. *Radiology* 1997;203:151–157.

27. Liberman L, Cohen MA, Dershaw DD, et al. Atypical ductal hyperplasia diagnosed at stereotaxic core biopsy of breast lesions: and indication for surgical biopsy. *AJR Am J Roentgenol* 1995;164:1111–1113.

28. Liberman L, Smolkin JH, Dershaw DD, et al. Calcification retrieval at stereotactic, 11-gauge, directional, vacuum-assisted breast biopsy. *Radiology* 1998;208:251–260.

29. Fisher ER, Costantino J, Fisher B, et al. Pathologic findings from the National Surgical Adjuvant Breast Project (NSABP) protocol B-17: Intraductal carcinoma (ductal carcinoma in situ). *Cancer* 1995;75:1310–1319.

30. Arnesson L-G, Smeds S, Fagerberg G, et al. Follow-up of two treatment modalities for ductal cancer in situ of the breast. *Br J Surg* 1989;76:672–675.

31. Silverstein MJ, Lagios MD, Groshen S, et al. The influence of margin width on local control of ductal carcinoma in situ of the breast. *N Engl J Med* 1999;340:1455–1461.

32. Rosai J. Borderline epithelial lesions of the breast. *Am J Surg Pathol* 1991;15:209–215.

33. Kinne DW, Petrek JA, Osborne MP, et al. Breast carcinoma in situ. *Arch Surg* 1989;124:33–36.

34. Hidalgo DA, Borgen PI, Petrek JA, et al. Immediate reconstruction after complete skin-sparing mastectomy with autologous tissue. *J Am Cancer Soc* 1998;187:17–21.

35. Kroll SS, Khoo A, Singletary SE, et al. Local recurrence risk after skin-sparing and conventional mastectomy: a 6-year follow-up. *Plast Reconstr Surg* 1999;104:421–425.

36. Klauber-Demore N, Tan LK, Liberman L, et al. Sentinel lymph node biopsy: is it indicated in patients with high-risk DCIS and DCIS with microinvasion? *Ann Surg Oncol* 2000;7:636–642.

37. Pendas S, Dauway E, Giuliano R, et al. Sentinel node biopsy in ductal carcinoma in situ patients. *Ann Surg Oncol* 2000;7:15–20.

38. Gallagher W, Koerner FC, Wood WC. Treatment of intraductal carcinoma with limited surgery: long-term follow-up. *J Clin Oncol* 1989;7:376–380.

39. Temple WJ, Jenkins M, Alexander F, et al. Natural history of in situ breast cancer in a defined population. *Ann Surg* 1989;210:653–657.

40. Price P, Sinnett HD, Gusterson B, et al. Duct carcinoma in situ: predictors of local recurrence and progression in patients treated by surgery alone. *Br J Cancer* 1990;61:869–872.

41. Lagios MD. Duct carcinoma in situ: pathology and treatment. *Surg Clin North Am* 1990;70:853–871.

42. Graham MD, Lakhani S, Gazet J-C. Breast conserving surgery in the management of in situ breast carcinoma. *Eur J Surg Oncol* 1991;17:258–264.

43. Van Zee KJ, Liberman L, Samli B, et al. Long term follow-up of women with ductal carcinoma in situ treated with breast-conserving surgery. *Cancer* 1999;86:1757–1767.

44. Ringberg A, Idvall I, Ferno M, et al. Ipsilateral local recurrence in relation to therapy and morphological characteristics in patients with ductal carcinoma in situ of the breast. *Eur J Surg Oncol* 2000;26:444–451.

45. Delouche G, Bachelot F, Premont M, et al. Conservation treatment of early breast cancer: long term results and complications. *Int J Radiat Oncol Biol Phys* 1987;13:29–34.

46. Stotter AT, McNeese M, Oswald MJ, et al. The role of limited surgery with irradiation in primary treatment of ductal in situ breast cancer. *Int J Radiat Oncol Biol Phys* 1990;18:283–287.

47. Bornstein BA, Recht A, Connolly JL, et al. Results of treating ductal carcinoma in situ of the breast with conservative surgery and radiation therapy. *Cancer* 1991;67:7–13.

48. Ringberg A, Andersson I, Aspegren K, et al. Breast carcinoma in situ in 167 women-incidence, mode of presentation, therapy and follow-up. *Eur J Surg Oncol* 1991;17:466–476.

49. Ray GR, Adelson J, Hayhurst E, et al. Ductal carcinoma in situ of the breast: results of treatment by conservative surgery and definitive irradiation. *Int J Radiat Oncol Biol Phys* 1994;28:105–111.

50. White J, Levine A, Gustafson G, et al. Outcome and prognostic factors for local recurrence in mammographically detected ductal carcinoma in situ of the breast treated with conservative surgery and radiation therapy. *Int J Radiat Oncol Biol Phys* 1995;31:791–797.

51. Haffty BG, Perrotta PL, Ward B, et al. Conservatively treated breast cancer: outcome by histologic subtype. *Breast J* 1997;3:7–14.

52. Vicini FA, Kestin LL, Goldstein NS, et al. Impact of young age on outcome in patients with ductal carcinoma-in-situ treated with breast-conserving therapy. *J Clin Oncol* 2000;18:296–306.

53. Recht A, Connolly JL, Schnitt SJ, et al. The effect of young age on tumor recurrence in the treated breast after conservative surgery and radiotherapy. *Int J Radiat Oncol Biol Phys* 1988;14:3–10.

54. Kurtz JM, Spitalier J-M, Amalric R, et al. Mammary recurrences in women younger than forty. *Int J Radiat Oncol Biol Phys* 1988;15:271–276.

55. Stotter AT, McNeese MD, Ames FC, et al. Predicting the rate and extent of locoregional failure after breast conservation therapy for early breast cancer. *Cancer* 1989;64:2217–2225.

56. Nemoto T, Patel J, Rosner D, et al. Factors affecting recurrence in lumpectomy without irradiation for breast cancer. *Cancer* 1991;67:2079–2082.

57. Veronesi U, Luini A, Del Vecchio M, et al. Radiotherapy after breast-preserving surgery in women with localized cancer of the breast. *N Engl J Med* 1993;328:1587–1591.

58. McCready DR, Hanna W, Kahn H, et al. Factors associated with local breast cancer recurrence after lumpectomy alone. *Ann Surg Oncol* 1996;3:358–366.

59. Neff PT, Bear HD, Pierce CV, et al. Long-term results of breast conservation therapy for breast cancer. *Ann Surg* 1996;223:709–717.

60. Fisher B, Constantino JP, Wickerham LD, et al. Tamoxifen for prevention of breast cancer: report of the National Surgical Adjuvant Breast and Bowel Project P-1 study. *J Natl Cancer Inst* 1998;90:1371–1388.

61. Fisher B, Dignam J, Wolmark N, et al. Tamoxifen in treatment of intraductal breast cancer: National Surgical Adjuvant Breast and Bowel Project B-24 randomised controlled trial. *Lancet* 1999;353:1993–2000.

62. Liberman L, Van Zee KJ, Dershaw DD, et al. Mammographic features of local recurrence in women who have undergone breast conserving therapy for ductal carcinoma in situ. *AJR Am J Roentgenol* 1997;168:495–499.

63. Ho G, Calvano J, Bisogna M, et al. In microdissected ductal carcinoma in situ, HER-2/neu amplification but not p53 mutation is associated with high nuclear grade and comedo histology. *Cancer* 2000;89:2153–2160.

29

THE VAN NUYS/UNIVERSITY OF SOUTHERN CALIFORNIA EXPERIENCE BY TREATMENT

MELVIN J. SILVERSTEIN

Patient data from the Van Nuys Breast Center and the Harold E. and Henrietta C. Lee Breast Center at the University of Southern California in Los Angeles has been used in numerous other chapters in this volume. In Chapter 17, the development of the Van Nuys Pathologic Classification was detailed and the results updated through 2000. In Chapter 21, prognostic factors that might contribute to local recurrence of ductal carcinoma in situ (DCIS) were analyzed (Fig. 21.6). Four of those factors (tumor size, margin width, pathologic classification, and age) were shown to be independent predictors of both local recurrence and local invasive recurrence by multivariate analysis. In Chapter 45, those four factors were used to modify the Van Nuys Prognostic Index. None of those chapters, however, deals with outcome by treatment. This chapter details our results by treatment so that they can more easily be compared with the results of others. The reader must always keep in mind that treatment was not randomized.

PATIENTS

The patient population consists of 909 patients with DCIS; 326 patients were treated with mastectomy, 237 with excision plus radiation therapy, and 346 with excision alone. Treatment was not randomized. Patients with large lesions (>40 mm), multicentricity, or involved margins not amenable to re-excision were advised to undergo mastectomy (usually with immediate breast reconstruction). Patients with smaller lesions (≤40 mm) and microscopically clear surgical margins were generally treated with excision alone or excision plus radiation therapy. However, some patients with larger lesions elected breast preservation and others with lesions 40 mm or smaller elected mastectomy. After the patient had been thoroughly counseled, she made the final decision regarding her treatment.

Until 1988, all patients with DCIS who elected breast conservation were advised to add breast irradiation to their treatment. Most patients accepted this recommendation; a small number refused and were treated with careful clinical follow-up without radiation therapy. Beginning in 1989, we were no longer convinced of the overall value of radiation therapy for DCIS, and all patients treated with breast conservation with uninvolved biopsy margins (clear by 1 mm or more) were offered the option of careful clinical follow-up without radiation therapy. Many patients accepted this option; some refused and were treated with breast irradiation. Outside patients with DCIS referred to our radiation oncologists for radiation therapy continued to be treated with radiation therapy in accord with the wishes of their referring physicians. The details and outcome of our radiation therapy treatment protocol are presented in Chapter 37.

Level I and II axillary dissections were done routinely until 1988, thereafter, a lower axillary node sampling was performed in some patents treated with mastectomy. Beginning in 1995, sentinel lymph node biopsies were performed for patients undergoing mastectomy, and no attempt was made to take any axillary nodes in conservatively treated patients with DCIS if it required a separate incision. Disease-free survival rates for each group were estimated by the Kaplan-Meier method. The statistical significance between survival curves was determined by the log-rank test.

RESULTS

Table 29.1 details a number of similarities and differences among the three treatment groups. Because we arbitrarily stopped recommending radiation therapy in the late 1980s without changing the criteria for breast preservation, there is a great deal of similarity between the excision plus radiation therapy and the excision alone groups.

MASTECTOMY

As expected, the patients treated with mastectomy had larger tumors than patients treated with breast conservation

TABLE 29.1. TUMOR CHARACTERISTICS BY TREATMENT: 909 PATIENTS WITH DUCTAL CARCINOMA IN SITU

	Mastectomy	Excision + RT	Excision Only
No. of patients	326	237	346
Average follow-up (mo)	81	106	70
Average size (mm)	42	18	15
No. of nonpalpable tumors (%)	248 (76%)	210 (87%)	325 (94%)
No. of margins <1 mm (%)	260 (80%)	83 (35%)	66 (19%)
No. of margins ≥1 mm (%)	66 (20%)	154 (65%)	280 (81%)
No. of margins ≥10 mm (%)	7 (2%)	45 (19%)	134 (39%)
No. of clear NSABP margins (%)	98 (30%)	208 (88%)	315 (91%)
No. of meeting Lagios et al. Criteria	70 (21%)	124 (52%)	240 (69%)
Average nuclear grade	2.32	2.24	2.19
No. of nuclear grade 3 (%)	141 (43%)	94 (40%)	147 (42%)
No. of predominantly comedo	136 (42%)	91 (38%)	105 (30%)
No. of local recurrences	2 (0.6%)	48 (20%)	61 (18%)
No. of invasive recurrences	2/2 (100%)	22/48 (46%)	25/61 (41%)
Median time to recurrence	Too few recurrences	57 mo	25 mo
5/10-yr LRFS	99%/99%	88%/80%	81%/72%
5/10-yr LRFS (Lagios et al. criteria)	100%/100%	92%/88%	88%/81%
No. of patients with metastases	1	6	1
No. of deaths	0	4	1
5/10-yr BCSS rate	100%	99.5%/97.8%	100%/99.3%
5/10-yr overall survival rate	99%/90%	97%/91%	95%/91%

RT, radiation therapy; NSABP, National Surgical Adjuvant Breast Project; LRFS, local recurrence–free survival; BCSS, breast cancer–specific survival.

that averaged 42 mm (versus 16.5 mm for patients treated with breast conservation). Because of this, a greater percentage of patients undergoing mastectomy had palpable tumors (24%) compared with patients treated with breast preservation (8%). Only 20% of patients treated with mastectomy had clear margins according to the original Van Nuys Breast Center standards (≥1 mm). If the National Surgical Adjuvant Breast Project (NSABP) definition of clear margins was used (nontransection of the tumor), this number increased to 30%. Only 21% of patients treated with mastectomy met the criteria of Lagios et al. (1) (i.e., DCIS 25 mm or smaller, nonpalpable, discovered mammographically by calcifications, margins clear by 1 mm or more). Of 326 patients treated with mastectomy, there were two local recurrences;

an actuarial local recurrence rate of only 1% at 10 years. There were no breast cancer–related deaths in the mastectomy group. The 10-year actuarial overall fatality rate owing to death from any cause was 10% (Table 29.2).

Breast Preservation

Although the patients were not randomized, there was a great deal of similarity between those treated with excision plus radiation therapy and those treated with excision alone. This is to be expected because of the evolution of the treatment policy at the Van Nuys Breast Center. Before 1988, virtually all patients treated with breast preservation received radiation therapy. After 1988, almost all were treated

TABLE 29.2. TYPES OF RECURRENCES BY TREATMENT: 909 PATIENTS WITH DUCTAL CARCINOMA IN SITU

	Mastectomy (n = 326)	Excision + RT (n = 237)	Excision Only (n = 346)	Total (n = 909)
Local only	1	42	60	103
Local + distant	1	6	1	8
Distant only	0	0	0	0
Total	2	48	61	111
Invasive	2	22	25	49
DCIS only	0	26	36	62
Total	2	48	61	111

RT, radiation therapy; DCIS, ductal carcinoma in situ.

with excision only. Because of this, the average follow-up times are shorter for patients treated with excision only (70 versus 106 months). In addition, as diagnostic abilities improved, tumor size became smaller. Other than that, the two groups are quite similar, particularly in two important categories: percentage of nonpalpable lesions and nuclear grade.

When patients treated with radiation therapy were compared with patients treated with excision only (Table 29.1), the average tumor size differed (18 mm for patients treated with radiation therapy versus 15 mm for patients treated with excision alone). Approximately 90% of each treatment group had nonpalpable tumors, and the average nuclear grade for patients treated with radiation therapy and those not treated with radiation therapy was similar.

The major difference between the two treatment groups is found in the category that reflects the adequacy of surgical excision: tumor margin status. Using our original definition of clear margins ($\geq$1 mm), which we used extensively during the 1980s, 81% of the patients treated with excision only and 65% of the patients treated with radiation therapy had clear margins ($p = 0.02$). The percentage of patients with widely clear margins ($\geq$10 mm) was higher in the excision-only group: 39% versus 19% for patients treated with radiation therapy ($p < 0.01$). These findings reflect the fact that close or focally involved margins were not routinely re-excised in the early 1980s when most of the patients treated with radiation therapy were accrued, whereas in the later years of this study, when most of the excision only patients were accrued, re-excision was routine for close margins. Using the NSABP definition of clear margins (nontransection), approximately 90% of both breast-preservation treatment groups had uninvolved margins (88% of the patients treated with excision plus radiation therapy and 92% of the patients treated with excision alone; $p = $ NS).

Recurrences

Forty-eight of 237 patients (20%) treated with excision and radiation therapy had a local recurrence, whereas 61 of 346 (18%) patients treated with excision only had a local recurrence. The raw recurrence percentages, which are similar, are misleading because the average follow-up for patients treated with excision only is 36 months less than for patients treated with radiation therapy. The actuarial recurrence rates yield more information. The local recurrence rates are 12% and 20% at 5 and 10 years, respectively, for patients treated with radiation therapy and 19% and 28% at 5 and 10 years, respectively, for patients treated with excision only ($p = 0.06$) (Fig. 29.1). The median time to local recurrence was 4.8 years for patients treated with excision plus radiation therapy, a result similar to that of Solin et al. (2,3). It was only 2.1 years for patients treated with excision alone ($p < 0.01$).

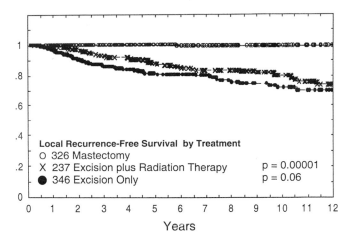

FIGURE 29.1. Probability of local recurrence–free survival by treatment for 909 patients with ductal carcinoma in situ.

Because half of all local recurrences after excision plus radiation therapy occur more than 4.8 years after treatment, these patients must be followed closely for more than the usual 5 years recommended by some authors. We performed mammography every 6 months for 10 years on the involved breast and every year on the contralateral breast. Physical examination is done twice a year for 10 years and yearly thereafter.

The 5-year recurrence rate for our patients treated with excision only (19%) is higher than that reported by the NSABP (4–8) and higher than that reported by Schwartz et al. (9) (Chapter 26) and Lagios et al. (1,10). This is to be expected because 6% of our patients treated with excision only had palpable lesions and 19% had margins less than 1 mm (Table 29.1), whereas both Schwartz et al. and Lagios et al. limited their patients treated with excision only to nonpalpable lesions with margins of 1 mm or more. Twenty percent of the lesions in the NSABP B-17 trial were palpable and as noted above, the NSABP had a more liberal definition of what constitutes a clear margin. In addition, Schwartz et al. and Lagios et al. limited their DCIS lesions to 25 mm or smaller and the NSABP accepted lesions 40 mm or smaller, whereas we had no size limitation on breast conservation. In fact, 8% (28 of 346) of patients treated with excision only in our series had tumors greater than 40 mm.

When the analysis of our patients is limited to those patients that meet the criteria of Lagios et al., the outcome, in terms of local recurrence, is similar to both that of Lagios et al. and Schwartz et al. and somewhat better than that of the NSAPB trial; moreover, there is no statistical advantage for patients who received postoperative radiation therapy in that select group (Fig. 29.2). The 5- and 10-year recurrence rates for Van Nuys Breast Center patients meeting the criteria of Lagios et al. treated with radiation therapy were 8% and 12%, respectively; for those treated with excision alone, they were 12% and 19%, respectively.

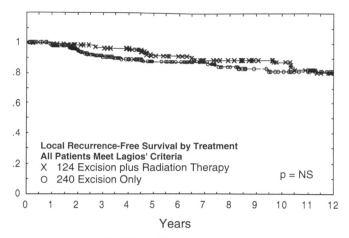

FIGURE 29.2. Probability of local recurrence–free survival by treatment for 364 patients treated with breast conservation who meet the criteria of Lagios et al. (*p* = NS).

The difference seen in Figure 29.1 between patients treated with radiation therapy and those not treated with radiation therapy bears comment. Although it is not quite significant using the log-rank test (*p* = 0.06), the benefit of radiation therapy is significant if one uses a statistic weighted more toward the earlier years (Gehan's Wilcoxon *p* =

0.008). There is no doubt that radiation therapy decreases the probability of local recurrence. This has been well proven in prospective randomized trials (4–8,11–14). Our own data clearly show a similar, approximately 50%, relative reduction in the probability of local recurrence if radiation therapy is added (Fig. 29.3) (Chapter 21). This effect is seen in all subgroups of patients. The question pending is in which patients is the effect worthwhile? For example, if a subgroup with a 30% local recurrence rate after excision alone received radiation therapy, the recurrence rate can be reduced to 15% (a relative reduction of about 50%). This is probably worthwhile and the benefits outweigh the risks. Conversely, if a subgroup with a 6% local recurrence rate after excision alone can be identified, radiation therapy will again reduce the risk of local recurrence by 50%, from 6% to 3%. With an absolute benefit of only 3%, the risks probably outweigh the benefits.

When subgroup analysis on our patients is performed by margin width and treatment, those patients with margin widths less than 1 mm (Fig. 29.4) obtain the greatest benefit from radiation therapy (*p* = 0.0009). Patients with intermediate margin widths of 1 to 9 mm receive an intermediate benefit (Fig. 29.5), which approaches significance (*p* = 0.07) when the log-rank test is used. The difference is sig-

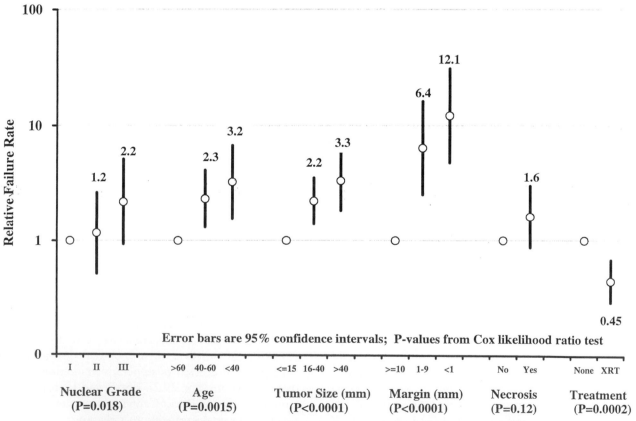

FIGURE 29.3. Multivariate analysis shows various important factors that play a role in local recurrence. The addition of radiation therapy after excision of the primary lesion reduces the risk of local recurrence by 55%.

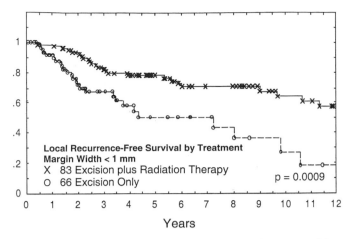

FIGURE 29.4. Probability of local recurrence–free survival by treatment for 149 patients treated with breast conservation with margin widths less than 1 mm ($p = 0.009$).

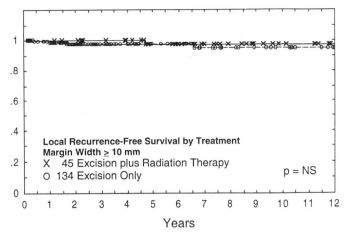

FIGURE 29.6. Probability of local recurrence–free survival by treatment for 179 patients treated with breast conservation with wide margin widths of greater than 10 mm or more ($p = NS$).

nificant if a statistical test that is weighted toward the earlier part of the curve is used. For patients with margins of 10 mm or more, there is no difference in the probability of local recurrence whether or not postoperative radiation therapy is given (Fig. 29.6) ($p = NS$).

Margin Width

The results of the NSABP protocol B-17 (4–8) (Chapter 42), the European Organization for Cancer Research and Treatment) protocol 10853 (11,12) (Chapter 43), and the United Kingdom, Australia, and New Zealand DCIS Trial (13,14) (Chapter 44) clearly show that radiation therapy after excision of DCIS reduces the risk of local recurrence. Previously published data (15), data presented in this chapter, and data presented by Blamey et al. (Chapter 27) suggest that margin width is a key factor in predicting local re-

currence; the narrower the margin, the greater the absolute effect of radiation therapy. (For a more detailed discussion of margin width, see Chapter 47.)

COMMENT

All prospective randomized trials for DCIS published to date have shown a benefit of radiation therapy in decreasing the rate of local recurrence (4–8,11–15) (Chapters 42, 43, 44). Unlike studies for invasive cancer, none of the studies limited to DCIS has shown the benefit of decreasing mortality from breast cancer. Because at present, there is no mortality benefit from radiation therapy, clinicians must be secure that the benefits of radiation therapy in terms of improved local recurrence–free survival significantly outweigh the side effects, complications, inconvenience, and costs for a given subgroup of patients.

Radiation therapy is not without side effects, and it should not be routinely added to the therapeutic plan of every patient treated with breast preservation. Careful consideration must be given to its risks versus its potential benefits (16–18). Radiation therapy is expensive and time-consuming and is accompanied by significant side effects in a small percentage of patients (e.g., cardiac, pulmonary). Radiation fibrosis of the breast is a more common side effect, particularly with the type of radiation therapy given during the 1980s. Radiation fibrosis changes the texture of the breast and skin, makes mammographic follow-up somewhat more difficult, and may result in delayed diagnosis if there is a local recurrence. The use of radiation therapy for DCIS precludes its use if an invasive recurrence develops at a later date. The use of radiation therapy with its accompanying skin and vascular changes make skin-sparing mastectomy, if needed in the future, more difficult to perform. Radiation therapy is not the answer to poor surgery and shoddy

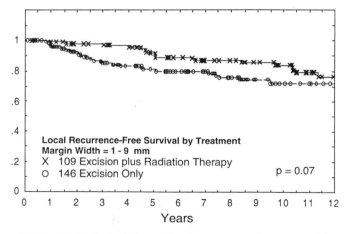

FIGURE 29.5. Probability of local recurrence–free survival by treatment for 255 patients treated with breast conservation with intermediate margin widths of 1 to 9 mm ($p = 0.07$).

pathology. It should be prescribed for patients who are likely to benefit from it, after having undergone carefully performed surgery and complete histopathologic specimen evaluation. The benefits, risks and costs of radiation therapy should be factored into the decision-making process along with the potential costs of local recurrence.

If we are about to enter an era in medicine in which surgery is marginal, no attempt is made to perform a complete excision, specimen radiography is not performed, only a small amount of tissue rather than the entire specimen is submitted for histologic processing, and intraoperative consultation among surgeon, pathologist, and radiologist is unusual, then I agree that radiation therapy will be indicated for most patients with DCIS who elect breast-preservation therapy. If surgeons, pathologists, and radiologists continue to work together, then I believe that various subsets of patients with DCIS can be defined, including those in whom the absolute benefit of radiation therapy is so small that they can be safely treated with excision alone, those who will clearly benefit from the addition of radiation therapy, and finally, those whose local recurrence rate will be so high with any form of breast preservation that mastectomy is indicated.

REFERENCES

1. Lagios MD, Westdahl PR, Margolin FR, et al. Duct carcinoma in situ: relationship of extent of noninvasive disease to the frequency of occult invasion, multicentricity, lymph node metastases, and short-term treatment failures. *Cancer* 1982;50:1309–1314.
2. Solin LJ, Yeh I, Kurtz J, et al. Ductal carcinoma in situ (intraductal carcinoma) of the breast treated with breast-conserving surgery and definitive irradiation. *Cancer* 1993;71:2532–2542.
3. Solin LJ, Kurtz J, Fourquet A, et al. Fifteen year results of breast conserving surgery and definitive breast irradiation for the treatment of ductal carcinoma in situ (intraductal carcinoma of the breast). *J Clin Oncol* 1996;14:754–763.
4. Fisher B, Costantino J, Redmond C, et al. Lumpectomy compared with lumpectomy and radiation therapy for the treatment of intraductal breast cancer. *N Engl J Med* 1993;328:1581–1586.
5. Fisher ER, Constantino J, Fisher B, et al. Pathologic finding from the National Surgical Adjuvant Breast Project (NSABP) Protocol B-17: intraductal carcinoma (ductal carcinoma in situ). *Cancer* 1995;75:1310–1319.
6. Fisher B, Dignam J, Wolmark N, et al. Lumpectomy and radiation therapy for the treatment of intraductal breast cancer: findings from National Surgical Adjuvant Breast and Bowel Project B-17. *J Clin Oncol* 1998;16:441–452.
7. Fisher ER, Dignam J, Tan-Chiu E, et al. Pathologic findings from the National Surgical Adjuvant Breast Project (NSABP) eight-year update of protocol B-17: intraductal carcinoma. *Cancer* 1999;86:429–438.
8. Fisher B, Land S, Mamounas E, et al. Prevention of invasive breast cancer in women with ductal carcinoma in situ: an update of the National Surgical Adjuvant Breast and Bowel Project Experience. *Semin Oncol* 2001;28:400–418.
9. Schwartz GF, Finkel GC, Garcia JC, et al. Subclinical ductal carcinoma in situ of the breast. Treatment by local excision and surveillance alone. *Cancer* 1992;70:2468–2474.
10. Lagios MD, Margolin FR, Westdahl PR, et al. Mammographically detected duct carcinoma in situ. Frequency of local recurrence following tylectomy and prognostic effect of nuclear grade on local recurrence. *Cancer* 1989;63:618–624.
11. Julien JP, Bijker N, Fentiman I, et al. Radiotherapy in breast conserving treatment for ductal carcinoma in situ: first results of EORTC randomized phase III trial 10853. *Lancet* 2000;355;528–533.
12. Bijker N, Peterse JL, Duchateau L, et al. Risk factors for recurrence and metastasis after breast conserving therapy for ductal carcinoma in situ: analysis of European Organization for Research and Treatment of Cancer Trial 10853. *J Clin Oncol* 2001;19: 2263–2271.
13. George WD, Houghton J, Cuzick J, et al. Radiotherapy and tamoxifen following complete local excision (CLE) in the management of ductal carcinoma in situ (DCIS): preliminary results from the UK DCIS trial. *Proc Am Soc Clin Oncol* 2000;19:70(abst).
14. George W, Houghton J, Cuzick J. et al. Radiotherapy and tamoxifen following complete local excision (CLE) in the management of ductal carcinoma in situ (DCIS): preliminary results from the UK DCIS trial. *Proc Am Soc Clin Oncol.* 2000;19:70A.
15. Silverstein MJ, Lagios MD, Groshen, S, et al. The influence of margin width on local control in patients with ductal carcinoma in situ (DCIS) of the breast. *N Engl J Med* 1999:340:1455.
16. Recht A. Side effects of radiation therapy. In: Silverstein MJ, ed. *Ductal carcinoma in situ of the breast.* Baltimore: Williams & Wilkins, 1997:347–352.
17. Early Breast cancer Trialists' Collaborative Group. Favorable and unfavorable effects on long-term survival of radiotherapy for early breast cancer. *Lancet* 2000;355:1757–1770.
18. Kurtz JM. Radiotherapy for early breast cancer: was a comprehensive overview of trials needed? *Lancet* 2000;355:1739–1740.

30

DUCTAL CARCINOMA IN SITU: THE EDINBURGH EXPERIENCE

J. MICHAEL DIXON

Between 1988 and 1996, in the Edinburgh Breast Unit, 133 women were treated with breast conserving surgery for ductal carcinoma in situ. The age range of patients was 29 to 89 years, with a mean age of 58, and a median age of 59.3 years. Follow-up was to the end of 1999, and the median follow-up was 6.3 years.

TREATMENT

From 1988 to 1992, initial treatment in the unit was complete, wide, local excision alone. Complete wide excision was defined as excision of the mammographic lesion as assessed postoperatively in a multidisciplinary meeting, and clear lateral margins of excision with 1 mm or more of tissue present at the lateral margin. Specimens were orientated with ligaclips, and the cavity in the breast was also marked with ligaclips. More recently patients were entered into the United Kingdom (U.K.) DCIS trial. The U.K. DCIS trial randomized patients to receive treatment by wide local excision alone, wide local excision + tamoxifen, wide local excision + radiotherapy, or wide local excision + radiotherapy + tamoxifen (Chapter 44). Patients who did not enter the trial were treated by wide local excision alone. The treatments received by patients in Edinburgh during the study period are outlined in Table 30.1.

Following treatment, patients were seen in the outpatient clinic every six months for regular review and had annual mammograms. Data presented included ipsilateral breast recurrences. All recurrences were subject to a detailed review of the pathology and mammograms, and were classified into the following categories:

- Residual disease—in these patients, a review of the specimen radiograph and the original mammograms demonstrated that the wide local excisions had not removed a small number of flecks of calcification from the breast. In retrospect, one or two flecks of calcium were visible on the mammogram one year following the surgery; however, these were visible only when using a magnifying glass to closely examine the area where the recurrence occurred, which is difficult to know prior to recurrence.
- True local recurrence—recurrence around the site of the original complete wide local excision (marked with ligaclips).
- New primary—invasive cancer that occurred at a distance of more than 2 cm from the cavity of the previous wide excision (visualized by ligaclips).

RESULTS

There were 20 ipsilateral breast "recurrences" in the group of 133 women, 11 of which were DCIS, and nine of which were invasive. Of the 11 so-called DCIS recurrences, five were considered to be residual DCIS, five were true in situ recurrences, and one was a second primary. Of the nine invasive recurrences, seven were true recurrences, and two were second primaries. The time to ipsilateral local breast recurrence for the entire series is shown in Figure 30.1.

The distribution of the different types of recurrence related to treatment is shown in Table 30.2. From these data, it can be seen that there were no true invasive or in situ recurrences in patients treated by radiotherapy alone or radiotherapy + tamoxifen. The only disease seen in these patients was either residual disease or a second primary.

FACTORS AFFECTING LOCAL RECURRENCE
Age

Patients under 50 had a higher rate of local recurrence than older patients (Fig. 30.2) but because of the small numbers of young women, this difference was not quite statistically significant, $p = 0.06$.

Margins

Following surgery, all patients were considered to have clear margins and a complete excision of the mammographic le-

TABLE 30.1. TREATMENT FOR PATIENTS WITH DUCTAL CARCINOMA IN SITU

Treatment	Number	% of Total
WLE alone	67	50.4
WLE + tamoxifen	28	21.0
WLE + radiotherapy	22	16.6
WLE + radiotherapy + tamoxifen	16	12.0
Total	133	100.0

WLE, wide local excision.

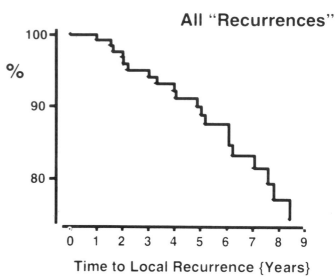

FIGURE 30.1. Actuarial plot of all local recurrences. Y axis represents recurrence free percentage.

sion. Following review of original mammograms, specimen x-ray films, and pathology specimens, two groups of patients were identified. The first group was defined as patients with confirmation of clear margins based on pathologic assessment and specimen x-rays (≥ 1 mm of normal tissue around all lateral margins). The second group consisted of patients with close or uncertain margins. This later group of patients generally had calcification present in more than one portion of breast tissue removed during surgery; it was therefore difficult to ascertain that all lateral margins were clear of disease by at least 1 mm. Specimen radiography of these margins revealed evidence of calcification very close to at least one apparent lateral margin. The majority of patients with uncertain margins had DCIS lesions extending over 4 cm (as measured by the pathologist).

Of the 133 patients, 117 were considered to have clear margins, and 16 had uncertain or close margins. The type of recurrence compared with margin status is shown in Table 30.3.

The actuarial time to local recurrence for patients with clear or uncertain margins is shown in Figure 30.3. Patients with clear margins showed a significantly lower rate of local recurrence ($p = 0.045$). When second primaries were excluded, the curves were not significantly altered (Fig. 30.4), and the difference between the two curves remained significant ($p = 0.04$).

Treatment

Because of small numbers in each group, patients with a wide local excision alone were compared with those receiving any adjuvant treatment. The actuarial recurrence rate for these two groups is shown in Figure 30.5. The difference between the two curves did not quite reach statistical significance ($p = 0.07$).

As noted above, in the group of 38 patients who received radiotherapy, either alone or with tamoxifen, no true inva-

TABLE 30.2. RECURRENCE VERSUS ADJUVANT THERAPY

Treatment	Number	Recurrence	Invasive	In Situ	Residual	2nd Primaries
Nil	67	12	5	4	3	0
Tamoxifen	28	4	2	1	0	1
Radiotherapy	22	2	0	0	1	1
Radiotherapy + tamoxifen	16	2	0	0	1	1
Total	133	20	7	5	5	3

TABLE 30.3. RECURRENCE VERSUS MARGINS

Margins	Number	True Recurrence	Residual	2nd Primaries
Indeterminate	16	6	3	0
Clear	117	6	2	3

Time to Local Recurrence: <=50 years vs >50 years

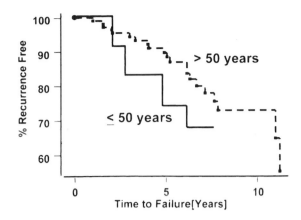

FIGURE 30.2. Local recurrence related to age.

sive recurrences and no in situ recurrences were found. The only ipsilateral breast tumor recurrences suffered by these patients related either to residual disease or development of a second primary.

Grade

There were 85 high-grade lesions and 48 intermediate or low-grade lesions (Table 30.4). All three second primaries occurred in non–high-grade lesions. Plotting the time to recurrence for high-grade and non–high-grade lesions showed that high-grade lesions had a significantly higher rate of recurrence, $p = 0.03$ (Fig. 30.6). Although the curves appear to come together later, there are smaller numbers of women at risk at later time points. However, it does appear that non–high-grade lesions still recur, although the time span over which recurrence develops may be longer than that seen in high-grade lesions.

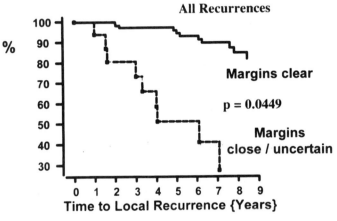

FIGURE 30.3. Local recurrences actuarial plot subdividing patients on the basis of margin status. Y axis is recurrence free %.

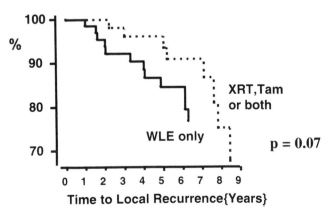

FIGURE 30.5. Local recurrence rate subdivided by adjuvant treatment received. Y axis is recurrence free %.

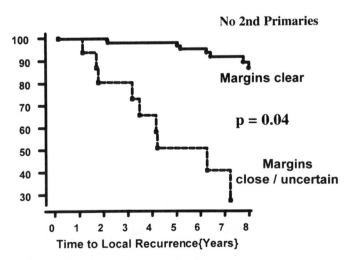

FIGURE 30.4. Recurrence rate (excluding second primary cancers) in patients with clear or close/uncertain margins. Y axis is recurrence free %.

TABLE 30.4. RECURRENCE VERSUS GRADE

Grade	Number	True Recurrence	Residual	2nd Primaries
High	85	8	2	0
Other	48	4	3	3

Size

Forty-five lesions were less than 15 mm, and 88 measured 15 mm or more. Twenty-five patients had lesions over 40 mm in size. Table 30.5 shows the relationship of type of recurrence to size. There were only two true recurrences in lesions measuring less than or equal to 15 mm, compared with 10 true recurrences in lesions greater than or equal to 15 mm. When analyzed actuarially this difference was significant, $p = 0.049$.

SUMMARY OF FINDINGS

Age is important: there was a greater rate of local recurrence in younger women. Margin size was the major predictor of residual disease and recurrence, but grade and size were also related to recurrence in this study. Following adequate wide local excision, radiotherapy seems to reduce true recurrence. Not all disease diagnosed in a treated breast following surgery for DCIS is actually recurrence; some so-called recurrence represents residual disease.

DISCUSSION

The results of the Edinburgh series are disappointing, because 20% of patients developed local recurrence over the 7- to 8-year period following treatment. There are explanations for this, however. During the early part of the U.K. breast screening program, the majority of DCIS cases detected were large and high grade. This is reflected by the fact that in the current Edinburgh series, two-thirds of lesions are over 15 mm in size, and 25 of the 133 cases of DCIS measure over 4 cm. It is evident that these larger lesions are best treated by mastectomy, because this group has high rates of incomplete excision and local recurrence (1,2).

Younger women in the Edinburgh series had a higher rate of local recurrence, although this did not quite reach statistical significance due to the small number of subjects. This is consistent with the findings of other groups (3), and supports the inclusion of age as an important determinant of treatment and outcome.

Margin status was the major factor associated with recurrence. Our study supports others' findings on the importance of complete excision with this disease (4,5). A

DCIS: Local Recurrence vs Grade

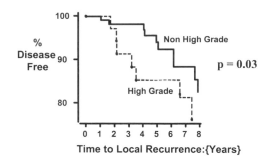

FIGURE 30.6. Local recurrence rates in high-grade or non–high-grade lesions.

number of patients in the Edinburgh series had margins that, on review, were classified as uncertain or close. These were mainly in women with large DCIS lesions wherein the calcification was often removed in more than one piece. Removal of DCIS in multiple pieces makes assessment of excision completeness difficult. All patients in the Edinburgh series had only a single wire inserted in the breast, and the calcification was not always well localized by the radiologist. The use of digital mammography and multiple wires has improved our ability to excise microcalcification in a single piece of tissue. Following single wire placement, a number of women with DCIS lesions over 4 cm did have complete wide excision alone (leaving margins clear of disease), and these women remain disease-free eight years or more. Although it is possible to excise even large DCIS lesions by breast-conserving surgery, it is necessary to balance an excision of adequate size to maintain local control with a smaller excision that limits cosmetic deformity. Although there is some evidence that performing a wide excision with a 1 cm margin might limit local recurrence rate, such excisions certainly have an impact on cosmesis (6). Doubt also remains about the need for such wide lateral margins; because some suggest that 1 mm (not 1 cm) is the critical point below which local recurrence increases (2). Data from the Edinburgh series support complete excision with clear margins rather than very wide excision.

With regard to grade of DCIS, two-thirds of patients treated in the Edinburgh series were high grade. When one

TABLE 30.5. RECURRENCE VS TUMOR SIZE

Size	Number	True Recurrence	Residual	2nd Primaries
<15 mm	45	2	1	0
≥15 mm	88	10	4	3

also considers that some patients who had high-grade lesions also had large lesions with doubtful or close margins, it is evident that a number of women in the Edinburgh series would have had Van Nuys scores of eight or nine (1). This almost certainly explains the high recurrence rate observed in this series. A greater recurrence rate in high-grade DCIS is consistent with the observation of a number of studies in the literature (1,4,7). Low- or intermediate-grade DCIS lesions are being diagnosed with increasing frequency. Whether there are differences in behavior between groups of non–high-grade lesions, and whether they are best classified on the basis of nuclear grade or on the presence or absence of necrosis requires further study (1).

Extent of DCIS within the breast as measured by the pathologist was found to be related to local recurrence. A major reason for this was that almost one-third of patients with a lesion over 4 cm developed local recurrence. There were only two recurrences in patients with lesions measuring less than 15 mm. In Edinburgh, extensive lesions are now treated by mastectomy, and there should therefore be a reduction in the recurrence rate following breast-conserving treatment of DCIS.

Ipsilateral breast tumor recurrence after surgery for DCIS includes at least three separate categories; residual DCIS, true local recurrence, and second primaries. These are not greatly different from the patient's perspective, but each treatment modality is likely to impact the various types of recurrence differently. For instance, wide excision alone will not stop a second breast primary. In contrast, tamoxifen and radiotherapy would be expected to influence the frequency of second breast primaries. Because of the small numbers of patients in different groups in this study from Edinburgh, it is difficult to make a comment about the effectiveness of various treatments on different types of recurrence. It is interesting that there were no true invasive or in situ recurrences in patients who received postoperative radiotherapy. Both the NSABP B-17 and the EORTC trials have shown a significant reduction in breast recurrence following radiotherapy (8,9). The value of radiotherapy has also been confirmed by the U.K. DCIS study. Following presentation and publication of these studies, it has become routine practice in Edinburgh to give radiotherapy to the majority of patients after wide local excision for DCIS. The exceptions are patients who are either unfit for radiotherapy or where the DCIS measures less than 15 mm

and is of low or intermediate grade. This treatment plan is supported by the results of both the EORTC and U.K. studies, which suggest a lesser effect of radiotherapy in reducing the recurrence rate of low-grade and some intermediate-grade lesions.

Even in the small series of patients treated in Edinburgh, the importance of patient age, margins, grade, and size of DCIS have been confirmed. The results indicate that factors besides margin status are important in relation to DCIS recurrence, and we continue to use these other factors to plan treatment. The Edinburgh data support the continued use of a prognostic index such as that proposed by the USC/Van Nuys group to incorporate all factors rather than basing management on distance to nearest margin alone (1).

REFERENCES

1. Silverstein MD, Lagios MD, Craig PH, et al. A prognostic index for ductal carcinoma in situ of the breast. *Cancer* 1996;77:2267–2274.
2. Holland R, Hendriks JHCL, Verbeek ALM, et al. Extent, distribution, and mammographic/histological correlation of breast ductal carcinoma in situ. *Lancet* 1990;335:519–522.
3. Vicini FA, Kestin LL, Goldstein NS, et al. Impact of young age on outcome in patients with ductal carcinoma in situ treated with breast-conserving therapy. *J Clin Oncol* 2000;18:296–306.
4. Silverstein MJ, Lagios MD, Groshen S, et al. The influence of margin width on local control of ductal carcinoma in situ of the breast. *N Engl J Med* 1999;340:1455–1461.
5. Chan KC, Knox WF, Sinha G, et al. Extent of excision margin width required in breast conserving surgery for ductal carcinoma in situ. *Cancer* 2001;91:9–16.
6. Al-Ghazal SK, Blamey RW. Cosmetic assessment of breast-conserving surgery for primary breast cancer. *The Breast* 1999;8:162–168.
7. Lagios MD, Westdahl PR, Margolin FR, et al. Duct carcinoma in situ: relationship of extent of noninvasive disease to the frequency of occult invasion, multicentricity, lymph node metastases and short-term treatment failures. *Cancer* 1982;50:1309–1314.
8. Fisher ER, Dignam J, Tan-Chiu E, et al for the National Surgical Adjuvant Breast & Bowel Project (NSABP) Collaborating Investigators. Pathologic findings from the national surgical adjuvant breast project (NSABP) eight year update of protocol B-17. *Cancer* 1999;86:429–438.
9. Julien JP, Bijker N, Fentiman IS, et al on behalf of the EORTC Breast Cancer Cooperative Group and EORT Radiotherapy Group. Radiotherapy in breast conserving treatment for ductal carcinoma in situ: first results of the EORTC randomised phase III trial 10853. *Lancet* 2000;355:528–533.

31

THE FLORENCE EXPERIENCE

LUIGI CATALIOTTI
VITO DISTANTE
LORENZO ORZALESI
SIMONETTA BIANCHI
STEFANO CIATTO
ROBERTA SIMONCINI
CALOGERO SAIEVA

The incidence of ductal carcinoma in situ (DCIS) is increasing due to the increase in mammographic screening programs (1,2). Before the advent of mammography, very few breast tumors were diagnosed as DCIS (3,4), and most patients presented with palpable masses or nipple discharge. In more recent studies, the proportion of DCIS found among all cancers ranges from 10% to 40% (5,6), with the majority of cases being found only through mammography.

Although mastectomy has been the "standard" DCIS treatment for many years, the current trend is toward treating patients with breast-preserving surgery with or without radiotherapy. Although available data suggest that conservative surgery plus radiotherapy is a reliable method of treatment for many patients (7,8), uncertainties remain about the most appropriate treatment, and numerous studies of it are ongoing (9–12).

In this chapter, we review our experience with DCIS over the last 25 years. New technologies have become available, and our knowledge of the natural history and classification of the disease have progressively improved. We believe such advances justify the changes in therapeutic policies made over time, but they also make it difficult to evaluate the impact of any single factor on patient outcome.

PATIENTS AND METHODS

From March 1975 to December 2000, 380 consecutive cases of DCIS were referred to and treated at the Departments of Surgery and Radiotherapy of the University and General Hospital of Florence. The patients ranged in age from 28 to 83 years old (mean and median age, 56 years). Synchronous bilateral breast cancer was present in 17 patients (bilateral DCIS in two patients, and invasive carcinoma and DCIS in 15 patients). Five patients had been previously treated for a contralateral breast cancer (four

invasive, one DCIS). Twelve patients developed a subsequent contralateral invasive breast cancer.

For the total series of 380 cases, clinical examination was negative in 202 cases (53%), and findings were present but considered benign in 29 cases (8%). Physical findings were considered "suspicious" in 63 cases (17%) and "positive" (unequivocally demonstrating malignancy) in 86 cases (23%). The sensitivity of clinical examination was therefore 0.39. The proportion of nonpalpable cases has increased over time, and was 79% during the last 3 years of the study period.

Mammography was performed in 378 of the 380 cases. Microcalcifications, with or without a concomitant mass, were present in 250 cases (76%). (Microcalcification without a mass was present in 67% of cases.) A mass without microcalcifications was detected in 61 cases (19%) and parenchymal distortion was found in seven cases (2%). Suspicious galactography was found in 10 patients (3%). Overall, mammography was negative in 34 cases (9%), benign in 11 (3%), suspicious in 34 (9%), positive in 283 (75%), and not interpretable in 16 (4%). The sensitivity of mammography was therefore 0.87, and that of clinical examination plus mammography was 0.96.

Fine-needle aspiration (FNA) was performed in 280 cases. The results were clearly malignant in 155 (55%), suspicious in 44 (16%), benign in 41 (15%), and in inadequate due to hypocellularity in 40 cases (14%). The sensitivity of fine-needle cytology was therefore 0.71, and that of clinical examination plus mammography plus cytology was 0.98.

Microscopic slides of 326 cases were reviewed. Subtypes were classified according to the predominant pattern. With regard to architecture, the distribution of cases was: 133 comedo (41%), 54 solid (16.6%), 83 cribriform (25%); 44 micropapillary (13%), 8 papillary (2.4%), and 4 clinging (1%). Nuclear grade was grade I in 91 cases (30%), grade II

TABLE 31.1. DISTRIBUTION OF CASES AND TYPE OF TREATMENT BY DATES OF ACCRUAL

Dates	Number of Cases	Conservative Surgery	Axillary Dissection	RT Given after Conservative Surgery
1975–1979	41	12%	80%	20%
1980–1984	50	40%	68%	20%
1985–1989	61	69%	54%	48%
1990–1995	166	73%	23%	47%
1996–2000	62	74%	16%	76%

RT, radiotherapy.

in 100 cases (33%), grade III in 108 cases (36%), and not recorded in 81 cases. The incidence of grade III tumors by histologic subtypes was 73 of 133 comedo (54.8%), 13 of 54 solid (24%), six of 83 cribriform (7.2%), nine of 43 micropapillary (20.9%), four of eight papillary (50%), and three of four clinging (75%).

Pathologic margin status was assessed in 198 out of 234 conservative surgery cases. The final margins were positive in 18 patients (9%). Multifocality was present in 76 of 350 evaluated patients (22%), and multicentricity in 41 out of 146 evaluated patients (28%).

Of the 380 cases, 146 (38%) were treated with various types of mastectomy (70 cases modified radical mastectomy, 25 radical mastectomy, 51 simple mastectomy), and 234 (62%) with breast preservation (119 with excision plus radiation therapy; 111 with excision only; and 4 with excision but whether postoperative radiation therapy was used is unknown). One hundred thirty-nine patients (37%) underwent axillary dissection. Radiation therapy consisted of a dose to the entire breast of 50 gray (Gy) delivered through tangential fields using a cobalt unit or a linear accelerator. In most cases, a 10-Gy boost dose to the surgical bed was also given, using an electron beam. Eighteen patients with microscopically positive specimen margins received a boost dose of 14 to 16 Gy. Surgical treatment and radiotherapy varied over time (Table 31.1).

The results were analyzed according to the type of surgical procedure and the use of radiotherapy. Analysis with regard to recurrence and survival was restricted to 332 patients treated before the end of 1998. All patients with a previous or synchronous contralateral cancer and four patients with no information about radiotherapy were also excluded. The mean follow-up time was shorter in the conservatively treated group (mean follow-up, 8.5 years; median, 7.6 years; range, 0.3 to 22.9 years) than in the mastectomy group (mean follow-up, 11.4 years; median, 12 years; range, 0.8 to 22.9 years). Overall and disease-free survival (DFS) rates were calculated using the Kaplan-Meier method. The statistical significance of differences was analyzed by means of the log-rank test (13). Multivariate analysis was performed using a Cox regression model.

RESULTS

Five of 130 patients (4%) treated with mastectomy developed chest wall recurrences (1 in situ, 4 invasive) at 15, 56, 91, 126, and 176 months after surgery, and one patient developed an axillary recurrence. In the conservatively treated group of 202 patients, 27 breast recurrences (13%) were detected: 7 recurrences (all invasive) in 97 patients treated by excision plus radiation therapy (7%), and 20 recurrences (11 invasive) in 105 patients treated by excision only (19%). Overall, a total of 23 of 33 (70%) local-regional recurrences were invasive. The mean and median times to relapse were 7.3 and 6.4 years in the irradiated patients, and 7.8 and 6.6 years in the patients treated by excision alone. There were two breast recurrences (both invasive) among the 12 patients with positive specimen margins.

Overall survival rates, including deaths due to all causes, were 97.5% at 5 years and 92% at 10 years for all patients. The respective five and ten-year rates for the conservatively treated patients were 97% and 94.0%, and for the mastectomy patients 98% and 90.5% ($p = 0.35$). Freedom from local recurrence is listed in Table 31.2. Conservatively treated patients who received radiation therapy recurred at a lower rate (11% at 10 years) than patients treated with excision alone (22%). The difference was statistically significant ($p = 0.03$).

The results of univariate and multivariate analysis for the impact of different prognostic factors on the risk of local recurrence in the conservatively treated group are shown in Table 31.3.

TABLE 31.2. ACTUARIAL FREEDOM FROM LOCAL RELAPSE BY TREATMENT

Treatment	No. Patients	5 Years	10 Years	p
Mastectomy	130	98%	96%	—
Excision + RT	97	94%	89%	0.0001
Excision alone	105	87%	78%	—

RT, radiotherapy.

TABLE 31.3. CONSERVATIVE TREATMENT: UNIVARIATE ANALYSIS OF 10-YEAR LOCAL RECURRENCE RATES AND MULTIVARIATE HAZARD RATIOS

Characteristic	No. Patients	Relapse	10-Yr Rate	Univariate p	HR (95% CI)
Age (years)					
≤50	67	7	0.13	0.40	1.0
>50	135	19	0.19	—	1.5 (0.5–5.0)
Grade					
I	56	5	0.14	0.80	1.0
II	56	4	0.08	—	1.0 (0.3–3.7)
III	60	7	0.15	—	0.8 (0.2–2.8)
Grade					
I + II	112	9	0.12	0.60	1.0
III	60	7	0.15	—	0.8 (0.2–2.8)
Microcalcifications					
No	62	9	0.18	0.60	1.0
Yes	140	17	0.17	—	0.9 (0.2–3.6)
Multifocal					
No	153	19	0.17	0.5	1
Yes	37	7	0.22	—	2.2 (0.7–6.6)
Margins					
Negative	157	24	0.18	0.9	1
Positive	12	2	0.55	—	1.0 (0.1–7.7)
Histology					
Others	115	10	0.12	0.3	1
Comedo	72	10	0.20	—	2.8 (0.6–13.2)
Size (mm)					
<10	29	2	0.07	—	1
10–19	91	13	0.19	0.6	2.6 (0.3–22.0)
20–29	49	7	0.18	—	4.2 (0.5–37.3)
>29	23	4	0.28	—	5.5 (0.5–63.0)
Radiotherapy					
No	105	19	0.22	0.03	1
Yes	97	7	0.11	—	0.4 (0.1–1.3)
Total	202	26	0.17	—	—

HR, hazard ratio; CI, confidence interval.
Note: Patients with missing information for a particular variable excluded.

DISCUSSION AND RECOMMENDATIONS

Mammography is undoubtedly the most important test for detecting DCIS, as 75% of cases present with nonpalpable microcalcifications. Masses and parenchymal distortion are less frequent presentations. The accuracy of mammography in defining the extent of the lesion is improved by using magnification views, which we obtain in all cases. The radiologist should indicate the exact site of the suspected lesion in both the craniocaudal and mediolateral mammographic projections, and comment on the presence of multifocality and multicentricity. Sonography can visualize microcalcification in only a small proportion of cases (14,15), and is therefore a poor screening tool for detecting DCIS. Rarely, lesions present with a bloody nipple discharge with or without suspicious cytology. In these cases, galactography can indicate the exact site of the lesion and is helpful in planning the surgical approach.

Fine-needle aspiration cytology is less sensitive for diagnosing DCIS compared with its sensitivity for diagnosing invasive carcinoma, because in situ lesions sometimes have a lesser degree of cytologic atypia. They are also less likely to form discrete lesions, which are easier to sample (15). When the cytology reading shows DCIS, core biopsy or open surgical biopsy is still needed to definitively distinguish between an in situ or invasive lesion. However, when a malignant cytology is present, the positive predictive value for cancer is 97% (16). Definitive surgical treatment of the breast can then proceed based on the cytology results. When cytology is inadequate, benign, atypical, suspicious, or not available, core biopsy or open surgical biopsy is necessary to confirm cancer.

Although aspiration cytology is usually accurate, it is rapidly being replaced by percutaneous core biopsy. When microcalcifications are present at mammography, percutaneous core biopsy allows preoperative diagnosis and subtyping of DCIS. Biological characterization of the lesion can be performed on the tissue sampled. The rate of inadequate specimens on core biopsy is low. Recent reports have shown a high degree of concordance between the results of the core biopsy specimens and the final histopathologic diagnosis in cases of DCIS.

The diagnostic accuracy of the 11-gauge vacuum-assisted device is better than that of the 14-gauge automated gun, probably due to the greater volume of tissue obtained. Burbank reported that invasive tumor was found at subsequent excision in 9 of 55 cases (16%) of DCIS performed with the automated biopsy device; although none of the 32 cases of DCIS diagnosed with the directional, vacuum-assisted device were found to have invasion at definitive surgery (17). Similarly, Lee et al. (18) reported the risk of having invasive disease at final biopsy with the two methods to be 44% and 18%, respectively.

Accurate localization methods are essential for performing breast-preserving treatment of nonpalpable DCIS. Such techniques must allow the lesion to be completely excised with a minimum of distortion to the breast. We have used a number of different localization methods. Hooked wires were used extensively in the past. The disadvantage of this method is that the procedure must be carried out shortly before surgery, which requires accurate planning. The hooked wire may move away from its original position; in our experience, this happens more frequently in fatty breasts.

Currently, our preferred method is to inject a sterile charcoal suspension at the same time that fine-needle aspiration cytology or core biopsy is performed. Surgery can be performed many days after the injection, if necessary. The use of the charcoal dye method requires close cooperation between the radiologist and the surgeon.

Lately we have been using a new localization method employing technetium-99m labeled colloid albumin (19). This is particularly useful for cases with clustered microcalcification, parenchymal distortion, or a single density. The radioactive tracer is injected into the center of the lesion the day before surgery under stereotactic mammographic or ultrasound guidance. At surgery, the lesion is localized by means of a γ-detecting probe. This is a very accurate method that allows a targeted excision of the tumor. After excision, the surgeon ensures that residual areas of radioactivity are not present in the resection bed.

Open surgical biopsy is rarely used to obtain the initial diagnosis, because we attempt to obtain a preoperative cytologic or core biopsy diagnosis. When performed, the biopsy incision is chosen with regard to the degree of clinical suspicion and the localization method used. The incision is usually placed directly over the lesion. We think that as little tissue as possible should be removed to allow a diagnosis to be made. Our quality control guidelines recommend that 80% of biopsies for lesions that ultimately prove to be benign should weigh less than 30 grams.

However the lesion is localized, it is extremely important to x-ray the specimen. For orientation, we strongly recommend using clips on the specimen. Orthogonal x-ray films should be obtained when the excision does not include the whole thickness of the parenchyma (from skin to fascia.)

Even if the lesion appears widely excised, the possibility of multifocality or multicentricity cannot be excluded by specimen radiography. Microscopic evidence of DCIS extending beyond the mammographic abnormality has been demonstrated by Holland et al. (20) in a substantial number of DCIS cases. This finding is more frequent with well-differentiated, noncomedo-type DCIS than with high-grade comedo-type DCIS. The characteristics of the mammographic microcalcifications suggest the subtype of DCIS likely to be found, and may help to select cases at low risk of having DCIS extending beyond the radiographically abnormal area. However, although there is a significant association of the mammographic calcification pattern with the DCIS subtype, this correlation is not sufficiently reliable for use in clinical decision making (21,22).

In most patients, the characteristics of the DCIS and the patient's wishes are the deciding factors in the choice of therapy. Mastectomy has the lowest rate of local recurrence, but may be an overtreatment in as many as 80% of patients diagnosed by current methods. However, certain special situations warrant attention. Bilateral presentation clearly influences the choice of therapy. A bilateral skin-sparing mastectomy is very often a good solution. There are numerous alternatives for patients with metachronous cancers. Those previously treated with mastectomy can undergo a new mastectomy with bilateral reconstruction. Patients previously treated with conservative surgery can undergo either new conservative surgery or bilateral mastectomy and reconstruction. After full discussion and obtaining informed consent, we suggest bilateral skin-sparing mastectomy for young patients with dense mammograms who present with unilateral DCIS and a strong family history of breast cancer.

Our general policy is to perform skin-sparing mastectomy when the tumor is multicentric, quadrantectomy when it is multifocal, and wide excision if it is unifocal. Plastic remodeling of the breast sometimes allows conservative surgery to be performed with good cosmetic results in women with larger breasts, even when extensive lesions are present. The good results achieved with skin-sparing mastectomy suggest it should be used more frequently for patients when performing adequate conservative surgery is not compatible with good cosmetic results.

Our series (Table 31.1) confirms the trend toward performing conservative surgery rather than mastectomy that has also been reported by others (1,6,7). During the last ten years, the proportion of patients treated with conservative treatment has not increased, probably because the use of mammographic screening reached a plateau. Following the recommendations of Silverstein et al. (23), we try to obtain clear margins of 1 to 1.5 cm in all directions around the lesion. We are convinced that performing the excision correctly at the time of the first surgery, with the tumor located at the center of the specimen with as uniform a margin as possible, is extremely important (11,24). Performing a re-operation due to initially positive margins usually decreases the chance of achieving a good cosmetic result.

Radial incisions are recommended in the presence of multifocal microcalcifications when it is important to excise the entire ductal tree, including the retroareolar region. In this case, the removal of a skin island can be useful both for cosmetic reasons and for orientation of the pathologic examination. Additionally, this guarantees that the anterior margins will be clear. Curvilinear incisions give better cosmetic results and are generally used for smaller, focal lesions that do not require wide radial parenchymal excision. The periareolar incision has the best cosmetic results and is the best approach when the lesion is at, or near, the retroareolar region.

Following the directives of the European Guidelines for Quality Assurance in Mammography Screening (25), we do not currently perform a frozen section examination if microcalcifications are present. (We previously performed frozen section examinations in the presence of microcalcifications only when the lesion was evident on a gross inspection of the surgical specimen (26,27).)

Reoperation may be necessary after incomplete wide excision. Such surgery was performed in 15% of our cases. The indications for re-excision or mastectomy are the extent of tumor in the surgical specimen and the involvement of the margins. A "negative" margin is defined as a margin with no tumor extending to it. Re-excision is performed in all cases where the margin is focally involved (28). Mastectomy is performed in the presence of multifocality with involvement of more than one margin. Reoperation is usually performed a few days after the definitive pathology report is available. In cases when re-excision still shows involved margins, mastectomy is suggested.

We do not perform mammography immediately after surgery (to find residual microcalcifications) if the intraoperative specimen radiography confirms the complete excision of the microcalcifications with a good margin. Using this technique, we have found only one case of residual microcalcifications at first mammography one year after operation.

After conservative surgery, we generally suggest radiotherapy in accordance with results of published clinical trials (7,8). The use of radiotherapy has significantly increased in the last 5 years. Overall survival is not affected by the addition of radiotherapy, but its use substantially reduces the risk of local recurrence at 10 years (hazard ratio, 0.40). More than half these recurrence (67%) were invasive (7,34,35). The exact time-course of local failure in patients treated conservatively is not well established, but in most studies conservatively treated patients who do not receive radiation therapy recur earlier than those treated with breast irradiation. However, in our experience, no such difference was found.

The risk factors increasing the likelihood of local recurrence are not completely known (6,36,37). The only statistically significant factor for local recurrence in our data was the use of radiotherapy. This treatment seemed more effective in reducing the risk of in situ recurrences than invasive recurrences. Prognostic factors such as tumor size and comedo subtype also appeared to influence the risk of local recurrence, although they did not reach statistical significance in the multivariate analysis.

Radiotherapy definitively reduces the risk of intramammary relapses after conservative surgery. However, there are probably groups of patients for whom radiotherapy can be avoided (23,29–32,38). We recommend excision without radiotherapy for patients older than 60 years with small, well-differentiated tumors as defined by the EORTC classification (38) with a margin width greater than 1 cm. The decision to omit radiotherapy is based on the patient's choice rather than standard practice (11).

Axillary dissection is useless for DCIS, does not contribute to either the diagnosis or treatment, and should not be performed. Nevertheless, a certain percentage of patients (16%) underwent axillary dissection in the last 5 years. This is because some surgeons in our group prefer to perform axillary dissection at the same time as mastectomy for patients with a large DCIS, due to the possibility that an unsuspected invasive cancer might be found that would later require reoperation. This consideration is especially important when immediate reconstruction is performed.

Recently, based on the results of the NSABP B-24 trial (33), we have advised patients with positive hormonal receptors to take tamoxifen when risk factors such as young age and a positive family history are present.

Local recurrence may appear in the same quadrant as the first tumor or in a different quadrant, and may be in situ or invasive. For local recurrence after conservative treatment, we usually perform mastectomy. Salvage mastectomy for recurrent DCIS generally results in a cure rate of nearly 100%. However, salvage surgery for recurrent invasive tumors may be less effective. When recurrence is in the same quadrant as the first tumor and no radiotherapy has been performed, we perform further conservative surgery, if cosmetically acceptable, followed by radiotherapy, regardless of the histology of the recurrence. In cases of invasive recurrence, axillary dissection is always performed.

REFERENCES

1. Van Dongen JA, Holland R, Peterse JL, et al. Ductal carcinoma in situ of the breast; second EORTC consensus meeting. *Eur J Cancer* 1992;28:626–629.
2. Ernster VL, Barclay J, Kerlikowske K, et al. Incidence of and treatment for ductal carcinoma in situ of the breast. *JAMA* 1996; 275:913–918.
3. Rosner D, Bedwani RN, Vana J, et al. Noninvasive breast carcinoma: results of a national survey by the American College of Surgeons. *Ann Surg* 1980;192:139–147.

4. Lagios MD, Westdahl PR, Margolin FR, et al. Ductal carcinoma in situ: relationship of extent of noninvasive disease to the frequency of occult invasion, multicentricity, lymph-node metastases, and short-term treatment failures. *Cancer* 1982;50:1309–1314.

5. Silverstein MJ, Barth A, Poller DM, et al. Ten-year results comparing mastectomy to excision and radiation therapy for ductal carcinoma in situ of the breast. *Eur J Cancer* 1995;31A:1425–1427.

6. Carty NJ, Royle GT, Carter C, et al. Management of ductal carcinoma in situ of the breast. *Ann R Coll Surg Engl* 1995;77:163–167.

7. Fisher B, Dignam J, Wolmark N, et al. Lumpectomy and radiation therapy: findings from National Surgical Adjuvant Breast and Bowel Project B-17. *J Clin Oncol* 1998;16:441–452.

8. Julien JP, Bijker N, Fentiman IS, et al. Radiotherapy in breast-conserving treatment for ductal carcinoma in situ: first results of the EORTC randomised phase III trial 10853. *Lancet* 2000;355:528–533.

9. Goldhirsch A, Wood WC, Senn HJ, et al. International consensus panel on the treatment of primary breast cancer. *Eur J Cancer* 1995;31A:1754–1759.

10. Hetelekidis S, Schnitt SJ, Morrow M, et al. Management of ductal carcinoma in situ. *Cancer J for Clinicians* 1995;45:244–253.

11. Fisher ER, Dignam J, Tan-Chiu E, et al. Pathologic Findings from the National Surgical Adjuvant Breast Project (NSABP) Eight-year update of Protocol B-17 Intraductal Carcinoma. *Cancer* 1999;86:429–438.

12. Vicini FA, Goldstein NS, Kestin LL. Pathologic and technical considerations in the treatment of ductal carcinoma in situ of the breast with lumpectomy and radiation therapy. *Ann Oncol* 1999;10:883–890.

13. Kaplan EL, Meier P. Nonparametric estimation from incomplete observations. *J Am Stat Assoc* 1958;135:185–198.

14. Ciatto S, Catarzi S, Morrone D, et al. Fine-needle aspiration cytology of nonpalpable breast lesions: US versus stereotactic guidance. *Radiology* 1993;188:195–198.

15. Schwartz GF, Solin LJ, Olivotto IA, et al. Consensus conference on the treatment of in situ ductal carcinoma of the breast, April 22–25, 1999. *Cancer* 2000;88:945–954.

16. Ciatto S, Rosselli Del Turco M, Ambrogetti D, et al. Solid nonpalpable breast lesions. Success and failure of guided fine-needle aspiration cytology in a consecutive series of 2,444 cases. *Acta Radiol* 1997;38:815–820.

17. Burbank F. Stereotactic breast biopsy of atypical ductal hyperplasia and ductal carcinoma in situ lesions: improved accuracy with directional, vacuum-assisted biopsy. *Radiology* 1997;202:843–847.

18. Lee CL, Carter D, Philpotts LE, et al. Ductal carcinoma in situ diagnosed with stereotactic core needle biopsy: can invasion be predicted? *Radiology* 2000;217:466–470.

19. Gennari R, Galimberti V, De Cicco C, et al. Use of technetium-99m–labeled colloid albumin for preoperative and intraoperative localization of nonpalpable breast lesions. *J Am Coll Surg* 2000;10:692–698.

20. Holland R, Hendricks JHCL, Verbeek ALM, et al. Extent, distribution, and mammographic/histological correlations of breast ductal carcinoma in situ. *Lancet* 1990;335:519–522.

21. Ciatto S, Bianchi S, Vezzosi V. Mammographic appearance of calcifications as a predictor of intraductal carcinoma histologic subtype. *Eur Radiol* 1994;4:23–26.

22. Dinkel HP, Gassel AM, Tschammler A. Is the appearance of microcalcifications on mammography useful in predicting histological grade of malignancy in ductal cancer in situ? *Br J Radiol* 2000;73:938–944.

23. Silverstein MJ, Lagios MD, Groshen S, et al. The influence of margin width on local control of ductal carcinoma in situ of the breast. *N Engl J Med* 1999;340:1455–1461.

24. Chan KC, Knox WF, Sinha G, et al. Extent of excision margin width required in breast-conserving surgery for ductal carcinoma in situ. *Cancer* 2001;91:9–16.

25. European Commission. European Guidelines for Quality Assurance in Mammography Screening. June, 1996.

26. Bianchi S, Palli D, Ciatto S, et al. Accuracy and reliability of frozen section. Diagnosis in a series of 672 nonpalpable breast lesions. *J Clin Pathol* 1995;103:199–205.

27. Ferreiro JA, Gisvold J, Bostwick DG. Accuracy of frozen-section diagnosis of mammographically directed breast biopsies. Results of 1,490 consecutive cases. *Am J Surg Pathol* 1995;19:1267–1271.

28. Schnitt SJ, Abner A, Gelman R, et al. The relationship between microscopic margins of resection and the risk of local recurrence in patients with breast cancer treated with breast-conserving surgery and radiation therapy. *Cancer* 1994;74:1746–1751.

29. Lagios MD, Page DL. Radiation therapy for in situ or localized breast cancer. *N Engl J Med* 1993;329:1577–1578.

30. Page DL, Lagios MD. Pathologic analysis of the National Surgical Adjuvant Breast Project (NSABP) B-17 trial: unanswered questions remaining unanswered considering current concepts of ductal carcinoma in situ. *Cancer* 1995;75:1219–1222.

31. Morrow M. Understanding ductal carcinoma in situ. A step in the right direction. *Cancer* 1999;86:375–377.

32. Boyages J, Delaney G, Taylor R. Predictors of local recurrence after treatment of ductal carcinoma in situ. A meta-analysis. *Cancer* 1999;85:616–628.

33. Fisher B, Dignam J, Wolmark N, et al. Tamoxifen in treatment of intraductal breast cancer: National Surgical Adjuvant Breast and Bowel Project B-24 randomized controlled trial. *Lancet* 1999;353:1993–2000.

34. Kestin LL, Goldstein NS, Martinez AA, et al. Mammographically detected ductal carcinoma in situ treated with conservative surgery with or without radiation therapy. *Ann Surg* 2000;231:235–245.

35. Warneke J, Grossklaus D, Davis J, et al. Influence of local treatment on the recurrence rate of ductal carcinoma in situ. *J Am Coll Surg* 1995;180:683–688.

36. White J, Levine A, Gustafson G, et al. Outcome and prognostic factors for local recurrence in mammographically detected ductal carcinoma in situ of the breast treated with conservative surgery and radiation therapy. *Int J Radiat Oncol Biol Phys* 1995;31:791–797.

37. Vicini FA, Kestin LL, Goldstein NS, et al. Impact of young age on outcome in patients with ductal carcinoma in situ treated with breast-conserving therapy. *J Clin Oncol* 2000;18:296–306.

38. Holland R, Deterse JL, Millis RR, et al. Ductal carcinoma in situ: a proposal for a new classification. *Semin Diagn Pathol* 1994;11:167–180.

32

BAYREUTH-ERLANGEN EXPERIENCE OF "RISK-ADAPTED" THERAPY OF DUCTAL CARCINOMA IN SITU

AGUSTINUS H. TULUSAN
MICHAEL BUEHNER
NORBERT LANG

Ductal carcinoma in situ (DCIS) is a heterogeneous group of diseases that constitutes approximately 30% of all breast cancers found in populations undergoing regular mammographic screening, as compared with 12.5% from the pre-screening era (1,2). The average size of the DCIS lesion at diagnosis has also decreased. Because breast-conserving therapy (BCT) has become commonly used for patients with invasive breast cancer, it has become increasingly difficult to justify the routine use of mastectomy for DCIS. As a result, the use of mastectomy for DCIS declined by half from 1983 to 1992 (2).

Nonetheless, there are risks associated with BCT. That is, while patients with DCIS have very high rates of breast cancer–specific survival, no matter how they are treated initially, retrospective studies and prospective trials of BCT for DCIS have shown local relapse rates of 6% to 45% (3–13). Approximately 50% of these local failures are invasive.

Because the mortality of patients with DCIS following mastectomy is 0% to 4% (4,8,14–16), the goal of BCT must be to keep local failure rates very low, so as to expose patients to as small a chance of developing invasive breast cancer as is reasonably possible. Recognition of the heterogeneity of DCIS has led to the realization that close cooperation among surgeons, radiologists, pathologists, and radiation oncologists is needed to optimize treatment. Such multispecialist collaboration also opens the possibility of better tailoring therapy to the individual.

There are reasons to believe that some patients may be cured of DCIS by excision without radiotherapy. For example, one series in which patients were followed after biopsy for an initially undiagnosed DCIS showed that only a minority developed a subsequent in situ or invasive breast cancer (17). In a similar study performed in Erlangen, three invasive breast cancers developed in the ipsilateral breast in nine patients with DCIS (all of noncomedo type) who had a breast biopsy in the 1950s for which the pathologic diagnosis had been missed after a follow-up time of 6 to 10 years. However, no cancers developed in those cases where the lesions were small (and therefore presumably excised with clear margins). Conversely, there is no doubt that breast irradiation can lower the local recurrence rate of patients treated with wide local excision when patients are not carefully selected (5,6).

The development of the Bayreuth-Erlangen scheme for tailored treatment (or "risk-adapted therapy") of DCIS was also influenced by pathologic considerations. In the mid-1970s, several reports revealed the terminal duct lobular unit to be the primary location of breast carcinoma development (18–20) and the importance of the ductal system for the subsequent spread of cancer within the breast (15,21). Meticulous serial sectioning in combination with specimen radiography of mastectomy specimens from 343 patients with invasive and 75 patients with in situ cancer in our institution showed DCIS to spread along the radially-branching segments of the ductal system. In 60% of the mastectomy specimens, neither invasive nor in situ cancer was detected outside a simulated segmental resection area. This was especially true for DCIS smaller than 4 cm in size. In particular, fewer than 4% of patients with DCIS smaller than 1 cm had in situ disease located more than 1cm from the location of the primary tumor. Lesions that measured 2.5 to 4 cm or larger commonly had intraductal spread to the adjacent segment of the ductal tree, and sometimes occupied an entire quadrant (defined as "multifocal") or even multiple quadrants of the breast ("multicentric").

STUDY DESIGN

We classified four types of DCIS based on their patterns of spreading: focal (1 cm or less in maximum extent beyond

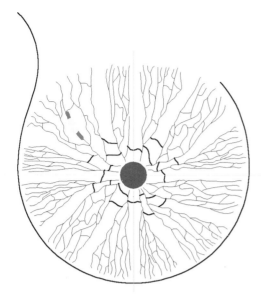

FIGURE 32.1. Focal ductal carcinoma in situ.

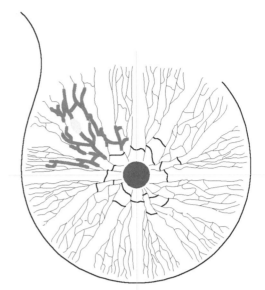

FIGURE 32.3. Multifocal ductal carcinoma in situ.

the apparent primary lesion); segmental (1.1 to 2.5 cm), multifocal (2.6 to 4 cm), and multicentric (> 4 cm) (Figs. 32.1 through 32.4).

Four risk groups (RGs) of patients were then defined based on the pathologic size of the DCIS, extension, and the margin status (Table 32.1). Other factors, such as histologic subtype, grade hormonal receptors, or proliferation rate were not incorporated into the risk group system (non-comedo micropapillary DCIS usually had a greater extent than comedo-type DCIS, perhaps because the latter was diagnosed earlier due to its characteristic microcalcifications). Mammographic and other imaging findings, clinical examination, specimen radiography, and pathologic findings had

to be assessed before definitively categorizing the patients to a particular RG. Complete semiserial histologic giant sections were used in processing the surgical specimen in 90% of the cases so the whole distension of the DCIS could easily be reconstructed (Fig. 32.5).

Patients with RG I and II were considered at "low risk," and patients with RG III and IV at "high risk" for local recurrence after BCT without radiotherapy. Radiation therapy was given only to high-risk patients (dose to the entire breast of 50 gray (Gy), followed by a 10 Gy boost). After informed consent of the study and viewing the results of the surgery pathologic report, mastectomy was also an option for high-risk patients.

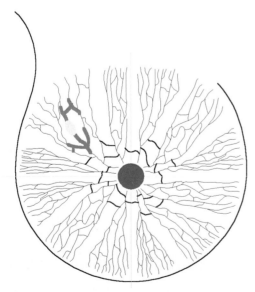

FIGURE 32.2. Segmental ductal carcinoma in situ.

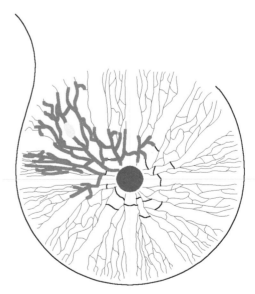

FIGURE 32.4. Multicentric ductal carcinoma in situ.

TABLE 32.1. RISK GROUPS, RECURRENCE RISK, AND TREATMENT OPTIONS

Risk Group	Definition	Risk of Local Recurrence	Treatment
I	<10 mm size, widely clear margins	Low	BCT without irradiation
II	10–25 mm, tumor-free margins	Low	BCT without irradiation
III	>25 mm, multifocal growth, close or uncertain margins	High	BCT with irradiation, or mastectomy
IV	Very extensive disease, multifocal or multicentric growth, involved margins	Very high	Mastectomy

BCT, breast-conserving therapy.

To remove the DCIS within the ductal tree of the involved breast parenchyma, surgery involved a radial segmental resection with simultaneous reconstruction of the defect using a parenchymal flap technique (Fig. 32.6). Other "oncoplastic" surgical techniques, such as the latissimus dorsi myocutaneous flap, were not used. For patients with extensive DCIS, lower axillary dissection or axillary node sampling was performed.

Patients were followed by clinical examination, annual or biannual mammography, and other imaging techniques as necessary. Suspicious findings were confirmed by open or core biopsy.

Patients with recurrence who had not previously undergone radiotherapy were eligible to undergo a second wide local excision followed by radiotherapy. Patients who had already been irradiated usually underwent mastectomy.

POPULATION AND RESULTS

From January 1985 through mid-1996, 118 patients with 122 cases of DCIS (four patients had bilateral disease) were accrued (87 from Erlangen, 31 from Bayreuth). Most patients had their DCIS diagnosed by mammography during an annual medical checkup, not by mammography performed as part of a screening program. The mean patient age was 51.9 years (range 28.2 to 78.0 years). In 19 cases, both DCIS and lobular carcinoma in situ were present.

Compliance with the protocol treatment guidelines was high. Only four patients (3%) were treated in ways that constituted major deviations from the protocol. These patients were not included in the analysis.

Of the eligible patients treated according to the protocol, 27 were in RG I, 44 in RG II, 44 in RG III, and three in RG IV. All patients in RG I and II were treated by segmental resection only; 21 patients in RG III were treated by segmental resection with breast irradiation. Twenty-three of the 44 patients in RG III and all three patients in RG IV decided to be treated with mastectomy. The mean follow-up time was 68 months (range, 12 to 141 months). No patients were lost to follow-up.

The crude local recurrence rate in patients treated with BCT was 8% (seven of 92). Four of these recurrences were DCIS and three were invasive recurrences. All seven recur-

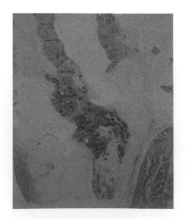

FIGURE 32.5. Histologic giant section.

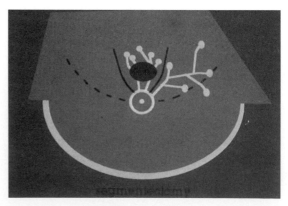

FIGURE 32.6. Segmental resection with reconstruction by parenchymal flap technique.

rences occurred near the vicinity of the primary DCIS. Local recurrence rates correlated closely with risk group (Fig. 32.7). The rate was 0% for RG I (zero of 27), 9% for RG II (four of 44), and 6% (four of 71) when combined. The rate was 14 % for RG III (three of 21, all of whom had radiotherapy in addition to surgery). The median time to local recurrence was 28 months (range, 6 to 60 months) for all patients combined, and it was not different for unirradiated (median 32 months, range 11 to 60 months) and irradiated patients (median 24 months, range 6 to 39 months).

We also retrospectively analyzed our results according to the Van Nuys Prognostic Index (VNPI). Forty-one patients in RG I (27 patients) and RG II (14 patients) were classified as having VNPI grade 3 to 4. None of the patients in this group were irradiated, and their local recurrence rate was 5% (two of 41). A total of 43 cases (30 from RG II and 13 from RG III) were classified as VNPI grade 5 to 7. Of these, the local failure rate was 7% (two of 30) for those patients not irradiated and 8% (one of 13) for those receiving radiotherapy. Finally, 8 patients from RG III were classified as being in VNPI grade 8 to 9; all received radiotherapy, with a local recurrence rate of 25% (two of eight).

Three of the four patients who had not previously been irradiated and two of the three irradiated patients who had a local recurrence were treated with breast-conserving surgery reoperation. The other patients were treated by mastectomy. One patient with an invasive recurrence also developed a stage III ovarian cancer; she died of the breast cancer.

No invasive cancer or positive axillary nodes were found in the 26 patients treated initially by mastectomy. None recurred or died of breast cancer.

DISCUSSION

The heterogeneity of DCIS implies that no single treatment plan can be the optimum for treating all patients. The aim of our prospective study was to confirm the possibility of selecting appropriate therapy for patients with DCIS according to their estimated risk for local recurrence. We were particularly concerned to determine if some patients could be treated without radiotherapy with a low risk of recurrence, and thereby avoid the possible side effects of radiotherapy.

In our study, margin status and the extent of the DCIS were the most important factors predicting for risk of local recurrence. The re-evaluation of our study results according to the VNPI again highlighted the significance of these factors.

Thus, careful assessment of the disease pattern and extent, shaping surgical resection according to the mammography findings and anatomical branching of the ductal tree, routine specimen radiography, and meticulous workup of the pathologic specimen can allow treatment to be tailored to each individual case. This can only be achieved through an interdisciplinary approach. In the future, the role of oncoplastic surgery for the treatment of larger DCIS should be explored, as more tissue can be removed without cosmetic defects. Breast irradiation can be applied for those cases with a high risk of recurrence with surgery alone. However, the high rate of recurrence seen in RG III (or VNPI grade 7 to 9 groups) in our study shows that radiotherapy does not compensate for inadequate surgical excision, as has also been recently pointed out by others (22).

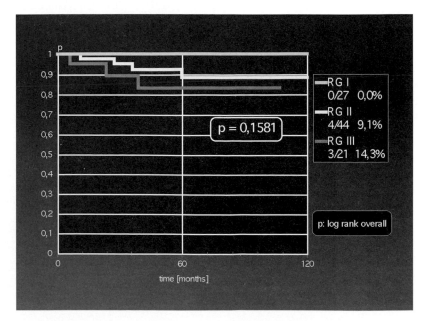

FIGURE 32.7. Kaplan-Meier estimates of local recurrence rates for risk groups *(RG)*.

REFERENCES

1. Ernster VL, Barclay J, Kerlikowske K, et al. Incidence of and treatment for ductal carcinoma in situ of the breast. *JAMA* 1996; 275:913–918.
2. Ernster VL. Epidemiology and natural history of ductal carcinoma in situ. In: Silverstein MJ, ed. *Ductal Carcinoma in Situ of the Breast.* Baltimore: Williams & Wilkins, 1997:23–33.
3. Arnesson LG, Olsen K. Linköping Experience. In: Silverstein MJ, ed. *Ductal Carcinoma in Situ of the Breast.* Baltimore: Williams & Wilkins, 1997:373–377.
4. Fisher ER, Leeming R, Anderson S, et al. Conservative management of intraductal carcinoma (DCIS) of the breast. *J Surg Oncol* 1991;47:139–147.
5. Fisher B, Costantino J, Redmond C, et al. Lumpectomy compared with lumpectomy and radiation therapy for the treatment of intraductal breast cancer.*N Engl J Med* 1993;328:1581–1586.
6. Fisher B, Dignam J, Wolmark N, et al. Lumpectomy and radiation therapy for the treatment of intraductal breast cancer: findings from National Surgical Adjuvant Breast and Bowel Project B-17. *J Clin Oncol* 1998;16:441–452.
7. Fisher B, Dignam J, Wolmark N, et al. Tamoxifen in treatment of intraductal breast cancer: National Surgical Adjuvant Breast and Bowel Project B-24 randomized controlled trial. *Lancet* 1999;353:1993–2000.
8. Fisher ER, Dignam J, Tan-Chiu E, et al. Pathologic findings from the National Surgical Adjuvant Breast Project (NSABP) eight-year update of protocol B-17: intraductal carcinoma. *Cancer* 1999;86:429–438.
9. Lagios MD, Margolin FR, Westdahl PR, et al. Mammographically detected duct carcinoma in situ. Frequency of local recurrence following tylectomy and prognostic effect of nuclear grade on local recurrence. *Cancer* 1989;63:618–624.
10. Lagios MD. Lagios Experience. In: Silverstein MJ, ed. *Ductal Carcinoma in Situ of the Breast.* Baltimore: Williams & Wilkins, 1997:361–365.
11. Schwartz GF, Schwarting R, Cornfield DB, et al. Sub-clinical duct carcinoma in situ of the breast: treatment by local excision and surveillance alone. *Breast J* 1996;2:41–44.
12. Silverstein MJ, Lagios MD, Craig PH, et al. A prognostic index for ductal carcinoma in situ of the breast. *Cancer* 1996;77:2267–2274.
13. Solin LJ, Kurtz J, Fourquet A, et al. Fifteen-year results of breast-conserving surgery and definitive breast irradiation for the treatment of ductal carcinoma in situ of the breast. *J Clin Oncol* 1996; 14:754–763.
14. Bradley SJ, Weaver DW, Bouwman DL. Alternatives in the surgical management of in situ breast cancer. A meta-analysis of outcome. *Am Surg* 1990;56:428–432.
15. Lagios MD, Westdahl PR, Margolin FR, et al. Duct carcinoma in situ. Relationship of extent of noninvasive disease to the frequency of occult invasion, multicentricity, lymph node metastases, and short-term treatment failures. *Cancer* 1982;50:1309–1314.
16. Silverstein MJ, Cohlan BF, Gierson ED, et al. Duct carcinoma in situ: 227 cases without microinvasion. *Eur J Cancer* 1992;28: 630–634.
17. Page DL, Dupont WD, Rogers LW, et al. Intraductal carcinoma of the breast: follow-up after biopsy only. *Cancer* 1982;49:751–758.
18. Gallager HS, Martin JE. Early phases in the development of breast cancer. *Cancer* 1969;24:1170–1178.
19. Wellings SR, Jensen HM. On the origin and progression of ductal carcinoma in the human breast. *J Natl Cancer Inst* 1973;50: 1111–1118.
20. Wellings SR, Jensen HM, Marcum RG. An atlas of subgross pathology of the human breast with special reference to possible precancerous lesions. *J Natl Cancer Inst* 1975;55:231–273.
21. Evans A, Pinder S, Wilson R, et al. Ductal carcinoma in situ of the breast: correlation between mammographic and pathologic findings. *AJR Am J Roentgenol* 1994;162:1307–1311.
22. Chan KC, Knox WF, Sinha G, et al. Extent of excision margin width required in breast-conserving surgery for ductal carcinoma in situ. *Cancer* 2001;91:9–16.

33

AN INTERNATIONAL COLLABORATIVE STUDY: A 15-YEAR EXPERIENCE

LAWRENCE J. SOLIN
FRANK A. VICINI
MARSHA D. MCNEESE
WILLIAM BARRETT
I-TIEN YEH
JOHN KURTZ
IVO OLIVOTTO

BERYL MCCORMICK
BRUCE HAFFTY
ROBERT R. KUSKE, JR.
BARBARA FOWBLE
ABRAM RECHT
JUNG-SOO KIM
JACQUES BORGER

ALAIN FOURQUET
MARIE TAYLOR
LORI PIERCE
BRUCE A. BORNSTEIN
CHRISTINE LANDMANN
ANNE DE LA ROCHEFORDIERE
DELRAY J. SCHULTZ

The growing use of screening mammography has been associated with an increasing detection of ductal carcinoma in situ (DCIS; intraductal carcinoma) of the breast. This increase in detection has led to the awareness of DCIS as an important disease entity, separate and distinct from early-stage, invasive carcinoma of the breast.

By the 1980s, breast-conserving surgery and definitive breast irradiation had been well established as treatment of early-stage, invasive breast carcinoma, with outcomes reported from both prospective, randomized trials and retrospective, single institution studies. Because of the accepted efficacy of breast-conservation treatment for early-stage, invasive breast carcinoma, continuing the use of mastectomy for in situ cancer breast cancer seemed illogical, although the lack of long-term outcome data was well recognized. Based on experience from early-stage, invasive breast carcinoma, breast-conservation treatment was increasingly used for women with DCIS of the breast. By the late 1980s, a number of investigators had reported early results of the outcome of this treatment for DCIS. However, these reports were limited by small numbers of patients and short follow-up.

In an effort to better understand the role of radiation in this disease, a group of institutions collaborated by combining data for patients with DCIS treated with breast-conservation surgery and definitive breast irradiation. The objective of this collaborative effort was to obtain sufficient numbers of patients to be able to determine long-term outcome and to evaluate end points that could not be assessed from smaller studies (e.g., outcome of salvage treatment, risk of development of contralateral breast carcinoma). A number of studies from this collaborative, multi-institutional database have been reported from 1991 through 1996 (1–6), and over time, several other institutions joined the initial group. Most recently, the group members opted to increase the number of patients in the database by extending the defined treatment date cut-off to 1990. In an effort to focus on the type of DCIS most commonly seen in current practice, only cases with mammographic detection were selected for data entry.

MATERIALS AND METHODS: EARLY GROUP

Member institutions in Europe and the United States have combined patient data from women treated with breast-conserving surgery and definitive breast irradiation for DCIS of the breast. To obtain long-term follow-up information for the study, only patients treated from 1967 to 1985 were initially entered into the database. The 10 institutions participating in this first collaboration were:

(i) University Hospital, Basel, Switzerland;
(ii) Institut Curie, Paris, France;
(iii) Cancer Institute, Marseille, France;
(iv) Joint Center for Radiation Therapy, Harvard University, Boston, Massachusetts;
(v) Memorial Sloan-Kettering Cancer Center, New York, New York;
(vi) University of Cincinnati, Cincinnati, Ohio;
(vii) University of Pennsylvania School of Medicine, Philadelphia, Pennsylvania;
(viii) University of Texas M.D. Anderson Cancer Center, Houston, Texas;
(ix) Mallinckrodt Institute of Radiology, St. Louis, Missouri; and
(x) Yale University, New Haven, Connecticut.

Many of the patients included in the present study have been reported in prior studies from one or two institutions (7–18).

All women included in this collaborative database had DCIS of the breast at the time of presentation. Not included were patients with:

(i)   prior or concurrent invasive carcinoma of the breast;
(ii)   microinvasive carcinoma of the breast;
(iii)   Paget's disease of the nipple;
(iv)   intraductal carcinoma of the breast plus associated Paget's disease of the nipple; or
(v)   prior or concurrent malignancy other than breast carcinoma.

The median patient age at presentation was 50 years (mean, 50 years; range, 26 to 82 years).

The analysis of this early collaborative effort reported the data on 268 women with 270 intraductal breast carcinomas (3). Two of the 268 women presented with synchronous bilateral intraductal carcinoma at diagnosis. The local treatment of the breast for all women was breast-conserving surgery followed by definitive breast irradiation. The surgical treatment of the primary tumor site included complete gross excision of the primary tumor in all cases. Because of the era during which these patients were treated, only 15% (40 of 270) of the cases underwent a re-excision of the primary tumor site. Additionally, pathologic staging to confirm negative axillary lymph nodes was performed in 32% (86 of 270) of the cases, although it should be recognized that pathologic axillary lymph node staging is no longer considered standard practice.

Forty-two percent of the breast cancers were diagnosed by mammography only, 36% by physical examination, and 22% by both. With regard to presentation, this early group is quite different from the later "mammographically detected" group.

After breast-conserving surgery, definitive breast irradiation was delivered to the whole breast for each patient in accordance with the policy of the institution where treated. The median dose per fraction for the whole-breast irradiation was 2.0 gray (Gy) (mean, 1.94 Gy; range, 1.6 to 2.45 Gy). The median dose delivered to the whole breast was 50.0 Gy (mean, 51.31 Gy; range, 31.2 to 64.0 Gy). After whole-breast radiation, a boost to the primary tumor site was delivered in 65% of the cases (176 of 270). The boost was delivered using electrons in 109 cases, an implant in 30 cases, and photons in 37 cases. The total dose to the primary tumor bed was defined as the sum of the dose from the whole-breast treatment plus the dose from the breast boost. The median total dose to the primary tumor bed was 60.0 Gy (mean, 61.17 Gy; range, 31.2 to 85.0 Gy). The total dose was greater than 50.0 Gy in 96% of the cases (258 of 270), and greater than 60.0 Gy in 61% of the cases (165 of 270).

In addition to radiation of the breast, regional nodal radiation was delivered to one or more regional nodal site(s) in 99 cases (37%). The regional nodal area(s) treated were the axilla (n = 85), the supraclavicular region (n = 78), and/or the internal mammary nodal region (n = 62).

Adjuvant systemic therapy was delivered after definitive breast irradiation in 4% of the patients (12 of 268). The adjuvant systemic therapy used was perioperative or intraoperative thiotepa in six cases, oophorectomy in three cases, tamoxifen in one case, megestrol acetate (Megace) in one case, and perioperative thiotepa plus tamoxifen in one case.

Actuarial curves for survival and local control were calculated using the Kaplan-Meier method (19). The time period was calculated beginning at the start of definitive breast irradiation, not at the time of diagnosis of intraductal carcinoma. Statistical comparisons between curves were determined using the Mantel-Cox test (20).

One of the strengths of this collaborative study is that long-term follow-up information is available. The median follow-up time for this early patient group was 10.3 years (mean, 10.7 years; range, 0.9 to 26.8 years). The median follow-up time for surviving patients was 10.4 years (mean, 11.0 years; range, 0.9 to 26.8 years).

A central pathology review was performed for 191 cases (71%) for which the pathology slides were available for review (6). Nine of the 10 institutions participated in the central pathology review; one institution elected not to participate. The central pathology review was performed by one pathologist (I-Tien Yeh) without knowledge of the clinical outcome. A detailed description of the methodology for this central pathology review has previously been reported (6). Architectural pattern, nuclear grade, and amount of necrosis were scored separately. However, insufficient information was available from the central pathology review to determine the status of the final pathology margins from the primary tumor excision. Therefore, the margins were determined from retrospective review of the patient records.

MATERIALS AND METHODS: MAMMOGRAPHICALLY DETECTED GROUP

The members of this collaboration decided to create a second database, limited to women with mammographically detected DCIS (21, 22). This project was initiated in response to the growing awareness that the diagnosis of DCIS encompassed a range of disease patterns that varied in clinical presentation, pathologic characteristics, and likely outcome to available treatment interventions.

Institutions participating in this second project include:

(i)   University of Pennsylvania, Philadelphia, Pennsylvania;
(ii)   Institut Curie, Paris, France;
(iii)   William Beaumont Hospital, Royal Oak, Michigan;
(iv)   Yale University, New Haven, Connecticut;
(v)   Mallinckrodt Institute of Radiology, St. Louis, Missouri;

(vi)   Memorial Sloan-Kettering Cancer Center, New York, New York;

(vii) University of Texas M.D. Anderson Cancer Center, Houston, Texas;

(viii) University of Michigan, Ann Arbor, Michigan;

(ix)   University Hospital, Basel, Switzerland;

(x)   British Columbia Cancer Agency, Vancouver, Canada; and

(xi)   Netherlands Cancer Institute, Amsterdam, The Netherlands.

As in the early collaborative group database, many of the patients included in the present study have been reported in previous single or limited institution studies, including the early database discussed above.

To increase the number of mammographically detected intraductal breast cancers in the database, this study expanded the time interval to include patients treated through 1990. Criteria for inclusion in this cohort included:

(i)   clinically occult, mammographically detected DCIS,

(ii)   no physical findings, such as breast mass or bloody nipple discharge,

(iii) treatment of breast-conserving surgery followed by definitive breast irradiation to a dose of 4000 cGy or more,

(iv)   treatment date of 1990 or before,

(v)   no adjuvant systemic chemotherapy or hormone therapy,

(vi)   no Paget's disease of the nipple,

(vii) no prior or concurrent invasive or microinvasive carcinoma of the ipsilateral or contralateral breast, and

(viii) no prior or concurrent malignancy other than DCIS, except for non-melanoma skin cancer.

A total of 422 mammographically detected cases of DCIS in 418 women were available for analysis. The surgical treatment included complete gross excision of the primary tumor site, generally using mammographic needle localization. Re-excision of the primary tumor site was performed in 153 cases (36%). As in the early group, 30% of the cases had a pathologic axilla node staging, and the lymph nodes were negative in all cases.

Each patient received radiation treatments to the whole breast in accordance with the policy of the institution where treated. The median whole-breast dose was 50 Gy, with a range of 40 to 66 Gy. A boost dose to the primary tumor site was delivered in 72% of all cases (303 of 442). Electrons were used in 219 cases, photons in 38 cases, and an implant boost in 46 cases. The median total dose to the tumor bed, including the contribution from the whole-breast irradiation and the boost dose, was 60 Gy (range, 41 to 76 Gy). Ninety-seven percent of all cases received a total dose of 50 Gy or more and 64% received a total dose of 60 Gy or more. In 32 cases (8%), regional radiation was also prescribed to the axilla ($n = 22$), the supraclavicular region ($n = 21$), and/or the internal mammary node region ($n = 24$).

The same statistical methods were used as in the early cohort, including the Kaplan-Meier method to calculate actuarial curves for survival, freedom from distant disease, local control, and contralateral breast events (19). The Mantel-Cox test was used for statistical comparison between groups (20). Confidence intervals were obtained using the logistic transform method (23), and the Cox proportional hazards multivariable regression model was used to evaluate the independent prognostic significance of the variables (24).

Median follow-up for this cohort was 9.4 years (mean, 9.6 years, range, 0.1 to 19.8 years), reflecting the additional patients treated between 1985 and 1990.

Margin information was recognized as important, but because inking of breast biopsy specimens was not routinely performed during the earlier years of this study, many of the cases with long-term follow-up have unknown margins of resection. The margin width was not routinely specified for cases in this study. Pathology margins, when known, were scored as negative, positive, or close according to the policy of each participating institution. The final margin was defined as the margin from the re-excision (if performed), or otherwise from the original specimen.

The margin information was determined from a review of the patient records. The majority of institutions ($n = 6$) defined the margin as negative when all tumor identified was more than 2 mm from the ink, and close when the tumor was 2 mm or less (but not at the margin). Two institutions used a 3 mm distance to define negative, and "close" margins, and one used a distance of 1 mm. The remaining two institutions did not use specific criteria for this definition. At all centers, an involved margin meant that the DCIS was at the inked margin of resection.

RESULTS: EARLY GROUP

A number of studies of the long-term outcome after treatment from this collaborative database have been previously reported (1–6). The most recent study reports 15-year outcome after treatment (3). Table 33.1 details the 5-year, 10-year, and 15-year outcome after breast-conserving surgery and definitive breast irradiation. Figure 33.1 shows the curves for overall survival and cause-specific survival, and Figure 33.2 shows the curve for local failure.

Figure 33.3 shows the curves for local failure as a function of pathology of the primary tumor on central pathology review. Although the curves split early, they come together by 10 years. Lesions with the combination of comedo subtype plus nuclear grade 3 tend to recur earlier than lesions without this combination (median time to recurrence of 3.1 years vs. 6.5 years, respectively), and tend to recur less commonly with invasive carcinoma [30% (3 of 10) vs. 67% (12 of 18), respectively].

Table 33.2 details the characteristics of the 45 local recurrences in the treated breast. The time to local recurrence

TABLE 33.1. ACTUARIAL OUTCOME DATA

Characteristic	At 5 Years (%)	At 10 Years (%)	At 15 Years (%)
Survival			
Overall	98	94	87
Cause-specific	99	97	96
Freedom from distant metastases	99	97	96
Local failure	7	16	19
Contralateral breast cancer	2	6	9

From Solin LJ, Kurtz J, Fourquet A, et al. Fifteen-year results of breast-conserving surgery and definitive breast irradiation for the treatment of ductal carcinoma in situ of the breast. J Clin Oncol 1996;14:754–763, with permission.

is protracted, with local failures detected at prolonged intervals after initial treatment. While 67% (30 of 45) of the local failures were in field or marginal, 29% (13 of 45) were elsewhere in the treated breast.

Analysis of the method of detection for the local failures according to method of initial presentation is shown in Table 33.3. Patients initially presenting with mammographic findings alone are more likely to have mammographic findings alone at the time of local failure.

Salvage treatment is one important consideration in the initial management of patients using breast-conservation treatment for DCIS. Table 33.4 details the salvage treatment for the 45 patients with local failure. Of the 44 patients without metastatic disease at the time of local failure, 42 (95%) underwent salvage mastectomy with curative intent, and 34 (81%) of the 42 did not receive adjuvant sys-

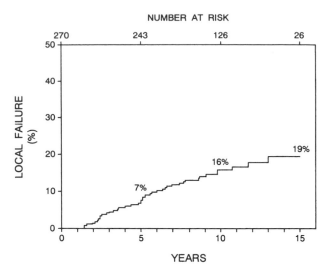

FIGURE 33.2. Actuarial local failure. From Solin LJ, Kurtz J, Fourquet A, et al. Fifteen-year results of breast-conserving surgery and definitive breast irradiation for the treatment of ductal carcinoma in situ of the breast. *J Clin Oncol* 1996;14:754–763, with permission.

temic therapy at the time of salvage treatment. With a median follow-up of 4.2 years (mean, 4.8 years; range, 0.2 to 11.4 years) after salvage treatment, 38 patients (84%) were alive without evidence of disease, two patients (4%) were alive with evidence of disease, four patients (9%) were dead of disease, and one patient (2%) was dead without evidence of disease.

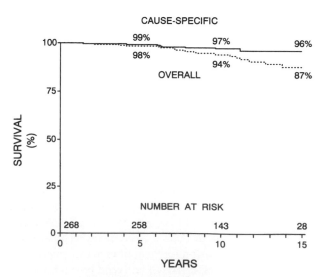

FIGURE 33.1. Actuarial overall survival and cause-specific survival. From Solin LJ, Kurtz J, Fourquet A, et al. Fifteen-year results of breast-conserving surgery and definitive breast irradiation for the treatment of ductal carcinoma in situ of the breast. *J Clin Oncol* 1996;14:754–763 with permission.

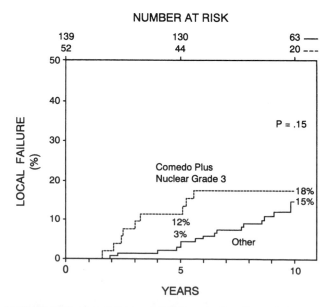

FIGURE 33.3. Actuarial local failure as a function of the presence *(dotted line)* versus the absence *(solid line)* of comedo subtype plus nuclear grade 3 on central pathology review. The curves separate early, but come together by 10 years. From Solin LJ, Kurtz J, Fourquet A, et al. Fifteen-year results of breast-conserving surgery and definitive breast irradiation for the treatment of ductal carcinoma in situ of the breast. *J Clin Oncol* 1996;14:754–763, with permission.

TABLE 33.2. CHARACTERISTICS OF 45 LOCAL RECURRENCES IN THE TREATED BREAST

Characteristic	Number	%
Histology of recurrence		
Infiltrating ductal carcinoma	24	53
Ductal carcinoma in situ[a]	21	47
Location of recurrence		
In field or marginal	30	67
Elsewhere	13	29
Diffuse or multifocal	2	4
Time to recurrence (years)		
≤5.0	20	44
5.1–10.0	19	42
10.1–15.0	3	7
>15.0	3	7
Method of detection		
Mammography	21	47
Physical examination	7	16
Both	16	36
Other[b]	1	2

From Solin LJ, Kurtz J, Fourquet A, et al. Fifteen-year results of breast-conserving surgery and definitive breast irradiation for the treatment of ductal carcinoma in situ of the breast. J Clin Oncol 1996;14:754–763.
[a] Includes one case with associated Paget's disease.
[b] One patient with nipple discharge.

RESULTS: MAMMOGRAPHICALLY DETECTED GROUP

In this patient cohort, 48 local regional failures occurred in 422 breasts, for a failure rate of 11% at ten years, in contrast to 16% in the early cohort. The median time to local recurrence was 5.0 years, (mean, 5.7 years; range, 1.0 to 15.2 years), which was similar to the early group median of 5.2 years. Again, approximately 50% of the local failures were invasive disease, and 50% were intraductal disease; one patient failed locally with an angiosarcoma of the breast (time = 6.3 years).

A number of factors were evaluated as potentially associated with an increased risk of local failure. These are listed in Table 33.5. Patient age at the time of diagnosis was strongly associated with risk of local failure, with the

TABLE 33.4. SALVAGE TREATMENT FOR 45 LOCAL RECURRENCES IN THE TREATED BREAST

Treatment	Number	%
Mastectomy[a]		
No adjuvant systemic therapy	34	76
Adjuvant chemotherapy	2	4
Adjuvant tamoxifen	4	9
Adjuvant tamoxifen and oophorectomy	1	2
Adjuvant chemotherapy and tamoxifen	1	2
Local excision		
Adjuvant tamoxifen	1	2
Local excision and axillary lymph node dissection		
No adjuvant systemic therapy	1	2
Other[b]	1	2

From Solin LJ, Kurtz J, Fourquet A, et al. Fifteen-year results of breast-conserving surgery and definitive breast irradiation for the treatment of ductal carcinoma in situ of the breast. J Clin Oncol 1996;14:754–763.
[a] With or without an axillary lymph node dissection.
[b] One patient with simultaneous local and distant first failure.

youngest patients having the highest failure rate, and the oldest patients, the lowest local failure rate. A final positive pathology margin (in those cases where it was known) was also associated with local failure. Interestingly, this was true only for in situ local failures, but not for invasive failures. In the multivariable Cox regression model, age less than or equal to 39 years and positive margins remained independent predictors for local failure in this cohort ($p = 0.0006$ and $p = 0.023$, respectively). In the same Cox model, age of 40 to 49 years and unknown margins were "borderline" for statistical significance.

The rate of distant failure in these 418 patients was also similar to the early group, and occurred in 11 patients (3%). Ten of these 11 distant failures were associated with either an invasive local recurrence or a new invasive cancer in the contralateral breast or elsewhere (non-breast).

Of the 48 local-regional failures, 42 were not associated with distant disease and were operable for salvage, with the outcome data shown in Table 33.6. Of these 42 women,

TABLE 33.3. METHOD OF DETECTION OF LOCAL RECURRENCE ACCORDING TO METHOD OF INITIAL PRESENTATION FOR 44 LOCAL RECURRENCES[a]

Method of Initial Presentation[b]	Method of Detection		
	Mammography	Physical Examination	Both
Mammography	10	1	3
Physical examination	7	2	2
Both	4	4	11

[a] One case excluded because of detection with nipple discharge at the time of local recurrence.
[b] $p = .032$ using the chi-square test.

TABLE 33.5. LOCAL FAILURE CORRELATED WITH VARIOUS POTENTIAL PROGNOSTIC PARAMETERS

	Number Treated	Local Failure[a] (%) At 5 Years	At 10 Years	p Value[b]
Patient age (years)				0.0001
≤39	31	20	31	
40–49	158	6	13	
50–59	114	3	8	
≥60	119	5	6	
Final pathology margin				0.030
Negative	222	6	9	
Positive	40	13	24	
Close	45	5	7	
Unknown	115	4	12	
Institution where treated				0.14
Date of treatment				0.85
1985 and before	107	7	12	
1986–1990	315	5	11	
Location of the primary tumor[c]				0.82
Outer quadrant	246	5	13	
Inner quadrant	78	7	9	
Central location	94	6	10	
Total radiation dose				0.89
<6000 cGy	154	4	9	
6000–6600 cGy	223	7	11	
>6600 cGy	45	4	17	
Mammographic findings[d]				0.59
Microcalcifications	360	6	11	
Mass	25	0	5	
Microcalcifications and mass	35	3	13	
Clinical tumor size[e]				0.61
≤2.0 cm	197	4	12	
2.1–5.0 cm	37	9	12	

[a] Any local failure.
[b] Mantel-Cox test (34).
[c] Excludes cases with unknown information.
[d] Excludes cases with other clinical presentations.
[e] Excludes cases with unknown information or tumor size >5.0 cm.

mammography was the most common method of detection of both intraductal (78%) and invasive (71%) local recurrences. The time from initial treatment to local failure was similar (4.8 versus 4.7 years) for both types of failures. Thirty-seven women had mastectomy as the salvage procedure, and the remaining five had a wide local excision.

Twenty women also had a surgical evaluation of the axillary nodes, with only one yielding positive nodes. Postoperatively, three women received chemotherapy, eight received tamoxifen, and one received both.

As expected, patients with an intraductal recurrence did better than those with an invasive recurrence; similarly,

TABLE 33.6. FIVE-YEAR AND EIGHT-YEAR ACTUARIAL OUTCOME DATA AFTER SALVAGE TREATMENT FOR ALL 42 PATIENTS

	At 5 Years (%)	95% C.I.	At 8 Years (%)	95% C.I.
Overall survival	92	(77, 97)	92	(77, 97)
Cause-specific survival	92	(77, 97)	92	(77, 97)
Freedom from distant metastases	89	(73, 96)	89	(73, 96)

C.I., confidence intervals.

those women whose recurrence was palpable did worse than those whose recurrence was only detectable by mammogram.

The one patient with an angiosarcoma was treated with a salvage mastectomy and no adjuvant systemic therapy. She is alive and well 7.2 years from her salvage procedure.

DISCUSSION

The present report summarizes the results from an international collaborative study of women with ductal carcinoma in situ of the breast treated with breast-conserving surgery and definitive breast irradiation. As retrospective studies, these data have a number of strengths and weaknesses. Significant strengths of these data include the large number of patients and the long-term follow-up information, such that 15-year outcome data have been reported. Important, but rarely reported end points have been analyzed and include the determination of the risk of development of contralateral breast cancer, an in-depth analysis of local failures, and outcome after salvage treatment for local failure. However, the data are limited by the fact that some of the tumor and treatment characteristics would be considered suboptimal by contemporary standards. Further, some of these cases were treated in an era during which mammographic-pathologic correlation of surgical specimens was not commonly performed. To some extent, these limitations have been addressed by the second cohort of patients, limited to those with mammographic-only detection. The rate of local failure is lower in this group, when compared with the early group. However, once the local failure was diagnosed, the two patient cohorts were remarkable similar.

An important lesson learned from these data is that DCIS of the breast has a long natural history, and that the results of breast conservation treatment (with or without radiation) should not be judged without adequate follow-up after treatment. In particular, the time course to local failure is protracted, with local failures seen more than 10 to 15 years after treatment (Tables 33.1 and 33.2, and Fig. 33.2). The curve for local failure rises steadily through 10 years of follow-up, but the rate of rise may be somewhat less in years 10 to 15 (Fig. 33.2). The late local failures may represent new tumors in the breast, or they may indicate a very long natural history of this disease. Although there is minimal decline in cause-specific survival and freedom from distant metastases observed in these data, the fact remains that half of these local failures are invasive disease with the potential for distant metastases.

Although these studies document a large experience with effective salvage surgery, no clear role for adjuvant chemotherapy or hormone therapy emerges from either cohort of women. The role of systemic treatment after local failure is yet to be determined, therefore, assessing the individual clinical situation is appropriate for the present.

Thus, careful and prolonged follow-up after initial treatment with breast conservation is critical to detect local failures early and to afford the opportunity to treat such failures with curative intent.

While retrospective data do not supplant the need for data from prospective trials, data from the present studies have provided long-term, 15-year outcome from women with DCIS treated with breast-conserving surgery and definitive breast irradiation

REFERENCES

1. Solin L, Fourquet A, McCormick B, et al. Intraductal carcinoma of the breast: long-term results with breast-conserving surgery and definitive irradiation. *Eur J Cancer* 1993;29A(Suppl 6): 66(abst).
2. Solin LJ, Fourquet A, McCormick B, et al. Salvage treatment for local recurrence following breast-conserving surgery and definitive irradiation for ductal carcinoma in situ (intraductal carcinoma) of the breast. *Int J Radiat Oncol Biol Phys* 1994;30:3–9.
3. Solin LJ, Kurtz J, Fourquet A, et al. Fifteen-year results of breast-conserving surgery and definitive breast irradiation for the treatment of ductal carcinoma in situ of the breast. *J Clin Oncol* 1996;14:754–763.
4. Solin LJ, McCormick B, Recht A, et al. Mammographically detected, clinically occult ductal carcinoma in situ treated with breast-conserving surgery and definitive breast irradiation. *Cancer J* 1996;2:158–165.
5. Solin LJ, Recht A, Fourquet A, et al. Ten-year results of breast-conserving surgery and definitive irradiation for intraductal carcinoma (ductal carcinoma in situ) of the breast. *Cancer* 1991;68: 2337–2344.
6. Solin LJ, Yeh I-T, Kurtz J, et al. Ductal carcinoma in situ (intraductal carcinoma) of the breast treated with breast-conserving surgery and definitive irradiation: correlation of pathologic parameters with outcome of treatment. *Cancer* 1993;71:2532–2542.
7. Bornstein BA, Recht A, Connolly JL, et al. Results of treating ductal carcinoma in situ of the breast with conservative surgery and radiation therapy. *Cancer* 1991;67:7–13.
8. Findlay P, Goodman R. Radiation therapy for treatment of intraductal carcinoma of the breast. *Am J Clin Oncol* 1983;6:281–285.
9. Fowble BL, Solin LJ, Goodman RL. Results of conservative surgery and radiation for intraductal noninvasive breast cancer. *Am J Clin Oncol* 1987;10:110–111(abst).
10. Haffty BG, Peschel RE, Papadopoulos D, et al. Radiation therapy for ductal carcinoma in situ of the breast. *Conn Med* 1990;54: 482–484.
11. Hiramatsu H, Bornstein BA, Recht A, et al. Local recurrence after conservative surgery and radiation therapy for ductal carcinoma in situ: possible importance of family history. *Cancer J* 1995;1:55–61.
12. Kurtz JM, Jacquemier J, Torhorst J, et al. Conservation therapy for breast cancers other than infiltrating ductal carcinoma. Cancer 1989;63:1630–1635.
13. Kuske RR, Bean JM, Garcia DM, et al. Breast conservation therapy for intraductal carcinoma of the breast. *Int J Radiat Oncol Biol Phys* 1993;26:391–396.
14. McCormick B, Rosen PP, Kinne D, et al. Duct carcinoma in situ of the breast: an analysis of local control after conservation surgery and radiotherapy. *Int J Radiat Oncol Biol Phys* 1991;21: 289–292.

15. Recht A, Danoff B, Solin LJ, et al. Intraductal carcinoma of the breast: results of treatment with excisional biopsy and irradiation. *J Clin Oncol* 1985;3:1339–1343.

16. Solin LJ, Fowble BL, Schultz DJ, et al. Definitive irradiation for intraductal carcinoma of the breast. *Int J Radiat Oncol Biol Phys* 1990;19:843–850.

17. Stotter AT, McNeese M, Oswald MJ, et al. The role of limited surgery with irradiation in primary treatment of ductal in situ breast cancer. *Int J Radiat Oncol Biol Phys* 1990;18:283–287.

18. Zafrani B, Fourquet A, Vilcoq JR, et al. Conservative management of intraductal breast carcinoma with tumorectomy and radiation therapy. *Cancer* 1986;57:1299–1301.

19. Kaplan EL, Meier P. Nonparametric estimation from incomplete observations. *J Am Stat Assoc* 1958;53:457–481.

20. Mantel N. Evaluation of survival data and two new rank order statistics arising in its consideration. *Cancer Chemother Rep* 1966; 50:163–170.

21. Solin LJ, Fourquet A, Vicini FA, et al. Mammographically detected ductal carcinoma in situ of the breast treated with breast-conserving surgery and definitive breast irradiation: Long-term outcome and prognostic significance of patient age and margin status. *Int J Radiat Oncol Biol Phys* 2001;50:991–1002.

22. Solin LJ, Fourquet A, Vicini FA, et al. Salvage treatment for local recurrence after breast-conserving surgery and radiation as initial treatment for mammographically detected ductal carcinoma in situ. *Cancer* 2001;91:1090–1097.

23. Lawless J. *Statistical models and methods for lifetime data.* New York: John Wiley and Sons, 1982:401–407.

24. Kalbfleisch J, Prentice R. *The Statistical analysis of failure time data.* New York: John Wiley and Sons, 1980:70–141.

34

BREAST-CONSERVING SURGERY PLUS RADIATION THERAPY IN DUCTAL CARCINOMA IN SITU: THE INSTITUT CURIE EXPERIENCE

ALAIN FOURQUET
BRIGITTE SIGAL-ZAFRANI
KRISHNA B. CLOUGH

The first observations suggesting that ductal carcinoma in situ (DCIS) could be treated with breast preservation were published in the 1980s (1–5). These retrospective studies were based on small series of selected patients treated with excision alone or with local excision followed by breast irradiation. Large multicentric trials comparing treatment by excision alone with excision plus radiotherapy in patients with limited tumor extension have demonstrated that breast irradiation reduces the risk of recurrence by 50% or more, depending on the length of follow-up (6,7). Breast radiotherapy decreases both invasive and in situ recurrences.

In 1986, we published our experience in a small series of patients with DCIS treated with wide excision plus radiotherapy at the Institut Curie in Paris (4). The results suggested that the rate of local recurrence was low, and that the outcome was favorable in these selected patients. Because of the increasing use of screening mammography, the rate of diagnosis of new DCIS cases increased substantially at our institution. Therefore, in late 1989, we designed a prospective management policy for DCIS (8) based on evaluation of pathologic and clinical features (9).

In this chapter, we will report our experience over a 30-year period (1967 to 1996) treating patients with DCIS of the breast.

MATERIALS AND METHODS

Patients

From 1967 to 1996, 601 patients who had intraductal breast cancer without evidence of invasion were treated at the Institut Curie. Very few patients were treated with wide excision alone during this time period (23 patients, 4%); these patients and those who presented with synchronous bilateral disease are excluded from this report. Beginning in 1990, treatment decisions were based on the status of the excision margins and on the results of postoperative mam-

mography (in patients who initially had microcalcifications). Before 1990, 100 patients were treated with mastectomy (40%), and 153 patients (60%) were treated with wide excision plus radiotherapy. Between 1990 and 1996, 190 patients (57%) were treated with wide excision plus radiotherapy, and 145 (43%) were treated with mastectomy. This study will focus on the comparison of mastectomy with wide excision plus radiotherapy in the patients treated before 1990, and on the outcome and risk factors for recurrence in the 343 patients treated with wide excision plus radiotherapy over the whole period of study.

Pathology

The diagnosis of DCIS was initially based on incisional or excisional biopsy specimens. For the present study, we reviewed slides of all patients treated before 1990 (except eight for whom materials were unavailable). The following pathologic features were prospectively recorded in patients treated from 1990 onward:

architectural type (papillary, micropapillary, cribriform, solid, or comedo);

nuclear grade (low, intermediate, or high; respectively, 1, 2, or 3);

amount of necrosis (none, small, moderate, or extensive);

lobular extension;

associated lobular carcinoma in situ;

the presence of microcalcifications in the pathologic specimen; and

the overall histologic classification (well differentiated, intermediately differentiated, or poorly differentiated) according to the EORTC draft schema (10).

Treatment

Before 1990, 100 patients underwent mastectomy, and 153 patients received breast irradiation following wide excision.

After 1990, 190 patients underwent wide excision plus radiotherapy. Only 17 of 343 patients (5%) treated with wide excision plus radiotherapy had their initial surgery outside our institution. All other treatments were done at the Institut Curie.

Axillary node dissection was performed in 92% of patients treated with mastectomy, but in only 5% of patients treated with breast conservation. Involved axillary nodes were found in 1.3% of patients; all were treated with mastectomy.

Breast radiation was delivered using the supine position technique in 20% of patients and the lateral decubitus position [according to our previously described technique (11)] in 80% of patients. The median whole-breast dose was 54 gray (Gy) (range, 45 to 66 Gy). Additional radiation to the tumor bed was given to 54% of the patients, for a median total dose in the tumor bed of 61 Gy (range, 45 to 83 Gy). Axillary, supraclavicular, and internal mammary lymph nodes were irradiated in 17% of patients.

Statistical Analysis

Comparison of the distribution of clinical and pathologic factors between different treatment groups was performed using the chi-squared test. Comparison of survival and recurrence rates were carried out for the 253 patients treated between 1967 and 1989. The median follow-up for surviving patients was 108 months (range, 7 to 323 months). The data for the 190 patients treated between 1990 and 1996 with wide excision and radiotherapy were updated for the present study, allowing us to perform the risk factors analysis on 343 patients, treated between 1967 and 1996, at a median follow-up of 92 months (range, 5 to 323 months).

The time to events was measured starting from the date of first surgery. Actuarial rates were estimated using the Kaplan-Meier method (12). Survival time was calculated in two ways: either as "overall survival" (scoring death due to any cause), or as "cancer-specific survival" (scoring only deaths due to cancer, not concurrent illnesses). Patients were censored for the calculations of ipsilateral local-regional recurrence rates and contralateral breast cancer development rates at the time of discovery of distant metastases or death. Patients were also censored without being scored as having a recurrence if they had no evidence of disease at the time of last follow-up. Comparisons between actuarial curves were performed with the log-rank test. The effects of different risk factors for local recurrence were tested for independence using a forward-stepping Cox proportional hazards model, and included patients with missing data (13).

RESULTS

Comparison of Mastectomy with Wide Excision plus Radiotherapy Groups

One hundred patients were treated with mastectomy and 153 were treated with wide excision plus irradiation. The patients treated with mastectomy were significantly older than patients treated with breast conservation. All other clinical and pathologic features were comparable between both groups (Table 34.1).

Residual disease after initial biopsy that could be retrospectively evaluated was found in 66 of 93 mastectomy specimens (71%). Of the 66 specimens with residual disease, 60 (91%) had pure DCIS, and six had both DCIS and invasive cancer.

Actuarial 10-year results for the retrospective cohort (patients treated from 1967 to 1989) are presented in Table 34.2. Cancer-specific survival rates were 98% ($\pm$ 3%) in both the mastectomy and breast-conservation groups. Metastasis-free survival rates were also similar. Five of 100 patients (5%) in the mastectomy group had a local recurrence or regional nodal recurrence, compared with 25 of 153 patients (16%) in the breast-conserving group. The actuarial rate of local-regional recurrence was also significantly lower in the mastectomy group ($p = 0.02$). Two of the five recurrences in the mastectomy group occurred as isolated axillary node recurrences, whereas no isolated nodal recurrences were observed in the breast-conservation group.

Risk Factors for Local Failure Following Wide Excision plus Radiotherapy

Various clinical and pathologic factors were tested for their influence on the risk of recurrence following wide excision plus radiation therapy in the 343 patients treated between 1967 and 1996. Median follow-up was 92 months (range, 5 to 323 months). Thirty-nine local recurrences were observed during the period of study. The results of the univariate analysis are presented in Table 34.3. Young age (defined as 40 years of age or younger at diagnosis), the absence of microcalcifications on pathologic examination, the presence of necrosis in any amount, and having an intermediate or poorly-differentiated tumor were all significantly associated with an increased risk of recurrence. Other pathologic factors, such as the histologic subtype of DCIS, did not influence the risk of recurrence. Histologic subtype and amount of necrosis were correlated: necrosis was absent in 57% of clinging or micropapillary subtypes, whereas it was not present in 33% of other subtypes ($p = 0.004$). In this study, the margins of excision status did not influence the rate of recurrence. A radiation dose to the tumor bed of more than 66 Gy decreased the recurrence rate, but this trend did not reach conventional statistical significance.

A Cox multivariate analysis was performed for all 343 patients treated with excision plus radiotherapy, and therefore included patients with missing data on some of the parameters studied (Table 34.4). The presence of necrosis, patient age younger than 41, and the absence of microcalcifications on pathologic examination independently increased the risk of developing a recurrence. Of note, there was a strong cor-

TABLE 34.1. COMPARISON OF CLINICAL AND PATHOLOGIC FEATURES OF PATIENTS TREATED BY MASTECTOMY OR WIDE EXCISION AND RADIOTHERAPY IN THE RETROSPECTIVE COHORT (1967–1989)

Feature	Mastectomy	Excision and Radiotherapy	p
Number of patients	100	153	—
Age (years)	—	—	0.0003
Median	52	48	—
Range	30–85	32–78	—
Premenopausal (%)	54	68	0.0002
Presentation (%)	—	—	NS
Palpable mass	27	25	—
Nipple discharge	20	11	—
Mammographic only (microcalcifications)	52	63	—
Microcalcifications (pathologic)(%)	—	—	NS
Absent	29	23	—
Present	71	77	—
Nuclear grade (%)	—	—	NS
1	16	22	—
2	39	40	—
3	45	38	—
Necrosis (%)	—	—	NS
Absent	38	42	—
Present	62	58	—
Comedo-type necrosis (%)	29	23	NS
Histologic classification	—	—	NS
Well-differentiated	17	22	—
Intermediate	39	44	—
Poor	44	34	—

NS, not significant.

relation between histologic classification (as well as nuclear grade, data not shown), and the presence of necrosis. Necrosis was present in 69.5% of grade 2 and 3 tumors, but in only 14.5% of grade 1 tumors ($p = 0.0001$).

A rough measure of the size of the excised specimen was calculated by multiplying its two largest diameters. This area was correlated with the presence or absence of microcalcifications. The mean area was 2,070 square millimeters when microcalcifications were absent, compared with 2,630 square millimeters when microcalcifications were present ($p = 0.065$).

The influence of the radiation dose to the tumor bed (adding the dose to the whole breast and the boost dose) was then analyzed in the multivariate model. The relative risk of recurrence was 0.5 (95% confidence interval, 0.2 to 1.1) when a dose of more than 66 Gy was delivered ($p = 0.07$).

Finally, the influence of different combinations of the absence or presence of both microcalcifications and necrosis on recurrence rates was evaluated. The low-risk group comprised the 75 patients older than 41 whose tumors contained microcalcifications but not necrosis. Only two recurrences (3%) were found in this group, at 109 months and 201 months after diagnosis, respectively. Both were invasive recurrences. The former was in the same quadrant than the primary tumor, and the latter was in another quadrant. The other group comprised 268 patients who had at least one risk factor, or for whom there was missing data on the presence of microcalcifications or necrosis. There were 37 recurrences (14%) in this group. The 8-year actuarial recurrence rates in these two groups were 0% and 14.5%, respectively ($p = 0.003$).

TABLE 34.2. ACTUARIAL 10-YEAR RESULTS IN THE RETROSPECTIVE COHORT (1967–1989)

Result (%)	Excision + Radiotherapy (153)	Mastectomy (100)
Overall survival	98	95
Cancer-specific survival	98	98
Metastasis-free survival	97	98
Local-regional recurrence	17	3
Contralateral breast cancer	7	10
Breast preservation	84	0

TABLE 34.3. UNIVARIATE ANALYSIS OF RISK FACTORS FOR RECURRENCE IN PATIENTS TREATED WITH WIDE EXCISION PLUS RADIOTHERAPY (343 PATIENTS: 1967–1996)

Factor	No. Patients	No. Recurrences	Actuarial 8-Year Recurrence Rate (%)	p
Age (years)	—	—	—	0.0002
≤40	29	10	28	—
>40	314	29	9	—
Margins	—	—	—	0.76
Free (>2 mm)	145	10	11	—
Close (1–2 mm)	72	6	12	—
Focally involved	52	5	12	—
Not determined	74	18	13	—
Histologic microcalcifications	—	—	—	0.0003
Absent	49	15	23	—
Present	261	19	18	—
Necrosis	—	—	—	0.01
Absent	112	9	3	—
Present	182	28	17	—
Histologic classification	—	—	—	0.02
Well differentiated	49	2	3	—
Intermediate or poor	151	29	14	—
Dose to tumor bed	—	—	—	0.08
≤66 Gy	243	32	13	—
>66 Gy	100	7	6	—

Time-Course of Development, Location, and Histology of Ipsilateral Recurrences in the Wide Excision plus Radiotherapy Group

Thirty-nine ipsilateral recurrences were reported among the 343 patients treated with wide excision plus radiotherapy during the entire period of observation. The 8-year actuarial rate of recurrence was 11% (± 4%). Twenty-one con-tralateral breast cancers occurred. The 8-year contralateral breast cancer rate was 5% (± 3%). The median interval between the time of the first surgery and the ipsilateral recurrence was 74 months (range, 25 to 250 months). The annual hazard of recurrence in the treated breast averaged 1.5%, which was higher than the average annual hazard of developing a contralateral breast cancer (0.7%). Twenty-four recurrences (63%) were in the same quadrant as the primary lesion after a median interval of 64 months (range, 24 to 201 months). Fourteen recurrences (37%) were in another quadrant of the breast after a median interval of 82 months (range, 36 to 250 months).

Nine recurrences consisted histologically of DCIS only, 14 were invasive cancer, and 13 contained both DCIS and invasive cancer. (The histology of recurrence was not known in two patients.) Seventeen of 24 recurrences (71%) in the same quadrant as the first lesion, contained DCIS (either alone or in association with invasive cancer), whereas seven of 14 (50%) recurrences that appeared in another quadrant contained DCIS (with or without areas of invasion). Two patients with ipsilateral recurrence also had concomitant axillary lymph node involvement.

Ten patients developed distant metastases. Metastases were preceded by an invasive ipsilateral or contralateral recurrence in nine patients. Only one patient developed distant disease without first having an invasive new primary or local recurrence.

TABLE 34.4. MULTIVARIATE ANALYSIS OF RISK FACTORS FOR RECURRENCE IN PATIENTS TREATED WITH WIDE EXCISION AND RADIOTHERAPY (343 PATIENTS: 1967–1996)

	Relative Risk	95% Confidence Interval	p
Histologic microcalcifications	—	—	0.001
Present	1	—	—
Absent	4.4	2.2–8.6	—
Necrosis	—	—	<0.001
Absent	1	—	—
Present	3.9	1.8–8.4	—
Age (years)	—	—	0.022
>40	1	—	—
≤40	2.4	1.1–5	—

Salvage Therapy in the Wide Excision plus Radiotherapy Group

Mastectomy was carried out in 37 of the 39 patients (95%) who had a recurrence. Thus, the 8-year rate of preserving the breast in the breast-conservation group was 89% (± 4%).

The median follow-up of patients after ipsilateral recurrence was 43 months (range, 1 to 175 months). Seven of these 39 patients (18%) subsequently developed distant metastases. All seven had recurrences that histologically contained invasive cancer; two of the seven had lymph node recurrences, and one had an invasive contralateral cancer, prior to distant metastases.

DISCUSSION

This study of a large group of consecutively treated patients with DCIS from a single institution showed that the local control rate was higher after mastectomy than wide excision plus radiotherapy. However, this difference did not lead to differences in metastasis-free, cancer-specific survival, or overall survival rates. Cancer-specific survival rates were very high for both treatments (98% at 10 years). Local-regional recurrences occurred in 3% of patients treated with mastectomy, which is consistent with the results of other retrospective studies (2,14,15). This study confirmed our previous observations, as well as those of others, that breast-conserving treatment of DCIS does not adversely impact on survival.

The estimated 8-year cumulative risk of recurrence in the 343 patients treated with breast-conserving surgery plus irradiation was 11%, comparable to that observed in a multi-center study on patients with mammographically detected DCIS that included 95 patients from the current population (16). Recurrences were found in the same quadrant as the primary tumor slightly more often than in other quadrants. Of note, the interval between surgery and recurrence was shorter when patients relapsed near the primary tumor site, but recurrences located elsewhere in the breast more frequently had invasive histology. This observation suggests that "recurrences" located some distance from the original tumor site could represent new primary tumors rather than a clinical return of the first lesion.

In this study, the risk of developing a recurrence was increased when the patient was young, when necrosis was present, and when there were no microcalcifications. These risk factors were statistically independent of one another.

The effect of young age (40 years or younger) on recurrence confirms the results from other studies (16–18).

The presence of necrosis of any amount was the risk factor most strongly associated with recurrence, which also confirms other observations (19,20). Some authors have suggested that necrosis may reflect tumor death resulting from apoptosis in high-grade tumors (21). Necrosis might also be associated with the presence of hypoxia, which would make these tumors less radiosensitive. This would, perhaps, explain how an increase of the radiation dose over 66 Gy to the tumor bed would decrease the rate of local failure. Moreover, a dose-effect relationship could exist in young patients with DCIS, as well as in young patients with invasive cancer, as suggested in an EORTC trial (22).

The increased risk of recurrence found in patients without microcalcifications on pathologic examination may indirectly reflect inadequate surgery. It would seem more difficult to appreciate the full extent of the lesion when its presence is not marked by microcalcifications. (This is the case when DCIS presents as a bloody ductal discharge or is incidentally found after a cyst or fibroadenoma is excised.) Indeed, we found that the size of the surgical specimen was significantly smaller when microcalcifications were absent than when they were present. Similarly, failure to appreciate the full extent of the tumor may result in a partial "miss" when one tries to give an additional radiation dose or "boost" to the tumor.

In contradiction to other studies, microscopic margin involvement was not found to be a risk factor for recurrence in this study (16,18,19, 23). Information on margins status was unavailable for 21% of patients, which represents a strong limitation of this study, as well as of other retrospective studies. On the other hand, it has long been the policy at our institution that breast-conserving surgery for either intraductal or invasive cancer should be performed only when wide margins could be obtained. Consequently, in this study, patients with extensive margin involvement underwent either a surgical re-excision or mastectomy (40% of the 601 patients with DCIS had a mastectomy). Therefore, only those patients with focal margin involvement were treated with breast-conserving surgery plus radiotherapy, with satisfactory results. The probability that tumor extends beyond the margins of resection is substantial (even in small tumors) unless wide margins are removed, and this risk increases with increasing tumor size (24). Thus, difficulty in accurately assessing tumor extension probably represents the major risk factor for recurrence in DCIS treated with wide excision plus radiotherapy.

Intermediate or poorly differentiated histologic type (according to the European classification), as well as nuclear grade, was associated with an increased risk of recurrence in our experience. However, this effect disappeared on multivariate analysis when the effect of necrosis was taken into account.

SUMMARY

Breast-conserving treatment for localized DCIS, consisting of excision followed by irradiation, provides a high level of local control, particularly in patients who present with microcalcifications. In tumors with focal margin involvement, radiation therapy may still represent an acceptable alternative to mastectomy, provided that improvements in diagnostic imaging help target the tumor more precisely. The very low rate of local failure after wide excision plus radiotherapy that was observed in patients older than 40 whose tumors had microcalcifications but not necrosis is particularly noteworthy. Whether radiotherapy can be safely omitted in such cases remains to be demonstrated. Currently, there is no statistical difference in breast cancer-specific or overall survival regardless of how the patient is treated.

ACKNOWLEDGMENTS

The authors would like to thank Dr. Benedicte Royer for help in reviewing the histologic slides and Mrs. Chantal Gautier for assistance in collecting the data and preparing the manuscript.

REFERENCES

1. Lagios MD, Westdahl PR, Margolin FR, et al. Ductal carcinoma in situ. Relationship of extent of noninvasive disease to the frequency of occult invasion, multicentricity, lymph node metastases, and short-term treatment failures. *Cancer* 1982;50:1309–1314.
2. Lagios NM, Margolin FR, Westdahl PR, et al. Mammographically detected duct carcinoma in situ. Frequency of local recurrence following tylectomy and prognostic effect of nuclear grade on local recurrence. *Cancer* 1989;63:619–624.
3. Recht A, Danoff BS, Solin LJ, et al. Intraductal carcinoma of the breast: results of treatment with excisional biopsy and irradiation. *J Clin Oncol* 1985;3:1339–1343.
4. Zafrani B, Fourquet A, Vilcoq JR, et al. Conservative management of intraductal breast carcinoma with tumorectomy and radiation therapy. *Cancer* 1986;57:1299–1301.
5. Kurtz J, Jacquemier J, Torhorst J, et al. Conservation therapy for breast cancers other than infiltrating ductal carcinoma. *Cancer* 1989;63:1630–1635.
6. Fisher B, Costantino J, Redmond C, et al. Lumpectomy and radiation therapy for the treatment of intraductal breast cancer: findings from National Surgical Adjuvant Breast and Bowel Project B-17. *J Clin Oncol* 1998;16:441–452.
7. Julien JP, Bijker N, Fentiman I, et al. Radiotherapy in breast-conserving treatment for ductal carcinoma in situ: first results of the EORTC randomised phase III trial 10853. EORTC Breast Cancer Cooperative Group and EORTC Radiotherapy Group. *Lancet* 2000;355:528–533.
8. Fourquet A, Zafrani B, Campana F, et al. Breast-conserving treatment of ductal carcinoma in situ. *Semin Radiat Oncol* 1992;2:116–124.
9. Zafrani B, Leroyer A, Fourquet A, et al. Mammographically detected ductal in situ carcinoma of the breast analyzed with a new classification. A study of 127 cases: correlation with estrogen and progesterone receptors, p53 and c-erbB-2 proteins, and proliferative activity. *Semin Diagn Pathol* 1994;11:208–214.
10. Holland R, Peterse JL, Millis RR, et al. Ductal carcinoma in situ: a proposal for a new classification. *Semin Diagn Pathol* 1994;11:167–180.
11. Fourquet A, Campana F, Rosenwald JC, et al. Breast irradiation in the lateral decubitus position: technique of the Institut Curie. *Radiother Oncol* 1991;22:261–265.
12. Kaplan EL, Meier P. Nonparametric estimation from incomplete observations. *J Am Stat Assoc* 1958;53:457–481.
13. Cox DR. Regression models and life table (with discussion). *J R Stat Soc B* 1972;34:187–220.
14. Silverstein MJ, Barth A, Poller DN, et al. Ten-year results comparing mastectomy to excision and radiation therapy for ductal carcinoma in situ of the breast. *Eur J Cancer* 1995;31A:1425–1427.
15. Contesso G, Petit JY. Les adenocarcinomes intracanalaires non infiltrants du sein. *Bull Cancer* 1979;66:1–8.
16. Solin LJ, Fourquet A, Vicini FA, et al. Mammographically detected ductal carcinoma in situ of the breast treated with breast-conserving surgery and definitive breast irradiation: long-term outcome and prognostic significance of patient age and margin status. *Int J Radiat Oncol Biol Phys* 2001;50:991–1002.
17. Van Zee KJ, Liberman L, Samli B, et al. Long-term follow-up of women with ductal carcinoma in situ treated with breast-conserving surgery: the effect of age. *Cancer* 1999;86:1757–1767.
18. Bijker N, Peterse JL, Duchateau L, et al. Risk factors for recurrence and metastasis after breast-conserving therapy for ductal carcinoma in situ: analysis of European Organization for Research and Treatment of Cancer trial 10853. *J Clin Oncol* 2001;19:2263–2271.
19. Fisher ER, Dignam J, Tan-Chiu E, et al. Pathologic findings from the National Surgical Adjuvant Breast Project (NSABP) eight-year update of protocol B-17. Intraductal carcinoma. *Cancer* 1999;86:429–438.
20. Silverstein MJ, Lagios MD, Craig PH, et al. A prognostic index for ductal carcinoma of the breast in situ. *Cancer* 1996;77:2267–2274.
21. Bodis S, Siziopikou KP, Schnitt SJ, et al. Extensive apoptosis in ductal carcinoma in situ of the breast. *Cancer* 1996;77:1831–1835.
22. Collette L, Fourquet A, Horiot JC, et al. Impact of a boost dose of 16 Gy on local control in patients with early breast cancer: the EORTC "Boost versus non boost" trial. *Radiother Oncol* 2000;56(Suppl 1):S46.
23. Silverstein MJ, Lagios MD, Groshen S, et al. The influence of margin width on local control of ductal carcinoma in situ of the breast. *N Engl J Med* 1999;340:1455–1461.
24. Holland R, Hendricks JHCL, Verbeek ALM, et al. Extent, distribution, and mammographic/histological correlations of breast ductal carcinoma in situ. *Lancet* 1990;335:519–522.

35

JOINT CENTER FOR RADIATION THERAPY EXPERIENCE

CATHERINE C. PARK
STUART J. SCHNITT
ABRAM RECHT

For many years, patients with ductal carcinoma in situ (DCIS) have been treated at the Joint Center for Radiation Therapy (JCRT) with breast-conserving therapy (BCT), either with or without radiotherapy. Such treatment is now widely accepted as an option for many women with DCIS. However, it is still unclear how to:

1) optimally select patients who are candidates for breast-conserving therapy; and
2) select patients who may be treated with conservative surgery alone.

We will summarize the JCRT publications on this subject in chronologic order, as they reflect the evolution of our understanding of these problems over the last twenty years.

BREAST-CONSERVING SURGERY AND RADIATION THERAPY

In 1985, Recht et al. (1) published a retrospective analysis of 40 women with DCIS treated at either the JCRT (20 patients) or Fox Chase Cancer Center/Hospital of the University of Pennsylvania (20 patients) between 1976 and 1983. Twenty-seven patients presented with a palpable mass (10 also had an abnormal mammogram), and 13 presented with an abnormal mammogram only. Four of the women also had bloody nipple discharge at presentation. All patients underwent gross excision of the tumor mass to include a rim of normal breast tissue, and this was done without regard to the microscopic margins. (Margins were not routinely examined during that era.) The breast and adjacent chest wall were treated with radiation therapy using opposed tangent portals to between 46 and 50 gray (Gy), with a further 10 to 20 Gy boost to the primary tumor bed in 26 patients (2). With a median follow-up time of 44 months, four patients developed a recurrence in the treated breast (two with non-invasive and two with invasive cancer). The 5-year actuarial rate of local recurrence was 10%. All four patients were suc-

cessfully salvaged with mastectomy. Three of the recurrences were in the four patients who presented with nipple discharge and a central primary tumor. Resection of the nipple-areola complex was not performed in these patients. Because of the small number of patients, no specific factors could be associated with the development of local failure. However, we suspected that incomplete excision of the tumor was responsible for the four recurrences seen in this series.

At approximately the same time of this publication, we found that patients with invasive breast tumors containing an extensive intraductal component (EIC) had a higher rate of local recurrence than patients without an EIC (3,4). An EIC was defined as a tumor having a prominent component of intraductal carcinoma within the invasive tumor (originally defined as 25% or more of the tumor mass), and having some DCIS in the adjacent grossly normal breast tissue. It was hypothesized that, in many of these patients, a significant amount of residual intraductal carcinoma remained within the breast near or beyond the margins of resection. This hypothesis was later confirmed by pathologic studies of mastectomy specimens (5). A similar situation was thought to apply to patients with pure DCIS without invasion.

Bornstein and colleagues (6) updated the JCRT series in 1991. By this time, it included 38 patients, all of whom were treated solely at the JCRT between 1976 and 1985. Twenty patients had lesions identified only by mammography. The median follow-up was now 81 months. Eight of the 38 patients (21%) experienced recurrence in the breast. Seven of the recurrences were at or near the primary tumor site. All seven underwent salvage mastectomy and were alive without further recurrence. One patient had a recurrence elsewhere in the breast at 83 months; a chest wall recurrence appeared 6 months after mastectomy, and she subsequently developed bone metastasis. No patient developed isolated distant metastasis. The 5-year and 8-year actuarial rates of tumor recurrence in the breast were 8% and 27%, respectively. The rate of recurrence was not significantly associated with any clinical and pathologic factors, but the study population was small. Five of the eight recurrences in the breast were after 5 years. We concluded that the time course to local recurrence after conservative surgery and radiotherapy may be protracted.

The rate of recurrence in the breast in our series was higher than that of most other results published at that time (7–15). We believe this was related to a lack of adequate pretreatment evaluation, as well as to the long follow-up time in our series. For instance, mammograms were not done in eight of the 18 patients who presented with abnormal physical examinations. Therefore, lesions may have been more extensive than we thought. Furthermore, histologic margins were not routinely inked and could be adequately evaluated in only 15 patients (39%). Tumor recurred in the breast in one of five patients with positive margins, and in two of 10 patients with negative margins. Re-excision for tumor involvement at the margins was not routinely performed.

Results from this study confirmed our earlier observation that the frequency, pattern, and time-course of recurrence of patients with DCIS are similar to those of patients with EIC-positive invasive breast tumors (3). The observation that most recurrences after conservative therapy are located at or near the original biopsy site supported the belief that in the majority of patients, DCIS is not multicentric and lesions can be potentially encompassed by a cosmetically acceptable excision. At about this time, Holland and colleagues (16) examined 82 mastectomy specimens of patients with DCIS using serial subgross sections and correlated the extent of DCIS with radiographs. They found that 81 of 82 cancers involved one region of the breast without large areas of uninvolved breast tissue between foci of DCIS.

After this study, we still advocated the use of BCT for selected individuals after careful mammographic and pathologic assessment to determine the adequacy of excision (17); however, we had no firm evidence that such an approach would be effective until the JCRT experience was updated by Hiramatsu and colleagues (18). Between 1976 and 1990, the number of patients in the JCRT series had grown to 76. This report included further follow-up on 36 of 38 patients

previously reported by Bornstein et al. (Two of the original 38 patients in that study were subsequently reclassified as having invasive breast cancer and were excluded.) There were 71 survivors at the time of analysis with a median follow-up time of 74 months (range, 27 to 213 months). No patients were lost to follow-up. The median age at diagnosis was 48 years, with a range of 28 to 76 years.

DCIS was detected by mammography alone in 54 patients (71%), by mammogram and physical examination in 13 patients (17%), and by physical examination alone (with a normal mammogram) in four patients (5%); five other patients who presented with an abnormal physical examination did not have mammograms performed. The most common physical examination finding was a palpable mass (13 of the 22 patients with positive physical examinations), followed by thickening or induration (five patients), and nipple discharge (four patients, of whom three had bloody discharge). For the 67 patients with abnormal mammograms, microcalcifications alone were found in 32, an area of increased density without a definite margin in 21 (20 of the 21 had associated microcalcifications), 10 had a mass (7 of 10 also had microcalcifications), and for the remaining four patients, the findings were unknown.

Table 35.1 demonstrates the change in patients and treatment characteristics between the cohort of patients treated from 1976 through 1985 reported previously by Bornstein et al., and those treated between 1986 and 1990. Fifty-nine percent of the patients in the earlier cohort had an abnormality detectable on physical examination compared with only 7% in the more recent cohort. Improvements in the quality of mammography together with an increase in routine screening during the time period spanned by the later cohort may be responsible for more patients being diagnosed with nonpalpable mammographically detected lesions. Guidelines for the evaluation of patients with mammographically detected nonpalpable lesions with microcalcifications, published by Schnitt et al. (17), were commonly followed during the period of the recent time cohort. These guidelines stressed the importance of re-excision of positive margins and the value of specimen radiographs and postex-

TABLE 35.1. CHARACTERISTICS OF TIME COHORTS OF BREAST-CONSERVING THERAPY WITH RADIATION THERAPY

Characteristic	1977–1985 Cohort	1986–1990 Cohort	1991–1995 Cohort
No. of patients	34	42	64
Nonpalpable	14 (41%)	39 (93%)	56 (89%)[a]
Re-excision	11 (32%)	39 (93%)	51 (80%)
Margins			
Positive	2 (6%)	9 (21%)	8 (12%)
Close/negative	12 (35%)	33 (79%)	44 (69%)
Unknown	20 (59%)	0	12 (19%)
Median TTV (cm³)	31.6	74.0	79.1

[a] Includes nonpalpable or unknown.

cision mammography. In the more recent cohort, 93% of patients had a re-excision compared with only 32% in the earlier cohort. Moreover, specimen radiographs and postexcision mammograms were rarely done prior to 1986, but were often obtained for the recent cohort.

The total tissue volume (TTV) of grossly excised breast tissue was significantly larger for patients in the later cohort than those in the earlier one. The TTV was calculated by multiplying thickness by width by length of the specimen using the maximum dimensions of the gross specimen from the pathology report (19). In cases in which multiple specimens or fragments were removed, the volume of each fragment was calculated, and all volumes were summed. If there was a re-excision after an initial biopsy, then the volumes of both excisions were added. Sixty-three patients had gross pathologic descriptions adequate to permit the calculation of TTV. The median TTV for the patients treated from 1986 to 1990 was 74 cm^3, compared with only 31.6 cm^3 for the group treated from 1976 to 1985.

Radiation therapy consisted of 45 to 50 Gy given to the entire breast using daily fractions of 1.8 to 2.0 Gy. Seventy-two patients (95%) had a boost to the primary site. The median total radiation dose to the primary site was 61 Gy (range, 46 to 71). Sixty-six patients (87%) received 60 Gy or more. The median time interval between the last breast surgery and the start of radiation therapy was 6 weeks, with a range of 2 to 14 weeks. No patients received adjuvant systemic therapy.

Seven patients (9%) recurred in the treated breast at 16, 18, 41, 63, 72, 83, and 104 months after treatment. Three recurrences were DCIS, and four were invasive breast cancer. The 5- and 10-year actuarial rates of local recurrence were 4% and 15%, respectively. Three patients had a "true recurrence" (within the boost area or at the site of the primary tumor), three a "marginal miss" (just outside the borders of the boost), and one lesion (described earlier) recurred elsewhere in the breast. All recurrences were detected by mammogram; one patient also had an abnormal physical examination. All seven patients underwent salvage mastectomy. Contralateral invasive breast cancer was eventually diagnosed in two patients. No patient developed isolated distant metastasis. The 5-and 10-year cause-specific survival rates for the entire population were 100% and 96%, respectively.

We examined several factors that may be related to the rate of recurrence in the breast (Table 35.2). The first was the method of initial tumor detection. Four local recurrences (7%) were found in the 54 patients who presented with mammographically detected DCIS with negative physical examinations. One of four was an invasive breast cancer. Three (14%) of 22 patients with an abnormal physical examination (regardless of mammographic findings) developed a breast recurrence; all three were invasive.

The number of recurrences in each time cohort was examined. Six of seven recurrences were seen in patients from the earlier cohort treated between 1976 and 1985. At 6.5 years, the actuarial local recurrence rate was 12% for the earlier cohort, compared with 2% for the later cohort ($p = 0.3$). Of note, the follow-up time for the recent cohort was still relatively short, with a median of 55 months.

We examined the rate of local recurrence in relation to the total volume of tissue excised. The median TTV was 60 cm^3, and this was used to divide patients into two groups. The 10-year actuarial local recurrence rate was 25% in the group with a TTV less than 60 cm^3 and 0% for those with a TTV of 60 cm^3 or greater ($p = 0.04$). Therefore, patients with DCIS appeared to benefit from wide, rather than limited, resection. Similarly, we and others have found that a larger excision volume is associated with better local control for EIC-positive invasive tumors (19,20).

Margin status did not appear to significantly influence the risk of recurrence. There were no recurrences in the 11 patients with positive margins (defined as tumor at an inked edge), one recurrence in 11 patients (9%) with close margins (defined as tumor being present within 1 mm of the resection margins), two recurrences in 34 patients (6%) with negative margins (wider than 1 mm), and four recurrences among 20 patients (20%) with unknown margins.

We also examined the relationship between a family history of breast cancer and patient outcome in 75 patients for whom such information was available. The 10-year actuarial rate of local recurrence was 37% in the 17 patients with a positive family history of breast cancer (a first-degree or second-degree relative), compared with 9% in the 58 patients with a negative family history ($p = 0.008$). Of note, one patient who recurred without a family history at initial diagnosis had a daughter who subsequently developed breast cancer. McCormick and coworkers (10) also reported an association between a family history of breast cancer and recurrence in patients treated with conservative surgery and radiation therapy. Forty percent of patients with a local recurrence had a positive family history in a first-degree relative, compared with 11% of patients without a local recurrence. These data are provocative, and more work is needed in this area.

Other factors, such as the interval from last breast surgery to the start of radiation therapy or age at diagnosis, did not significantly affect the rate of recurrence in the breast.

In summary, our results showed improvement over time, and the volume of resected tissue was the major factor associated with the rate of recurrence.

We next updated and expanded our series in 2000 (21). This study included 136 patients treated at the JCRT from 1976 to 1994, with updated outcome on 68 of the 74 patients included in the report by Hiramatsu et al. Patients eligible for this study had a minimum potential follow-up of 5 years with a median follow-up time of 8.7 years. The median radiotherapy dose delivered to the primary tumor bed was 60 Gy (range, 46 to 71 Gy).

In this cohort, DCIS was detectable by mammography in 122 patients (89%), and 30 patients (22%) had a palpable mass. The incidence of a palpable mass correlated with the

TABLE 35.2. LOCAL RECURRENCE RATES: CORRELATION WITH CLINICAL AND TREATMENT CHARACTERISTICS

Clinical Factor	No. of Pts.	No. of LR	Actuarial LR Rates 5-Year	Actuarial LR Rates 10-Year
Age at diagnosis (yr)				
<49	39	4	8%	12%
>50	37	3	0%	17%
Family history				
Positive	17	4	12%	37%[a]
Negative	58	3	2%	9%[a]
Unknown	1	0	—	—
Detection mode of primary tumor				
MMG(+), PE(−)	54	4	2%	23%
Any MMG, PE (+)	22	3	9%	14%
Re-excision				
Yes	50	3	7%	7%
No	26	4	0%	17%
Margins (by report)				
Positive	11	0	0%	0%
Close	11	1	9%	9%
Negative	34	2	4%	11%
Unknown	20	4	5%	20%
Total excision volume				
<59.9 cm	32	6	9%	25%[b]
>60.0 cm	31	0	0%	0%[b]
Unknown	13	1	—	—
Surgery-radiotherapy interval				
<42 days	33	3	6%	11%
>43 days	41	3	2%	14%
Unknown	2	1	—	—
Time cohort				
1976–1985	34	6	6%	12%[c]
1986–1990	42	1	2%	3%[c]

From Hiramatsu H, Bornstein BA, Recht A, et al. Local recurrence after conservative surgery and radiation therapy for ductal carcinoma in situ—possible importance of family history. *Cancer J Sci Am* 1995;1:55–61, with permission.
[a] $p = 0.008$.
[b] $p = 0.04$.
[c] Percent at 6.5 years, $p = $ NS.
MMG, mammography; PE, physical examination; LR, local recurrence.

era in which the patient presented, showing a progressive decrease over time (Table 35.1). Among the 62 patients treated between 1991 and 1994, 7 (11%) had a palpable mass on physical exam. Twenty-two patients (29%) treated between 1986 and 1990 presented with a palpable mass. In contrast, 20 patients (59%) treated between 1976 and 1985 (prior to the era of routine mammographic screening) presented with a palpable mass.

TTV in the most recent cohort was 79.1 cm³, with 61 patients (98%) undergoing re-excision.

Because of the shorter length of follow-up in the most recently treated cohort, we limited the analysis to results at five years. At that point, 130 (95%) patients were alive without evidence of disease; there were no distant failures or deaths. There were four ipsilateral local recurrences (3%).

The times to development of local recurrence were 16, 18, 41, and 57 months. This low rate of local recurrence after BCS and RT was consistent with reported actuarial results at 5 years from other modern series that ranged from 1% to 11% (15,22–24). Of the four ipsilateral recurrences, three were invasive carcinomas and one was DCIS. Three of the four ipsilateral recurrences were marginal misses and one was in an undetermined site within the breast. Two patients (1%) developed contralateral breast cancers that occurred 16 and 30 months after diagnosis.

All recurrences were among patients diagnosed at younger than age 50. Contemporary reports by other groups with relatively long follow-up have also reported an increased risk of recurrence among younger women (22,24–27). We examined this subgroup for possible factors associated with recurrence. In a logistic regression model performed among patients younger than 50 years old, patients with TTV less than 60 cm³ had a local recurrence rate of 11% (three of 26), compared with 11% (one of nine) among patients with TTV greater than 60 cm³. However, the number of events in any subgroup was small; hence, the reliability of these findings may be limited.

The histologic specimen slides from 97 patients are currently under review.

In summary, our results showed that improvement in local failure rates occurred as we gained experience in managing patients with DCIS. In the report by Hiramatsu, TTV was a major factor associated with the rate of recurrence. In our most recent report, TTV was not found to be a major factor; however, this may be due to the small number of events that occurred. Young patient age appears to have emerged as an important risk factor.

WIDE EXCISION ALONE

The National Surgical Adjuvant Breast and Bowel Project (NSABP) Trial B-17 randomized patients with DCIS with "negative" margins (defined as a one parenchymal cell or more between the tumor and the inked specimen edge) to radiation or no further therapy following excision. Radiotherapy caused a statistically significant reduction in local recurrence at 8 years (28). Similar reductions in local recurrence were more recently reported in another randomized trial performed by the European Organization for the Treatment and Research of Cancer (EORTC) (29). However, because the NSABP B-17 trial was relatively unselective with regard to patient entry (especially the tumor-free margin width), we did not feel that the question of whether highly selected patients can undergo excision alone without radiation therapy had been settled. Other improvements were also made in the diagnosis and management of patients with DCIS after the creation of the B-17 trial. For example, the use of magnification views in mammographic evaluation was shown to more accurately delineate the extent of the lesion (16). In addition, factors consistently found to be associated with increased risk for recurrence in single-institution series included the size and grade of the lesion, as well as pathologic margin status (8,11,30–34).

To address this question, we retrospectively evaluated the outcome of 59 patients who were treated with excision alone between 1985 and 1990 by our collaborating surgeons in the hospital in the Longwood Medical Area served by the JCRT. As reported by Hetelekidis et al. (35), patients in this study had available follow-up, histologic slides for central review, and negative histologic margins. The median age was 54 years at the time of diagnosis (range, 37 to 83 years). At the time of analysis, there were 56 survivors with a median follow-up time of 95.5 months (range, 34 to 141 months).

DCIS was detected by mammographic findings only in 54 (96%) of the 56 patients who were evaluated for method of detection. Further information regarding the number of patients with magnification views, specimen radiographs, or post-biopsy mammograms was unavailable.

All histologic slides were centrally reviewed. Pathologic margin status was scored "negative" when tumor cells were seen more than 1 mm from the inked surface and "close" when tumor cells were within 1 mm or less of the margin. Lesion size was determined by the number of low-power fields (LPF) where DCIS was present using a microscope with a $4\times$ objective and a $10\times$ ocular field (field diameter, 5 mm; field area, 19.6 mm²).

Ten lesions recurred in the breast at intervals ranging from 5 to 132 months after excision. The 5-year actuarial rate of local recurrence was 10%. Six of ten patients had mammographically detected recurrences, and the method of detection was unknown in the remaining four patients. Six recurrences were DCIS only, and four recurrences were invasive carcinoma. No patients developed systemic metastases or died of breast cancer. Four patients were censored upon diagnosis of contralateral breast cancer, and none of these patients had an ipsilateral recurrence.

Several factors were evaluated for association with increased risk for recurrence (Table 35.3). On univariate analysis, lesion size was the only factor significantly associated with local recurrence. The 5-year actuarial recurrence rate among patients with lesions measuring larger than 5 LPF was 17% compared with 3% among patients with smaller lesions ($p = 0.02$). Although no other factors were statistically significant, several trends were observed. Patients with a histologically negative resection margin had a local recurrence rate of 8% compared with 25% among patients with close margins. Among patients with a negative re-excision, the local recurrence rate was 6%, compared with 14% among patients with residual disease present in the re-excision. Local recurrence was more frequent among patients with nuclear grade (NG) 3 lesions, compared with NG 1 or 2 lesions. Of note, there were no local recurrences among the 19 patients with tumors less than 2.5 cm in size that were NG 1 or 2 and that had tumor-free margin widths of greater than 1 mm.

CONCLUSIONS AND CURRENT MANAGEMENT POLICY

The reports discussed illustrate the development in the JCRT clinical practice over the last two decades and demonstrate how patient selection, techniques of evaluation, and treatment policies have changed substantially over this period. As a result of these ongoing investigations at our institutions and others, we have begun to understand which factors are associated with an increased risk for recurrence following BCT with or without radiotherapy.

TABLE 35.3. PROGNOSTIC FACTORS FOR RECURRENCE IN PATIENTS WITH DUCTAL CARCINOMA IN SITU TREATED WITH EXCISION ALONE

Factor	No. Patients	Actuarial 5-Yr Local Failure Rate (%)	p Value
Patient age			
≤54	28	11	0.84
>54	31	10	
Family history			
Positive	15	0	0.44
Negative	31	13	
Unknown	13		
Residual in re-excision			
Present	22	14	0.22
Absent	35	6	
Unknown	2		
Lesion size			
≤5 LPF	31	3	0.02
>5 LPF	24	17	
Unknown	(4)		
Nuclear grade			
1	16	6	0.27
2	21	5	
3	22	18	
Final margin status			
Negative	51	8	0.40
Close (≤1 mm)	8	25	
Total tissue volume			
≤73 cm³	24	13	0.98
>73 cm³	23	13	
Unknown	12		
Predominant architectural pattern	11	18	0.15
Comedo	48	9	
Other			
Necrosis			
Absent	16	6	0.81
Central	29	14	
Small foci	13	8	
Mixed	1	0	

From Hetelekidis S, Collins L, Silver B, et. al. Predictors of local recurrence following excision alone for ductal carcinoma in situ. *Cancer* 1999;85:427–431, with permission.
LR, Local Recurrence; LPF, low-power field

These efforts have substantially reduced the risk of local failure. We expect that further clinical trials and retrospective studies will further improve our results. In addition, DCIS appears to be a heterogeneous group of lesions, and an optimal histologic and biologic classification still needs to be established. We have great hopes that the discovery and development of genetic and biologic markers and other new tools will help guide clinicians and patients in making treatment choices.

We believe that the keystone of optimal management of patients with DCIS is a multidisciplinary approach requiring close and constant collaboration between the surgeon, radiation oncologist, pathologist, and diagnostic radiologist.

Patients interested in breast-conserving therapy should undergo careful mammographic and pathologic evaluation. This includes the use of magnification views to determine the extent of microcalcifications, routine specimen mammography of needle-localization specimens, and the selective use of post-biopsy mammograms to confirm that all the suspicious microcalcifications have been removed. Pathologic evaluation requires inking of the margins of the excised specimen and a careful gross description of the specimen. The microscopic description should state the relationship between the calcifications and the DCIS or benign breast tissue and the distance between the DCIS and the inked margin. A re-excision is often necessary to achieve adequate margins if the tumor microscopically involves the margins of resection or if residual microcalcifications are seen on post-biopsy mammograms. The relative importance of meticulous mammographic and pathologic evaluation compared with large excision volumes is still uncertain. Because of the very small risk of axillary node metastasis, axillary dissection is reserved for patients with extensive lesions treated with mastectomy or those whose tumors contain foci suggestive of invasion.

Mastectomy is usually recommended for patients with lesions larger than 4 to 5cm in maximum diameter, tumors that spread diffusely through one or more quadrants of the breast, or patients with positive margins on re-excision. We do not use family history as a selection factor favoring mastectomy due to the presence of contradictory results on this subject from other investigators. We also have not yet felt that patient age should modify the management of patients with DCIS.

Radiotherapy consists of a dose of 44 to 46 Gy given to the entire breast in 22 to 25 fractions over 4.5 to 5 weeks. A boost of 16 Gy in eight fractions is given to the involved quadrant, usually with electrons of appropriate energy (prescribed to the 80% isodose line).

The use of tamoxifen has been reported in a single randomized trial (NSABP B-24) to reduce the risk of recurrence in women receiving BCS and radiation therapy for DCIS (36). This effect was seen predominantly for patients younger than age 50 and for those with positive or unknown margins. Tamoxifen will also clearly reduce the risk of development of contralateral primaries or new ipsilateral primaries. However, we do not feel that tamoxifen should as yet be considered "standard" treatment for all patients with DCIS because of the lack of long-term follow-up (especially with regard to overall and breast cancer–specific survival rates), adequate subgroup analysis, and the absence of corroborating data from other trials. Given the available data, we believe tamoxifen may reasonably be given to individuals who are adequately informed about the risks of such treatment as well as the limitations of our understanding of its long-term benefits.

We continue to be interested in whether some patients can avoid radiation therapy after BCS. We therefore created an observational protocol for patients treated in the Harvard teaching hospitals several years ago. To be eligible, patients must have low or intermediate–nuclear grade DCIS clinically measuring 2.5 cm or smaller, high-quality mammograms with magnification views (ideally done prior to excision), no evidence of diffuse microcalcifications, a specimen mammogram showing complete removal of all suspicious microcalcifications, and histologically negative margins of at least 1 cm. This study has nearly reached its accrual goal. Based on our own past results and those of other investigators, we believe that excision alone is reasonable treatment for such highly selected individuals outside a protocol setting as well.

REFERENCES

1. Recht A, Danoff BS, Solin LJ, et al. Intraductal carcinoma of the breast: results of treatment with excisional biopsy and irradiation. *J Clin Oncol* 1985;3:1339–1343.
2. Harris JR, Botnick L, Bloomer WD, et al. Primary radiation therapy for early breast cancer: the experience at The Joint Center for Radiation Therapy. *Int J Radiat Oncol Biol Phys* 1981;7:1549–1552.
3. Harris JR, Connolly JL, Schnitt SJ, et al. The use of pathologic features in selecting the extent of surgical resection necessary for breast cancer patients treated by primary radiation therapy. *Ann Surg* 1985;201:164–169.
4. Schnitt SJ, Connolly JL, Harris JR, et al. Pathologic predictors of early local recurrence in Stage I and II breast cancer treated by primary radiation therapy. *Cancer* 1984;53:1049–1057.
5. Holland R, Connolly JL, Gelman R, et al. The presence of an extensive intraductal component following a limited excision correlates with prominent residual disease in the remainder of the breast. *J Clin Oncol* 1990;8:113–118.
6. Bornstein BA, Recht A, Connolly JL, et al. Results of treating ductal carcinoma in situ of the breast with conservative surgery and radiation therapy. *Cancer* 1991;67:7–13.
7. Fourquet A, Zafrani B, Campana F, et al. Breast-Conserving Treatment of Ductal Carcinoma In Situ. *Semin Radiat Oncol* 1992;2:116–124.
8. Fisher B, Costantino J, Redmond C, et al. Lumpectomy compared with lumpectomy and radiation therapy for the treatment of intraductal breast cancer [see comments]. *N Engl J Med* 1993;328:1581–1586.
9. Kurtz JM, Jacquemier J, Torhorst J, et al. Conservation therapy for breast cancers other than infiltrating ductal carcinoma. *Cancer* 1989;63:1630–1635.
10. McCormick B, Rosen PP, Kinne D, et al. Duct carcinoma in situ of the breast: an analysis of local control after conservation surgery and radiotherapy. *Int J Radiat Oncol Biol Phys* 1991;21:289–292.
11. Silverstein MJ, Cohlan BF, Gierson ED, et al. Duct carcinoma in situ: 227 cases without microinvasion [see comments]. *Eur J Cancer* 1992;28:630–634.
12. Solin LJ, Yeh IT, Kurtz J, et al. Ductal carcinoma in situ (intraductal carcinoma) of the breast treated with breast-conserving surgery and definitive irradiation. Correlation of pathologic parameters with outcome of treatment. *Cancer* 1993;71:2532–2542.
13. Stotter AT, McNeese M, Oswald MJ, et al. The role of limited surgery with irradiation in primary treatment of ductal in situ breast cancer. *Int J Radiat Oncol Biol Phys* 1990;18:283–287.
14. Ray GR, Adelson J, Hayhurst E, et al. Ductal carcinoma in situ of the breast: results of treatment by conservative surgery and definitive irradiation. *Int J Radiat Oncol Biol Phys* 1994;28:105–111.
15. Kuske RR, Bean JM, Garcia DM, et al. Breast conservation therapy for intraductal carcinoma of the breast [see comments]. *Int J Radiat Oncol Biol Phys* 1993;26:391–396.
16. Holland R, Hendriks JH, Vebeek AL, et al. Extent, distribution, and mammographic/histological correlations of breast ductal carcinoma in situ. *Lancet* 1990;335:519–522.
17. Schnitt SJ, Silen W, Sadowsky NL, et al. Ductal carcinoma in situ (intraductal carcinoma) of the breast. *N Engl J Med* 1988;318:898–903.
18. Hiramatsu H, Bornstein BA, Recht A, et al. Local Recurrence After Conservative Surgery and Radiation Therapy for Ductal Carcinoma in Situ. *Cancer J* 1995;1:55.

19. Vicini FA, Eberlein TJ, Connolly JL, et al. The optimal extent of resection for patients with stages I or II breast cancer treated with conservative surgery and radiotherapy. *Ann Surg* 1991;214:200–204; discussion 204–205.

20. Veronesi U, Luini A, Galimberti V, et al. Conservation approaches for the management of stage I/II carcinoma of the breast: Milan Cancer Institute trials. *World J Surg* 1994;18:70–75.

21. Park CC, Recht A, Gelmon R, et al. The impact of young age on outcome after breast-conserving surgery and radiation therapy for carcinoma in situ of the breast. Proceeding of the American Society for Therapeutic Radiology and Oncology, (Abs. 2058), 2000.

22. Kestin LL, Goldstein NS, Lacerna MD, et al. Factors associated with local recurrence of mammographically detected ductal carcinoma in situ in patients given breast-conserving therapy. *Cancer* 2000;88:596–607.

23. Fowble B, Hanlon AL, Fein DA, et al. Results of conservative surgery and radiation for mammographically detected ductal carcinoma in situ (DCIS). *Int J Radiat Oncol Biol Phys* 1997;38:949–957.

24. Van Zee KJ, Liberman L, Samli B, et al. Long-term follow-up of women with ductal carcinoma in situ treated with breast-conserving surgery: the effect of age. *Cancer* 1999;86:1757–1767.

25. Solin LJ, Kurtz J, Fourquet A, et al. Fifteen-year results of breast-conserving surgery and definitive breast irradiation for the treatment of ductal carcinoma in situ of the breast. *J Clin Oncol* 1996;14:754–763.

26. Vicini FA, Kestin LL, Goldstein NS, et al. Impact of young age on outcome in patients with ductal carcinoma-in-situ treated with breast-conserving therapy. *J Clin Oncol* 2000;18:296–306.

27. Fisher ER, Dignam J, Tan-Chiu E, et al. Pathologic findings from the National Surgical Adjuvant Breast Project (NSABP) eight-year update of Protocol B-17: intraductal carcinoma [see comments]. *Cancer* 1999;86:429–438.

28. Fisher B, Dignam J, Wolmark N, et al. Lumpectomy and radiation therapy for the treatment of intraductal breast cancer: findings from National Surgical Adjuvant Breast and Bowel Project B-17. *J Clin Oncol* 1998;16:441–452.

29. Julien JP, Bijker N, Fentiman IS, et al. Radiotherapy in breast-conserving treatment for ductal carcinoma in situ: first results of the EORTC randomised phase III trial 10853. EORTC Breast Cancer Cooperative Group and EORTC Radiotherapy Group [see comments]. *Lancet* 2000;355:528–533.

30. Arnesson LG, Smeds S, Fagerberg G, et al. Follow-up of two treatment modalities for ductal cancer in situ of the breast. *Br J Surg* 1989;76:672–5.

31. Carpenter R, Boulter PS, Cooke T, et al. Management of screen detected ductal carcinoma in situ of the female breast. *Br J Surg* 1989;76:564–567.

32. Fisher ER, Leeming R, Anderson S, et al. Conservative management of intraductal carcinoma (DCIS) of the breast. Collaborating NSABP investigators. *J Surg Oncol* 1991;47:139–147.

33. Lagios MD, Margolin FR, Westdahl PR, et al. Mammographically detected duct carcinoma in situ. Frequency of local recurrence following tylectomy and prognostic effect of nuclear grade on local recurrence. *Cancer* 1989;63:618–624.

34. Schwartz GF, Finkel GC, Garcia JC, et al. Subclinical ductal carcinoma in situ of the breast. Treatment by local excision and surveillance alone [see comments]. *Cancer* 1992;70:2468–2474.

35. Hetelekidis S, Collins L, Silver B, et al. Predictors of local recurrence following excision alone for ductal carcinoma in situ. *Cancer* 1999;85:427–431.

36. Fisher B, Dignam J, Wolmark N, et al. Tamoxifen in treatment of intraductal breast cancer: National Surgical Adjuvant Breast and Bowel Project B-24 randomised controlled trial [see comments]. *Lancet* 1999;353:1993–2000.

36

THE IMPACT OF YOUNG AGE ON OUTCOME IN PATIENTS WITH DUCTAL CARCINOMA IN SITU: THE WILLIAM BEAUMONT HOSPITAL EXPERIENCE

FRANK A. VICINI
LARRY KESTIN
JOHN INGOLD
ALVARO A. MARTINEZ

The influence of age at diagnosis on the success of breast-conserving therapy (BCT) in patients with ductal carcinoma in situ (DCIS) of the breast has not been extensively studied. Although the association between young age and the prognosis of patients with invasive breast cancer suggests a poorer overall outcome, published results in patients with DCIS have not been conclusive (1–5). Recent data from our institution document a significantly higher rate of local recurrence in younger patients with DCIS that is independent of previously defined prognostic factors (6–11). Since the publication of our data, larger national studies have corroborated our initial observations (12). Both the National Surgical Adjuvant Breast and Bowel Project (NSABP) B-24 randomized trial of over 1,800 women with DCIS treated with BCT (12) and a collaborative study of pooled cases of mammographically detected DCIS treated with BCT at 11 institutions in North America and Europe recently published by Solin et al. (13) substantiate the potential differences in outcome attributable to age at diagnosis. At the present time, these data suggest that young age is an additional risk factor that should be taken into consideration when determining the acceptability of a patient for BCT. However, it remains uncertain if this increased risk of local recurrence is related to an inherently worse biologic behavior in younger patients or to treatment-related factors that can be overcome with meticulous attention to detail. It is important to point out that differences in outcome with mastectomy have also not been extensively analyzed based on patient age. More importantly, it does not appear that cancer-specific survival is compromised in younger patients undergoing BCT. In this chapter, we will review the body of literature addressing the influence of patient age on outcome with the goals of defining potential differences in clinical, pathologic, biologic, and treatment-related factors based on patient age.

SUMMARY OF THE LITERATURE

The body of literature addressing the impact of patient age at diagnosis on outcome with BCT for DCIS has been relatively inconsistent. This is due to the fact that:

(i) the definition of young age has been variable from study to study ranging in years from less than or equal to 39 to less than or equal to 45 or less than or equal to 50;
(ii) many older series consist of few patients with relatively short follow-up;
(iii) most studies do not have complete pathologic reviews;
(iv) the methods of statistical analysis have varied significantly between studies; and
(v) the definitions of critical pathologic variables (e.g., histology, grade, margins, etc.) have not been consistently applied.

Table 36.1 lists the major studies that have addressed this issue. Although there are a few exceptions, larger trials seem to suggest a significant difference in outcome based on age. Results from several of the most important series will be reviewed below.

National Surgical Adjuvant Breast and Bowel Project Protocol B-24

One of the largest studies of patients with DCIS treated with BCT that reported outcome based on patient age was the recently published NSABP B-24 randomized trial (12). This well-designed study randomized 1,804 women with DCIS (including those whose resection margins were involved with DCIS) to either lumpectomy, radiation therapy

TABLE 36.1. STUDIES ADDRESSING PATIENT AGE AT DIAGNOSIS VERSUS OUTCOME WITH BREAST-CONSERVING THERAPY

Series (Ref.)	Age Group (Years)	No. Patients	No. Recurrences	Recurrence Rate 5-Year	Recurrence Rate 10-Year
Institut Curie (36)	≤40	24	7	—	30[b]
	>40	129	18	—	14
Fowble et al. (18)	≤40	8	1	25[c]	—
	>40	102	2	0	—
Hiramatsu et al. (17)	≤49	39	4	8[c]	12
	>50	37	3	0	17
NSABP B-17 (14)	≤49	137	21	15[c]	—
	50–59	115	12	11[d]	—
	≥60	151	14	9[d]	—
NSABP B-24 (12)	≤49	602	79	13.2[b]	—
	≥50	1,196	63	5.3	—
Solin et al. (13)	≤39	31	10	20[a]	31[a]
	≥60	391	38	5	6
Van Zee et al. (15)	<40	15	6	47.2[b]	—
	40–69	103	19	14.0	—
	≥70	39	3	10.8	—
Vicini et al. (6)	<45	31	7	21[a]	26[a]
	≥45	117	10	7	9
Szelei-Stevens et al. (21)	≤50	44	4	9%[c]	—
	>50	84	2	2%	—
Harris et al. (20)	≤39	12	1	8%[c]	—
	40–49	39	5	13%	—
	≥50	92	8	9%	—

[a] Statistically significant on multivariate analysis; [b] Statistically significant on univariate analysis; [c] Not statistically significant; [d] Crude recurrence rate.

(RT), and placebo (*n* = 902), or lumpectomy, RT, and tamoxifen (20 mg daily for 5 years, *n* = 902). With a median follow-up of 74 months, 150 local recurrences were noted in the ipsilateral breast (both invasive and noninvasive). Young age at diagnosis (defined as < 49 years) was significantly associated with recurrence of the ipsilateral breast tumor. Younger patients in both treatment groups were at higher risk than older patients for such an event. The crude rate of local recurrence in women < 49 years of age receiving placebo (and treated with lumpectomy plus RT) was 16% (48 of 300) versus 6.5% in patients age 50 or older (39 of 599) treated in a similar fashion. Likewise, the crude rate of local recurrence in patients treated with tamoxifen (plus lumpectomy and RT) was 11% (32 of 302) in patients less than or equal to 49 years of age versus 5.2% (31 of 597) in older patients (≥ 50 years). These differences were statistically significant. The annual rate of ipsilateral breast tumor per 1000 women age 49 years or younger who received placebo was 33.3 and was 13.03 for those age 50 or older. Tamoxifen administration resulted in a 38% reduction in ipsilateral breast tumors in women younger than 50 years and a 22% reduction in women older than 50 years.

No attempt was made to determine if young age was an independent risk factor for local recurrence in the NSABP B-24 trial. Positive margins, the presence of comedo necrosis, and the method of detection were also associated with local recurrence. It remains uncertain how each of these variables independently affected results. In addition, the type of local recurrence [e.g., true recurrence/marginal miss (TR/MM) versus elsewhere (E)] was not discussed. Despite the obvious negative effect young age had on outcome, it is difficult to determine if the incidence and/or type of local recurrence were a direct result of incomplete surgical excision or of a biologically more aggressive tumor in younger patients. Unlike the previous NSABP B-17 trial that did *not* demonstrate a statistically significant difference in outcome based on patient age (see Table 36.1), the B-24 trial enrolled women with more extensive DCIS (14). Whether this explains, *in part*, the significant difference in local recurrence due to patient age remains uncertain. We recently demonstrated that younger patients with DCIS undergoing BCT have smaller initial excision volumes (65% versus 45% < 25 cm³, *p* = 0.06), more frequent close or positive margins, a greater proportion of high–nuclear grade DCIS, and central necrosis (6,10). Each of these variables has been reported in several other studies as being associated with the development of tumor recurrence after BCT. It is likely, although certainly not proven, that the less stringent enrollment criteria in the B-24 trial may have accounted for *part* of the higher incidence of local failure in a subset of patients (younger age) with a greater incidence of risk factors for the development of this event.

Collaborative Ductal Carcinoma in Situ Study

Solin et al. (13) recently published the results of one of the largest databases of patients treated with BCT for mammographically detected DCIS from 11 institutions in North America and Europe. A total of 422 cases in 418 women were retrospectively analyzed, and risk factors for local recurrence were studied (see Chapter 33). With a median follow-up of 9.4 years, a total of 48 local failures were detected for a 15-year rate of 16%. Young patient age (defined as ≤ 39 years) at the time of treatment and positive margin status from the primary tumor were both significantly associated with local failure ($p = 0.0006$ and $p = 0.023$, respectively) in a multivariate Cox regression model. Age 40 to 49 years was associated with an increased risk of local recurrence that was borderline for statistical significance ($p = 0.098$). The 10-year rate of local failure was 31% for patient age less than or equal to 39 years, 13% for age 40 to 49 years, 8% for age 50 to 59 years, and 6% for age greater than or equal to 60 years ($p = 0.0001$). Analysis by type of local failure showed significant differences by age for invasive local recurrence and DCIS local recurrence. The 10-year rate of invasive local recurrence was 15% for patients less than or equal to 39 years old, 4% for age 40 to 49 years, 4% for age 50 to 59 years, and 6% for patients greater than or equal to 60 years old ($p = 0.015$). The 10-year rate of DCIS local recurrence was 19% for patients less than or equal to 39 years old, 9% for age 40 to 49 years, 4% for age 50 to 59 years, and 1% for patients greater than or equal to 60 years old ($p = 0.0008$).

The crude incidence of local failure for women less than or equal to 39 years old in the Solin study was 2 of 18 (11%) when margins of resection were negative, 4 of 5 (80%) when margins were positive, 2 of 3 (67%) when the margins were close, and 2 of 5 (40%) when the margins of resection were unknown. Although these crude rates of local recurrence were based on small patient numbers, they suggest that obtaining negative margins of resection may be especially important in younger patients, because only 2 of 18 patients (≤ 39 years of age) with negative margins failed. Unfortunately, the authors were unable to analyze outcome based on the type (location) of the local recurrence. As a result, their results are somewhat clouded by the fact that their rates of local recurrence are based on failures of both the index lesion (e.g., TR/MM failure) and of *de novo* cancers (e.g., E failures) not necessarily related to treatment of the primary DCIS lesion. We have previously shown that different risk factors for local recurrence can be obtained if these two types of local recurrences are analyzed together or separately (6,11). Even without this critical method of analysis, however, it is interesting to note the profoundly negative, independent effect young age had on the rate of local recurrence.

Memorial Sloan-Kettering Cancer Center

Van Zee et al. (15) recently updated their experience in patients with DCIS undergoing BCT at Memorial Sloan-Kettering Cancer Center (MSKCC). From 1978 to 1990, 171 cases of DCIS were treated either with lumpectomy alone or lumpectomy plus postoperative RT, of which 157 were available for analysis. Factors that were significantly associated with a lower recurrence rate were older age, noncomedo subtype, lower nuclear grade, negative margins, and postoperative RT. Comparison of patients of ages greater than or equal to 70, 40 to 69, and less than 40 years revealed a significantly lower risk of recurrence with increasing age. Actuarial 6-year local relapse rates were 10.8%, 14.0%, and 47.2%, respectively ($p = 0.047$). A benefit from radiation therapy was suggested for each age group.

Despite the significant differences in local recurrence based on age noted in the MSKCC study, it should be pointed out that margin status was unknown in 53% of patients, patients not receiving RT were analyzed together with those that did, and on multivariate analysis, only margin status was associated with local recurrence ($p = 0.05$). As a result, it is difficult to determine the independent influence young age had on outcome. Nonetheless, these results also attest to the importance of accounting for patient age when considering a patient with DCIS for BCT.

William Beaumont Hospital Experience

We recently published our experience in treating patients with DCIS with BCT and analyzed the risk factors for local recurrence (6). From 1980 to 1993, 146 patients were managed with lumpectomy followed by postoperative RT to a median total tumor bed dose of 60.4 gray (Gy). Slides on every patient were reviewed by one pathologist. The median follow-up period was 7.2 years.

Seventeen patients developed an ipsilateral recurrence for 5- and 10-year actuarial rates of 10.2% and 12.4%, respectively (Table 36.2). The 10-year rate of ipsilateral failure was 26.1% in patients younger than 45 years of age versus 8.6% in older patients ($p = 0.03$). On multivariate analysis, young age was independently associated with recurrence of the index lesion (TR/MM failure), regardless of how it was analyzed (e.g., < 45 years of age or as a continuous variable). Other variables that were independently associated with the development of local recurrence included the number of slides with DCIS, margin status, the number of DCIS or cancerization of lobules (COL) foci less than or equal to 5 mm from the margin, and the absence of pathologic calcifications (Table 36.3). Similar to the Solin study, younger patients had a dramatically higher 10-year rate of invasive TR/MM failures (19.2% versus 3.2%). When a separate multivariate analysis was performed only for the development of invasive TR/MM failures, patient age and the predominant nuclear grade were the only factors associated

TABLE 36.2. FAILURE CHARACTERISTICS BASED ON PATIENT AGE–WILLIAM BEAUMONT HOSPITAL EXPERIENCE

Type of Recurrence	Age <45		Age ≥45		p Value[a]
	5 Years	10 Years	5 Years	10 Years	
Ipsilateral breast failure	20.8%	26.1%	7.3%	8.6%	0.03
Non-invasive	3.3%	3.3%	2.8%	2.8%	0.83
Invasive	17.5%	22.7%	4.5%	5.8%	0.02
TR/MM failure	18.0%	23.5%	4.8%	6.1%	0.009
Non-invasive	3.3%	3.3%	2.8%	2.8%	0.83
Invasive	14.7%	19.9%	1.9%	3.2%	0.003
Elsewhere failure[b]	3.2%	3.2%	2.6%	2.6%	0.96

[a] log-rank; [b] all elsewhere failures were invasive; TR/MM, true recurrence/marginal miss.

with the development of recurrence. Interestingly, when the results were then analyzed solely in the 95 patients who underwent a re-excision, the total volume of re-excision was the greatest factor associated with outcome. On multivariate analysis in these 95 patients, age was no longer associated with local recurrence (Table 36.4). Also, when we restricted our analysis to the 31 patients who were less than or equal to 45 years of age, a total excision volume less than 60 cc^3 and the predominant nuclear grade were the only variables associated with TR/MM failures (multivariate analysis). These findings clearly suggest that young age must be taken into consideration when recommending a patient for BCT, and that adequacy of excision (as represented by the total volume of excision) may be *partly* responsible for the success or failure of treatment in these patients. The importance of volume of resection is further addressed below.

Additional Studies

Several additional studies have addressed patient age as it relates to the success of BCT in patients with DCIS. Studies

that did *not* show a statistically significant increased risk of local recurrence include:

the UCLA group (16),
the NSABP B-17 trial (14),
the Joint Center for Radiation Therapy (JCRT) (17),
a combined study from the Fox Chase Cancer Center and the University of Pennsylvania (18),
a collaborative multi-institutional study from northeast Italy (19),
a report on 146 patients from the University of Pennsylvania (20),
a study from the Ochsner Clinic (21),
a study of predictors of local recurrence following excision alone from the JCRT (22),
a report from Toronto on 124 patients (23),
a small study of 41 women with DCIS from M.D. Anderson (24)
and previous publications from the collaborative DCIS studies published by Solin et al. (25,26).

It should be noted, however, that in many of these trials, recurrence rates in younger patients were actually higher,

TABLE 36.3. FACTORS ASSOCIATED WITH IPSILATERAL FAILURE AND TR/MM FAILURE (COX PROPORTIONAL HAZARDS MODEL)

Factor	Ipsilateral Breast Failure		TR/MM Failure	
	p Value	Hazard Ratio	p Value	Hazard Ratio
No calcifications with DCIS vs calcs	0.02	3.57	0.06	3.57
Age at diagnosis (years)	0.06	0.96	0.007	0.93
No. of slides with DCIS	0.09	1.09	0.02	1.29
Margin status–close/(+) vs. (−)	0.09	2.49	0.03	4.47
No. of DCIS or COL foci ≤5 mm from margin	0.57	—	0.06	1.05
Maximum tumor dimension (mm)	0.50	—	0.11	—
Predominant nuclear grade	0.23	—	0.13	—
Total volume of excisions <60 cc vs. >60 cc	0.07	2.69	0.06	2.89

TR/MM, true recurrence/marginal miss; COL, cancerization of lobules; DCIS, ductal carcinoma in situ.

TABLE 36.4. COX PROPORTIONAL HAZARDS MODEL IN 95 PATIENTS WHO UNDERWENT RE-EXCISION

Factor	Ipsilateral Failure		TR/MM Failure		Invasive TR/MM	
	p Value	Hazard Ratio	p Value	Hazard Ratio	p Value	Hazard Ratio
No calcifications with DCIS vs. calcifications	0.43	—	0.04	4.76	0.41	—
Age at diagnosis (years)	0.08	0.94	0.23	—	0.11	—
No. of slides with DCIS	0.31	—	0.48	—	0.68	—
Margin status close/(+) vs. (−)	0.04	3.78	0.01	7.78	0.06	3.26
Maximum tumor dimension (mm)	0.26	—	0.50	—	0.40	—
Predominant nuclear grade	0.32	—	0.17	—	0.02	8.86
Comedo vs. noncomedo	0.97	—	0.30	—	0.64	—
Volume of re-excision: <40 cc vs. >40 cc	0.08	2.92	0.005	15.68	0.02	6.33

TR/MM, true recurrence/marginal miss; DCIS, ductal carcinoma in situ.

but most studies did not have the statistical power (due to small patient numbers) to detect significant differences in outcome or simply had inadequate follow-up. This point is demonstrated by an update of the northeast Italy study by Amichetti et al. (19). Their original study published in 1997 did not demonstrate a significant difference in outcome based on age. However, a more recent update with an extended follow-up and addition of cases from five more institutions (and with the analysis restricted to nonpalpable lesions) did demonstrate that the average age at diagnosis (45.5 years) was the only prognostic factor found to be statistically significant on univariate analysis ($p = 0.003$) (27). It is unfortunate that the European Organization for Research and Treatment of Cancer (EORTC) 10583 trial that randomized patients after lumpectomy to either no further treatment or to radiotherapy did not initially analyze age as a potential prognostic factor for outcome (28). Hopefully, further analyses of this extraordinary database and trial will provide additional insight into this critical issue.

CLINICAL/PATHOLOGIC AND TREATMENT-RELATED DIFFERENCES BASED ON PATIENT AGE

Although it has been demonstrated that younger patients with invasive breast cancer generally have a greater proportion of tumor characteristics associated with an adverse outcome, studies in patients with DCIS have been minimal. We have recently shown, however, that younger patients with DCIS do indeed have a spectrum of pathologic and treatment-related characteristics generally considered to be associated with an increased risk of local recurrence (10). In our recent analysis, excised specimens from 177 breasts in 172 patients with DCIS treated with BCT were studied. All slides from all specimens were reviewed by one pathologist. Patients were divided into three age groups: less than 45 years, 45 to 59 years, and greater than or equal to 60 years. Patients less than 45 years old at the time of diagnosis more

frequently had higher nuclear grade DCIS (highest nuclear grade 3: 69%, 60%, and 39%, respectively; $p = 0.003$) and central necrosis (72%, 62%, and 44%, respectively; $p = 0.01$). Although not statistically significant, younger patients tended to have comedo subtype DCIS more often (31%, 23%, and 18%, respectively; $p = 0.35$) (Table 36.5). Younger patients also had smaller initial biopsy specimen maximum dimensions more often (4.3 cm, 5.2 cm, and 5.7 cm, respectively; $p = 0.004$), with close or positive margins (89%, 61%, and 64%; $p = 0.03$) and more terminal duct lobular units (TDLUs) with cancerization of lobules (COL) in the 0.42 cm rim of tissue adjacent to the margin (5.2, 3.6, and 1.9, respectively; $p = 0.23$). No other features, including the amount of DCIS when classified as greater than 50% or greater than 75% of ducts, calcifications within DCIS ducts, pattern of DCIS involvement, number of slides examined, number of slides with DCIS, and mean number of DCIS ducts near the margin were found to occur more frequently in younger patients. These differences in pathologic and treatment-related features based on age are further analyzed in Tables 36.6 and 36.7.

Similar to the William Beaumont Hospital experience, Hwang et al. (29) also demonstrated a difference in the volume of resection in younger patients. In 173 cases of histologically confirmed DCIS treated at MSKCC with BCT, data on volumes of resection (VRs) were available in 126 cases. The VRs obtained were divided into two groups: less than 60 cm^3 and greater than 60 cm^3. Patients were then divided into three groups by age at diagnosis: younger than 40 years, 40 to 69 years, and 70 years or older. The eldest group had a significantly greater proportion of large VRs (30%) as compared with the middle group (11%) and the younger group (9%) ($p = 0.03$, x^2). Although not statistically significant, the large VR group had a lower 6-year actuarial local recurrence rate (5.6%) than did the small VR group (21.3%) ($p = 0.16$, log-rank test). This trend was observed even though adjuvant radiotherapy was used less often in patients who had large VRs. In a more recent update of the MSKCC experience, Van Zee et al. (15) were not able to

TABLE 36.5. PATHOLOGIC FEATURES BASED ON AGE

Feature	Age <45 No. Cases	Age <45 % Cases	Age 45–59 No. Cases	Age 45–59 % Cases	Age ≥60 No. Cases	Age ≥60 % Cases	p Value
Predominant nuclear grade 3	12	38%	19	32%	20	24%	0.08[a]
Highest nuclear grade 3	22	69%	36	60%	33	39%	0.003[a]
Any central necrosis	23	72%	37	62%	37	44%	0.01
Central necrosis >50% ducts	12	38%	18	30%	16	19%	0.08
Predominantly comedo	10	31%	14	23%	16	18%	0.35
Any comedo	13	41%	21	35%	23	27%	0.32
Dispersed DCIS pattern		44%		33%		43%	NS
Tumorous DCIS pattern		31%		47%		30%	NS
Mean No. slides with DCIS		4.5		4.1		4.5	NS
Mean max. tumor dimension (mm)		9.1		6.8		6.5	0.03
Mean No. DCIS ducts ≤0.42 cm from margin		5.8		3.8		7.0	NS
≥5 DCIS ducts ≤0.42 cm from final margin		31%		18%		29%	0.28
≥5 COL TDLUs ≤0.42 cm from final margin		31%		17%		8%	0.008

[a] Excludes 71 patients with immeasurable tumor.
DCIS, ductal carcinoma in situ; TDLU, terminal duct lobular units; COL, cancerization of lobules; NS, not significant.

TABLE 36.6. DISTRIBUTION OF SPECIMEN FEATURES BY PATIENT AGE GROUP

Feature	Age <45	Age 45–59	Age ≥60	p Value
Initial biopsy specimen				
Mean specimen volume (cc)	42.2	72.8	117.6	0.08
Close or positive margin	89%	61%	64%	0.03
Re-excision specimen				
Re-excision performed (Yes)	75%	65%	59%	0.26
Residual DCIS at re-excision	58%	49%	58%	0.63
Mean specimen volume (cc)	121.9	60.1	76.7	0.22
Close or positive margin	26%	21%	14%	0.44
Final status				
Mean total specimen volume (cc)	164.1	132.9	194.3	0.48
Close or positive final margin	38%	25%	30%	0.45

TABLE 36.7. 5-YEAR ACTUARIAL RATES OF LOCAL RECURRENCE (TR/MM) BASED ON VOLUME OF EXCISION

Group	No. of Patients	Excision Volume <60 cc	Excision Volume >60 cc	p Value
No. of slides with DCIS				
≤5	101	5%	0%	0.15
≥6	47	28%	13%	0.15
All patients	148	11%	5%	0.13
Tumor size (cm)				
<0.7	49	9%	4%	0.50
≥0.7	34	33%	9%	0.05
All patients	83[a]	16%	7%	0.15

[a] Excluded patients with immeasurable tumor size (predominantly dispersed).
TR/MM, true recurrence/marginal miss.

demonstrate a statistically significant correlation between age group and any histologic factor.

Imamura et al. (30) studied the relationships between the morphologic and biologic characteristics of intraductal components accompanying invasive ductal breast carcinoma and patient age. Three hundred twenty-four cases were divided into three age groups ($\leq$ 39, 40 to 64, and $\geq$ 65), and differences in proliferative activity of the intraductal components (as measured using the MIB1 antibody) and extension of the intraductal components through the breast were recorded based on patient age. Patients less than or equal to 39 years of age had a significantly higher maximum distance of intraductal spread compared with the other two age groups ($p = 0.0028$). This trend was more pronounced in patients with non–high grade DCIS without necrosis ($p = 0.0045$). The proliferative activity in younger patients (referred to as the MLI- MIB-1 labeling index) with high-grade DCIS was significantly higher compared with older patients ($p = 0.0269$). Associations between age groups and margin status in the 143 patients treated with BCT found that patients less than or equal to 39 years had higher margin-positive rates in their lumpectomy specimens compared with the older age groups ($p = 0.0362$) for both high and low-grade DCIS. Although these results were seen in patients with *invasive* breast cancer, the study suggested that younger patients may have a higher probability of residual carcinoma after lumpectomy due to a greater maximum distance of intraductal spread. They also pointed out that it may be more difficult to evaluate margins in younger patients because of the controversy as to the differential diagnosis between low-grade DCIS and atypical hyperplasia (30).

Ohtake et al. (31) also reported that the intraductal extension was greater in younger patients with invasive breast cancer. In an elegant study of 20 patients with primary breast cancer undergoing quadrantectomy, the authors used a subgross and stereomicroscopic technique to visualize intraductal tumor extension. Serial, 2 mm–thick sections were subjected to two-dimensional tumor mapping measuring the distances and angles of extension and to three-dimensional reconstruction of the mammary duct-lobular systems by means of computer graphics. The distances of tumor extension were greatest in younger patients and decreased with age. Patients between 30 and 39 years of age had intraductal extension of 33.7 mm versus 14.3 mm for patients 40 to 50 years of age, and 6.7 to 7.7 mm for patients greater than 50 years of age. Again, although these results were obtained in patients with *invasive* breast cancer, they probably can be extrapolated to patients with DCIS, and point out the potential problems associated with obtaining and defining adequate tumor excision in younger patients.

Ikeda et al. (32) analyzed the frequency of positive initial surgical margins in 66 cases of DCIS treated with BCT at seven institutions in Japan. Young age was the most significant factor correlated with a positive surgical margin. Un-

fortunately, the authors did not look at the initial volumes of resection in younger patients or in the probability of finding residual disease at re-excision in these patients. Wazer et al. (33) recently studied the influence of age and extensive intraductal component histology on the lumpectomy margin assessment as a predictor of residual tumor in 265 cases of stage I/II breast cancer. Criteria for the study was an initial excision margin that was less than or equal to 2 mm, or indeterminate, that then underwent re-excision. Age less than or equal to 45 years was associated with a greater incidence of a positive re-excision compared with patients greater than 45 years of age. This was most pronounced when the initial margins of excision were focally positive. In younger patients, the probability of a positive re-excision was 60% versus 18% for patients greater than 45 years of age ($p = 0.05$).

Collectively, the studies discussed above point out the concerns in managing younger patients with BCT. First, for reasons that are unclear, there appears to be a greater tendency to perform more conservative initial surgeries in these patients. Second, because of these limited surgeries, younger patients are more likely to have positive margins after their initial definitive cancer operation. Third, the evaluation of margins in younger patients appears to be more difficult and less precise. Finally, younger patients also have a tendency for more extensive involvement of their ductal system, which leaves the breast at a potentially greater risk of harboring significant unappreciated residual disease after lumpectomy. Given these findings, it is clear that younger patients treated with BCT need to be managed more meticulously to account for these unique characteristics, and appropriate steps should be taken to minimize their potential negative influence on treatment outcome (see below).

Other groups have also explored differences in pathologic characteristics at diagnosis based on age. Although Solin et al. demonstrated a statistically significant difference in local recurrence in younger patients treated with BCT for mammographically detected DCIS, no difference was seen by age group for the final pathology margin status ($p = 0.82$) or mammogram findings at presentation. Unfortunately, these results must be tempered by the fact that no central pathology or mammography review was conducted. Similarly, although Fisher et al. (12) also demonstrated a statistically significant difference in outcome in the NSABP B-24 trial based on age, no attempt was made to look at the frequency of any clinical, pathologic, or treatment-related characteristics based on age.

As noted above, it appears that younger patients with DCIS potentially have a greater likelihood of more widespread/extensive disease at diagnosis, yet also appear to undergo more conservative initial (and possibly total) excisions. The factors responsible for these generally more limited surgeries are not clear. However, the importance of total excision volume on outcome appears to be real. For example, at our institution, we recently analyzed the treat-

TABLE 36.8. 5-YEAR ACTUARIAL RATES OF LOCAL RECURRENCE (TR/MM) BASED ON VOLUME OF EXCISION AND MARGIN STATUS

Group	No. of Patients	Excision Volume <60 cc			Excision Volume >60 cc		
		Margin ≤2 mm	Margin >2 mm	p Value	Margin ≤2 mm	Margin >2 mm	p Value
Slides with DCIS							
≤5	99	0%	4%	0.27	0%	0%	0.85
≥6	46	18%	50%	0.35	19%	5%	0.30
All patients	145[a]	8%	10%	0.65	11%	2%	0.02
Tumor size							
<0.7 cm	48	0%	7%	0.42	25%	0%	0.03
≥0.7 cm	33	40%	25%	0.55	0%	6%	0.55
All patients	81	11%	8%	0.77	10%	3%	0.35

[a] Excluded three patients due to uncertain margin status.
TR/MM, true recurrence/marginal miss.

ment of 146 patients with DCIS with BCT focusing on the interrelationships between excision volume, margin status, and tumor size with local recurrence (9). As demonstrated in our previous work (discussed above), multivariate analysis of patient age, margin status, the number of slides containing DCIS, the number of DCIS/COL foci (< 5mm) near the margin, and a smaller volume of excision (< 60cm^3) showed that each factor is independently associated with outcome. Although the local recurrence rate generally decreased as margin distance increased, these differences did not achieve statistical significance unless the volume of excision was taken into consideration.

Tables 36.7 and 36.8 clearly illustrate the points above. Patients with smaller total excision volumes (< 60 cm^3) generally had higher rates of local recurrence. These differences in local recurrence were more pronounced as tumor size (≥ 0.7 cm versus < 0.7 cm, 33% versus 9%; $p = 0.05$) or the number of slides with DCIS increased (≥ 6 versus ≤ 5, 28% versus 13%; $p = 0.15$). When controlling for volume of excision, no consistent trends in local recurrence

were noted based solely on margin status (e.g., ≤ 2 versus τ 2 mm).

Because patient numbers in all of the above subcategories were quite small and the statistical associations were weak, we then analyzed the ratio of tumor volume (as represented by the number of slides with DCIS or cubic centimeters of tumor) divided by the total excision volume. To eliminate potential bias in selecting an appropriate ratio, patients were either divided into two or three roughly equal groups of patients (e.g., either halves or thirds). As noted in Table 36.9, statistically significant differences in the rates of local recurrence were noted at 5 and 10 years as this ratio increased. Patients with a ratio less than or equal to 0.02 had a 10-year rate of local recurrence of 0% compared with 16% for patients with ratios greater than or equal to 0.08 ($p = 0.04$). Because this ratio appeared to correlate well with outcome, it was then entered into a separate multivariate analysis. When analyzed in this fashion, this ratio was the only *treatment*-related variable independently associated with 5-year TR/MM failure. Margins

TABLE 36.9. ACTUARIAL RECURRENCE RATES BASED ON RATIO OF TUMOR/EXCISED VOLUME

Measurement	No. of Patients	No. of TR/MM	5-Yr TR/MM	10-Yr TR/MM	p Value
No. Slides with DCIS/total excision volume (cc)					
≤0.03	70	1	0%	2%	0.01
≥0.04	78	11	14%	16%	
≤0.02	48	0	0%	0%	
0.03–0.07	49	5	9%	11%	0.04
≥0.08	51	7	13%	16%	
Tumor volume (cc)/excision volume (cc)					
≤0.002	49	3	6%	6%	0.17
≥0.003	34	5	16%	16%	

TR/MM, true recurrence/marginal miss; DCIS, ductal carcinoma in situ.

were no longer significantly associated with outcome (TR/MM failure).

The above findings serve to emphasize the critical importance of adequacy of excision (along with margin assessment and tumor size) in ensuring excellent local control in patients with DCIS treated with BCT. This concern is only magnified in younger patients, and most likely accounts for *part* of the higher rates of local recurrence observed.

RESULTS IN PATIENTS TREATED WITH MASTECTOMY

Limited information exists regarding the influence of patient age at diagnosis on the success of mastectomy in patients with DCIS. Although total mastectomy is considered definitive treatment for DCIS, there is still a 0% to 8% incidence of local recurrence noted in the literature. It has been suggested that total mastectomy should be associated with cure rates approaching 100% because DCIS is more frequently detected as a nonpalpable, mammographic abnormality in most patients. However, even in this setting, recurrence of DCIS after mastectomy is still possible. The mechanism(s) by which DCIS recurs after mastectomy is probably a function of several variables, including the fact that approximately 1% to 5% of breast tissue can remain after surgery. There is currently no uniform method for determining the risk of recurrence after mastectomy for DCIS.

Certainly factors such as age, extent of DCIS, positive versus negative margins, mitotic index, nuclear grade, proliferative index, and ploidy may be important but are currently unproven.

Table 36.10 lists studies that have investigated the risk of local and distant recurrence after mastectomy in patients treated for DCIS (37–59). Unfortunately, the majority of these reports consist of small groups of patients, and consequently, only a handful of recurrences. As a result, the ability to identify risk factors for recurrence is nearly impossible. It is interesting to note, however, that the majority of recurrences discussed in the 23 trials identified in Table 36.10 (where age at recurrence was provided) developed in patients less than 50 years of age. In addition, of the seven case report studies discussing local recurrences after mastectomy for DCIS, the vast majority occurred in patients who were less than 50 years of age at diagnosis (Table 36.11). Although no conclusions can or should be derived from these interesting observations, it may be possible that younger patients are at an increased risk of recurrence, even after total mastectomy (60–66). Hopefully, groups that have published their results with mastectomy for DCIS will address this issue in their data sets and provide some meaningful numbers to this potential concern. Until then, it certainly should not be concluded that younger patients do not fare as well as older patients when treated with mastectomy, or that mastectomy offers any additional advantage to BCT in younger patients.

TABLE 36.10. RECURRENCE AFTER MASTECTOMY IN PATIENTS WITH DUCTAL CARCINOMA IN SITU

Author (Reference)	Follow-Up	No. Patients	Recurrences	Patient Ages
Sunshine et al. (37)	10 years	70	3 (4%)	52, 46, 78
Schuh et al. (38)	5.5 years	51	1 (2%)	49
Warneke et al. (39)	3.6 years	75	1 (1.3%)	54
Silverstein et al. (40)	3.8 years	97	2 (2%)	31, 33
Bedwani et al. (41)	5 years	112	1 (1%)	NS
Brown et al. (42)	1–15 years	40	0	—
Carter and Smith (43)	15 years	38	3 (8%)	NS
Lagios et al. (44)	10 years	53	3 (6%)	NS
Millis and Thyme (45)	20 years	20	0	—
Westbrook and Gallager (46)	20 years	60	2 (3%)	NS
Howard et al. (47)	1.5–12 years	55	3 (5%)	NS
Kinne et al. (48)	5–17 years	82	1 (1%)	NS
Fisher et al. (49)	5–95 months	27	1 (4%)	NS
Ashikari et al. (50)	0–11 years	74	0	—
Ashikari et al. (51)	1–10 years	110	7 (6%)	NS
Farrow (52)	5–20 years	200	6 (3%)	NS
Wulsin and Schreiber (53)	NS	12	0	—
Lewis and Geschickter (54)	2–36 years	36	7 (19%)	NS
Arnesson et al. (55)	6 years	28	0	—
Simpson et al. (56)	NS	34	0	—
Rosner et al. (57)	5 years	182	0	—
Fentiman et al. (58)	5 years	76	1 (1%)	NS
Ciatto et al. (59)	5.5 years	210	3 (1%)	NS

NS, not stated.

TABLE 36.11. CASE REPORTS OF PATIENTS RECURRING AFTER MASTECTOMY FOR DUCTAL CARCINOMA IN SITU

Author	No. of Cases Reported	Age at Diagnosis (Years)	Type of Recurrence	Status at Last P/U
Clark et al. (60)	1	42	DCIS	NED
Deutsch (61)	2	38	Invasive	NED
		46	DCIS	NED
Finkelstein et al. (62)	1	40	Invasive	NED
Fisher et al. (63)	1	40	DCIS	NED
de Jong (64)	3	33	Invasive	Metastases
		42	Invasive	Metastases
		53	Invasive	NED
Salas et al. (65)	2	47	Invasive	NED
		48	Invasive	NED
Helvie et al. (66)	6	(<48 mean)	All Invasive	Unknown

NED, no evidence of disease.

OVERALL OUTCOME BASED ON PATIENT AGE

The most important issue facing patients with a diagnosis of DCIS is which treatment alternative will provide the greatest probability of cancer cure. At the present time, the accumulated body of data does not indicate any difference in outcome based on the method of treatment or patient age at diagnosis. However, the amount of information on this issue is limited. In our series of 146 patients treated with BCT, the actuarial 10-year cause-specific survival (CSS) rate for all patients was 99.1%. No statistically significant difference in the CSS rate was observed in younger patients despite a local recurrence rate that was three times greater than in older patients (26.1% versus 8.6%, $p = 0.03$) and despite the fact that the majority of recurrences in younger patients were invasive. In the Solin study discussed previously, a 15-year CSS rate of 98% was observed for all patients (13). Although not reported in their work, differences in CSS based on patient age were not analyzed due to small patient numbers.

Although the data discussed above do not show an increased rate of cancer-specific death based on age at diagnosis, these results must be tempered by the fact that patient numbers were small. Differences in outcome might actually exist, which is suggested by the fact that younger patients appear to have a higher rate of invasive local recurrences that can potentially lead to a higher risk of cancer death. Silverstein et al. (34) clearly emphasized this point in one of their recent analyses. A total 35 invasive recurrences after treatment for DCIS were collected. Fifty-one percent of these patients recurred with stage I disease. Overall, for patients with invasive local recurrence, the 8-year breast cancer–specific mortality and distant-disease probability were 14.4% and 21.7%, respectively.

Similar results were observed in the collaborative DCIS study by Solin et al. (35). Forty-two patients with local failure after treatment of mammographically detected DCIS treated with BCT were analyzed. Twenty-two of these patients (52%) had an invasive recurrence. The 4-year rate of CSS and freedom from distant metastases in these patients were 78% and 67%, respectively. The implications of these findings for younger patients are obvious (36). If the substantially higher rates of invasive local recurrence noted in younger patients in both the Vicini et al. study and the Solin et al. study are substantiated in the larger national trials, further methods to optimize outcome (local control) in these patients may need to be considered (6,13).

CONCLUSIONS AND RECOMMENDATIONS

The implications of young age at diagnosis in patients with DCIS treated with BCT are inconclusive due to a lack of sufficient clinical, pathologic, and treatment-related data addressing this issue. However, in the handful of studies that have specifically investigated the influence of patient age on outcome, the following observations can be made:

i) The majority of studies with large numbers of patients and sufficient follow-up indicate that younger patients with DCIS treated with BCT have a statistically significant higher rate of local recurrence that appears to be independent of previously defined prognostic factors compared with older patients. Although insufficient data are available addressing the issue, young age at diagnosis may also have an adverse impact in patients treated with excision alone.

ii) In two large studies, younger patients treated with BCT were found to have higher rates of invasive local recurrences compared with older patients. The implications of this observation are uncertain. This finding needs to be corroborated in larger studies before definitive conclusions and recommendations can be made.

iii) In the few studies that addressed the issue, younger patients appeared to have a higher incidence of several adverse prognostic factors, including higher nuclear grade, central necrosis, and comedo histology. In addition, although younger patients are more likely to have DCIS extending over a greater distance in the breast, they appear to undergo more conservative excisions. As a consequence of this, younger patients are more likely to have close/positive surgical margins after the initial excisional biopsy.

iv) Insufficient data are available that indicate whether younger patients with DCIS treated with mastectomy have a higher rate of recurrence compared with older patients.

v) Despite the higher rates of local recurrence observed in younger patients treated with BCT, overall cancer-specific survival appears to be indistinguishable from that of older patients or those treated with mastectomy.

vi) When margins of resection are negative and an adequate surgical excision (e.g., volume of resection) has been performed, it appears that younger patients can be safely treated with BCT and expect control rates in the breast comparable to those of older patients.

Based on the observations noted above, the following statements regarding patient age at diagnosis can be made.

First, young age at diagnosis is not a contraindication to BCT but needs to be taken into consideration when determining the acceptability of a patient with DCIS for conservative management. Given the potential for a significantly greater risk of failure (which may be invasive), meticulous attention needs to be given to the adequacy of excision as defined by surgical margins, volume of resection, and post-excision mammography. It cannot be overemphasized that younger patients represent a group where adequacy of excision is absolutely critical, and where it may actually be more difficult to ensure acceptable tumor removal.

Second, there are no data that indicate that younger patients with DCIS are better treated by mastectomy. Cancer-specific survival appears equivalent between breast-conservation and radical surgery. In addition, there is a suggestion (although certainly not proven) that younger patients may actually fare worse when treated with mastectomy compared with older patients.

Finally, given the potential implications of this issue, it is hoped that data from the larger national and international studies on DCIS are analyzed with respect to age at diagnosis. The large number of patients treated in these trials, the length of follow-up, and the complete pathologic reviews should help to conclusively establish the importance of patient age at diagnosis and to generate meaningful treatment recommendations in these patients.

ACKNOWLEDGMENTS

The authors would like to thank members of the Departments of Radiation Oncology, Pathology, Surgery, and Medical Oncology for their assistance in the management of these patients and for providing excellent follow-up information, and to Ms. Vicky Dykes for her secretarial assistance in preparation of this manuscript.

REFERENCES

1. Yildirim E, Dalgic T, Berberoglu U. Prognostic significance of young age in breast cancer. *J Surg Oncol* 2000;74:267–272.
2. Kroman N, Jensen MB, Wohlfahrt J, et al. Factors influencing the effect of age on prognosis in breast cancer: population based study. *BMJ* 2000;320:474–478.
3. Winchester DP. Breast cancer in young women. *Surg Clin North Am* 1996;76:279–287.
4. Nixon AJ, Neuberg D, Hayes DF, et al. Relationship of patient age to pathologic features of the tumor and prognosis for patients with stage I or II breast cancer. *J Clin Oncol* 1994;12:888–894.
5. Elkhuizen PH, van Slooten HJ, Clahsen PC, et al. High local recurrence risk after breast-conserving therapy in node-negative premenopausal breast cancer patients is greatly reduced by one course of perioperative chemotherapy: A European Organization for Research and Treatment of Cancer Breast Cancer Cooperative Group Study. *J Clin Oncol* 2000;18:1075–1083.
6. Vicini FA, Kestin LL, Goldstein NS, et al. Impact of young age on outcome in patients with ductal carcinoma-in-situ treated with breast-conserving therapy. *J Clin Oncol* 2000;18: 296–306.
7. Kestin LL, Goldstein NS, Lacerna MD, et al. Factors associated with local recurrence of mammographically detected ductal carcinoma in situ in patients given breast-conserving therapy. *Cancer* 2000;88:596–607.
8. Kestin LL, Goldstein NS, Martinez AA, et al. Mammographically detected ductal carcinoma in situ treated with conservative surgery with or without radiation therapy: patterns of failure and 10-year results. *Ann Surg* 2000;231:235–245.
9. Vicini F, Kestin LL, Goldstein NS, Baglan KL, Pettinga J, Martinez A. The relationship between excision volume, margin status, and tumor size with the development of local recurrence in patients with ductal carcinoma-in-situ treated with breast conserving therapy. *J Surg Oncol* 2001;76:245–254.
10. Goldstein NS, Vicini FA, Kestin LL, et al. Differences in the pathologic features of ductal carcinoma in situ of the breast based on patient age. *Cancer* 2000;88:2553–2560.
11. Vicini FA, Goldstein NS, Kestin LL. Pathologic and technical considerations in the treatment of ductal carcinoma in situ of the breast with lumpectomy and radiation therapy. *Ann Oncol* 1999;10:883–890.
12. Fisher B, Dignam J, Wolmark N, et al. Tamoxifen in treatment of intraductal breast cancer: National Surgical Adjuvant Breast and Bowel Project B-24 randomized controlled trial. *Lancet* 1999;353:1993–2000.
13. Solin LJ, Fourquet A, Vicini F, et al. Mammographically detected ductal carcinoma in situ of the breast treated with breast-conserving surgery and definitive breast irradiation: Long-term outcome and prognostic significance of patient age and margin status. *Int J Radiat Oncol Biol Phys* 2001;50:991–1002.
14. Fisher B, Dignam J, Wolmark N, et al. Lumpectomy and radiation therapy for the treatment of intraductal breast cancer: findings from National Surgical Adjuvant Breast and Bowel Project B-17. *J Clin Oncol* 1998;16:441–452.

15. Van Zee KJ, Liberman L, Samli B, et al. Long-term follow-up of women with ductal carcinoma in situ treated with breast-conserving surgery: the effect of age. *Cancer* 1999;86:1757–1767.

16. Weng EY, Juillard GJ, Parker RG, et al. Outcomes and factors impacting local recurrence of ductal carcinoma in situ. *Cancer* 2000;88:1643–1649.

17. Hiramatsu H, Bornstein BA, Recht A, et al. Local Recurrence after Conservative Surgery and Radiation Therapy for Ductal Carcinoma in Situ. *Cancer J* 1995;1:55.

18. Fowble B, Hanlon AL, Fein DA, et al. Results of conservative surgery and radiation for mammographically detected ductal carcinoma in situ (DCIS). *Int J Radiat Oncol Biol Phys* 1997;38:949–957.

19. Amichetti M, Caffo O, Richetti A, et al. Ten-year results of treatment of ductal carcinoma in situ (DCIS) of the breast with conservative surgery and radiotherapy. *Eur J Cancer* 1997;33:1559–1565.

20. Harris EE, Schultz DJ, Peters CA, et al. Relationship of family history and outcome after breast conservation therapy in women with ductal carcinoma in situ of the breast. *Int J Radiat Oncol Biol Phys* 2000;48:933–941.

21. Szelei-Stevens KA, Kuske RR, Yantsos VA, et al. The influence of young age and positive family history of breast cancer on the prognosis of ductal carcinoma in situ treated by excision with or without radiation therapy or by mastectomy. *Int J Radiat Oncol Biol Phys* 2000;48:943–949.

22. Hetelekidis S, Collins L, Silver B, et al. Predictors of local recurrence following excision alone for ductal carcinoma in situ. *Cancer* 1999;85:427–431.

23. Fish EB, Chapman JA, Miller NA, et al. Assessment of treatment for patients with primary ductal carcinoma in situ in the breast. *Ann Surg Oncol* 1998;5:724–732.

24. Sneige N, McNeese MD, Atkinson EN, et al. Ductal carcinoma in situ treated with lumpectomy and irradiation: histopathological analysis of 49 specimens with emphasis on risk factors and long term results. *Hum Pathol* 1995;26:642–649.

25. Solin LJ, Yeh IT, Kurtz J, et al. Ductal carcinoma in situ (intraductal carcinoma) of the breast treated with beast-conserving surgery and definitive irradiation: correlation of pathologic parameters with outcome of treatment. *Cancer* 1993;71:2532–2542.

26. Solin LJ, McCormick B, Recht A, et al. Mammographically detected clinically occult ductal carcinoma in situ (intraductal carcinoma) treated with breast conserving therapy and definitive breast irradiation. *Cancer J* 1996;2:158–165.

27. Amichetti M, Caffo O, Richetti A, et al. Subclinical ductal carcinoma in situ of the breast: treatment with conservative surgery and radiotherapy. *Tumori* 1999;85:488–493.

28. Julien JP, Bijker N, Fentiman IS, et al. Radiotherapy in breast-conserving treatment for ductal carcinoma in situ: first results of the EORTC randomised phase III trial 10853. EORTC Breast Cancer Cooperative Group and EORTC Radiotherapy Group. *Lancet* 2000;355:528–533.

29. Hwang E, Samili B, Tran K, et al. Volume of resection in patients treated with breast conservation for ductal carcinoma in situ. *Arch Pathol Lab Med* 1998;5:757–763.

30. Imamura H, Haga S, Shimizu T, et al. Relationship between the morphological and biological characteristics of intraductal components accompanying invasive ductal breast carcinoma and patient age. *Breast Cancer Res Treat* 2000;62:177–184.

31. Ohtake T, Abe R, Kimijima I, et al. Intraductal extension of primary invasive breast carcinoma treated by breast-conserving surgery. Computer graphic three-dimensional reconstruction of the mammary duct-lobular systems. *Cancer* 1995;76:32–45.

32. Ikeda T, Akiyama F, Hiraoka M, et al. The Current Status of the Treatment of Ductal Carcinoma In Situ of Japanese Women, Es-

pecially Breast Conserving Operation in Relation to the Surgical Margin and Short Term Outcome. *Breast Cancer* 1998;5:53–58.

33. Wazer DE, Schmidt-Ullrich RK, Ruthazer R, et al. The influence of age and extensive intraductal component histology on breast lumpectomy margin assessment as a predictor of residual tumor. *Int J Radiat Oncol Biol Phys* 1999;45:885–891.

34. Silverstein MJ, Lagios MD, Martino S, et al. Outcome after invasive local recurrence in patients with ductal carcinoma in situ of the breast. *J Clin Oncol* 1998;16:1367–1373.

35. Solin LJ, Fourquet A, Vicini F, et al. Salvage treatment for local recurrence after breast-conservation surgery and radiation as initial treatment for mammographically-detected ductal carcinoma in situ of the breast. *Cancer* 2001; 91:1090–1097.

36. Fourquet A, Zafrani B, Campana F, et al. Institut Curie experience. In: Silverstein MJ, ed. *Ductal Carcinoma In Situ of the Breast.* Baltimore: Williams & Wilkins, 1997:391–397.

37. Sunshine JA, Moseley HS, Fletcher WS, et al. Breast carcinoma in situ. A retrospective review of 112 cases with a minimum 10 year follow-up. *Am J Surg* 1985;150:44–51.

38. Schuh ME, Nemoto T, Penetrante RB, et al. Intraductal carcinoma. Analysis of presentation, pathologic findings, and outcome of disease. *Arch Surg* 1986;121:1303–1307.

39. Warneke J, Grossklaus D, Davis J, et al. Influence of local treatment on the recurrence rate of ductal carcinoma in situ. *J Am Coll Surg* 1995;180:683–688.

40. Silverstein MJ, Barth A, Poller DN, et al. Ten-year results comparing mastectomy to excision and radiation therapy for ductal carcinoma in situ of the breast. *Eur J Cancer* 1995;31A:1425–1427.

41. Bedwani R, Vana J, Rosner D, et al. Management and survival of female patients with "minimal" breast cancer: as observed in the long-term and short-term surveys of the American College of Surgeons. *Cancer* 1981;47:2769–2778.

42. Brown PW, Silverman J, Owens E, et al. Intraductal "noninfiltrating" carcinoma of the breast. *Arch Surg* 1976;111:1063–1067.

43. Carter D, Smith RR. Carcinoma in situ of the breast. *Cancer* 1977;40:1189–1193.

44. Lagios MD, Westdahl PR, Margolin FR, et al. Duct carcinoma in situ. Relationship of extent of noninvasive disease to the frequency of occult invasion, multicentricity, lymph node metastases, and short-term treatment failures. *Cancer* 1982;50:1309–1314.

45. Millis RR, Thynne GS. In situ intraduct carcinoma of the breast: a long term follow-up study. *Br J Surg* 1975;62:957–962.

46. Westbrook KC, Gallager HS. Intraductal carcinoma of the breast. A comparative study. *Am J Surg* 1975;130:667–670.

47. Howard PW, Locker AP, Dowle CS, et al. In situ carcinoma of the breast. *Eur J Surg Oncol* 1989;15:328–332.

48. Kinne DW, Petrek JA, Osborne MP, et al. Breast carcinoma in situ. *Arch Surg* 1989;124:33–36.

49. Fisher ER, Sass R, Fisher B, et al. Pathologic findings from the National Surgical Adjuvant Breast Project (protocol 6). I. Intraductal carcinoma (DCIS). *Cancer* 1986;57:197–208.

50. Ashikari R, Huvos AG, Snyder RE. Prospective study of non-infiltrating carcinoma of the breast. *Cancer* 1977;39:435–439.

51. Ashikari R, Hajdu SI, Robbins GF. Intraductal carcinoma of the breast (1960–1969). *Cancer* 1971;28:1182–1187.

52. Farrow JH. Current concepts in the detection and treatment of the earliest of the early breast cancers. *Cancer* 1970;25:468–477.

53. Wulsin JH, Schreiber JT. Improved prognosis in certain patterns of carcinoma of the breast. *Arch Surg* 1962;85:111–120.

54. Lewis RD, McBride CM. Role of simple mastectomy in treating patients with breast cancer. *South Med J* 1977;70:931–934.

55. Arnesson LG, Smeds S, Fagerberg G, et al. Follow-up of two treatment modalities for ductal cancer in situ of the breast. *Br J Surg* 1989;76:672–675.
56. Simpson T, Thirlby RC, Dail DH. Surgical treatment of ductal carcinoma in situ of the breast. 10- to 20-year follow-up. *Arch Surg* 1992;127:468–472.
57. Rosner D, Bedwani RN, Vana J, et al. Noninvasive breast carcinoma: results of a national survey by the American College of Surgeons. *Ann Surg* 1980;192:139–147.
58. Fentiman IS, Fagg N, Millis RR, et al. In situ ductal carcinoma of the breast: implications of disease pattern and treatment. *Eur J Surg Oncol* 1986;12:261–266.
59. Ciatto S, Bonardi R, Cataliotti L, et al. Intraductal breast carcinoma. Review of a multicenter series of 350 cases. Coordinating Center and Writing Committee of FONCAM (National Task Force for Breast Cancer), Italy. *Tumori* 1990;76:552–554.
60. Clark L, Ritter E, Glazebrook K, et al. Recurrent ductal carcinoma in situ after total mastectomy. *J Surg Oncol* 1999;71:182–185.
61. Deutsch M. Ductal carcinoma in situ recurrent on the chest wall after mastectomy. *Clin Oncol (R Coll Radiol)* 1999;11:61–62.
62. Finkelstein SD, Sayegh R, Thompson WR. Late recurrence of ductal carcinoma in situ at the cutaneous end of surgical drainage following total mastectomy. *Am Surg* 1993;59:410–414.
63. Fisher DE, Schnitt SJ, Christian R, et al. Chest wall recurrence of ductal carcinoma in situ of the breast after mastectomy. *Cancer* 1993;71:3025–3028.
64. de Jong E, Peterse JL, Van Dongen JA. Recurrence after breast ablation for ductal carcinoma in situ. *Eur J Surg Oncol* 1992;18:64–66.
65. Salas AP, Helvie MA, Wilkins EG, et al. Is mammography useful in screening for local recurrences in patients with TRAM flap breast reconstruction after mastectomy for multifocal DCIS? *Ann Surg Oncol* 1998;5:456–463.
66. Helvie MA, Wilson TE, Roubidoux MA, et al. Mammographic appearance of recurrent breast carcinoma in six patients with TRAM flap breast reconstructions. *Radiology* 1998;209:711–715.

BREAST-CONSERVING THERAPY FOR DUCTAL CARCINOMA IN SITU: THE VAN NUYS EXPERIENCE WITH EXCISION PLUS RADIATION THERAPY

BERNARD S. LEWINSKY
OSCAR E. STREETER, JR.
MELVIN J. SILVERSTEIN

The incidence of ductal carcinoma in situ (DCIS) of the breast has increased significantly in the last 15 years, paralleling increases in the use of screening mammography. DCIS now represents 25% to 30% of mammographically detected breast cancer and poses a considerable challenge to the clinician (1). This challenge continues to evolve as new facts are discovered about the natural history, biology, pathology, genetics, and treatment of DCIS and as new techniques evolve for minimally invasive breast biopsy and image acquisition.

Breast-conserving therapy with radiation therapy became established as a treatment option for early-stage invasive breast cancer in the 1980s (2–7). In the years following, it became increasingly difficult to justify the continued use of mastectomy for patients with DCIS when patients with invasive breast cancers were being treated and cured with breast-conserving therapy. Subsequently, numerous retrospective reviews and multiple randomized trials (8–16) have been published regarding the efficacy of excisional biopsy plus radiation therapy for patients with DCIS. These studies demonstrate that breast-conserving therapy is practical for the majority of patients with DCIS, and that overall, radiation therapy reduces the probability of local recurrence by approximately 50% in all subgroups. Patients and physicians, however, must be willing to accept a risk of local recurrence of approximately 10% to 20% and a theoretical long-term 1% to 2% risk of mortality.

There are two important issues concerning the use of breast-conserving surgery plus radiation therapy for patients with DCIS that we will focus on in this chapter.

First, whether the same weekly dose of irradiation necessary to eradicate invasive cancer of the breast should be used for patients with DCIS. Two studies have examined the total weekly radiation dose delivered for invasive breast cancer (17,18); however, no study has reported local recurrence data with different weekly radiation doses for patients with DCIS. In this chapter, we will examine different weekly doses of irradiation as well as alternate fractionation schedules for patients with DCIS.

The second issue focuses on a technical aspect of radiation therapy. Is a boost to the tumor bed necessary? Most published reports used a boost; however, the prospectively randomized National Surgical Adjuvant Breast and Bowel Project (NSABP) protocol B-17 (8) utilized a whole-breast dose of 5,000 centigray (cGy) without a boost, as did the European Organization for Research and Treatment of Cancer (EORTC) (13). If a boost is necessary, the optimal type of boost has not been clearly defined. This chapter will also address the role of the boost in Patients with DCIS. As knowledge increases regarding biologic and pathologic differences between DCIS and invasive cancer, various boost types, or no boost at all, may be indicated for different type of lesions.

PATIENTS AND METHODS

The data presented in this chapter are derived from 237 patients with DCIS treated with local excision plus radiation therapy between 1979 and 2000. All 237 patients underwent excisional biopsy. Close or involved margins were generally not re-excised prior to 1985. After 1985, re-excision was routine. Nonpalpable lesions were excised using multiple wire excision biopsy techniques.

Until 1990, all patients with DCIS who underwent breast irradiation were treated with 200 cGy per day, 4 days per week to a total dose of 4,600 or 5,000 cGy. Radiation therapy was delivered with 4 or 6 MV photons to the whole breast. All patients were treated with non-coplanar, tangential fields with the deep beam edge of the tangent field coincident to minimize dose to lung. Every effort was made to assure the demagnified perpendicular distance from the posterior field edge to the posterior part of the chest wall was less than 3 cm. Regional nodal irradiation generally was not performed. All fields were treated during each treatment session.

All patients received a boost of 1,000 to 2,000 cGy, with the majority delivered via Iridium-192 implant. In the early years, clips to outline the biopsy cavity were not placed by most surgeons. Thus, the treatment depth in the majority of patients was to the chest wall; the nipple was generally included. Implants were performed simultaneously at the time of lymph node dissection (which was routine until the late 1980s) and were a minimum of two planes. The entire involved quadrant was included in the boost field.

By 1990, our radiation oncologists had switched to 180 cGy per day, 5 days per week, to a total whole-breast dose of 4,500 to 5,040 cGy. The technique of radiation therapy delivery remained unchanged. Most patients received a photon boost between 1,080 and 1,860 cGy, which also covered the quadrant of the excised lesion. Patients who underwent radiation therapy at other area irradiation facilities all received photons to the whole breast 5 days per week; the majority received an electron boost to the tumor bed.

Cosmetic results were assessed at follow-up appointments. A standard scoring system was used to evaluate telangiectasia, fibrosis, breast edema, pigmentation, and retraction. The overall cosmetic score was graded poor, fair, good, or excellent based on the combined score of the individual parameters.

Local recurrence-free survival rates for each group were estimated by the Kaplan-Meier method. The statistical significance of the differences between numerical values was calculated using the log rank test.

RESULTS

Patient characteristics are shown in Table 37.1. The median follow-up for all patients was 103 months. The average tu-

TABLE 37.1. PATIENT DEMOGRAPHICS

No. of patients	237
Median follow-up (months)	103
Median age (years)	53
Average tumor size (mm)	18
Median tumor size (mm)	15
No. of recurrences	48 (20%)
Invasive recurrences	22 (46%)
Median time to recurrence (months)	57
Axillary dissection	126—all negative
Physical examination	
Palpable	27 (11%)
Nonpalpable	210 (89%)

TABLE 37.2. LOCAL RECURRENCE BY NUCLEAR GRADE

Nuclear Grade	No. of Patients	Recurrences (%)	Deaths (%)
1	36	4 (11%)	0 (0%)
2	107	21 (20%)	1 (0.9%)
3	94	23 (24%)	3 (3.2%)
Total	237	48 (20%)	4 (1.7%)

mor diameter was 18 mm. The vast majority of patients (89%) had nonpalpable lesions; 126 axillary dissections were negative. Forty-eight patients (20%) developed recurrence in the treated breast, of which 22 (46%) were invasive breast cancer; six developed distant metastases, and four died.

The pattern of recurrence is somewhat different when radiotherapy patients are compared with patients treated with excision only. Ninety-three percent (57 of 61) of excision-only patients recurred in the same quadrant as the index tumor, whereas 83% (40 of 48) of radiotherapy patients recurred in the same quadrant. Although the difference is not significant ($p = 0.09$), there is a trend in favor of better local control for the patients treated with radiation therapy. The median time to local recurrence is also different: 57 months for radiotherapy patients compared with only 25 months for excision-only patients ($p = 0.03$). Therefore, it takes longer for radiotherapy patients to recur, and they are somewhat more likely to recur in different quadrants.

The risk of local recurrence was analyzed by nuclear grade of the primary tumor. A trend of increasing local recurrence is seen as the nuclear grade of the primary tumor increased (Table 37.2). Local recurrence is analyzed by margin width in Table 37.3 and by tumor size in Table 37.4. As margin widths increased, the risk of local recurrence decreased; as tumor size increased, the risk of local recurrence increased.

Local control as a function of subtype (predominantly comedo versus noncomedo) of DCIS is shown in Figure 37.1. The curves separate and are statistically different. Tumors containing predominantly comedo histology continue to have increased local recurrence rates through 12 years of follow-up. The actuarial local recurrence curves do not begin to approach one another in the later years as experienced

TABLE 37.3. LOCAL RECURRENCE BY MARGIN WIDTH

Margin Width	No. of Patients	Recurrences	Percentage
≥10 mm	45	1	2%
1–9 mm	109	20	18%
<1 mm	83	27	33%
Total	237	48	20%

TABLE 37.4. LOCAL RECURRENCE BY TUMOR SIZE

Tumor Size	No. of Patients	Recurrences	Percentage
≤15 mm	129	17	13%
16–40 mm	89	25	28%
≥41 mm	19	6	32%
Total	237	48	20%

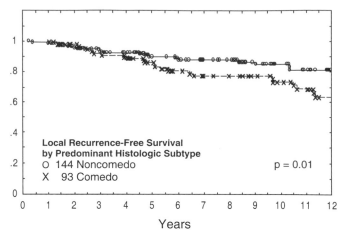

FIGURE 37.1. Probability of local recurrence–free survival for 237 radiation therapy patients grouped by predominant histologic subtype, comedo versus noncomedo architecture (*p* = 0.01).

by Solin et al. (19). However, the patients in the series of Solin et al. have been followed a median of 124 months, which is 21 months longer than our study.

Patients treated with radiation therapy 4 days per week were compared with patients treated 5 days per week (Table 37.5). The median time to local recurrence was 61 months for patients treated 4 days per week compared with 54 months for patients treated 5 days per week (*p* = not significant). The probability of local recurrence–free survival for patients treated with irradiation 4 days per week versus 5 days per week is shown in Figure 37.2. No statistical difference was found between the curves, although they began to trend apart in the later years to favor those treated 4 days per week. It was surprising that patients treated 5 days per week had a somewhat higher local recurrence rate, because those treated 4 days per week had 71 more months of median follow-up. The majority of patients treated 4 days per week were boosted with interstitial iridium implants, although patients treated 5 days per week were boosted with external beam. The overall cosmetic result was good, and all sub-categories of cosmetic outcome were equivalent between the patients treated 4 days per week and those treated 5 days per week.

The local recurrence–free survival rate was analyzed for the 237 patients in the study. At 12 years, the actuarial local recurrence rate was 26% (Fig. 37.3). The recent NSABP B-17 update reported a 16% local recurrence rate at 12 years (12). The 10% difference may be explained by the fact that

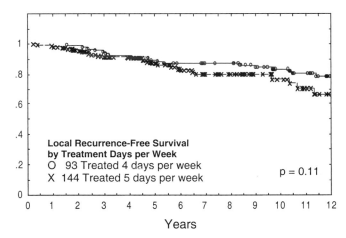

FIGURE 37.2. Probability of local recurrence–free survival for 237 radiation therapy patients grouped by treatment schedule, 4 days per week versus 5 days per week (*p* = 0.11).

TABLE 37.5. TREATMENT FOUR DAYS/WEEKS VERSUS FIVE DAYS/WEEK

	4 Days/Week	5 Days/Week	*p* Value
Number of patients (*n* = 237)	93	144	
Median follow-up (months)	147	76	<0.0001
Average age (years)	53	53	NS
Median tumor size	15	15	NS
Average nuclear grade	2.15	2.31	NS
Clear margins (≥1 mm)	69%	63%	NS
Clear margins (nontransection)	92%	85%	NS
Nonpalpable	86%	90%	NS
Local recurrence	21 (23%)	27 (19%)	NS
Invasive local recurrence	12 (57%)	10 (37%)	NS
Median time to recur (months)	61	54	NS
5-Yr recurrence-free survival	89%	87%	NS
10-Yr recurrence-free survival	83%	77%	NS

NS, not significant.

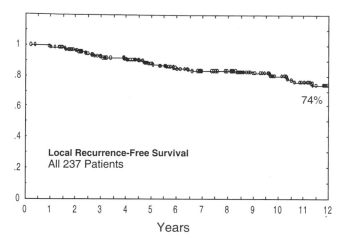

FIGURE 37.3. Probability of local recurrence–free survival for 237 radiation therapy patients.

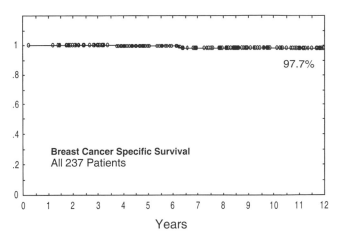

FIGURE 37.5. Probability of local recurrence–free survival for 143 radiation therapy patients.

there was no size limitation on DCIS lesions that could be treated with radiation therapy. In our study, 8% of patients (19 of 237) had tumors 41 mm or greater in size, whereas, the NSABP had none. In our series, only 36% (86 of 237) of the patients had tumors less than or equal to 10 mm in largest dimension. The NSABP had a much higher percentage of small tumors. In the 2001 update, they reported that 75% of their B-17 patients had tumors 10 mm in extent or less (12). Previously, they reported that as many as 85% to 90% of B-17 patients had tumors that small (9–11). In our series, patients with involved and close margins were treated, whereas, the NSABP required clear margins for inclusion in B-17. These differences are sufficient to explain the higher local recurrence rate in our series. When a Kaplan-Meier analysis is run limiting our patients to those with tumors 40 mm in size or smaller and with margins clear by 1 mm or more (*n* = 143), the result is identical to the NSABP: a local recurrence rate of 16% at 12 years (Fig. 37.4).

The overall higher local recurrence rate (26% at 12 years) had no effect on the probability of breast cancer–specific fatality. At 12 years, the breast cancer–specific fatality for our series was 2.3% (Fig. 37.5) compared with 3.7% for the NSABP. In our series, no patient developed regional or distant disease without first developing a local invasive recurrence. In the NSABP B-17 trial, at least seven irradiated patients developed regional or distant disease as the first event.

In our series, the patients were further subdivided by whether or not they met the criteria of Lagios (20,21) (Fig. 37.6). Essentially, to meet the Lagios criteria, a lesion had to be nonpalpable, discovered mammographically by microcalcifications, less than 25 mm in diameter, and completely excised with margins of 1 mm or more. Patients who met those criteria had an actuarial local recurrence rate of 8% at 5 years and 12% at 10 years; patients who did not meet the Lagios criteria had 5- and 10-year recurrence rates of 16% and 30%, respectively.

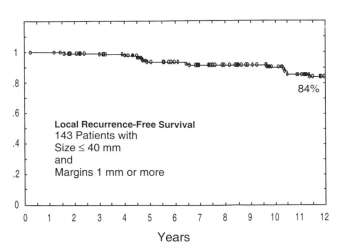

FIGURE 37.4. Probability of breast cancer–specific survival for 237 radiation therapy patients.

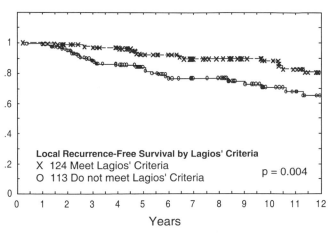

FIGURE 37.6. Probability of local recurrence–free survival for 237 radiation therapy patients grouped by whether they meet the Lagios criteria for breast preservation without radiation therapy (*p* = 0.004).

DISCUSSION

Since the mid 1980s, radiation therapy has routinely been used as part of breast-conserving therapy for patients with DCIS. The NSABP protocol B-17, which was the first prospective randomized study published that examined post-excision radiation therapy versus observation in patients with DCIS, concluded that postoperative radiation therapy was more appropriate than excision alone for conservatively treated patients with DCIS (8). The initial publication lacked a subset analysis that could have defined patients who might not benefit from radiation therapy. In defense of the NSABP, this study was designed to answer a more global question, that is, does radiation therapy decrease the local recurrence rate for patients with DCIS? The answer was clear and affirmative. Radiation therapy decreased local recurrence of both DCIS and invasive breast cancer, and the decreases were statistically significant. These results have been confirmed by prospective randomized trials conducted by the EORTC (13,14) and the U.K. (15,16).

It is now recognized that postoperative radiation therapy may not significantly benefit all patients with DCIS (12,22,23), and efforts are currently underway to determine which subsets of patients are best treated with wide excision followed by careful observation and which will require radiation therapy. Once these studies have been completed, many patients will continue to require radiation therapy, but not all patients will require post-excisional radiation therapy. Until these studies have matured, the information obtained from retrospective reviews and observational trials will aid in making treatment decisions about the growing DCIS population and will help to formulate new avenues for prospective trials. Earlier and earlier diagnosis and total excision by stereotactic biopsy will introduce a new subset of patients about which there is no data at this time.

The data presented in this chapter summarize our experience in treating patients with DCIS with excision plus definitive radiation therapy. Almost 90% of the patients in this series had nonpalpable lesions. Microcalcifications were the most common finding on mammography (> 80%). The rate of local recurrence in the breast increased as the nuclear grade of the primary tumor increased. The probability of local recurrence increased as tumors got larger, and decreased as margin width increased. Finally, no differences between radiation therapy delivered 4 days per week compared with 5 days per week was apparent as measured by time to first local recurrence, local recurrence–free survival, or cosmetic result.

An analysis regarding the weekly irradiation dose given to the breast has never been done for patients with DCIS. Other studies have examined weekly doses for infiltrating ductal carcinoma (17,18). These series suggest that doses less than 800 cGy per week may lead to increased local recurrence rates in the breast. However, in the study of Kurtz et al. (17), patients were treated with a protracted treatment course (τ 10 weeks) and weekly dose rates as low as 400 to 600 cGy. Furthermore, these older series did not assess margin status, nuclear grade, tumor size, or mammographic findings (parameters routinely used to guide current treatment decisions); therefore, their results are not comparable with the current series.

The present analysis examined a weekly dose of 800 cGy (200 cGy per fraction 4 days per week) in patients with DCIS and found no difference in local disease free–survival and cosmetic result when compared with 900 cGy per week (180 cGy 5 days per week). There may be several reasons why this study did not find a difference in outcome for these two different methods of treatment.

The patients treated 4 days per week were generally boosted with 2,000 cGy by iridium implant. The 5 days per week patients usually underwent external beam boost, and the average boost dose was approximately 1,600 cGy. Therefore, the type of boost and total boost dose differed between the two groups.

Two studies have examined outcome in patients given various boost modalities as part of breast-conserving therapy for invasive breast cancer. Ray et al. (24) compared electron beam with Iridium-192 boosts in 130 patients and reported no significant differences in local control or overall cosmesis. Vicini et al. (25) analyzed the implant experience of William Beaumont Hospital for 402 patients. After excisional biopsy and whole-breast irradiation, patients received at least 6,000 cGy to the tumor bed with photons, electrons, or interstitial implant that used either Iridium-192 or I-125. After a median follow-up of 60 months, no significant differences were noted between the boost modalities with regard to local control or cosmetic outcome. These two studies provide evidence suggesting that boost method does not affect local control or cosmesis with appropriate overall dose to the tumor bed.

The results of the above studies are similar to our findings in patients with DCIS. However, our 4-days-per-week patients were given a slightly higher median dose to the tumor bed than the 5-days-per-week patients. Literature regarding the optimal dose of irradiation for patients undergoing breast-conserving therapy comes from studies on invasive ductal cancers. Nobler et al. (26) reported increased local control with doses exceeding 6,000 cGy. Van Limbergen (27) also reported the existence of a dose-response relationship. Clarke et al. (5) reported a dose-response relationship: an increased local recurrence rate was seen when a nominal standard dose of less than 1,840 ret (rad equivalent therapy) was given to the tumor bed. Our patients received a minimum of 6,000 cGy to the tumor bed, and most implant patients received 7,000 cGy. It is possible that a dose-response relationship exists between 6,000 cGy and 7,000 cGy that accounts for the equivalent local control seen in patients treated 4 days per week compared with 5 days per week. Based on these data, we conclude that patients with DCIS who miss treatments because of travel considerations or medical reasons are not compromised by treatment given 4 days per week as long as an appreciable boost to the tumor bed is delivered.

No comment can be made, based on our data, regarding the need for a boost. Both the NSABP and EORTC DCIS trials treated to 5,000 cGy without a boost. Their 4- to 12-year recurrence rates are similar to ours and to other published studies (most of which used a boost). For invasive breast cancer, the EORTC has recently reported a statistically significant lower local recurrence rate when a boost was used (28).

In summary, the increasing incidence of DCIS necessitates that current treatment options undergo continuous re-evaluation. Although it is likely that subsets of low-risk patients will be adequately treated with excision and observation, it is equally likely that patients at high risk for local recurrence will require radiation therapy as part of their management. Our data suggest that histologic factors may aid in treatment decisions: large size, narrow margin width, high nuclear grade, and comedo architecture were all statistically associated with increased local recurrence rates.

REFERENCES

1. Ernster VL, Barclay J, Kerlikowske K, et al. Incidence and treatment for ductal carcinoma in situ of the breast. *JAMA* 1996;275: 913–918.
2. Sarrazin D, Le MG, Arriagada R, et al. Ten year results of a randomized trial comparing a conservative treatment to mastectomy in early breast cancer. *Radiother Oncol* 1989;14:177–184.
3. Fisher B, Anderson S. Conservative surgery for the management of invasive and noninvasive carcinomas of the breast: NSABP trials. *World J Surg* 1994;18:63–69.
4. Blichert-Toft M, Rose C, Anderson JA, et al. Danish randomized trial comparing breast conservation therapy with mastectomy: six years of life-table analysis. *J Natl Cancer Inst Monogr* 1992;11:19–25.
5. Clarke DH, Le MG, Sarrazin D, et al. Analysis of local regional relapse in patients with early breast cancers treated by excision and radiotherapy: experience of the Institut Gustave-Roussy. *Int J Radiat Oncol Biol Phys* 1985;11:137–145.
6. Lichter AS, Lippman ME, Danforth DN, et al. Mastectomy versus breast-conserving therapy in the treatment of stage I and II carcinoma of the breast: A randomized trial at the National Cancer Institute. *J Clin Oncol* 1992;10:976–983.
7. Veronesi U. Rationale and indications for limited surgery in breast cancer: Current data. *World J Surg* 1987;11;493–498.
8. Fisher B, Costantino J, Redmond C, et al. Lumpectomy compared with lumpectomy and radiation therapy for the treatment of intraductal breast cancer. *N Engl J Med* 1993;328:1581–1586.
9. Fisher B, Dignam J, Wolmark N, et al. Lumpectomy and radiation therapy for the treatment of intraductal breast cancer: Findings from National Surgical Adjuvant Breast and Bowel Project B-17. *J Clin Oncol* 1998;16:441–452.
10. Fisher ER, Constantino J, Fisher B, et al. Pathologic Finding from the National Surgical Adjuvant Breast Project (NSABP) Protocol B-17: Intraductal Carcinoma (Ductal Carcinoma In Situ). *Cancer* 1995;75:1310–1319.
11. Fisher ER, Dignam J, Tan-Chiu E, et al. Pathologic findings from the National Surgical Adjuvant Breast Project (NSABP)
eight-year update of Protocol B-17: Intraductal Carcinoma. *Cancer* 1999;86:429–438.
12. Fisher B, Land S, Mamounas E, et al. Prevention of invasive breast cancer in women with ductal carcinoma in situ: An update of the National Surgical Adjuvant Breast and Bowel Project Experience. *Semin Oncol* 2001;28:400–418.
13. Julien JP, Bijker N, Fentiman I, et al. Radiotherapy in breast-conserving treatment for ductal carcinoma in situ: First results of EORTC randomised phase III trial 10853. *Lancet* 2000;355; 528–533.
14. Bijker N, Peterse JL, Duchateau L, et al. Risk factors for recurrence and metastasis after breast conserving therapy for ductal carcinoma in situ: Analysis of European Organization for Research and Treatment of Cancer Trial 10853. *J Clin Oncol* 2001; 19:2263–2271.
15. George WD, Houghton J, Cuzick J, et al. Radiotherapy and tamoxifen following complete local excision (CLE) in the management of ductal carcinoma in situ (DCIS): preliminary results from the U.K. DCIS trial. *Proc Am Soc Clin Oncol* 2000;19: 70a(abst).
16. George W, Houghton J, Cuzick J et al. Radiotherapy and tamoxifen following complete local excision (CLE) in the management of ductal carcinoma in situ (DCIS): preliminary results from the UK DCIS trial. *Proc Am Soc Clin Oncol* 2000; 19:70A.
17. Kurtz JM, Amalrick R, Brandone H, et al. How important is adequate radiotherapy for the long-term results of breast-conserving treatment? *Radiother Oncol* 1991;20:84.
18. Osborne MP, Ormiston N, Harmer CL, et al. Breast conservation in the treatment of early breast cancer. *Cancer* 1984;53:349.
19. Solin LJ, Kurtz J, Fourquet A, et al. Fifteen-year results of breast-conserving surgery and definitive breast irradiation for the treatment of ductal carcinoma in situ of the breast. *J Clin Oncol* 1996; 14:754–763.
20. Lagios MD, Westdahl PR, Margolin FR, et al. Duct carcinoma in situ: Relationship of extent of noninvasive disease to the frequency of occult invasion, multicentricity, lymph node metastases, and short-term treatment failures. *Cancer* 1982;50:1309–1314.
21. Lagios MD, Margolin FR, Westdahl PR, et al. Mammographically detected duct carcinoma in situ. Frequency of local recurrence following tylectomy and prognostic effect of nuclear grade on local recurrence. *Cancer* 1989;63:618–624.
22. Silverstein MJ, Lagios M, Craig P, et al. A prognostic index for ductal carcinoma in situ of the breast. *Cancer* 1996;77:2267–2274.
23. Silverstein MJ, Lagios MD, Groshen S, et al. The influence of margin width on local control in patients with ductal carcinoma in situ (DCIS) of the breast. *N Engl J Med* 1999:340:1455–1461.
24. Ray GR, Fish VJ. Biopsy and definitive radiation therapy in stage I and II adenocarcinoma of the female breast: Analysis of cosmesis and the role of electron beam supplementation. *Int J Radiat Oncol Biol Phys* 1983;9:813.
25. Vicini FA, White J, Gustafson G, et al. The use of Iodine-125 seeds as a substitute for Iridium-192 seeds in temporary interstitial breast implants. *Int J Radiat Oncol Biol Phys* 1993;27:561–566.
26. Nobler MP, Venet L. Prognostic factors in patients undergoing curative irradiation for breast cancer. *Int J Radiat Oncol Biol Phys* 1985;11:1323–1331.
27. Van Limbergen E, van den Bogaert W, van der Schueren E, et al. Tumor excision and radiotherapy as primary treatment of breast cancer analysis of patient and treatment parameters and local control. *Radiother Oncol* 1987;8:1–9.
28. Bartelink H, Collette L, Forquet A, et al. Impact of a boost of 16GY on the local control and cosmesis in patients with early breast cancer: The EORTC "Boost versus no boost" trial. *Int J Radiat Oncol Biol Phys* 2000;48(3)S:111.

38

DUCTAL CARCINOMA IN SITU: COLLECTED EXPERIENCE OF THE FRENCH REGIONAL COMPREHENSIVE CANCER CENTERS

BRUNO CUTULI
HERVÉ MIGNOTTE
RENAUD FAY
SYLVIA GIARD

CHRISTINE COHEN-SOLAL-LE NIR
VIRGINIE FICHET
CLAIRE LEMANSKI
CLAIRE CHARRA-BRUNAUD
JEAN-CHRISTOPHE CHARPENTIER

BRIGITTE DE LAFONTAN
VÉRONIQUE SERVENT
FRÉDÉRIQUE PENAULT-LLORCA
HUGUES AUVRAY

Approximately 35,000 new cases of breast cancer are diagnosed in France each year, of which about 3,500 are ductal carcinoma in situ (DCIS). With the increasing use of mammography, it is estimated that the proportion of DCIS will rise to 20% over the next decade (1,2,3).

The regional comprehensive cancer centers treat approximately 25% of all breast cancer patients in France. We pooled our experience for patients with DCIS treated at nine centers from January 1985 to December 1995 by either mastectomy or breast-conserving therapy (with or without radiotherapy). In this chapter, we summarize our findings and discuss their implications.

PATIENTS AND METHODS

Patients with DCIS treated at nine cancer centers were identified by querying a common tumor registry (the "Enquete Permanente Cancer"). Patients with microinvasive cancers or axillary nodal involvement were excluded. A total of 882 cases were treated during the study period of 1985 to 1995: 177 patients (20%) underwent mastectomy, 190 patients (22%) had conservative surgery without radiotherapy (CS), and 515 patients (58%) were treated with conservative surgery plus radiotherapy (CS + RT). Breast-conserving surgery was generally used for tumors smaller than 3 cm, but the use of radiation therapy following CS varied widely between the centers. Axillary dissection was performed routinely in the mastectomy group and in 36% and 53% of patients treated with breast-conserving therapy who had nonpalpable or palpable lesions, respectively.

Patient characteristics for each treatment subgroup are listed in Table 38.1. The mean age of the study population was 53.5 years. Sixty-four percent of lesions were nonpalpable, 21% were palpable, and the means of detection were not specified in 15% of cases. The size of the lesion was precisely assessed in only 50% of patients. The mean tumor size was largest in the mastectomy group and smallest in the CS group. Histological subtype was known in 91% of cases.

The recurrence-free interval was defined by the period between the date of the first surgery and the date of disease recurrence. Actuarial recurrence rates were calculated by the Kaplan-Meier method and compared using the log-rank test. A Cox proportional-hazards model was used to assess the relationship of outcome to the use of radiotherapy, tumor stage, age at diagnosis, margin status, and family history of breast cancer in the breast-conserving therapy group.

RESULTS

With a mean follow-up of 7 years, there were 129 local recurrences (15%). The crude local failure rates in the three treatment subgroups are shown in Table 38.2. These were 2%, 31%, and 13% among the mastectomy, CS, and CS + RT groups, respectively ($p < 0.0001$) (Fig. 38.1). The median times to development of local recurrence were 53, 41, and 55 months, respectively. Nodal recurrence was found in only 2% of the conservatively treated patients (3 patients in the CS group and 9 in the CS + RT group). Distant metastases occurred in 1%, 3%, and 1% of the three treatment groups.

The risk of recurrence was substantially reduced by the addition of radiotherapy for the 501 patients with mammographically detected tumors treated with conservative

TABLE 38.1. PATIENT CHARACTERISTICS

Characteristic	Mastectomy	Conservative Surgery	Conservative Surgery Plus Radiotherapy
No. of patients	177	190	515
Mean age (years)	53.6	54.1	53.4
Mean follow-up (years)	6.4	7.2	7.3
Nonpalpable	37%	65%	73%
Size, palpable lesions			
<2 cm	9%	17%	13%
2–5 cm	11%	4%	8%
Unknown	43%	14%	6%
Positive family history	38%	25%	26%
Histological tumor size			
<10 mm	2%	22%	26%
>10 mm	25%	17%	36%
Not specified	73%	61%	37%
Mean size (mm)	30.7	9.9	14.5
Architectural subtype			
Cribriform	12%	18%	12%
Papillary	4%	3%	7%
Cribriform + papillary	22%	34%	28%
Solid	6%	3%	8%
Clinging	2%	2%	3%
Comedo	49%	17%	37%
Not specified	6%	20%	5%

surgery. Local failure rates were 37% and 11% without and with RT, respectively ($p < 0.000001$) (Fig. 38.2).

The other two most important factors influencing the risk of local failure in patients treated with breast-conserving therapy as a group were patient age and margin status. Among women treated with CS, 7-year local failure rates were 36%, 31%, and 30% among women age 40 years or younger, 41 to 60, and 61 or older, respectively. The differences were not statistically significant. For women treated with CS + RT, local failure rates in these age subgroups were 33%, 13% and 8%, respectively ($p < 0.001$) (Fig. 38.3). Patients with negative, positive, or uncertain margins

had 7-year local failure rates of 26%, 56%, and 29%, respectively if treated with CS ($p = 0.02$) and 11%, 23%, and 9% if treated with CS + RT ($p = 0.008$) (Fig. 38.4).

Tumor size did not influence local failure rates in either the CS or CS + RT groups (Table 38.3). For "favorable" patients (those having complete excision of tumors smaller than 10 mm), radiotherapy decreased the local failure rate, regardless of patient age (Table 38.4). The type of surgery performed (quadrantectomy or tumorectomy) did not significantly influence failure rates in either the CS group (23% and 32% local failure rates, respectively) or among patients treated with CS + RT (15% versus 12%).

TABLE 38.2. TREATMENT RESULTS

Result	Mastectomy (177)	Conservative Surgery (190)	Conservative Surgery Plus Radiotherapy (515)	p
Local recurrence (total)	4 (2%)	59 (31%)	66 (13%)	<0.0001
Noninvasive	0	28 (15%)	26 (5%)	<0.0001
Invasive	4	31 (16%)	40 (8%)	<0.001
Mean time to local failure (months)	52.8	40.8	55.2	NS
Nodal recurrence	0	3 (2%)	9 (2%)	NS
Distant metastases	3 (1%)	5 (3%)	7 (1%)	NS

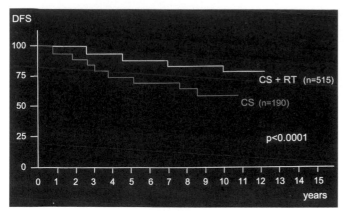

FIGURE 38.1. Disease-free survival after breast-conserving therapy. (*CS, conservative surgery; CS + RT, conservative surgery and radiotherapy.*)

Table 38.5 shows the results in relation to histologic subtype. Radiotherapy reduced the local recurrence rates in all subgroups, but particularly in those with comedocarcinoma (59% versus 17% in the CS and CS + RT groups, respectively; $p < 0.0001$) and those patients with mixed cribriform/papillary tumors (31% versus 9%; $p < 0.0001$). The presence of necrosis, atypical hyperplasia, mastosis, or lobular carcinoma in situ had no influence on the risk of local recurrence in either the irradiated or unirradiated patients.

In the multivariate Cox model, when all patients undergoing breast-conserving therapy were grouped together, the most significant parameter affecting the local recurrence rate was the use of radiotherapy. The relative risk in the CS + RT group compared with the CS group was 0.35 (95% confidence interval, 0.25 to 0.51; $p = 0.0001$). When patients treated with CS were analyzed separately, the only significant risk factor was margin status, with a relative risk of 1.64 (95% confidence interval, 1.08 to 2.49) for patients with positive or uncertain margins compared with patients with negative margins. For the CS + RT group, young age (40 years or younger) was the most significant predictor of local failure ($p = 0.0012$). The second most significant parame-

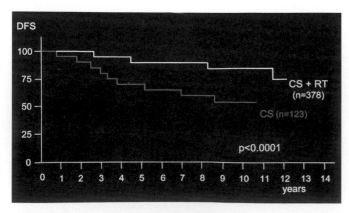

FIGURE 38.2. Disease-free survival after breast-conserving therapy in patients with mammographically detected lesions.

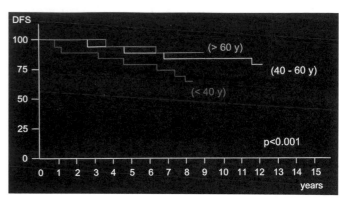

FIGURE 38.3. Disease-free survival in relation to patient age, conservative surgery + radiotherapy group.

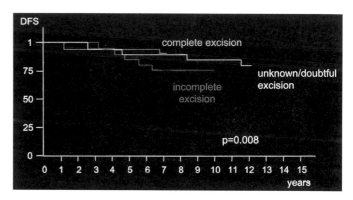

FIGURE 38.4. Disease-free survival in relation to margin status, conservative surgery + radiotherapy group.

TABLE 38.3. LOCAL RECURRENCE IN RELATION TO TUMOR SIZE AND TREATMENT

Treatment	Size <10 mm	Size >10 mm	Not Specified
CS	30%	31%	31%
CS + RT	11%	13%	14%

CS, conservative surgery; CS + RT, conservative surgery + radiotherapy.

TABLE 38.4. LOCAL RECURRENCE IN RELATION TO AGE AND TREATMENT FOR LESIONS SMALLER THAN 10 MM WITH NEGATIVE MARGINS

Treatment	Age <50 Years	Age >50 Years
CS	33% (3/9)	32% (6/19)
CS + RT	9% (4/43)	12% (9/73)
p value	0.09	0.07

CS, conservative surgery; CS + RT, conservative surgery + radiotherapy.

TABLE 38.5. LOCAL RECURRENCE IN RELATION TO HISTOLOGICAL SUBTYPE IN PATIENTS TREATED BY BREAST-CONSERVING THERAPY

Subtype	Conservative Surgery	Conservative Surgery + Radiotherapy	p
Cribriform	14% (5/35)	6% (4/62)	NS
Papillary	17% (1/6)	8% (3/36)	NS
Mixed[a]	31% (21/68)	9% (13/146)	0.0001
Solid + clinging	40% (4/10)	16% (9/56)	NS
Comedocarcinoma[b]	59% (19/32)	17% (32/156)	0.0001
Not specified	23% (9/39)	19% (5/26)	NS

[a] Cribiform plus papillary.
[b] Pure comedo carcinoma or comedo mixed with one or more other subtypes.
NS, not significant.

ter was (again) margin status, with a relative risk of 1.39 (95% confidence interval, 1.06 to 1.82; $p = 0.016$).

For patients in the CS group who suffered a local failure, 34 were treated with mastectomy (including axillary dissection in 25 cases) and 25 with further breast-conserving therapy (including radiotherapy in 20 cases). Further local recurrences occurred in five of these 25 latter cases, and these were then treated with salvage mastectomy.

For the patients who recurred locally following CS + RT, 54 underwent mastectomy (including axillary dissection in 18 cases). Only 14 women underwent breast-conserving surgery, and a second local recurrence developed in four of them, requiring mastectomy.

The local recurrences in all four patients initially undergoing mastectomy were invasive, compared with 53% and 61% of patients initially in the CS and CS + RT groups, respectively. The risk of developing distant failure after an invasive local failure was 16% and 18% in the CS and CS + RT groups, respectively.

Thirty of the 882 study patients (3%) had been previously treated for a contralateral invasive or in situ breast cancer by either mastectomy or breast-conserving therapy. Another 19 patients (2%) were found to have a synchronous invasive breast cancer at the time of diagnosis of DCIS. Finally, 108 patients (12%) developed a contralateral breast cancer. Rates of contralateral breast cancer in the three treatment groups are shown in Table 38.6.

DISCUSSION

Mastectomy remained the safest treatment for women with DCIS, with a 7-year control rate of 98% (3–6). However, breast-conserving therapy has become increasingly popular, as shown by our series collected over a 10-year period, which reflects the routine daily practice in nine French regional comprehensive cancer centers. We observed some minor differences between these centers in patient and tumor characteristics (for example, an increased proportion of nonpalpable DCIS in the regions with an organized mammographic screening program) and in the treatment approach (i.e., different proportions of women treated with breast-conserving therapy, especially without radiotherapy). However, we believe it unlikely that such differences had a substantial impact on the results of the combined population.

Women treated with CS and CS + RT in our series were similar in age, in the proportion of nonpalpable tumors, and in family history of breast cancer. They differed in the mean histologic size of the lesions (9.9 mm and 14.5 mm in CS and CS + RT groups, respectively) and in histologic subtypes, with a higher proportion of comedocarcinoma forms (pure or mixed) in the CS + RT group (37% versus 17%). Despite the lack of random treatment assignment, our results were very similar to those of the NSABP B-17 and EORTC 10853 trials (7–10).

TABLE 38.6. INCIDENCE OF CONTRALATERAL BREAST CANCER BEFORE, SYNCHRONOUS WITH, AND AFTER DIAGNOSIS OF DUCTAL CARCINOMA IN SITU

Treatment (n)	Before	Synchronous[a]	After	Total
Mastectomy (177)	5 (3%)	5 (3%)	11 (7%)	21 (12%)
CS (190)	14 (7%)	4 (2%)	13 (8%)	31 (16%)
CS + RT (515)	11 (2%)	10 (2%)	35 (7%)	56 (11%)
Entire population (882)	30 (3%)	19 (2%)	59 (7%)	108 (12%)

[a] Rates of synchronous and later contralateral breast cancers calculated by excluding patients with prior or synchronous contralateral cancers, respectively.
CS, conservative surgery; CS + RT, conservative surgery plus radiotherapy.

TABLE 38.7. IMPACT OF PATIENT AGE AT DIAGNOSIS ON LOCAL RECURRENCE RATES IN PATIENTS TREATED WITH CONSERVATIVE SURGERY AND RADIOTHERAPY

Series (Reference)	Age	Crude LR Rate	5-Year Actuarial LR	10-Year Actuarial LR
Fourquet (24)	<40	29% (7/24)	—	30%
	>40	14% (18/129)	—	14%
Solin (23)	<50	25% (14/56)	—	25%
	>50	2% (1/54)	—	2%
Hiramatsu (26)	<50	8% (4/39)	—	12%
	>50	8% (3/37)	—	17%
Vicini (25)	<45	23% (7/31)	21%	26%
	>45	9% (10/117)	7%	9%
Van Zee (13)	<40	33% (2/6)	33%	—
	40–69	8% (4/49)	8%	—
	>70	0% (0/10)	0%	—
Fisher (9)	<50	15% (21/137)	15%	—
	50–59	10% (12/115)	11%	—
	>60	9% (14/151)	9%	—
Bijker (10)	<40	23% (5/22)	23%	—
	>40	12% (49/415)	12%	—
Present series	<40	32% (13/40)	—	32%
	40–59	13% (42/334)	—	13%
	>60	8% (11/141)	—	8%

LR, local recurrence.

The most important histologic parameter correlated with the risk of local recurrence is margin status (2,5,11–14). Silverstein and colleagues (12) retrospectively analyzed results in 469 women treated conservatively for DCIS, 256 without and 213 with radiotherapy. With mean follow-up times in these two groups of 72 and 92 months, respectively, local recurrence rates were 15% and 17%, respectively. Radiotherapy substantially reduced the risk of local recurrence in the group with margins of less than 1 mm ($p = 0.01$); whereas only a small benefit of radiotherapy was found for patients with margin widths of 1 to 10 mm, and no difference in local recurrence was seen when the margin width was greater than 10 mm. However, the two groups were not strictly comparable, because patients in the radiotherapy group had a significantly larger median tumor size and a higher percentage of lesion with comedo-type necrosis (10,12). In addition, several investigators consider the fact that "optimal" margin width has not yet been clearly defined (e.g., is it 1, 2, 5, or 10 mm?), and that the optimal width may depend on the surgical procedure used (e.g., whether or not re-excision is performed) and the accuracy of pathologic evaluation (8,12,15–19).

The relationship of tumor size to treatment outcome is uncertain. Tumor size is difficult to assess in multi-institutional studies. For example, in the EORTC trial, the original pathology report only described tumor size 23% of the time (178 of 775 cases) (2,10,15,17). With this consideration in our study, tumor size (smaller or larger than 1 cm) did not influence local recurrence rates in either the CS or CS + RT group.

The impact of histologic features on the risk of local failure is also unclear. There are currently several different schemes for subtyping DCIS (2,15,18,20,21). The more recent classifications use nuclear grade and the presence of necrosis to define "high-risk" groups, but significant problems with interobserver variability still remain in classifying lesions (2). Interpreting the impact of histology has also been difficult because of the frequent finding of two or more architectural patterns in the same lesion. These difficulties may explain, in part, why several series found a higher local recurrence rate among patients with comedo subtypes, but others have shown that with longer follow-up, recurrence rates became similar for all histologic subtypes (2,3,11,22). For example, in the international collaborative multicentric study (which included 270 patients treated with CS + RT), the local failure rate was 18% at 10 years in patients with comedo carcinomas with nuclear grade 3 compared with 15% for patients with other subtypes (22,23). In our study, radiotherapy reduced local recurrence rates for all histologic subgroups with a high significance ($p < 0.0001$ in both cases) among 214 mixed (cribriform plus papillary) and 188 comedocarcinoma lesions.

Our data confirm that young age is an independent risk factor for local recurrence following breast-conserving therapy for DCIS, as it is for patients with invasive breast cancer (7,10,13,22–26). Its impact was especially prominent in the CS + RT group, with a 32% local failure rate in women younger than 40 years old, compared with 11% in older women ($p = 0.001$). In the latest report by Vicini and colleagues (25), 31 women younger than 45 years who were treated with CS + RT had a 10-year local failure rate of 26%, compared with 9% for older patients ($p = 0.03$). The randomized EORTC trial (10) and another two series (13,23) found similar results, as detailed in Table 38.7.

The risk of developing a metachronous contralateral breast cancer (either in situ or invasive) in our series was 7%, 8%, and 7% in the mastectomy, CS, and CS + RT groups, respectively, excluding the 49 women with a previous or simultaneous contralateral invasive breast cancer (Table 38.6). This is consistent with other studies. Singletary (27) noted 2% and 6% rates of synchronous and metachronous contralateral breast cancers, of which 60% were invasive. In a recent study in Bordeaux, 4% of patients (25 of 572) developed a subsequent contralateral breast cancer (5). In the EORTC trial, the rates of contralateral breast cancer in the CS and CS + RT groups were 2% and 4%, respectively ($p = 0.01$) (9). However, the incidences of contralateral breast cancer development were the same in both arms of the NSABP B-17 trial (5%) (7,8). Tamoxifen reduced this risk from 4% to 2% in the NSABP B-24 trial ($p = 0.01$) (28). The majority of contralateral breast cancers in patients in our study were invasive, again consistent with the findings of others.

The outcome of women with local recurrence following breast-conserving treatment for DCIS treatment has not been well studied (29,30). According to Silverstein (30), 15% to 20% of patients with an invasive local recurrence will develop distant metastases. However, other risk factors associated with developing distant metastases are unknown. The EORTC trial results suggest that poorly differentiated DCIS significantly increased this risk (10).

CONCLUSIONS

Our results are based on "clinical current practice" in highly specialized centers that regularly employ a multidisciplinary approach to treat breast diseases with strict quality control procedures (31). We found that radiotherapy strongly reduces local recurrence rates, in accordance with the findings in the NSABP B-17 and EORTC 10853 randomized trials. We confirm the importance of performing complete excision (i.e., having negative margins), both in the CS and the CS + RT groups, and the unfavorable influence of young age at diagnosis on local recurrence rates.

REFERENCES

1. Silverstein MJ. Ductal carcinoma in situ of the breast. *Annu Rev Med* 2000;51:17–32.
2. Schwartz GF, Solin LJ, Olivotto IA, et al. Consensus Conference on the treatment of in situ ductal carcinoma of the breast, April 22–25, 1999. *Cancer* 2000;88:946–954.
3. Winchester DP, Jeske JM, Goldschmidt RA. The diagnosis and management of ductal carcinoma in situ of the breast. *CA Cancer J Clin* 2000;50:184–200.
4. Ringberg A, Idwall I, Fernö M, et al. Ipsilateral local recurrence in relation to therapy and morphological characteristics in patients with ductal carcinoma in situ of the breast. *Eur J Surg Oncol* 2000;26:444–451.
5. Tunon de Lara C, de Mascarel I, MacGrogan G, et al. Analysis of 676 ductal carcinoma in situ (DCIS) of the breast from 1971 to 1995: Diagnosis and treatment; the experience of one institute. *Am J Clin Oncol* 2001;24:531–536.
6. Boyages J, Delaney G, Taylor R. Predictors of local recurrence after treatment of ductal carcinoma in situ. A meta-analysis. *Cancer* 1999;85:616–628.
7. Fisher B, Dignam J, Wolkmar N, et al. Lumpectomy and radiation therapy for the treatment of intraductal breast cancer: findings from National Surgical Adjuvant Breast and Bowel Project B-17. *J Clin Oncol* 1998:16:441–452.
8. Fisher ER, Dignam J, Tan-Chiu E, et al. Pathologic findings from National Surgical Adjuvant Breast Project (NSABP). Eight-year update of Protocol B-17. Intraductal Carcinoma. *Cancer* 1999;86:429–438.
9. Julien JP, Bijker N, Fentiman IS, et al. Radiotherapy in breast-conservative treatment for ductal carcinoma in situ: first results of the EORTC randomised phase III trial 10853. *Lancet* 2000;355: 528–533.
10. Bijker N, Peterse JL, Duchateau L, et al. Risk factors for recurrence and metastasis after breast-conserving therapy for ductal carcinoma in situ: Analysis of European Organisation for Research and Treatment of Cancer trial 10853. *J Clin Oncol* 2001; 19:2263–2271.
11. Hwang ES, Esserman LJ. Management of ductal carcinoma in situ. *Surg Clin North Am* 1999;79:1007–1030.
12. Silverstein MJ, Lagios MD, Groshen S, et al. The influence of margin width on local control of ductal carcinoma in situ of the breast. *N Engl J Med* 1999;340:1455–1461.
13. Van Zee KJ, Liberman L, Samli B, et al. Long-term follow-up of women with ductal carcinoma in situ treated with breast-conserving surgery. The effect of age. *Cancer* 1999;86:1757–1767.
14. Bonnier P, Body G, Bessenay F, et al. Prognostic factors in ductal carcinoma in situ of the breast: results of a retrospective study of 575 cases. The Association for Research in Oncologic Gynecology. *Eur J Obstet Gynecol Reprod Biol* 1999;84:27–35.
15. Recht A, Van Dongen JA, Fentiman IS, et al. Third meeting of the DCIS Working Party of the EORTC (Fondazione Cini, Isola S. Giorgio, Venezia, 28 February 1994)—conference report. *Eur J Cancer* 1994;30A:1895–1901.
16. Holland R, Hendriks JHCL. Microcalcifications associated with ductal carcinoma in situ: mammographic-pathologic correlation. *Semin Diagn Pathol* 1994;11:181–192.
17. Faverly DRG, Burgers L, Bult P, et al. Three-dimensional imaging of mammary ductal carcinoma in situ: clinical implications. *Semin Diagn Pathol* 1994;11:193–198.
18. Zafrani B, Contesso G, Eusebi V, et al. Guidelines for the pathological management of mammographically detected breast lesions. *Breast* 1995;4:52–56.
19. Vicini FA, Lacerna MD, Goldstein NS, et al. Ductal carcinoma in situ detected in the mammographic era: an analysis of clinical, pathologic, and treatment-related factors affecting outcome with breast-conserving therapy. *Int J Radiat Oncol Biol Phys* 1997;39: 627–365.
20. Holland R, Peterse JL, Millis RR, et al. Ductal carcinoma in situ: a proposal for a new classification. *Semin Diagn Pathol* 1994;11: 167–180.
21. Silverstein MJ, Poller DN, Waisman JR, et al. Prognostic classification of breast ductal carcinoma in situ. *Lancet* 1995;345: 1154–1157.
22. Solin LJ, Yeh IT, Kurtz J, et al. Ductal carcinoma in situ (intra-

ductal carcinoma) of the breast treated with breast-conserving surgery and definitive irradiation. Correlation of pathologic parameters with outcome of treatment. *Cancer* 1993;71:2532–2542.

23. Solin LJ, Kurtz J, Fourquet A, et al. Fifteen-year results of breast-conserving surgery and definitive breast irradiation for the treatment of ductal carcinoma in situ of the breast. *J Clin Oncol* 1996; 14:754–763.

24. Fourquet A, Zafrani B, Campana F, et al. Institut Curie experience. In: Silverstein MJ, ed. *Ductal Carcinoma In Situ of the Breast*. Baltimore: Williams & Wilkins, 1997:391–397.

25. Vicini FA, Kestin LL, Golstein NS, et al. Impact of young age on outcome in patients with ductal carcinoma in situ treated with breast-conserving therapy. *J Clin Oncol* 2000;18:296–306.

26. Hiramatsu H, Bornstein BA, Recht A, et al. Local recurrence after conservative surgery and radiation therapy for ductal carcinoma in situ: possible importance of family history. *Cancer J* 1995;1:55–61.

27. Singletary SE. Management of the contralateral breast. In: Silverstein MJ, ed. *Ductal Carcinoma In Situ of the Breast*. Baltimore: Williams & Wilkins, 1997:563–567.

28. Fisher B, Dignam J, Wolmark N, et al. Tamoxifen in treatment of intraductal breast cancer: National Surgical Adjuvant Breast and Bowel Project B-24 randomised controlled trial. *Lancet* 2000;353:1993–2000.

29. Hillner BE, Desch CE, Carlson RW, et al. Trade-offs between survival and breast preservation for three initial treatments of ductal carcinoma in situ of the breast. *J Clin Oncol* 1996;14:70–77.

30. Silverstein MJ, Lagios MD, Martino S, et al. Outcome after invasive local recurrence in patients with ductal carcinoma in situ of the breast. *J Clin Oncol* 1998;16:1367–1373.

31. Rutgers EJ. Quality control in the locoregional treatment of breast cancer. *Eur J Cancer* 2001;37:447–453.

39

SHOULD ALL DUCTAL CARCINOMA IN SITU PATIENTS RECEIVE RADIATION THERAPY AND IS PARTIAL BREAST IRRADIATION AN OPTION?

ROBERT R. KUSKE, JR.

SHOULD ALL DUCTAL CARCINOMA IN SITU PATIENTS RECEIVE BREAST IRRADIATION?

The role of radiation therapy after breast-conserving surgery is to reduce the risk of future recurrence by eradicating occult foci of malignant cells remaining after lesionectomy. Therefore, to address this question, four issues are paramount:

1. What is the chance that ductal carcinoma in situ (DCIS) remains after surgery?
2. Is radiation therapy effective in eliminating these malignant cells?
3. What is the threshold risk above which radiation therapy will be recommended?
4. Are there subsets of DCIS with a low risk of recurrence after surgery without radiation therapy?

The chance that DCIS remains after surgery depends on how extensive the surgery has been. Patients undergoing a total mastectomy have a risk of recurrence generally less than 2% in most studies. Patients having a limited excision of the lesion, with varying margin width, at a minimum of "no ink on tumor," have a recurrence rate of at least 30% at 8 years (1). Patients with microscopic margin involvement may have a risk of recurrence greater than 30%.

Numerous studies have demonstrated the effectiveness of radiation therapy in reducing the risk of either noninvasive or invasive recurrence after breast-conserving surgery. Two randomized trials have directly compared lesionectomy alone versus lesionectomy followed by radiation therapy (1,2). In the National Surgical Adjuvant Breast Project (NS-ABP) trial B-17, whole-breast external beam irradiation reduces the risk of an invasive recurrence by a factor of 3 and noninvasive recurrence by a factor of 2.

Somewhere between the 30% or greater risk of recurrence after limited excision of DCIS and the 0% to 2% risk of recurrence after total mastectomy, there is an in-between risk with a more generous excision below which radiation therapy would not be recommended for most patients. Above this threshold, most patients would receive radiation therapy. This threshold risk is controversial and may vary based on the priorities of individual patients but generally is approximately 15%. If one assumes that half of the recurrences are likely to be invasive carcinoma and accepts the risk reduction for breast irradiation, then the 7.5% of invasive recurrences would be reduced to 2.5% and the noninvasive recurrences would be reduced to 7.5% divided by 2, or 3.7%. For a woman at this presumptive threshold risk of 15%, her overall risk would be reduced to 6.2% by breast irradiation, for an absolute risk reduction of 8.8%. These figures are illustrative and based on critical assumptions, but the process can be helpful in deciding which patients should be offered breast irradiation. Of course, clinical judgment would prevail when other factors such as age older than 70 years come into play.

The difficult task is determining the recurrence risk for an individual patient based on minimum margin width, lesion size, and perhaps other clinical or pathologic features. It seems certain that subsets of patients with DCIS can safely avoid whole-breast irradiation. Defining this subset should be the focus of future clinical trials.

If margin width is the critical factor in avoiding radiation therapy, there are two major concerns that should be considered. First, the pathologist must report accurate and reliable assessment of margin width. This is not simple, and how the specimen is processed and sectioned can affect the result. Second, cosmetic outcome may be adversely affected by surgical attention to achieving generous margins. In many women, a 5-mm minimum margin without re-excision, followed by radiation therapy, may be cosmetically preferable to a 10-mm margin without breast irradiation, especially if re-excision is required. Small increases in the amount of tissue removed can have a large impact on the volume of breast tissue remaining. For example, if an additional 1 cm of tissue is excised after an initial specimen measuring $5 \times 4 \times 2.5$ cm, the additional volume removed is more than double (105 cc versus 50 cc). Thus, there can be a significant cosmetic price to pay for surgical attempts to achieve generously negative margins to avoid radiation therapy in patients with DCIS.

CONCEPT OF PARTIAL BREAST IRRADIATION: ACCELERATED HYPERFRACTIONATED RADIATION THERAPY TO 2 CM BEYOND THE SURGICAL BED IN SELECT BREAST CANCERS

Once the decision has been made to lower the risk of breast cancer relapse by offering breast irradiation, whole-breast external beam radiation therapy has been the standard of care, using tangential fields to minimize lung and heart dose. Does the entire breast require treatment in every case of breast cancer? Traditionally, the answer to this question has been an unequivocal yes. Beginning with the Halstead radical and evolving to the modified radical and simple (total) mastectomies, the surgical teaching has been predicated on removal of all breast tissue. With the advent of breast-preserving approaches, this underlying philosophy remained constant because the remaining breast tissue was comprehensively irradiated. Indeed, the switch from mastectomy to breast-conservation therapy was not the radical departure from tradition as the concept discussed in this chapter. The rationale for treating less than the total breast is presented in the next section.

Biologically, there is a theoretical advantage to dose-intense radiation therapy. All the techniques described below deliver the radiation dose over 5 days instead of the traditional 6 weeks of whole-breast external beam treatment. Using a linear quadratic model, the dose of radiation is calculated to be equivalent with respect to tumor cell kill to 6 weeks of traditional external beam radiation therapy. This model also predicts that the late normal tissue effects will be similar. The goal is to deliver the equivalent of a conventional fractionation (180 to 200 cGy per day over 5 weeks) total dose of 45 Gy to the periphery of the target volume, with higher central doses, providing a boost to the breast tissue closest to the surgical edge. The prescription point receives 340 to 400 cGy twice daily. The second daily fraction is given 6 or more hours after the first one to allow time for the repair of sublethal DNA damage in normal tissues. With a 4-day regimen, 32 Gy is given in eight fractions of 400 cGy over 4 days. With a 5-day regimen, 34 Gy is given in ten fractions of 340 cGy over 5 days. This treatment is hyperfractionated, meaning that more than one fraction is given per day and accelerated because the entire treatment course is completed within 1 week.

The goal of radiation therapy is to eradicate subclinical microscopic disease remaining after surgical excision of the gross tumor. Regions at low risk of residual carcinoma are to be avoided, whereas the most likely sites should be treated. The ideal radiation delivery system seems to conform the dose around the most peripheral cancer cell, sparing normal tissue as much as possible.

A key issue is defining the correct target volume. The Milan investigators performed surgical quadrantectomies, with tumor control rates better than tumorectomies, but still inferior to quadrantectomy followed by whole breast irradiation (3). It is clear that many patients benefit from the treatment of more than a simple quadrant. We hypothesized that the breast tissue harboring any remaining cancer cells was within 2 cm of a clean excision margin. This definition usually exceeds a quadrant of the breast. For example, if an average lumpectomy specimen measures $5 \times 4 \times 2.5$ cm and 2 cm is added to each of these dimensions, the resulting volume is 189 cm^3, clearly more than a simple quadrant of most breasts.

There are many methods for delivering partial-breast irradiation:

1. Wide-volume breast interstitial brachytherapy,
2. Intracavitary brachytherapy,
3. Conformal external beam radiation therapy,
4. Intensity-modulated radiation therapy,
5. Intracavitary soft x-rays,
6. Electron beam radiation therapy.

Brachytherapy, from the Greek root meaning "from a short distance," is the placement of radioactive sources within tissue. For interstitial brachytherapy, iridium 192 seeds are popular because they emit gamma rays, which have a favorable energy and specific activity to treat to a proper depth over a reasonable period of time. Iodine 125 has also been used. The seeds typically measure 3×1 mm so they can be conveniently placed inside plastic catheters or 17-gauge needles. The radiation dose falls off rapidly as the distance away from the source increases, according to the inverse square law of physics. With proper intercatheter separations, a geometric array of catheters encompassing the target volume will deliver a relatively hot central dose, presumably where the greatest density of malignant clonogenic cells is likely to reside, the prescribed dose to the periphery of the target volume, and lower doses to the surrounding normal breast tissue, skin, muscle, ribs, lung, heart, and so on. Because of this ability to control the dose distribution, brachytherapy is considered the ultimate conformal radiation therapy.

Both low and high dose rate brachytherapy have been investigated for accelerated partial-breast irradiation, as described later. Low dose rate source trains are left inside the catheters for the duration of the treatment, typically 45 Gy over 4 to 5 days, 24 hours per day. Low dose rate brachytherapy can be envisioned as an infinite number of

TABLE 39.1. SITE OF RECURRENCE AFTER CONSERVATIVE SURGERY AND BREAST IRRADIATION (INVASIVE CANCER)

Study	% of Recurrence that is Local (same quadrant)	% of Recurrence that is Remote (different quadrant)	% of All Treated Patients with Remote Recurrences
Fisher et al., 1989 (5)	100	0	0
Clark, 1992 (6)	83	17	1.0
Recht et al., 1988 (7)	80	20	2.0
Fowble et al., 1990 (8)	65	35	2.2
Kurtz et al., 1990 (9)	79	21	2.3
Veronesi et al., 1990 (10)	55	45	2.5
Haffty et al., 1989 (11)	67	33	3.6

tiny radiation doses. Because they are manually loaded and require an in-patient stay in isolation, there are radiation safety issues with low dose rate brachytherapy. High dose rate brachytherapy delivers 340 to 400 cGy over approximately 12 to 15 minutes to the prescription point as an outpatient while the patient is in a shielded room, avoiding many radiation safety problems. Between fractions, the patient can work, stay at home with her family, and eliminate the cost associated with an in-patient hospital stay.

There is recent work exploring the possibility of delivering similar doses and dose distribution with external beam techniques. Using multiple fields and special beam shaping, conformal radiation therapy may be a noninvasive alternative to brachytherapy. A more complex technique, intensity-modulated radiation therapy can contour radiation dose curves of virtually any shape. Conceivably, intensity-modulated radiation therapy would be capable of treating 2 cm around the lesionectomy cavity. Practical difficulties include chest wall motion during breathing and exposure of a significant portion of the body to a small radiation dose. It also remains to be seen whether clinical outcomes with a homogeneous dose distribution of these external beam systems will match the results of brachytherapy, where there is an inherent dose gradient.

RATIONALE FOR PARTIAL-BREAST IRRADIATION

When mastectomy specimens are fixed and analyzed slice by slice using the Egan serial subgross method, the distribution of breast cancer cells within the breast can be determined.

Holland et al. (4) examined mastectomy specimens from 264 patients with cancers 4 cm or smaller, all considered candidates for breast-conservation therapy. True multicentric breast cancer was rarely seen; the disease was noted to be interconnected, spreading outward from the epicenter. The chance of finding cancer decreases as the distance from the primary cancer increases.

Most true recurrences after breast-conservation therapy develop within and surrounding the original tumor site. In Table 39.1, data are presented from studies in which recurrences are divided between local (in the immediate vicinity of the surgical site) and remote (at a distance from the surgical site or in a different quadrant).

Thus, the percentage of patients receiving whole-breast irradiation who fail in a remote location of the breast, possibly not covered by partial-breast irradiation, ranges from 0% to 3.6%. Is this low rate attributable to sterilization of the other quadrants of the treated breast by radiation therapy? If so, then one would expect the rate of remote relapse to increase dramatically in studies in which no radiation therapy is given. Table 39.2 presents the location of breast failure in patients treated with lumpectomy alone.

The percentage of patients who fail in a portion of the breast that may not be covered by partial-breast irradiation is approximately the same, 0% to 3.5% or 3.6%, whether whole-breast irradiation is given or not. Because remote relapses tend to occur more than 5 years after treatment (7), they follow a time pattern similar to that of second primary breast cancers in the contralateral breast. These data cast doubt on the belief that remote recurrences originate from multicentric carcinoma present at the time of the index lesion. It is more plausible that a remote relapse originates

TABLE 39.2. SITE OF RECURRENCE AFTER LUMPECTOMY ALONE (INVASIVE CANCER)

Study	% of Recurrence that is Local (same quadrant)	% of Recurrence that is Remote (different quadrant)	% of All Treated Patients with Remote Recurrences
Fisher et al., 1986 (12)	100	0	0
Crile & Esselstyn, 1990 (13)	84	16	1.7
Liljegren et al., 1994 (14)	85	15	3.0
Clark et al., 1992 (6)	86	14	3.5

from a new primary tumor developing in another part of the breast after treatment of the index lesion.

The above studies do not exclude patients with a higher likelihood of multicentric disease, who have been incorporated into trials of partial-breast irradiation (see section on Selection Criteria). The rate of remote relapse may be even lower when patients with these features are not offered partial-breast irradiation. In addition, newer diagnostic modalities such as breast magnetic resonance imaging may detect patients with pre-existing multicentric carcinoma, further mitigating concerns about partial-breast irradiation missing disease within the breast.

Although these data are from studies of invasive carcinoma, there is no evidence that DCIS deviates from this pattern of failure. Recurrence after lesionectomy alone for pure DCIS or lesionectomy followed by radiation therapy also occurs primarily in the vicinity of the original lesion.

POTENTIAL BENEFITS FOR PATIENTS

Despite data from seven randomized prospective clinical trials for invasive breast cancer comparing breast-conservation therapy with mastectomy showing equal survival rates, it is estimated that fewer than 50% of women in the United States receive breast-conserving surgery and radiation therapy. The main obstacle to women who are otherwise candidates for breast-conservation therapy receiving breast irradiation is the inconvenience of 5 to 7 weeks of external beam radiation therapy. Patients who live far from a radiation oncology center, who depend on a relative or friend for transportation, or who are working women, may prefer an accelerated 4- or 5-day treatment regimen. The frail, elderly, or infirmed patient may also benifit. Table 39.3 highlights some of the potential advantages of accelerated partial-breast irradiation.

SELECTION CRITERIA

Patients considered for accelerated partial-breast irradiation should have solitary breast cancers with a low probability of having malignant cells outside the target volume. Table 39.4 highlights many of the factors to be considered in selecting patients with either invasive breast cancer or DCIS.

CLINICAL EXPERIENCE: TUMOR CONTROL, TOXICITY, COSMESIS, AND QUALITY OF LIFE

There are no studies of partial-breast irradiation specifically for DCIS. In my experience at the Ochsner Clinic and the University of Wisconsin, with a total of 210 patients treated by wide-volume interstitial catheter or intracavitary balloon breast brachytherapy, 15% have had pure DCIS. No patient with pure DCIS has failed within the breast, nodes, or distant sites. In the entire cohort of 210 patients, there has been one breast relapse and four nodal recurrences, with a median follow-up interval of 4.5 years and a range of 6 months to 10 years. The principal toxicity has been fat necrosis, which occurred in 10% of the first 51 breasts treated but in less than 2% of the subsequent 159 patients treated. Long-term results from the original pilot trial were published (15). Fifty-one patients receiving brachytherapy were matched with 94 patients receiving external beam irradiation treated by the same physicians over the same time interval. At a median follow-up of 75 months, the two groups were similar for grade 3 toxicities, breast and nodal relapses, and cosmesis scores. Grade 1 and 2 toxicities, mostly acute skin reactions, were significantly less common with brachytherapy (11 of 51, 22%) than with external beam irradiation (75 of 94, 80%). Grade 3 toxicities requiring surgical intervention were approximately the same as for brachytherapy (four of 51, 8%) versus external beam irradiation (five of 94, 5%). There were one breast recurrence (2%) and three nodal recurrences (6%) in the brachytherapy group compared with five breast recurrences (5%) and no nodal recurrence in the external beam irradiation group. Distant disease developed in four patients in each group. Excellent or good cosmetic outcomes were obtained in 75% of the patients receiving brachytherapy and 84% of the patients receiving external beam irradiation ($p = $ NS)

TABLE 39.3. ADVANTAGES OF ACCELERATED PARTIAL BREAST IRRADIATION OVER CONVENTIONAL EXTERNAL BEAM THERAPY

Accelerated Partial Breast Radiation Therapy	Conventional External Beam Radiation Therapy
4- or 5-day treatment duration	5 to 7 wk
Less burdensome travel required	25–35 trips to the department
Much easier on the elderly, frail, or infirm	Frequently prohibitive for these patients
Convenient for the working woman	Disruptive to schedule
May increase % BCT	Some BCT candidates choose mastectomy
Reduced cost (?)	Expensive
Less radiation exposure to normal tissues	Must pass through skin, normal breast, chest wall, and a portion of lung and possibly heart

BCT, breast-conservation therapy.

TABLE 39.4. SELECTION CRITERIA FOR ACCELERATED PARTIAL BREAST IRRADIATION (INVASIVE AND NONINVASIVE CASES)

Absolute exclusion criteria
  Lesions >4 cm in maximum diameter
  Four or more positive axillary lymph nodes
  One to three positive lymph nodes with extracapsular extension
  Postlumpectomy mammography demonstrating suspicious microcalcifications that have not been biopsied
  Positive surgical margins
  More than one breast cancer within the breast
  Patients who are pregnant or nursing
  Locally advanced or inflammatory breast cancer

Relative contraindications
  Lesions between 3 and 4 cm
  Invasive cancers with an extensive intraductal component
  Lobular type of breast cancer
  Patients with systemic lupus erythematosus, scleroderma, or dermatomyositis with an elevated CPK level or erythrocyte sedimentation rate
  Patients who have little chance of obtaining a good cosmetic outcome
  Patients whose surgeon or medical oncologist is opposed to this therapy
  Delay of more than 6 wk from surgery
  Technically difficult
  Silicone prosthesis
  Very small breasts
  Lesions in the tail of the breast near the axilla
  Tumors very close to the skin or nipple
  Tumors adjacent to the chest wall
  Neither surgical clips nor a seroma are present to define the target volume

Special cases
  Prior radiation therapy including any portion of the breast
  Local recurrence after breast conservation therapy
  Mantle irradiation for Hodgkin's lymphoma
  Chemotherapy before consultation

Vicini et al. (16) has an 8-year experience with wide-volume breast brachytherapy. Pure DCIS has been excluded from their studies. Between 1993 and January 2000, 174 cases of early-stage invasive breast cancer were managed with lumpectomy followed by an interstitial implant. An external beam radiation therapy case was matched to each brachytherapy case. At a median follow-up of 36 months, no statistically significant differences were noted in the 5-year actuarial rates of ipsilateral breast treatment failure, 2% external beam versus 1% brachytherapy. Distant metastasis rates (6% versus 3%), disease-free survival (87% versus 91%), overall survival (90% versus 93%), and cause-specific survival (97% versus 99%) were all not significantly different. Excellent or good cosmetic outcomes were achieved in 83% of patients receiving external beam irradiation and 90% of patients receiving brachytherapy. No adverse sequelae were noted.

The Radiation Therapy Oncology Group initiated a multi-institutional phase II cooperative group trial, Radiation Therapy Oncology Group study 95-17, of wide-volume breast brachytherapy. DCIS was excluded from this trial for the purpose of study purity. The first patient was entered in August 1997 and the last in March 2000; 103 patients were treated per protocol. Quality control was excellent in this study with ten institutions accruing patients into the study. The results are currently being analyzed.

Fentiman and colleagues (17) reported a negative study for brachytherapy alone for operable breast cancer. Twenty-seven patients received a 55-Gy low dose rate over 5 days after tumorectomy and axillary clearance. After 6 years median follow-up, breast relapse occurred in ten of 27 patients (37%). Patient selection differed from the above studies; three patients had a tumor larger than 4 cm, 15 had positive margins, three had lymphatic permeation, 12 had positive axillary nodes, and 11 had an extensive intraductal component. Because the median number of catheters inserted was only nine (e.g., five in a deep plane and four in a superficial plane), the volume treated was significantly less than in the U.S. studies quoted above.

TECHNIQUE

This section focuses on brachytherapy techniques because conformal and intensity-modulated radiotherapy methods are still under development.

1. Intraoperative catheter placement with the lesionectomy wound open. After the surgeon has removed the lesion, the radiation oncologist is called to the operating suite. With a finger in the surgical cavity, a deep plane of catheters is guided underneath the excision site, and a superficial plane is inserted in front of it (Fig. 39.1). Care must be taken to encompass tissue 2 cm beyond the cavity in all directions. Because the pathology report is not yet available, a delay in loading the radiation sources is necessary. In some cases, the patient will be declared ineligible for brachytherapy (e.g., positive microscopic margins), and the catheters pulled before treatment.

2. Ultrasonographic guidance. A diagnostic radiologist and breast-imager uses ultrasonography to identify the seroma that fills the surgical cavity. The junction between the water density of the seroma and the fat density of breast tissue is easily seen for the first 5 to 6 weeks after surgery, providing that the surgeon does not close the cavity. Using a sterile paint marker, the projection of the seroma onto the skin surface is mapped, and the thickness from the skin to the superficial and deep edges of the cavity is noted. Each needle can be guided real-time through the breast at selected depths, so as to encompass the target volume (Fig. 39.2).

3. Mammographic guidance in the prone position on the stereotactic core biopsy table. This procedure is usually performed 2 to 6 weeks after surgery. Using ultrasonography, 3 to 5 mL of nonionic contrast is injected into the le-

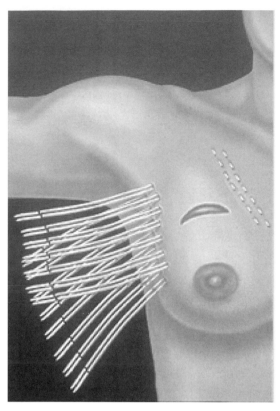

FIGURE 39.1. The original New Orleans and national RTOG 95-17 trials employed 2-plane implants, bracketing the lumpectomy site between superficial and deep planes of catheters. The current multiplane volume implants more reliably encompass an irregularly-shaped excision cavity.

sionectomy cavity. After positioning the patient prone on the stereotactic table, a template with pre-drilled holes is attached to the breast. A mammographic image is taken, aligned with direction of the holes in the template. Needles are inserted through the holes corresponding to the target volume (Fig. 39.3).

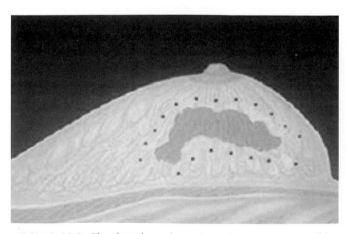

FIGURE 39.2. The dots show the points where catheters will be inserted.

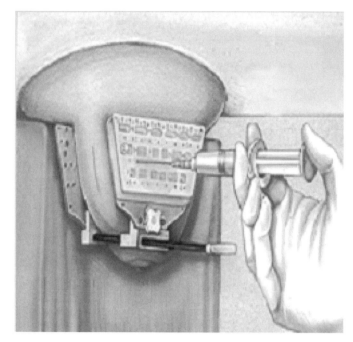

FIGURE 39.3. The breast under each hole is completely anesthetized prior to catheter insertion.

4. **Balloon intracavitary brachytherapy.** At the time of lesionectomy, a balloon catheter is inserted into the cavity. The balloon is inflated, filling and distending the cavity. A catheter through the center of the balloon centers the iridium 192 source within the target volume. Because it is only one catheter and essentially a point source, the treatment is simplified.

5. **Soft x-rays.** With the surgical excision cavity exposed, a device capable of generating soft x-rays is inserted directly into the cavity. Again, the pathology report is not yet available. Only one large fraction is delivered, which theoretically should produce more late effects such as fibrosis.

6. **Electron beam.** Ribeiro and colleagues (18,19) from the Christie Hospital (Manchester, U.K.) delivered multiple fractions of electrons after surgery directly through the skin. The Milan group delivers a single large fraction at the time of surgery with the skin wound open (Veronesi, personal communication, 2002).

FUTURE INVESTIGATIONS: SIMPLIFYING THE TECHNIQUE AND MAKING TARGET VOLUME COVERAGE REPRODUCIBLE

One major concern with all the above techniques of accelerated partial-breast irradiation is the skill dependence. If only a few institutions can provide this treatment, it is unlikely to improve breast cancer care worldwide. Schools to teach these techniques will be necessary, and credentialing criteria established.

The evolution of techniques trends toward image guidance, which should make target volume coverage reproducible and feasible for any well-trained radiation oncologist/surgeon team to accomplish.

SUMMARY

In this chapter, two important questions were considered: Do all patients with DCIS require breast irradiation, and is there a select subset of women who may receive accelerated partial-breast irradiation?

It is unlikely that all women with DCIS require breast irradiation, but choosing those who can be treated by surgery alone is not easy. In general, the more generous the surgical margins, the less important radiotherapy becomes. Surgeons striving for large margins, however, especially when re-excision is required, may pay a price in terms of worsening cosmetic outcome because of tissue volume loss.

Accelerated partial-breast irradiation requires meticulous attention to detail in selecting patients and covering the target volume. The results from Fentiman et al. (17) and Ribeiro et al. (18,19) illustrate the potential problems with both of these critical issues. Their results diverge dramatically from the U.S. studies of wide-volume breast brachytherapy and are very similar to published studies of patients treated with lumpectomy alone.

The experience with accelerated partial-breast irradiation is primarily derived from experience with invasive carcinoma. We do not know whether outcomes will be similar for DCIS. Given the similar pattern of recurrence with DCIS, with the majority being in the vicinity of the index lesion and surgery site, it would be surprising to see a difference in results.

REFERENCES

1. Fisher B, Dignam J, Wolmark N, et al. Lumpectomy and radiation therapy for the treatment of intraductal breast cancer: findings from National Surgical Adjuvant Breast and Bowel Project B-17. *J Clin Oncol* 1998;16:441–452.
2. Julien JP, Bijker N, Fentiman IS, et al. Radiotherapy in breast-conserving treatment for ductal carcinoma in situ: first results of the EORTC randomized phase III trial 10853. *Lancet* 2000;355: 528–533.
3. Veronesi U, Luini A, Galimberti V, et al. Conservation approaches for the management of stage I/II carcinoma of the breast: Milan Cancer Center Trials. *World J Surg* 1994;18:70.
4. Holland R, Veling SH, Matrunac M, et al. Histologic multifocality of Tis, T1-2 breast carcinomas: implications for clinical trials on breast conserving therapy. *Cancer* 1985;56:979–991.
5. Fisher B, Redmond C, Poisson R, et al. Eight year results of a randomized clinical trial comparing total mastectomy and lumpectomy with or without irradiation in the treatment of breast cancer. *N Engl J Med* 1989;320:822–828.
6. Clark RM, McCulloch PB, Levine MN, et al. Randomized clinical trial to assess the effectiveness of breast irradiation following lumpectomy and axillary dissection for node-negative breast cancer. *J Natl Cancer Inst* 1992;84:683–689.
7. Recht A, Silver B, Schnitt S, et al. Time course of local recurrence following conservative surgery and radiotherapy for early stage breast cancer. *Int J Radiat Oncol Biol Phys* 1988;15:255–261.
8. Fowble B, Solin LJ, Schultz DJ, et al. Breast recurrence following conservative surgery and radiation: patterns of failure, prognosis, and pathologic findings from mastectomy specimens with implications for treatment. *Int J Radiat Oncol Biol Phys* 1990;19:833–842.
9. Kurtz JM, Spitalier JM, Amalric R, et al. The prognostic significance of late local recurrence after breast-conserving therapy. *Int J Radiat Oncol Biol Phys* 1990;18:87–93.
10. Veronesi U, Salvadori B, Luini A, et al. Conservative treatment of early breast cancer: long-term results of 1232 cases treated with quadrantectomy, axillary dissection, and radiotherapy. *Ann Surg* 1990;211:250–259.
11. Haffty BG, Goldberg NB, Rose M, et al. Conservative surgery with radiation therapy in clinical stage I and II breast cancer. Results of a 20-year experience. *Arch Surg* 1989;124:1266–1270.
12. Fisher ER, Sass R, Fisher B, et al. Pathologic findings from the National Surgical Adjuvant Breast Project (protocol 6). II. Relation of local breast recurrence to multicentricity. *Cancer* 1986;57: 1717–1724.
13. Crile G Jr, Esselstyn CB Jr. Factors influencing local recurrence of cancer after partial mastectomy. *Cleve Clin J Med* 1990;57: 143–146.
14. Liljegren G, Holmberg L, Adami HO, et al. Sector resection with or without postoperative radiotherapy for stage I breast cancer: five-year results of a randomized trial. Uppsala-Orebro Breast Cancer Study Group. *J Natl Cancer Inst* 1994;86:717–722.
15. King TA, Bolton JS, Kuske RR, et al. Long-term results of wide-field brachytherapy as the sole method of radiation therapy after segmental mastectomy for Tis,1,2 breast cancer. *Am J Surg* 2000; 180:299–304.
16. Vicini FA, Baglan KL, Kestin LL, et al. Accelerated treatment of breast cancer. *J Clin Oncol* 2001;19:1993–2001.
17. Fentiman IS, Poole C, Tong D, et al. Inadequacy of iridium implant as sole radiation treatment for operable breast cancer. *Eur J Cancer* 1996;32A:608–611.
18. Ribeiro GG, Magee B, Swindell R, et al. The Christie Hospital breast conservation trial: an update at 8 years from inception. *Clin Oncol (R Coll Radiol)* 1993;5:278–283.
19. Ribeiro GG, Dunn G, Swindell R, et al. Conservation of the breast using two different radiotherapy techniques: interim report of a clinical trial. *Clin Oncol (R Coll Radiol)* 1990;2:27–34.

40

RANDOMIZED TRIAL OVERVIEW

ABRAM RECHT

Only well-designed, randomized clinical trials can firmly establish the benefits of alternative treatment approaches for patients with ductal carcinoma in situ (DCIS) because of bias in patient selection in retrospectively analyzed series. This chapter describes and contrasts currently open and completed national and international trials examining the roles of postoperative radiotherapy and tamoxifen in patients treated with breast-conserving surgery. (There are no trials that include a mastectomy control arm.) More detailed descriptions of some of these trials with updated results may be found in Chapters 41 to 44. In particular, issues that affect the interpretation of individual studies and comparisons between trials are discussed.

RANDOMIZED TRIALS COMPARING SURGERY ALONE WITH SURGERY PLUS RADIOTHERAPY

Several randomized trials comparing breast-conserving surgery alone with breast-conserving surgery combined with radiation therapy have been started in North America and Europe (Table 40.1). With the exception of the Swedish trial, they require histologically negative margins as an entry criterion. Unfortunately, similar trials in Germany and Denmark were closed owing to insufficient accrual rates.

The earliest of these trials (conducted from 1985 to 1990) was the National Surgical Adjuvant Breast and Bowel Project (NSABP) B-17 trial (1–4). Radiotherapy consisted of 50 Gy in 25 fractions given to the whole breast. An optional external beam boost of 10 Gy was given to only 9% of the patients receiving radiotherapy. The most recent report of this trial showed that the 8-year actuarial risk of local failure was 12.1% for the 411 patients treated with surgery plus radiotherapy compared with 26.8% for the 403 patients treated with surgery alone, with a mean follow-up time of 90 months (range, 67 to 130 months) (3). Irradiation reduced the risk of both invasive (8.2% versus 13.4%) and noninvasive (3.9% versus 13.4%) recurrences. (However, these results were not subdivided by margin status; see below.) The crude incidences of contralateral breast cancer

developing at any time during follow-up through 8 years were 6% (20 of 411) and 5% (19 of 403) in the radiotherapy and observation arms, respectively. Overall survival rates at 8 years in the two arms were 95% and 94%, respectively. There were ten deaths owing to breast cancer in the patients who received radiotherapy compared with four in the patients who did not. No explanation of this difference was given.

Similar reductions in the relative risk of ipsilateral breast tumor recurrence (IBTR) were seen for all subgroups, whether defined by mammographic characteristics, tumor size, the method of detection, or patient age (3). The absolute risk of recurrence varied only modestly between such subgroups in each arm. The greatest variation (and the only one that was statistically significant) was seen with regard to the extent of calcifications found on central mammographic review. The crude incidence of IBTR for patients who received radiotherapy with clustered calcifications (without a mass) of 1.0 cm or smaller, clustered calcifications larger than 1.0 cm, or scattered calcifications (not clearly defined) were 9% (17 of 181 patients), 16% (12 of 77), and 27% (seven of 26), respectively. For patients who did not receive radiotherapy, the respective incidences of IBTR were 20% (39 of 194), 44% (27 of 62), and 37% (ten of 27).

Patients entered in this study were required to have negative resection margins (defined as the absence of tumor at an inked specimen edge). However, central pathology review resulted in some patients some patients being scored as having positive or unknown margins. The most recent analysis of margin effect showed that the risk of IBTR for patients with negative margins was 13% (34 of 267 patients) in the irradiated arm compared with 29% (73 of 249) in the observation arm. For patients with positive or uncertain margins, the respective IBTR rates were 17% (nine of 53) and 39% (21 of 54), respectively (4). Radiotherapy substantially reduced the risk of IBTR for all patient subgroups defined by histologic features. The most important pathologic factor in predicting the risk of recurrence (aside from margin status) was the degree of comedonecrosis. For patients whose tumors had little or no necrosis, the risks of IBTR were 13% (23 of 178) and 23% (38 of 164) in the ir-

TABLE 40.1. NATIONAL AND INTERNATIONAL PROSPECTIVE TRIALS OF CONSERVATIVE SURGERY WITH OR WITHOUT RADIOTHERAPY FOR DUCTAL CARCINOMA IN SITU

Trial	Dates	Actual or Planned Accrual	Coexisting LCIS Allowed?	Nonpalpable Tumors	Size Limits	Refs.
NSABP B-17[a]	1985–1990	790	Yes	83%	None	1–4
EORTC 10853[b]	1986–1996	1,010	No	71%	≤5 cm	5,6
Sweden[c]	1987–?	1,000	?	?	≤1 quadrant	7,8
Norway[d]	1990–?	?	?	?	0.5–3 cm	
NBCG-4		—				
U.K.-Australia-New Zealand[e]	1990–1998	1,011	Yes	?	None	9–11

[a] Patients with LCIS only were registered separately. Axillary dissection was optional. Negative margins were required for entry but were not always present (see text).
[b] Patients refusing randomization or not eligible were registered and followed. Original size limitation of 3 cm was changed to 5 cm in late 1989. Axillary dissection was optional.
[c] No formal requirement that margins be microscopically negative, although they must be free by 1 cm or more clinically or radiologically. No size limit, but tumor must be less than one quadrant of the breast. Includes the South Swedish trial begun in September 1987, which was integrated into the national trial begun in 1988.
[d] Patients with atypical ductal hyperplasia or DCIS less than 0.5 cm undergo excision alone and are registered. Patients with DCIS larger than 3 cm or diffuse disease have mastectomy and are registered.
[e] A total of 1,694 patients accrued to the entire trial, which used a 2 × 2 factorial design. Patients could be randomized to receive radiation therapy (504 patients) or not (507 patients) and to receive tamoxifen (791 patients) or not (786 patients). Not all centers participated in both randomizations.
LCIS, lobular carcinoma in situ; NSABP, National Surgical Adjuvant Breast Project; EORTC, European Organization for Research and Treatment of Cancer; NBCG, Norwegian Breast Cancer Group; DCIS, ductal carcinoma in situ.

radiated and unirradiated arms, respectively. For patients whose tumors had moderate or marked necrosis, the respective incidences were 14% (20 of 142) and 40% (56 of 139). However, the impact of necrosis was not reported in subgroups of different margin status.

The European Organization for Research and Treatment of Cancer conducted a similar trial (10853) from 1986 to 1996 (56). One thousand ten patients with DCIS excised with negative margins (using the same definition as the NSABP) were randomized either to receive whole-breast radiotherapy (50 Gy in 5 weeks; only 5% of patients received a boost) or to be observed. With a median follow-up time of 4.25 years (maximum, 12.0 years), the 4-year actuarial local failure rates in the two arms were 9% and 16%, respectively. Approximately half of the recurrences in each arm were invasive. The risk of contralateral breast cancer development was higher in the irradiated patient arm (3% or 21 patients) than in the unirradiated arm (1% or eight patients) ($p = 0.01$); no reasons for this difference could be found by the investigators. Overall survival rates at 4 years were the same in both arms (99%). There were four deaths owing to breast cancer in the radiotherapy group and seven in the observation group. No results from the central pathologic review of this trial are yet available.

From 1990 to 1998, cooperative trials groups in the United Kingdom, New Zealand, and Australia conducted a joint trial with a 2 × 2 factorial design, in which patients could be randomized to receive radiotherapy or not and/or to receive tamoxifen or not (9–11). (Clinicians were allowed to elect whether their patients would be entered in only one

of these randomizations or both.) Although designed primarily for patients with screening-detected lesions, patients with palpable tumors were also eligible. Histologically negative margins (defined as no tumor seen directly at an inked surface) were required for entry. Early results were scheduled for oral presentation at the annual meeting of the American Society of Clinical Oncology in May 2000. However, the presentation was withdrawn for unstated reasons, although the abstract was published (11). A total of 1,011 patients was entered in the radiotherapy comparison; an unstated number of them thus received tamoxifen. With a median follow-up time of 3 years, radiotherapy reduced the risk of IBTR by 59%. However, the exact failure rates in each arm were not reported.

The Radiation Therapy Oncology Group opened a trial (9804) in December 1999, comparing excision plus tamoxifen to excision plus tamoxifen plus radiotherapy for patients with tumors of nuclear grades 1 to 2 measuring 2.5 cm or smaller with minimum tumor-free margin widths of 3 mm or greater. The accrual goal for this trial is 1,900 patients.

RANDOMIZED TRIALS OF THE ROLE OF TAMOXIFEN

Two trials have examined the value of tamoxifen for patients with DCIS. The NSABP B-24 trial, conducted from 1991 to 1995, accrued 1,804 patients (12). All patients were irradiated using the same approach as in the B-17 trial. Patients were randomized to receive either a placebo or tamoxifen for 5 years. Tamoxifen and radiotherapy were given concurrently. With a median follow-up time of 74 months (range, 57 to 93 months), the 5-year cumulative incidence of IBTR was 9.3% in the placebo arm compared with 6.0% in the tamoxifen arm. The impact of tamoxifen was proportionally greater in preventing invasive local failures (rates of 4.2% and 2.1% in the placebo and tamoxifen arms, respectively) than for noninvasive cancer (rates of 5.1% and 3.9%, respectively). Tamoxifen also reduced the number of contralateral breast cancers (either invasive or noninvasive), with 5-year incidences of 3.4% and 2.0% in the two arms, respectively. The overall survival rate at 5 years was 97% for both groups; causes of death were not reported.

Unlike all previous NSABP breast-conservation studies, patients with unknown or positive margins, as well as negative margins (defined as in the B-17 trial), were eligible for this trial. The crude local failure rate in patients with negative margins (assessed by the pathologist at the treating institution, not by central review) who received a placebo was 8.0% (54 of 675 patients). Tamoxifen reduced this rate to 6.3% (42 of 666). However, patients with positive or unknown margins on the placebo arm had a local failure rate of 14.7% (33 of 224) compared with 9.0% (21 of 233) among patients randomized to tamoxifen. Patient age also was related to the absolute benefit that tamoxifen yielded. Patients aged 49 or younger in the placebo arm had a 16.0% risk of local failure (48 of 300 patients) compared with 10.6% (32 of 302) in the tamoxifen arm. In contrast, for patients 50 years and older, the local failure rates were only 6.5% (39 of 599) and 5.2% (31 of 597) in the two arms, respectively. (Unfortunately, no analysis was performed of the impacts of age and margin status in combination.) Tamoxifen also reduced the rate of IBTR for patients whose tumors had comedonecrosis from 12.9% (56 of 433) to 9.4% (39 of 414). For patients whose tumors did not contain necrosis, the respective IBTR rates were 6.5% (29 of 446) and 5.1% (24 of 469), respectively.

In the United Kingdom-Australia-New Zealand trial, 791 patients were randomly allocated to receive tamoxifen for 5 years and 786 patients to receive a placebo (11). With a median follow-up time of 3 years, there was no statistical difference in the risk of an event (either ipsilateral or contralateral breast cancer) between the two arms (relative risk for tamoxifen to placebo, 0.92, with a 95% confidence interval of 0.77 to 2.08). However, results were not reported separately for the patients with and without radiotherapy.

CRITIQUE

The Critical Role of Margin Definition and Assessment

Radiotherapy decreased the risk of local failure in patients treated with breast-conserving surgery in the three reported trials examining this question. However, these trials were designed and started when much less information was available about DCIS than there is now. In particular, none of these three trials recorded the actual tumor-free margin width, which has since become widely recognized to be perhaps the most critical parameter in treatment results, particularly for patients who do not receive radiotherapy (13). Hence, the relevance of their results to current practice is uncertain.

Several investigators examined the impact of margin width in relation to the risk of IBTR after conservative surgery alone. For example, a Joint Center for Radiation Therapy/Harvard retrospective study of patients who did not receive radiotherapy found (with a median follow-up of 62 months) that the 5-year actuarial risk of local failure was 8% among 51 patients in whom the tumor was more than 1 mm from the resection margins compared with 25% (of nine patients) in whom the tumor-free margin width was 1 mm or less (14) (see also Chapter 35). In a study from Linköping, Sweden, the 5-year IBTR rate was 38% for eight patients with tumor-free margins of less than 5 mm compared with 6% for 33 patients with wider margins (15). The combined Van Nuys/Children's Hospital of San Francisco series found 8-year actuarial IBTR rates of 20% (23 of 124 patients) for those individuals with margins of 1 to 9 mm and 3% (two of 93) for patients with margins of 10 mm or greater, respectively, with a median follow-up of 72 months (16). Finally, a study from Nottingham, England, found a recurrence rate of 6% among 48 patients with margin widths greater than 10 mm, with median follow-up time of 77 months (17).

Unfortunately, no two groups have analyzed their data using the same break point for defining narrow versus wide margins, nor have the distributions of margin widths and results been reported according to narrow intervals (e.g., 0 to 1 mm, 1.1 to 2 mm, 2.1 to 3 mm) in a standardized fashion. This was performed by Park et al. for patients with invasive disease treated with lumpectomy and radiotherapy (18), but not for patients with DCIS. Hence, we cannot tell from these studies what the critical minimum margin width is, beyond which having additional uninvolved tissue will have negligible impact on outcome. (The size of the critical minimum width might also vary according to other factors; see below.)

This definition of the critical minimum width has important implications. First, cosmetic results are strongly influenced by the volume of tissue removed (19). Second, the wider the definition of the critical minimum width is, the fewer will be the patients who will qualify for treatment with surgery alone. For example, the Nottingham breast surgery group was able to achieve a minimum 10-mm tumor-free margin in 81% (48 of 59) of patients whom they initially thought were candidates for this approach preoperatively (20). However, these 48 patients constituted only 35% of all patients with DCIS treated in their unit from 1988 to 1993.

It is also unclear whether the results in the radiotherapy arms of these trials are truly representative of those achievable in current practice. Several retrospective series have substantially lower local recurrence rates than in the randomized trials (see Chapter 24). I would venture (without the availability of data on the subject) that this may partly be owing to the patients in these series having (on average) wider tumor-free margin widths than the patients in the randomized trials. (Another reason may be radiotherapy techniques; see below.) For example, in the Joint Center for Radiation Therapy series, the actuarial 5-year local failure rate was 2% for 34 patients with margins wider than 1 mm compared with 9% for 11 patients with narrower margins, with a median follow-up time of 74 months (21). In a study from Fox Chase Cancer Center, Philadelphia, with a median follow-up time of 64 months, 1% (one of 68) of patients with tumor more than 2 mm from the inked edge developed a local failure compared with 8% (one of 12) of patients with closer, but still uninvolved, margins (22). In a series of patients treated with breast-conserving surgery and radiotherapy at William Beaumont Hospital near Detroit with a median follow-up time of 78 months, the risk of local failure was 27% (four of 15) among patients with tumor-free margin widths of 0 to 2 mm and 6% (five of 82) for patients with margins wider than 2 mm (23). (However, three of the five local recurrences in the latter patient group were actually located in other portions of the breast, so that the risk of failure at or near the tumor bed was only 2% in this group.) Finally, in the Van Nuys experience, with a median follow-up time of 92 months, patients with margins 10 mm or wider had a lower 8-year actuarial risk of failure (4% or one of 40 in crude terms) than patients with margins of 1 to 9 mm (12% or 15 of 100) (16).

A subtler problem in assessing the applicability of the randomized trials for routine patient care is their methodology for margin assessment and coding. There has clearly been great variability in these procedures between participating institutions. For example, in the NSABP B-17 trial, no information was available on how many blocks were sampled or slides cut by the hospital pathologists, but the number of slides sent for central review ranged from one to 70 (median, nine slides) (2). On central review, 18% of eligible cases (101 of 573) were reclassified as having involved or inevaluable margins. As part of the quality control effort for the United Kingdom-Australia-New Zealand trial, six coders independently reviewed the same hospital pathology and National Health Service reports for 50 patients (24). All six coders agreed on margin status for only 16% of the study patients!

DIFFERENCES IN PATHOLOGIC ANALYSIS AND SUBTYPING

Interobserver variability in distinguishing DCIS from microinvasion or atypical ductal hyperplasia can be substantial (see Chapter 22). In many, if not most, cooperative group

trials, it is impractical for biopsy material to be submitted for central review before enrolling patients. As a result, some patients may be erroneously entered in the study. For example, in the NSABP B-17 trial, the central reviewer considered the lesion to be atypical hyperplasia in 7% (58 patients) and invasive cancer in 2% of cases (17 patients) (2). In the European Organization for Research and Treatment of Cancer trial, central review of 845 cases found a benign lesion in 5% (44 patients), atypical hyperplasia in 7% (62 patients), definite invasion in 3% (26 patients), and a suspicion of invasion in 1% (12 patients) (25). The results in such patients have not always been clearly analyzed and reported separately from those with true DCIS.

Several classification schemes have been proposed for DCIS. In the past, each cooperative group has used its own preferred scheme to analyze the results of its own trials. These schemes are similar but not identical, and hence it may be difficult to compare or combine pathologic subgroups from one trial with another. However, encouraging steps have been taken toward analyzing trial materials using multiple classification systems. For example, the NSABP B-17 trial results have been examined using the modified Lagios classification (4).

SURGICAL TECHNIQUE

Differences in surgical practice and technique within and between trials (and retrospective series) are likely to be substantial. For example, in one registry series, 11% of patients (four of 38) treated with wide excision developed local recurrence compared with 3% of patients (two of 65) treated with quadrantectomy (26). The total volume of the excision specimen(s) was also an important factor in the risk of recurrence in patients treated with radiation therapy at the Joint Center for Radiation Therapy (21) and for patients younger than age 45 in the William Beaumont series (27). However, the relationship between tumor histology and margin status was not reported in these series.

As yet, there is no agreement on how to assess or quantify surgical technique. Recording excision volumes is a start but is a blunt instrument at best. Beyond a certain point, it probably matters little how much tissue is taken, if it is taken from the wrong place. Anatomic parameters (the location and orientation of the surgical specimen) may also be critical, but it is not clear how these can be integrated into a useful measure of the adequacy of surgical technique.

RADIOTHERAPY DOSE

There are almost no data available to untangle the effects of radiotherapy dose from those of histology, margin width, and the type of surgical procedure for patients with either invasive or noninvasive cancers treated with breast-conserving therapy. Two randomized trials for patients with invasive cancer found improvements in local control when a "boost" dose was used (28, 29). One series of patients with DCIS suggested there was a higher risk of failure with a dose of less than 63 Gy to the tumor bed (30), but this was not been confirmed in other studies (25,26). Doses of approximately 50 Gy have resulted in excellent local control rates in several series of patients with invasive cancers in which all patients had negative resection margins (19). Nonetheless, there has been concern among radiation oncologists that 50 Gy may not be sufficient for patients with DCIS, particularly those with close margins. Whether such differences in outcome truly result from differences in radiotherapy dose is, however, unknown.

TAMOXIFEN: MARGIN WIDTH AND ESTROGEN-RECEPTOR PROTEIN STATUS

The NSABP B-24 trial showed that tamoxifen reduces the risk of both ipsilateral recurrence and the development of contralateral breast cancers in patients treated with lumpectomy and radiotherapy for DCIS. This is not surprising, given all the information previously known about tamoxifen's effects with regard to these end points. However, as noted above, the absolute magnitude of tamoxifen's impact was greatest in patients with positive or unknown margin status.

There are few data on how tamoxifen affects patients with known tumor-free margin width. In a nonrandomized study conducted in Manchester, England, patients with uninvolved microscopic margins were treated with wide excision with or without radiotherapy (33). Tamoxifen had little impact on the risk of local failure in patients with or without radiotherapy. However, the risk of local failure was closely related to the tumor-free margin width. For patients with tumor-free margin widths of 1 mm or less, the rates of local failure for patients treated with excision alone or excision plus tamoxifen were 40% (17 of 43) and 33% (five of 15), respectively. For patients treated with excision plus radiotherapy or excision plus radiotherapy plus tamoxifen, the rates were 33% (two of six) and 50% (one of two), respectively. For patients with margin widths greater than 1 mm, the respective local failure rates for patients treated with excision alone or excision plus tamoxifen were 8% (seven of 86) and 0% (none of 12). For patients receiving radiotherapy or radiotherapy plus tamoxifen, the rates were 0% (none of 12) and 0% (none of seven), respectively. (The median length of follow-up in this series was 47 months.)

Finally, the value of tamoxifen (at least with regard to its effect on the index lesion) may depend on the estrogen receptor protein status of the tumor. Not all DCIS display the estrogen receptor protein (34,35). It is not clear what steps will be taken to evaluate the potential effects of estrogen receptor protein status in the NSABP B-24 and United Kingdom-Australia-New Zealand trials.

CONCLUSIONS

Within the next few years, a wealth of additional data should become available from the first generation of randomized clinical trials described here. Although there may yet be much to learn from them, their relevance to daily practice is likely to be very limited. Variability in specimen processing and pathologic assessment, heterogeneity of surgical technique, possibly suboptimal radiotherapy doses, and problems of eligibility and physician and patient bias of who entered these studies (7,30,31) certainly affect the generalizability of their results. Their most important shortcoming, however, is the lack of data on the actual tumor-free margin width. This is a crippling flaw that it is now too late to correct.

The reality is that the consensus regarding the critical treatment issues for patients with DCIS (obtained mainly from retrospective analyses) has moved far beyond that existing when these trials were developed. Some of the lessons learned (e.g., the need for a minimum tumor-free margin width greater than a few cells for patients treated with excision without radiotherapy) have been incorporated into the most recent of these trials (Radiation Therapy Oncology Group trial 9804).

REFERENCES

1. Fisher B, Constantino J, Redmond C, et al. Lumpectomy compared with lumpectomy and radiation therapy for the treatment of intraductal breast cancer. *N Engl J Med* 1993;328:1581–1586.
2. Fisher ER, Constantino J, Fisher B, et al. Pathologic findings from the National Surgical Adjuvant Breast Project (NSABP Protocol B-17: intraductal carcinoma (ductal carcinoma in situ). *Cancer* 1995;75:1310–1319.
3. Fisher B, Dignam J, Wolmark N, et al. Lumpectomy and radiation therapy for the treatment of intraductal breast cancer: findings from the National Surgical Adjuvant Breast and Bowel Project B-17. *J Clin Oncol* 1998;16:441–452.
4. Fisher ER, Dignam J, Tan-Chiu E, et al. Pathologic findings from the National Surgical Adjuvant Breast Project (NSABP) eight-year update of protocol B-17. *Cancer* 1999;86:429–438.
5. Fentiman IS, Julien J-P, van Dongen JA, et al. Reasons for non-entry of patients with DCIS of the breast into a randomized trial (EORTC 10853). *Eur J Cancer* 1991;27:450–452.
6. Julien J-P, Bijker N, Fentiman IS, et al. Radiotherapy in breast-conserving treatment for ductal carcinoma in situ: first results of the EORTC randomised phase III trial 10853. *Lancet* 2000; 355:528–533.
7. Ringberg A. Accrual rate limiting factors in a Swedish randomized DCIS trial. *Eur J Cancer* 1994;30A[Suppl 2]:S33(abst).
8. Ringberg A, Möller T. Accrual rate-limiting factors in a Swedish randomised ductal carcinoma in situ (DCIS)—a demographic study. *Eur J Cancer* 2000;36:483–488.
9. Fentiman IS. Treatment of screen detected ductal carcinoma *in situ*: a silver lining within a grey cloud? [Editorial]. *Br J Cancer* 1990;61:795–796.
10. Spittle M, Stewart HJ. Non-surgical management of early breast cancer in the United Kingdom: ductal carcinoma in situ. *Clin Oncol* 1995;7:217–218.

11. George WD, Houghton J, Cuzick J, et al. Radiotherapy and tamoxifen following complete local excision (CLE) in the management of ductal carcinoma in situ (DCIS): preliminary results from the UK DCIS trial. *Proc Am Soc Clin Oncol* 2000;19: 70a(abst).

12. Fisher B, Dignam J, Wolmark N, et al. Tamoxifen in treatment of intraductal breast cancer: National Surgical Adjuvant Breast and Bowel Project B-24 randomised controlled trial. *Lancet* 1999;353:1993–2000.

13. Recht A, Rutgers EJJ, Fentiman IS, et al. The Fourth EORTC DCIS consensus meeting (Château Marquette, Heemskerk, The Netherlands, 23–24 January 1998) conference report. *Eur J Cancer* 1998;34:1664–1669.

14. Hetelekidas S, Collins L, Silver B, et al. Predictors of local recurrence following excision alone for ductal carcinoma in situ. *Cancer* 1999;85:427–431.

15. Arnesson L-G, Smeds S, Fagerberg G, et al. Follow-up of two treatment modalities for ductal carcinoma in situ of the breast. *Br J Surg* 1989;76:672–675.

16. Silverstein MJ, Lagios MD, Groshen S, et al. The influence of margin width on local control of ductal carcinoma in situ. *N Engl J Med* 1999;340:1455–1461.

17. Waheda Y, Sibbering DM, Pinder SE, et al. Local excision with a 10mm margin as sole treatment for DCIS of the breast. *Eur J Surg Oncol* 1998;24:629(abst).

18. Park C, Mitsumori M, Nixon A, et al. Outcome at 8 years following breast-conserving surgery and radiation therapy for invasive breast cancer: influence of margin status and systemic therapy on local recurrences. *J Clin Oncol* 2000;18:1668–1675.

19. Recht A. Breast carcinoma: in situ and early-stage invasive cancers. In: Gunderson LL, Tepper JE, eds. *Clinical radiation oncology.* New York: Churchill-Livingstone, 2000:968–998.

20. Sibbering DM, Blamey RW. Nottingham experience. In: Silverstein MJ, Lagios MD, Poller DN, et al., eds. *Ductal carcinoma in situ of the breast.* Baltimore: William & Wilkins, 1997:367–372.

21. Hiramatsu H, Bornstein B, Recht A, et al. Local recurrence after conservative surgery and radiation therapy for ductal carcinoma-in-situ: the possible importance of family history. *Cancer J Sci Am* 1995;1:55–61.

22. Fowble B, Hanlon AL, Fein DA, et al. Results of conservative surgery and radiation for mammographically detected ductal carcinoma in situ (DCIS). *Int J Radiat Oncol Biol Phys* 1997;38: 949–957.

23. Vicini FA, Lacerna MD, Goldstein NS, et al. Ductal carcinoma *in situ* detected in the mammographic era: an analysis of clinical, pathologic, and treatment-related factors affecting outcome with breast-conserving therapy. *Int J Radiat Oncol Biol Phys* 1997;39: 627–635.

24. Houghton J, Moritz S, Douglas A. Pathological reporting of ductal carcinoma in situ (DCIS) in the UK trial. *Breast* 1997;6: 229(abst).

25. Bijker N, Peterse JL, van de Vijver MJ, et al. Classification of ductal carcinoma in situ of the breast in the EORTC 10853 trial: do subtypes predict the risk of recurrence? *Breast* 1999;8:243–244(abst).

26. Ciatto S, Bonardi R, Cataliotti L, et al. Intraductal breast carcinoma: review of a multicenter series of 350 cases. *Tumori* 1990; 76:552–554.

27. Vicini FA, Kestin LL, Goldstein NS, et al. Impact of young age on outcome in patients with ductal carcinoma-in-situ treated with breast-conserving therapy. *J Clin Oncol* 2000;18:296–306.

28. Romestainy P, Lehingue Y, Larrie C, et al. Role of a 10-Gy boost in the conservative treatment of early breast cancer: Results of a randomized clinical trial in Lyon, France, *J Clin Oncol* 1997;15:963–968.

29. Bertelink M, Collette L, Fourquet A, et al. Impact of a boost dose of 16 Gy on the local control and cosmesis in patients with early breast cancer: The EORTC boost vs. no boost trial (Abst.). *Int J Radial Oncol Biol Phys* 2000;486(suppl. 1):111.

30. Fourquet A, Zafrani B, Campana F, et al. Breast conserving treatment of ductal carcinoma in situ. *Semin Radiat Oncol* 1992;2: 116–124.

31. Kuske RR, Bean JM, Garcia DM, et al. Breast conservation therapy for intraductal carcinoma of the breast. *Int J Radiat Oncol Biol Phys* 1993;26:391–396.

32. Solin L, Kurtz J, Fourquet A, et al. Fifteen-year results of breast-conserving surgery and definitive breast irradiation for the treatment of ductal carcinoma in situ of the breast. *J Clin Oncol* 1996; 14:754–763.

33. Chan KC, Knoz WF, Sinha G, et al. Extent of excision margin width required in breast conserving surgery for ductal carcinoma in situ. *Cancer* 2001;91:9–16.

34. Chaudhuri B, Crist KA, Mucci S, et al. Distribution of estrogen receptor in ductal carcinoma in situ of the breast. *Surgery* 1993;113:134–137.

35. Poller DN, Snead DRJ, Roberts EC, et al. Oestrogen receptor expression in ductal carcinoma in situ of the breast: relationship to flow cytometric analysis of DNA and expression of the c-*erb*B-2 oncoprotein. *Br J Cancer* 1993;68:156–161.

41

PROSPECTIVE CLINICAL TRIALS: THE NATIONAL SURGICAL ADJUVANT BREAST PROJECT EXPERIENCE

RICHARD G. MARGOLESE

In a sense, ductal carcinoma in situ (DCIS) is a relatively new disease, and we are still grappling with uncertainties and misunderstanding. The reasons for this are easier to see when we compare this disease with one with no controversy such as acute appendicitis. Here, the natural history of the process is well understood, and there is no controversy about management because the treatment is close to 100% successful with no significant downside, especially compared with the nontreatment options. In the case of DCIS, however, the natural history is not completely understood. Not all cases evolve into cancer. Radiologists have not reached unanimity on when biopsy is indicated. Pathologists cannot agree on which features are prognostically important. There are four different classification systems proposed. All have a similar base or foundation, but there is no consensus on details. Furthermore, these all depend on morphologic characteristics, at a time when it is becoming clear that a more biologically based evaluation will be more accurate.

Treatment options are even more unsettled. There are several different options, all of which have essentially similar outcomes, with slightly different undesirable effects (risks), and the final choice becomes one of value judgments. In different centers and with different surgeons, patients with essentially similar disease are receiving very different treatments—from mastectomy to lumpectomy with radiation therapy to lumpectomy only. When experts can cite evidence to support all these approaches, it is time to examine the evidence and the methodology of the studies. A review of the different chapters in this volume illustrates the variety of studies and methodologies, and this can give the discerning reader some insight in interpreting the evidence.

BACKGROUND

Although DCIS was first described in the 1930s, it was a relatively rare disease, and little attention was paid until the advent of widespread use of mammography in the 1970s. To-

day, more than 80% of cases are mammographically detected, but in the days before mammography, DCIS could only be discovered when it had grown large enough to be clinically detectable, Very often there were foci of early invasion, and the entity became known as minimal breast cancer or early breast cancer. All the cases were treated by Halsted radical mastectomy, as were all presentations of breast neoplasia, and this helped give that operation its reputation as a highly curative procedure. The struggle to escape from the tenets of the Halsted mastectomy for invasive breast cancer (IBC) lasted from the 1950s to the mid-1980s when the National Surgical Adjuvant Breast Project (NSABP) (1) and others (2–4) published the results of definitive prospective clinical trials demonstrating that breast-conserving surgery (BCS) is the appropriate operation. At almost the same time, mammography became available in a widespread and effective fashion, allowing the discovery of preclinical cases of DCIS. During these years, DCIS increased from 3% of breast cancer presentations to 30% (5). With the increase in incidence, there was a surge of interest, especially in addressing questions relating to management. In particular, the landmark studies of BCS in IBC now led to consideration of this approach for DCIS. With modern screening equipment, subclinical DCIS is now seen frequently, and new approaches to treatment and even prevention are required (Fig. 41.1).

Throughout the 1980s and 1990s, the debates on the management of DCIS mirrored the debates that had taken place two decades earlier for invasive cancer and led up to the definitive clinical trials that provided reliable guidelines for treatment of IBC. In the case of DCIS, the issues were not exactly the same. It was proposed that total mastectomy could completely remove all foci of DCIS and therefore prevent the development of IBC. It was recognized that BCS was equally effective and appropriate for IBC, but it could be argued that total breast removal, although a severe treatment for noninvasive cancer, should cure all cases, whereas BCS may fail to adequately control DCIS. Local recurrence

Breast Cancer Incidence Rates, 1973-1996 by Age, In Situ vs. Malignant All Races, Female

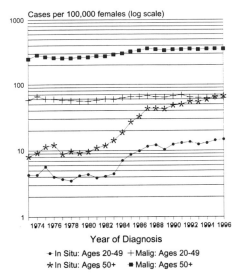

Cases per 100,000 females (log scale)

Year of Diagnosis

• In Situ: Ages 20-49   + Malig: Ages 20-49
✳ In Situ: Ages 50+   ■ Malig: Ages 50+

FIGURE 41.1. Increasing incidence of ductal carcinoma in situ, 1973–1996. (Surveillance, Epidemiology, and End Results program, National Cancer Institute).

exposes the patient to the possibility of invasive cancer and metastases. In other words, BCS for invasive cancer is no worse than mastectomy, but this may not be true for DCIS. These two issues, that total mastectomy cures 100% of DCIS and that breast cancer mortality might be worse with BCS, need to be carefully considered before they are accepted as true.

After two decades of research, controversy continues. Two randomized prospective studies of DCIS treatment have now been published (6,7). The use of BCS in place of total mastectomy seems to be more commonly accepted, but in many centers, this practice seems to be confined to cases of small tumors with wide clear margins. Many women are still being advised to accept mastectomy or very wide local excision because of the fear that DCIS might recur and especially might recur as IBC. We remain with the paradox that the less threatening disease (DCIS) often receives the more radical surgery (total mastectomy).

A specific problem stems from the surgical treatment of women after the identification of DCIS, which is not biologically important. How aggressive should surgery be in cases that include a large number of women who do not really need it? With the widespread use of mammography, we may be discovering histologic abnormalities that would not otherwise become apparent or important in that woman's lifetime. Autopsy studies have shown that the frequency of histologic DCIS exceeds the clinical incidence of DCIS in the general population. In a study of 110 autopsies on young and middle-aged women without known breast cancer, Nielsen et al. (8) found an incidence of unsuspected IBC of 2%, which is close to the detection rate in mam-

mography screening programs. DCIS, however, was present in 20% of the subjects, which is much higher than the rate of clinical DCIS. This is similar to historic studies in IBC that documented a high incidence of residual multicentricity (usually DCIS) found after serial sectioning of mastectomy specimens (9). This suggests that there should be a much higher expectation of local recurrence than actually occurs in patients treated with BCS. In the case of IBC, this difference has been recognized and many unnecessary mastectomies have been avoided. The evidence is mounting that the same will be true for DCIS. This will be important for all DCIS cases. Understanding that total mastectomy is not always necessary will lessen the dilemma of choosing appropriate surgical treatment (Fig. 41.2).

Changes in our approach to the treatment of IBC came about through the twin scientific principles of accumulation of biologic evidence and testing resultant ideas in randomized clinical trials. In fact, fundamental changes in our understanding of cancer biology come from clinical trial results because a good clinical trial is not simply a collection of statistical outcomes; rather the trial itself is a probe to uncover elements of the biology of the disease and apply them in designing the next clinical trial to learn even more. This concept represents a major reason for the advantages of randomized clinical trials over retrospective case reviews. The keystone belief supporting the Halsted mastectomy, the role of regional nodes, was removed as a result of NSABP protocol B-04 (10). The Halsted approach stood on the concept that breast cancer was an expansive disease, and there were direct connections from its origin first to regional nodes and then to all the metastatic elements present in that woman's body. By showing that mastectomy with or without axillary node dissection had the same long-term outcome, it became clear that axillary lymph nodes did not serve as the source of distant metastasis. Removing them did not provide any additional therapeutic benefit, and leaving them untreated did not result in poorer survival. This led to a much more dynamic biologic concept of breast cancer and allowed us to

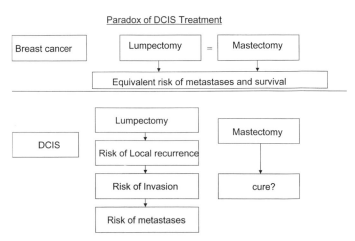

FIGURE 41.2. The apparent dilemma in matching treatment with the underlying problem of ductal carcinoma in situ.

TABLE 41.1. MORTALITY REPORTS FOR COLLECTED SERIES OF DUCTAL CARCINOMA IN SITU CASES TREATED WITH TOTAL MASTECTOMY

Study	Year	No. of Cases	% Mortality
Ashikari (28)	1971	182	0.9
Lagios (29)	1982	53	1.9
Rosner (30)	1980	182	2.0
Fisher et al. (10)	1991	27	3.7
Schuh (31)	1986	51	2.0
Farrow (33)	1970	181	2.0
Bradley (11)[a]	1990	588	1.7
Silverstein (Ch. 29)	2002	326	0

[a] Meta-analysis.

focus on two different strategies: one involved treatments aimed at local/regional control and the other at systemic application of anticancer drugs to try to control established micrometastases. For the past 20 years, guided by evolving biologic understanding and effective use of randomized clinical trials, we have witnessed a de-emphasizing of surgery and a rise in the use of adjuvant therapies for IBC. BCS is now common, and mortality rates have declined as a result of adjuvant therapies. It is important that we now maintain a biologic approach to DCIS to learn more about the disease as we grapple with treating it in the present day.

It is probably true that total mastectomy will cure almost every patient with this disease and so, probably, will very wide local excision, approaching quadrantectomy. However, the evidence is clear that even with total mastectomy, the long-term cure rate is not 100%. From the perspective of the biologic model of this disease, it is not difficult to understand that microscopic foci of invasive cancer may exist and may have metastasized, explaining the 1% to 2% mortality that occurs even with total mastectomy (11) (Table 41.1). Indirect support for this concept comes from considering the cases of occult breast cancer—the discovery of metastatic breast cancer in axillary lymph nodes when there is no evident primary tumor in the breast. In most cases, the primary tumor is eventually found and the mystery evaporates. Similarly, when axillary node dissection is performed in DCIS, approximately 1% to 2% of cases show involved nodes, although invasive cancer is not seen in the breast tissue.

RETROSPECTIVE STUDIES OF BREAST-CONSERVING SURGERY

Throughout the 1980s and 1990s, many investigators contributed their ideas and experiences with breast-conserving management of the new presentations of DCIS: mammographically discovered cases that were usually subclinical in size. These studies were all retrospective, and most were small and lacked comprehensive pathologic review. Differ-

ent treatments and different types of case selection hamper interpretation of these. Nevertheless, there was a constant theme that showed that limited breast surgery was reasonable and had a local recurrence rate that was acceptable. Those studies that combined lumpectomy with radiation therapy had even lower local recurrence rates than lumpectomy alone, and this evidence together with results of 76 patients with DCIS from the NSABP B-06 lumpectomy trial led to the planning of prospective clinical trials in DCIS.

Surgery Only

There is a relatively large number of collected personal series, or retrospective studies, that have been used to suggest treatment guidelines in the absence of large prospective trials. A small number of patients has been followed after simple local excision by Lagios et al. (12) and Schwartz et al. (13). Patients in these series were carefully selected for having small tumors and favorable histopathology. Even in these highly selected patients, recurrence rates were disappointingly high: 21% at 15 years for Lagios et al. and 25% at 10 years for Schwartz et al. A third study by Fisher et al. (14) was not limited to favorable patients but provided a similar outcome in a small set of unselected patients treated with lumpectomy. In a subset analysis, Lagios et al. (12) found that nearly all local recurrences were of the high-grade type. Although 10% of cases were IBC, there were no deaths attributable to breast cancer in the 10 years of follow-up.

Surgery and Radiation Therapy

At this time, the randomized clinical trials carried out by the NSABP and others (1–4) established that BCS (lumpectomy plus radiation therapy) was appropriate for IBC. The retrospective reports of BCS with and without radiation therapy for DCIS showed that local recurrence rates were similar to those obtained with these treatments in invasive cancer (Table 41.2). In those reports in which DCIS was treated with lumpectomy combined with radiation therapy, better rates of local control were obtained. The debates of the 1970s about BCS for IBC, which preceded the prospective clinical trials, are recalled by these studies, which are similarly retrospective, usually contain small numbers of patients, and are often difficult to evaluate because of selection features and other variables. Nevertheless, these studies of lumpectomy and radiation therapy in DCIS indicate a relatively low rate of local breast recurrence and at least set the stage for conducting a definitive, prospective, randomized clinical trial.

PROSPECTIVE TRIALS: B-17

Because of concerns that the retrospective reports may not be accurate because they involved highly selected cases and the

TABLE 41.2. RETROSPECTIVE REPORTS: RESULTS OF TREATMENT WITH LUMPECTOMY AND RADIATION THERAPY (DUCTAL CARCINOMA IN SITU: LUMPECTOMY + RADIATION THERAPY)

Study	Year	No. of Cases	No. of Patients (%) with Local Recurrence	No. of Patients (%) with Invasion
Bornstein (34)	1991	38	8 (21%)	1 (13%)
Kurtz (35)	1989	43	3 (7%)	3 (100%)
Fisher et al. (10)[a]	1986	29	2 (7%)	1 (50%)
Stotter (36)	1990	42	4 (10%)	4 (100%)
Zafrani (37)	1986	54	3 (6%)	1 (33%)
Solin (38)	1993	172	16 (9%)	7 (44%)
Fisher (6)[a]	1993	399	28 (7%)	8 (29%)
Kuske (39)	1993	70	6 (9%)	4 (67%)
Silverstein (Ch. 37)	2002	237	48 (20%)	22 (46%)

[a] Randomized trial.

question that radiation therapy might not be as effective in DCIS as it is in IBC, the NSABP embarked on a prospective clinical trial comparing lumpectomy only with lumpectomy and radiation therapy. The NSABP protocol B-17 is the first large-scale, prospective study of DCIS treatments. This study was preceded by some information derived from protocol B-06, the trial of lumpectomy with or without radiation therapy in IBC. Among the 1,835 patients randomized in this protocol, 76 patients were found on pathologic review after surgery to have had DCIS and not IBC. These participants had been randomized into the three treatment groups of protocol B-06: total mastectomy, lumpectomy, or lumpectomy with radiation therapy. Analysis of this small patient subset showed that radiation therapy was effective in minimizing local recurrence in patients with DCIS treated with lumpectomy (16). One patient in the total mastectomy group and one patient in the lumpectomy group died of breast cancer. It is interesting that, as has been reported in many other studies, patients treated with total mastectomy do have a measurable rate of death caused by breast cancer. This is an important point and must be considered when evaluating recommendations for primary surgical treatment.

Because of its small sample size, this report is not definitive. It is, however, the only randomized, prospective evidence comparing total mastectomy with BCS, and it is worth noting that the number of patients evaluated exceeds that reported for most of the retrospective, nonrandomized treatment reports in the literature at that time (Table 41.2).

NSABP protocol B-17 (16) was designed to assess the value of radiation therapy after BCS. The trial compared lumpectomy only with lumpectomy and postoperative breast irradiation. Women who had DCIS resected with pathologically free margins (defined as no tumor present at the physical margin) were eligible. Consenting patients were then randomly assigned to receive either ipsilateral breast irradiation or no radiation therapy. Initially, all women underwent axillary node dissection, but in June 1987, this in-

tervention became optional because of the low probability of positive nodes in women with DCIS. Radiation therapy was similar to that in protocol B-06 and consisted of a 50-Gy dose given over 25 days. No interstitial or regional node irradiation was given. In this trial, the same simple definition of clear margins from B-06 was used: a clear margin is one that does not transect tumor. No minimum width is required.

Results

There were 818 women enrolled in this trial. The results of protocol B-17 were published in 1993 (16) and updated in 1998 (6) and 2001 (17). The mean duration of follow-up when this trial was first reported in 1993 was 43 months (range, 11 to 86 months). At the 8-year update published in 1998, the mean follow-up time was 90 months, and in 2001, it was 128 months. The benefit of adding radiation therapy to lumpectomy was virtually unchanged between 5 and 12 years of follow-up and was owing to a reduction in

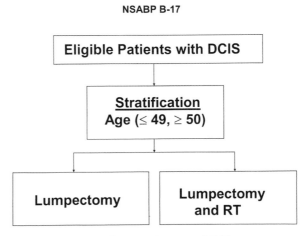

FIGURE 41.3. Scheme for NSABP protocol B-17.

both invasive and noninvasive ipsilateral breast tumors (IBTs). The frequency of IBC was reduced from 32% to 16% overall at 12 years by the addition of radiation therapy.

Mortality attributable to breast cancer for the entire group was found to be 1.6% at 8 years. The absolute incidence of noninvasive IBT was reduced from 13.4% to 8.2% ($p = 0.007$). Invasive IBT was reduced from 13.4% to 3.9% ($p < 0.0001$). This is a reduction of 59% for IBT of any type ($p < 0.00005$); a 47% reduction of noninvasive cancer ($p = 0.007$) and a 71% reduction of invasive cancer ($p = 0.000005$) (Fig. 41.4 and 41.5). Overall long-term survival rates were similar to those obtained with total mastectomy in historical studies. It was concluded that mastectomy was not generally warranted in women with DCIS (16).

This was the first large-scale prospective study of DCIS management to be reported, and it confirmed the preliminary evidence of the benefit of radiation therapy suggested in the analysis of the patients in the B-06 trial (14). It is noteworthy that the initial 5-year results were confirmed at the 8-year follow-up analysis. The evidence is clear that radiation therapy is effective in reducing the incidence of both invasive and noninvasive recurrences in the treated breast. The similar benefit in reducing local recurrence seen in the B-17 and B-06 trials is not surprising because primary DCIS and the zone of DCIS surrounding an invasive tumor are probably similar biologic processes. The B-17 trial has now defined and documented these issues for DCIS.

Treatment and Outcome of Patients with Ipsilateral Breast Tumor

One hundred four patients whose primary DCIS was treated with lumpectomy only subsequently developed an

IBT. Fifty-four (51.9%) of these women were treated with a second lumpectomy. Only 14 of these received additional radiation therapy. The other 50 patients (47.2%) were treated with mastectomy (Fig. 41.4).

In the 411 women treated with excision plus radiation therapy, 47 had local recurrences. Of these, 17 were invasive and 30 were noninvasive. In the latter group, 50% were treated with repeat lumpectomy. Among the 17 women with invasive cancers, three were retreated with lumpectomy and 14 had mastectomies.

In women with recurrent tumors, 77% were within the same quadrant; 13% showed second tumors at different sites in the same breast. The other 10% were at the edge of the index quadrant or were retroareolar recurrences. This is similar to the outcome patterns in B-06 where it is believed that residual DCIS was responsible for most recurrences.

Treatment by Type of Recurrence

For patients with IBT that was not invasive, approximately half underwent a second lumpectomy. Thus, a second operation was equally likely to be lumpectomy plus radiation therapy or mastectomy in all categories except those women in the lumpectomy plus radiation therapy group who developed an invasive cancer. For this group, 82% had mastectomy. It is likely that surgeons treating a recurrence in a woman who did not receive radiation therapy were often comfortable with re-excision when they were free to add radiation therapy, but when radiation therapy had previously been used, the option of re-excision only usually gave way to a recommendation for mastectomy. Of 54 women who had a second lumpectomy, three developed a second IBT, all of whom had DCIS as their first recurrence. One of these pa-

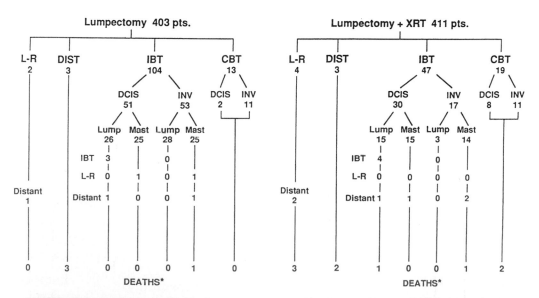

FIGURE 41.4. Outcomes in National Surgical Adjuvant Breast Project protocol B-17. L-R, local recurrence; DIST, distant recurrence; IBT, invasive breast tumors; CBT, contralateral breast tumor; INV, invasive breast cancer. (Reprinted with permission from *J Clin Oncol* 1998;16:441–452.)

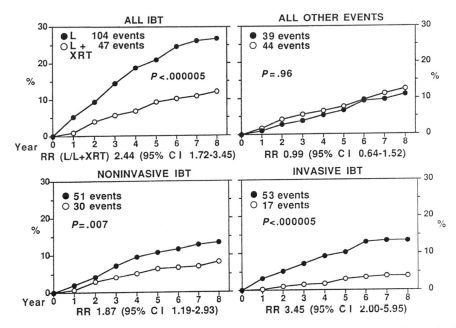

FIGURE 41.5. Cumulative incidence of all breast cancer events, invasive, non-invasive, and other first events. (Reprinted with permission from *The Lancet*.1999;253:1993–2000.)

tients developed distant metastases and is still alive. One of the patients whose DCIS had been treated with mastectomy developed subsequent local regional disease. Another patient who had a local regional invasive recurrence was treated with mastectomy and subsequently developed metastases and died. None of the 54 women whose first IBT was treated with lumpectomy has died.

Location of Ipsilateral Breast Tumor

The location of the primary DCIS and the IBT was similar in 84% of the 126 women in whom the site of these tumors was known. This concordance was greater in the group who showed an IBT of DCIS (80.3%) than in the group who had invasive IBT (51.7%). This was true for patients with and without radiation therapy.

Regional and Distant Recurrences

There were three women with regional lymph node metastases. Two of them originally had DCIS detected mammographically (microcalcifications) and were treated with lumpectomy and radiation therapy. Lymph node metastases developed subsequently but without evidence of disease in the breast. The third woman with regional metastases was initially treated with lumpectomy only and had nodal metastases 5 years later.

Two women developed distant metastases. One had bone metastases with no evidence of recurrence in the breast; the other developed an extensive IBC recurrence with simultaneous widespread metastases.

Other Events

As might be expected, excluding ipsilateral tumor recurrence, the cumulative incidence of other events was not significantly different between the irradiated and nonirradiated groups.

Survival

Through 8 years of follow-up, the overall survival rate was 94% for women in the lumpectomy group and 95% for those in the radiation therapy group. There were 15 deaths from causes unrelated to breast cancer, mainly owing to diabetes and cardiovascular or pulmonary problems. Fourteen deaths were attributable to breast cancer; four of these oc-

NSABP B-24

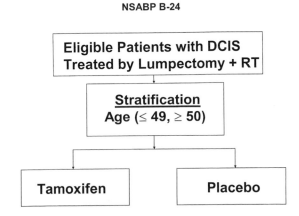

FIGURE 41.6. Schema for NSABP protocol B-24.

curred in those treated with lumpectomy only and ten in the group treated with lumpectomy and radiation therapy. Five patients who died had distant failures as the first event, three in the lumpectomy only group and two in the radiation therapy group. Among the 151 women with IBT, there were three deaths from metastatic disease. One patient was in the lumpectomy only group who died after removal of an IBT. The other two deaths were patients who received radiation therapy, one after removal of an noninvasive IBT and the other after mastectomy for an invasive IBT. Two women with contralateral breast tumor also died.

Predictors

The size of the mammographically detected tumor was not a significant predictor of an IBT. Dividing the initial tumor size into 1 cm or smaller or larger than 1 cm yielded no significant difference (rr = 0.86). There was a reduction in the rate of IBT after radiation therapy in both tumor size categories. However, in women with no mass whose mammograms showed suspicious calcifications larger than 1 cm in maximum diameter had a greater rate of IBT than those whose mammogram showed clustered calcifications 1 cm or smaller.

The most important finding was that the cumulative incidence of an invasive IBT was only 3.9% in patients treated with lumpectomy and radiation therapy compared with 13.4% in the lumpectomy only group, and there was a similar decrease for patients with noninvasive IBTs. Also important is the finding that the benefit does not decrease with longer follow-up. Retrospective studies have shown that the incidence of IBT appears to double between 5 and 8 years of follow-up in women who received radiation therapy after lumpectomy. Findings from this prospective study show only a slight increase in the cumulative incidence of invasive (from 3.8% to 3.9%) and noninvasive cancers (from 6.4% to 8.2%) over this interval.

Who Should Have Radiation Therapy?

For both invasive and noninvasive tumors treated with BCS, there has always been an interest in identifying a cohort of patients who could safely be treated with lumpectomy only. In another report (18), the NSABP examined nine pathologic characteristics traditionally believed to possibly contribute predictive information on local recurrence. In each of the subcategories, an overall benefit from the use of radiation therapy was observed. In a univariate analysis, only nuclear grade, comedonecrosis, specimen margin status, and histologic tumor type were significant prognostic variables for an IBT. However, in a multivariate analysis, only slight or marked comedonecrosis and uncertain or involved tumor margins were independent predictors of IBT. However, at the 8-year follow-up, margin status was no longer found to be a predictor of local recurrence (19). It was clear, however, that the use of radiation therapy bene-

fited both good and poor risk patients, and outcomes of all subgroups were essentially similar among those who received radiation therapy. Thus, there was no clear discriminant that identified patients with DCIS who should not receive postoperative radiation therapy.

Effect on Survival

The low incidence of metastatic disease and death from breast cancer observed in this trial makes it impossible to study predictive factors for these events. When it is remembered that regional treatment failures, distant disease, and death occur even after mastectomy is performed for DCIS (Table 41.1), the few deaths seen in the B-17 trial fall into perspective. It is likely that the same women would have had metastases even if treated with mastectomy. It is noteworthy that metastatic events occurred most often in women who failed to demonstrate an IBT when the distant events were discovered. Two patients who experienced distant disease died within 12 months after treatment of their primary tumor. In several patients, local regional disease developed only 7 to 15 months after removal of the primary tumor. The frequency of metastatic disease and deaths was similar in both treatment groups, indicating that radiation therapy did not influence the occurrence of distant metastases and death. From this, it is reasonable to infer that residual disease, attributable to BCS rather than mastectomy or very wide local excision, was not the source of the metastases. If it had been the source, then radiation therapy to the breast would have decreased or delayed the appearance of metastases and death in many cases. Thus, arguments about margin control lose their importance in the face of this observation. The same outcome and conclusion were seen when these issues were studied in IBC (20). Thus, for both IBC and DCIS, there is no evidence to suggest that a reduction in the occurrence of IBT was associated with better or worse distant disease–free survival or survival, and the IBT is seen as a marker for, and not the source of, the metastases.

Despite this evidence that BCS provided excellent control, controversy continued in two areas. Many women, especially those whose mammograms suggested more diffuse tumors, were still being advised to accept mastectomy. For those women with smaller tumors easily removed by BCS, the advantages of radiation therapy were clear, and it seemed that lumpectomy only should be abandoned. Further research could then be directed at biologic interventions to reduce local and distant failures even more. However, another avenue of thought emerged that suggested that wide local excision only would be preferable and that radiation therapy could be omitted in selected cases. It was argued that many women did not need radiation therapy and that evaluating the width of free margin surrounding the tumor could identify this group. Furthermore, there was a concern, raised by results from a European study that radiation therapy increased the risk of contralateral cancer.

EUROPEAN ORGANIZATION FOR RESEARCH AND TREATMENT OF CANCER STUDY

The European Organization for Research and Treatment of Cancer (EORTC) conducted a trial similar to B-17 (7). Beginning in 1986, they recruited 1,002 patients randomized to excision only or excision plus radiation therapy. Their report corroborates the main conclusion of B-17 that radiation therapy decreases local recurrence, both invasive and noninvasive. A central pathology review has yet to be reported so that information on possible predictors for local recurrence is not yet available. The main difference in outcome between the two studies is the apparently increased rate of contralateral breast cancer in the radiation cohort. One concern is that this increased incidence is a result of scatter of ionizing radiation given to the ipsilateral breast. The EORTC technique included compensatory filters or wedges that can increase the scatter dose to the contralateral breast. However, a comparison with the NSABP study can be instructive. In B-17, there were 16 contralateral breast cancers in the excision only group and 12 in the combined radiation therapy group. In the EORTC study, there were only five cases in the excision only group and 16 in the radiotherapy group. Thus, a possible explanation for this difference is a spuriously low incidence of contralateral breast cancer in the EORTC excision only group suggesting an apparent but not a real increase for the radiation therapy group. In response to this questionable anomaly in the EORTC study, Brenner et al. (21) examined Surveillance, Epidemiology, and End Results program data on 32,000 women treated for breast cancer with postoperative radiation therapy between 1973 and 1993 and did not detect an increase attributable to irradiation-induced tumors. In addition, the apparent increase in irradiation-induced tumors is highly improbable given the short latency period, the low scatter dose to the contralateral breast, and the lack of such an effect in numerous other studies in which radiation therapy has been used.

Another area of potential controversy between the two randomized studies concerns the differential reduction in invasive cancer (from 10.5% to 2.9% in the NSABP study and from 8% to 4% in the EORTC study). Although the relative differences seem to be important, the absolute rates are not that different, and it appears that both studies show a meaningful decrease in IBC. The base rate was confirmed in B-24 in which both groups received radiation therapy, but the incidence of local recurrence in the B-24 placebo (lumpectomy plus radiation therapy) group was no higher than in the B-17 lumpectomy plus radiation therapy group.

B-24 RATIONALE

Although the B-17 and EORTC results indicate that mastectomy is not usually warranted, many women with DCIS were not eligible for this treatment because they either had mammographic evidence of diffuse calcifications or pathologically positive margins.

In previous adjuvant studies of tamoxifen after BCS for IBC, the NSABP reported that tamoxifen, among its other benefits, decreased the incidence of tumor recurrences in the ipsilateral breast to less than 5% and reduced the rate of new primary tumors in the contralateral breast by 50% (22). Tamoxifen was thus shown to interfere with the development of primary invasive cancer or with the progression of DCIS to invasive cancer. It is known that tamoxifen has anti-initiator and antipromoter actions on breast cells. Therefore, in B-24, patients received 5 years of adjuvant tamoxifen or placebo after standard lumpectomy and radiation therapy. It was postulated that tamoxifen would be more effective than radiation therapy only in preventing recurrences of DCIS or IBC. To learn more about the biology of breast cancer and to extend the benefits of BCS for women who were ineligible for breast-conserving treatment in B-17 because of pathologic or clinical features, the NSABP undertook a second DCIS protocol, B-24 (Fig. 41.6).

Results of B-24

A total of 1,804 women was randomly assigned to one of the two groups (Fig. 41.6). This study was first reported after 5 years of follow-up and has been recently updated to 7 years (17). Eligibility requirements matched those of B-17 except for the inclusion in B-24 of patients with diffuse suspicious calcifications and those with positive margins. Median follow-up was 74 months. Patient characteristics were similar in both groups, 65% were postmenopausal. More than 80% of tumors were smaller than 1 cm and detected by mammography only.

The incidence of all cancer events at 7 years decreased from 11.1% in the placebo group to 7.7% in the tamoxifen group ($p = 0.0009$). The cumulative incidence of all invasive cancers decreased from 5.3% in the placebo group to 2.6% in the tamoxifen group. The invasive recurrences in the tamoxifen group were further broken down to 2.1% in the ipsilateral breast, 1.8% in the contralateral breast, and 0.2% at regional and distant sites. The rate of noninvasive IBT showed a lower trend, which was nonsignificant (18%, $p = 0.43$) (Fig. 41.7).

The type of surgery after IBT was similar in two groups; 68% of women who received placebo and 59% of those who received tamoxifen underwent mastectomy. However, as was also seen in B-17, in women who had received lumpectomy plus radiation therapy, mastectomy was more frequently used in women with invasive cancer (75% versus 56%). There was a 52% reduction in contralateral breast tumors in patients who received tamoxifen, although the absolute rate of contralateral breast tumors was not high. The cumulative incidence was 3.4% in the placebo group and 2.0% in the tamoxifen group.

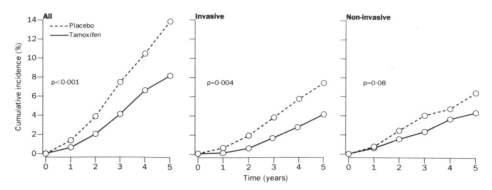

FIGURE 41.7. Cumulative incidence of all, invasive, and noninvasive events and ipsilateral and contralateral breast tumors in the National Surgical Adjuvant Breast Project B-17 and B-24 studies. (Reprinted with permission from *Lancet* 1999;353:1993–2000.)

Other Cancers

There was no difference in the rate of occurrence of cancers other than breast or endometrial. There was a nonsignificant increase in endometrial cancer similar to that seen in other tamoxifen trials.

Predictive Characteristics

The chance of developing an IBT was significantly related to age at diagnosis. The annual rate of IBT at 7 years was 29.2% for women aged 49 years or younger and 13.3% for those older than 50. Tamoxifen reduced these by 32% and 30%, respectively.

Pathologically positive tumor margins were associated with an increased risk of invasive or noninvasive IBT. Similarly, clinically palpable tumors carried an increased risk for local recurrence. This risk was decreased among women who received tamoxifen regardless of margin status. The rate was 21% lower in the tamoxifen group in those whose margins were negative and 45% lower in those whose margins were positive.

In B-17, the presence of comedonecrosis pathologically carried an increased risk of local recurrence. In B-24, there

was a similar increase if this feature was present, although it was more predictive for noninvasive than invasive recurrence. The rate of IBT was lowered by tamoxifen in both groups (29% lower in those who had no comedonecrosis and 28% lower in those who did). In the multivariate analysis of B-17 (18), positive margins and comedonecrosis were both associated with an increased risk of ipsilateral tumors, although the radiation therapy reduced the risk in both categories. Tamoxifen further reduced the incidence of such events, whether comedonecrosis or positive margins were present. More recently, an update of the B-17 pathologic findings shows that comedonecrosis continues to be a predictor of IBT, but margin status is not a strong predictor (19).

Survival

After 5 years of follow-up, the survival rate was 97% overall for both groups. At 7 years, it was 95% for both groups. There were 44 deaths in the placebo group and 42 in the group receiving tamoxifen. In the placebo group, ten deaths were attributed to breast cancer, whereas in the group who received tamoxifen, the deaths of five women were attributable to breast cancer ($p = $ NS).

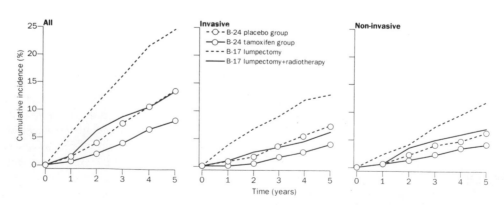

FIGURE 41.8. Cumulative incidence of all, invasive, and non-invasive events in ipsilateral and contralateral breast; comparison of B-17 and B-24.

Interpretation

The addition of tamoxifen to lumpectomy and radiation therapy decreased the rate of invasive cancer, especially in the ipsilateral breast. There was a significantly lower cumulative incidence of all breast cancer–related events compared with the placebo group. In this regard, it can be useful to compare B-17 and B-24 because they share a common arm of lumpectomy and radiation therapy (Fig. 41.8). Comparison with B-17 is possible because of the similarity of the eligibility requirements and patient characteristics in the two lumpectomy and radiation therapy arms. The only differences were the inclusion in B-24 of women with more extensive DCIS, and the fact that 16% of patients in the B-24 trial had pathologically positive margins. Nevertheless, the cumulative incidences of all breast cancer events in the two radiation therapy and lumpectomy arms were similar, confirming the assumption that comparative, cross-protocol comparisons can be made. This also confirms the advantage of radiation therapy. The cumulative incidence of all events in women treated with lumpectomy only was 25% at 5 years (5). This fell to 13% after the radiation therapy in the two trials and to 7% in the group given tamoxifen in B-24. The benefit is owing to the low rate of recurrences at ipsilateral, contralateral, regional, and distant sites in women treated with tamoxifen. Overall, the addition of tamoxifen led to a 68% lower cumulative incidence of all breast cancer events at 5 years compared with women treated with lumpectomy only in B-17. For ipsilateral breast cancer only, there was a 77% reduction and approximately a 64% reduction for all noninvasive events.

Although the benefit from additional treatment with tamoxifen was derived largely from the decrease in the incidence of invasive cancer, especially in the ipsilateral breast, there was benefit in the reduction of contralateral breast cancer and in regional and distant disease categories. These findings show that focusing on the frequency of ipsilateral recurrence only is too narrow a strategy. The possible effect that a biologic treatment such as tamoxifen has on all invasive and noninvasive cancers at any site seems more important. The non-Halstedian model recognizes that cancer is a disorder of growth and that simple mastectomy or very wide local excision is a less sophisticated approach than those that consider a more biologic approach. The benefits of this approach are a reduction in the overall incidence of all breast cancer events, ipsilateral, contralateral, and distant, and a reduction in the extent and severity of surgery required.

FUTURE CONSIDERATIONS

The low cumulative incidence of IBC events in the ipsilateral breast at 5 years in B-24 (2.1%) indicates excellent control. It is unlikely that this can be reduced to zero because having a breast present carries some mathematical risk for future cancer. Even with total mastectomy, local recurrence may be almost completely eliminated, but freedom from mortality is not achieved. The one report in the literature of zero mortality (23) stands against the entire world experience, which shows approximately a 1% to 2% mortality rate even with breast ablation. This is understandable from the biologic standpoint. The same biology explains the small but reproducible incidence of cancer after prophylactic mastectomy and the phenomenon of occult breast cancer. The achievement of zero mortality in one retrospective report, even with total mastectomy, must be explained either as a spurious finding or a function of case selection. Nevertheless, the success of tamoxifen in lowering all types of recurrence stimulates the search for more effective and safer agents to control the stimulation and growth of precancerous and cancerous cells in the breast.

MARGINS, BIOLOGY, RADIATION, AND MASTECTOMY

The search for a group with very low risk of recurrence who might be safely treated without radiation therapy is always a worthwhile effort. Swedish studies testing radiation therapy in patients with small invasive tumors showed that radiation therapy is still of benefit compared with treatment with lumpectomy only. Furthermore, NSABP B-21 specifically addressed this question in patients with invasive tumors smaller than 1 cm who also received tamoxifen. Analysis of this study shows that postoperative radiation therapy plus tamoxifen is superior to tamoxifen only or radiation therapy only in controlling local recurrence.

Most of the studies in the literature are not randomized, and, therefore, attempts to identify risk factors for relapse face potential selection bias. At present, radiation therapy has been proven to reduce the risk of IBT recurrence by 50% to 71% in two randomized trials. The proposal by Silverstein and colleagues (24, 25) that radiation therapy may not be necessary provided clear margins of 10 mm or more are obtained has not been confirmed in any prospective study. The NSABP reports on B-17 and B-24 indicate a remarkable freedom from local recurrence with radiation therapy when margins are clear by the NSABP definition (no transection of tumor microscopically).

In an editorial, Silverstein and Lagios acknowledged that radiation therapy is beneficial for patients with DCIS (40). Their criticism is that these protocols have not answered the question of which subgroups will truly benefit from radiation therapy and by how much. Two pathologic reviews of the NSABP data failed to demonstrate a subgroup that does not benefit from radiation therapy. Much controversy accompanied the publication of these reviews, but the arguments concern concepts, which may not continue to be seen as important in the future as we develop more biologic predictors and move away from classifications based on microscopic anatomy. The NSABP randomized studies show that all patients benefit from radiation therapy. Although in patients with clear margins and favorable nuclear grade, the benefit is small, it is still real.

Some authors favor the goal of obtaining margins of 10 mm or more and omitting radiation therapy (24,25). The evidence that wide margins carry better freedom from recurrence comes from retrospective reviews of material obtained over a 20-year span in which substantial changes in diagnostic mammography, biopsy approach, and other important variables have occurred. These studies involve a relatively small number of patients who were not randomized so that we have no idea of the comparability of the two groups for other factors that might be important in changing the outcome. Such studies lack the confidence that the outcome is owing to the difference in the variable being cited.

The main evidence for the 10-mm margin comes from retrospectively dividing the overall group (with a 27% local recurrence rate) into three groups: less than 1 mm, 1 mm to 10 mm, and larger than 10 mm. Those with a margin less than 1 mm had a 58% recurrence rate. For those with a margin larger than 10 mm, the rate was 3%. Was the size of the surgical margin the reason for the favorable result or was the nature of the tumor the reason for the fortuitously wide margin and the low local recurrence rate? Because surgeons tend to attempt to grossly encompass the lesion in a standard fashion, it is probable that thin margins are more likely in tumors with more extensive intraductal proliferation and extension. Small compact lesions are easily excised and found to have wide margins, whereas expansile lesions with extensive proliferation along ducts will likely show narrow margins. If so, then margin width may simply be a marker for the more expansile, aggressive type of DCIS.

Support for this comes from the examining issue of the extensive intraductal component in invasive cancer. In the 1980s, it was shown, in retrospective reviews that the extensive intraductal component was a predictor of local recurrence in patients treated with lumpectomy plus radiation therapy. Subsequently, it became clear that the extensive intraductal component was only a marker for the likelihood of positive margins (27). With negative margins, and even with focally positive margins, the extensive intraductal component was not associated with a higher incidence of local recurrence (27). Furthermore, local recurrence itself was demonstrated to be simply a marker for the presence of aggressive disease and the likelihood of metastases but was shown not to be the source of those metastases (20). Perhaps the most important fact in all this is that in all studies, the most important outcome measurement, overall survival, is the same regardless of what treatment is initially used.

Thus, the issue is to choose between two different treatment regimens: wide local excision or traditional lumpectomy and radiation therapy. The decision is made all the more complicated by the fact that the evidence in favor of

radiation therapy is based on randomized clinical trials, whereas the 10-mm margin evidence is retrospective. This is not a trivial point. It is worthwhile remembering that issues like multicentricity provided arguments against the use of BCS for invasive cancer in all retrospective studies but became a "nonissue" when evidence from prospective studies was presented. Similarly, for decades, retrospective reviews from respected authorities like Haagensen showed results for the Halsted radical mastectomy to be better than those from centers reporting on more limited surgery, but when randomized clinical trials were reported, all differences disappeared. Retrospective observations cannot be used to definitively answer the question of the choices that we now face, but they can be used to remind us of the need for scientific discipline as we seek the answers. Perhaps a more modern research agenda for new clinical trials would be to seek to identify more specific growth-controlling factors that could be used to prevent the development of neoplasia in either breast or at distant sites. The combination of BCS, radiation therapy, and tamoxifen is not the ultimate answer, but it is a step in the direction that we need to go.

REFERENCES

1. Fisher B, Bauer M, Margolese R, et al. Five-year results of a randomized clinical trial comparing total mastectomy and segmental mastectomy with or without radiation in treatment of breast cancer. *N Engl J Med* 1985;312:665–673.
2. Veronesi U, Sacrozi R, DelVecchio M, et al. Comparing radical mastectomy with quadrantectomy, axillary dissection and radiotherapy in patients with small cancers of the breast. *N Engl J Med* 1981;305:6–11.
3. Jacobson JA, Cowan KH, D'Angelo T, et al. Ten-year results of a comparison of conservation with mastectomy in the treatment of stage I and II breast cancer. *N Engl J Med* 1995;332:907–911.
4. Blichert-Toft M, Rose C, Anderson JA, et al. Danish randomized trial comparing breast conservative therapy with mastectomy. *J Natl Cancer Inst Mongr* 1992;11:19–25.
5. Fisher B, Dignam J, Wickerham DL, et al. Tamoxifen in treatment of intraductal breast cancer: National Surgical Adjuvant Breast and Bowel Project B-24 randomized controlled trial. *Lancet* 1999;353:1993–2000.
6. Fisher B, Dignam J, Wolmark N, et al. Lumpectomy and radiation therapy for the treatment of intraductal breast cancer: findings from National Surgical Adjuvant Breast and Bowel Project B-17. *J Clin Oncol* 1998;16:441–452.
7. Julien JP, Bijker N, Fentiman IS, et al. Radiotherapy in breast-conserving treatment of ductal carcinoma in situ: first results of the EORTC randomized phase III trial 10853. EORTC breast cancer cooperative group and EORTC radiotherapy group. *Lancet* 2000;355:528–533.
8. Nielsen M, Thomsen JL, Primdahl S, et al. Breast cancer and atypia among young and middle-aged women: a study of 110 medicolegal autopsies. Breast cancer in younger women. Need *Br J Cancer* 1987;56:814–819.
9. Rosen P, Fracchia AA, Urbain JA, et al. Residual mammary carcinoma following simulated partial mastectomy. *Cancer* 1975;35:739–747.
10. Fisher B, Redmond C, Fisher ER, et al. Ten-year results of a randomized clinical trial comparing radical mastectomy and total

mastectomy with or without radiation. *N Engl J Med* 1985; 312:674–681.

11. Bradley SJ, Weaver DW, Bouwman DL. Alternatives in the surgical management of in situ breast cancer. A meta-analysis of outcome. *Am Surg* 1990;56:428–432.

12. Lagios MD, Margolin FR, Westdahl PR, et al. Mammographically detected duct carcinoma in situ: frequency of local recurrence following tylectomy and prognostic effect of nuclear grade on local recurrence. *Cancer* 1989;63:618–624.

13. Schwartz GF, Finkel GC, Garcia JC, et al. Subclinical ductal carcinoma in situ of the breast. *Cancer* 1992;70:2468–2474.

14. Fisher ER, Leeming R, Anderson S, et al. Conservative management of intraductal carcinoma DCIS of the breast. Collaborating NSABP investigators. *J Surg Oncol* 1991;47:139–147.

15. Bonadonna G, Veronesi U, Brambilla C, et al. Primary chemotherapy to avoid mastectomy in tumors with diameters of three centimeters or more. *J Natl Cancer Inst* 1990;82:1539–1545.

16. Fisher B, Constantino J, Redmond C, et al. Lumpectomy compared with lumpectomy and radiation therapy for the treatment of intraductal breast cancer. *N Engl J Med* 1993;328:1581–1586.

17. Fisher B, Land S, Mamounas E, et al. Prevention of invasive breast cancer in women with ductal carcinoma in situ: an update of the National Surgical Adjuvant Breast and Bowel Project Experience. *Semin Oncol* 2001;28:400–418.

18. Fisher ER, Constantino J, Fisher B, et al. Pathologic findings from the National Surgical Adjuvant Breast Project (NSABP) Protocol B-17. *Cancer* 1995;75:1310–1319.

19. Fisher ER, Dignam J, Tan-Chiu E, et al. Pathologic findings from the National Surgical Adjuvant Breast Project (NSABP). Eight-year update of protocol B-17. *Cancer* 1999;86:429–438.

20. Fisher B, Anderson S, Fisher ER, et al. Significance of ipsilateral breast tumor recurrence after lumpectomy. *Lancet* 1991;8763:327–331.

21. Brenner DJ, Schiff PB, Zablotska LB. Adjuvant radiotherapy for DCIS. *Lancet* 2000;355:2071.

22. Fisher B, Constantino J, Redmond C, et al. A randomized clinical trial evaluating tamoxifen in the treatment of patients with node-negative breast cancer who have estrogen-receptor-positive tumors. *N Engl J Med* 1989;320:479–484.

23. Silverstein MJ. Van Nuys experience by treatment. In: Silverstein MJ, ed. *Ductal carcinoma in situ of the breast.* Baltimore: Williams & Wilkins, 1997:443–447.

24. Silverstein MJ. Ductal carcinoma in situ of the breast: a surgeon's disease. *Ann Surg Oncol* 1999;6:802–810.

25. Silverstein MJ, Lagios MD, Groshen S, et al. The influence of margin width on local control in patients with ductal carcinoma in situ (DCIS) of the breast. *N Engl J Med* 1999;340:1455–1461.

26. Holland R, Connolly JI, Gelman R, et al. The presence of an extensive intraductal component following a limited excision correlates with prominent residual disease in the remainder of the breast. *J Clin Oncol* 1990;8:113–118.

27. Schnitt SJ, Abner A, Gelman R, et al. The relationship between microscopic margins of resection and the risk of local recurrence in patients with breast cancer treated with breast-conserving surgery and radiation therapy. *Cancer* 1994;74:1746–1751.

28. Ashikari R, Hadju S, Robbins G. Intraductal carcinoma of the breast. *Cancer* 1971;28:1182–1187.

29. Lagios M, Westdahl P, Margolin F, et al. Duct Carcinoma in situ: Relationship of extent of noninvasive disease to the frequency of occult invasion, multicentricity, lymph node metastases, and short-term treatment failures. *Cancer* 1982;50:1309–1314.

30. Rosner D, Bedwani R, Vana J, et al. Noninvasive breast carcinoma. Results of a national survey of The American College of Surgeons. *Ann Surg* 1980;192:139–147.

31. Schuh M, Nemoto T, Penetrante R, et al. Intraductal carcinoma: analysis of presentation, pathologic findings, and outcome of disease. *Arch Surg* 1986;121:1303–1307.

32. Deleted in press.

33. Farrow, J. Current concepts in the detection and treatment of the earliest of the breast cancers. *Cancer* 1970;25:468–477.

34. Bornstein B, Recht A, Connolly J, et al. Result of treating ductal carcinoma in situ of the breast with conservative surgery and radiation therapy. *Cancer* 1991;67:7–13.

35. Kurtz J, Jacquemier J, Torhorst J, et al. Conservation therapy for breast cancers other than infiltrating ductal carcinoma. *Cancer* 1989;63:1630–1635.

36. Stotter A, McNeese M, Oswald M, et al. The role of limited surgery with irradiation in primary treatment of ductal carcinoma in situ breast cancer. *Int J Radiat Oncol Bio Phys* 1990;18:283–290.

37. Zafrani B, Fourquet A, Vilcoq J, et al. Conservative management of intraductal breast carcinoma with tumorectomy and radiation therapy. *Cancer* 1986;57:1299–1301.

38. Solin L, Yeh I, Kurtz J, et al. Ductal carcinoma in situ (intraductal carcinoma) of the breast treated with breast-conserving surgery and definitive irradiation. Correlation of pathologic parameters with outcome of treatment. *Cancer*, 1993;71:2532–2542.

39. Kuske R, Bean J, Garcia D, et al. Breast conservation therapy for intraductal carcinoma of the breast. *Int J Radiat Oncol Biol Phys* 1993;26:391–396.

40. Silverstein MJ, Lagios MD. Benefits of Irradiation for DCIS: a Pyrrhic Victory. *Lancet* 2000;355:510–511.

PREVENTION OF INVASIVE BREAST CANCER IN WOMEN WITH DUCTAL CARCINOMA IN SITU: AN UPDATE OF THE NATIONAL SURGICAL ADJUVANT BREAST AND BOWEL PROJECT EXPERIENCE*

BERNARD FISHER
STEPHANIE LAND
ELEFTHERIOS MAMOUNAS
JAMES DIGNAM
EDWIN R. FISHER
NORMAN WOLMARK

The National Surgical Adjuvant Breast and Bowel Project (NSABP) conducted two sequential randomized clinical trials to aid in resolving uncertainty about the treatment of women with small, localized, mammographically detected ductal carcinoma in situ (DCIS). After removal of the tumor and normal breast tissue so that specimen margins were histologically tumor-free (lumpectomy), 818 patients in the B-17 trial were randomly assigned to receive either radiation therapy to the ipsilateral breast or no radiation therapy. B-24, the second study, which involved 1,804 women, tested the hypothesis that, in DCIS patients with or without positive tumor specimen margins, lumpectomy, radiation, and tamoxifen (TAM) would be more effective than lumpectomy, radiation, and placebo in preventing invasive and noninvasive ipsilateral breast tumor recurrences (IBTRs), contralateral breast tumors (CBTs), and tumors at metastatic sites. The findings in this report continue to demonstrate through 12 years of follow-up that radiation after lumpectomy reduces the incidence rate of all IBTRs by 58%. They also demonstrate that the administration of TAM after lumpectomy and radiation therapy results in a significant decrease in the rate of all breast cancer events, particularly in invasive cancer. The findings from the B-17 and B-24 studies are related to those from the NSABP prevention (P-1) trial, which demonstrated a 50% reduction in the risk of invasive cancer in women with a history of atypical ductal hyperplasia (ADH) or lobular carcinoma in situ (LCIS) and a reduction in the incidence of both DCIS and LCIS in women without a history of those tumors. The B-17 findings demonstrated that patients treated with lumpectomy alone were at greater risk for invasive cancer than were women in P-1 who had a history of ADH or LCIS and who received no radiation therapy or TAM. Although women who received radiation benefited from that therapy, they remained at higher risk for invasive cancer than women in P-1 who had a history of LCIS and who received placebo or TAM. Thus, if it is accepted from the P-I findings that women at increased risk for invasive cancer are candidates for an intervention such as TAM, then it would seem that women with a history of DCIS should also be considered for such therapy in addition to radiation therapy. That statement does not imply that, as a result of the findings presented here, all DCIS patients should receive radiation and TAM. It does suggest, however, that, in the treatment of DCIS, the appropriate use of current and better therapeutic agents that become available could diminish the significance of breast cancer as a public health problem.

INTRODUCTION

Until the1980s, when mammography began to be used more frequently, fewer than 3% of newly diagnosed breast cancers were ductal carcinoma in situ (DCIS). Because those lesions were generally treated with mastectomy, there was little opportunity for evaluating the natural history of DCIS or for determining the incidence of invasive or non-invasive ipsilateral breast tumors (IBTs) that might have occurred subsequent to a diagnostic biopsy. Moreover, the limited amount of information that was available (1–6) had been collected retrospectively. Two studies, one by Betsill et al. and the other by Page et al., were instrumental in formulating opinion about the way in which DCIS should be treated. In 1978, Betsill et al. reported that 25 women with untreated DCIS among 8,609 patients at Memorial Sloan-Kettering Cancer Center in New York had had breast biopsies between 1940 and 1950 and that the results initially had been determined to be benign (2). An examination of clinical records, which were available for 15 of the patients, showed that 10 had long-term follow-up. After an average interval of 9.7 years from biopsy, seven of these 10 developed an IBT. In 1982, Page et al. reported that a histologic review of 11,760 breast biopsies that had been performed at Vanderbilt Hospital in Nashville, TN, between 1950 and 1968 revealed 28 cases of DCIS that had been treated by biopsy alone (3). Twenty-five of these women (28%) were followed for more than 3 years; seven developed an IBT. It is of interest that, although many of the tumors in these studies were considered to be free of comedonecrosis and were well-differentiated types, there was a higher mortality rate among women with these tumors than would have been expected as a result of the current view that such lesions indicate a good prognosis.

Almost all of the DCIS diagnosed before the widespread use of mammography was discovered in women who visited their physicians with an obvious mass or with nipple discharge. DCIS was infrequently found in women who had a focus of the disease that had been detected during the removal of a benign lesion. Evidence of associated invasive breast cancer was observed in many women with large tumors. Consequently, the high rate of tumor recurrence that was found subsequent to the management of the tumor by "biopsy" is not surprising, and, as a result, there could have been little, if any, justification for considering breast conservation as a treatment for DCIS. It might be concluded that the information about DCIS that was obtained during that era has little relevance to the treatment of the nonclinically detectable DCIS free of an invasive component that is being diagnosed with increasing frequency as the result of mammography (DCIS currently comprises 35% or more of mammographically detected tumors).

Despite the shortcomings of the premammographic era, there did arise, during that time, an awareness of biologic issues that continue to be unresolved with regard to the management of DCIS. The question of whether DCIS is an obligatory step in the progression of biologic events that ultimately result in the development of invasive breast cancer or is merely a marker of risk remains unanswered. Similarly, uncertainty persists about whether all DCIS will eventually become invasive cancer. If the latter is the case, such a change could be the result of a somatic genetic event, and the factor(s)

responsible for such an occurrence might be speculated upon. In addition to the persistence of these and other biologic uncertainties, physicians and their patients are currently faced with a more pragmatic concern, ie, the issue of how to treat DCIS that has been mammographically detected.

The National Surgical Adjuvant Breast and Bowel Project (NSABP) has made an effort to obtain information about the biology, natural history, and treatment of the occult version of DCIS as the result of a paradoxical situation that arose in 1985. As a consequence of the first report of findings from NSABP B-06 (7), a randomized clinical trial which demonstrated that lumpectomy followed by radiation therapy was as effective as modified radical mastectomy in the treatment of invasive breast cancer, breast preservation began to be advocated for the management of invasive disease, while non-invasive disease continued to be treated with mastectomy. That circumstance, which resulted in uncertainty about how women with small, localized, mammographically detected DCIS should be treated, prompted the NSABP to initiate the B-17 trial, the first randomized trial related to DCIS. The purpose of that study was to determine whether excision of localized DCIS with tumor-free margins of removed tissue (a procedure referred to as lumpectomy, although most women had no palpable mass) followed by radiation therapy was more effective than lumpectomy alone in the prevention of an IBT, particularly one that was invasive. Regardless of whether DCIS is a precursor of invasive breast cancer or a marker for increased risk for that disease, the primary purpose of any treatment for DCIS is the prevention of the subsequent occurrence of an invasive cancer.

The findings from the B-17 study, which were first reported in 1993, demonstrated that, after 5 years of follow-up, lumpectomy and postoperative breast irradiation were more appropriate than lumpectomy alone for the prevention of both invasive and noninvasive IBT (8). A subsequent analysis after 8 years of follow-up confirmed the worth of lumpectomy and radiation therapy for the treatment of localized, mammographically detected DCIS (9). Additional findings showed that there were no pathologic, clinical, mammographic, or biologic discriminants to identify which of the patients enrolled in the trial either did or did not need radiation therapy after lumpectomy (10).

During the conduct of the B-17 trial, several circumstances led the NSABP to initiate the B-24 study, a second randomized clinical trial involving women with DCIS. One of these circumstances related to the observation that many women with DCIS had been ineligible for B-17 because their mammograms showed scattered calcifications that were thought to be either benign or associated with unremoved DCIS, or because, despite several excisions, the margins of resected breast tissue continued to be involved with DCIS. Consequently, these women were treated with mastectomy because of concern that unremoved DCIS might progress to invasive cancer or because a small, unidentified focus of invasive tumor associated with DCIS might have remained unremoved.

Another circumstance that led us to conduct the B-24 trial related to information that demonstrated the importance of tamoxifen (TAM) for the treatment of invasive breast cancer. Because it had been shown that TAM had anti-initiator and antipromoter properties (11–13), reduced the incidence of IBT (14), and prevented second primary tumors in the contralateral breast (CBTs) (15–19), we considered it appropriate to initiate the B-24 study to test the hypothesis that, in DCIS patients who had tumors removed with or without positive specimen margins or whose mammograms showed evidence of scattered calcifications that were unlikely to be associated with invasive cancer, lumpectomy, radiation therapy, and TAM would be more effective than lumpectomy, radiation therapy, and placebo in preventing invasive and noninvasive IBTs and CBTs, as well as tumors at metastatic sites. Through 5 years of follow-up, the findings from B-24 supported that hypothesis (20).

Of significance is the fact that the B-17 and B-24 findings are inter-related with those reported from the NSABP Breast Cancer Prevention Trial (P-1), which demonstrated that TAM reduced, by 50%, the occurrence of invasive and noninvasive breast cancer in women at increased risk for such tumors (21). The observation in P-1 that TAM dramatically reduced the rate of invasive breast cancer in women with a history of either atypical ductal hyperplasia (ADH) or lobular carcinoma in situ (LCIS), also considered to be pathologic markers or precursors of invasive breast cancer, was particularly relevant to the finding in B-24 that TAM reduced the incidence of that pathologic entity in women with a history of DCIS. This report provides an update of the major findings from B-17 through 12 years of follow-up and from B-24 through 7 years of follow-up; in addition, it presents the relation between the findings from B-24 and those from B-17 and P-1.

CONDUCT OF THE TWO TRIALS

A detailed description of patient eligibility requirements, study design, surgery and radiation therapy used, follow-up,

study end points, and statistical analyses appears in both the 5- and 8-year reports of B-17 (8,9) and in the initial report of the 5-year findings from B-24 (20). Because many of the same investigators and institutions implemented and conducted the B-24 trial after completion of the B-17 study, and because most aspects of the two protocols that governed the studies were comparable, any perceived disparities between them were related to factors necessary to achieve their individual objectives. Patients with small, localized foci of DCIS that had been detected by mammography were eligible for the B-17 study. Women with a histologic diagnosis of DCIS whose mammograms showed scattered calcifications were also eligible if no tumor was demonstrated when the tissue that contained the calcifications was examined and if radiologists considered such findings to be unrelated to invasive or noninvasive cancers. All women in B-17 were required to have a lumpectomy with removal of both the tumor and a sufficient amount of normal breast tissue so that specimen margins were histologically tumor-free. The eligibility requirements for women admitted to the B-24 study were similar to those for women in B-17, except that women whose tumor specimen margins were positive or whose mammograms showed findings that were unlikely to be invasive cancer were also eligible for B-24.

After they had undergone lumpectomy and had given written consent, women in B-17 were randomly assigned between October 1, 1985, and December 31, 1990, to receive either radiation therapy to the ipsilateral breast or no radiation therapy. Women in B-24 were randomly assigned between May 9, 1991, and April 13, 1994, to receive either placebo and radiation therapy to the ipsilateral breast or radiation therapy and TAM. Although axillary dissection was obligatory at the onset of the B-17 study, it subsequently became optional on the basis of evidence that it was not necessary in the treatment of DCIS. B-24 patients did not undergo axillary dissection. In the B-17 study, 818 patients were randomly assigned; 19 (2.3%) of these women were ineligible and five (0.6%) had no follow-up (Table 42.1). Of the 1,804 women randomly assigned in B-24, 30 (1.7%) were ineligible and six (0.3%) had no follow-up.

TABLE 42.1. STUDY INFORMATION

Variable	B-17 L	B-17 L + XRT	B-24 L + XRT + Placebo	B-24 L + XRT + TAM
Patients				
Randomly assigned	405	413	902	902
Ineligible	6	13	12	18
With no follow-up	2	3	3	3
Included in analysis	403	410	899	899
Duration of follow-up (mo)				
Mean	128		82	
Median	129		83	

L, lumpectomy; XRT, radiation therapy; TAM, tamoxifen.

In both studies, radiation therapy (50 Gy) was begun no later than 8 weeks after surgery. The technique used was similar to that which has been described in previous NSABP studies (22). In the B-24 trial, placebo or TAM, 10 mg twice daily, was administered within 56 days of lumpectomy and given continuously for 5 years. No dose modifications were made for either agent. Patients in both trials underwent physical examination every 6 months and had a mammogram once a year. The primary end point in both studies was the occurrence of invasive or noninvasive IBT or CBT. Lesions detected at local or regional sites were accepted as events only if they were found to be tumor-positive on pathologic examination. Tumors detected at distant sites, i.e., before local or regional invasive cancer was noted, were considered to be events if clinical, radiographic, or pathologic findings showed evidence of metastatic breast cancer. IBTs or CBTs, regional or distant metastases, second primary tumors other than breast tumors that occurred as a first event, or deaths in the absence of evidence of recurrent breast cancer were included in the determination of event-free survival (EFS).

Statistical Analyses

In both trials, data for analyses were from all randomly assigned patients with follow-up, regardless of their eligibility status (the intention-to-treat principle) (Table 42.1). The mean duration of follow-up was 128 months in B-17 and 82 months in B-24. The median duration was 129 months in the former study and 83 months in the latter. Before this report, all previous NSABP publications have referred to the length of follow-up as being the time from randomization to the time of analyses, regardless of whether or not a subject was still being followed. For this study, the median follow-up time was computed by use of the Kaplan-Meier method, using each patient's most recently reported follow-up as the event of interest and death as the censoring event. Findings reflect follow-up information reported through June 30, 2000.

EFS and overall survival were determined by Kaplan-Meier life-table estimates (23), and the two treatment groups were compared by use of a two-sided log-rank test (24). Comparisons adjusted for stratification variables were computed by means of the Cox proportional hazards model (25). Findings did not differ from those obtained by use of the unstratified analysis. The Cox model was also used to evaluate interactions among treatment and covariates. Average annual rates of occurrence for specific events were computed and compared by exact binomial tests. Relative risks and 95% confidence intervals (CIs) were derived from the Cox model for the event-specific end points (26). The cumulative probability of specific events comprising EFS was determined by means of cumulative incidence functions (27) that correctly accounted for competing risks. All P values reported are two-sided.

RESULTS

The similarity of the patients in the two studies is supported by the concordant distribution of patient age, race, method of detection, and tumor type among the treatment groups, both within and across the studies (Table 42.2). Although the tumor sizes in B-17 patients were slightly greater than those of the women enrolled in B-24, and although there was some disparity in the status of comedonecrosis observed in women in the two studies, the distribution of all characteristics was equivalent among treatment groups within a study. As anticipated, the incidence of specimen margins that contained tumor in B-24 was greater than that in B-17, where eligibility criteria required that the margins be tumor-free.

Benefit From Radiation Therapy After Lumpectomy In The B-17 Trial

EFS

It was observed that women treated with lumpectomy followed by radiation therapy to the ipsilateral breast continued to have a significantly better EFS through 12 years of follow-up than did women treated with lumpectomy alone (Fig. 42.1). The EFS of the two treatment groups was 63.6% versus 50.4%, respectively (P = .00004). A relative risk of failure of 0.63 (95% CI, 0.50 to 0.78) for patients treated with lumpectomy alone as compared with those treated with lumpectomy and breast irradiation confirmed the beneficial effect of radiation therapy.

Site, Rate, Rate Ratio, 95% CI, And Cumulative Incidence Of First Events

There was a 37.4% reduction in the average annual incidence rate (per 1,000 women) for all events among patients who received radiation therapy (59.9 for the group treated with lumpectomy alone v 37.5 for the group treated with lumpectomy plus radiation therapy; rate ratio [RR] = 0.63; 95% CI, 0.50 to 0.78; P = .00004; Table 42.3). The rate of all (invasive and noninvasive) breast cancer events was 47.7 and 28.2 for the two groups, respectively (RR = 0.59; 95% CI, 0.46 to 0.76; P = .00005). The average annual incidence rate of all IBTs was reduced by 57% as a consequence of radiation therapy (39.7 and 17.1 per thousand patients per year in the lumpectomy group and in the group treated with lumpectomy and radiation therapy, respectively; P < .000005). The rate of noninvasive IBTs was reduced by 51% (18.3 and 8.9 per thousand patients per year in the two treatment groups, respectively; P < .001) and the rate of invasive IBTs was reduced by 62% (21.1 and 8.1 per thousand patients per year, respectively; P = .00001). No significant reductions in the annual incidence rates of first events at

TABLE 42.2. PATIENT AND TUMOR CHARACTERISTICS IN B-17 AND B-24

	B-17		B-24	
	L (n = 403) %	L + XRT (n = 410) %	Placebo (n = 899) %	TAM (n = 899) %
Age (yr)				
≤49	34	33	33	34
50–59	29	32	31	30
≥60	37	35	36	37
Detection				
Mammogram	81	80	84	82
Clinical	8	8	8	9
Both	11	12	8	9
Tumor size (cm)				
≤1.0	74	75	83	85
1.1–2.0	15	13	12	9
≥2.1	8	9	4	5
Unknown	3	3	2	1
Tumor type				
DCIS	94	97	94	96
DCIS + LCIS	6	3	6	4
Specimen margins				
Tumor free			75	74
Not free	<1	<1	16	16
Unknown			9	10
Comedonecrosis				
Absent	35	34	50	52
Present	47	50	48	46
Unknown	19	16	2	2
Race				
White	88	88	85	86
Black	6	6	8	6
Other	4	5	6	6
Unknown	2	1	2	1

L, lumpectomy; XRT, radiation therapy; TAM, tamoxifen; DCIS, ductal carcinoma in situ; LCIS, lobular carcinoma in situ.

sites other than in the ipsilateral breast occurred from the use of radiation therapy subsequent to lumpectomy. A total of 17 local-regional and distant first events occurred in the 813 randomized patients with follow-up data; this total was only five more than were noted in the 8-year report. The number of CBTs that occurred as first events or subsequent

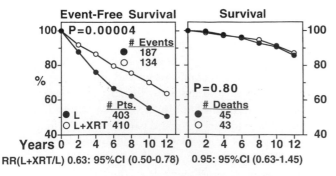

FIGURE 42.1. EFS and survival of women in B-17 who were treated with lumpectomy alone (L) or with lumpectomy and radiation therapy (L+XRT).

to an IBT were about equal. This updated report shows that 48 CBTs (5.9%) occurred as first events when the two treatment groups were combined. The rates of CBT occurring as a first event were 5.8 and 8.4 per thousand patients per year in the two treatment groups, respectively (P = .26). Fifteen of the 18 (83%) CBTs in the lumpectomy-treated group and 18 of 30 (60%) in the group that received lumpectomy and radiation therapy were invasive breast cancers. As reported after 8 years of follow-up, there continued to be no significant difference between the two treatment groups in the rate of occurrence of second primary cancers (other than CBT) (P = 1.0). Four years earlier, 10 and 14 second cancers, exclusive of cancer in the contralateral breast, had been reported. In this report, there were 18 and 20 in the groups treated with lumpectomy alone and lumpectomy and radiation therapy, respectively.

The cumulative incidence of the occurrence of an IBT of any type through 12 years of follow-up in women whose primary tumors were treated with lumpectomy alone was 31.7%; in women treated with lumpectomy followed by ra-

TABLE 42.3. SITE, RATE, AND RATE RATIOS OF FIRST EVENTS (B-17)

Type of Event	L (n = 403) No.	L (n = 403) Rate[a]	L + XRT (n = 410) No.	L + XRT (n = 410) Rate[a]	RR[b]	95% CI	Exact p
All events	187	59.9	134	37.5	0.63	0.50–0.78	0.00004
All breast cancer events	149[e]	47.7	101	28.2	0.59	0.46–0.76	0.00005
Invasive[c]	88[e]	28.2	57	15.9	0.57	0.41–0.79	0.0009
Noninvasive[d]	60	19.2	44	12.3	0.64	0.43–0.94	0.03
Ipsilateral breast cancer	124[e]	39.7	61	17.1	0.43	0.32–0.58	<0.000005
Invasive	66	21.1	29	8.1	0.38	0.25–0.59	0.00001
Noninvasive	57	18.3	32	8.9	0.49	0.32–0.76	0.001
Local, regional, and distant metastases	7	2.2	10	2.8	1.25	0.47–3.28	0.84
Contralateral breast cancer	18	5.8	30	8.4	1.46	0.81–2.61	0.26
Invasive	15	4.8	18	5.0	1.05	0.53–2.08	1.00
Noninvasive	3	1.0	12	3.4	3.49	0.99–12.38	0.06
Second primary cancer (other than breast cancer)	18	5.8	20	5.6	0.97	0.51–1.83	1.00
Endometrial	3	1.0	2	0.6	0.58	0.10–3.48	0.87
Other	15	4.8	18	5.0	1.05	0.53–2.08	1.00
Deaths, NED	20	6.4	13	3.6	0.57	0.28–1.14	0.15

[a] Rate per 1,000 patients per year.
[b] Rate in the group treated with lumpectomy and radiation therapy divided by the rate in the group treated with lumpectomy alone.
[c] Includes ipsilateral breast cancer, contralateral breast cancer, and local, regional, and distant disease.
[d] Includes noninvasive tumors in the ipsilateral and contralateral breast.
[e] Includes one case that was not classified as invasive or noninvasive.
L, lumpectomy; XRT, radiation therapy; RR, rate ratio; CI, confidence interval; NED, no evidence of disease.

diation therapy, it was 15.7% (P < .000005; Fig. 42.2). The cumulative incidence of the occurrence of a noninvasive IBT was 14.6% in women treated with lumpectomy alone and 8.0% in women treated with lumpectomy and radiation therapy (P = .001). The cumulative incidence of the occurrence of an invasive IBT was 16.8% in the former group and 7.7% in the latter group (P = .00001). Just as was observed at 8 years, the cumulative incidence of all first events other than IBT was not significantly different in the two treatment groups: 17.9% in the group treated with lumpectomy alone and 20.7% in the group treated with lumpectomy and radiation therapy (P = .99). When the two groups were combined, the cumulative incidence of the occurrence of any CBT was 6.6%; 4.7% were invasive and 1.9% were noninvasive cancers through 12 years of follow-up (Fig. 42.3).

Survival And Causes Of Death

Through 12 years of follow-up, the overall survival was 86% for women treated with lumpectomy alone and 87% for women who received radiation therapy after lumpectomy (RR = 0.95; 95% CI, 0.63 to 1.45; P = .80; Fig. 42.1). There were 45 deaths in the group of patients treated with lumpectomy alone and 43 deaths in patients who received radiation therapy after lumpectomy. Twenty-six (58%) of

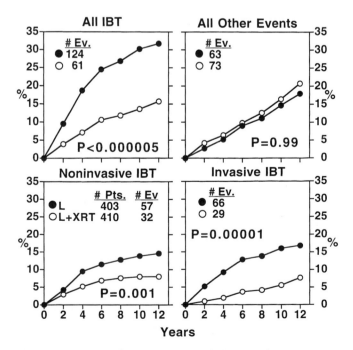

FIGURE 42.2. Cumulative incidence of all IBTs, of invasive and noninvasive IBTs, and of all other events in B-17 patients treated with lumpectomy (L) or with lumpectomy and radiation therapy (L+XRT). P values are comparisons of annual rates of failures.

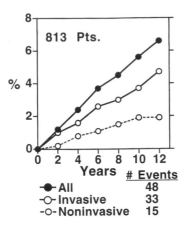

FIGURE 42.3. Cumulative incidence of all invasive or noninvasive CBTs occurring in B-17 patients, both treatment groups combined.

the deaths in the former group and 25 (58%) of the deaths in the latter group occurred before any breast cancer event. There were 19 deaths in lumpectomy-treated patients who had either an invasive or noninvasive breast cancer event that occurred before death. Of the 19 deaths, 12 were attributed to invasive breast cancer. In the group of patients who received radiation therapy after lumpectomy, 18 had a breast cancer event before death. Fifteen of these were attributed to invasive breast cancer.

Benefit From TAM In Addition To Lumpectomy And Radiation Therapy In The B-24 Trial

EFS

As observed after 5 years of follow-up, evidence of a benefit from the use of TAM following lumpectomy and radiation therapy has persisted through 7 years. The EFS was 83.0% in the former group versus 77.1% in the group that received lumpectomy, radiation therapy, and placebo (RR = 0.72; 95% CI, 0.59 to 0.89; P = .002; Fig. 42.4).

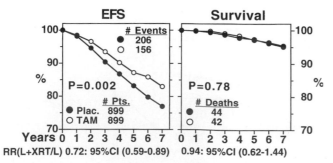

FIGURE 42.4. EFS and survival of women in B-24 who were treated with lumpectomy and radiation therapy (L+XRT) + placebo (Plac.) or with L+XRT + TAM.

Site, Rate, RR, 95% CI, And Cumulative Incidence Of First Events

There was a 27% reduction in the average annual incidence rate (per 1,000 women) for all events among patients who received TAM in addition to lumpectomy and radiation therapy when this group was compared with women who received placebo after lumpectomy and radiation therapy. The incidence rate was 37.9 in the placebo group and 27.6 in the TAM group (RR = 0.73; 95% CI, 0.59 to 0.90; P = .003). The rate of all breast cancer events was 28.2 in the placebo group versus 17.7 in the group that received TAM (RR = 0.63; 95% CI, 0.48 to 0.81; P = .0003; Table 42.4). The average annual incidence rate of IBT was reduced by 31% as a consequence of TAM administration (18.4 in the placebo group and 12.8 in the TAM-treated group; P = .02). The rate of invasive IBT was reduced by 47% (9.0 and 4.8 per 1,000 patients per year in the two treatment groups, respectively; P = .01) and the rate of noninvasive IBT by 15% (9.4 and 8.0 in the two groups, respectively; P = .48). Too few events occurred at local-regional or distant sites for meaningful findings to be obtained; there were, however, fewer such events in women who received TAM. The administration of TAM after lumpectomy and radiation therapy resulted in a significant reduction in the annual incidence rate not only of IBT but also of CBT (8.3 to 4.4 per 1,000 patients per year in the two groups, respectively; P = .01; Table 42.4). As reported after 5 years of follow-up, there continued to be no significant difference between the two treatment groups relative to the occurrence of second primary tumors other than CBTs (P = .94; Table 42.4).

At 7 years of follow-up, the cumulative incidence of any (invasive or noninvasive) IBT occurring in women whose primary tumors were treated with lumpectomy, radiation therapy, and placebo was 11.1%; in women treated with lumpectomy, radiation therapy, and TAM, the cumulative incidence was 7.7% (P = .02; Fig. 42.5). The cumulative incidence of an invasive IBT was 5.3% in the placebo group and 2.6% in the group that received TAM (Fig. 42.5). The cumulative incidence of noninvasive IBT was unaffected by TAM administration (5.8% in the placebo group and 5.0% in the group that received TAM) (P = .48; data not shown). The cumulative incidence of all contralateral breast tumors that occurred as first events at 7 years was 4.9% in the placebo group and 2.3% in the TAM-treated group, a reduction of 53% (Table 42.4; P = .01). The reduction in invasive contralateral breast tumors from 3.2% to 1.8% was not significant (P = .16). There was, however, a significant reduction in noninvasive contralateral breast cancers (P = .03; data not shown). When the cumulative incidence of all IBTs and that of all CBTs were combined, a 39% reduction (from 16.9% in the placebo group to 10% in the TAM group) was observed as the result of TAM administration. There was a 48% reduction (from 8.5% to 4.4%) in invasive cancer.

TABLE 42.4. SITE, RATE, AND RATE RATIOS OF FIRST EVENTS (B-24)

Type of First Event	L + XRT + Placebo (n = 899)		L + XRT + TAM (n = 899)		RR[b]	95% CI	Exact *p*
	No.	Rate[a]	No.	Rate[a]			
All events	206	37.9	156	27.6	0.73	0.59–0.90	0.003
All breast cancer events	153	28.2	100	17.7	0.63	0.48–0.81	0.0003
Invasive[c]	87	16.0	50	8.8	0.55	0.38–0.79	0.0009
Noninvasive[d]	66	12.2	50	8.8	0.73	0.49–1.07	0.11
Ipsilateral breast tumor	100	18.4	72	12.8	0.69	0.50–0.95	0.02
Invasive	49	9.0	27	4.8	0.53	0.32–0.86	0.01
Noninvasive	51	9.4	45	8.0	0.85	0.56–1.29	0.48
Local, regional, and distant (invasive cancer)	8	1.5	3	0.5	0.36	0.06–1.50	0.20
Contralateral breast cancer	45	8.3	25	4.4	0.53	0.31–0.89	0.01
Invasive	30	5.5	20	3.5	0.64	0.35–1.17	0.16
Noninvasive	15	2.8	5	0.9	0.32	0.09–0.93	0.03
Second primary (other than breast) cancer	34	6.3	37	6.6	1.05	0.66–1.67	0.94
Endometrial	3	0.6	7	1.2	2.24	0.51–13.44	0.38
Other	31	5.7	30	5.3	0.93	0.54–1.56	0.88
Deaths, NED	19	3.5	19	3.4	0.96	0.48–1.92	1.00

[a] Rate per 1,000 patients per year.
[b] Rate in the group treated with TAM divided by rate in the placebo group.
[c] Includes ipsilateral breast cancer, contralateral breast cancer, and local, regional, and distant disease.
[d] Includes noninvasive tumors in the ipsilateral and contralateral breast.
L, lumpectomy; XRT, radiation therapy; TAM, tamoxifen; RR, rate ratio; CI, confidence interval; NED, no evidence of disease.

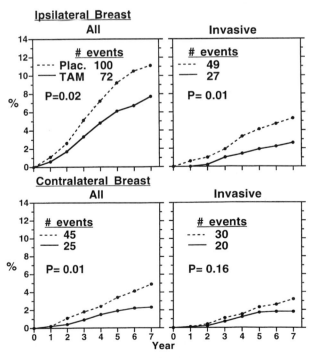

FIGURE 42.5. Cumulative incidence of all events and of invasive events in the ipsilateral breast (IBT) and in the contralateral breast (CBT) of women in B-24. Plac., placebo; TAM, tamoxifen.

Relation Between Selected Characteristics and Rates and Relative Risks of IBT

Age at diagnosis was significantly associated with the occurrence of an IBT. Younger patients in the two groups were at higher risk for such an event than were older patients (Table 42.5). The annual rate of IBT per 1,000 women aged 49 years or younger and 50 years or older who received placebo was 29.2 and 13.3, respectively. TAM administration resulted in a 32.7% reduction in IBTs in women younger than 50 years of age and a 30.1% reduction in those older than 50 years.

The presence of positive tumor margins after surgery was also associated with an increased rate of invasive and noninvasive IBT. Similar findings were observed in patients in both treatment groups whose DCIS was clinically palpable compared with those whose disease had been diagnosed by mammography alone. The risk of IBT was lower among women who received TAM; this was irrespective of margin status (21.1% lower in women in the TAM-treated group who had negative tumor-margins and 45.1% lower in women whose tumor margins were either positive or unknown). For the relatively few patients whose DCIS was clinically apparent at study entry, failure rates were higher in the two groups than was the case in patients whose DCIS was not clinically apparent.

TABLE 42.5. RELATIONSHIP BETWEEN SELECTED CHARACTERISTICS OF PATIENTS AND TUMORS AND RATES AND RELATIVE RISKS OF IPSILATERAL BREAST TUMORS

Characteristic	Placebo Group			Tamoxifen Group			Covariate RR (95% CI)[c]
	Patients	IBT[a]	Rate[b]	Patients	IBT[a]	Rate[b]	
All patients	899	100	18.42	899	72	12.75	
Age (yr)							
≤49	300	51	29.24	302	37	19.67	1.00
≥50	599	49	13.29	597	35	9.29	0.46 (0.34–0.62)
Sample margins							
Negative	676	60	14.52	668	47	11.27	1.00
Positive[d]	223	40	30.84	231	25	16.94	1.84 (1.35–2.51)
Comedonecrosis[e]							
Absent	446	37	13.23	469	28	9.36	1.00
Present	433	61	23.86	414	44	16.98	1.82 (1.33–2.47)
Method of tumor detection							
Mammography	755	80	17.49	733	45	9.67	1.00
Clinical examination and mammography	144	20	23.38	166	27	27.09	1.90 (1.36–2.65)

[a] Invasive and noninvasive.
[b] Rate per 1,000 patients per year.
[c] RR for patients in given covariate stratum, relative to reference (first) stratum, adjusted for treatment.
[d] Includes unknown (77 and 92 patients in the placebo and TAM groups, respectively). These patients had failure rates similar to those in women whose tumor margins were positive.
[e] No information was available for 20 patients in the placebo group and 16 patients in the TAM group.
IBT, ipsilateral breast tumor; RR, relative risk; CI, confidence interval.

Women whose initial DCIS showed comedonecrosis, as found by institutional pathologists, were almost twice as likely to develop an IBT as women whose DCIS showed no evidence of that pathologic entity. The rate of IBT was lower in women in the TAM-treated group who had no comedonecrosis (29.2% lower), as well as in women whose DCIS showed evidence of comedonecrosis (28.8% lower).

Survival and Causes of Death

Through 7 years of follow-up, the overall survival was 95% in women who received placebo and 95% in those treated with TAM (RR = 0.94; 95% CI, 0.62 to 1.44; P = .78; Fig. 42.4). There were 44 deaths in lumpectomy-treated patients who received radiation therapy and placebo and 42 deaths in patients who received TAM after lumpectomy and radiation therapy. Thirty-three (75%) of the deaths in the placebo group and 32 (76%) of the deaths in the TAM group occurred before any breast cancer event. There were 11 deaths in women who received placebo and who had either an invasive or noninvasive breast-cancer event that occurred before death. Ten of the 11 deaths were attributed to breast cancer. Ten of the patients who received TAM had a breast cancer event before death; five of these were attributed to breast cancer.

Relationship Between the B-17 and B-24 Trials and the Relationship Between Those Trials and the NSABP Prevention Trial (P-1)

Relationship Between B-17 And B-24

Because the B-17 and B-24 studies were similar, except for the inclusion in B-24 of women who had more extensive DCIS (16% had specimen margins involved with tumor and, in an additional 10%, the margins could have been involved), the findings from the B-24 trial may be considered within the context of the B-17 findings. The fact that the cumulative incidence of all breast cancer events at 7 years in the group of patients in B-24 who underwent lumpectomy followed by radiation therapy and placebo was almost identical to that of women in B-17 who were treated with lumpectomy and radiation therapy (Fig. 42.6) further indicates the propriety of interrelating the two studies. When related to cumulative incidence of invasive cancer, the spectrum of results from the two studies depicts the advantage from radiation therapy, as well as the added benefit from TAM. In the B-17 study, the cumulative incidence of all breast cancer-related events in the ipsilateral and contralateral breasts of women with DCIS that were treated with lumpectomy alone was 30.3% at 7 years. After radiation

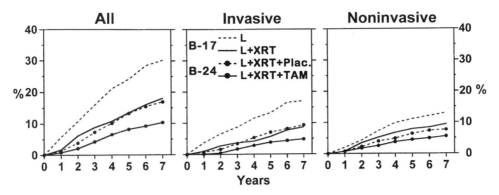

FIGURE 42.6. Cumulative incidence of all, and of invasive and noninvasive, events in the ipsilateral and contralateral breast in B-17 and B-24. L, lumpectomy; XRT, radiation therapy; Plac., placebo; TAM, tamoxifen.

therapy in B-17, the cumulative incidence of all breast cancer events was 18.0%; it was 16.9% in B-24. When TAM was given in B-24, the cumulative incidence was 10.3%. This benefit was due not only to a reduction in the rate of IBT but also partly to the lower rate of both CBT and invasive cancer at regional and distant sites in TAM-treated women. Thus, TAM and radiation therapy led to a 66% lower cumulative incidence of all breast cancer events at 7 years of follow-up than was observed in women treated with lumpectomy alone in B-17. Compared with women who underwent lumpectomy alone, the TAM-treated group showed about an 84% reduction in the rate of all invasive breast cancer events and about a 62% reduction in noninvasive breast cancer events.

Relationship of the B-17 and B-24 Studies to the P-1 Trial

As has been previously emphasized, the findings from the B-17 and B-24 studies in this report are closely related to those from the NSABP P-1 trial (21), which showed that TAM administration not only reduced the incidence of invasive cancer but also decreased the incidence of both DCIS and LCIS. Of particular significance were the observations from the B-17 study that women with a history of DCIS treated with lumpectomy alone were at about a two times greater risk for invasive cancer (28.2/1,000 women/year) than were women in P-1 who received placebo and who had a history of LCIS (13.0/1,000 women/year) and about three times at greater risk than were those with atypical duct hyperplasia (ADH) (10.2/1,000 women/year). Also of relevance is the finding from both the B-17 and B-24 studies that the rates of invasive cancer in women with DCIS who received radiation therapy alone remained higher than the rates in patients with a history of either LCIS or ADH who had been treated with TAM alone (Fig. 42.7).

DISCUSSION

Through 12 years of follow-up, the findings from the B-17 trial continue to demonstrate that radiation therapy after the removal of localized, mammographically detected DCIS by lumpectomy so that resected specimen margins are tumor-free markedly reduces the incidence of ipsilateral breast tumor recurrence (IBTR). The reduction in the average annual incidence rate of all IBTRs (invasive or noninvasive) in B-17 remained similar (58%) to that observed after 5 years of follow-up (59%). These findings continue to repudiate the contention of Lagios that, although radiation therapy may result in a short-term advantage, the benefit is apt to decrease with longer follow-up (28). Results from the only other randomized clinical trial to evaluate the worth of radiation therapy for the treatment of DCIS, which were recently reported by the European Organization for Research and Treatment of Cancer (EORTC), confirm our findings (29). When compared at an equivalent follow-up time, our findings, as well as those from the EORTC, were similar, in that a similar reduction in the local recurrence rate was

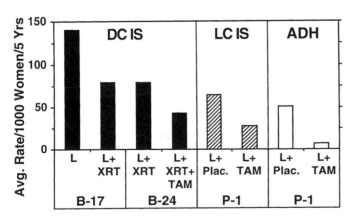

FIGURE 42.7. Rates of invasive breast cancer in women with a history of DCIS treated with lumpectomy (L), lumpectomy and radiation therapy (L+XRT) or with L + XRT + tamoxifen (TAM) compared with women who had a history of lobular carcinoma in situ (LCIS) or atypical ductal hyperplasia (ADH) who received placebo or TAM.

noted in both studies when the group that underwent lumpectomy was treated with radiation therapy.

In this report we also continue to affirm our previous findings of an additional benefit from the administration of TAM after lumpectomy and radiation therapy to the breast. As we have noted previously (20), TAM administration resulted in a significant decrease in the rate of all breast cancer events. Although there was a reduction in the rate of noninvasive cancers, the advantage from TAM was due mainly to a decrease in the rate of invasive cancer, at any site. As we have stated previously (20), these findings suggest that merely focusing on the frequency with which IBTs occur after lumpectomy for DCIS is apt to be too limited, particularly when systemic therapy such as TAM is administered. In that regard, the effect that treatment strategies for DCIS have on all invasive or noninvasive breast cancer events at any site should receive consideration. Therefore, while insufficient to allow for drawing firm conclusions, the number of metastases that were detected at regional and distant sites in the B-24 study cannot be dismissed, especially in view of the fact that TAM administration resulted in fewer such events.

Similarly, although the mortality from invasive breast cancer in DCIS patients may be low, the fact that deaths do occur cannot be ignored. Through 12 years of follow-up in the B-17 study, 3% of all patients in the lumpectomy group and 4% of all women treated with radiation therapy after lumpectomy died of breast cancer. Perhaps a more accurate impression of the impact of breast cancer mortality among DCIS patients is derived from the fact that 27% (12 of 45 deaths) of the lumpectomy patients and 35% (15 of 43 deaths) of the lumpectomy patients who received radiation therapy after lumpectomy and who died had their cause of death attributable to breast cancer. These findings justify the consideration of adjuvant therapy in at least some of these patients. At this time, information about the long-term cause-specific mortality of women with a history of DCIS such as that encountered in B-17 and B-24 who were treated with surgery alone is tenuous, at best. The retrospective derivation of dubious information and the relatively short follow-up times prohibit quantifying breast cancer mortality in such patients. Paradoxically, it has recently been reported by Page et al. (30) and commented upon by Silverstein (31) that 40% of untreated low-grade lesions develop into invasive breast cancer after 25 to 30 years of follow-up and that about half of the patients ultimately die of breast cancer. It is speculated that, for high-grade lesions, the invasive rate is probably much higher than 40%, "but no study evaluating this exists" (31).

We have considered the B-17 findings in context with those from the B-24 trial. The characteristics of patients in both studies were similar, except for the inclusion in B-24 of some women who had more extensive DCIS, as was evidenced by the fact that their specimen margins were involved with tumor. Most important, the findings from B-17 in women who were treated with lumpectomy and radiation therapy were almost identical to those of women in B-24 who received radiation therapy and placebo after lumpectomy. Therefore, we deemed it appropriate to relate the spectrum of results obtained in the two studies. When patients were examined according to the cumulative incidence of breast cancer or according to average annual incidence rates, from the standpoint of the magnitude of the reductions in those parameters, there can be little disagreement that radiation therapy and TAM can alter the natural history of women with the kind of DCIS that was treated in those trials. However, just as has been observed after each demonstration of a therapeutic benefit, be it the result of a surgical, radiologic, chemotherapeutic, or hormonal intervention, controversy has emerged to challenge the application of the findings from our two trials for the treatment of patients with DCIS. The issues are always the same. Is the prognosis of patients being considered for treatment sufficiently unfavorable to warrant administration of the therapy? Are the benefits of the therapy sufficient to justify acceptance of the side effects and costs that occur as a result of the treatment? Are there prognostic factors that can indicate whether or not an individual patient needs to be treated, and are there predictive factors that indicate whether or not she will benefit from the therapeutic intervention? It seems most appropriate to consider the last question first because the answer to it will likely affect the response to the other questions.

In an effort to identify pathologic discriminants predictive of IBT, a central review of pathologic information from patients enrolled in B-17 was performed by the NSABP Headquarters pathologist, E.R. Fisher, and the findings were initially reported in 1995 (32). Of nine pathologic features that were evaluated individually by univariate Cox proportional hazards regression modeling adjusted for treatment, only nuclear grade, comedonecrosis, margin status, and histologic tumor type were found to be statistically significant prognostic variables for IBT. The highest hazard rates for IBT were noted for poor nuclear grade, moderate/marked comedonecrosis, uncertain/involved margins, and solid tumor type. When these variables were examined by multivariate analysis, only moderate/marked comedonecrosis and uncertain/involved tumor margin status were independent predictors of IBT. The findings demonstrated that, when comedonecrosis and tumor margin status were combined, patients with tumor-free specimen margins and with slight comedonecrosis had less chance of developing an IBT than did patients whose margins were involved with tumor and demonstrated moderate-to-marked comedonecrosis. However, not only did both good-risk and poor-risk patients benefit from radiation therapy, but their outcomes also became similar after the therapy. Of particular significance were the findings demonstrating that the average annual hazard rate of IBT was lower for all pathologic characteristics in the group that received radiation therapy.

A recent update of the pathologic findings from B-17 was carried out because of the occurrence of a greater number of events during the past several years (33). As previously was observed, the average annual hazard rates for IBT were lower for all nine pathologic characteristics in the group treated with lumpectomy and radiation therapy than in the group treated with lumpectomy alone. Unlike what had been observed in the first pathology report, margin status was of borderline significance in relation to frequency of IBT (P = .06). Nuclear grade also had only a borderline effect (P = .07).

Patients whose tumors exhibited both absent/slight comedonecrosis and tumor-free specimen margins had the lowest annual rates of IBT, whereas those who had moderate/marked comedonecrosis and uncertain/involved margins had the highest. Patients with moderate/marked comedonecrosis and free margins exhibited an incidence of IBT similar to that of patients whose tumors exhibited both unfavorable features. When margins were uncertain/involved and comedonecrosis was absent/slight, the hazard rate of IBT was higher than that observed when both characteristics were favorable and lower than that observed when both characteristics were unfavorable. In the B-24 study, just as in the B-17 trial, positive margins and comedonecrosis were associated with an increased risk for IBT. TAM reduced the incidence of such tumors, irrespective of the presence or absence of comedonecrosis or of margin involvement with tumor.

Just as occurred with pathologic features, when the rates of IBT in B-17 were evaluated according to selected mammographic and clinical characteristics at the time of diagnosis of the primary DCIS, we failed to identify a discriminant that selected DCIS patients who did not require postoperative radiation therapy and patients who had a particular characteristic whose hazard rate for an IBT was not lowered after radiation therapy (10). Thus, these and other findings from our studies have led us to conclude that we are, as yet, unable to clearly identify a pathologic, mammographic, or clinical discriminant that might be used to indicate with certitude if an individual patient, or a particular cohort of patients, with the type of DCIS encountered in our studies will not benefit from radiation therapy or from radiation therapy and TAM. The compelling need for elucidating prognostic and predictive markers to resolve the issues of who will or will not require therapy and who will or will not benefit is demonstrated by a "short list" of some of the prognostic factors that have been or are now being considered important in that regard (Table 42.6). To our knowledge, none have been judged effective enough to justify their use for therapeutic decision making in patients with DCIS.

Some investigators have made a concerted effort to determine which patients should or should not receive radiation therapy after lumpectomy for DCIS (34–36). Their formulation of the Van Nuys Prognostic Index (VNPI) and their more recent findings associating the influence of specimen margin width on local control of DCIS have received considerable attention and are purported to have provided

TABLE 42.6. PUTATIVE PROGNOSTIC FACTORS FOR THE OCCURRENCE OF AN IPSILATERAL BREAST TUMOR AFTER THE REMOVAL OF DUCTAL CARCINOMA IN SITU

Age	Multifocality
Angiogenesis	Myeloepithelial cells
Apoptotic index	nm23
Architecture of the tumor	NSABP margins
Bcl-2 expression	Nottingham Classification
Clinical palpable versus nonpalpable	Nucleolar grade
	Nuclear grade
Comedonecrosis	p21ras
Cyclin D1	p53
DNA ploidy	pS2
E-cadherin expression	Progesterone receptor
Estrogen receptor	Residual tumor at excised specimen margin
Fibrosis	
HER-2/neu	S phase
Histologic subtypes	Suspicious margins
Lagios criteria	Tumor DNA
Lymphocyte infiltrate	Tumor fibrosis
Margin width	Tumor necrosis
Metallothionein	Tumor size
Microcalcification	Van Nuys Classification

Adapted from Predicting local recurrences in patients with ductal carcinoma in situ. In: Silverstein MJ, ed. *Ductal carcinoma in situ of the breast*. Baltimore: Williams & Wilkins, 1997:271–283, with permission.

definitive information that resolves the uncertainty about the use of radiation therapy and of TAM for DCIS. In the VNPI, three categories of tumor size (≤15 mm, 16 to 40 mm, and ≥41 mm), three of tumor-free specimen margins (≤10 mm, 1 to 9 mm, and <1 mm), and three levels of pathologic tumor type (nuclear grade [NG] 3, NG 1 or 2 with comedonecrosis, and NG 1 or 2 without comedonecrosis) are incorporated into a scoring scheme that is purported to identify which patients should be treated with either lumpectomy, lumpectomy and radiation therapy, or mastectomy. The shortcomings of the VNPI have been the subject of extensive criticism (33,37,38). We have concluded that this schema cannot be applied to patients in B-17 because it was derived from patients with all sizes of DCIS, including those whose tumors were ≥4.1 cm. Particularly because the VNPI has not been validated by appropriate prospective studies, there is lack of justification for its use as part of a strategy for the treatment of DCIS.

Another retrospective analysis by the same investigators who employed much of the same patient population that was used to formulate the VNPI has provided information that is purported to demonstrate that the width of tumor-free specimen margins is an important determinant of local recurrence in patients with DCIS (36). These investigators concluded that, when DCIS was excised with a tumor-free margin width of 10 mm in every diameter, postoperative breast irradiation was unnecessary. After an extensive review of their report, we have decided that, while we commend research efforts that are directed toward obtaining better local control after DCIS and identifying patients for whom radiation therapy should be omitted, their study has merely provided a reason for conducting a prospective evaluation, with appropriate study design, to test their premise. Moreover, we take umbrage with the veiled statement made by the investigators (36) and echoed by others (39) that "radiation, though highly effective, simply cannot compensate for inadequate surgery." Our views with regard to both the VNPI and the article related to margin width after local excision of DCIS are generally shared by Julien et al. in the EORTC report (29). Thus, in answer to the third question that we proposed earlier in this discussion, it seems that we are faced with the reality that there is currently no acceptable quantitative information to indicate the existence of either a single or a combination of prognostic or predictive markers that can unequivocally indicate, a priori, which patient with DCIS requires no treatment and which one is unlikely to benefit from a particular therapeutic intervention. That conclusion does not conflict with the fact that, for a majority of such patients, lumpectomy alone with tumor-free specimen margins may be adequate therapy and that radiation therapy, either alone or with the addition of TAM, is of benefit for other patients. This conclusion does, however, make answering the other two questions that we previously posed more difficult. Whether or not the prognosis of the DCIS patients in our studies is sufficiently unfavorable to justify administration of the therapy to all patients, including those who either do not need it or will not benefit from it, becomes a matter for contention, as are the concerns about the benefits versus the side effects and cost of the treatment.

More than a decade ago, when we reported the first findings from randomized trials that demonstrated the value of chemotherapy for node-negative patients with estrogen receptor (ER)-negative tumors (40), and TAM for patients with ER-positive tumors (41), the same questions arose relative to the clinical application of those findings. At that time, and on numerous other occasions, we expressed our views about those issues. Those comments are also germane to the controversy that has been generated by the findings described in this report. In a report that we published in 1989 about the applicability of the findings from our studies, we pointed out that there are no absolute criteria for deciding how great the benefit must be for a therapy to be considered appropriate for general use. We also emphasized that there are no rules for evaluating the benefit in relation to the toxicity, the cost of treatment, and other variables. We continue to be forced to rely on value judgments and ethical imperatives when there are no firm criteria for making such a decision. In our report we also remarked that, until better markers become available for selecting those patients who require and who will respond to a therapy, physician bias should not be a reason to deny patients the opportunity to receive the benefit that has been demonstrated. It has been

reported that many patients are willing to accept the toxicity of a therapy even if it is accompanied by what many would consider to be a "small" benefit (42–44). We also stated that, because the number of patients who could be candidates for such therapy "is increasing with the use of mammography, the employment of a treatment resulting in a moderate benefit could, by affecting a considerable number of patients, have important public health consequences."

Currently, there is an even more compelling reason for considering that therapy be made available to patients with the kind of DCIS that was evaluated in B-17 and B-24. As a result of the findings from the NSABP Breast Cancer Prevention Trial (P-1) (21), it seems imperative that DCIS be viewed from a different perspective. The present concept that DCIS is a surgical disease that can be eradicated by more extensive operations (31) relies on the Halstedian paradigm of the early twentieth century and is, at best, retrogressive, particularly when that thesis is related to the more localized, mammographically detected DCIS that is currently being encountered with greater frequency. It is apt to be counterproductive for clinicians to continue to debate the treatment of DCIS on the basis of the need to know the precise millimeter of margin width that is tumor free or the size of the tumor. It is equally imprudent to attempt to apply experimental methodologies in everyday clinical practice to the processing of tumors and to argue over the need for precise classification and correlations of a large number of pathologic characteristics. It is now appropriate to view DCIS, a phenotypically expressed pathologic entity, within the rubric of breast cancer prevention.

The findings from the P-1 trial demonstrated that, when treated with TAM, women at increased risk for breast cancer because they (i) were 60 years of age or older, (ii) were 35 to 59 years of age with a 5-year predicted risk for breast cancer of at least 1.66%, or (iii) had a history of LCIS or ADH had about a 50% reduction in the risk of invasive breast cancer overall, as well as in both age groups. Particularly germane to this discussion is the finding in P-1 of a 50% reduction in the risk of invasive cancer in women who had a history of either ADH or LCIS and a reduction in the incidence of both DCIS and LCIS in women without a history of those tumors. The reason that patients with a history of DCIS were not included in the P-1 study was that the B-17 study was in progress at the same time. Thus, the studies would have competed for the same tumor population. Most important was the observation that women in B-17 who had a history of DCIS treated with lumpectomy alone were at greater risk for invasive cancer than were women in P-1 who had a history of either ADH or LCIS and who had not received radiation therapy or TAM (Fig. 42.7). Findings from the B-17 and B-24 studies showed that the rates of invasive cancer in DCIS patients who were treated with radiation therapy alone were higher than the rates in those patients in P-1 who had a history of LCIS and who had received placebo or TAM. In most categories of high-risk patients in P-1 who received placebo, when the rate of invasive cancer was evaluated according to age or 5-year predicted breast cancer risk or according to number of first-degree relatives with breast cancer, it was lower than the rates that were observed in DCIS patients. Thus, the findings from the B-17 and B-24 studies indicate that patients with DCIS in those trials who received radiation therapy were at higher risk for invasive breast cancer than were most of the women with LCIS or ADH in the P-1 study.

It remains unclear as to whether ADH, LCIS, and DCIS are precursors of invasive breast cancer or are markers that indicate biologically perturbed breast tissue that is capable of giving rise to a spectrum of phenotypically expressed lesions, one of which is invasive cancer. Despite that uncertainty, however, it has been proven that TAM and radiation therapy are capable of markedly reducing the rate of clinical expression of all of these phenotypes. If it is accepted from the P-1 findings that women at increased risk for invasive breast cancer are candidates for the use of an intervention, i.e., TAM, then women with a history of DCIS, who are at even higher risk than the P-1 participants, should also be considered for such therapy, even if they have also been treated with radiation therapy. At this time, the effectiveness of TAM in treating DCIS without radiation therapy is speculative. Until information is available to resolve that issue, it would seem that, in view of the magnitude of the benefit from its effect, the use of TAM in conjunction with radiation therapy is more appropriate than is TAM administration alone. The results from another trial, NSABP B-21, which has evaluated the use of TAM both with and without radiation therapy for the prevention of IBT after lumpectomy in women with small invasive breast cancers, support that thesis (45). As has been previously speculated, radiation therapy as used in the treatment of DCIS may play a role as a preventive agent, in that it may not only destroy residual cancer cells but may also affect the precursors of those cells. The biologic basis for the use of TAM is more certain. The P-1 findings demonstrated that TAM lowered the rate of invasive cancer overall because of an effect on tumors that were ER-positive (21). TAM also lowered rates of invasive cancer in P-1 participants who had a history of either ADH or LCIS (46,47), both of which are frequently ER-positive. TAM could have led to lower rates of invasive cancer in patients with DCIS because that lesion is also associated with tumor cells that are ER-positive (46–50).

In conclusion, the updated findings from the B-17 and B-24 randomized trials continue to demonstrate that the benefit attained from radiation therapy and from TAM for the treatment of mammographically and pathologically detected DCIS persists. And, as a result of our contention that DCIS should now be considered within the rubric of breast cancer prevention in women at increased risk for invasive cancer as in NSABP P-1, we believe that any decision to deny women the opportunity of receiving a therapy from which they might benefit must be extremely circumspect in view of the fact that thousands of women with invasive breast cancer die each year despite receiving effective treatment or because they have received either inadequate treatment or no treatment at all. However, that statement does not imply, as has too often been asserted by others, that we contend ipso facto that all patients with DCIS should receive radiation therapy and TAM, nor have we recommended that all women who meet the requirements of the P-1 study should receive TAM, or that all patients with invasive breast tumors equal to or less than 1 cm should be given chemotherapy and/or TAM. We do affirm our contention, however, that, with the increased use of those therapies and of better therapeutic agents that may become available to treat women with a history of DCIS, with invasive tumors 1 cm or smaller, and with an increased risk for breast cancer, progress will be made in ameliorating the breast cancer problem.

ACKNOWLEDGMENT

Supported by Public Health Service grant nos. U10-CA-12027, U10-CA-69651, U10-CA-37377, and U10-CA-69974 from the National Cancer Institute, National Institutes of Health, Department of Health and Human Services.

REFERENCES

1. Farrow JH: Current concepts in the detection and treatment of the earliest of the early breast cancers. Cancer 25:468–477, 1970
2. Betsill WL Jr, Rosen PP, Lieberman PH, et al: Intraductal carcinoma. Long-term follow-up after treatment by biopsy alone. JAMA 239:1863–1867, 1978
3. Page DI, DuPont WD, Rogers LW, et al: Intraductal carcinoma of the breast: Follow-up after biopsy only. Cancer 49:751–758, 1982
4. Carter D, Smith RRL: Carcinoma in situ of the breast. Cancer 40:1189–1193, 1977
5. Rosen PP, Braun DW, Kinne DE: Clinical significance of pre-invasive breast carcinoma. Cancer 46:919–925, 1980
6. Lagios MD, Westdahl PR, Margolin FR, et al: Duct carcinoma in situ. Cancer 50:1309–1314, 1982
7. Fisher B, Bauer M, Margolese R, et al: Five-year results of a randomized clinical trial comparing total mastectomy and segmental mastectomy with or without radiation in the treatment of breast cancer. N Engl J Med 312:665–673, 1985
8. Fisher B, Costantino J, Redmond C, et al: Lumpectomy compared with lumpectomy and radiation therapy for the treatment of intraductal breast cancer. N Engl J Med 328:1581–1586, 1993
9. Fisher B, Dignam J, Wolmark N, et al: Lumpectomy and radiation therapy for the treatment of intraductal breast cancer: Findings from National Surgical Adjuvant Breast and Bowel Project B-17. J Clin Oncol 16:441–452, 1998
10. Fisher ER, Costantino J, Fisher B, et al: Pathologic findings from the National Surgical Adjuvant Breast and Bowel Project (NSABP) Protocol B-17: Intraductal carcinoma (duct carcinoma in situ). Cancer 75:1310–1319, 1995

11. Terenius L: Effect of anti-oestrogens on initiation of mammary cancer in the female rat. Eur J Cancer 7:65–70, 1971

12. Jordan VC: Effect of tamoxifen (ICI 46,474) on initiation and growth of DMBA-induced rat mammary carcinomata. Eur J Cancer 12:419–424, 1976

13. Jordan VC, Allen KE: Evaluation of the antitumour activity of the nonsteroidal antioestrogen monohydroxytamoxifen in the DMBA-induced rat mammary carcinoma model. Ear J Cancer 16:239–251, 1980

14. Fisher B, Dignam J, Bryant J, et al: Five versus more than five years of tamoxifen therapy for breast cancer patients with negative lymph nodes and estrogen receptor-positive tumors. J Natl Cancer Inst 88:1529–1542, 1996

15. Adjuvant tamoxifen in the management of operable breast cancer: The Scottish Trial. Report from the Breast Cancer Trials Committee, Scottish Cancer Trials Office (MRC), Edinburgh. Lancet 2:171–175, 1987

16. Fisher B, Costantino J, Redmond C, et al: A randomized clinical trial evaluating tamoxifen in the treatment of patients with node-negative breast cancer who have estrogen-receptor-positive tumors. N Engl J Med 320:479–484, 1989

17. CRC Adjuvant Breast Trial Working Party: Cyclophosphamide and tamoxifen as adjuvant therapies in the management of breast cancer. Br J Cancer 57:604–607, 1988

18. Rutqvist LE, Cedermark B, Glas U, et al: Contralateral primary tumors in breast cancer patients in a randomized trial of adjuvant tamoxifen therapy. J Natl Cancer Inst 83:1299–1306, 1991

19. Fisher B, Redmond C: New perspective on cancer of the contralateral breast: A marker for assessing tamoxifen as a preventive agent. J Natl Cancer Inst 83:1278–1280, 1991 (editorial)

20. Fisher B, Dignam J, Wolmark N, et al: Tamoxifen in treatment of intraductal breast cancer: National Surgical Adjuvant Breast and Bowel Project B-24 randomised controlled trial. Lancet 353:1993–2000, 1999

21. Fisher B, Costantino JP, Wickerham DL, et al: Tamoxifen for prevention of breast cancer: Report of the National Surgical Adjuvant Breast and Bowel Project P-1 study. J Natl Cancer Inst 90:1371–1388, 1998

22. Fisher B, Wolmark N, Fisher ER, et al: Lumpectomy and axillary dissection for breast cancer: Surgical, pathological, and radiation considerations. World J Surg 9:692–698, 1985

23. Kaplan EL, Meier P: Nonparametric estimation from incomplete observations. J Am Stat Assoc 53:457–481, 1958

24. Mantel N: Evaluation of survival data and two new rank order statistics arising in its consideration. Cancer Chemother Rep 50:163–170, 1966

25. Cox DR: Regression models and life-tables. J R Stat Soc B 34:187–220, 1972

26. Prentice RL, Kalbfleish JD, Peterson AV, et al: The analysis of failure times in the presence of competing risks. Biometrics 34:541–554, 1978

27. Gaynor JJ, Feuer EJ, Tan CC, et al: On the use of cause-specific failure and conditional failure probabilities: Examples from clinical oncology data. J Am Stat Assoc 88:400–409, 1993

28. Lagios MD: Duct carcinoma in situ: Biological implications for clinical practice. Semin Oncol 23:6–11, 1996 (suppl 2)

29. Julien J-P, Bijker N, Fentiman IS, et al: Radiotherapy in breast-conserving treatment for ductal carcinoma in situ: First results of the EORTC randomised phase III trial 10853. Lancet 355:528–533, 2000

30. Page DL, Dupont WD, Rogers LW, et al: Continued local recurrence of carcinoma 15–25 years after a diagnosis of low grade ductal carcinoma in situ of the breast treated only by biopsy. Cancer 76:1197–1200, 1995

31. Silverstein MJ: Ductal carcinoma in situ of the breast: A surgeon's disease. Ann Surg Oncol 6:802–810, 1999

32. Fisher ER, Costantino J, Fisher B, et al: Pathologic findings from the National Surgical Adjuvant Breast and Bowel Project (NSABP) Protocol B-17: Intraductal carcinoma (duct carcinoma in situ). Cancer 75:1310–1319, 1995

33. Fisher ER, Dignam J, Tan-Chiu E, et al: Pathologic findings from the National Surgical Adjuvant Breast Project (NSABP) eight-year update of Protocol B-17. Cancer 86:429–438, 1999

34. Silverstein MJ, Poller DN, Waisman JR, et al: Prognostic classification of breast ductal carcinoma-in-situ. Lancet 345:1154–1157, 1995

35. Silverstein MJ, Lagios MD, Craig PH, et al: A prognostic index for ductal carcinoma in situ of the breast. Cancer 77:2267–2274, 1996

36. Silverstein MJ, Lagios MD, Groshen S, et al: The influence of margin width on local control of ductal carcinoma in situ of the breast. N Engl J Med 340:1455–1461, 1999

37. Fisher ER: Pathobiological considerations relating to the treatment of intraductal carcinoma (ductal carcinoma in situ) of the breast. CA Cancer J Clin 47:52–64, 1997

38. Schnitt SJ, Harris JR, Smith BL: Developing a prognostic index for ductal carcinoma in situ of the breast. Are we there yet? Cancer 77:2189–2192, 1996

39. Chan KC, Knox WF, Sinha G, et al: Extent of excision margin width required in breast conserving surgery for ductal carcinoma in situ. Cancer 91:9–16, 2001

40. Fisher B, Redmond C, Dimitrov NV: A randomized clinical trial evaluating sequential methotrexate and fluorouracil in the treatment of patients with node-negative breast cancer who have estrogen-receptor-negative tumors. N Engl J Med 320:473–478,1989

41. Fisher B, Costantino J, Redmond C: A randomized clinical trial evaluating tamoxifen in the treatment of patients with node-negative breast cancer who have estrogen-receptor-positive tumors. N Engl J Med 320:479–484, 1989

42. Coates AS, Simes RJ: Patient assessment of adjuvant treatment in operable breast cancer, in Williams CJ (ed): Introducing New Treatments for Cancer: Practical, Ethical, and Legal Problems. New York, NY, Wiley, 1992, pp 447–458

43. Ravdin PM, Siminoff IA, Harvey JA: Survey of breast cancer patients concerning their knowledge and expectations of adjuvant therapy. J Clin Oncol 16:515–521, 1998

44. Lindley C, Vasa S, Sawyer WT, et al: Quality of life and preferences for treatment following systemic adjuvant therapy for early-stage breast cancer. J Clin Oncol 16:380–387, 1998

45. Wolmark N, Dignam J, Margolese R, et al: The role of radiotherapy and tamoxifen in the management of node negative invasive breast cancer ≤1 cm treated with lumpectomy: Preliminary results of NSABP protocol B-21. Proc Am Soc Clin Oncol 19:70a, 2000 (abstr 271)

46. Giri DD, Dundas SA, Nottingham JF, et al: Oestrogen receptors in benign epithelial lesions and intraductal carcinomas of the breast: An immunohistological study. Histopathology 15:575–584, 1989

47. Barnes R, Masood S: Potential value of hormone receptor assay in carcinoma in situ of breast. Am J Clin Pathol 94:533–537, 1990

48. Zafrani B, Leroyer A, Fourquet A, et al: Mammographically detected ductal in situ carcinoma of the breast analyzed with a new classification: A study of 127 cases: Correlation with estrogen and progesterone receptors, P53 and c-erb B-2 proteins, and proliferative activity. Semin Diagn Pathol 11: 208–214,1994

49. Pallis L, Wilking N, Cedermark B, et al: Receptors for estrogen and progesterone in breast carcinoma in situ. Anticancer Res 12:2113–2115, 1992

50. Leal CB, Schmitt FC, Bento MJ, et al: Ductal carcinoma in situ of the breast: Histologic categorization and its relationship to ploidy and immunohistochemical expression of hormone receptors, p53, and c-erb B-2 protein. Cancer 75:2123–2131, 1995

43

AN UPDATE ON EUROPEAN ORGANIZATION FOR RESEARCH AND TREATMENT OF CANCER TRIAL 10853 FOR DUCTAL CARCINOMA IN SITU OF THE BREAST

IAN S FENTIMAN
NINA BIJKER

BACKGROUND

In the mid-1980s, because of the rarity of ductal carcinoma in situ (DCIS) of the breast, treatment had not been examined in any randomized clinical trials, causing a problem for breast surgeons and radiation oncologists. There was good evidence that breast-conservation therapy was a safe option for selected patients with invasive disease, but the standard treatment for DCIS was simple (total) mastectomy. This achieved an almost 100% cure rate, but it was becoming difficult to justify a mutilating operation for a non–life-threatening condition. Additionally, more cases of DCIS were being diagnosed as a result of mammographic screening so that there was an increasing need for evidence-based treatment.

Accordingly, the European Organization for Research and Treatment of Cancer (EORTC) Breast Cancer Cooperative Group decided to run a prospective trial of treatment options for DCIS. Because of changing medical and public attitudes toward informed consent, it would have been impossible to conduct a study randomizing between mastectomy and breast conservation for this disease. Evidence from follow-up of patients in whom DCIS had been missed in a biopsy specimen diagnosed as benign indicated that after 4 to 18 years, ipsilateral invasive carcinoma occurred in 34% (range, 18% to 70%) (1–6). Where a wide excision had been attempted, the incidence of ipsilateral invasive disease decreased to 19% (7–9). This indicated that wide excision (complete local excision) of DCIS should be prerequisite for trial entry and hence a certain proportion of cases would be ineligible because a mastectomy would be necessary to achieve clearance.

One object of the study was to determine whether the method of detection of DCIS (clinical lump, blood-stained nipple discharge, or mammography) would affect the extent of disease and likely the effectiveness of wide local excision. With regard to the axillary sampling/clearance, because of the low probability of nodal involvement from undetected invasive disease (10,11), it was thought that axillary surgery should not be a part of the surgical protocol but was permitted if a clinically suspicious node was palpable.

Because confirmation of complete local excision was a requirement for trial entry, it was recognized that pathologic quality assurance would be essential. A protocol for specimen handling, marking of margins, and appropriate sampling of the specimen was written. At that time, the histologic classification of DCIS was in flux, moving from the use of morphologic subtypes, often mixed, to tumor grade with or without comedonecrosis. Although it was assumed that the comedo variant was more aggressive than the non-comedo variant and therefore more likely to evolve into an invasive tumor, it was not thought that any histologic subtype should be excluded from entry, provided that clear margins had been achieved. Indeed, one aim of the study was to determine whether certain subtypes of DCIS might require different treatment. A minimum width of tumor-free margin was not specified to make the trial as inclusive as possible.

EUROPEAN ORGANIZATION FOR RESEARCH AND TREATMENT OF CANCER TRIAL 10853 STUDY DESIGN

Eligibility and exclusion criteria for the trial are given in Table 43.1. Patients fulfilling the entry criteria and agreeing to participate were randomized to either no further treatment or breast irradiation, with no axillary treatment or

TABLE 43.1. SELECTION CRITERIA FOR THE EUROPEAN ORGANIZATION FOR RESEARCH AND TREATMENT OF CANCER 10853

Eligibility Criteria	Exclusion Criteria
Any type of DCIS	Paget's disease of nipple
No evidence of microinvasion	Pregnant
Tumor-free margins	Prior malignancy
Lump or microcalcification ≤5 cm	Age ≥70 yr
Suitable for long-term follow-up	WHO performance status ≥2

DCIS, ductal carcinoma in situ; WHO, World Health Organization.

boost to the excision site. Randomization had to take place within a maximum of 12 weeks after histologic confirmation of complete excision and the absence of invasion.

Radiotherapy had to begin no later than 12 weeks after wide excision. The dose was 50 Gy in 25 fractions (2 Gy per fraction) in 5 weeks, treating patients five times a week. This trial was the first joint effort of the EORTC Breast Cancer Cooperative Group and the EORTC Radiotherapy Group. Because of its multicenter nature, it was deemed necessary to include quality assurance as an intrinsic part of the protocol, using site visits when necessary to confirm that the specified doses had been delivered.

Timing of follow-up visits was at the discretion of the participating centers, but follow-up forms were completed annually. All patients had a clinical examination at each follow-up visit and annual bilateral, single-view mammograms. Suspected recurrences found clinically or radiologically were confirmed histologically. Recurrence within an irradiated breast was treated with mastectomy with an axillary clearance if the recurrence was invasive. Recurrence within a nonirradiated breast, if completely excised, could be treated with breast irradiation.

At closure in mid-1996, the trial had accrued 1,010 cases from 46 centers in 13 countries. There were 503 cases who had no radiotherapy and 507 who received breast irradiation.

QUALITY ASSURANCE

From October 1995 until March 1996, 30 institutes were site visited and the medical files of 824 patients were reviewed (12). Reasons for nonreview were geographic (82), nonavailability (18), randomization after the site visit (67), and inadequate documentation (19). The purpose of the review was to check the accuracy of the original data entered on the on-study forms and to determine the manner in which the cases were detected, i.e., by screening or because of symptoms. Detailed data about clinical presentation, mammographic findings, the surgical procedures, the pathologic findings, and the dosage of radiation delivered were collected.

Mammography reports were screened for the type of abnormality, lesion diameter, and whether excision adequacy had been checked by specimen x-ray. Detailed information about the surgical procedure was retrieved from the surgical report, including the number of excisions and procedures performed. From the pathology reports, data on frozen-section procedures, inking of the specimen, sectioning and radiography of the sliced specimen, number of blocks, gross and microscopic diameter of the lesion, and the margin status were obtained. Radiotherapy specification was checked for the total dosage, the number of fractions, and whether a boost dose had been given. By collecting the missing follow-up forms, the quality assurance exercise increased the median length of follow-up by 214 days.

Table 43.2 shows that only 28% of the patients were symptomatic and 72% were mammographically detected. In the early years of the trial, approximately half of the lesions were x-ray–detected, increasing to almost 80% in the final years. Mammograms were part of population-based screening programs in 31%, and individual screening was the basis in the remainder. Microcalcifications were found in 77% (Table 43.2), and of these, 14% had an associated density. A specimen x-ray was taken to check the presence of the mammographic abnormality in 90% of mammographically detected lesions. In the symptomatic patients, a mammographic abnormality was found in 71%. In only 49% was an estimation of the diameter of the mammographic abnormality given, and in these cases, the mean mammographic diameter was 20.2 mm (Table 43.3). The mean di-

TABLE 43.2. METHODS OF DETECTION OF DUCTAL CARCINOMA IN SITU IN EUROPEAN ORGANIZATION FOR RESEARCH AND TREATMENT OF CANCER 10853

Method of Detection	No. (%)
Palpable lesion	161 (20)
Nipple discharge	64 (8)
Nipple/skin retraction	6 (1)
Mammography alone	591 (72)
Unknown	1
Mammographic abnormality	
Microcalcifications	521 (63)
Microcalcifications and density	115 (14)
Density	83 (10)
No abnormality	58 (7)
Abnormality on ultrasound	15 (2)
Not classified/unknown	32 (5)
Magnification view	
Yes	74 (12)
No	562 (88)
Specimen x-ray (mammographic lesions only)	
Yes	531 (90)
No	56 (9)
Unknown	4 (1)

TABLE 43.3. LESION DIAMETER OF THE DUCTAL CARCINOMA IN SITU IN EUROPEAN ORGANIZATION FOR RESEARCH AND TREATMENT OF CANCER 10853

	No. Reported (%)	Mean (Range) in mm
Clinical measurement	163 (84)	21.1 (4–80)
Mammographic size	385 (49)	20.2 (4–70)
Pathologic size		
Macroscopic	228 (28)	11 (2–50)
Microscopic	138 (17)	6.5 (1–70)
Summary	94 (11)	10 (1–30)
Microscopic or summary	187 (23)	8 (1–70)
Any size reported	368 (45)	10 (1–70)

ameter of the palpable lesions was 21 mm. The pathologic extent of the lesion was not well reported. For nonpalpable lesions, a gross size was reported in 22% compared with 47% of palpable lesions (Table 43.3). A microscopic diameter of the lesion was reported in only 17% and a size of the lesion was given in the conclusion of 11% of the reports.

Various surgical procedures were performed with only 36% of the patients undergoing a single wide excision (Table 43.4). In 29%, the surgeon performed multiple excisions in one procedure, mostly by immediate re-excision of the biopsy cavity after a diagnostic excision by shaving. After this, the margins were considered free if no DCIS was found in the re-excision specimens. This policy was standard in a number of institutes, including three large institutes, responsible for the entry of more than one-third of the patients. Frozen-section procedures were performed in 45% of all patients, but in 73% with palpable lesions and 40% of those with nonpalpable, screen-detected lesions. In 62%, the diagnosis of DCIS was confirmed, and in 38%, another diagnosis was made (Table 43.5).

Among cases in which the diagnosis of malignancy was made by frozen section, an axillary dissection was performed in 90%. When the DCIS was confirmed by frozen section,

TABLE 43.4. SURGICAL TREATMENT IN EUROPEAN ORGANIZATION FOR RESEARCH AND TREATMENT OF CANCER 10853

Treatment	No. of Patients (%)
Surgical procedures	
One wide excision	299 (36)
Biopsy cavity shaving	239 (29)
Two-step procedure	279 (34)
More than two steps	7 (1)
Axillary dissection	166 (20)
Sampling	105 (63)
Complete	52 (31)
Unknown	9 (5)

TABLE 43.5. PATHOLOGIC PROCEDURES IN EUROPEAN ORGANIZATION FOR RESEARCH AND TREATMENT OF CANCER 10853

Procedure	No. of Patients (%)
Frozen section	
Yes	372 (45)
No	449 (54)
Unknown	3
Frozen section diagnosis	
DCIS	231 (62)
Malignant	20 (5)
Benign	71 (19)
Deferred	41 (11)
Unknown	9 (3)
Inking specimen	
No	594 (72)
Yes	206 (25)
Unknown	24 (3)
Sectioning and radiography (for mammographically detected lesions only)	
No	495 (84)
Yes	78 (13)
Unknown	18 (3)
Margins free	213 (26)
Exact distance reported	38 (5)
Re-excision, no residual tumor	179 (22)
surrounded by normal breast tissue	7 (1)
shaving of biopsy cavity	208 (25)
Margins near/doubtful/not sure/not evaluable	37 (4)
Margins involved	4 (0.5)
Margins not reported	116 (14)
Margins unknown	22 (3)

an axillary dissection was performed in 33%, but when no frozen-section procedure was performed, an axillary dissection was carried out in only 6% of cases. This does indicate the inadvisability of frozen section in the attempted diagnosis of DCIS/invasive disease because it may lead to overtreatment (axillary dissection) in many cases.

The median histologic size tended to be smaller than the mammographic size (5 mm versus 13 mm) (Wilcoxon signed-rank test, $p < 0.001$). Margin status was reported with large variability, and in only 38 cases (5%) was an exact distance of the DCIS given (Table 43.5). The DCIS was reported to be surrounded by normal breast tissue in only seven cases (1%).

Twenty-two patients did not receive the treatment to which they were randomized: 16 patients in the radiotherapy arm did not receive radiotherapy and six in the local excision arm were irradiated. Twelve patients assigned to the radiotherapy arm did not receive the prescribed 50 Gy (range, 47 to 55 Gy) and 19 received a booster dose to the tumor bed.

OUTCOME

A total of 1,010 patients was accrued, but no data were available for eight of them, so the analysis was conducted on 500 patients randomized to wide local excision alone and 502 randomized to wide local excision and breast irradiation (13). The median follow-up time was 4.25 years. The event-free survival of irradiated and nonirradiated groups was similar (86% and 82%, respectively, $p = 0.20$). This masks some important findings in event subtypes. As Table 43.6 shows, radiotherapy reduced significantly the risk of local relapse, particularly invasive recurrence. This was counterbalanced by the finding of significantly more contralateral tumors in the irradiated group. In a more recent analysis, the significant difference between the arms with respect to contralateral disease disappeared (14 versus 24 events, $p = 0.09$).

NSABP B-17 was a trial of similar design, with early results were reported in 1993 (14). There were 790 evaluable women with DCIS that had been completely excised (not transected) who were randomized to observation (391 patients) or whole-breast irradiation (399).

After a median follow-up of 43 months, ipsilateral breast cancer developed in 64 patients in the nonirradiated group (32 DCIS and 32 invasive) and in 28 of the irradiated group (20 DCIS and eight invasive). The 5-year cumulative breast relapse rate was reduced from 10% to 7.5% for DCIS and from 10.5% to 3% for invasive cancers, and these differences were statistically significant. The NSABP found a much greater reduction in invasive disease after radiother-

apy: a relative risk of 0.20 compared with no radiotherapy. Although the overall local relapse rates do not appear to differ greatly in the two trials, the EORTC study does not show a similar magnitude of reduction of progression to invasive disease from breast irradiation as found in NSABP B-17. In two other large, nonrandomized studies, half of the reported relapses after local excision plus radiotherapy were invasive breast cancers (15,16).

HISTOPATHOLOGIC REVIEW

The pathology review was performed by Dr. J. L. Peterse and focused on the diagnosis and classification of the lesions (17). Specimen slides of 889 patients (88%) were available for review. In 20 cases, inadequate material was sent, and in six cases, the quality of the slides did not allow a reliable diagnosis, leaving 863 cases (85%) for analysis. The distribution of the clinical characteristics was similar for reviewed and nonreviewed cases.

Because the extent of the lesion and margin status could not reliably be assessed by review of the histologic slides, the pathology reports were reviewed for the extent of the lesion and margin status. Only those measurements mentioned in the report were used for determination of size. It was recorded whether margin status was reported, whether it was considered free (>1 mm), close (≤1 mm), or involved, and whether an exact measurement of the minimal width of the tumor-free margin was given. When re-excision was performed and no residual DCIS was found, this was recorded separately. For cases of DCIS, the histologic features assessed are shown in Table 43.7.

At the time of analysis, the median follow-up was 5.4 years. Because too few events were available, only overall tests between the two treatment arms were performed. The diagnosis of DCIS was confirmed in 775 of 863 lesions (90%). In 45 cases (5%), benign proliferative lesions were diagnosed, comprising epithelial hyperplasia without atypia (22) and complex sclerosing lesions (23). Invasive tumor

TABLE 43.6. RELAPSE-FREE INTERVALS AND HAZARD RATES IN RELATION TO TREATMENT

	WLE	WLE + RT	Hazard Ratio	p Value
Local relapse				
Events	83	53	0.62	0.005
4-yr RFI	84%	91%		
DCIS relapse				
Events	44	29	0.65	0.06
4-yr RFI	92%	95%		
Invasive relapse				
Events	40	24	0.60	0.04
4-yr RFI	92%	96%		
Distant metastases				
Events	12	12	0.98	0.96
4-yr RFI	98%	99%		
Deaths				
Events	12	12	0.97	0.94
4-yr RFI	99%	99%		
Contralateral disease				
Events	8	21	2.57	0.01
4-yr RFI	99%	97%		

WLE, wide local excision; RT, radiation therapy; RFI, recurrence-free interval; DCIS, ductal carcinoma in situ.

TABLE 43.7. HISTOLOGIC FEATURES DETERMINED IN CENTRAL PATHOLOGIC REVIEW

Feature	Comment
Correct diagnosis of DCIS	Invasion defined as carcinoma of at least 1 mm outside the periductal stromal cuff
Cytonuclear grade	Low, moderate, high
Necrosis	None or moderate/marked (559)
Architectural growth pattern	Clinging, micropapillary, cribriform, solid/comedo
Grade	Well, intermediately, and poorly differentiated

DCIS, ductal carcinoma in situ.

was found in 27 cases (3%), and in another 13 (1.5%), there was suspicion of invasion. In three cases, the lesion was classified as lobular carcinoma in situ.

A pathologic diameter was reported in 178 cases (25%). Size was reported as less than 1 cm in 121 (68%), 1 to 2 cm in 41 (23%), and greater than 2 cm in 16 cases (9%). Margin status was unspecified in 88 cases (12%) and reported free without further specification in 350 cases (49%), an exact distance was given in 36 cases (5%), no residual DCIS was found at surgical re-excision in 147 (21%), and the margins were reported close/involved in 62 cases (9%). At review, of 775 cases of DCIS, 284 (37%) were classified as well-differentiated DCIS, 198 (25%) as intermediately differentiated, and 293 (38%) as poorly differentiated.

OUTCOME IN RELATION TO REVIEWED PATHOLOGY

After a median follow-up of 5.4 years, 137 of the 863 patients (16%) developed a local recurrence, 71 DCIS and 66 invasive carcinomas. The diagnosis at review was significantly related to the risk of recurrence. Of the 45 women with benign proliferative lesions, only one developed an invasive lesion in an area of the breast remote from the original biopsy. In one of three patients with lobular carcinoma in situ, DCIS was found in another quadrant 2 years later. In the group of 27 with invasive lesions on review, there were four invasive and four DCIS recurrences, and two invasive relapses occurred in the 13 with suspicion of invasion. All subsequent analyses were performed on the 775 patients with a confirmed histologic diagnosis of DCIS. Of these, 125 developed a local recurrence, 66 DCIS and 60 invasive carcinomas (one patient had an invasive recurrence after DCIS relapse).

The multivariate analysis (Table 43.8) shows that risk factors for local recurrence include young age, symptomatic detection, cribriform or solid/comedo architecture, nonspecified or close/involved margins, and local excision without radiotherapy.

Some of the variables used in the multivariate analysis were correlated: symptomatic patients showing a trend toward more extensive lesions ($p < 0.01$) and younger patients were more likely to be symptomatic compared with older patients (63% versus 24%, $p = 0.001$ by the chi-squared test). Radiotherapy reduced the risk of local relapse in all subgroups of patients with DCIS.

Although patients with involved/nonspecified margins had a longer median local recurrence–free interval when treated with radiotherapy compared with local excision alone, a high local recurrence rate is still observed in the group treated with radiotherapy (16 of 81, 20%), implying that radiotherapy cannot compensate for inadequate surgery.

The risk of distant metastasis was significantly higher in poorly differentiated DCIS compared with well-differentiated DCIS (1% versus 5%, hazard ratio 6.65, $p = 0.008$).

TABLE 43.8. MULTIVARIATE ANALYSIS OF RISK FACTORS RELATED TO LOCAL RECURRENCE

Variable	Hazard Ratio (95% CI)	p Value
Histologic type		
Well differentiated	1	
Intermediately differentiated	1.39 (0.75–2.58)	0.56
Poorly differentiated	1.30 (0.61–2.77)	
Age (yr)		
>40	1	
≤40	2.14 (1.17–3.91)	0.02
Architecture		
Clinging/micropapillary	1	
Cribriform	2.67 (0.28–5.59)	0.012
Solid/comedo	2.69 (1.12–6.47)	
Treatment		
Excision + RT	1	
Excision alone	1.74 (1.13–2.68)	0.009
Method of detection		
X-ray finding only	1	
Symptomatic	1.80 (1.16–2.78)	0.008
Margins		
Free	1	
Nonspecified/close/involved	2.07 (1.35–3.16)	0.0008

CI, confidence interval.

In an analysis comparing the histology of the primary DCIS with its invasive local recurrence, it was found that well-differentiated DCIS usually recurs as grade 1 invasive carcinoma and poorly differentiated DCIS as grade 3 invasive breast cancer (18).

FUTURE STUDIES

The major question asked in the 10853 trial was the effect of radiotherapy after apparent complete local excision of DCIS. The answer is that there is a reduction in risk of relapse of DCIS and a reduced rate of progression to invasive disease. The major risk factors for local relapse or progression to invasive disease are margin status, symptomatic disease, withholding radiotherapy, DCIS architecture, and young age. Although radiotherapy reduces the risk of recurrence for all subgroups of patients with DCIS, in some cases, such as young patients or those with incompletely excised lesions, even with radiotherapy, the risk of recurrence is unacceptably high. This underlines the need for close cooperation between radiologist, surgeon, and pathologist and suggests that breast-conserving treatment for DCIS should only be attempted within a multidisciplinary setup. Future trials will require more stringent entry criteria so that effects of treatments being tested are not diluted by DCIS characteristics such as involvement of margins.

Because systemic therapies have been shown to be very useful in invasive disease, studies of the role of tamoxifen have been reported or are underway. As with invasive disease, it is unlikely that estrogen receptor–negative disease will respond to DCIS, and this is more likely to be the case in high-grade DCIS, which carries the highest risk of progression to invasive disease that is most likely to be grade 3. Newer approaches using DNA methylation inhibitors such as 5-aza-2^1-deoxy-cytidine may be worthwhile investigating, particularly in those with more extensive estrogen receptor–negative DCIS.

ACKNOWLEDGMENT

The following centers have collaborated in the trial: Istituto Nazionale dei Tumori, Milano; Institut Bergoni, Bordeaux; CRLC Val D'Aurelle, Montpellier; Centre Henri Becquerel, Rouen; Institut Jules Bordet, Brussels; Radiotherapeutisch Instituut, Arnhem; UZ Gasthuisberg, Leuven; The Netherlands Cancer Institute/Antoni van Leeuwenhoek Huis, Amsterdam; RRTI, Rotterdam; Ospedale Civile, Geneva; IKW, Leiden; Policlinico di Careggi, Firenze; Dr. Bernard Verbeeten Instituut, Tilburg, AZ Leiden; De Wever Ziekenhuis, Heerlen; Guy's Hospital, London; AZ Utrecht; St. Radboud Ziekenhuis, Nijmegen; IKA, Amsterdam; Centre Eugene Marquis, Rennes; IPO, Oporto; St. Savas Hospital, Athens; AMC, Amsterdam Longmore Hospital, Edinburgh; Centre Georges-Francois Leclerc, Dijon; Hopital Jean Minjoz, Besancon; Istituto de Ginecologia e Ostetrica, Torino; Universitatsklinik fur Chirurgie, Graz; Marika Eliadi Hospital, Athens; I Universitatsklinik fur Chirurgie, Innsbruck; Istituto Europeo di Oncologia, Milano; Radiotherapeutisch Instituut Friesland, Leeuwarden; Policlinico di Borgo Roma, Verona; Hopital Cantonale, Geneve; CHU Vaudois, Lausanne; University of Stellenbosch, Tijgerberg; Ospedale de Noale, Venezia; Rambam Medical Centre, Haifa; Inst Oncol, San Sebastian; Onze Lieve Vrouw Gasthuis, Amsterdam; Diaconessenhuis, Utrecht; Ninewells Hospital, Dundee; Dijkzigt Ziekenhuis, Rotterdam; Andreas Ziekenhuis, Amsterdam; Streekziekenhuis, Blaricum; Universitatsklinik, Gottingen.

REFERENCES

1. Betsill WL, Rosen PP, Lieberman PH, et al. Intraductal carcinoma. Long-term follow-up after treatment by biopsy alone. *JAMA* 1978;239:1863–1866.

2. Rosen PP, Braun DW, Kinne DF. The clinical significance of non-invasive breast carcinoma. *Cancer* 1980;46:919–925.

3. Page DL, Dupont WD, Rogers LW, et al. Intraductal carcinoma of the breast: follow-up after biopsy alone. *Cancer* 1982;49: 751–758.

4. Farrow JH. Current conception. The detection and treatment of early breast carcinomas. *Cancer* 1970;47:2928–2937.

5. Ashikari R, Huvos AG, Snyder RE. Prospective study of non-infiltrating carcinoma of the breast. *Cancer* 1977;39:435–439.

6. Carter D, Orr SL, Merino MJ. Intracystic papillary carcinoma of the breast after mastectomy, radiotherapy or excisional biopsy alone. *Cancer* 1983;52:14–19.

7. Millis RR, Thynne GSJ. In situ intraduct carcinoma of the breast: a long-term follow-up study. *Br J Surg* 1975;62:957–962.

8. Lagios MD, Westdahl PR, Margolin FR, et al. Duct carcinoma in situ: relationship of non-invasive disease to the frequency of occult invasion, multicentricity, lymph node metastases, and short-term treatment failures. *Cancer* 1982;50:1309–1314.

9. Fisher ER, Sass R, Fisher B, et al. Pathologic findings from the National Surgical Adjuvant Breast Project (protocol 6). 1. Intraductal carcinoma (DCIS). *Cancer* 1986;57:197–208.

10. Silverstein MJ, Rosser RJ, Gierson ED, et al. Axillary node dissection for intraductal breast carcinoma—is it indicated? *Cancer* 1987;59:1819–1824.

11. Fentiman IS. *Detection and treatment of breast cancer*, 2nd ed. Chapter 17. London: Martin Dunitz, 1998.

12. Bijker N, Rutgers EJT, Peterse JL, et al. Variations in diagnostic and therapeutic procedures in a multicentre randomised clinical trial (EORTC 10853) investigating breast-conserving treatment for DCIS. *Eur J Cancer* 2001;27:135–140.

13. Julien J-P, Bijker N, Fentiman IS, et al. Radiotherapy in breast-conserving treatment for ductal carcinoma in situ: first results of the EORTC randomised phase III trial 10853. *Lancet* 2000;355:528–523.

14. Fisher B, Costantino J, Redmond C, et al. Lumpectomy compared with lumpectomy and radiation therapy for treatment of intraductal breast cancer. *N Engl J Med* 1993;328:1581–1586.

15. Solin LJ, Kurtz J, Fourquet A, et al. Fifteen year results of breast-conserving surgery and definitive breast irradiation for the treatment of ductal carcinoma in situ of the breast. *J Clin Oncol* 1996;14:754–763.

16. Silverstein MJ, Barth A, Poller DN, et al. Ten-year results comparing mastectomy to excision and radiation therapy for ductal carcinoma in situ of the breast. *Eur J Cancer* 1995;31A: 1425–1427.

17. Bijker N, Peterse JL, Duchateau L, et al. Risk factors for recurrence and metastasis after breast-conserving therapy for ductal carcinoma in situ: analysis of EORTC trial 10853. *J Clin Oncol* 2001;19:2263–2271.

18. Bijker N, Peterse JL. Duchateau L, et al. Histological type and marker expression of the primary tumour compared with its local recurrence after breast-conserving therapy for ductal carcinoma in situ. *Br J Cancer* 2001;84:539–544.

44

RADIOTHERAPY AND TAMOXIFEN AFTER COMPLETE EXCISION OF DUCTAL CARCINOMA IN SITU OF THE BREAST

JOAN HOUGHTON
W. DAVID GEORGE*

The United Kingdom Ductal Carcinoma in Situ (DCIS) trial was launched in May 1990 to evaluate the roles of radiotherapy and tamoxifen after breast-conserving surgery for mammographically detected DCIS. The primary objective was to determine whether complete local excision (CLE) followed by radiotherapy (recommended dose was 50 Gy in 25 fractions over 5 weeks) to the residual ipsilateral breast or CLE followed by tamoxifen (20 mg daily for 5 years) reduced the incidence of subsequent ipsilateral invasive breast cancer. The secondary objective was to determine the incidence of subsequent DCIS in the ipsilateral and contralateral breasts of patients treated with CLE alone or with CLE followed by radiotherapy or tamoxifen. A 2 × 2 factorial design was used to allow evaluation of both treatments simultaneously. Randomization was independent for each of the two treatments (radiotherapy and tamoxifen) and stratified by screening assessment center. Individual participating clinicians could elect to enter patients into either the four-way randomization or one of two separate two-way randomizations. The two-way randomizations were CLE versus CLE plus randomization to radiotherapy or alternatively CLE versus CLE plus randomization for tamoxifen. Within the two separate two-way randomizations, the alternative treatment, i.e., radiotherapy or tamoxifen, could ei-

ther be given or withheld as an elective decision (but the analysis only makes comparisons between randomized patients and was stratified by any elective treatments given). Ethical approval was obtained from each local hospital ethics committee before participating in the trial.

Patients with unilateral or bilateral DCIS and deemed suitable for breast conservation were eligible. Complete excision as determined by free margins both on histologic examination and radiologic assessment by the local pathologist was mandatory. Re-excision of the tumor bed to achieve histologically clear margins was permitted if necessary.

Patients were recruited in the trial from May 1990 until August 1998. A total of 1,701 patients were randomized [radiotherapy versus control (n = 1,030), tamoxifen versus control (n = 1,576)]. Two hundred sixty-three women (15.5%) developed new breast disease during the follow-up period (median 52.6 months). Of these, 150 were cases of recurrent DCIS and 108 were invasive cancer (in an additional five patients, the type of new disease has yet to be confirmed). Of the 263 events, 223 were in the ipsilateral breast and 35 in the contralateral breast (laterality has yet to be confirmed in five patients). Results are summarized in Tables 44.1 and 44.2.

To date, 33 (2.0%) of the randomized patients have developed a new nonbreast cancer. Death has been reported for 45 patients; 23 patients of breast cancer or with breast cancer present at death. Of the remaining 22 deaths, nine were owing to cancers other than breast, four to cardiac failure, two to vascular events, and two to other causes. Too few deaths have occurred at the present time for meaningful analysis by treatment.

The results of the United Kingdom-Australia-New Zealand (UK/ANZ) trial confirm the previously reported benefit of radiotherapy after breast-conserving surgery for DCIS. Unresolved issues remain, particularly whether radiotherapy is necessary for patients at low risk of recurrence

* On behalf of the United Kingdom Co-ordinating Committee on Cancer Research DCIS Working Party and the DCIS trialists in the United Kingdom, Australia, and New Zealand. Members of the Working Party of the trial are W. David George (Chairman), Western Infirmary, Glasgow; Joan Houghton (Secretary) CRC and UCL Cancer Trials Centre, London; Joan Austoker, Institute of Health Sciences, Oxford University; Hugh Bishop, Royal Bolton Hospital; Jack Cuzick (Statistician), ICRF, London; Catherine Duggan, ICRF, London; Ian S. Fentiman, Guy's Hospital; John F. Forbes, Mater Misericordiae Hospital, Newcastle, Australia; Elizabeth Foster, Scottish Cancer Therapy Network Central Office, Edinburgh; Ian Ellis, Nottingham City Hospital; Samuel Leinster, University of East Anglia; Margaret Spittle, The Middlesex Hospital and Norman Williams CRC and UCL Cancer Trials Centre, London.

TABLE 44.1. RESULTS FOR RADIATION THERAPY

End Point	RT (n = 522)	No RT (n = 508)	Hazard Ratio	95% CI	p Value
All events[a]	38	82	0.43	0.29–0.63	<0.0001
Total invasive	24	36	0.62	0.37–1.04	0.07
Total DCIS	14	44	0.31	0.17–0.56	<0.0001
Ipsilateral invasive/DCIS	29	69	0.38	0.25–0.59	<0.0001
Ipsilateral invasive	15	30	0.45	0.24–0.85	0.01
Ipsilateral DCIS	14	38	0.36	0.19–0.66	0.0004

[a] For five patients, the laterality of the tumor was unknown, and for two, the invasive status was unknown.
RT, radiation therapy; CI, confidence interval; DCIS, ductal carcinoma in situ.

(i.e., those with low-grade tumors and/or a wide excision margin). Further studies are indicated to answer this question. Our results with tamoxifen in women with DCIS over the age of 50 do not currently support the use of this agent outside of prospective randomized trials. Longer follow-up may clarify the situation. Further trials of tamoxifen or newer endocrine agents such as the aromatase inhibitors, perhaps with the randomization stratified by hormone receptor status, are needed to evaluate the true role of endocrine agents in this situation in terms of both prevention of ipsilateral recurrence and the prevention of contralateral disease. These are important questions because in the United Kingdom, approximately 20% of the disease found with the screening program is DCIS.

EDITOR'S COMMENTS ON THE UNITED KINGDOM DUCTAL CARCINOMA IN SITU TRIAL: ABRAM RECHT

The impact of radiotherapy on the risk of ipsilateral breast tumor recurrence (IBTR) (either invasive or invasive) in the 1,030 patients in the UK/ANZ trial appears comparable with those of other randomized trials (see Chapters 40–43). The risk of IBTR was substantially reduced in those patients randomized to receive radiotherapy, with a hazard ratio of 0.38. However, unlike the findings of the National Surgical Adjuvant Breast and Bowel Project (NSABP) B-24 trial (1), there was no impact of tamoxifen on the risk of IBTR among the 523 patients actually receiving radiotherapy (15 events in patients randomized to tamoxifen and 15 in those randomized not to receive it). Tamoxifen use also had very little impact on the risk of IBTR in those 1,053 patients not receiving radiotherapy either (with 87 events in patients randomized to receive tamoxifen compared to 97 in those randomized not to receive it, i.e., an absolute crude difference of approximately 2%).

This apparent discrepancy between the NSABP B-24 trial and the UK/ANZ trial on the impact of tamoxifen in patients receiving radiotherapy can be resolved by considering the different eligibility requirements of the trials. Patients entered in the UK/ANZ trial were required to have clear margins, whereas the NSABP B-24 trial accepted patients with positive or unknown margins (257 patients) or patients with negative margins (1,341 patients). In the NSABP B-24 trial, margin status had a substantial impact on results. The crude local failure rate in the patients with negative margins who received a placebo was 8.0%, compared with 6.3% in the tamoxifen arm. However, patients with positive or unknown margins on the placebo arm had a lo-

TABLE 44.2. RESULTS FOR TAMOXIFEN

End Point	Tamoxifen (n = 794)	No Tamoxifen (n = 782)	Hazard Ratio	95% CI	p Value
Total invasive/DCIS	114	137	0.83	0.64–1.06	0.13
Total invasive	55	50	1.11	0.76–1.63	0.59
Total DCIS	58	84	0.68	0.49–0.96	0.03
Ipsilateral DCIS/invasive[a]	102	114	0.90	0.69–1.17	0.42
Ipsilateral invasive	45	35	1.31	0.84–2.03	0.23
Ipsilateral DCIS	57	77	0.74	0.52–1.04	0.08
Contralateral invasive/DCIS[a]	11	21	0.52	0.25–1.07	0.07
Contralateral invasive	10	15	0.66	0.30–1.46	0.30

[a] For four patients, the laterality and/or the invasive status of the tumor were unknown.
CI, confidence interval; DCIS, ductal carcinoma in situ.

cal failure rate of 14.7%, compared with 9.0% among patients randomized to tamoxifen. Given the small absolute amount of benefits of tamoxifen treatment in patients who received radiotherapy that we might therefore expect from the B-24 trial, the absence of an effect in the UK/ANZ trial (which has many fewer patients who received radiotherapy and a shorter follow-up) is not surprising.

The most important finding of the UK/ANZ trial may be the minimal effect of tamoxifen on IBTR in patients not receiving radiotherapy. However, as pointed out in Chapter 40, in the randomized trials, there was no minimum tumor-free margin width required for these patients. It seems likely that tamoxifen may be most useful for those individuals with a minimal residual postoperative tumor burden (i.e., with widely negative margins). (This hypothesis is being tested in the Radiation Therapy Oncology Group trial, which requires a minimum margin of 3 mm.) Unfortunately, margin width data were not collected in the initial data entry. Also, tamoxifen may be more effective for low-grade lesions, which are usually estrogen receptor positive, rather than high-grade lesions, which are often estrogen receptor negative. Hence, the central pathologic review of materials from this trial will be critical in assessing the true value of tamoxifen.

It should be noted that the interpretation of the trial is potentially complicated by its unusual design. Patients could be entered either into a conventional 2 × 2 randomization (resulting in assignment to one of four arms: radiotherapy alone, tamoxifen alone, both, or neither) or at the discretion of the entering physician into one of two 2 × 1 randomizations (either to receive tamoxifen or not or to receive radiotherapy or not), with other treatment being allowed as desired. The characteristics of the patients in these three different subtrials are not given, but it seems likely that they were substantially different. Data are not presented for these subtrials individually, unfortunately. This makes it all the more critical to perform detailed a central pathology review and subgroup analyses before using their results with assurance.

REFERENCE

1. Fisher B, Dignam J, Wolmark N, et al. Tamoxifen in treatment of intraductal breast cancer: National Surgical Adjuvant Breast and Bowel Project B-24 randomised controlled trial. *Lancet* 1999;353:1993–2000.

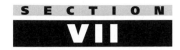

TOOLS FOR SELECTING PATIENTS FOR BREAST CONSERVATION WITH AND WITHOUT RADIATION THERAPY

45

THE UNIVERSITY OF SOUTHERN CALIFORNIA/VAN NUYS PROGNOSTIC INDEX

MELVIN J. SILVERSTEIN

The Van Nuys Prognostic Index (VNPI), as originally described in 1996 (1), is a tool that quantifies four measurable prognostic factors (tumor size, margin width, nuclear grade, and the presence or absence of comedonecrosis) that are currently being used in the treatment decision-making process for patients with ductal carcinoma in situ (DCIS). It is based on tumor morphology and recurrence data in a large series of patients with DCIS and was developed as a numerical aid to be used in conjunction with clinical experience. The University of Southern California/Van Nuys Prognostic Index (USC/VNPI) adds a fifth factor (patient age) that has now been shown by numerous investigators to be of clinical importance (2–5) (see also Chapter 21).

As we have seen in numerous chapters throughout this text, DCIS represents a broad biologic spectrum of disease (6,7) with a wide range of treatment approaches. The lack of clear and universally accepted treatment criteria has resulted in a diverse range of confusing clinical recommendations, distressing to both patients and clinicians (8).

Are there patients with DCIS whose local recurrence rate with breast preservation is so high that mastectomy is clearly the most appropriate treatment? If so, how can they be identified? For those patients who do not require mastectomy, must radiation therapy always be added to their breast-preservation regimen? These are the questions that are addressed in this chapter.

With mastectomy, the ipsilateral breast is no longer at risk, and local recurrence of DCIS or progression to invasive disease is uncommon (9–13). Mastectomy is, by far, the most effective treatment available for DCIS if our goal is simply to prevent local recurrence. Figure 45.1 reveals a statistically significant lower probability of local recurrence when mastectomy is compared with either form of breast preservation (excision alone or excision plus radiation therapy) for patients with DCIS. Mastectomy is also a superior operation when patients with DCIS are compared with patients with invasive cancer breast cancer and the probability of local recurrence is the end point. Figure 45.2 shows a less

than 1% local recurrence probability for DCIS patients treated with mastectomy compared with a 10% local recurrence probability at 12 years for patients with invasive cancer treated with mastectomy. The lower curve on Figure 45.2 represents the spectrum of invasive breast cancer and includes patients with T3 and T4 lesions treated with primary (neoadjuvant) chemotherapy before mastectomy. If the patients with invasive cancer are limited to those with T1 lesions, the probability of local recurrence drops to less than 5% at 12 years, but it is still significantly worse than for those with DCIS.

Although mastectomy is clearly a superior operation in terms of local recurrence, it is an aggressive form of treatment for patients with DCIS and provides only a theoretical survival benefit. No prospective randomized trial to date has reported a survival benefit (14–23), regardless of treatment nor have our data shown any survival benefit by any form of treatment (Fig. 45.3). It is, therefore, often difficult to justify mastectomy, particularly for otherwise healthy women with screen-detected DCIS, during an era of increasing utilization of breast conservation for more aggressive invasive breast carcinoma.

As our knowledge of DCIS has evolved during the past decade, the treatment decision-making process has become much more complex and controversial. There are numerous ongoing prospective randomized trials that are attempting to simplify the treatment selection process. Three have been published: one performed by the National Surgical Adjuvant Breast Project (NSABP) (protocol B-17) (14), one performed by the European Organization for Cancer Research and Treatment EORTC 10853 (20), and one performed by the United Kingdom Co-ordinating Committee on Cancer Research (generally referred to as the UK Trial) (see Chapter 44) (22).

The results of NSABP B-17 were updated in 1995 (15), 1998 (16), 1999 (17), and 2001 (18). In this study, more than 800 patients with DCIS excised with clear surgical margins were randomized into two groups: excision only

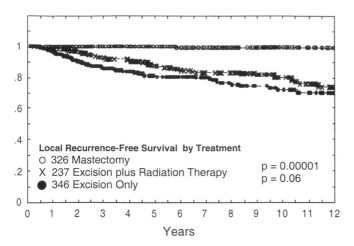

FIGURE 45.1. Probability of local recurrence–free survival by treatment for 909 patients with ductal carcinoma in situ.

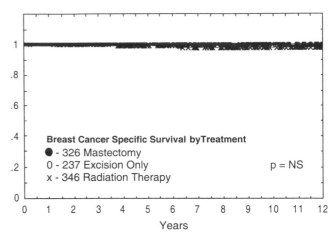

FIGURE 45.3. Probability of breast cancer–specific survival by treatment for 909 patients with ductal carcinoma in situ (*p* = NS).

versus excision plus radiation therapy. The main end point of the study was local recurrence, invasive or noninvasive (DCIS).

After 12 years of follow-up, there was a statistically significant 50% decrease in local recurrence of both DCIS and invasive breast cancer in patients treated with radiation therapy. The overall local recurrence rate for patients treated with excision only was 32% at 12 years. For patients treated with excision plus irradiation, it was 16%, a 16% difference in favor of those treated with radiation therapy (18). These updated data led the NSABP to reaffirm their 1993 position and to continue to recommend postoperative radiation therapy for patients with DCIS who chose to save their breasts. The early results of B-17, in favor of radiation therapy for patients with DCIS, led the NSABP to perform protocol B-

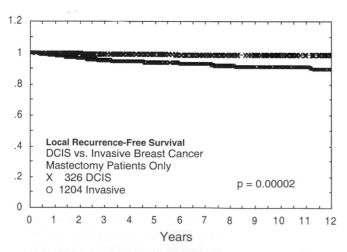

FIGURE 45.2. Probability of local recurrence–free survival by treatment for 1,530 patients treated with mastectomy: 326 with ductal carcinoma in situ and 1,204 with invasive breast cancer. The reason that the local recurrence rate after mastectomy is so high (approximately 10% at 12 years) is because this curve includes patients with locally advanced breast cancer who received neoadjuvant chemotherapy before mastectomy.

24. In this trial, more than 1,800 patients with DCIS were treated with excision and radiation therapy, then randomized to receive either tamoxifen or placebo. After 7 years of follow-up, 11.1% of patients treated with placebo recurred locally, whereas only 7.7% of those treated with tamoxifen had a recurrence (18). The difference, although small, was statistically significant for invasive local recurrence but not for noninvasive (DCIS) recurrence.

The EORTC results were published in *The Lancet* in February 2000 (20). This study was virtually identical to B-17 in design and included more than 1,000 patients. At 4 years of follow-up, 9% of patients treated with excision plus radiation therapy had a local recurrence compared with 16% of patients treated with excision only, results similar to those obtained by the NSABP at the same point in their trial. After 6 years of follow-up, the local recurrence rates were 11% for those treated with radiation and 20% for those treated with excision only. In distinction to the NSABP, one-half of the recurrences in each group were invasive, and there was a statistically significant increase in contralateral breast cancer in patients who were randomized to receive radiation therapy. This increase in contralateral breast cancer cannot be easily explained and is considered by most to be a statistical aberration. There was no survival benefit for either arm of the trial.

The UK Trial was first published in abstract form in 2000 (22), and the full paper was submitted in 2002 (23). This trial had a 2 × 2 design. Patients were randomized to excision only versus excision plus radiation therapy and/or to tamoxifen or placebo. At the time of publication, 1,694 patients were evaluable: 544 received excision only, 567 excision plus tamoxifen, 267 excision plus radiation therapy, and 316 excision plus radiation therapy plus tamoxifen. Like the NSABP and EORTC trials, the UK Trial showed a substantial and statistically significant approximately 50% reduction in local recurrence for patients who received radiation therapy. Unlike the NSABP B-24 trial, there was no statistically significant benefit in the reduction of local recurrence for those who received tamoxifen. Again, there was no benefit in terms of survival in any of the arms of the study.

WHY NOT GIVE RADIATION THERAPY TO EVERY CONSERVATIVELY TREATED PATIENT WITH DUCTAL CARCINOMA IN SITU?

Before simply giving radiation therapy to all conservatively treated patients with DCIS, a number of issues should be considered. Radiation therapy is expensive, time-consuming, and accompanied by significant side effects in a small percentage of patients (e.g., cardiac, pulmonary) (24). Radiation fibrosis of the breast is a more common side effect, particularly with the type of radiation therapy given during the 1980s. Radiation fibrosis changes the texture of the breast and skin, makes mammographic follow-up somewhat more difficult, and may result in delayed diagnosis if there is a local recurrence. The use of radiation therapy for DCIS precludes its use if an invasive recurrence develops at a later date. The use of radiation therapy with its accompanying skin and vascular changes make skin-sparing mastectomy, if needed in the future, more difficult to perform. There may be some identifiable subgroups of DCIS patients in whom radiation therapy offers little improvement in local recurrence–free survival. Also, we must understand why there was a statistically significant increase in contralateral breast cancer among patients who received radiation therapy in the EORTC study.

Recently, the Early Breast Cancer Trialists' Collaborative Group published a meta-analysis of the 10- and 20-year results from 40 unconfounded, randomized trials of radiation therapy for early breast cancer (25). Radiation therapy regimens routinely produced a reduction in local recurrence along with a reduction in 20-year breast cancer–specific mortality in the range of 2% to 4%. However, cardiovascular mortality was increased in those patients who received radiation therapy. Because of this, the absolute survival gain with radiation therapy was only 1.2% (26). The studies reported in the meta-analysis were conducted between 1961 and 1990. More modern radiation therapy techniques are designed to minimize cardiopulmonary exposure, but long-term cardiovascular mortality data do not exist. The NSABP 1999 update reported four breast cancer deaths among the excision-only group and seven among the excision plus radiation therapy group (16) (p = NS). By the time the 2001 update was published, there were 12 deaths attributed to invasive breast cancer among the excision-only group and 15 among the excision plus radiation therapy group (p = NS) (18). The EORTC study and the UK Trial also failed to show a difference in breast cancer–specific survival between any of the treatment arms. If we cannot show a benefit in

survival when radiation therapy is added to the treatment plan of patients with DCIS and there is potential mortality with the use of radiation therapy, then we must be extremely careful when prescribing radiation therapy for patients with DCIS. Physicians must be secure that the benefits of radiation therapy significantly outweigh the potential side effects, complications, inconvenience, and costs for a given subgroup of patients, particularly those with relatively nonlethal malignancies such as DCIS.

COMPLEX CLINICAL DECISIONS

Consider the following two patients. Patient 1 is a 54-year-old woman with a 13-mm focus of highly suspicious microcalcifications on mammography. A wire-directed excision revealed an 11-mm, high-grade DCIS with extensive comedonecrosis. The lesion extended tenuously close to the lateral margin (0.3 mm) but was clear by NSABP standards (the tumor was not transected).

Patient 2 is a 65-year-old woman with minimally suspicious calcifications on mammography. A wire-directed excision revealed an 8-mm low-grade DCIS without comedonecrosis. The margins were widely clear (>10 mm) in all directions.

Using the recommendations developed from the results of NSABP B-17, it would be appropriate to treat both of these patients with radiation therapy and without further surgery. Because all the published prospective randomized trials show a benefit for radiation therapy, many physicians would consider the NSABP results and recommendations as the standard of care in their community and would treat both of these patients with breast irradiation and no additional surgery.

However, despite the results of all three prospective randomized trials, there continues to be debate regarding the treatment decision-making process in patients with DCIS. According to the 1997 National Cancer Institute's Surveillance, Epidemiology, and End Results (SEER) data, approximately one-third of all patients with DCIS in the United States are being treated with excision only. Clearly, American physicians and patients are not accepting the results of B-17 as the standard of care (The EORTC trial and UK Trial were not published when the 1997 SEER data were analyzed) for every case of DCIS.

In the shadow of this ongoing debate, many physicians might approach these two cases differently. If I were treating these patients, I would allow approximately 3 months of healing for the first patient with the high-grade lesion close to margins. I would then re-excise the excision cavity in an attempt to obtain widely clear margins before making a final decision on definitive therapy. Significant residual disease approaching the new margins would earn a recommendation for mastectomy and immediate reconstruction; widely clear new margins with little or no residual DCIS would earn a recommendation for careful clinical follow-up without the addition of radiation therapy, although most physicians would probably feel more comfortable with the addition of radiation therapy. The final recommendation would, of course, depend on the patient's preference and her ability to tolerate an increased risk in the probability of local recurrence if radiation therapy were withheld.

For the second patient with the small, non–high-grade lesion that was widely excised, I would advise no additional therapy. I would be satisfied with excision alone as the treatment for a small, low-grade DCIS with margins greater that 10 mm in every direction. In the pages that follow, I try to shed light on the thought processes that led me to those therapeutic recommendations.

THE ORIGINS OF THE VAN NUYS PROGNOSTIC INDEX

Our research (13,27–29) (see also Chapters 17 and 21) and the research of others (2–5,30–40), including the NSABP in their 1995 update of protocol B-17 (15), have shown that various combinations of nuclear grade, the presence of comedonecrosis, tumor size, margin width, and age are all important factors that can be used to predict local recurrence in conservatively treated patients with DCIS. Combinations of these factors can be used to select subgroups of patients whose recurrence rate is theoretically so high, even with breast irradiation, that mastectomy is preferable or to select patients who do not require radiation therapy in addition to complete excision if breast conservation is selected.

Previously, my colleagues and I analyzed 30 prognostic factors and found that nuclear grade, tumor size, margin width, and comedonecrosis were all significant predictors of local recurrence by univariate analysis (27,41,42). All statistically significant predictors of local recurrence by univariate analysis were evaluated using a Cox multivariate regression analysis. In 1996, only three prognostic factors, Van Nuys Classification (which is made up by a combination of grade and necrosis), tumor size, and margin width, were significant predictors of local recurrence and invasive local recurrence by multivariate analysis in patients treated with breast preservation (1). The Cox multivariate regression analysis held up when it was rerun for each treatment group separately (excision only or excision plus radiation therapy). Again, tumor size, margin width, and pathologic classification were all statistically significant independent predictors of local recurrence for either form of treatment (all $p < 0.05$).

The Van Nuys DCIS Pathologic Classification (28) has been described in detail in Chapter 17. Nuclear grade and comedonecrosis, which make up the Van Nuys DCIS Pathologic Classification (28) (henceforth, referred to simply as pathologic classification), are closely related to the biology of the lesion, but neither is adequate as the sole guide-

line for deciding treatment. A very large, low-grade lesion without necrosis (group 1) may require mastectomy because its size makes complete excision with an acceptable cosmetic result almost impossible. Whereas a small, high-grade lesion with necrosis (group 3), well marked by mammographic microcalcifications, may be completely excised easily with nearly perfect cosmesis.

Tumor size and margin width, both independent predictors of local recurrence, reflect the extent of disease, the adequacy of surgical treatment, and, therefore, the likelihood of residual disease and are clearly extremely important. The results of the multivariate analysis of prognostic factors performed on our patients confirm the importance of these variables (Fig. 45.4) (Chapter 21).

THE ORIGINAL VAN NUYS PROGNOSTIC INDEX

In 1995, my colleagues and I began to quantify these variables, trying to make them clinically useful. The factors needed to be more than simply positive or negative results used in an anecdotal fashion. The VNPI (1,43,44) was devised by combining three statistically significant independent predictors of local tumor recurrence in patients with DCIS: tumor size, margin width, and pathologic classification (determined by nuclear grade and necrosis). The challenge was to devise a system that would be clinically valid, therapeutically useful, and user friendly. The concept was to assign a score for each of the prognostic variables based on its relative contribution as defined by the multivariate analysis. Numerous models were tried and thoroughly analyzed.

Ultimately, a score ranging from 1 for lesions with the best prognosis to 3 for lesions with the worst prognosis was given for each of the three prognostic predictors. The objective with all three predictors was to create three statistically different subgroups for each, using local recurrence as the marker of treatment failure. Cutoff points (for example, what size or margin width constitutes low, intermediate, or high risk of local recurrence) were determined statistically, using the log-rank test with an optimal p-value approach.

Size Score

A score of 1 was given for small tumors 15 mm or less, 2 was given for intermediate sized tumors 16 to 40 mm, and 3 was given for large tumors 41 mm or more in diameter.

Margin Score

A score of 1 was given for widely clear, tumor-free margins of 10 mm or more. This was most commonly achieved by re-excision with the finding of no residual DCIS or only focal residual DCIS in the wall of the biopsy cavity. A score of

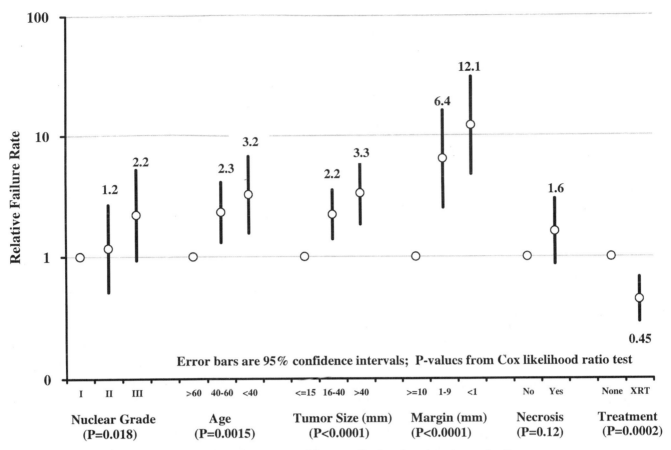

FIGURE 45.4. Cox multivariate analysis of factors affecting ductal carcinoma in situ recurrence-free survival (conservatively treated patients only).

2 was given for intermediate margins of 1 to 9 mm and a score of 3 for margins less than 1 mm (involved or close margins).

Pathologic Classification Score (28) (Chapter 17)

A score of 3 was given for tumors classified as group 3 (all high-grade lesions with or without necrosis), 2 for tumors classified as group 2 (non–high-grade lesion with comedonecrosis), and a score of 1 for tumors classified as group 1 (non–high-grade lesion without comedonecrosis). The classification is diagrammed in Figure 45.5 (see Chapter 17) (28).

Tissue Processing

Tissue processing is extremely important if a prognostic index dependent on pathologic variables is going to work. During tumor excision, every effort was made to completely excise all suspicious lesions. Needle localization, intraoperative specimen radiography, and correlation with the preoperative mammogram were performed in every nonpalpable case. Margins were inked or dyed, and speci-

mens were serially sectioned at 2- to 3-mm intervals. The tissue sections were arranged and processed in sequence. Pathologic evaluation included the subtype by pathologic classification, the size or extent of the lesion, and the margin width.

Tumor size was determined by direct measurement or ocular micrometry from stained slides for smaller lesions.

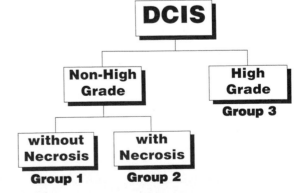

FIGURE 45.5. Van Nuys Classification of ductal carcinoma in situ (DCIS). Patients with DCIS are separated into high nuclear grade and non-high nuclear grade. Non-high nuclear grade cases are then separated by the presence or absence of necrosis. Lesions in group 3 (high nuclear grade) may or may not show necrosis. (From Silverstein MJ, Poller DN, Waisman JR, et al. Prognostic classification of breast ductal carcinoma in situ. *Lancet* 1995;345:1154–1157, with permission.)

For larger lesions, a combination of direct measurement and estimation, based on the distribution of the lesion in a sequential series of slides, was used. The proximity of DCIS to an inked margin was determined by direct measurement or ocular micrometry. The closest single distance between DCIS and an inked margin was the margin width used to calculate the margin score.

Calculating the Original Van Nuys Prognostic Index

The original VNPI formula was determined by using the beta values obtained from the initial multivariate analysis (1,27). The beta values reflect the relative contribution of each factor in the estimation of the likelihood of local recurrence (1,28,45) and were similar for all three factors. This method yielded a relatively user-unfriendly formula with 27 possible VNPI scores. The 27 subgroups naturally divided into three prognostic subgroups. One with a low risk of recurrence, one with an intermediate risk of recurrence, and one with a high risk of local recurrence. Because the beta values for the three factors were similar, additional analyses revealed that the formula could be simplified, without compromising validity, by omitting the beta weighting, suggested by the multivariate analysis, and by readjusting the numerical range for each of the three subgroups. The final formula for the original VNPI became VNPI = pathologic classification score + margin score + size score. This formula yielded a total of seven groups with whole-number scores ranging from 3 to 9. The best possible VNPI score was 3, a score of 1 for each predictor [e.g., a 5-mm, low-grade lesion with widely clear margins (≥10 mm) would earn a score of 3]. The worst possible score was 9; a score of 3 for each predictor [e.g., a 50-mm, high-grade lesion with close or involved margins (<1 mm) would earn a score of 9]. When patients were subdivided into those with scores of 3 or 4 versus 5, 6, or 7 versus 8 or 9, the results were identi-

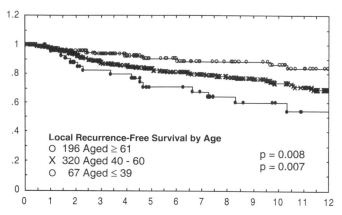

FIGURE 45.7. Probability of local recurrence–free survival by age for 583 patients treated with breast conservation (all *p* = 0.01).

cal when compared with the more complicated beta-weighted version and the VNPI was much easier to use.

The Modified University of Southern California/Van Nuys Prognostic Index

In 1997, we noted that when age was analyzed as a continuous variable, there was an inverse relationship between increasing age and local recurrence. In other words, the older a patient was when diagnosed with DCIS, the less likely she was to recur with all other factors being equal. Figure 45.6 is an updated version of that analysis. In addition, numerous other authors began to report that age was an important factor in predicting local recurrence in patients with DCIS (see Chapter 36) (2–5). Early in 2001, multivariate analysis at USC revealed that age was an independent prognostic factor (Fig. 45.4) and that it should be added to the VNPI with a weight equal to that of the other factors.

An analysis of our local recurrence data by age revealed that the most appropriate break points for our data were between ages 39 and 40 and between ages 60 and 61 (Fig. 45.7). Based on this, a score of 3 was given to all patients 39 years old or younger, a score of 2 was given to patients aged 40 to 60, and a score of 1 was given to patients 61 or older. The new scoring system for the modified USC/VNPI is shown in Table 45.1. The final formula for the modified USC/VNPI became pathologic classification score + margin score + size score + age score.

RESULTS

Patients treated with mastectomy are not included in this analysis. Five hundred eighty-three patients were treated with breast conservation, 346 with excision only, and 237 with excision plus radiation therapy. The patients were divided into three groups with differing probabilities for local recurrence as determined by USC/VNPI score (4, 5, or 6

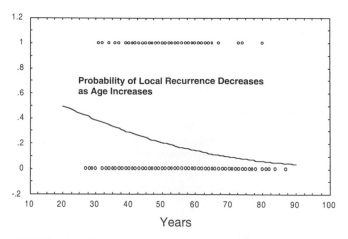

FIGURE 45.6. Using age as a continuous variable, the probability of local recurrence decreases as age increases.

TABLE 45.1. THE UNIVERSITY OF SOUTHERN CALIFORNIA/VAN NUYS PROGNOSTIC INDEX SCORING SYSTEM

	Score		
	1	**2**	**3**
Size (mm)	≤15	16–40	≥41
Margin width (mm)	≥10	1–9	<1
Pathologic classification	Non-high grade without necrosis (nuclear grade 1 or 2)	Non-high grade with necrosis (nuclear grade 1 or 2)	High grade with or without necrosis (nuclear grade 3)
Age (yr)	>60	40–60	<40

One to three points are awarded for each of four different predictors of local breast recurrence (size, margin width, pathologic classification, and age). Scores for each of the predictors are totaled to yield a Van Nuys Prognostic Index score ranging from a low of 4 to a high of 12.

versus 7, 8, or 9 versus 10, 11, or 12). Table 45.2 shows the clinical parameters for each group. The average follow-up for all patients was 83 months.

One hundred nine patients experienced local failure; 48 were treated with excision plus breast irradiation and 61 were treated with excision alone. Of 109 local recurrences, 47 (43%) were invasive; 22 of 48 (46%) in patients treated with excision plus irradiation and 25 of 61 (41%) in patients treated with excision alone (p = NS). Six patients treated with radiation therapy developed local recurrences followed by distant metastases, four of whom have died. One patient treated with excision only developed local and metastatic disease and died of breast cancer. There is no statistical difference in breast cancer–specific survival when patients treated with excision only are compared with those treated with excision plus irradiation (Fig. 45.3). There is no statistical difference in breast cancer–specific survival when patients are compared by USC/VNPI groupings (Fig. 45.8).

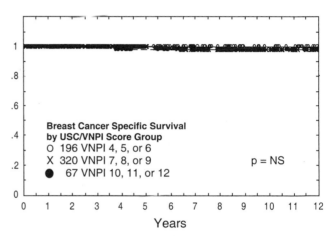

FIGURE 45.8. Probability of breast cancer–specific survival for 583 patients treated with breast conservation grouped by modified University of Southern California/Van Nuys Prognostic Index score (4, 5, or 6 versus 7, 8, or 9 versus 10, 11, or 12) (p = NS).

TABLE 45.2. TUMOR CHARACTERISTICS, RECURRENCES, AND BREAST CANCER DEATHS BY MODIFIED VAN NUYS PROGNOSTIC INDEX GROUPS

	VNPI 4, 5 or 6	VNPI 7, 8, or 9	VNPI 10, 11, or 12	Total
No. of patients treated with breast conservation	196	320	67	583
Average size of tumor (mm)	8.6	17.3	36.0	16.5
Average nuclear grade	1.63	2.43	2.88	2.21
No. of recurrences (%)	4 (2)	70 (22)	35 (52)	109
No. of invasive recurrences (%)	0 (0)	32 (46)	15 (43)	47 (43)
5- & 10-yr local recurrence–free survival (%)	99/96	83/73	54/37	85/77
Breast cancer deaths	0	4	1	5
5- & 10-yr breast cancer–specific survival (%)	100/100	100/97.7	97.6/97.6	99.7/98.5

Patients treated with mastectomy are not included in this table because they are at limited risk of local recurrence.

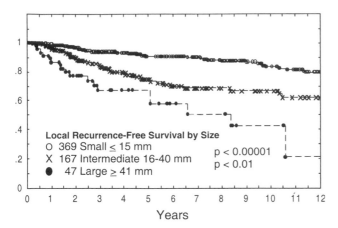

FIGURE 45.9. Probability of local recurrence–free survival by tumor size for 583 patients treated with breast conservation (all p = 0.01).

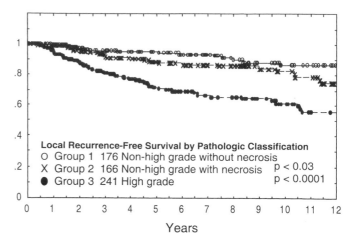

FIGURE 45.11. Probability of local recurrence–free survival for 583 patients treated with breast conservation using Van Nuys ductal carcinoma in situ pathologic classification (all $p < 0.05$).

Fifty additional patients have died of other causes without evidence of recurrent breast cancer. The 12-year actuarial overall survival rate, including deaths owing to all causes, is 90%

The local recurrence–free survival for all 583 patients is shown by tumor size in Figure 45.9, by margin width in Figure 45.10, by pathologic classification in Figure 45.11, and by age in Figure 45.7. The differences between every local disease–free survival curve for each of the four predictors that make up the USC/VNPI are statistically significant.

Figure 45.12 shows all patients by USC/VNPI score (4 to 12), and Figure 45.13 groups patients with low (USC/VNPI score of 4, 5, or 6), intermediate (USC/VNPI score of 7, 8, or 9), or high (USC/VNPI score of 10, 11, or 12) risks of local recurrence together. Each of these three groups is statistically different from one another.

Patients with a USC/VNPI score of 4, 5, or 6 do not show a local disease–free survival benefit from breast irradi-

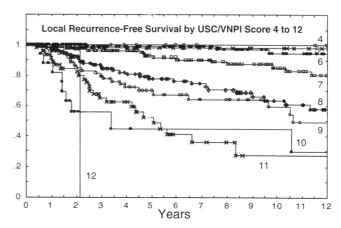

FIGURE 45.12. Probability of local recurrence–free survival for 583 patients treated with breast conservation by modified University of Southern California/Van Nuys Prognostic Index score of 4 to 12.

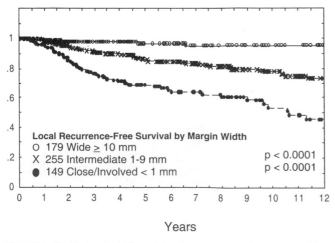

FIGURE 45.10. Probability of local recurrence–free survival by margin width for 583 patients treated with breast conservation (all $p < 0.001$).

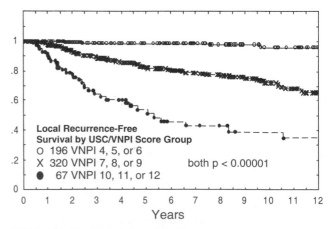

FIGURE 45.13. Probability of local recurrence–free survival for 583 patients treated with breast conservation grouped by modified University of Southern California/Van Nuys Prognostic Index score (4, 5, or 6 versus 7, 8, or 9 versus 10, 11, or 12) (all $p < 0.00001$).

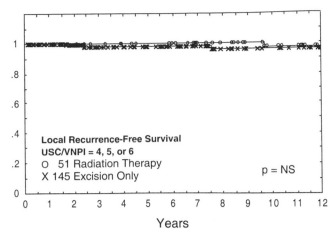

FIGURE 45.14. Probability of local recurrence–free survival by treatment for 196 patients treated with breast conservation with University of Southern California/Van Nuys Prognostic Index scores of 4, 5, or 6 (*p* = NS).

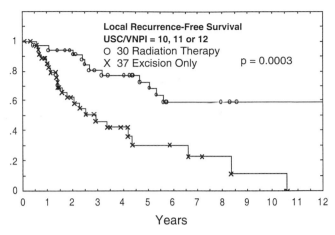

FIGURE 45.16. Probability of local recurrence–free survival by treatment for 67 patients treated with breast conservation with modified University of Southern California/Van Nuys Prognostic Index scores of 10, 11, or 12 (*p* = 0.0003).

ation (Fig. 45.14) (*p* = NS). Patients with an intermediate rate of local recurrence (USC/VNPI score of 7, 8, or 9) benefit from irradiation (Fig. 45.15). There is a statistically significant decrease in local recurrence rate, averaging approximately 10% to 15% throughout the curves, for patients who received radiation therapy with intermediate USC/VNPI scores compared with those treated with excision alone (*p* = 0.03). Figure 45.16 divides patients with USC/VNPI scores of 10, 11, or 12 into those treated with excision plus irradiation and those treated with excision alone. Although the difference between the two groups is highly significant (*p* = 0.0003), conservatively treated patients with DCIS with USC/VNPI scores of 10, 11, or 12 recur at an extremely high rate even with radiation therapy.

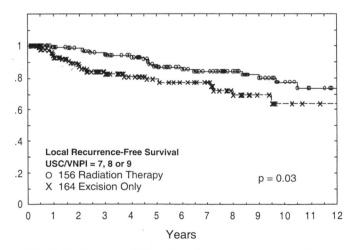

FIGURE 45.15. Probability of local recurrence–free survival by treatment for 320 patients treated with breast conservation with modified University of Southern California/Van Nuys Prognostic Index scores of 7, 8, or 9 (*p* = 0.03).

DISCUSSION

DCIS is a heterogeneous group of lesions, and a uniform approach to treatment is not appropriate. Some patients require no treatment other than excisional biopsy; others benefit from complete excision plus radiation therapy, and some will require mastectomy. The challenge is to use available clinical and pathologic data to select the most appropriate therapy for each patient. The USC/VNPI quantifies the evolving knowledge of prognostic factors in DCIS to define specific subsets of patients for whom treatment with excision alone, excision plus radiation, or mastectomy could be recommended.

Although mastectomy is curative for approximately 99% of patients with DCIS (9–13), mastectomy represents significant overtreatment for most cases detected by current methods. When breast conservation is elected rather than mastectomy, radiation therapy statistically decreases the likelihood of local recurrence compared with excision only (16,20,23), but radiation therapy, like mastectomy, may also represent overtreatment for a significant number patients who elect breast preservation.

The broad recommendation by the NSABP that radiation therapy is appropriate for all patients with DCIS who are treated with breast preservation, although clearly correct based on their data, does not take into account the heterogeneity of DCIS nor the differences in subsets demonstrated by our data (1,13,28) and those of others (29–40) including their own (15,17).

Radiation therapy is not without side effects (24). It changes the texture of the breast, makes subsequent mammography more difficult to interpret, and its use precludes additional radiation therapy and breast conservation should a metachronous invasive breast cancer develop. Radiation therapy should only be offered to those patients with DCIS likely to obtain a substantial benefit.

Subsets of patients who are not likely to receive any significant benefit from radiation therapy can be identified, e.g., those with USC/VNPI scores of 4, 5, or 6 in the series presented here, low-grade lesions in the series of Lagios et al. (30,31,35), small, noncomedo lesions with uninvolved margins in the series of Schwartz (39), or the well-differentiated lesions of Zafrani et al (40). Such patients may account for more than 30% of the total number of patients diagnosed with DCIS (13,29,35,36,39,40,46–48).

Patients in this series with USC/VNPI scores of 10, 11, or 12 present a different problem. Although these patients show the greatest absolute benefit from postexcisional radiation therapy, their local recurrence rate continues to be extremely high and a recommendation for mastectomy should be considered.

Treatment recommendations for the intermediate group (patients with USC/VNPI scores of 7, 8, or 9) are the most difficult. For patients with intermediate USC/VNPI scores and margin scores of 2 or 3, re-excision may improve local disease–free survival. If the score remains intermediate after re-excision, radiation therapy should be considered. However, some patients with scores of 9 may be better treated with mastectomy (e.g., a 50-year-old patient with a large, nuclear grade 2 lesion without necrosis with less than 1 mm margins after re-excision), whereas some patients with scores of 7 (e.g., a 56-year-old patient with widely clear margins, small tumor size, but high nuclear grade) may elect no further treatment. These are independent judgments that must be made by the patient and her physician. I would hope that the USC/VNPI would be a helpful adjunct as these difficult decisions are discussed.

To date, no study of patients with DCIS has shown a statistically significant difference in mortality when the three available treatments (mastectomy, excision only, and excision plus radiation therapy) are compared. However, there are clear differences in local recurrence rates, and they are of extreme importance. Local recurrences in patients who have struggled to save their breasts are both demoralizing and theoretically, if invasive, a threat to life (34,49). In this series (44%) and in most other reported series (3,31,34,39), approximately one-half of all local recurrences are invasive.

Treatment selection bias is not an important factor when using the USC/VNPI because it does not compare different treatments. Rather, the USC/VNPI is based on measured parameters and compares patients who have achieved similar scores. Although the patient and her clinician control treatment selection, neither can influence final margin measurement, tumor size, pathologic classification, or age. The fact that some patients opted for suboptimal treatments that were not recommended (e.g., 67 patients with USC/VNPI scores of 10, 11, or 12 who selected breast-conservation therapy were all advised to undergo mastectomy) was actually helpful in developing and evaluating the USC/VNPI.

Counseling patients with DCIS in a rational manner can be extremely difficult when the range of treatment options is extreme. The USC/VNPI allows a scientifically based discussion with the patient, using the parameters of the lesion obtained after an initial excision. Thus, in some cases, a patient can choose re-excision in an effort to "downscore" her lesion. Successful downscoring of a patient with a USC/VNPI score of 10 or 11 could result in substantial reduction in the risk of local recurrence, perhaps changing a recommendation from mastectomy to radiation therapy. Similarly, patients with close or involved margins, with USC/VNPI scores of 7 or 8 after initial excision could opt for re-excision. Successful downscoring by achieving widely clear margins could result in a final USC/VNPI score sufficiently low to avoid breast irradiation.

Downscoring can be achieved only by re-excising patients with margin scores of 2 or 3. Re-excision will not lower the pathologic classification score nor will it reduce the size of the tumor. In some cases, re-excision will "upscore" the tumor, increasing the USC/VNPI score by revealing a larger tumor size, a higher nuclear grade, the presence of previously undetected comedonecrosis, or an involved margin.

The USC/VNPI may be useful to clinicians because it divides DCIS into three groups with statistically significant different risks for local recurrence after breast-conservation therapy. Although there is an apparent treatment choice for each group (Table 45.3), excision alone for patients with scores of 4, 5, or 6, excision plus radiation therapy for patients with scores of 7, 8, or 9, and mastectomy for patients with scores of 10, 11, or 12, the USC/VNPI is offered only as a guideline, a starting place in the discussions with patients.

This work suggests that patients with DCIS can be stratified into specific subsets based on age, the pathologic classification (using nuclear grade and necrosis), the size of the lesion, and the adequacy of surgical treatment as determined by histologic margin assessment. The USC/VNPI is an attempt to quantify the known important prognostic factors in DCIS, making them clinically useful in the treatment decision-making process.

The validity of the USC/VNPI must be independently and prospectively confirmed by other groups with access to

TABLE 45.3. TREATMENT GUIDELINES: MODIFIED UNIVERSITY OF SOUTHERN CALIFORNIA/VAN NUYS PROGNOSTIC INDEX

Score	Treatment
4–6	Excision alone
7–9	Excision + radiation therapy
10–12	Mastectomy

large numbers of patients with DCIS. In the future, other factors, such as molecular markers, may be integrated into the index when they are shown to be statistically important predictors of local recurrence.

CASE PRESENTATIONS USING THE UNIVERSITY OF SOUTHERN CALIFORNIA/VAN NUYS PROGNOSTIC INDEX AS AN AID IN TREATMENT SELECTION

Case 1: Downscoring (University of Southern California/Van Nuys Prognostic Index Score 8 to 6)

Suspicious branching microcalcifications were noted on screening mammography in a 49-year-old woman. Stereotactic core biopsy revealed low-grade DCIS with necrosis. Multiple wire-directed excision yielded a 12-mm, low-grade cribriform DCIS with comedonecrosis. The lesion was not transected but approached tenuously close to one margin. The USC/VNPI score was 8 (size score = 1, pathologic classification score = 2, margin score = 3, age score = 2). Re-excision was performed and a 2-mm focus of residual DCIS was found adjacent to the excision cavity wall. The re-exci-

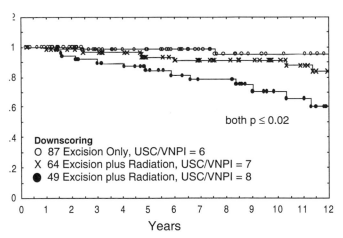

both p ≤ 0.02

Downscoring
O 87 Excision Only, USC/VNPI = 6
X 64 Excision plus Radiation, USC/VNPI = 7
● 49 Excision plus Radiation, USC/VNPI = 8

FIGURE 45.17. The potential benefit of downscoring is illustrated: 49 patients with a University of Southern California/Van Nuys Prognostic Index (USC/VNPI) score of 8 treated with excision plus radiation therapy have a probability of local recurrence–free survival at 12 years of 60%. The probability of local recurrence–free survival for 64 patients with a USC/VNPI score of 7 treated with excision plus radiation therapy was 84%. The probability of local recurrence–free survival for 87 patients with a USC/VNPI score of 6 treated with excision alone was 95%. Re-excision of a patient with a margin less than 1 mm and a USC/VNPI score of 8 can change the USC/VNPI score from 8 to 6, eliminating the need for additional radiation therapy while yielding a statistically significant 35% local recurrence–free survival benefit. If re-excision had achieved clear margins of only 3 to 4 mm rather than more than 10 mm, the patient would have been downscored to a USC/VNPI score of 7. The benefit in local recurrence–free survival with the additional of radiation therapy would be 24% ($p = 0.006$).

sion margins were judged to be clear by more than 10 mm in all directions. This procedure downscored the lesion by converting the margin score from 3 to 1. The pathologic classification score, size score, and age score remained unchanged. The patient now has a USC/VNPI score of 6 and can be considered for no further therapy (Fig. 45.17).

Case 2: Upscoring (University of Southern California/Van Nuys Prognostic Index Score 8 to 10)

A 55-year-old woman presented with mammographically detected microcalcifications and no palpable abnormalities. Wire-directed excision revealed a 5-mm solid DCIS of intermediate grade with focal comedonecrosis. One margin was transected. The USC/VNPI score was 8 (size score = 1, pathologic classification score = 2, margin score = 3, age score = 2). Re-excision revealed extensive residual disease measuring 45 mm. In addition, four foci of high-grade DCIS were found. The margins, however, were clear. The closest margin was now 4 mm. The final USC/VNPI score was 10 (size score = 3, pathologic classification score = 3, margin score = 2, age score = 2). Re-excision upscored the patient's size score to 3 and her pathologic classification score to 3. It downscored her margin score to 2. The patient now has a USC/VNPI score of 10 and would be best treated with mastectomy. An alternative treatment plan would allow the re-excision site to heal for 3 to 6 months and then to re-excise it one more time in the hope of obtaining widely clear margins. If this were to happen, the patient's margin score would become 1 and her USC/VNPI score would become 9. At that point, radiation therapy would be an alternative to mastectomy. However, in this case, I would clearly prefer a mastectomy with immediate breast reconstruction.

This case illustrates that the size score may be unreliable when the lesion is transected or the margin is close. This should be taken into account when considering conservative treatment for patients with involved/close margins. The preoperative mammograms should be reviewed and the size of the lesion estimated from them. This should be factored into the USC/VNPI score.

Case 3: A Random Finding

A 7-mm, low-grade micropapillary DCIS without necrosis was found inadvertently within a breast reduction specimen in a 52-year-old woman. Because this was a reduction, margins were not marked and tissue was not serially sectioned and sequentially processed. Microscopically, the margins appeared widely clear, but the pathologist could not be certain. Prereduction mammography was negative. The USC/VNPI score was 5 or 6 (size score = 1, pathologic classification score = 1, margin score = 1 or 2, age score = 2).

The pathologist cut in the remaining tissue, and no additional foci of DCIS were found. The patient has a final

USC/VNPI score of 5 or 6. I would not treat this patient with radiation therapy. Reduction mammoplasty causes significant postoperative mammographic scarring. Radiation therapy added to this would make future mammography even more difficult. Additionally, this DCIS was found inadvertently without mammographic signs. Under the best of circumstances, mammographic follow-up will be difficult. This patient should be fully apprised that this is a less than optimal circumstance because margins could not be properly evaluated. However, Schwartz et al. (47) reported no local recurrences in 12 similar patients with incidental DCIS treated with excision alone.

Case 4: A University of Southern California/Van Nuys Prognostic Index Score of 7 That Does Not Require Radiation Therapy

The patient was an 81-year-old woman with a screen-detected 15-mm area of microcalcifications. Stereotactic core biopsy revealed high-grade DCIS. Multiple wire–directed excision revealed a 17-mm, high-grade comedo DCIS. The margins were widely clear (>10 mm in all directions). The USC/VNPI score was 7 (size score = 2, pathologic classification score = 3, margin score = 1, age score = 1). Patients in the intermediate group (7, 8, or 9) generally require more thought and discussion. Some patients with scores of 7 may be better served by omitting radiation therapy. Some patients with scores of 9 may be better served by mastectomy. In this particular case, I would not irradiate for the following reasons. The lesion was well marked by calcifications. It measured 15 mm on mammography and 17 mm on the microscopic slides, so in this case, mammography is a good predictor of the extent of the lesion. Postoperative mammography showed no residual microcalcifications. The margins were widely clear and, finally, the patient is 81 years old. Overall, the likelihood of recurrence if radiation therapy is not added is small in this patient. I prefer to omit radiation therapy in a patient of this age whenever possible. If this patient were 45, her USC/VNPI score would increase to 8, and I would be more inclined to treat her with radiation therapy.

Case 5: Downscoring (University of Southern California/Van Nuys Prognostic Index Score 8 to 7)

The patient was a 57-year-old woman with a screen-detected 22-mm area of microcalcifications. Wire-directed excision revealed a 25-mm, intermediate-grade DCIS with comedonecrosis. The closest margin measured 3 mm. The USC/VNPI score was 8 (size score = 2, pathologic classification score = 2, margin score = 2, age score = 2). This patient could be treated with radiation therapy. However, I would prefer to re-excise first. If widely clear margins were obtained, she would be downscored to a USC/VNPI

score of 7. Radiation therapy would continue to be indicated, but the probability of local recurrence would be less than for a patient with a USC/VNPI score of 8. This patient does meet the criteria of Lagios et al. (30), and some physicians might elect to omit postoperative radiation therapy.

Case 6: A University of Southern California/Van Nuys Prognostic Index Score of 9 That is Better Treated with Mastectomy

The patient was a 51-year-old woman with a vaguely palpable upper outer quadrant thickening. Mammography showed a nondiagnostic architectural distortion. Fine needle aspiration revealed moderately atypical cells, and biopsy was suggested. A core biopsy revealed a low-grade DCIS without necrosis (micropapillary architecture). The patient was strongly motivated for breast conservation. A four-wire bracketed upper outer quadrant segmental resection was done. A 70-mm DCIS identical to the core biopsy, extending tenuously close to three margins, was found. The USC/VNPI score was 9 (size score = 3, pathologic classification score = 1, margin score = 3, age score = 2).

In this particular case, a skin-sparing mastectomy with immediate Tranverse Rectus Abdominus Myocutaneous (TRAM) flap reconstruction would be my preference. I would choose this because the lesion is large and extends to multiple margins. Because it is not marked by microcalcifications, it is more difficult to completely excise and will be more difficult to follow postoperatively if breast preservation is elected. If the patient refused mastectomy, I would allow the wound to heal for 3 to 6 months and follow this with a formal quadrantectomy resection. With a low-grade micropapillary lesion, there is little risk in delaying definitive treatment for 6 months. If margins became clear after quadrantectomy, consideration should be given to adding radiation therapy to the treatment plan.

Case 7: The First Excision is the Best Chance to Get Both Clear Margins and A Good Cosmetic Result

The patient was a 52-year-old woman with microcalcifications measuring 48 mm on mammography. A core biopsy revealed high-grade DCIS with comedonecrosis. The patient had a large breast and was strongly motivated for breast preservation if possible. A four-wire directed segmental resection revealed a 52-mm, high-grade DCIS with widely clear margins (>12 mm in all directions). The USC/VNPI score was 9 (size score = 3, pathologic classification score = 3, margin score = 1, age score = 2). She is a candidate for breast preservation with radiation therapy.

At another facility not using stereotactic core biopsy or multiple wires, the case might have been handled somewhat differently. The scenario might have gone like this. A single-wire directed biopsy was performed. A 36-mm, high-grade DCIS with involved margins was found. The USC/VNPI score was 10 (size score = 2, pathologic classification score = 3, margin score = 3, age score = 2). Postoperative mammography revealed residual microcalcifications. The patient continued to be strongly motivated for breast preservation, and a quadrant type re-excision was done. Residual DCIS was found, but the margins were now clear by more than 10 mm in all directions. The USC/VNPI score was 9 (size score = 3, pathologic classification score = 3, margin score = 1, age score = 2). The score is the same as with the first scenario, but it took two operations. Because a formal quadrantectomy was done, the cosmetic result was not quite as good.

Another possibility, using the second scenario, also exists. With a USC/VNPI score of 8 and residual microcalcifications on postoperative mammography, many surgeons would prefer to proceed directly to mastectomy and reconstruction rather than re-excision. I likely would have suggested that.

Case 8: A Young Woman with a University of Southern California/Van Nuys Prognostic Index Score of 6 and a Family History of Breast Cancer

The patient was a 35-year-old woman whose mother and maternal grandmother had both had premenopausal breast cancer. The patient's mother died of breast cancer 5 years after diagnosis. Because of her family history, this patient had her first screening mammogram at age 30. No abnormalities were seen, but her breasts were dense and difficult to evaluate both by physical examination and mammography. She had her second mammogram at age 33, and it showed no abnormalities. This was her third screening mammogram, and this time it revealed worrisome microcalcifications measuring 26 mm in diameter in the upper outer quadrant of her left breast. Stereotactic core biopsy revealed a high-grade lesion with comedonecrosis. No invasion was seen. Because high-grade, comedo-type lesions are generally well marked by microcalcifications, the surgeon thought that by using multiple wires, the entire lesion could be completely excised. If this had happened, the USC/VNPI score would have equaled 9 (size score = 2, pathologic classification score = 3, margin score = 1, age score = 3), and the patient could have been treated with radiation therapy.

She sought numerous additional opinions while wrestling with an extremely difficult decision. Because she was so young, she desperately wanted to save her breast, but because she had so much more time to live, she felt that an invasive recurrence, at some time in the future, was a worrisome possibility. She was concerned that careful clinical and mammographic follow-up would be difficult because she had mam-mographically dense breasts, and radiation therapy would make mammography more difficult. In addition, if she developed a recurrence after radiation, skin-sparing mastectomy would be more difficult to perform successfully. Most of all, she was affected by her mother's premature death, which occurred when the patient was still a teenager. This patient decided to undergo a unilateral mastectomy and immediate reconstruction. She planned to undergo a contralateral prophylactic mastectomy 5 years later regardless of whether any abnormalities developed.

Not all patients would have made this choice. Some might have opted for immediate bilateral mastectomies with or without reconstruction, whereas others might have chosen breast preservation with careful follow-up. The choices for this patient would have been clearer if genetic testing had been available at the time that this patient was treated.

SUMMARY

There is controversy and confusion regarding therapy for patients with DCIS of the breast. The USC/VNPI was developed to aid in the complex treatment selection process. The USC/VNPI combines four significant predictors of local recurrence: tumor size, margin width, age, and pathologic classification (derived from nuclear grade and the presence or absence of comedonecrosis). Scores of 1 (best) to 3 (worst) were assigned for each of the three predictors and then totaled to give an overall USC/VNPI score ranging from 4 to 12.

Five hundred eighty-three patients with pure DCIS treated with breast preservation (346 with excision only and 237 by excision plus radiation therapy) were studied with local recurrence as the marker of treatment failure. There was no statistical difference in the 12-year local recurrence–free survival in patients with USC/VNPI scores of 4, 5, or 6, regardless of whether radiation therapy was used (p = NS). Patients with USC/VNPI scores of 7, 8, or 9 received a statistically significant average 10% to 15% local recurrence–free survival benefit when treated with radiation therapy (p = 0.03). Patients with scores of 10, 11, or 12, although showing the greatest absolute benefit from radiation therapy, experienced local recurrence rates of almost 50% at 5 years.

Patients with DCIS with USC/VNPI scores of 4, 5 or 6 can be considered for treatment with excision only. Patients with intermediate scores (7, 8, or 9) show an average 15% decrease in local recurrence rates with radiation therapy and should be considered for treatment with that modality. Patients with USC/VNPI scores of 10, 11, or 12 exhibit extremely high local recurrence rates, regardless of irradiation, and should be considered for mastectomy, generally with immediate reconstruction.

REFERENCES

1. Silverstein MJ, Lagios MD, Craig PH, et al. A prognostic index for ductal carcinoma in situ of the breast. *Cancer* 1996;77: 2267–2274.
2. Vicini FA, Kestin LL, Goldstein NS, et al. Impact of young age on outcome in patients with ductal carcinoma-in-situ treated with breast-conserving therapy. *J Clin Oncol* 2000;18:296–306.
3. Solin LJ, Kurtz J, Fourquet A, et al. Fifteen year results of breast conserving surgery and definitive breast irradiation for the treatment of ductal carcinoma in situ of the breast. *J Clin Oncol* 1996;14:754–763.
4. Szelei-Stevens KA, Kuske R, Yantos VA, et al. The influence of young age and positive family history of breast cancer on the prognosis of ductal carcinoma in situ treated with excision with or without radiation therapy or mastectomy. *Int J Radiat Oncol Biol Phys* 2000;48:943–949.
5. Goldstein NS, Vicini FA, Kestin LL, et al. Differences in the pathologic features of ductal carcinoma in situ of the breast based on patient age. *Cancer* 2000;88:2552–2560.
6. Patchefsky AS, Schwartz GF, Finkelstein SD, et al. Heterogeneity of intraductal carcinoma of the breast. *Cancer* 1989;63: 731–741.
7. Lennington WJ, Jensen RA, Dalton LW, et al. Ductal carcinoma in situ of the breast. Heterogeneity of individual lesions. *Cancer* 1994;73:118–124.
8. Silverstein MJ. Intraductal breast carcinoma: two decades of progress? *Am J Clin Oncol* 1991;14:534–537.
9. Ashikari R, Hadju SI, Robbins GF. Intraductal carcinoma of the breast. *Cancer* 1971;28:1182–1187.
10. Fentiman IS, Fagg N, Millis RR, et al. In situ ductal carcinoma of the breast: implications of disease pattern and treatment. *Eur J Surg Oncol* 1986;12:261–266.
11. Bradley SJ, Weaver DW, Bouwman DL. Alternative in the surgical management of in situ breast cancer. *Am Surg* 1990; 56:428–432.
12. Rosner D, Bedwani RN, Vana J, et al. Noninvasive breast carcinoma. Results of a national survey of The American College of Surgeons. *Ann Surg* 1980;192:139–147.
13. Silverstein MJ, Barth A, Poller DN, et al. Ten-year results comparing mastectomy to excision and radiation therapy for ductal carcinoma in situ of the breast. *Eur J Cancer* 1995;31: 1425–1427.
14. Fisher B, Costantino J, Redmond C, et al. Lumpectomy compared with lumpectomy and radiation therapy for the treatment of intraductal breast cancer. *N Engl J Med* 1993;328:1581–1586.
15. Fisher ER, Constantino J, Fisher B, et al. Pathologic finding from the National Surgical Adjuvant Breast Project (NSABP) protocol B-17: intraductal carcinoma (ductal carcinoma in situ). *Cancer* 1995;75:1310–1319.
16. Fisher B, Dignam J, Wolmark N, et al. Lumpectomy and radiation therapy for the treatment of intraductal breast cancer: findings from National Surgical Adjuvant Breast and Bowel Project B-17. *J Clin Oncol* 1998;16:441–452.
17. Fisher ER, Dignam J, Tan-Chiu E, et al. Pathologic findings from the National Surgical Adjuvant Breast Project (NSABP) eight-year update of protocol B-17: intraductal carcinoma. *Cancer* 1999;86:429–438.
18. Fisher B, Land S, Mamounas E, et al. Prevention of invasive breast cancer in women with ductal carcinoma in situ: an update of the National Surgical Adjuvant Breast and Bowel Project experience. *Semin Oncol* 2001;28:400–418.
19. Fisher B, Dignam J, Wolmark N. Tamoxifen in treatment of intraductal breast cancer: National Surgical Adjuvant Breast and Bowel Project B-24 randomized controlled trial. *Lancet* 1999;353:1993–2000.
20. Julien JP, Bijker N, Fentiman I, et al. Radiotherapy in breast conserving treatment for ductal carcinoma in situ: first results of EORTC randomized phase III trial 10853. *Lancet* 2000; 355:528–533.
21. Bijker N, Peterse JL, Duchateau L, et al. Risk factors for recurrence and metastasis after breast conserving therapy for ductal carcinoma in situ: analysis of European Organization for Research and Treatment of Cancer Trial 10853. *J Clin Oncol* 2001;19:2263–2271.
22. George WD, Houghton J, Cuzick J, et al. Radiotherapy and tamoxifen following complete local excision (CLE) in the management of ductal carcinoma in situ (DCIS): preliminary results from the UK DCIS trial. *Proc Am Soc Clin Oncol* 2000;19: 70a(abst).
23. UKCCCR DCIS Working Party. The UK, Australian and New Zealand randomized trial comparing radiotherapy and tamoxifen in women with completely excised ductal carcinoma in situ of the breast. (Submitted for publication).
24. Recht A. Side effects of radiation therapy. In: Silverstein MJ, ed. *Ductal carcinoma in situ of the breast.* Baltimore: Williams & Wilkins, 1997:347–352.
25. Early Breast Cancer Trialists' Collaborative Group. Favorable and unfavorable effects on long-term survival of radiotherapy for early breast cancer. *Lancet* 2000;355:1757–1770.
26. Kurtz JM. Radiotherapy for early breast cancer: was a comprehensive overview of trials needed? *Lancet* 2000;355:1739–1740.
27. Silverstein MJ, Barth A, Waisman JR, et al. Predicting local recurrence in patients with intraductal breast carcinoma (DCIS). *Proc Am Soc Clin Oncol* 1995;14:117.
28. Silverstein MJ, Poller DN, Waisman JR, et al. Prognostic classification of breast duct carcinoma in situ. *Lancet* 1995;345: 1154–1157.
29. Silverstein MJ, Lagios MD, Groshen, S, et al. The influence of margin width on local control in patients with ductal carcinoma in situ (DCIS) of the breast. *N Engl J Med* 1999;340:1455–1461.
30. Lagios MD, Westdahl PR, Margolin FR, et al. Duct carcinoma in situ: relationship of extent of noninvasive disease to the frequency of occult invasion, multicentricity, lymph node metastases, and short-term treatment failures. *Cancer* 1982;50:1309–1314.
31. Lagios MD. Duct carcinoma in situ: pathology and treatment. *Surg Clin North Am* 1990;70:853–871.
32. Solin LJ, Yeh I, Kurtz J, et al. Ductal carcinoma in situ (intraductal carcinoma) of the breast treated with breast-conserving surgery and definitive irradiation. *Cancer* 1993;71:2532–2542.
33. Bellamy COC, McDonald C, Salter DM, et al. Noninvasive ductal carcinoma of the breast. The relevance of histologic categorization. *Hum Pathol* 1993;24:16–23.
34. Solin LJ, Fourquet A, McCormick B, et al. Salvage treatment for local recurrence following breast conserving surgery and definitive irradiation for ductal carcinoma in situ (intraductal carcinoma) of the breast. *Int J Radiat Oncol Biol Phys* 1994;30:3–9.
35. Lagios MD, Margolin FR, Westdahl PR, et al. Mammographically detected duct carcinoma in situ. Frequency of local recurrence following tylectomy and prognostic effect of nuclear grade on local recurrence. *Cancer* 1989;63:618–624.
36. Lagios MD. Ductal carcinoma in situ: controversies in diagnosis, biology, and treatment. *Breast J* 1995;1:68–78.
37. Ottesen GL, Graversen HP, Bilcher-Toft M, et al. Ductal carcinoma in situ of the female breast: short term results of a prospective nationwide study. *Am J Surg Pathol* 1992;16:1183–1196.
38. Poller DN, Silverstein MJ, Galea M, et al. Ductal carcinoma in situ of the breast: a proposal for a new simplified histological classification association between cellular proliferation and c-erbB-2 protein expression. *Mod Pathol* 1994;7:257–262.
39. Schwartz GF. The role of excision and surveillance alone in subclinical DCIS of the breast. *Oncology* 1994;8:21–26.

40. Zafrani B, Leroyer A, Fourquet A, et al. Mammographically-detected ductal carcinoma in situ of the breast analysed with a new classification. A study of 127 cases: correlation with estrogen and progesterone receptors, p53 and c-erbB-2 proteins and proliferative activity. *Semin Diagn Pathol* 1994;11:208–213.

41. Silverstein MJ. Prognostic factors that predict recurrence of DCIS. In: Silverstein MJ, ed. *Ductal carcinoma in situ of the breast*. Baltimore: Williams & Wilkins, 1997:271–284.

42. Silverstein MJ. Prognostic factors and local recurrence in patient with ductal carcinoma of the breast. *Breast J* 1998;4:349–362.

43. Silverstein MJ, Lagios MD, Craig PH, et al. The Van Nuys Prognostic Index for ductal carcinoma in situ. *Breast J* 1996;2:38–40.

44. Silverstein MJ, Poller DN, Craig PH, et al. A prognostic index for breast ductal carcinoma in situ. *Breast Cancer Res Treat* 1996;37[Suppl]:34(abst).

45. Galea MH, Blamey RW, Elston CE, et al. The Nottingham Prognostic Index in primary breast cancer. *Breast Cancer Res Treat* 1992;22:207–219.

46. Ottesen GL, Graversen HP, Blichert-Toft M, et al. Ductal carcinoma in situ of the female breast. Short-term results of a prospective nationwide study. *Am J Surg Pathol* 1992;16:1183–1196.

47. Schwartz GF, Finkel GC, Garcia JC, et al. Subclinical ductal carcinoma in situ of the breast. Treatment by local excision and surveillance alone. *Cancer* 1992;70:2468–2474.

48. Solin LJ, Recht A, Fourquet A, et al. Ten-year results of breast-conserving surgery and definitive irradiation for intraductal carcinoma of the breast. *Cancer* 1991;68:2337–2344.

49. Silverstein MJ, Lagios MD, Martino S, et al.. Outcome after invasive local recurrence in patients with ductal carcinoma in situ of the breast. *J Clin Oncol* 1998;16:1367–1373.

46

PROBLEMS WITH THE USE OF THE VAN NUYS PROGNOSTIC INDEX

CONSTANTINOS YIANGOU
MARGARET J. JEFFREY

The management of ductal carcinoma in situ (DCIS) remains one of the most controversial areas in breast cancer. With the introduction of widespread mammographic screening, DCIS has been diagnosed with increasing frequency. In the prescreening era, DCIS accounted for about 5% of breast cancers (1–3); but recently, this has risen to approximately 25% of all newly diagnosed (3–5) and up to 30% of screen-detected breast cancers (6).

The major risk for women with DCIS is local recurrence, not metastatic disease (7,8). The rare occurrence of the latter is usually due to an occult focus of microinvasive carcinoma or residual DCIS progressing to invasive carcinoma. Axillary lymph node metastases are detected in less than 1% of cases of DCIS; and therefore, axillary dissection is not routinely performed in these patients (9,10). Treatment of DCIS should be planned to achieve a near 100% cure from the disease at a time when this is possible, i.e., at presentation. Failure to achieve a cure a presentation results in local recurrence and, in many cases, shorter survival, because approximately 50% of recurrences are invasive carcinomas (11–15). In the past, mastectomy was the preferred treatment for patients with DCIS, resulting in nearly 100% cure rates; but the introduction of breast-conserving surgery for invasive cancers has put extreme pressure on surgeons to apply the same principles when treating DCIS. Prospective randomized trials comparing breast-conserving procedures with radiotherapy and mastectomy showed similar local recurrence rates and survival outcomes in patients with invasive carcinomas (16–19). However, there have only been three randomized prospective trials with DCIS (14,20,21) (see Chapter 44), and some of the evidence comes from retrospective and non-randomized trials (for an overview see Chapters 23 and 24). The results of ongoing prospective randomized trials addressing these points are keenly awaited.

DCIS is not one disease entity, but rather a spectrum of diseases. The various types differ in their pathologic characteristics and mammographic appearances (see Chapter 10) as well as in their biologic behavior (3,22–24). At one end of the spectrum, low-grade DCIS can be difficult to distinguish from atypical ductal hyperplasia (ADH). At the other end, the presentation of large, high-grade lesions may be similar to invasive carcinoma. These fundamental differences must be recognized when diagnosing and treating DCIS. Studies that fail to address these differences and group all types of DCIS together are likely to produce misleading results.

PATHOLOGIC CLASSIFICATION OF DUCTAL CARCINOMA IN SITU

As mentioned above, DCIS is a spectrum of diseases with different histologic architecture, mammographic appearance, molecular characteristics, and clinical behavior. Any pathologic classification system must be based on important histologic features, easy to use, and reproducible. It must correlate with the clinical behavior of DCIS, and predict prognosis and risk of local recurrence, especially after breast-conserving procedures. It must provide help not only to the pathologist during histologic diagnosis but also to the clinician when deciding appropriate treatment.

Several classification systems for DCIS have been devised (see Chapter 63). The pathologic features used in these systems are:

architecture,
presence or grade of necrosis,
cell size,
nuclear grade,
cytoarchitecture,
nucleolar grade,
pattern of microcalcification,
presence of coexisting ADH,
three-dimensional studies of DCIS distribution,
expression of estrogen and progesterone receptors,
c-erbB-2 and p53,
DNA ploidy,
and proliferation fraction (3,11,25–29).

Traditionally, DCIS was classified according to its architectural pattern into

papillary,
micropapillary,
solid,
cribriform,
comedo, and
other rarer special types.

It was soon realized, however, that most DCIS lesions are heterogeneous and consist of a mixture of architectural patterns. Moreover, architecture does not show strong correlation with prognosis. For these reasons, pathologists have moved away from this classification system. In 1990, Lagios (3) described a system dividing DCIS into low, intermediate, and high grade, based on nuclear grade and presence and grade of necrosis. In 1992, the Edinburgh group (25) devised a system based on nuclear grade and architecture, and Ottensen (26) looked at 112 cases and grouped them according to nuclear grade, architecture, cell size, presence of necrosis, and mode of presentation. In 1994, the European Pathologists Working Group (27) used similar criteria to divide DCIS into poorly, intermediately, and well-differentiated groups, and showed clear association between several molecular markers and the degree of differentiation of the tumor. In the same year, the Nottingham group devised a new system based on the presence and degree of necrosis and divided lesions into pure comedo, non-pure comedo, and DCIS without necrosis (28). A retrospective clinical analysis confirmed the validity of this system and showed correlation with expression of molecular markers, DNA ploidy, and proliferation fraction.

The Van Nuys DCIS classification was introduced in 1995 (see Chapter 17). It uses high or non-high nuclear grade and the presence or absence of comedo-type necrosis to divide DCIS into three categories (11). Both parameters have been shown to be significant independent predictors of local recurrence (11,27,30–32). Its superiority over other classification systems is due to its simplicity and reproducibility, and the fact that it uses two parameters easily recognizable by pathologists. Its superiority over the Nottingham classification is in the use of nuclear grade, which puts high nuclear grade lesions without necrosis into the high-risk category; whereas in the Nottingham system, these lesions will be in the best prognostic group. Identification of the intermediate nuclear grade can be difficult, and can cause interobserver variation; however, in the Van Nuys system, this is not a problem because low- and intermediate-grade lesions are grouped together. It also uses necrosis in a qualitative way that makes it easier to apply, because quantitative assessment of necrosis may lead to significant interobserver variation. There is disagreement between pathologists as to how much comedo-type necrosis should be present before classifying a lesion as comedo DCIS. For example, in the Nottingham system, 75% of comedo necrosis

is required to classify a lesion as pure comedo DCIS and 5% to 74% classifies it as non-pure comedo. In the NSABP B-17 study using a cut-off figure of 33%, the DCIS lesions were divided into two groups: those with absent/slight and those with moderate/marked comedo necrosis (20).

The Van Nuys classification has been applied to a large series of patients with DCIS (see Chapter 17), and statistical analyses show clear differences between the three groups in the risk of local recurrence, the expression of various molecular markers, and the effect of radiotherapy on local recurrence rates when used in addition to excision (33,34). This system has also been validated by other groups, and its superiority has been confirmed in comparison with other systems (35).

VAN NUYS PROGNOSTIC INDEX

The above-mentioned classification systems, and in particular the Van Nuys DCIS classification system, provide prognostic information about the different types of DCIS. However, when planning treatment for patients with DCIS, other important prognostic factors should be taken into consideration.

The Van Nuys Prognostic Index (VNPI) was developed for this reason. It does not replace the Van Nuys classification; it incorporates it. The VNPI is based on three important parameters: pathologic classification (per the Van Nuys system), tumor size, and margin width (34,36). This provides a more comprehensive assessment of the risk of local recurrence of DCIS and helps with the planning of treatment. These three factors are significant predictors of local recurrence by univariate as well as multivariate analyses (33). The modified USC/Van Nuys prognostic index adds a fourth factor, age (see Chapter 45).

Over the years, clinical experience played an important part in planning treatment. A high-grade lesion close to the margin was further treated with surgery, radiotherapy, or both; whereas a well-defined, low-grade lesion with good margins was suitable for observation after a breast-conserving procedure. Non-randomized trials (3,12,15,26,31,37, 38) also provided some guidance, but the two randomized, prospective trials—although showing the importance of radiotherapy—did not provide us with detailed subset analysis (14,20,21,39,40).

The results of ongoing randomized trials (41) will hopefully present useful information about different treatment strategies for various subsets of DCIS. In the meantime, the VNPI appears to be the most useful aid in deciding the best treatment options in patients with DCIS and helps standardize the treatment that is offered in different institutions.

The validity of the VNPI depends on careful assessment of its three constituent factors. This is an area where the expertise of the surgeon, radiologist, and pathologist play a crucial role in the preoperative assessment of the patient as well as the preoperative and postoperative assessment of the specimen. In any given case of DCIS, correlation of mammograms with operative findings and specimen analysis is vital in the accurate estimation of the VNPI. Mammographically detected DCIS is completely different from symptomatic breast cancer, and should be managed by specialists who have been trained in the use of the above methods.

We have already discussed the Van Nuys DCIS classification, which defines three different groups of DCIS based on two pathologic parameters. We would now like to discuss the other two factors of the VNPI, namely, tumor size and excision margins.

EXCISION MARGINS

When discussing excision margins of breast cancer, and DCIS in particular, three questions must be addressed:

(i)   what is an adequate margin?,
(ii) preoperative assessment of excision margins, and
(iii) pathologic examination of excision margins.

What is an Adequate Margin?

There is strong disagreement among surgeons and pathologists as to what constitutes an adequate margin after wide excision of DCIS. This failure to agree on a figure has led to wide variation in both surgical practice and in the margin that a surgeon aims to achieve and is prepared to accept as adequate. The concept of multifocality and multicentricity of DCIS with incidence varying from 0% to 80% (42–45) complicates the issue further and has serious implications on margin adequacy. Multifocality or extensive disease within the same quadrant is quite common, and true multicentricity is uncommon. In our practice (and that of others), the vast majority of local recurrences are near the site of the original tumor and are rarely in a different quadrant (20,31,37,46). In the majority of cases, "recurrence" is due to persistent residual disease. Unfortunately, the lack of a uniform definition has led to different studies reporting quite different results. Moreover, by simply failing to identify connections between these apparently separate tumor foci, "inadequate" pathologic examination of specimens using standard two-dimensional plane assessment may overestimate the incidence of multifocal DCIS. Whole-organ studies using a three dimensional technique and stereomicroscopy (described in Chapter 22) provide a more accurate assessment of multifocality by looking at the pattern of growth of a given tumor and establishing whether it is continuous or discontinuous (47). The study of Faverly et al. (47) shows that multifocality is more often present in the better-differentiated tumors (around 70% of well-differen-

tiated DCIS versus 10% of the poorly differentiated DCIS), and that gaps less than 5 mm between different foci were present in 63% of the tumors. In this study on a series of 60 patients, a 5 mm margin of excision would have been adequate in 82% of the cases and a 10 mm margin in 92%. Similar results have been reported by two other groups. Silverstein et al. (46), showed that when the margin was less than 1 mm, the incidence of residual disease was 76%, compared with 43% when the margin was 1 mm or greater. In a small retrospective study of 79 patients, Lagios et al. (30) showed that recurrence rates were 68% and 20% for margins less than 1 mm and 1 to 9 mm, respectively. Arnesson et al. (48) showed in a small number of patients treated with excision and radiotherapy, that the risk of local recurrence was 38% when the margin was less than 5 mm and only 6% for margins greater than 5 mm. Moreover, the results of the Nottingham group and the Lagios/Van Nuys series clearly demonstrated that margins of at least 10 mm were associated with very low recurrence rates (4% to 6%) (49,50).

The VNPI margin scoring system divides patients into three groups: margin greater than or equal to 10 mm, margin 1 to 9 mm, and margin less than 1 mm with scores of 1, 2, and 3, respectively. This, perhaps, is an oversimplification of a complex issue. The middle category is too wide and, although it has been shown that recurrence-free survival for this group of patients is somewhere between the other two groups, a 2 mm margin is unlikely to have the same prognostic value as an 8 mm margin. The adequacy of a 5 mm margin has been addressed above, and Faverly et al. (47) have shown that gaps of 5 mm or greater between DCIS foci were present in seven of 27 well-differentiated lesions but only in one of 19 poorly differentiated tumors. Assuming that a well-differentiated tumor corresponds to groups 1 or 2 and a poorly differentiated tumor to group 3 of the Van Nuys classification, margin scoring for these groups should be different. Dividing the 1 to 9 mm group into two groups (1 to 5 mm, and 6 to 9 mm) would allow changes to be made to the scoring system that would take into account the nuclear grade of the tumor. Based on this new scheme, a high-grade tumor with a 7 mm margin would be given a lower score than a low-grade tumor with the same margin (1 and 2, respectively). This suggestion would need to be validated with a large series of patients with DCIS, of course.

Preoperative Margin Assessment

Frozen section examination has no place in the assessment of DCIS excision margins (40,51). Specimen radiography, however, is mandatory for all cases of screening-detected DCIS. Careful surgery aims at removing the tumor in one piece and avoiding displacement of the guide-wire, which should remain in situ and act as a marker during specimen radiography. The surgeon may place sutures or staples to help further orient the specimen. High-quality, digital radiographic equipment should be used, and the surgeon, radiologist, and pathologist should review the radiographs together. Single-plane specimen radiography, as advocated by the Nottingham group, concentrates on the circumferential margin of the cylindrical specimen (49). Two-plane radiography should increase the specificity of margin assessment; however, a study by Graham et al. (52) showed that on pathologic examination, 38 of 56 patients with radiographically clear margins actually had involved margins.

This is due to the fact that conventional mammography and specimen radiography usually underestimate the extent of the tumor and overestimate the excision margins. DCIS sometimes extends beyond the area of microcalcifications (MCC). In the absence of a mammographic mass or distortion, it is virtually impossible to estimate the distance from the nearest excision plane. Using whole-organ studies in a small series of patients with DCIS, Holland et al. (53) demonstrated that if the surgeon aims for a 2 cm margin beyond the mammographic MCC, complete excision of the tumor will be achieved in 83% of cases. Compression and magnification views may increase the accuracy of this method, but also may cause significant disruption of the specimen.

Three-plane specimen radiography that assesses all six excision margins may prove superior to previously described methods. There is no doubt that the thoroughness of the surgeon in excising the tumor in one piece, proper orientation of the specimen, and correlation with the appropriate radiographs provide the pathologist with the best opportunity to accurately assess margins. Failure to do so results in the calculation of a misleading VNPI score for the patient.

Pathologic Examination of Excision Margins

Numerous methods have been described for the assessment of excision margins (49,54) (Chapters 16 and 20). Different techniques are used by different pathologists (sometimes with different results), and this has significant clinical implications.

Sequential processing of the whole specimen, as described by Lagios in Chapter 16, must be considered the gold standard. The specimen is inked either with one color (but preferably with a different color for each margin) and then cut in 2 to 3 mm slices. Radiographs are then obtained and correlated with pre- and perioperative radiographs. Ideally, the entire specimen should be examined to allow accurate assessment of excision margins. In reality, however, this approach generates a significant increase in the workload of breast pathologists who must examine multiple sections in the case of large specimens. The use of large tissue blocks and macrosections can be very helpful, but is time consuming and expensive (54). Therefore, a selective approach has

been adopted by most pathologists in the United Kingdom who examine segments of the specimen that are selected after careful correlation with the relevant radiographs.

The Nottingham group advocates a method that involves the "onion skinning" of margins (49). The excision margins of the cylindrical specimen are assessed by taking radial blocks that include tumor and margin and shaving blocks from the circumferential margins.

There is no doubt that a selective approach to specimen processing may result in the incomplete assessment of margins and, therefore, the information used to calculate the VNPI score can be inaccurate. Close cooperation between surgeon and pathologist is essential.

TUMOR SIZE

Tumor size is a significant prognostic indicator of local recurrence in patients treated with breast conservation for DCIS. In a combined series of 394 patients, Silverstein and Lagios (30,33,55,56) showed that the chance of local recurrence increases as tumor size increases. Using a statistical model as described in Chapter 45, the tumors were divided in three groups according to their size: small (up to 15 mm), medium (16 to 40 mm), and large (> 40 mm). As the probability of local recurrence is significantly different in the three groups (7%, 24%, and 55% for small, medium, and large tumors, respectively), this grouping system is used in the VNPI (34). In Lagios' original series, all 79 patients had tumors up to 25 mm in diameter and were treated with breast-conserving procedure without radiotherapy. They were divided into two groups according to tumor size: those with tumors up to 15 mm, and those with tumors measuring 16 to 25 mm, and recurrence rates were 15% and 50%, respectively. However, the NASBP B-17 trial found that tumor size was not a significant predictor of local recurrence (39).

The size of a palpable, usually invasive breast cancer refers to the maximum diameter of the tumor. This approach, however, is not very useful in the vast majority of patients with DCIS who have impalpable lesions. Radiologic and pathologic methods are therefore used for measuring the extent of DCIS. The size of a focus of DCIS can sometimes be estimated by measuring the area of MCC on the mammogram. However, this approach can over- or underestimate the extent of the disease in some cases if the DCIS extends beyond the area of MCC or if MCC due to benign disease are present adjacent to the focus of DCIS. Holland and Hendriks (53) showed that mammography generally underestimates the true size of DCIS by an average of 1 to 2 cm; whereas in the EORTC trial 10853, the mammographic diameter tended to be larger than the histologic diameter of the DCIS (40). When the MCC is linear, branching, or coarse, the extent of the disease can be estimated with greater accuracy. Estimation of size tends to be inaccurate in well-differentiated DCIS, which is associated with fine granular MCC (57). Specimen radiography is also useful, but its accuracy is similar to that of preoperative mammography. The presence of several foci of MCC further complicates the issue. The use of multiple stereotactic core biopsies both of areas of MCC and of the surrounding areas may give a better estimate of the extent and multifocality of the disease so that decisions about the most appropriate treatment option can be made preoperatively.

Pathologic estimation of the size of DCIS can be very difficult and is often inaccurate. Macroscopic measurement of the lesion is often not possible in screening-detected DCIS because of the absence of a palpable or visible mass when processing the specimen. The first Philadelphia DCIS Consensus Conference in 1997 concluded that the whole specimen should be sliced into 2 to 3 mm–thick slices, with the size of DCIS estimated from the number of slices that contain tumor (58). For small DCIS lesions that are present on only one slide, a direct microscopic measurement can be made of its maximum diameter. Careful correlation of the serial slices with preoperative mammograms and specimen radiographs allows three-dimensional reconstruction of the lesion, which then helps with the microscopic measurement of the lesion.

True multifocality and the discontinuous growth of some DCIS lesions, especially low-grade lesions, make tumor size measurement very difficult. Holland and colleagues' whole-organ study (47) with a three-dimensional technique clearly showed that ductal connections exist between some foci of DCIS; therefore, what appears as multifocal disease in two dimensions may actually be unifocal disease in three dimensions. This obviously has serious implications in estimating tumor size.

There is no doubt that tumor size is an independent predictor of local recurrence in patients with DCIS treated with breast-conserving procedures (30,33,34,55,56). As such, it is one of the three parameters of the VNPI. However, in order to calculate the index, the value of any prognostic index is based on the accuracy of the information entered. Unfortunately, pathologic techniques have not been standardized and vary from department to department. In the EORTC trial 10853, pathologic size was only given in 45% of cases and microscopic size in only 17% of cases (40). As previously mentioned, because of the large workload they generate, serial sectioning and microscopic assessment of the whole specimen have not been adopted by many pathology departments. This may lead to unreliable results and the calculation of a misleading VNPI score.

SUMMARY

The management of DCIS remains a challenge. The principles used in the treatment of invasive breast carcinoma cannot, on the whole, be applied to DCIS. What makes treatment selection difficult is

first, the heterogeneity of DCIS lesions,

second, the fact that as a preinvasive disease, DCIS is potentially curable, and

third, the fact that its natural history is not fully known.

Prognostic indices for DCIS (the VNPI, in particular) are designed to help in decision making and selection of the most appropriate treatment for each patient. The choice, of course, is between complete excision alone, complete excision and radiotherapy, and mastectomy.

Undertreatment may result in local recurrence and even decreased survival if the recurrent carcinoma is invasive. Overtreatment may be associated with significant morbidity. Radiotherapy can have side effects and can only be given once; whereas mastectomy may be associated with significant psychological morbidity. In the era of breast-conserving surgery for invasive carcinoma, it is very difficult to justify to asymptomatic patients the need for a more aggressive approach to their mammographically detected preinvasive cancer.

The suggestion that patients with DCIS can be divided into three groups according to their VNPI score and each group allocated one of the above treatments is an oversimplification of a difficult problem and does not take clinical experience into account. Treating patients with VNPI scores 3 or 4 with excision alone and those with scores 8 or 9 with mastectomy is reasonable. However, the middle group with scores 5, 6, or 7 is more diverse and, therefore, treating all these patients with excision and radiotherapy may be inappropriate. In this group, the relative contribution of the three components of the VNPI should be taken into consideration, because a large, low-grade lesion with necrosis (group 2 of the Van Nuys DCIS classification) with good margins may be treated adequately with complete excision followed by observation.

For any prognostic index to achieve universal acceptance, it must be simple to use and reproducible. On the surface, the VNPI fulfills these criteria. However, for the reasons mentioned above, we doubt whether reliable and reproducible results can be achieved for all patients with DCIS, especially in the assessment of nuclear grade, margins of excision, and tumor size. The way margins and tumor size were reported in the two randomized trials supports this view (39,40). Moreover, in their series of 367 patients with DCIS, de Mascarel et al. (13) found an unexpectedly high percentage of low-grade lesions without necrosis and lower VNPI. Although they used the same histologic criteria as Silverstein, this finding raises questions about the pathologic interpretation of their specimens. What is very interesting is the high local recurrence rate in their low VNPI group (4.5 times higher than the one reported by Silverstein et al.), which could be due to the narrower margins in this series, although, perhaps, some of the intermediate VNPI tumors were underscored and placed in the low VNPI group (13,56).

The fact that multifocality varies according to the degree of differentiation of the tumor (with high nuclear grade lesions showing more continuous growth) indicates that scoring systems for excision margins should be modified to take nuclear grade into consideration.

There is no clear definition of what constitutes a clear margin. It appears that a 1 mm margin is inadequate, whereas achieving a 10 mm margin while maintaining good cosmesis is not always possible. Therefore, identifying lesions that do not require a 10 mm margin would be useful.

Meticulous pathologic examination of the specimen by looking at, on average, more than 30 tissue sections will have serious implications on the workload of busy pathology departments. It is very doubtful that many units could currently provide such a detailed assessment of margin status and tumor size. This may lead to gross inaccuracies in calculating the VNPI.

The predictive power of the VNPI depends on the standardization of surgical and pathologic practices. This will hopefully eliminate the variation in the management of DCIS that currently exists between different institutions. The recently published report on the diagnostic and therapeutic procedures in the EORTC 10853 trial clearly showed the variations in surgical practice and pathologic processing and analysis of the DCIS specimens. A high percentage of the reports were incomplete, because exact margin status was stated in only 5% of cases, no margin status was mentioned in 14%, and less than half of the reports stated pathologic size of the tumor (40). In some cases of DCIS, estimation of tumor size may be difficult; de Mascarel et al. (13) suggested that the percentage of positive blocks should be used instead.

The three constituent factors of the VNPI are very important and, as mentioned above, are linked to local recurrence. However, it is very likely that age or other biologic factors may be as (or more) important in predicting clinical outcome (59,60).

The challenge now is to identify both patients who need minimal treatment for their DCIS as well as a way of accurately predicting which lesions will progress to invasive malignancy.

KEY POINTS

- The management of DCIS remains controversial.
- The VNPI provides a more comprehensive assessment of the risk of local recurrence of DCIS and helps plan treatment.
- The value of any prognostic index is based on the accuracy of the information entered in order to calculate the index.

- True multifocality and the discontinuous growth of some DCIS tumors may lead to incomplete excision and make assessment of margins and tumor size difficult and inaccurate.
- Serial sectioning and microscopic assessment of the specimen, careful correlation with radiographs, and three dimensional reconstruction of the tumor make measurement of margin width and tumor size more accurate.
- The predictive power of the VNPI depends on the standardization of surgical and pathologic practices to eliminate the variation in the management of DCIS that currently exists between different institutions.

REFERENCES

1. Rosner D, Bedwani RN, Vana J, et al. Non-invasive breast carcinoma: results of a national survey by the American College of Surgeons. *Ann Surg* 1980;192:139–147.
2. Schnitt SF, Silen W, Sadowsky NL, et al. Ductal carcinoma in situ (intraductal carcinoma of the breast). *N Engl J Med* 1988;318:898–903.
3. Lagios MD. Duct carcinoma in situ: pathology and treatment. *Surg Clin North Am* 1990;70:853–871.
4. Schwartz GF, Feig SA, Patchefsky A. Significance and staging of nonpalpable carcinomas of the breast. *Surg Gynaecol Obstet* 1988;166:6–10.
5. Silverstein MJ, Gamagami P, Colburn WJ, et al. Nonpalpable breast lesions: diagnosis with slightly overpenetrated screenfilm mammography and hook wire–directed breast biopsy in 1,014 cases. *Radiology* 1989;171:633–638.
6. Ernster VL, Barclay J, Kerlikowske K, et al. Incidence of and treatment for ductal carcinoma in situ of the breast. *JAMA* 1996;275:913–918.
7. Lagios MD, Westdahl PR, Margolin FR, et al. Duct carcinoma in situ: relationship of extent of noninvasive disease to the frequency of occult invasion, multicentricity, lymph node metastases, and short-term treatment failures. *Cancer* 1982;50:1309–1314.
8. Silverstein MJ, Gierson ED, Colburn WJ, et al. Axillary lymphadenectomy for intraductal carcinoma of the breast. *Surg Gynaecol Obstet* 1991;172:211–214.
9. van Dongen J, Holland R, Peterse JL, et al. Ductal carcinoma in-situ of the breast; second EORTC consensus meeting. *Eur J Cancer* 1992;28:626–629.
10. Yiangou C, Shousha S, Sinnett HD. Primary tumor characteristics and axillary lymph node status in breast cancer. *Br J Cancer* 1999;80:1974–1978.
11. Silverstein MJ, Poller DN, Waisman JR. Prognostic classification of breast ductal carcinoma in situ. *Lancet* 1995;345:1154–1157.
12. Solin LJ, Kurtz J, Fourquet A, et al. Fifteen-year results of breast-conserving surgery and definitive breast irradiation for the treatment of ductal carcinoma in situ of the breast. *J Clin Oncol* 1996;14:754–763.
13. de Mascarel I, Bonichon F, MacGrogan G, et al. Application of the Van Nuys prognostic index in a retrospective series of 367 ductal carcinomas in situ of the breast examined by serial macroscopic sectioning: Practical considerations. *Breast Cancer Res Treat* 2000;61:151–159.
14. Julien J-P, Bijker N, Fentiman IS, et al, on behalf of the EORTC Breast Cancer Cooperative Group and EORTC Radiotherapy

Group. Radiotherapy in breast-conserving treatment for ductal carcinoma in situ: first results of the EORTC randomised phase III trial 10853. *Lancet* 2000;355:528–533.

15. Silverstein MJ, Barth A, Poller DN, et al. Ten-year results comparing mastectomy to excision and radiation therapy for ductal carcinoma in situ of the breast. *Eur J Cancer* 1995;31: 1425–1427.

16. Fisher B, Redmond C, Poisson R, et al. Eight-year results of a randomized clinical trial comparing total mastectomy and lumpectomy with or without irradiation in the treatment of breast cancer. *N Engl J Med* 1989;320:822–828.

17. Sarrazin D, Le MG, Arriagada R, et al. Ten-year results of a randomized trial comparing a conservative treatment to mastectomy in early breast cancer. *Radiother Oncol* 1989;14:177–184.

18. Veronesi U, Banfi A, Salvadori B, et al. Breast conservation is the treatment of choice in small breast cancer: long-term results of a randomized trial. *Eur J Cancer* 1990;26:668–670.

19. Jacobson JA, Danforth DN, Cowan KH, et al. Ten-year results of a comparison of conservation with mastectomy in the treatment of stage I and II breast cancer. *N Engl J Med* 1995;332:907–911.

20. Fisher B, Costantino J, Redmond C, et al. Lumpectomy compared with lumpectomy and radiation therapy for the treatment of intraductal breast cancer. *N Engl J Med* 1993;328:1581–1586.

21. Fisher B, Dignam J, Wolmark N, et al. Lumpectomy and radiation therapy for the treatment of intraductal breast cancer: findings from National Surgical Adjuvant Breast and Bowel Project B-17. *J Clin Oncol* 1998;16:441–452.

22. Poller DN, Ellis IO. Ductal carcinoma in situ (DCIS) of the breast. In: Kirkham N, Lemoine NR, eds. *Progress in Pathology*. Vol. 2. London: Churchill Livingstone, 1995:47–88.

23. Micale MA, Visscher DW, Gulino SE, et al. Chromosomal aneuploidy in proliferative breast disease. *Hum Pathol* 1994;25: 29–35.

24. Stratton MR, Collins N, Lakhani SR, et al. Loss of heterozygosity in ductal carcinoma in situ of the breast. *J Pathol* 1995;175:195–201.

25. Bellamy CO, McDonald C, Salter DM, et al. Noninvasive ductal carcinoma of the breast: the relevance of histologic categorization. *Hum Pathol* 1993;24:16–23.

26. Ottesen GL, Graversen HP, Blichert TM, et al. Ductal carcinoma in situ of the female breast. Short-term results of a prospective nationwide study. The Danish Breast Cancer Cooperative Group. *Am J Surg Pathol* 1992;16:1183–1196.

27. Holland R, Peterse JL, Millis RR, et al. Ductal carcinoma in situ: a proposal for a new classification. *Semin Diagn Pathol* 1994;11:167–180.

28. Poller DN, Silverstein MJ, Galea M, et al. Ideas in pathology. Ductal carcinoma in situ of the breast: a proposal for a new simplified histological classification association between cellular proliferation and c-erbB-2 protein expression. *Mod Pathol* 1994;7: 257–262.

29. Lennington WJ, Jensen RA, Dalton LW, et al. Ductal carcinoma in situ of the breast. Heterogeneity of individual lesions. *Cancer* 1994;73:118–124.

30. Lagios MD, Margolin FR, Westdahl PR, et al. Mammographically detected duct carcinoma in situ. Frequency of local recurrence following tylectomy and prognostic effect of nuclear grade on local recurrence. *Cancer* 1989;63:618–624.

31. Solin LJ, Yeh IT, Kurt J, et al. Ductal carcinoma in situ (intraductal carcinoma) of the breast treated with breast-conserving surgery and definitive irradiation: correlation of pathologic parameters with outcome of treatment. *Cancer* 1993;71:2532–2542.

32. Sneige N, McNesse MD, Atkinson EN, et al. Ductal carcinoma in situ treated with lumpectomy and irradiation: histopathological analysis of 49 specimens with emphasis on risk factors and long-term results. *Hum Pathol* 1995;126:642–649.

33. Silverstein MJ, Barth A, Waisman JR, et al. Predicting local recurrence in patients with intraductal breast carcinoma (DCIS). *Proc Am Soc Clin Oncol* 1995;14:117.

34. Silverstein MJ, Lagios MD, Craig PH, et al. A prognostic index for ductal carcinoma in situ of the breast. *Cancer* 1996;77:2 267–2274.

35. Douglas-Jones AG, Gupta SK, Attanoos RL, et al. A critical appraisal of six modern classifications of ductal carcinoma in situ of the breast (DCIS): correlation with grade of associated invasive carcinoma. *Histopathology* 1996;29:397–409.

36. Silverstein MJ, Lagios MD, Craig PH, et al. The Van Nuys Prognostic Index for ductal carcinoma in situ. *Breast J* 1996;2:38–40.

37. Schwartz GF, Finkel GC, Garcia JC, et al. Subclinical ductal carcinoma in situ of the breast. Treatment by local excision and surveillance alone. *Cancer* 1992;70:2468–2474.

38. Lagios MD. Ductal carcinoma in situ: controversies in diagnosis, biology, and treatment. *Breast J* 1995;1:68–78.

39. Fisher ER, Dignam J, Tan-Chiu E, et al. Pathologic findings from the National Surgical Adjuvant Breast Project (NSABP) eight-year update of Protocol B-17: intraductal carcinoma. *Cancer* 1999;86:429–438.

40. Bijker N, Rutgers EJT, Peterse JL, et al. Variations in diagnostic and therapeutic procedures in a multicentre, randomized clinical trial (EORTC 10853) investigating breast-conserving treatment for DCIS. *Eur J Surg Oncol* 2001;27:135–140.

41. Fowble B. The role of radiotherapy in the treatment of ductal carcinoma in situ: the challenge of the 1990s. *Breast J* 1996;2:45–51.

42. Patchefsky AS, Schwartz GF, Finkelstein SD, et al. Heterogeneity of intraductal carcinoma of the breast. *Cancer* 1989;63: 731–741.

43. Ashikari R, Haidu SI, Robbins GF. Intraductal carcinoma of the breast. *Cancer* 1971;28:1182–1187.

44. Alpers CE, Wellings SR. The prevalence of carcinoma in situ in normal and cancer-associated breasts. *Hum Pathol* 1985; 16; 796–807.

45. Posner MC, Wolmark N. Noninvasive breast carcinoma. *Breast Cancer Res Treat* 1992;21:155–164.

46. Silverstein MJ, Gierson ED, Colburn WJ, et al. Can intraductal breast carcinoma be excised completely by local excision? Clinical and pathologic predictors. *Cancer* 1994;73:2985–2989.

47. Faverly DRG, Burgers L, Bult P, et al. Three-dimensional imaging of mammary ductal carcinoma in situ: clinical implications. *Semin Diagn Pathol* 1994;11:193–198.

48. Arnesson LG, Smeds S, Fagerberg G, et al. Follow-up of two treatment modalities for ductal cancer in situ of the breast. *Br J Surg* 1989;76:672–675.

49. Sibbering DM, Pinder SE, Obuszko Z, et al. Local excision with a 10 mm margin as sole treatment for ductal carcinoma in situ of the breast. *Eur J Cancer* 1996;32A(Suppl 2):24.

50. Poller DN, Silverstein MJ, Lagios MD, et al. Use of a prognostic index for breast ductal carcinoma in situ: is excision margin status still the most crucial factor in predicting disease recurrence? *J Pathol* 1996;178(Suppl):6A.

51. Pinder SE, Elston CW, Ellis IO. The role of pre-operative diagnosis of breast cancer. *Histopathology* 1996;28:563–566.

52. Graham RA, Homer MJ, Sigler CJ, et al. The efficacy of specimen radiography in evaluating the surgical margins of impalpable breast carcinoma. *AJR Am J Roentgenol* 1994;162:33–36.

53. Holland R, Hendriks JHCL. Microcalcifications associated with ductal carcinoma in situ: mammographic-pathologic correlation. *Semin Diagn Pathol* 1994;11:181–192.

54. Jackson PA, Merchant W, McCormick CJ, et al. A comparison of large block macrosectioning and conventional techniques in breast pathology. *Virchows Arch* 1994;425:243–248.

55. Silverstein MJ, Poller DN, Craig PH, et al. A prognostic index for breast ductal carcinoma in situ. *Breast Cancer Res Treat* 1996;37[Suppl]:34(abst).

56. Silverstein MJ, Lagios MD. Ductal carcinoma in situ of the breast: factors predicting recurrence and how they can be used in treatment planning. *Oncology* 1997;11(3):393–410.

57. Holland R, Hendriks JHCL, Verbeek ALM, et al. Extent, distribution, and mammographic/histological correlations of breast ductal carcinoma in situ. *Lancet* 1990;335:519–522.

58. Schwartz GF, Lagios MD, Carter D, et al. Consensus conference of the classification of Ductal Carcinoma in Situ. *Hum Pathol* 1997;28(11):1221–1225.

59. Solin LJ, McCormick B, Recht A, et al. Mammographically detected, clinically occult ductal carcinoma in situ treated with breast-conserving surgery and definitive breast irradiation. *Cancer J* 1996;2:158–165.

60. Van Zee KJ, Liberman L, Samli B, et al. Long term follow-up of women with ductal carcinoma in situ treated with breast-conserving surgery: The effect of age. *Cancer* 1999;86:1757–1767.

47

MARGIN WIDTH AS THE SOLE PREDICTOR OF LOCAL RECURRENCE IN PATIENTS WITH DUCTAL CARCINOMA IN SITU OF THE BREAST

MELVIN J. SILVERSTEIN

INTRODUCTION

Radiation therapy for ductal carcinoma in situ (DCIS) works. The published prospective randomized trials (1–10) as well as our work (Fig. 47.1) (Chapter 21, Sposto, Epstein, Silverstein) reveal an approximate 50% reduction in local recurrence for patients treated with radiation therapy compared with those treated with excision alone. But is radiation therapy required in every case when breast conservation is the planned treatment? And if it is not, how can we select those patients that can be treated with excision alone?

Previously, we proposed the Van Nuys Prognostic Index (VNPI) as an aid in the treatment selection process (11). Earlier in this text (Chapter 45, Silverstein), we modified the VNPI to include age, another important predictive factor (6,12–16), and renamed it the USC/VNPI.

The VNPI has been criticized because two of its components, size and nuclear grade, may be difficult to reproduce for a given case from laboratory to laboratory (17). In this chapter, we explore the possibility of using margin width alone as the sole predictor of local recurrence. It is not likely that margin width alone will be as good as the USC/VNPI, because the latter is made up of five important factors, including margin width. But margin width is such an important factor (Fig. 47.1) that, even by itself, it is an excellent predictor of outcome as measured by local recurrence.

Why Not Let the Prospective Randomized Trials Answer the Question?

None of the three prospective randomized trials performed for DCIS [one performed by the National Surgical Adjuvant Breast Project (NSABP B-17) (1,3,6), one performed by the European Organization for Cancer Research and Treatment EORTC 10853 (7), and one performed by the United Kingdom Coordinating Committee on Cancer Re-

search (UKCCCR) (generally referred to at the U.K. trial) (9,10) (Chapter 44)] can answer the sophisticated questions that patients and doctors ask today. Precisely which subgroups of patients with DCIS will benefit from postexcisional radiation therapy and by exactly how much?

The problem with the three prospective randomized trials is that they were designed in the 1980s to answer a single broad question: does radiation therapy decrease local recurrence? These were all positive trials, and they have all clearly shown that radiation therapy decreases local recurrence. Moreover, the relative reduction seems to be about the same in all three trials—about 50% for all subgroups.

A word about relative reduction: if the absolute local recurrence rate is 30% at 10 years for a given subgroup of patients treated with excision alone, radiation therapy will reduce this rate by approximately 50%, leaving a group of patients with a 15% local recurrence rate at 10 years. Radiation therapy clearly seems indicated for this subgroup. But consider a more favorable subgroup, a group of patients with a 6% absolute recurrence rate at 10 years when treated with excision alone. A 50% reduction here yields a group of patients with a recurrence rate of only 3%. This is only a 3% absolute benefit, and 100 patients need to be treated with radiotherapy to achieve this benefit. Here, we must ask whether the benefits are worth the risks and costs incurred.

The NSABP has recently agreed that all patients with DCIS may not need postexcisional radiation therapy (6). The problem is how to accurately identify those patients. If we can identify subgroups of patients with DCIS where the risk of local recurrence after excision alone is low, they may be the patients where the costs, risks, and side effects of radiotherapy outweigh the benefits. How can patients with a risk of local recurrence so low that it may be reasonable to treat with excision alone be identified? This has been a key question for the last decade.

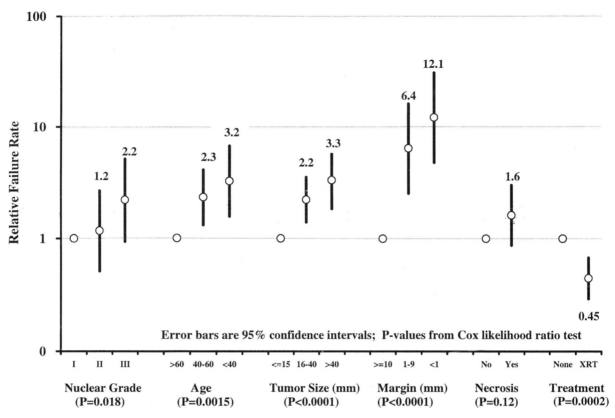

FIGURE 47.1. Cox multivariate analysis of factors affecting local recurrence–free survival.

Many of the parameters that are now considered important in predicting local recurrence (for example, size, margin width, nuclear grade, etc.) were not routinely collected prospectively during the randomized DCIS trials. The prospective trials did not specifically require the marking of margins nor the measurement of margin width. The exact measurement of margin width was present in only 5% of the EORTC pathology reports (8). The NSABP did not require size measurements, and much of their pathologic data have been determined by a retrospective review. In the initial NS-ABP report, more than 40% of patients had no size measurement (1). Unfortunately, if margins were not inked and tissue not completely sampled and sequentially submitted, then these data can never be accurately determined by retrospective review.

Predictors of Ductal Carcinoma in Situ Recurrence

Previously, the Van Nuys Prognostic Index, a quantitative algorithm based on three factors [tumor size, margin width, and histologic classification (based on nuclear grade and necrosis)], was developed as an aid to the complex treatment-selection process (11). A multivariate analysis performed in 1996, revealed near equal contributions to the likelihood of local recurrence from the three factors. In this text, we have introduced the USC/VNPI, which adds age to

the formula as a fourth factor (Chapter 45, Silverstein). However, the ability to accurately and consistently reproduce tumor size measurements by three-dimensional reconstruction has been questioned (17). This is clearly difficult. When the NSABP reviewed their pathologic material, they reported the largest diameter on a single slide. This may or may not be the true size of the lesion. By way of example, approximately 85% to 90% of the NSABP cases were measured at 10 mm or less in extent (in their 2001 update, this number was reduced to 75%) (2,4,6), whereas only 46% (269 of 583) of our conservatively treated cases measured 10 mm or less. It is unlikely that the NSABP has that many much smaller cases than a single facility devoted to diagnosing and treating DCIS. Rather, the explanation probably lies in the way tissue was processed and tumor size was measured. The NSABP used the largest dimension on a single slide as the size, whereas we used mammographic/pathologic correlation and three-dimensional reconstruction over a series of slides. In all likelihood, both groups treated tumors of similar size.

The reproducibility of histologic classification may also be difficult (18), although recent studies with defined criteria indicate a high degree of interobserver concordance (19–22). Douglas-Jones et al. (21) found the Van Nuys Classification the most easily reproduced of six tested.

This chapter explores various margin widths in patients stratified by nuclear grade, comedonecrosis, tumor size, and age, and uses these data to predict the likelihood of local recurrence with or without the addition of postoperative radiation therapy. The goal is to determine whether or not a subset of patients can be easily identified with a local recurrence rate so low that postexcisional radiation therapy is not justified.

PATIENTS AND METHODS

A total of 583 breast preservation patients were studied; 346 were treated with excision alone and 237 received excision plus radiation therapy. Data were accrued from 1970 through 2000. Every effort was made to completely excise all suspect lesions and to completely process all excised tissue. Needle localization, intraoperative specimen radiography, and correlation with the preoperative mammogram were performed in every nonpalpable case. Margins were inked or dyed, and specimens were serially sectioned at 2 to 3 mm intervals. Tissue sections were arranged and processed in sequence. Pathologic evaluation included histologic subtype, nuclear grade, the presence or absence of comedonecrosis, the maximum size of the lesion, and margin width.

Tumor size was determined by direct measurement or ocular micrometry from stained slides for smaller lesions. For larger lesions, a combination of direct measurement and estimation, based on the distribution of the lesion in a sequential series of slides (three-dimensional reconstruction), was used along with mammographic/pathologic correlation.

For example, a lesion that measured 5 mm on a single slide but extended across 10 sequential blocks was estimated to be 25 mm in extent (2.5 mm per block). Tumors were divided into two groups by size: small (less than 10 mm) and large (greater than 10 mm), similar to the NSABP. They were also analyzed by the three sizes used in the USC/VNPI: 15 mm or smaller, 16 to 40 mm, and 41 mm or larger. Margin width was determined by direct measurement or ocular micrometry. The closest single distance between DCIS and an inked margin was reported. Tumors were divided into three groups by margin width: close or involved (less than 1 mm), intermediate (1 to 9 mm), and wide (greater than 10 mm). Patients who underwent re-excision, and in whom no additional DCIS was found, were scored as having greater than 10 mm margins.

Tumors were divided into three groups by nuclear grade: nuclear grade 1 (low), nuclear grade 2 (intermediate), and nuclear grade 3 (high). Our method for nuclear grading has been previous reported (23) and is detailed in Chapter 16 (Lagios) and Chapter 17 (Poller and Silverstein).

Comedonecrosis was considered present for any architectural pattern of DCIS in which a central zone of necrotic debris with karyorrhexis was identified, no matter how limited. For a more detailed discussion of comedonecrosis see Chapter 17 (Poller and Silverstein). Tumors were divided into two groups by the presence or absence of any comedonecrosis.

Age was analyzed two different ways. Patients were divided into three groups as per the USC/VNPI: less than 40 years, 40 to 60 years, and more than 60 years. They were also analyzed as two groups: less than 50 years versus 50 and older.

All conservatively treated patients with DCIS were included in this analysis. Treatment was not randomized. In general, patients with lesions 40 mm or smaller and with margins clear by at least 1 mm were treated with breast preservation. Patients with lesions larger than 40 mm or with persistently positive surgical margins after re-excision were generally treated with mastectomy, usually with immediate reconstruction. These guidelines were not absolute, and some patients who could have been treated with breast preservation elected mastectomy and vice versa.

Radiation therapy was routinely added to most breast preservation patients' treatment regimen until 1989; thereafter most breast preservation patients were treated with excision alone. Whole-breast external beam irradiation (40 to 50 Gy) was performed on a 4 or 6 MeV linear accelerator with a boost of 10 to 20 Gy to the tumor bed by iridium 192 implant or external beam.

The outcome measure used in this study was local recurrence–free survival, which was calculated as the time from tumor excision to the date of local recurrence. There were 109 ipsilateral breast cancer events following initial conservative treatment, 97 of which (89%) were at or near the original lesion. Because it is impossible to determine with complete accuracy which lesions were true local recurrences and which were new cancers, all 109 were scored as local recurrences. Patients who did not experience a local recurrence were censored at the date of last follow-up. Eight patients developed metastatic breast cancer, all of whom had local recurrences. Five of these patients died of metastatic breast cancer; and 35 additional patients died of non–breast cancer related causes.

Kaplan-Meier plots (24) were used to estimate the probability of remaining free of local recurrence at 10 years; standard errors were based on Greenwood's formula (25). The Cox proportional hazards model (25) was used to evaluate the association of radiation therapy, margin width, comedonecrosis, tumor size, and nuclear grade with time to local recurrence—each alone and then jointly. The likelihood ratio test based on the Cox model was used to calculate p values (all two-sided), and standard errors based on the inverse of the information matrix were used to construct confidence intervals. Plots of the log (−log)–transformed Kaplan-Meier estimates were used to visually assess the assumption of proportional hazards. Within the strata formed by the three margin groups, the assumption of proportional hazards was not unreasonable.

The relative risk based on the Cox hazard model was defined as the ratio of the hazard of recurring for the patients who did not receive radiation therapy divided by the hazard of recurring for the patients who did.

TABLE 47.1. PATIENT DEMOGRAPHICS, TUMOR FACTORS, AND LOCAL RECURRENCES BY TREATMENT

Demographic	Excision + Radiation	Excision Alone	Total	p Value
No. of patients	237	346	583	
Average follow-up (months)	106	70		<0.001
No. of local recurrences	48	61	109	
Invasive	22	25	47	
Noninvasive (DCIS)	26	36	62	
Tumor size (mm)				
Median	15	10		0.01
Average	18	15		0.01
Comedonecrosis present	73%	61%		0.003
Nuclear grade (average)	2.24	2.19		NS
Average age (years)	53	54		NS
Margin width				
≥10	19%	39%		<0.001
1–9 mm	46%	42%		NS
<1 mm	35%	19%		<0.001

NS, not significant.

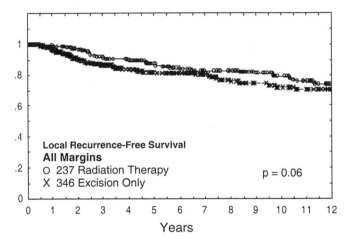

FIGURE 47.2. Local recurrence–free survival for 583 conservatively treated patients with ductal carcinoma in situ of the breast analyzed by treatment: excision plus radiation therapy versus excision alone.

RESULTS

Five hundred and eighty-three (583) patients were treated with breast conservation, 346 by excision alone and 237 by excision plus radiation therapy. Table 47.1 analyses patient demographics, tumor factors, and local recurrences by treatment (excision alone versus excision plus radiation therapy). There was a total of 109 local recurrences: 61 in excision alone patients (25 invasive, 36 DCIS) and 48 in irradiated patients (22 invasive, 26 DCIS). The mean follow-up for all patients was 84 months: 106 months for patients who received radiation therapy and 70 months for patients treated with excision alone. Figure 47.2 shows the local recurrence rate for all patients by treatment. The difference in favor of radiation therapy approaches significance ($p = 0.06$).

Table 47.2 and Figures 47.3 through 47.5 show the probability of local recurrence by treatment when patients

TABLE 47.2. ASSOCIATION OF RECURRENCE AND MARGIN WIDTH IN PATIENTS WITH DUCTAL CARCINOMA IN SITU

	No Radiation Therapy			Radiation Therapy			Statistical Analysis		
Margin	No. of Patients	No. of Local Recurrences	Probability of Recurring by 8 Years SE	No. of Patients	No. of Local Recurrences	Probability of Recurring by 8 Years SE	RR[a]	95% Confidence Interval	p Value[b]
≥10 mm	134	4	0.06 ± 0.04	45	1	0.03 ± 0.03	2.17	(0.24, 19.91)	0.46
1–9 mm	146	31	0.24 ± 0.04	109	20	0.13 ± 0.04	1.95	(1.09, 3.51)	0.023
<1 mm	66	26	0.57 ± 0.01	83	27	0.29 ± 0.06	2.60	(1.49, 4.53)	0.0007

[a] Relative risk of recurrence in non-radiation group compared to the patients who received radiation. The Relative Risk can be thought as the average increased chance of recurring at any point in time for patients who did not receive radiation therapy, compared to those who received radiation. If there is no association with recurrence, the relative risk should be close to 1.00.
[b] Based on likelihood ratio test from the Cox proportional hazards model.
RR, relative risk; SE, standard error.

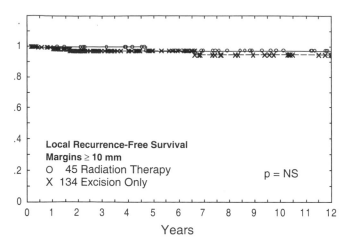

FIGURE 47.3. Local recurrence–free survival for 179 conservatively treated patients with ductal carcinoma in situ of the breast analyzed by treatment: excision plus radiation therapy versus excision alone. All patients have excision margins greater than or equal to 10 mm. There is no benefit from the addition of postexcisional radiation therapy.

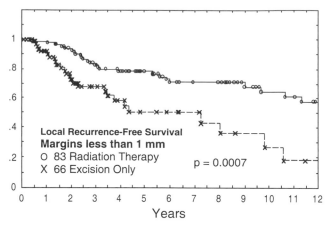

FIGURE 47.5. Local recurrence–free survival for 149 conservatively treated patients with ductal carcinoma in situ of the breast analyzed by treatment: excision plus radiation therapy versus excision alone. All patients have margins less than 1 mm. The benefit from the addition of radiation therapy is highly significant ($p = 0.0007$).

are stratified by margin width: wide (≥ 10 mm), intermediate (1 to 9 mm), and close/involved (< 1 mm). Only five of the 179 patients with greater than 10 mm margins experienced a local recurrence. Although the relative risk of local recurrence was decreased by 50% (from 6% to 3%) by adding radiation therapy, this reduction was not statistically significant, and because there are so few local recurrences in the group with 10 mm or greater margins, the effect of radiation therapy is of little practical importance (Fig. 47.3). In patients with 1 to 9 mm margins, those who did not receive radiation therapy experienced a 1.95-fold increase in the risk of local recurrence, compared with patients who received radiation therapy ($p = 0.023$) (Fig. 47.4). For pa-

tients whose surgical margins were less than 1 mm, the association of radiation therapy with decreased recurrence was strongly significant: patients who did not receive radiation therapy had a 2.60-fold increased risk of recurrence ($p = 0.0007$) (Fig. 47.5).

Because the decision to treat with radiation therapy was based on physician and patient choice rather than as part of a randomized trial, the data were further examined to see if the benefit from radiation therapy in patients with less than 1 mm margins and the lack of benefit in patients with greater than 10 mm margins could be explained by an imbalance in prognostic factors, such as patients with known adverse tumor characteristics that were more likely to receive radiation therapy. Table 47.3 summarizes baseline clinical values by treatment groups and margin width. Within the greater than 10 mm margin group, no statistically significant differences in nuclear grade or comedonecrosis were found between treatment groups, but patients who received radiation therapy had larger tumors. Among patients with 1 to 9 mm margins, those who received radiation therapy had larger tumors and were more likely to have comedonecrosis. In patients with less than 1 mm margins, there were no significant differences in baseline variables between treatment groups.

Table 47.4 recalculates the relative risk and p values after stratifying for comedonecrosis, tumor size, and nuclear grade. In all cases, the relative risks were not substantially changed after these adjustments. That is, regardless of the presence of comedonecrosis, large tumor size, or high nuclear grade, if wide margins are obtained, the probability of local recurrence remains small and there is no statistically significant benefit from the addition of radiation therapy, as measured by a decrease in local recurrence. With margins 1 to 9 mm, there is a significant trend toward a benefit from

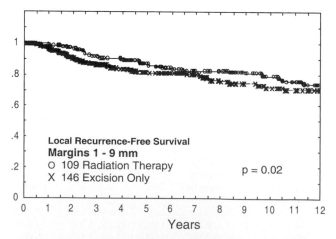

FIGURE 47.4. Local recurrence–free survival for 255 conservatively treated patients with ductal carcinoma in situ of the breast analyzed by treatment: excision plus radiation therapy versus excision alone. All patients have excision margins 1 to 9 mm. The benefit from the addition of radiation therapy is statistically significant ($p = 0.02$).

TABLE 47.3. COMPARISON OF BASELINE VALUES BY MARGIN WIDTH AND TREATMENT

Margins	No Radiotherapy	Radiotherapy	p Value
>10 mm			
n = 179	134	45	—
Median size (mm)	10	15	0.01
Nuclear grade (average)	2.21	2.15	0.67
% grade 3	41%	40%	0.90
% with comedonecrosis	63%	69%	0.45
1–9 mm			
n = 255	146	109	—
Median size (mm)	9	13	0.001
Nuclear grade (average)	2.05	2.17	0.22
% grade 3	36%	33%	0.67
% with comedonecrosis	47%	32%	0.02
<1 mm			
n = 149	66	83	—
Median size (mm)	20	20	0.30
Nuclear grade (average)	2.47	2.38	0.46
% grade 3	61%	48%	0.13
% with comedonecrosis	26%	18%	0.26

irradiation. With margins less than 1 mm, there is a highly significant decrease in the probability of local recurrence if radiation therapy is added.

Figures 47.6 through 47.8 look at some of these data in graphic form for patients with 10 mm margins. Figure 47.6 shows that if widely clear margins are obtained, the presence of comedonecrosis does not significantly increase the local recurrence rate. Figure 47.7 shows that if widely clear margins are obtained, that high nuclear grade (grade 3) does not

significantly increase the local recurrence rate. Figure 47.8 shows that if widely clear margins are obtained, that large size does not significantly increase the local recurrence rate, although there are very few lesions greater than or equal to 41 mm with 10 mm or more margins (n = 6).

Table 47.5 analyzes the 5- and 10-year probability of local recurrence by treatment for all patients and then subdivides the patients by margin widths: wide (10 mm or more), intermediate (1 to 9 mm), and narrow or involved (< 1

TABLE 47.4. ASSOCIATION OF RADIATION THERAPY WITH RECURRENCE STRATIFIED BY COMEDOTYPE NECROSIS, NUCLEAR GRADE, AND TUMOR SIZE

Margin	Un-Adjusted Analysis			Adjusted Analysis			
	RR[a]	95% CI[b]	p Value[c]	Stratified by	RR[a]	95% CI[b]	p Value[d]
≥10 mm	2.17	(0.24, 19.91)	0.46	Necrosis	2.31	(0.25, 21.59)	0.43
				Nuclear grade	2.07	(0.23, 18.60)	0.49
				Size	1.75	(0.18, 17.28)	0.62
1–9 mm	1.95	(1.09, 3.51)	0.023	Necrosis	1.96	(1.09, 3.50)	0.023
				Nuclear grade	1.94	(1.05, 3.57)	0.031
				Size	2.02	(1.10, 3.68)	0.021
<1 mm	2.60	(1.49, 4.53)	0.0007	Necrosis	2.55	(1.46, 4.45)	0.001
				Nuclear grade	2.27	(1.29, 3.98)	0.005
				Size	2.84	(1.57, 5.09)	0.001

[a] Relative risk of recurrence in non—radiation therapy group compared with patients who received radiation.
[b] 95% confidence interval for the relative risk.
[c] Based on likelihood ratio test from the Cox proportional hazard model.
[d] Based on likelihood ratio test from the Cox proportional hazard model stratifying for either necrosis (yes, no), nuclear grade (1, 2, 3), or tumor size (<10 mm, >10 mm).
CI, confidence interval; RR, relative risk.

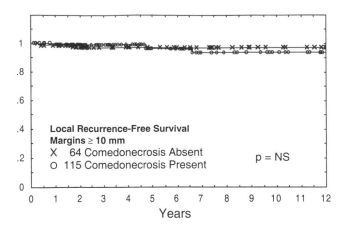

FIGURE 47.6. Local recurrence–free survival for 179 conservatively treated patients with ductal carcinoma in situ of the breast and margins greater than or equal to 10 mm analyzed by the presence or absence of comedonecrosis. With widely clear margins, the presence of comedonecrosis is not a factor.

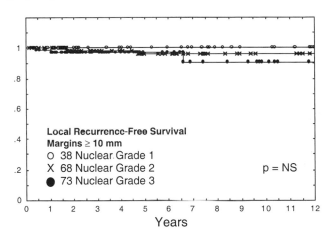

FIGURE 47.7. Local recurrence–free survival for 179 conservatively treated patients with ductal carcinoma in situ of the breast and margins greater than or equal to 10 mm analyzed by nuclear grade. With widely clear margins, high nuclear grade (grade 3) is not a factor.

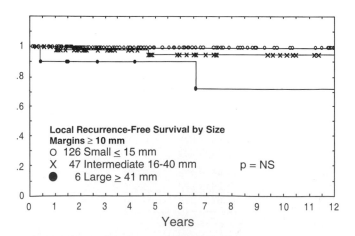

FIGURE 47.8. Local recurrence–free survival for 179 conservatively treated patients with ductal carcinoma in situ of the breast and margins greater than or equal to 10 mm analyzed by tumor size. With widely clear margins, size is not a factor, but there are too few lesions greater than 40 mm to draw any conclusions.

TABLE 47.5. 5 TO 10-YEAR PROBABILITY OF LOCAL RECURRENCE BY TREATMENT AND FURTHER SUBDIVIDED BY MARGIN WIDTH

Factor	Excision + Radiation	Excision Only	*p* Value
Number of patients (*n* = 583)	237	346	
Local recurrence rate (all patients)	13/21%	18/28%	0.06
Margins ≥10 mm (n = 179)	3/3%	3/6%	NS
Margins = 1–9 mm (n = 255)	8/16%	19/28%	0.05
Margins <1 mm (n = 149)	22/35%	50/73%	0.002

NS, not significant.

mm). For all patients with 10 mm or more margins (n = 179), no advantage in terms of decreased local recurrence is gained by adding postoperative radiation therapy. Tables 47.6, 47.7, and 47.8 further subdivide the patients by nuclear grade (Table 47.6), by the presence of absence of comedonecrosis (Table 47.7), and by tumor size (smaller, < 10, and larger, > 10 mm) (Table 47.8).

The relationship of nuclear grade and margins is shown in Table 47.6. These data reveal that if wide margins are obtained, the probability of local recurrence remains at 11% or less at 10 years, and there is no statistically significant benefit regardless of the nuclear grade (as measured by a decrease in local recurrence) from the addition of radiation therapy. With close or involved margins (< 1 mm), there is a marked decrease in the probability of local recurrence for high-grade lesions if radiation therapy is added. Due to small sample size, these differences are not significant in patients with nuclear grade 1 or 2 lesions.

The relationship of comedonecrosis and margins is shown in Table 47.7. These data reveal that regardless of the presence or absence of comedonecrosis, if wide margins are

TABLE 47.6. 5 TO 10-YEAR ACTUARIAL PROBABILITY OF LOCAL RECURRENCE BY NUCLEAR GRADE AND MARGIN WIDTH

	Excision + Radiation	Excision Only	*p* Value
Nuclear grade 1 (low nuclear grade) (n = 116)			
Margins ≥10 mm (n = 38)	0/0%	0/0%	NS
Margins = 1–9 mm (n = 61)	5/5%	2/5%	NS
Margins <1 mm (n = 17)	17/29%	44/100%	NS
Nuclear grade 2 (intermediate nuclear grade) (n = 226)			
Margins ≥10 mm (n = 68)	6/6%	3/3%	NS
Margins = 1–9 mm (n = 106)	6/13%	8/20%	NS
Margins <1 mm (n = 52)	17/26%	11/24%	NS
Nuclear grade 3 (high nuclear grade) (n = 241)			
Margins ≥10 mm (n = 73)	0/0%	4/11%	NS
Margins = 1–9 mm (n = 88)	15/27%	43/53%	0.01
Margins <1 mm (n = 80)	25/43%	67/84%	0.002

NS, not significant.

TABLE 47.7. 5/10-YEAR ACTUARIAL PROBABILITY OF LOCAL RECURRENCE BY COMEDONECROSIS AND MARGIN WIDTH

Necrosis/Margin Status	Excision + Radiation	Excision Only	p Value
Comedonecrosis present (n = 382)			
Margins ≥10 mm (n = 115)	4/4%	1/7%	NS
Margins = 1–9 mm (n = 150)	9/19%	32/43%	0.01
Margins <1 mm (n = 117)	20/35%	61/74%	0.0009
Comedonecrosis absent (n = 201)			
Margins ≥10 mm (n = 64)	0/0%	4/4%	NS
Margins = 1–9 mm (n = 105)	5/9%	5/11%	NS
Margins <1 mm (n = 32)	28/37%	19/100%	NS

NS, not significant.

obtained, the probability of local recurrence remains at 7% or less at 10 years and there is no statistically significant benefit (as measured by a decrease in local recurrence) from the addition of radiation therapy. With close or involved margins (< 1 mm), there is a marked decrease in the probability of local recurrence if radiation therapy is added. Due to small sample size, the difference is not significant in patients where comedonecrosis is absent.

The relationship of tumor size and margins is shown in Table 47.8. In this table, the patients have been divided into two groups: those with small lesions (10 mm in greatest diameter or less) and those with larger lesions (> 10 mm). These data reveal that regardless of size grouping, if wide margins are obtained, the probability of local recurrence remains at 17% or less at 10 years and there is no statistically significant benefit (as measured by a decrease in local recurrence) from the addition of radiation therapy. With close or involved margins (< 1 mm), there appears to be a marked decrease in the probability of local recurrence if radiation therapy is added.

Figures 47.9 and 47.10 look at age as a predictor of local recurrence in patients with wide margins greater than or

TABLE 47.8. 5/10-YEAR ACTUARIAL PROBABILITY OF LOCAL RECURRENCE BY TUMOR SIZE AND MARGIN WIDTH

Tumor Size/Margin Width	Excision + Radiation	Excision Only	p Value
Tumor size ≤10 mm (n = 269)			
Margins ≥10 mm (n = 98)	0/0%	0/0%	NS
Margins = 1–9 mm (n = 125)	8/12%	13/22%	NS
Margins <1 mm (n = 46)	12/29%	36/76%	0.02
Tumor size >10 mm (n = 314)			
Margins ≥10 mm (n = 81)	4/4%	7/17%	NS
Margins = 1–9 mm (n = 130)	8/19%	26/36%	0.03
Margins <1 mm (n = 103)	19/39%	57/72%	0.005

NS, not significant.

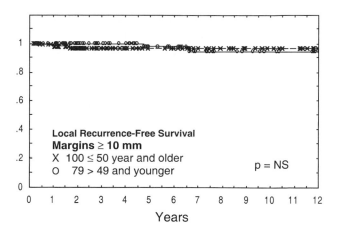

FIGURE 47.9. Local recurrence–free survival for 179 conservatively treated patients with ductal carcinoma in situ of the breast and margins greater than or equal to 10 mm analyzed by two age groups: 50 years and older versus 49 years and younger. With widely clear margins, age is not a factor.

equal to 10 mm. Figure 47.9 divides the patients into two age groups: less than 50 years versus 50 years and older. Figure 47.10 divides the patients into three age groups, as in the USC/VNPI: less than 40 years versus 40 to 60 years versus more than 60 years. In both of these analyses, age does not make a significant difference if wide margins have been achieved, although there are very few patients under age 40 with wide margins (n = 11).

DISCUSSION

The most likely cause of local recurrence after breast-conservation therapy for DCIS is inadequate surgery resulting in residual disease—a fractional persistence of the original

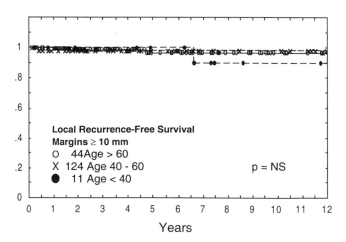

FIGURE 47.10. Local recurrence–free survival for 179 conservatively treated patients with ductal carcinoma in situ of the breast and margins greater than or equal to 10 mm analyzed by three age groups: 61 years and older versus 40 to 60 years versus 39 years and younger. With widely clear margins, age is not a factor.

490 Section VII: Tools for Selecting Patients for Breast Conservation with and without Radiation Therapy

lesion, for example. This statement is supported by the fact that most local recurrences after breast-conservation therapy for DCIS occur at or near the primary lesions. In our own series, 89% (97 of 109) of local recurrences after breast-conservation therapy were at or near the original lesion.

Additional evidence that surgeons commonly leave residual disease behind comes from our own data. We found that 43% of patients with clear margins (all margins 1 mm or more from the inked margin) had residual disease on re-excision or mastectomy. In addition, residual disease was found in 76% of patients with DCIS less than 1 mm from the inked original margins (26). The vast majority of these patients (94%) would have had clear margins if judged by NSABP standards (tumor not transected). An analysis of our data revealed that as margin width increased, the probability of local recurrence decreased, and at 10 mm or more, it was only about 5% to 6% (11). It quickly became apparent that 1 mm margins, although clear by most definitions, were woefully inadequate when it comes to achieving complete removal of DCIS.

If all local recurrences were noninvasive (DCIS), there would be little danger and, therefore, little indication for mastectomy as the initial procedure for patients with DCIS. In most reported series, approximately half of all local recurrences are invasive (27–29). Local recurrences are, therefore, extremely important. When they occur in patients who have struggled to save their breasts, they are both demoralizing and, theoretically, a threat to life (30). By avoiding mastectomy, we gain both psychological and physical advantages; but when there is an invasive recurrence, we have permitted an almost totally curable noninvasive lesion to advance to a potentially less curable form. An invasive recurrence represents a biologic worsening of the stage of disease, which may, in turn, ultimately translate into a higher mortality rate for patients initially treated conservatively.

Currently, there are three major treatment approaches for DCIS: mastectomy, excision with radiation therapy, and excision alone. After mastectomy, little breast tissue remains and there is little risk of local recurrence (either invasive or DCIS) (27,30–33). Breast preservation, with or without radiation therapy, yields a better cosmetic result and a sensate breast, but is accompanied by an increase in the probability of local failure (23,27,34–41). Approximately one-half of all local recurrences are invasive and, therefore, a potential threat to life (28,30,38,42).

The results of NSABP Protocol B-17 have shown a significant decrease in local recurrence, particularly in local invasive recurrence, for breast preservation patients treated with postoperative radiation therapy (1,3,6). More than 800 patients with DCIS excised with clear surgical margins (as defined by the criterion of nontransection) were prospectively randomized into two groups: excision only versus excision plus radiation therapy. After 5, 8, and 12 years of follow-up (1,3,6), there was a significant decrease in local recurrence of both DCIS and invasive breast cancer in pa-

tients treated with radiation therapy, leading the NSABP to initially recommend and to continue to recommend postexcisional radiation therapy for all patients with DCIS who chose to save their breasts.

The NSABP did not require marking of margins, complete tissue processing, specimen radiography, or margin width measurement. In the initial report, 40% of the patients did not have a size measurement (1,2). This lack of data makes it impossible for the NSABP study to answer some of the subset questions asked today. For example, exactly which subgroups benefit from radiation therapy and by how much? If the benefit in a particular subgroup is only a few percent, the advantage gained by radiation therapy may be offset by its cost and other potential disadvantages. Similar criticisms can be levied against the EORTC and U.K. DCIS trials. On the other hand, all three trials did what they set out to do: that is, prove the value of postexcisional radiation therapy across the board.

In other nonrandomized series, subsets of patients who are not likely to receive significant benefit from radiation therapy have been identified, such as those with small well-excised noncomedo lesions in the series of Schwartz et al. (37), or those with well-differentiated lesions as described by Zafrani et al. (43). Such patients may account for more than 30% of all patients with DCIS (23,37,42–44).

One of the most important questions in DCIS management today is: Which patients selected for breast preservation require postexcisional radiation therapy? Our reluctance to use radiation therapy in all patients led us initially to develop the Van Nuys Prognostic Index, a quantitative algorithm based on tumor size, margin width, and histologic classification (11), and then to modify it by adding age (USC/VNPI). However, the ability to accurately and consistently reproduce tumor size measurements has been questioned (17). In addition, the reproducibility of nuclear grading and classification may also be difficult (18,19). This led us to look for a simpler (and hopefully more reproducible) approach in selecting patients who might not require radiation therapy. The data presented here suggest that margin width is an excellent predictor of the probability of local recurrence and, therefore, of the likelihood of residual DCIS. With further corroboration, margin width could possibly be used as the sole determinant of the need for postoperative radiation therapy. However, the use of margins as a predictor requires complete tissue processing without which involved margins and invasive foci may go unrecognized. Standardized and reproducible methods of margin evaluation must be developed and prospectively tested.

Because most local recurrences occur at or near the primary lesion and are therefore likely a result of inadequate initial excision, lesions that are completely excised should require no additional treatment (such as radiation therapy). Evidence exists to suggest that complete excision is possible. The three-dimensional imaging of Faverly et al. (45) and the serial subgross work of Holland et al. (46,47) reveal that

DCIS is almost always unicentric (a single involved ductal unit) but commonly multifocal (multiple foci of disease within a single ductal unit). Holland et al. (46) showed that 118 of 119 (99.2%) patients with DCIS had lesions confined to a single segment of the breast (Chapter 19). DCIS was often larger than expected and extended beyond mammographic microcalcifications, and skip areas (gaps) were common. For both patients and surgeons, this is positive information. For years, the misconception that DCIS was commonly multicentric (involving multiple quadrants and, therefore, more than one ductal unit), forced many surgeons to suggest mastectomy as the treatment of choice for these lesions. The work of Lagios and associates (34,42), however, suggested that procedures far less than mastectomy could be safely performed.

In spite of its often large size, DCIS is a local disease that is lacking two important components of the fully expressed malignant phenotype: stromal invasion and distant metastasis. This information, combined with the fact that its distribution is almost always segmental (unicentric), makes complete excision and, therefore, surgical cure theoretically possible. That is not to say that it is easily accomplished.

In 1994, Faverly et al. (45) showed that 85% to 90% of DCIS lesions were completely excised if all margins were 10 mm or more, regardless of histologic type. In 1996 and 1997, Silverstein et al. (11,48) reported an 8% local recurrence rate for all conservatively treated DCIS lesions with margins of 10 mm or more. In 1997, Lagios et al. (49) showed a 5% local recurrence rate at 84 months for conservatively treated patients with margins 10 mm or more, and the Nottingham group reported a 6% local recurrence rate among 48 patients with 10 mm or greater margins treated with excision only after a median follow-up of 58 months (50). These data clearly show the increasing importance given to wider margin width in the recent literature.

In this chapter, we have taken these data one step farther, subdividing by margin width first and then analyzing outcome by nuclear grade (low to high), the presence or absence of comedonecrosis, tumor size (10 mm or smaller versus 11 mm or larger), and by age. In each and every case, there was no significant benefit to the addition of postoperative radiation therapy if margin width was 10 mm or more. Although there is no perfect tool, these data suggest that margin width is a good judge of complete excision. If complete excision cures the disease, how then does one accomplish this within the confines of obtaining an acceptable cosmetic result? (See Chapter 15 on oncoplastic breast surgery.)

Our data reveal a significant benefit when radiation therapy is given to patients with less than 1 mm margins (Table 47.1, Fig. 47.4). Although the probability of local recurrence at 8 years is nearly cut in half, from 57% to 29% (Table 47.2), the local recurrence rate remains too high. In many patients with less than 1 mm margins, radiation therapy, although highly effective, simply cannot overcome inadequate surgery.

The most important data in this chapter reveal that radiation therapy does not appear to benefit patients with margins greater than 10 mm, regardless of tumor size, nuclear grade, comedonecrosis, or age. Table 47.3 reveals that within the greater than 10 mm margin subgroup, there are no statistically significant differences between the baseline parameters of patients who received postexcisional breast irradiation and those who did not, other than larger size tumors in the irradiated group. These patients do well regardless of whether or not they receive radiation therapy, because with margins greater than 10 mm, there is little likelihood of residual DCIS (30,45–47). With little likelihood of residual disease, the potential impact of radiation therapy is minimized.

The results of NSABP Protocol B-24 were published in 1999 (5) and updated in 2001 (6). In this prospective randomized trial, more than 1,800 patients with DCIS were randomized to receive excision plus radiation therapy and either tamoxifen or placebo. At 5 years, the local recurrence rate was 6% for the tamoxifen group and 9.3% for the placebo group. After 7 years of follow-up, the cumulative incidence of ipsilateral recurrence was 7.7% for the tamoxifen group and 11.1% for the placebo group.

Our excision-only patients with greater than or equal to 10 mm margins had a comparable low local recurrence rate (6% ± 4% at 8 years) (Table 47.2) without either radiation therapy or tamoxifen. At 12 years, the local recurrence rate was unchanged. Our data suggest that additional therapy is unlikely to be of significant benefit in selected patients; for example, those with widely clear margins greater than or equal to 10 mm based on complete and sequential tissue processing.

Radiation therapy markedly improves the outcome of patients with close or involved margins (less than 1 mm) and to a lesser degree in patients with intermediate margins (1 to 9 mm) ($p = 0.02$). These data have been carefully collected prospectively but their weakness lies in the reality that they were not the result of a randomized clinical trial. These findings should be confirmed within the context of a future study that uses comparable thorough mammographic correlation and standardized pathology as described herein.

Subsets of patients who are not likely to receive any significant benefit from radiation therapy can be identified, e.g., those with VNPI scores of 3 or 4; those with wide margins (equal or greater than 10 mm), as in the series presented here; low-grade lesions in the series of Lagios et al. (42,44); small noncomedo lesions with uninvolved margins in the series of Schwartz, et al. (37); or the well-differentiated lesions of Zafrani et al. (43). Such patients may account for more than 30% of the total DCIS group (23,37,42–44).

To date, no study of patients with DCIS has shown a statistically significant difference in mortality when the three available treatments (mastectomy, excision alone, and excision plus radiation therapy) are compared. However, there are clear differences in local recurrence rates, and they are of extreme importance. Local recurrence in patients who have struggled to save their breasts are both demoralizing and theoretically, if invasive, a threat to life (30). In this series and in most other reported series (28,29), approximately one-half of all local recurrences are invasive.

In summary, these data, the result of an analysis of 583 conservatively treated patients with DCIS, suggest that excellent local control can be achieved when margin widths greater than 10 mm are obtained, regardless of high nuclear grade, the presence of comedonecrosis, large tumor size, or young age. The fact that there were so few recurrences (n = 5) among 179 patients with 10 mm or greater margins makes it unlikely that radiation therapy could have any significant impact on this subgroup.

Wide margin width increases the probability of complete excision, and it is an important predictor of good local control. DCIS lesions excised with 10 mm or greater margins do not significantly benefit from the addition of radiation therapy, regardless of high nuclear grade, the presence of comedonecrosis, or large tumor size. These factors are important when there is a high likelihood of residual disease: margins less than 1 mm, for example.

Margin width reflects the adequacy of excision. Aside from age, margin width, defined as the distance between DCIS and the closest inked margin, is the easiest measurement in the USC/VNPI to reproduce and, based on the multivariate analysis (Fig. 47.1), the most important predictor of local recurrence.

REFERENCES

1. Fisher B, Costantino J, Redmond C, et al. Lumpectomy compared with lumpectomy and radiation therapy for the treatment of intraductal breast cancer. *N Engl J Med* 1993;328:1581–1586.
2. Fisher ER, Constantino J, Fisher B, et al. Pathologic Finding from the National Surgical Adjuvant Breast Project (NSABP) Protocol B-17: Intraductal Carcinoma (Ductal Carcinoma In Situ). *Cancer* 1995;75:1310–1319.
3. Fisher B, Dignam J, Wolmark N, et al. Lumpectomy and radiation therapy for the treatment of intraductal breast cancer: Findings from National Surgical Adjuvant Breast and Bowel Project B-17. *J Clin Oncol* 1998;16:441–452.
4. Fisher ER, Dignam J, Tan-Chiu E, et al. Pathologic findings from the National Surgical Adjuvant Breast Project (NSABP) eight-year update of Protocol B-17: Intraductal Carcinoma. *Cancer* 1999;86:429–438.
5. Fisher B, Dignam J, Wolmark N. Tamoxifen in treatment of intraductal breast cancer: National Surgical Adjuvant Breast and Bowel Project B-24 randomised controlled trial. *Lancet* 1999;353:1993–2000.
6. Fisher B, Land S, Mamounas E, et al. Prevention of invasive breast cancer in women with ductal carcinoma in situ: An update of the National Surgical Adjuvant Breast and Bowel Project Experience. *Semin Oncol* 2001;28:400–418.
7. Julien JP, Bijker N, Fentiman I, et al. Radiotherapy in breast conserving treatment for ductal carcinoma in situ: First results of EORTC randomised phase III trial 10853. *Lancet* 2000;355:528–533.
8. Bijker N, Peterse JL, Duchateau L, et al. Risk factors for recurrence and metastasis after breast conserving therapy for ductal carcinoma in situ: Analysis of European Organization for Research and Treatment of Cancer Trial 10853. *J Clin Oncol* 2001;19:2263–2271.
9. George WD, Houghton J, Cuzick J, et al. Radiotherapy and tamoxifen following complete local excision (CLE) in the management of ductal carcinoma in situ (DCIS): preliminary results from the U.K. DCIS trial. *Proc Am Soc Clin Oncol* 2000; 19:70a(abst).
10. UKCCCR DCIS Working Party. The UK, Australian, and New Zealand randomised trial comparing radiotherapy and tamoxifen in women with completely excised ductal carcinoma in situ of the breast. (*Submitted*)
11. Silverstein MJ, Lagios MD, Craig PH, et al. A prognostic index for ductal carcinoma in situ. *Cancer* 1996;77:2267–2274.
12. Szelei-Stevens KA, Kuske R, Yantos VA, et al. The influence of young age and positive family history of breast cancer on the prognosis of ductal carcinoma in situ treated by excision with or without radiation therapy or mastectomy. *Int J Radiat Oncol Biol Phys* 2000;48:943–949.
13. Goldstein NS, Vicini FA, Kestin LL, et al. Differences in the pathologic features of ductal carcinoma in situ of the breast based on patient age. *Cancer* 2000;88:2552–2560.
14. Vicini FA, Kestin LL, Goldstein NS, et al. Impact of young age on outcome in patients with ductal carcinoma in situ treated with breast conserving therapy. *J Clin Oncol* 2000;18:296–306.
15. Kestin LL, Goldstein NS, Lacerna MD, et al. Factors associated with local recurrence of mammographically detected ductal carcinoma in situ in patients given breast conserving therapy. *Cancer* 2000;88:596–607.
16. Van Zee KJ, Liberman L, Samli B, et al. Long-term follow-up of women with ductal carcinoma in situ treated with breast conserving surgery. The effect of age. *Cancer* 1999;86:1757–1767.
17. Schnitt SJ, Harris JR, Smith BL. Developing a prognostic index for ductal carcinoma in situ of the breast: Are we there yet? *Cancer* 1996;77:2189–2192.
18. Rosai J. Borderline epithelial lesions of the breast. *Am J Surg Pathol* 1991;15:209–221.
19. Schnitt SJ, Connolly JL, Tavassoli FA, et al. Interobserver reproducibility in the diagnosis of ductal proliferative breast lesions using standardized criteria. *Am J Surg Pathol* 1992;16:33–43.
20. Scott MA, Lagios MD, Axelsson K, et al. Ductal carcinoma in situ of the breast: Reproducibility of histological subtype analysis. *Hum Pathol* 1997;28:967–973.
21. Douglas-Jones AG, Gupta SK, Attanoos RL, et al. A critical appraisal of six modern classifications of ductal carcinoma in situ of the breast (DCIS): Correlation with grade of associated invasive disease. *Histopathology* 1996;29:397–409.
22. Bethwaite P, Smith N, Delahunt B, et al. Reproducibility of new classification schemes for the pathology of ductal carcinoma in situ of the breast. *J Clin Pathol* 1998;51:450–454.
23. Silverstein MJ, Poller DN, Waisman JR, et al. Prognostic classification of breast duct carcinoma in situ. *Lancet* 1995;345:1154–1157.
24. Kaplan EL, Meier P. Nonparametric estimation from incomplete observations. *J Am Statist Ass* 1958;53:457–481.
25. Miller RG, Jr. *Survival Analysis.* New York: John Wiley & Sons, 1981.
26. Silverstein MJ, Gierson ED, Colburn WJ, et al. Can intraductal breast carcinoma be excised completely by local excision? *Cancer* 1994;73:2985–2989.
27. Silverstein MJ, Barth A, Poller DN, et al. Ten-year results comparing mastectomy to excision and radiation therapy for ductal carcinoma in situ of the breast. *Eur J Cancer* 1995;31:1425–1427.

28. Solin LJ, Fourquet A, Vicini FA, et al. Mammographically detected ductal carcinoma in situ of the breast treated with breast conserving surgery and definitive breast irradiation: Long-term outcome and prognostic significance of patient age and margin status. *Int J Radiat Oncol Biol Phys* 2001;50:991–1002.

29. Solin LJ, Kurtz J, Fourquet A, et al. Fifteen-year results of breast conserving surgery and definitive breast irradiation for the treatment of ductal carcinoma in situ of the breast. *J Clin Oncol* 1996;14:754–763.

30. Silverstein MJ, Lagios MD, Martino S, et al. Outcome after local recurrence in patients with ductal carcinoma in situ of the breast. *J Clin Oncol* 1998;16:1367–1373.

30. Ashikari R, Hadju SI, Robbins GF. Intraductal carcinoma of the breast. *Cancer* 1971;28:1182–1187.

31. Fentiman IS, Fagg N, Millis RR, et al. In situ ductal carcinoma of the breast: Implications of disease pattern and treatment. *Eur J Surg Oncol* 1986;12:261–266.

32. Bradley SJ, Weaver DW, Bouwman DL. Alternative in the surgical management of in situ breast cancer. *Am Surg* 1990;56:428–432.

33. Rosner D, Bedwani RN, Vana J, et al. Noninvasive breast carcinoma. Results of a national survey of The American College of Surgeons. *Ann Surg* 1980;192:139–147.

34. Lagios MD, Westdahl PR, Margolin FR, et al. Duct Carcinoma in situ: Relationship of extent of noninvasive disease to the frequency of occult invasion, multicentricity, lymph node metastases, and short-term treatment failures. *Cancer* 1982;50:1309–1314.

35. Lagios MD. Duct carcinoma in situ: Pathology and treatment. *Surg Clin North Am* 1990;70:853–871.

36. Ottesen GL, Graversen HP, Blichert-Toft M, et al. Ductal carcinoma in situ of the female breast. Short-term results of a prospective nationwide study. *Am J Surg Pathol* 1992;16:1183–1196.

37. Schwartz GF, Finkel GC, Garcia JC, et al. Subclinical ductal carcinoma in situ of the breast. Treatment by local excision and surveillance alone. *Cancer* 1992;70:2468–2474.

38. Solin LJ, Recht A, Fourquet A, et al. Ten-year results of breast-conserving surgery and definitive irradiation for intraductal carcinoma of the breast. *Cancer* 1991;68:2337–2344.

39. McCormick B, Rosen PP, Kinne D, et al. Duct carcinoma in situ of the breast: An analysis of local control after conservation surgery and radiotherapy. *Int J Radiat Oncol Biol Phys* 1991;21:289–292.

40. Kuske RR, Bean JM, Garcia DM, et al. Breast conservation therapy for intraductal carcinoma of the breast. *Int J Radiat Oncol Biol Phys* 1993;26:391–396.

41. Bornstein BA, Recht A, Connolly JL, et al. Results of treating ductal carcinoma in situ of the breast with conservative surgery and radiation therapy. *Cancer* 1991;67:7–13.

42. Lagios MD, Margolin FR, Westdahl PR, et al. Mammographically detected duct carcinoma in situ. Frequency of local recurrence following tylectomy and prognostic effect of nuclear grade on local recurrence. *Cancer* 1989;63:618–624.

43. Zafrani B, Leroyer A, Fourquet A, et al. Mammographically-detected ductal carcinoma in situ of the breast analyzed with a new classification. A study of 127 cases: Correlation with estrogen and progesterone receptors, p53 and c-erbB-2 proteins, and proliferative activity. *Semin Diagn Pathol* 1994;11(3):208–213.

44. Lagios MD. Ductal carcinoma in situ: Controversies in diagnosis, biology, and treatment. *The Breast Journal* 1995;1:68–78.

45. Faverly DRG, Burgers L, Bult P, et al. Three dimensional imaging of mammary ductal carcinoma in situ; clinical implications. *Semin Diagn Pathol* 1994;11:193–198.

46. Holland R, Hendriks JHCL, Verbeek ALM, et al. Extent, distribution and mammographic/histological correlations of breast ductal carcinoma in situ. *Lancet* 1990;335:519–522.

47. Holland R, Faverly DRG. Whole organ studies. In: Silverstein MJ, ed. *Ductal Carcinoma In Situ of the Breast*. Baltimore: Williams and Wilkins, 1997:233–240.

48. Silverstein MJ, Lagios MD. Ductal carcinoma in situ: Factors predicting recurrence and how they can be used in treatment planning. *Oncology* 1997;11(3):393–410.

49. Lagios MD, Silverstein MJ. Duct carcinoma in situ: The success of breast conservation therapy: A shared experience of two single institution nonrandomized prospective studies. *Surg Oncol Clin N Am* 1997;6(2):385–392.

50. Sibbering DM, Blamey RW. Nottingham Experience. In: Silverstein MJ, ed. *Ductal Carcinoma In Situ of the Breast*. Baltimore: Williams and Wilkins, 1997:271–84.

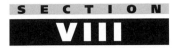

SECTION VIII

ADJUVANT THERAPY, PREVENTION, AND HORMONE REPLACEMENT THERAPY

48

CAN THE NEW PREVENTION STRATEGIES REDUCE THE INCIDENCE OF DUCTAL CARCINOMA IN SITU?

CSABA GAJDOS
JENNIFER I. MACGREGOR
DEBRA A. TONETTI
V. CRAIG JORDAN

Ductal carcinoma in situ (DCIS) can be considered a precursor of breast cancer. If untreated, the localized carcinoma will invade the surrounding tissues and, ultimately, travel to metastatic sites. A strategy to reduce the incidence of DCIS in the general population is, therefore, breast cancer prevention but must be made available, as a general health measure, to the whole population.

Estrogen replacement, on balance, provides enormous advantages for postmenopausal women but does not reduce the incidence of breast cancer or, by extrapolation, the incidence of DCIS. We briefly describe the progress that is being made with tamoxifen in the prevention of breast cancer; however, we believe that the current strategy of preventing breast cancer in high-risk women will ultimately be too narrow to produce a significant impact on the detection of DCIS. We propose a new, scientifically based strategy for the prevention of osteoporosis, coronary heart disease, and breast cancer that may also dramatically reduce the incidence of DCIS. Site-specific agents are already in clinical trials, and future drug designs hold the promise for further refinements in targeted preventive agents.

BENEFIT OF TAMOXIFEN TO TREAT DUCTAL CARCINOMA IN SITU

Until 1999, the standard treatment for localized DCIS was surgery and radiation therapy. The addition of tamoxifen is now known to decrease recurrence in patients with a diagnosis of DCIS (1). Tamoxifen is an approved part of the treatment plan for DCIS.

PROGRESS TOWARD A PREVENTION MAINTENANCE THERAPY

Tamoxifen has been tested as an agent for the prevention of breast cancer because

(i) there is clear evidence of potential efficacy,
(ii) there are ancillary physiologic benefits, and
(iii) the toxicities are modest compared with the development of breast cancer.

In 1986 at the Royal Marsden in London, Powles and coworkers (2–5) started to recruit high-risk women who would receive either tamoxifen or placebo for up to 8 years. This Vanguard study is now closed, and 2,018 women are enrolled. The group is a mixture of pre- and postmenopausal women who are also being evaluated for the effects of tamoxifen on bone density, circulating cholesterol, and gynecologic effects (4,5). Overall, tamoxifen has a beneficial effect on bone maintenance and lowers circulating cholesterol in postmenopausal women, but as expected, in premenopausal women there is a slight decrease in bone density and no effect on cholesterol measurements. The group has made a rigorous investigation of gynecologic changes, but found very little effect from tamoxifen other than an increase in polyps (4). However, recent analysis of these data showed no differences in the incidence of invasive breast cancer between tamoxifen and control arms (6). However, the statistical power of the study is probably too low to observe a definitive answer.

Presently there is general recruitment throughout the United Kingdom, Australia, and New Zealand to an international breast intervention study to provide more support

Potential Participants

>60 years old – with/without risk factors
35–59 years old – with risk factors

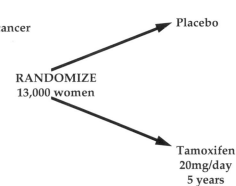

- LCIS
- First-degree relative with breast cancer
- Breast biopsies
- Atypical hyperplasia
- Over 25 years old before birth of first child
- No children
- Menarche before age 12

FIGURE 48.1. National Surgical Adjuvant Breast and Bowel Project-National Cancer Institute trial to test the worth of tamoxifen to prevent breast cancer in women. Women between the ages of 35 and 59 years had to present with risk factors to produce a cumulative risk equivalent to the risk for the 60-year-old woman. Recruitment of participants was completed in 1997 and results reported in 1998. From Fisher B, Costantino JP, Wickerham DL, et al. Tamoxifen for prevention of breast cancer: report of the National Surgical Adjuvant Breast and Bowel Project P-1 Study. *J Natl Cancer Inst* 1998;90:1371–1388, with permission.

for chemoprevention. The recruitment goal is 8,000 additional high-risk women to be randomized to tamoxifen or placebo for 5 years.

In the United States and Canada, the National Surgical Adjuvant Breast and Bowel Project has completed recruitment to a study of pre- and postmenopausal high-risk women. The design of the clinical trial is shown in Figure 48.1. Indeed, the volunteers were shown to be of such high-risk that the original goal of 16,000 women randomized to either tamoxifen or placebo for 5 years was reduced to 13,000 women. Tamoxifen produced a 49% decrease in invasive breast cancer and DCIS (7) in high-risk women. Side effects included an anticipated rise in endometrial cancer in postmenopausal women that was not life threatening. Premenopausal women treated with tamoxifen did not have an increase in endometrial cancer compared with control.

Finally, a study of tamoxifen as a preventive has been reported from Italy (8). Women over the age of 45 with no risk factors but who have already undergone a hysterectomy were recruited to determine the decrease in breast cancer with 5 years of therapy. Tamoxifen reduced the incidence of breast cancer in those women taking hormone replacement therapy but did not decrease incidence overall because only 3,000 normal risk women could be evaluated. These data are compared in Figure 48.2. In 1998, tamoxifen was approved by the Food and Drug Administration for the reduction of the risk of breast cancer in pre- and post-

menopausal high-risk women. However, the majority of breast cancer is sporadic and the affected women are usually not associated with high-risk factors. This reasoning lead us to suggest a more generalized strategy to prevent breast cancer in postmenopausal women.

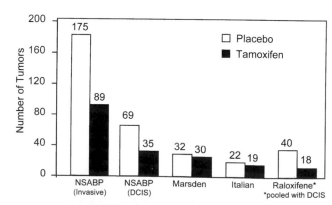

FIGURE 48.2. Results of the National Surgical Adjuvant Breast and Bowel Project-National Cancer Institute trial to test the worth of tamoxifen to prevent breast cancer in women. Women between the ages of 35 and 59 years had to present with risk factors to produce a cumulative risk equivalent to the risk for the 60-year-old woman. Recruitment of participants was completed in 1997 and results reported in 1998. From Fisher B, Costantino JP, Wickerham DL, et al. Tamoxifen for prevention of breast cancer: report of the National Surgical Adjuvant Breast and Bowel Project P-1 Study. *J Natl Cancer Inst* 1998;90:1371–1388, with permission.

A NEW STRATEGY

It is not possible to precisely predict who will develop breast cancer or, indeed, when the event occurs. Based on animal studies, it appears that the carcinogenic insult occurs early in life, before puberty (9). Therefore, any prevention strategy later in life really prevents promotion. As a women's health issue, it is clear that a very broad strategy is required if a general decrease in the incidence of breast cancer is to be achieved. To address this problem, in 1989 we suggested (10) that a new approach to the prevention of breast cancer could be achieved by developing agents to prevent osteoporosis and coronary heart disease in women. We wrote that, "Important clues have been garnered about the effects of tamoxifen on bones and lipids so it is possible that derivatives could find targeted applications to retard osteoporosis or atherosclerosis. The ubiquitous application of novel compounds to prevent diseases associated with the progressive changes after menopause, may, as a side effect, significantly retard the development of breast cancer. The target population would be postmenopausal women in general, thereby avoiding the requirement to select a high-risk group to prevent breast cancer." This was the start of a search for targeted antiestrogens to prevent the diseases of menopause in women (11–13).

DESIGN OF AN IDEAL TARGETED AGENT

The extensive clinical and laboratory database about tamoxifen now makes it possible to envision the properties of an ideal antiestrogen to provide the optimal clinical effects (Fig. 48.3). The agent should exhibit estrogenic effects in the central nervous system (CNS) and on endothelial cells to improve mood and decrease the frequency of postmenopausal symptoms. Similarly, the agent should have estrogen-like actions in the liver to lower low density lipoprotein (LDL) cholesterol and raise high density lipoprotein (HDL) cholesterol. This effect should translate to decreased atherosclerosis and coronary heart disease. It is now possible to design an agent to be free from DNA adducts in laboratory models so that there are no concerns about carcinogenesis during prolonged treatment. This is an important aspect of the design of a new agent, because indefinite therapy will be required to maintain bone density and prevent osteoporosis.

In contrast to the targeted estrogenic effects of the new agent, the compound should demonstrate inhibitory effects on growth and carcinogenesis in the uterus and breast so that there will be a decreased incidence of endometrial and breast cancer. Although there are many new compounds that exhibit the majority of properties needed in an ideal targeted antiestrogen, there is important new evidence to sup-

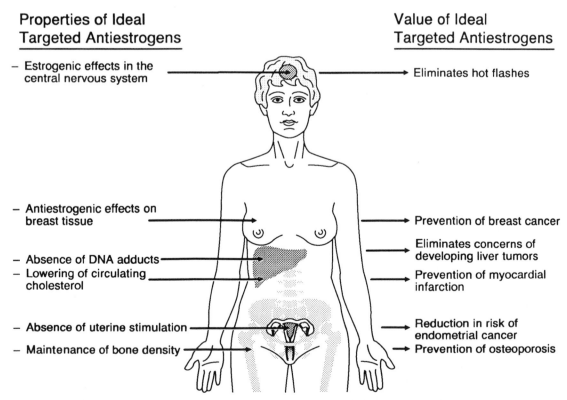

FIGURE 48.3. The design of a new target site–specific drug to selectively stimulate or inhibit estrogenic responses in target tissues. The novel agent will have the potential to control the development of several diseases associated with menopause.

port a rational approach to drug design. We survey the possible mechanisms for target site specificity before we consider the current status of strategies already in clinical trial.

SCIENTIFIC BASIS FOR TARGET SITE SPECIFICITY

The history of pharmacology is filled with examples of the use of drugs to elucidate the complex organization of signal transduction throughout the body. Targeted blocking drugs have helped to classify adrenergic receptors into a and b (1 and 2) types and to classify histamine receptors into H-1 and H-2 types. Additionally, the cholinergic system is organized into muscarinic and nicotinic receptors based on a clear cut pharmacologic classification. With this past experience as a guide, the unusual properties of nonsteroidal antiestrogens have raised the possibility that these compounds could be powerful tools to elucidate the organization of the estrogenic responses throughout the body.

At the subcellular level, it is now known that there is target site localization of different receptor molecules. The conventional estrogen receptor has been recognized for 30 years, but a novel estrogen receptor β (14) was just described. Alternatively, inhibitory or stimulatory factors could be located in different tissues that ultimately control whether a ligand receptor complex will be an inhibitory or stimulatory signal. These associated proteins are a topic of intense investigation (15). Finally, the genes in a target tissue may be activated or blocked specifically because a receptor ligand complex binds differentially to sites in a targeted promoter region. A raloxifene response element has been described in the promoter region of the TGF-β gene that might be responsible for differential bone stimulation (16). With all these possibilities, the actions of a targeted agent could be the result of one, several, or all mechanisms.

STRATEGIES TO DEVELOP A NOVEL PREVENTION MAINTENANCE THERAPY

The pharmaceutical industry has synthesized and tested thousands of novel antiestrogens and estrogens over the last 40 years. Numerous new compounds are now being tested for the treatment of breast cancer (17) but select agents are being developed further for the treatment of osteoporosis.

Raloxifene (Fig. 48.4), originally named keoxifene, was initially shown to maintain bone density in ovariectomized rats (18) and prevent rat mammary carcinogenesis (19). Raloxifene has subsequently been studied extensively in the laboratory to confirm the actions on bone (20–22) and to demonstrate that circulating cholesterol is reduced (20). Perhaps of importance is the observation that raloxifene has only a modest estrogenic action in the rodent uterus (23). This may be an advantage in developing an agent that has a

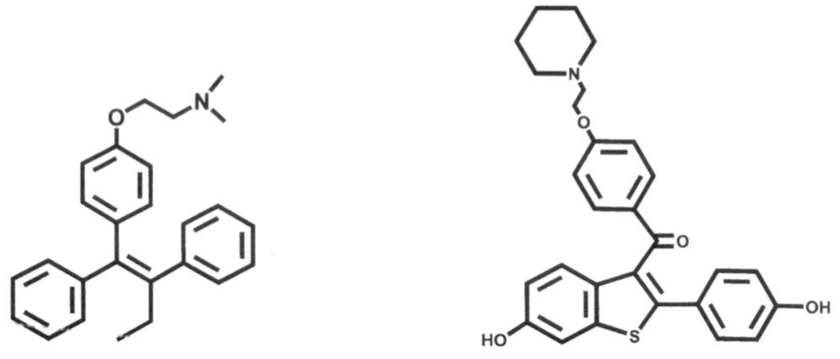

TAMOXIFEN **RALOXIFENE**

FIGURE 48.4. The formulae of tamoxifen and raloxifene.

less estrogenic effect on the growth of pre-existing endometrial carcinomas.

Raloxifene has been tested extensively in clinical trials to determine its worth in the treatment and prevention of osteoporosis. Raloxifene maintains bone density in postmenopausal women (24) and reduces fractures (25). The drug is approved by the Food and Drug Administration for the treatment and prevention of breast cancer. Breast safety was assessed in the osteoporosis trials, and a significant decrease in the incidence of invasive breast cancer was observed after 3 years of treatment. No decrease was observed in DCIS (26) (Fig. 48.2). These data provided the basis for the Study of Tamoxifen and Raloxifene (STAR) that is evaluating the worth of raloxifene to prevent breast cancer in high-risk women (Fig. 48.5).

SUMMARY

There are now exciting opportunities to develop a new prevention maintenance therapy for postmenopausal women (27). These strategies hold the promise of retarding the development of osteoporosis, coronary heart disease, and breast and endometrial cancer. An understanding of the molecular events involved in the target site–specific effects of estrogen through a novel ERβ system or the selective activation of genes by antiestrogen through novel response elements provides a basis for new drug discovery in the future.

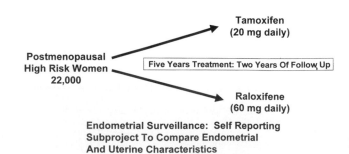

FIGURE 48.5. Study of Tamoxifen and Raloxifene trial endometrial surveillance: self reporting subproject to compare endometrial and uterine characteristics.

However, for the present, the well-documented clinical effects of estrogen coupled with the expanding database for tamoxifen has laid the foundation for the current clinical trials with raloxifene. Clinical studies with a large population of postmenopausal women have established the efficacy of the drug to treat and prevent osteoporosis (25), and ancillary studies will confirm the actions to prevent breast cancer and coronary heart disease (28). Raloxifene is the first of a whole series of new agents that hold the potential to revolutionize the approach to disease prevention in the majority of postmenopausal women (29). The general application of a prevention maintenance therapy will specifically reduce the development of breast cancer and reduce the detection of ductal carcinoma in situ.

ACKNOWLEDGMENT

We thank the Lynn Sage Breast Cancer Foundation and the Avon Products Foundation for supporting our program. Jennifer MacGregor is supported by DAMD 17-94-J-4466 in our Department of Defense Breast Cancer Training Program.

REFERENCES

1. Fisher B, Dignam J, Wolmark N, et al. Tamoxifen in treatment of intraductal breast cancer: National Surgical Adjuvant Breast and Bowel Project B-24 randomised controlled trial. *Lancet* 1999;353:1993–2000.
2. Powles TJ, Hardy JR, Ashley SE, et al. A pilot trial to evaluate the acute toxicity and feasibility of tamoxifen for prevention of breast cancer. *Br J Cancer* 1989;60:126–131.
3. Powles TJ, Tillyer CR, Jones AL, et al. Prevention of breast cancer with tamoxifen—an update on the Royal Marsden Hospital pilot programme. *Eur J Cancer* 1990;26:680–684.
4. Powles TJ, Jones AL, Ashley SE, et al. The Royal Marsden Hospital pilot tamoxifen chemoprevention trial. *Breast Cancer Res Treat* 1994;31:73–82.
5. Powles TJ, Hickish T, Kanis JA, et al. Effect of tamoxifen on bone mineral density measured by dual-energy x- ray absorptiometry in healthy premenopausal and postmenopausal women. *J Clin Oncol* 1996;14:78–84.
6. Powles T, Eeles R, Ashley S, et al. Interim analysis of the incidence of breast cancer in the Royal Marsden Hospital tamoxifen randomised chemoprevention trial. *Lancet* 1998;352:98–101.
7. Fisher B, Costantino JP, Wickerham DL, et al. Tamoxifen for prevention of breast cancer: report of the National Surgical Adjuvant Breast and Bowel Project P-1 Study. *J Natl Cancer Inst* 1998;90:1371–1388.
8. Veronesi U, Maisonneuve P, Costa A, et al. Prevention of breast cancer with tamoxifen: preliminary findings from the Italian randomised trial among hysterectomised women. Italian Tamoxifen Prevention Study. *Lancet* 1998;352:93–97.
9. Jordan VG, Morrow M. An appraisal of strategies to reduce the incidence of breast cancer. *Stem Cells* 1993;11:252–262.
10. Lerner LJ, Jordan VC. Development of antiestrogens and their use in breast cancer: Eighth Cain memorial award lecture. *Cancer Res* 1990;50:4177–4189.
11. Jordan VC. Alternate antiestrogens and approaches to the prevention of breast cancer. *J Cell Biochem Suppl* 1995;22:51–57.
12. Tonetti DA, Jordan VC. Targeted anti-estrogens to treat and prevent diseases in women. *Mol Med Today* 1996;2:218–223.
13. Tonetti DA, Jordan VC. Design of an ideal hormone replacement therapy for women. *Mol Carcinog* 1996;17:108–111.
14. Kuiper GG, Enmark E, Pelto-Huikko M, et al. Cloning of a novel receptor expressed in rat prostate and ovary. *Proc Natl Acad Sci U S A* 1996;93:5925–5930.
15. Baniahmad C, Nawaz Z, Baniahmad A, et al. Enhancement of human estrogen receptor activity by SPT6: A potential coactivator. *Mol Endocrinol* 1995;9:34–43.
16. Yang NN, Venugopalan M, Hardikar S, et al. Identification of an estrogen response element activated by metabolites of 17beta-estradiol and raloxifene [see comments] [published erratum appears in *Science* 1997;275(5304):1249]. *Science* 1996;273:1222–1225.
17. Gradishar WJ, Jordan VC. Clinical potential of new antiestrogens. *J Clin Oncol* 1997;15:840–852.
18. Jordan VC, Phelps E, Lindgren JU. Effects of anti-estrogens on bone in castrated and intact female rats. *Breast Cancer Res Treat* 1987;10:31–35.
19. Gottardis MM, Jordan VC. Antitumor actions of keoxifene and tamoxifen in the N-nitrosomethylurea-induced rat mammary carcinoma model. *Cancer Res* 1987;47:4020–4024.
20. Black LJ, Sato M, Rowley ER, et al. Raloxifene (LY139481 HCl) prevents bone loss and reduces serum cholesterol without causing uterine hypertrophy in ovariectomized rats. *J Clin Invest* 1994;93:63–69.
21. Evans G, Bryant HU, Magee D, et al. The effects of raloxifene on tibia histomorphometry in ovariectomized rats. *Endocrinology* 1994;134:2283–2288.
22. Sato M, Kim J, Short LL, et al. Longitudinal and cross-sectional analysis of raloxifene effects on tibiae from ovariectomized aged rats. *J Pharmacol Exp Ther* 1995;272:1252–1259.
23. Black LJ, Jones CD, Falcone JF. Antagonism of estrogen action with a new benzothiophene derived antiestrogen. *Life Sci* 1983;32:1031–1036.
24. Delmas PD, Bjarnason NH, Mitlak BH, et al. Effects of raloxifene on bone mineral density, serum cholesterol concentrations, and uterine endometrium in postmenopausal women [see comments]. *N Engl J Med* 1997;337:1641–1647.
25. Ettinger B, Black DM, Mitlak BH, et al. Reduction of vertebral fracture risk in postmenopausal women with osteoporosis treated with raloxifene: results from a 3-year randomized clinical trial. Multiple Outcomes of Raloxifene Evaluation (MORE) Investigators [see comments]. *JAMA* 1999;282:637–645.
26. Cummings SR, Eckert S, Krueger KA, et al. The effect of raloxifene on risk of breast cancer in postmenopausal women: results from the MORE randomized trial. Multiple Outcomes of Raloxifene Evaluation. *JAMA* 1999;281:2189–2197.
27. Jordan VC. Tamoxifen: the herald of a new era of preventive therapeutics [editorial; comment]. *J Natl Cancer Inst* 1997;89:747–749.
28. Jordan VC, Morrow M. Raloxifene as a multifunctional medicine? *BMJ* 1999;319:331–332.
29. Levenson AS, Jordan VC. Selective Oestrogen Receptor Modulation: Molecular pharmacology for the millennium. *Eur J Cancer* 1999;35:1628–1639.

49

TAMOXIFEN AND/OR HORMONE REPLACEMENT THERAPY AFTER TREATMENT FOR DUCTAL CARCINOMA IN SITU

CHRISTY A. RUSSELL

As a result of the increasing use of screening mammography, the incidence and prevalence of ductal carcinoma in situ (DCIS) in women 40 and older has steadily increased over the last decade in the United States. Because the risk of developing life-threatening metastatic breast cancer is rare in women with DCIS, other causes of premature morbidity and mortality for these women must be taken into consideration. Women with no prior history of breast cancer, either invasive or in situ, often face decisions regarding the use of hormone replacement therapy either for the acute symptoms of menopause or for the primary prevention of diseases of aging such as cardiovascular disease or osteoporotic fractures. The decision to initiate the use of hormone replacement therapy (HRT) is not easy, because the data supporting the benefits of these replacement hormones are not as clear as women have frequently been lead to believe. Healthy women have historically been undereducated regarding the true expected risks and benefits of HRT because of the lack of statistically meaningful randomized clinical trials assessing these benefits and risks. The picture is even murkier when considering women with a high risk of developing breast cancer or in those women with a personal history of DCIS. Their options for systemic therapy include the following: no HRT, HRT for a limited time (1 to 2 years) until the cessation of acute symptoms of menopause, long-term hormone therapy for primary prevention of non–breast related diseases, or tamoxifen therapy for breast cancer prevention. Women with a prior history of invasive breast cancer also have a similar dilemma but are faced with the potential risk of the hormones stimulating the growth of micrometastatic disease and hastening their demise.

There is very little data available on the safety of estrogen replacement therapy (ERT) or HRT in women with a prior invasive breast cancer. Certainly, no large, controlled randomized trial has been performed that will definitively answer the safety questions of replacement hormones in this patient population. All reports at this point have included a very small number of women in nonrandomized trials who have varying risks of metastatic recurrence and varying lengths of use of their HRT. For the large majority of women with invasive breast cancer, the greatest risk of premature mortality for the remainder of their lives will be from breast cancer. In fact, if HRT increases the risk of metastatic recurrence in any way, then the risks hugely outweigh the benefits. Unfortunately, as little as is known about the risks of HRT in women with invasive breast cancer, even less is known about the use of supplemental hormones after the diagnosis of DCIS. This chapter will discuss the known benefits and risks of HRT and the benefits and risks of tamoxifen hormonal therapy as they are currently described and as they affect morbidity and mortality from any cause in postmenopausal women.

HORMONE REPLACEMENT THERAPY: BENEFITS AND RISKS

Benefits

Two of the most distressing events of menopause are hot flashes and vaginal dryness. ERT is one of the most effective interventions to treat these symptoms (1).

The incidence of *vasomotor instability (hot flashes)* in perimenopausal and postmenopausal women is not well understood, as most reports have been self-described and not based on a reliable and reproducible hot flash scale. Symptoms of vasomotor instability appear to be described more frequently and more severely in breast cancer patients who are suddenly withdrawn from their HRT or who undergo a medical menopause as a result of chemotherapy. ERT is one of the most effective therapies for hot flashes. As moderate or severe hot flashes rarely last five years after onset, the use of ERT can be curtailed within a relatively short period of time. Progesterone in the form of megestrol acetate (Megace) may also be equally effective in controlling hot flashes, but is limited by the side effects of increased appetite and weight gain (2).

Urogenital atrophy is frequently a delayed sign of menopause and is manifested in multiple ways including vaginal dryness, dyspareunia, pruritis, urinary urgency, frequency, and incontinence (3). Estrogen is by far the most effective method of dealing with all of these symptoms. Extensive clinical trials have explored both oral and vaginal methods of delivering the estrogen, each with its advantages and disadvantages. Plasma levels of estradiol are lower when the estrogen is applied locally in the form of vaginal estrogen cream. However, this is at the expense of the inconvenience and messiness of a rather large bolus of fat-based emollient that must be delivered intravaginally in order to achieve adequate levels of estrogen to the vaginal tissues. To ameliorate these problems, a silastic vaginal ring that delivers small amounts of estrogen locally to the vaginal tissues and is replaced by the patient every 3 months has been developed.

With an aging population, morbidity from *osteoporotic fractures* is on the rise (4). It is recommended that women maintain adequate calcium intake (1,500 mg per day with vitamin D) and maintain a physical activity schedule that includes weight-bearing exercise. Estrogen has been shown in randomized and observational studies to preserve bone mineral density after menopause. In fact, estrogen has FDA approval for this indication. With the advent of bisphosphonate therapies, additional choices are now available for the treatment of osteoporosis. A commonly prescribed drug for women with osteoporosis is aledronate (Fosamax). A comparison between this bisphosphonate aledronate and ERT proved them to be essentially equivalent to one another, and both superior to calcium plus placebo. Both forms of therapy must be continued indefinitely to maintain bone density over long periods of time. The effectiveness of both estrogen and aledronate drop rapidly when either is discontinued.

Estrogen has been definitively shown to have a positive impact on *lipids* by decreasing LDL cholesterol levels and increasing both HDL cholesterol levels and triglyceride levels in postmenopausal women (1). This effect appears to be strongest during the first year of use, and may be somewhat dampened over time. The addition of progesterone to estrogen (HRT) is known to reduce some of the beneficial effects of estrogen on lipids, particularly when evaluating the increase in HDL. The beneficial impact of estrogen on *cardiovascular disease* is clearly more controversial. There is a myriad of both observational and case-control studies that suggest a significant reduction in coronary heart disease in women who use HRT or ERT. This "truth" has been spouted for some time. However, there is only one published randomized trial, which was in women with a preceding coronary event. The women were randomized to

HRT or placebo (5). The Heart and Estrogen-Progesterone Replacement Study (HERS) not only failed to show a benefit of the hormone therapy but suggested an increase in the incidence of nonfatal myocardial infarctions and cardiac deaths in the first year of hormone use when compared with placebo. Despite the known lipid benefits of hormones, it has been suggested that the apparent benefit of estrogen in the primary prevention of coronary artery disease may be more based on the underlying health of women who choose HRT rather than the effect of the therapy itself. A large, randomized clinical trial that evaluates the actual cardiovascular benefit in postmenopausal women has not been completed. Hopefully, the Women's Health Initiative Hormone Trial currently being run in the United States will dispel some of the myths and unequivocally prove the benefits of estrogen. This trial has been designed to enroll over 27,000 healthy women who will be blindly and randomly assigned to HRT, ERT, or placebo.

Observational studies and large-population studies have analyzed the relationship between *stroke* and estrogen therapy. Some of these studies have suggested an increased risk of stroke, although others have suggested the opposite. Investigators have recently published data on the first large randomized trial evaluating the benefit of ERT after an ischemic stroke. The Women's Estrogen for Stroke Trial (WEST) was initiated in December 1993, and randomized 664 women older than 44 years of age who had developed an ischemic stroke or transient ischemic attack. Women were assigned to receive 1 mg of estradiol-17B daily, or placebo (6). Women were given estrogen alone to reduce the potential antagonistic effects of progesterone. The primary end point of the study was death from any cause or the occurrence of a nonfatal stroke. Women were also observed for transient ischemic attack or nonfatal myocardial infarctions. With a reported mean of 2.8 years of follow-up, women randomized to the estradiol group did not have a reduction in the overall risk of death or risk of nonfatal strokes. Women randomized to estrogen actually had a higher risk of fatal strokes, and those with nonfatal strokes suffered worse neurologic and functional deficits. The authors suggested that their results, along with the results of the HERS trial indicate that ERT should not be initiated for the purpose of *secondary* prevention of cardiovascular disease.

There are two other potential benefits of ERT that await substantially more data and results from randomized clinical trials. Many observational studies have suggested a significant reduction in the incidence of *colorectal cancer* for women who take ERT, although others have reported no such effect. The second potential benefit is that of improved *cognitive function*, or the delay and prevention of dementia. At this point, there are far too many conflicting data with regard to this potential benefit to reach any meaningful conclusion. Clearly, further research is needed in this area (1).

Risks

The risk of *endometrial cancer* and benign hyperplasia of the uterus are both markedly increased in postmenopausal women who take unopposed estrogen (7). This effect is abrogated by the addition of progesterone. The primary indication for the addition of progesterone to estrogen in postmenopausal women is for the protection of the uterus. There is certainly no other known health benefit of progesterone in postmenopausal women.

Deep venous thrombosis, pulmonary emboli, and *cholecystitis* are also known complications of HRT. Each of these risks was magnified in the HERS study, which evaluated a group of women who tended to be older and had established underlying cardiovascular disease (5). Deep venous thrombosis and pulmonary emboli were increased by 300% and cholecystitis was increased by 40%. Healthy postmenopausal women continue to show an increase in these risks, but to a lesser degree.

Of all the risks discussed from HRT, the one that strikes the greatest fear in the heart of women is the risk of developing *breast cancer*. In a large number of studies and two meta-analyses, long-term use of ERT or HRT has been shown to increase the risk of development of breast cancer by approximately 30% (8,9). Another way of stating this statistic is that the risk of developing breast cancer increases by 3% per year of HRT use. This risk is likely influenced by the underlying risk factors for breast cancer in those women who take HRT, including genetic risk, endogenous exposure of estrogen related to reproductive factors, exercise, and body weight after menopause, to name a few. One recent large cohort study and a second case-control study have suggested strong evidence that the addition of progesterone to estrogen as HRT markedly increases the risk of development of breast cancer compared with women who use ERT alone (10,11). It has been stated that rather than implicating ERT or HRT as substantially increasing the risk of developing breast cancer in all women exposed, that we begin to better understand the specific subgroups at greatest risk from supplemental hormones. Perhaps this avenue of investigation will be more fruitful than studies that try to prove that ERT or HRT is indeed related to the development of breast cancer, and to what degree.

TAMOXIFEN: BENEFITS AND RISKS

Benefits

The benefits of tamoxifen in women with hormone receptor–positive, invasive breast cancer are well established not only in the metastatic but also in the adjuvant setting. As the theme of this chapter is the potential effect of HRT versus tamoxifen in the setting of DCIS, I will present only the benefit data that are gleaned from the two large randomized clinical trials in women with a high risk of developing breast cancer, or with DCIS.

NSABP P-1 Study

In 1992, the NSABP initiated a clinical trial evaluating the effects of tamoxifen in women at high risk of breast cancer as determined by the Gail model (12). The initial report published in 1998 presented data on 13,388 "high-risk" women who were randomly assigned to take either five years of tamoxifen or placebo. "High risk" was defined as any woman age 60 or older, any woman age 35 to 59 with the same high risk as a women age 60 (at least a 1.66% risk of breast cancer over the next 5 years), or any woman with a pathologic diagnosis of lobular carcinoma in situ or atypical ductal hyperplasia. Women could not have had a prior diagnosis of DCIS or invasive breast cancer. Median follow-up time of women on this study was 54.6 months at the time of the original publication. Tamoxifen reduced the incidence of *invasive breast cancer* by 49% with a comparative cumulative incidence of cancer of 43.4 versus 22 breast cancers per 1000 women in the placebo and tamoxifen groups, respectively. Incidence of new cancers was reduced regardless of age, previous histologic findings, or extent of increased risk. The incidence of *DCIS* was also reduced by 50% with a comparative cumulative incidence of 15.9 versus 7.7 per 1000 women in the placebo and tamoxifen groups, respectively. Of interest, tamoxifen did not alter the incidence of estrogen receptor–negative invasive breast cancer when compared with placebo.

Other than the previously described effects on the breast, tamoxifen also reduced the incidence of *osteoporotic bone fractures* by 19%, which was expectedly even higher in women in the trial over the age of 50. Although tamoxifen is known to improve the lipid profile in postmenopausal women, this did not translate into a reduction in manifestations of *ischemic heart disease*. There was no change in the numbers of myocardial infarctions, angina requiring CABG or angioplasty, or in the incidence of acute ischemic syndrome.

Risks

As expected, *endometrial cancer* was increased in women taking tamoxifen versus those taking placebo. This increase was only seen in women 50 years of age or older. The cumulative incidence of endometrial cancer through 66 months of follow-up was 5.4 versus 13.0 per 1000 women on placebo and tamoxifen, respectively. All of the endometrial cancers in the tamoxifen group and all but one in the placebo group were Fédération Internationale de Gunecologie et Obstetrique (FIGO) stage I, contrary to other case-control studies that have suggested a higher grade and higher stage incidence of uterine cancer in women exposed to tamoxifen. *Vascular events* were also significantly increased in women on tamoxifen. The cumulative incidence of stroke was 0.92 versus 1.45 per 1000 women in women on placebo and tamoxifen, respectively. Increased risk was only seen in women age 50 and older. The incidence of transient ischemic attacks was reduced from 25 to 19 in women on placebo versus tamoxifen. Neither the increased incidence of stroke nor the reduction in incidence of transient ischemic attacks was statistically significant. *Pulmonary emboli* and *deep venous thrombosis* were also significantly increased in women on tamoxifen. The increase in events was limited to women age 50 and older. There were 18 versus 6 pulmonary emboli and 35 versus 22 cases of deep venous thrombosis in women on tamoxifen versus placebo, respectively. New onset of *cataracts* was slightly increased in women taking tamoxifen. The rate of self-reported development of cataracts was 21.72 versus 24.82 per 1000 women on placebo and tamoxifen, respectively.

Toxicity

There were two symptoms that were significantly increased in women on tamoxifen: *hot flashes* and *vaginal discharge*. Extremely bothersome hot flashes were reported at rates of 45.7% and 28.7% in women on tamoxifen versus placebo, respectively. Vaginal discharge that was moderately bothersome or worse was reported at rates of 29% and 13% in women on tamoxifen and placebo, respectively. The incidence of *clinical depression* was not different between the two arms.

DUCTAL CARCINOMA IN SITU

Although the NSABP P-1 trial represents the largest double-blind randomized trial comparing tamoxifen with placebo in women at high risk for primary breast cancer, the trial is more instructive in assessing the toxicity of tamoxifen and the reduction in risk of primary breast cancer for this specific group of women. It can be questioned as to whether these data can be translated to predict benefits and risks of tamoxifen in women with DCIS. Prior to assessing the potential benefit of tamoxifen in women with a history of DCIS, it is important to understand the actual incidence of either ipsilateral or contralateral new breast cancers for these women. To our knowledge, the incidence of both ipsilateral and contralateral breast cancers after primary breast-conserving therapy for DCIS can be derived from two large randomized trials conducted by the NSABP in women with DCIS (13).

In 1985, **NSABP B-17** was initiated. The purpose of the study was to determine whether segmental mastectomy (lumpectomy) followed by radiation therapy was superior to segmental mastectomy alone when evaluating the incidence of ipsilateral breast tumor (IBT) recurrence. Between October 1, 1985 and December 31, 1990, 818 women were randomly assigned to one of the two treatment groups. The primary end point of this study was the recurrence IBT or the occurrence of contralateral breast tumors (CBTs), whether invasive or noninvasive. As recently reported, the mean duration of follow-up for this study was 128 months.

There were 124 IBT found in the 403 women randomized to the lumpectomy-alone arm, and 61 IBT found in the 410 women randomized to postsurgical radiation therapy. These recurrences were split fairly evenly between invasive and noninvasive recurrences. Thus, the incidence rate of all IBTs was reduced by 57% as a result of the post-lumpectomy radiation therapy. Through 12 years of follow-up, the cumulative incidence of IBT was 31.7% for those randomized to lumpectomy and 15.7% for those receiving radiation therapy after lumpectomy. Contralateral breast tumor occurrences were relatively low, and radiation therapy did not influence their statistical occurrence. There were 18 CBTs in the lumpectomy arm and 30 CBTs in the lumpectomy plus radiation therapy arm. Differently stated, there was an annual incidence of 5.8 CBT per 1000 patients versus 8.4 CBT per 1000 patients, respectively. The cumulative incidence of CBT for the combined group was 6.6% over the 12 years of follow-up. Through these 12 years of follow-up, 3% of the women treated with lumpectomy and 4% of those treated with lumpectomy plus radiation therapy died of breast cancer. These data give us an excellent baseline of risk for either CBT or IBT in women with a history of DCIS, and suggest a significantly higher risk of new invasive breast cancers for these women compared with the "high-risk" women participating in the P-1 trial, including those women with lobular carcinoma in situ or atypical ductal hyperplasia. Presuming that the new onset of invasive breast cancer is the most significant finding, the results comparing the B-17 data with the P-1 trial are as shown in Table 49.1.

In addition, the rates of invasive breast cancer in women on the B-17 trial who received radiation therapy still remained higher than those women in the P-1 trial with either lobular carcinoma in situ or atypical ductal hyperplasia who received placebo.

Because of the known benefit of tamoxifen in reducing both the risk of recurrent ipsilateral and contralateral breast cancers in women with invasive breast cancer undergoing breast-conservation therapy, the NSABP performed the **NSABP B-24** trial to assess whether tamoxifen can have a similar benefit in women with DCIS. Between May 9, 1991 and April 13, 1994, 1,804 women with the diagnosis of DCIS who had undergone lumpectomy were randomly assigned to radiation therapy to the ipsilateral breast in the same manner as was delivered in B-17 plus placebo versus radiation therapy with concurrent tamoxifen. All women

TABLE 49.1. B-17 VERSUS P-1 TRIAL RESULTS

Trial	Rates of Invasive Cancer (Per 1,000 Women/Year)
B-17 lumpectomy alone	28.2
P-1 placebo and LCIS	13.0
P-1 placebo and ADH	10.2

LCIS, lobular carcinoma in situ; ADH, atypical ductal hyperplasia.

randomized to the tamoxifen arm received tamoxifen 20 mg per day for a total of five years. In both the B-17 and B-24 trials, radiation therapy was initiated within 8 weeks of the lumpectomy. Tamoxifen was required to be initiated within 56 days of lumpectomy. The current mean duration of follow-up for NSABP B-24 is 82 months. Of interest, women with positive surgical margins were eligible for randomization in the B-24 trial.

There were 100 IBTs in the 899 women in the placebo arm and 72 IBTs in the 899 women in the tamoxifen arm. There was no difference in the rates of noninvasive tumors between the two groups, but there was a significant diminution in the incidence of invasive IBTs when tamoxifen was added. The rate of invasive IBTs in the placebo arm was 9.0 per 1000 women per year compared with 4.8 invasive IBTs per 1000 women per year. This represents a 47% reduction in invasive IBTs as a result of taking five years of tamoxifen. CBTs were also impacted by the use of tamoxifen. There were 45 versus 25 CBTs as the first event for women on placebo versus tamoxifen, respectively. At seven years, the cumulative incidence of invasive IBT was 5.3% in the placebo group and 2.6% in the tamoxifen group. The cumulative incidence of all CBTs at 7 years was 4.9% in the placebo group and 2.3% in the tamoxifen group. The reduction in invasive CBT from 3.2% to 1.8% was not statistically significant ($p = 0.16$). There was a significant reduction of noninvasive CBT ($p = .03$). Most significantly, there was a 48% reduction in all invasive cancers (IBT or CBT) by the use of tamoxifen compared with placebo.

Several prognostic factors for ipsilateral recurrence were seen from this trial. Age at diagnosis, the presence of positive tumor margins, palpable tumors, and the histologic finding of comedonecrosis were all predictive of IBT recurrence. Tamoxifen had a positive impact on all of the prognostic subgroups. None of these prognostic factors were predictive for the occurrence of contralateral breast cancer. There was an expected, but not statistically significant increase in incidence of endometrial cancer in women on tamoxifen (seven versus three, $p = 0.38$). There were no deaths from endometrial cancer. Through 7 years of follow-up, the overall survival is identical in the two groups (95%).

Conclusions: When considering the NSABP P-1, B-17, and B-24 trials, there is adequate information regarding the incidence of both contralateral and ipsilateral breast cancers in women at high risk due to reproductive history, histologic findings of lobular carcinoma in situ or atypical ductal hyperplasia, or from DCIS. There is also adequate information regarding the benefits and risks of tamoxifen hormonal therapy when compared with placebo for this group of women. There is no such randomized data available for women exposed to either ERT or HRT who are at high risk for breast cancer as described in the P-1 trial or for women with a preceding history of DCIS of the breast. It appears

quite clear that the use of tamoxifen after an episode of DCIS will reduce the incidence of subsequent ipsilateral and contralateral breast cancers. It is also quite clear that the use of ERT or HRT after the diagnosis of DCIS will not reduce either the incidence of ipsilateral or contralateral breast cancers. Whether it increases that risk and by what degree is unknown. If one compares the risk of ipsilateral breast cancer recurrence in a woman with a lumpectomy and radiation therapy after DCIS to that of a woman with a breast biopsy revealing either LCIS or ADH, the evidence shows that the woman with DCIS stands a much greater chance of ipsilateral breast cancer than either of the other histologic findings. As it is universally accepted that tamoxifen could be considered for chemoprevention for these high-risk findings, then clearly it must be considered and discussed with women with a history of DCIS.

Why would a physician consider anything other than tamoxifen in these circumstances? Of course, one must consider not only the benefits that tamoxifen provides, but also the toxicities. The common side effects of hot flashes and vaginal discharge with tamoxifen seem relatively unimportant when comparing them with the reduced risk of development of breast cancer with all of its associated morbidity and mortality. However, neither NSABP P-1 nor NSABP B-24 has shown an improvement in survival when comparing placebo with tamoxifen, despite the reduced incidence of invasive cancers. Although the risk of endometrial cancer must also be considered when prescribing tamoxifen, both the P-1 and the B-24 trials convincingly show that more breast cancers are prevented than endometrial cancers caused in these circumstances.

As with most large randomized double-blinded trials, more new questions are asked at the conclusion than are answered by the trial. What is it that women really want to know? Women want to know that if they have DCIS, and what their actual risk of developing another breast cancer might be. They wish to know whether it is better to do a mastectomy, a lumpectomy, or a lumpectomy with radiation therapy, and whether this decision will impact an eventual ipsilateral recurrence. They want to know if there are greater long-term benefits from tamoxifen or from HRT after their local therapy for DCIS. They want to know if they can take tamoxifen for five years and then follow it with HRT. They want to know if there is any harm in combining tamoxifen concurrently with HRT. Physicians cannot look to any randomized clinical trials to answer these questions or guide us in counseling our patients. It is imperative that all physicians treating women with DCIS become familiar with the known benefits and risks of ERT, HRT, and tamoxifen and use this knowledge to guide their patients toward a course that they are comfortable in accepting and living with. Tamoxifen and/or HRT after DCIS: good medicine or bad? At this time it still remains an informed judgment call.

REFERENCES

1. McNagny, SE. Prescribing hormone replacement therapy for menopausal symptoms. *Ann Intern Med* 1999;131(8):605–616.

2. Loprinzi CL, Michalak JC, Quella SK, et al. Megestrol acetate for the prevention of hot flashes. *N Engl J Med* 1994;331:347–352.

3. Swain S, Santen R, Burger H, et al. Treatment of estrogen deficiency symptoms in women surviving breast cancer. Urogenital atrophy, vasomotor instability, sleep disorders, and related symptoms. *Oncology* 1999;13(4):551–575.

4. Swain S, Santen R, Burger H, et al. Treatment of estrogen deficiency symptoms in women surviving breast cancer. Prevention of osteoporosis and CV effects of estrogens and antiestrogens. *Oncology* 1999;13(3):397–432.

5. Hulley S, Grady D, Bush T, et al. Randomized trial of estrogen plus progestin for secondary prevention of coronary heart disease in postmenopausal women. Heart and Estrogen/Progesterone Replacement Study (HERS) Research Group. *JAMA* 1998;280:605–613.

6. Viscoli CM, Brass LM, Kernan WN, et al. A clinical trial of estrogen-replacement therapy after ischemic stroke. *N Engl J Med* 2001;345(17):1243–1249.

7. Grady D, Gebretsadik T, Kerlikowske K, et al. Hormone replacement therapy and endometrial cancer risk: a meta-analysis. *Obstet Gynecol* 1995;85:304–313.

8. Collaborative Group on Hormonal Factors in Breast Cancer. Breast cancer and hormone replacement therapy: collaborative re-analysis of data from 51 epidemiological studies of 52,705 women with breast cancer and 108,411 women without breast cancer. *Lancet* 1997;350:1047–1059.

9. Steinberg KK, Thacker SB, Smith SJ, et al. A meta-analysis of the effect of estrogen replacement therapy on the risk of breast cancer. *JAMA* 1991;265:1985–1990.

10. Schairer C, Lubin J, Troisi R, et al. Menopausal estrogen and estrogen-progestin replacement therapy and breast cancer risk. *JAMA* 2000;283(4):485–491.

11. Ross RK, Paganini-Hill A, Wan PC, et al. Effect of hormone replacement therapy on breast cancer risk: estrogen versus estrogen plus progestin. *J Natl Cancer Inst* 2000;92(4):328–332.

12. Fisher B, Costantino JP, Wickerham DL, et al. Tamoxifen for prevention of breast cancer: Report of the National Surgical Adjuvant Breast and Bowel Project P-1 study. *J Natl Cancer Inst* 1998;90:1371–1388.

13. Fisher B, Land S, Mamounas E, et al. Prevention of invasive breast cancer in women with ductal carcinoma in situ: An update of the National Surgical Adjuvant Breast and Bowel Project Experience. *Semin Oncol* 2001;28:400–418.

50

TAMOXIFEN CHEMOPREVENTION FOR DUCTAL CARCINOMA IN SITU: MAGIC BULLET OR MISSTEP?

MICHAEL D. LAGIOS

The goal of nonsurgical therapies, including chemoprevention, for ductal carcinoma in situ (DCIS) remains a fiercely sought but elusive grail; successful chemotherapeutic intervention has yet to be achieved.

The use of tamoxifen and other antiestrogenic selective estrogen receptor modulators (SERMS) is predicated on the basis that estrogens are a major promoter of breast cancer carcinogenesis and growth, and that risk of recurrence and/or progression of DCIS can be diminished by their use. Yet evidence continues to accumulate to cast doubt on this traditional medical understanding of the role of estrogen in breast cancer.

This chapter reviews the size of the benefit for local control and contralateral tumor suppression with the adjuvant use of tamoxifen in the only randomized trial to claim a benefit, the NSABP B-24 trial. The perspective that emerges is that the benefits, if they are reproducible, are of minute size and statistically significant but clinically meaningless.

For more than 100 years, particularly since Beatson's (1) demonstration of tumor regression following ovarian ablation in 1896, estrogen has been classified as a causative agent and/or a promoting factor in breast cancer. During my residency 35 years ago, it was revealed truth that any patient with breast cancer must avoid any condition that increases estrogen exposure. Young women who had been successfully treated for early stage breast cancer were told to avoid pregnancy at all costs, because the hormonal titers in pregnancy might well provoke a recurrence.

It would take another 15 years for clinicians to tentatively accept pregnancy after breast cancer treatment as anything but a major provocation. Postmenopausal women generally, and those with a history of breast cancer in particular, then as they are today, were proscribed from taking hormone replacement therapy (HRT) to diminish the risk of recurrence. With the advent of mammography, noninvasive carcinomas such as duct carcinoma in situ and lobular carcinoma in situ and what came to be recognized as risk markers such as atypical duct and atypical lobular hyperplasia, were also included in the group that would sustain unacceptably high risk from HRT. As a result, almost all patients who might seek consultation with diagnoses of atypical hyperplasia, duct and lobular carcinoma in situ, and low-grade T1, N0 invasive carcinomas have been abruptly withdrawn from HRT. Moreover, for many of these patients, tamoxifen has been recommended as providing substantial improvement in disease-free survival based on the NSABP randomized trials P-1 (prevention trial), B-24, and B-20 (2–4). Despite this understanding, Dupont and Page (5,6) showed that HRT had no significant adverse effect on breast cancer risk, and Vassilopoulou-Sellin et al. (7) and Fowble et al. (8) showed no significant difference in outcome for women with invasive breast cancer subsequently placed on HRT or previously having received HRT, respectively.

Reevaluation of the role of HRT in breast cancer patients, particularly those at low risk, has been going on for nearly a decade, but there has been little inclination to change traditional belief for uncertainty in the absence of randomized trial data. Recently, O'Meara et al. (9) published a case-control study of HRT in patients with documented invasive breast cancer without evidence of distant metastases and without a prior history of in situ or invasive breast cancer. Their results challenged the existing paradigms about estrogen and breast cancer risk. Patients with HRT had approximately half the recurrence rate, and a third of the breast cancer mortality compared with case controls without HRT. Similar results had been demonstrated in other case-control studies by DiSaia et al. (10), Eden et al. (11), and Puthgraman et al. (12), all of which showed a decreased recurrence rate and mortality related to conventional HRT. In their outcome study, Fowble et al. (8) demonstrated a decrease in both locoregional and distant metastases and contralateral breast cancers in postmenopausal prior HRT users compared with nonusers.

Although estrogen has been touted in the recent past (13) as a significant promotor of breast cancer based on 10-year

HRT usage resulting in relative risks of 1.14, this does not jibe with the findings of O'Meara et al. (9) and others in which it actually reduced both recurrence and cause-specific mortality. Perhaps as discussed in a recent editorial, HRT is actually protective against recurrence after breast-conservation therapy. Without well-designed, prospective studies, this radical rethinking of the role of estrogen in breast cancer will never be confirmed; but, indeed, the benefits of tamoxifen in chemoprevention and as an adjuvant agent in postmenopausal women may well relate to its molecular similarity to estrogen itself rather than its antiestrogenic activity.

Let us review, assuming that local recurrences, both in situ and invasive, following breast-conservation therapy for DCIS can be suppressed with tamoxifen, what kind of benefit can be demonstrated on the basis of the NSABP B-24 and the United Kingdom-Australia-New Zealand (UK/ANZ) randomized trials (4,14).

The thesis that tamoxifen can reduce the frequency of in situ breast cancer in a treated population has been tested in several randomized trial settings. The best known of these are the NSABP B-24 trial of lumpectomy and radiation therapy with patients randomized to tamoxifen for DCIS, and the prevention trial for women defined by the Gail model as having a breast cancer risk equivalent to a 60-year-old.

In B-24, at a median 74-month follow-up, 37% fewer breast cancer events were reported for the tamoxifen arm. Breast cancer events in this tabulation include local in situ and invasive carcinomas in the ipsilateral breast, loco-regional and distant metastases, and contralateral carcinomas both in situ and invasive. This benefit amounts to an actual (as opposed to relative) difference of 5.1% at 74 months of follow-up or an approximate annualized reduction of all breast cancer events of 0.85% (calculated at 74 months). In this trial, approximately one in 20 women randomized to the tamoxifen arm actually is expected to benefit after 5 years of treatment!

Although contralateral breast cancer events do occur in patients with treated DCIS, most clinicians are primarily concerned with the ipsilateral breast (in which most of the risk lies). In B-24, the benefit of tamoxifen in reducing a noninvasive (in situ) recurrence in the ipsilateral breast was 0.778% at a median 74 months of follow-up or as presented in the table at 5 years. One in 128 women randomized to the tamoxifen arm would be expected to benefit at 5 years. The *p* value for this benefit was not significant (0.43), and the annualized benefit (predicated on 5 years) is 0.15% (Table 50.1).

In situ recurrences generally amount to half of all recurrences in the ipsilateral breast in all studies save those conducted by the NSABP (B-17 and B-24), and certainly this was the ratio observed in the placebo–radiation therapy arm in B-24 as well. This contrasts to the earlier study, B-17, in which there was a selective benefit of radiation therapy in preventing invasive recurrences, a finding not corroborated in the more recent EORTC 10853 randomized trial for DCIS (15). For the ipsilateral breast, tamoxifen produced a significant ($p = 0.03$) reduction in invasive recurrences, a benefit of 1.89% at 5 five years or an annualized benefit of 0.37%. Approximately one in 53 (Table 50.1) women randomized to tamoxifen in B-24 would be spared an invasive ipsilateral recurrence at 5 years.

The P-1 prevention trial showed that the reduction in invasive events in that trial was entirely confined to estrogen receptor–positive carcinomas, and this is likely true of B-24 as well. Such a reduction at 5 years most likely reflects the presence of undetected residual invasive breast cancer within the resected tissue or in the breast at the time of treatment, as it most likely does in the prevention trial. That invasive breast cancer could be pathologically overlooked in a protocol based on tissue sampling for DCIS should not be a surprise at this point (see Chapter 16), but clear evidence of this is seen from the percentages of first events at regional or distant sites (without an intervening local recurrence). This

TABLE 50.1. TAMOXIFEN BENEFIT AT 5 YEARS

Recurrence Type and Location	No. of Patients Benefitted	No. of Patients Needed to Prevent a Single Recurrence	*p* Value
Ipsilateral			
Invasive	17[a]	52	0.03
In situ	7	128	0.43
Contralateral			
Invasive	8	112	0.22
In situ	10	90	0.02
Locoregional/Distant	4	225	0.32

[a] Example: 17 fewer patients (40 − 23) in the Tamoxifen arm developed an ipsilateral invasive recurrence at 5 years = no. benefitted. The number of treated patients needed to prevent a single ipsilateral invasive recurrence at 5 years = 52 (899/17).
From Fisher B, Dignam J, Wolmark N, et al. Tamoxifen in treatment of intraductal breast cancer: National Surgical Adjuvant Breast and Bowel Project B-24 randomised controlled trial. *Lancet* 1999;353:1993–2000, with permission.

amounted to 1.47% of the entire group in B-17 at 8 years of follow-up (3) and 0.77% of the placebo arm in B-24 at 5 years. Not surprisingly, given its usefulness in patients with metastatic disease, tamoxifen reduced the risk of regional and distant events substantially in the tamoxifen arm in B-24. Prior studies of duct carcinoma in situ (16–19) have shown a great rarity of first events as distant or regional metastases. Only Solin et al. (19) reported a single case in 270 patients with 15 years of follow-up; none were reported in the other studies.

For the contralateral breast, no significant difference ($p = 0.22$) was found in preventing an invasive event, and only 8 patients benefitted (a benefit of 0.889% at five years, annualized to 0.178%); only one in 112 women randomized to tamoxifen would be spared an invasive contralateral cancer at 5 years in B-24. A significant difference was claimed for preventing a contralateral in situ carcinoma event ($p = 0.02$), but only 10 patients benefitted, a 1.1% benefit at 5 years or an annualized benefit of 0.22%. Only one patient in 90 randomized to the tamoxifen arm would have an in situ or invasive contralateral event prevented.

These tabulations suggest that the actual benefits of tamoxifen in the prevention of DCIS are minuscule as derived from the actual data of B-24. This compilation does not address the many adverse effects seen with tamoxifen use or the fact that of the three randomized trials using tamoxifen as a chemopreventative agent, only Fisher et al. (4) showed a significant benefit (20,21).

Indeed, the UK/ANZ trial (14), in which patients with DCIS were randomized to radiation therapy, tamoxifen, or radiation therapy and tamoxifen has shown no benefit for tamoxifen in a 53 month median follow-up. The trial required complete excision with careful mammographic-pathologic correlation, including specimen radiographs and postoperative mammography to confirm the excision. These requirements for radiology and pathology substantially reduced the rates of local recurrences in both treated and control arms relative to B-17 and B-24 (see Chapter 44), and no doubt reduced the likelihood of unrecognized invasive cancer in the breast and the resected tissue. Tamoxifen provided no significant reduction in ipsilateral invasive events ($p = 0.23$) or ipsilateral noninvasive recurrences ($p = 0.08$). Only by summing the benefits of ipsilateral and contralateral noninvasive events could a significant benefit for tamoxifen be demonstrated ($p = 0.03$).

In summary, only one of two published randomized trials has shown a significant benefit of tamoxifen in reducing breast cancer events following breast-conserving therapy in patients with DCIS. In B-24, the significant benefit is almost entirely derived from the reduction in ipsilateral local invasive recurrences that most likely reflect unrecognized invasive disease in the breast at the time of entry. The extraordinary number of loco-regional and distant metastases within 5 years (many occurring with 12 months of treat-

ment) are consistent with this evaluation. There was no significant benefit of tamoxifen in reducing noninvasive ipsilateral events, invasive contralateral events, or distant metastases in the trial. Moreover, the specific benefits are minute, and the 27% relative benefit of tamoxifen in reducing ipsilateral recurrences represents an actual benefit of 2.6% at 5 years. Only one in 37 women would achieve an ipsilateral benefit over that interval.

Many women trying to understand these benefits misunderstand the meaning of both the relative benefit and the actual benefit. Misunderstanding the relative benefit has been promoted by direct commercial appeals to potential "clients," even though misunderstanding the specific benefit results in women believing that a 2.6% ipsilateral benefit accrues to everyone treated. It is dismaying for the patient to learn that a 2.6% ipsilateral benefit at 5 years means that there is a one in 38 chance of benefitting in that time interval; a 2% contralateral benefit translates to a one in 50 chance of benefitting.

REFERENCES

1. Beatson GT. On the treatment of inoperable cases of carcinoma of the mamma. Suggestions for a new method of treatment with illustrative cases. *Lancet* 1896;2:104–107.
2. Fisher B, Dignam J, Wolmark N, et al. Tamoxifen and chemotherapy for lymph node–negative, estrogen receptor–positive breast cancer. *J Natl Cancer Inst* 1997;22:1673–1682.
3. Fisher B, Dignam J, Wolmark N, et al. Lumpectomy and radiation therapy for the treatment of intraductal breast cancer: Findings from National Surgical Adjuvant Breast and Bowel Project B-17. *J Clin Oncol* 1998;16:441–452.
4. Fisher B, Dignam J, Wolmark N, et al. Tamoxifen in treatment of intraductal breast cancer: National Surgical Adjuvant Breast and Bowel Project B-24 randomised controlled trial. *Lancet* 1999;353:1993–2000.
5. Dupont WD, Page DL, Rogers LW, et al. Influence of exogenous estrogens, proliferative breast disease, and other variables on breast cancer risk. *Cancer* 1989;63:948–957.
6. Dupont WD, Page DL, Parl FF, et al. Estrogen replacement therapy in women with a history of proliferative breast disease. *Cancer* 1999;85:1277–1283.
7. Vassilopoulou-Sellin R, Asmar L, Hortobagi GN, et al. Estrogen replacement therapy after localized breast cancer: Clinical outcome of 319 women followed prospectively. *J Clin Oncol* 1999;17:1482–1487.
8. Fowble B, Hanton A, Freedman G, et al. Postmenopausal hormone replacement therapy: Effect on diagnosis and outcome in early-stage invasive breast cancer treated with conservative surgery and radiation. *J Clin Oncol* 1999;17:1680–1688.
9. O'Meara ES, Rossing MA, Daling JR, et al. Hormone replacement therapy after a diagnosis of breast cancer in relation to recurrence and mortality. *J Natl Cancer Inst* 2001;93:764–762.
10. DiSaia PJ, Brewster WR, Ziogas A, et al. Breast cancer survival and hormone replacement therapy: A cohort analysis. *Am J Clin Oncol* 2000;23:541–545.
11. Eden JA, Bush T, Nand S, et al. A case-control study of combined continuous estrogen-progestin replacement therapy among women with a personal history of breast cancer. *Menopause* 1995;2:67–72.

12. Puthgraman K, Natrajan MD, Soumakis K, et al. Estrogen replacement therapy in women with previous breast cancer. *Am J Obstet Gynecol* 1999;181:288–295.

13. Grodstein F, Stampfer MJ, Colditz GA, et al. Postmenopausal hormone therapy and mortality. *N Engl J Med* 1997;63:948–957.

14. George WD, Houghton J, Cuzick J, et al. Radiotherapy and tamoxifen following complete local excision (CLE) in the management of ductal carcinoma in situ (DCIS): Preliminary results from the U.K. DCIS trial (*submitted*).

15. Julien JP, Bijker N, Fentiman IS, et al. Radiotherapy in breast-conserving treatment for ductal carcinoma in situ: First results of the EORTC randomized phase III trial 10853. EORTC Breast Cancer Cooperative Group and EORTC Radiotherapy Group. *Lancet* 2000;355:528–533.

16. Lagios MD, Margolin FR, Westdahl PR, et al. Mammographically detected duct carcinoma in situ. Frequency of local recurrence following tylectomy and prognostic effect of nuclear grade on local recurrence. *Cancer* 1989;63:619–624.

17. Silverstein MJ, Lagios MD, Craig PH, et al. A prognostic index for ductal carcinoma in situ of the breast. *Cancer* 1996;77:393–409.

18. Silverstein MJ, Lagios MD, Groshen S, et al. The influence of margin width on local control of ductal carcinoma in situ of the breast. *N Engl J Med* 1999;340:1455–1461.

19. Solin LJ, Kurtz J, Fourquet A, et al. Fifteen-year results of breast conserving surgery and definitive breast irradiation for the treatment of ductal carcinoma in situ of the breast. *J Clin Oncol* 1996;14:754–763.

20. Veronesi U, Maisonneuve P, Costa A, et al. Prevention of breast cancer with Tamoxifen. *Lancet* 1998;352:93–97.

21. Powles T, Eeles R, Ashley S, et al. Interim analysis of the incidence of breast cancer in the Royal Marsden Hospital tamoxifen randomized chemoprevention trial. *Lancet* 1998;352:98–101.

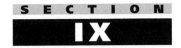

OTHER ISSUES

51

MASTECTOMY AND IMMEDIATE RECONSTRUCTION FOR EXTENSIVE DUCTAL CARCINOMA IN SITU OF THE BREAST

JAMES C. GROTTING
JAMES L. HENDERSON

Advancements in the surgical treatment of breast cancer are broadening the options available to the breast cancer patient. During the last decade, patients could choose between undergoing "breast-conserving" lumpectomy and radiation therapy or a "mutilating" mastectomy (1,2). Usually the mastectomy was reserved as a last resort in breast-conserving treatment failures. However, mastectomy with improvements in immediate glandular replacement using autogenous tissue has become an acceptable treatment option (3).

It is also interesting to note why certain patients prefer mastectomy to conservation treatment. Because mastectomy has long been considered "the gold standard" against which all other treatments are compared, many patients simply don't trust "new" types of treatment despite any logical argument to the contrary that their doctor might provide (2,3). Others fear radiation therapy because they cannot "see it," or the long-term effects are frightening to them. Practically speaking, some patients may not be able to travel and stay at or commute to the nearest radiation therapy center. Time off from work or time away from family may be considerations. Mastectomy, although more "extensive surgery," is more finite in terms of the time commitment necessary to reach the end point. Young women with a positive family history may also be better candidates for bilateral prophylactic procedures (26).

It is our premise that mastectomy does not necessarily need to be associated with the notion of failed preferable treatment. Granted, mastectomy by itself leaves a void of soft tissue on the chest wall that can profoundly affect a woman's self image, social and marital relationships, and ability to comfortably partake in certain sports, as well as properly fit in clothing (4). Although breast reconstruction cannot restore a perfectly normal breast, recent improvements in autogenous reconstruction, particularly when combined with skin-sparing mastectomy techniques, have resulted in many cases where the patients feel they look better after the operation than they did before! This brings the art and science of reconstructive breast surgery closer to the realm of elective aesthetic surgery. The overall size and shape of a woman's body has become one additional factor to consider in arriving at the best possible type of treatment for an individual patient.

DUCTAL CARCINOMA IN SITU

The incidence of ductal carcinoma in situ (DCIS) has increased over the last two decades due to improved methods of screening mammography (5). In 1985, the National Cancer Data Base showed that DCIS comprised 7% of all newly diagnosed breast cancers, and 10 years later, this number increased to 14%. DCIS accounts for 20% to 40% of all mammographically detected lesions (6,7). In 1993, DCIS was diagnosed in 23,275 cases, and 9,245 mastectomies were performed (5).

Using breast-conserving operations in a study of 333 patients, Silverstein (9) determined the relative risk of recurrence based on three factors: the size of the area involved with DCIS, the grade of the tumor, and the width of the closest margin. Silverstein stratified the results and developed the Van Nuys Prognostic Index (VNPI). Ninety-seven percent of the patients with a VNPI of 3 to 4 remained disease free, 77% disease free with a VNPI of 5 to 7, and only 20% disease free with a VNPI of 8 to 9 (8,9). In the lower VNPI risk group, wide excision without radiotherapy was found to be acceptable.

However, in the high-risk group (VNPI 8 to 9), local resection with or without radiotherapy had a high (80%) recurrence rate (10). Mastectomy yields a 0% to 2% local recurrence rate (11,12). Therefore, in the high-grade group, mastectomy with immediate reconstruction is an acceptable intervention.

BREAST RECONSTRUCTION

Surgical advancements in reconstruction of the breast using implants or autogenous tissue have refocused attention on reconstruction as an option. Free transverse rectus abdominis myocutaneous (TRAM) flap reconstruction is now considered the gold standard for breast reconstruction (13,14). With the advent of the skin-sparing mastectomy combined with TRAM flap reconstruction, it is now possible to recreate a very natural appearing and feeling reconstructed breast (Fig. 51.1).

The plastic surgeon should be involved in the preoperative planning if mastectomy with reconstruction is to be undertaken. Multiple factors will have an impact on the type of reconstruction planned for each individual patient (22). Some factors that can be detrimental to wound healing and increase the operative risk include obesity, smoking, diabetes, steroid use, a past medical history of lupus, and, most importantly, the use of adjuvant radiation therapy during the treatment of the breast cancer (15–17). Radiation therapy adversely affects the healing processes of the soft tissue and increases the need for autogenous tissue reconstruction.

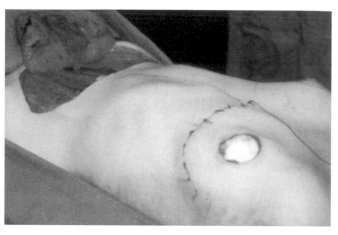

FIGURE 51.2. The oncologists and plastic surgeons work simultaneously with separate instruments. Completed skin-sparing mastectomy through the periareolar incision. Free transverse rectus abdominis myocutaneous ready for transfer.

The plastic surgeon and oncologic surgeon should work together in the operative planning to determine the location of the lines of incision and the position of the inframammary fold. The inframammary fold attachments should be preserved unless it is oncologically inadvisable. By working simultaneously with the general surgeon, the operative time can be decreased. The multidisciplinary team directs the postoperative management of the patient.

SKIN-SPARING MASTECTOMY

The most significant recent contribution to breast reconstruction is the incorporation of skin-sparing principles. The aesthetic result of the TRAM flap has been further improved by this technique.

We began maximally conserving mammary skin in 1986 as we gained more experience with immediate autogenous reconstruction. The concept evolved from the recognition that smaller lesions deep in the breast did not require the sacrifice of large amounts of skin to achieve adequate local control of the disease. The skin-sparing mastectomy is performed by excising the nipple-areola complex plus a thin rim of periareolar breast skin (Fig. 51.2). The circumferential superficial skin flaps are elevated over the breast mound, and the mastectomy is completed if the tumor is not in proximity to the skin. In addition, the biopsy site in invasive tumors should be resected. The incision for the skin-sparing mastectomy has been divided into four subtypes. In type I, only the nipple-areola complex is removed; in type II, the nipple-areola complex in continuity with the skin overlying superficial tumor or biopsy site is removed; in type III, the nipple-areola complex and skin overlying the biopsy site or superficial tumors is removed without removing the intervening skin; in type IV, the nipple-areola complex is removed with inverted T or reduction skin incision (20,21).

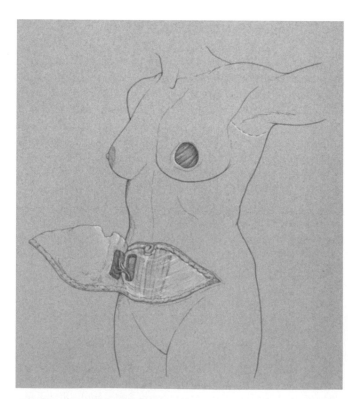

FIGURE 51.1. Free transverse rectus abdominis myocutaneous uses the deep inferior epigastric donor vessels. The recipient vessels are exposed through a separate axillary incision.

In a series of 95 patients diagnosed with DCIS, there were only three local recurrences over a 10-year period (18,19,23,25). Carlson's group (20,21,24) demonstrated that the local recurrence rate after skin-sparing mastectomy was 4.8% versus 9.5% in the non–skin-sparing mastectomy. However, in this series the surgical oncologist determined whether a skin-sparing or non–skin-sparing technique would be performed. Mastectomy skin flap loss following the skin-sparing technique has been shown to be equivalent to non–skin-sparing techniques at approximately 11%.

Nowhere has this been more applicable than in the treatment of early breast cancer or premalignant disease, such as DCIS. The recognition that saving the skin of the breast does not necessarily affect clearance of breast tissue allows skin coverage of the reconstructed breast to be identical to the opposite side in color and texture. When the skin envelope is filled with autogenous tissue of similar size and shape to the mastectomy specimen, superior results can be obtained. The final scar occupies only the periareolar circumference and can often be concealed by tattooing the areola. Creative incisions can also be used with this concept when the opposite breast requires alteration. Reduction mammaplasty and mastopexy incisions can be used for the mastectomy so that the ultimate scars appear as though the patient has had an aesthetic procedure rather than cancer treatment.

IMPLANT RECONSTRUCTION

Implant reconstruction is the most common method of breast reconstruction worldwide (27). However, patient selection is crucial when using implants as the sole method of reconstruction or in combination with autogenous tissue transfer. Patients with small breasts and minimal ptosis with adequate soft tissue coverage are the best candidates for implant reconstruction (28–30). The implant is placed deep to the anterior chest wall muscles, and the skin envelope is draped over the reconstruction and allowed to heal. Nipple reconstruction is performed at a subsequent operative setting. Satisfactory short-term results are achieved in 86% of patients at 2 years follow-up. However, at 5 years postreconstruction, the shortcomings of implant reconstruction become evident. Baker type III and IV capsular contracture occurs in 15% of the patients undergoing implant reconstruction without radiation therapy (27). Unfortunately, an overall satisfactory aesthetic result was achieved in only 54% of patients at five years (27). Advantages of implant reconstruction over other techniques include: simplicity of the surgical procedure and the use of adjacent tissue for skin color and texture matching, no donor site morbidity, and reduced postoperative recovery. The low cost of the initial surgical procedure is negated with the subsequent cost of future corrective surgical interventions. These costs approach

(and in some cases exceed) the cost of autogenous tissue reconstruction (32).

Several surgical options are available for breast reconstruction using implants and expanders (28–30). The reconstruction can be a single-stage operation using a standard implant or an adjustable implant. The second option available is a two-stage reconstruction in which an expander is placed; at a subsequent operation, the expander is removed and replaced with a permanent implant. In the context of DCIS, we prefer to place the tissue expander at the time of mastectomy. The expander is filled to 150% of the intended implant volume and then replaced with the permanent implant.

Complication rates are reported higher in the immediate reconstruction group of implant and expander reconstructions (31). These complications include seroma formation, skin necrosis, implant exposure and extrusion, valve malfunction, leakage and deflation, and rippling of the skin. Patients who have undergone or will undergo radiation therapy are not candidates for implant reconstruction. Expansion of the tissue envelope is difficult with irradiated tissue, and the risk of capsular contracture, implant extrusion, infection, and rib fractures is increased (14,17).

AUTOGENOUS TISSUE BREAST RECONSTRUCTION

Latissimus Dorsi Myocutaneous Flap

The latissimus dorsi myocutaneous pedicle flap has been a real "workhorse" of reconstruction due to its decreased cost, operative time, and technical ease. The latissimus dorsi myocutaneous flap provides a satisfactory result with or without an implant. The use of an implant in the submuscular pocket is necessary when the volume of subcutaneous back fat overlying the muscle is scant. However, in patients in whom radiation therapy is part of the adjuvant therapy, the addition of an implant is still plagued by the complications associated with radiation therapy. In patients with a relatively large tissue deficiency, the reconstruction of the mastectomy defect with the extended latissimus dorsi myocutaneous may provide adequate autogenous tissue (33). This extended version of the latissimus dorsi flap increases the volume of tissue harvested by elevating the entire latissimus dorsi muscle and all of the overlying fat with the flap. This dissection can be carried out through the skin island incision, and the flap is passed through a subcutaneous tunnel in the axilla. This technique has greatly improved the aesthetic result, and when it is combined with a skin-sparing mastectomy, the results are satisfactory.

The advantages of latissimus dorsi flap are its reliability, ease of harvest, and proximity to the mastectomy defect. If the mastectomy skin can be conserved, the flap can be completely buried to replace the resected mammary gland. The latissimus dorsi myocutaneous flap is very useful in the contouring of the breast when a defect is present due to breast-conserving surgery and post-radiation deformity. The disadvantages of the flap include its potentially large visible donor site scar, seroma formation, functional morbidity due to the loss of the muscle function at the donor site, and the fact that it frequently requires the use of an implant (which is contraindicated if radiation therapy is required) (23,32).

Pedicle Transverse Rectus Abdominis Myocutaneous

In 1982, Hartrampf and his colleagues (37) popularized the use of the single pedicled ipsilateral transverse rectus abdominis myocutaneous flap for glandular replacement after mastectomy. The pedicled TRAM flap receives its blood supply from the superior epigastric system through a series of choke vessels in the rectus muscle. The blood then enters the inferior epigastric system and passes up through the rectus muscle perforators and into the cutaneous circulation. This provides a sufficient amount of autogenous tissue to form a new breast mound. The cutaneous portion of the TRAM flap is divided into four regions. The more distal regions are prone to ischemia and subsequent fat necrosis. In all of its forms, the TRAM flap is a hardy flap that is capable of withstanding postoperative radiation therapy, and it can be used in previously irradiated fields (44). The pedicle TRAM suffers from several drawbacks, including medial inframammary fold fullness caused by the tunneling of the pedicle, distal flap ischemia, and fat necrosis. Fat necrosis can be decreased by performing a complete rectus muscle harvest and deletion of zone 4, and minimal use of tissue in zone 2 across the midline (43,45). The unipedicle ipsilateral TRAM has become the preferred type of pedicle flap configuration (40,41).

The use of a double-pedicled TRAM is safer for adequate flap blood supply if microsurgery is not an option. However, when soft tissue requirements are large, the double pedicle TRAM can provide more viable flap tissue. Subsequent to the delay of the single pedicle and the double pedicle TRAM flap, turbocharging or supercharging has been added to address the problem of inadequate inflow in the compromised patient, and has improved TRAM flap survival (40).

The rectus muscle fascial defect can be closed primarily or may require the use of synthetic mesh. The skin defect will be closed as in an abdominoplasty procedure or "tummy tuck," thereby leaving an aesthetically more pleasing scar (46). However the harvesting of the complete muscle does greatly increase the risk of the formation of abdominal wall donor site hernias. The double pedicled TRAM flap donor site is associated with an even higher rate of abdominal wall complications (13).

Microsurgery has further advanced the pedicle TRAM flap by making "turbocharging" and "supercharging" of the

flap possible. The turbocharged pedicled TRAM flap is a technique that uses a microsurgical anastomosis of the previously transected inferior epigastric vessels, forming a closed loop. This technique is designed to improve distal flap circulation. The supercharged pedicled TRAM flap uses the microsurgical anastomosis of the deep inferior epigastric vessels to donor vessels in the axial region while maintaining the superior circulation.

Free Transverse Rectus Abdominis Myocutaneous

The free TRAM uses the dominant inferior epigastric vessels, which feed directly into the inferior perforators, to supply blood flow directly to the TRAM flap. The donor pedicle vessels are then anastomosed to either the thoracodorsal vessels or the internal mammary vessels as recipients. The free TRAM provides a very reliable blood supply that yields a lower incidence of fat necrosis and partial flap loss (39). The free TRAM flap provides a very natural-appearing reconstruction result. At 2-year follow-up, 96% of patients were satisfied with the aesthetic results, and at 5-year follow-up, 94% of patients were satisfied with the aesthetic results (35). The free TRAM technique has been further refined by decreasing the portion of rectus muscle harvested with the flap. Only the length and width of muscle to accommodate and to protect the perforators is now harvested (34–36).

Advantages of the free TRAM include virtually no fat necrosis, minimal sacrifice of rectus muscle wall, and improvement in the aesthetics of the reconstructed breast and donor site (49). Recent studies have indicated that the cost of TRAM versus implant reconstruction is higher at the time of surgery. But at greater than 4 years follow-up, the total dollar cost, total number of hospital days, and total hours of operative time is equivalent between the two groups (38). The disadvantage of the free TRAM is the increased demands on the expertise of the plastic surgeon (42). Loss of the free TRAM flap occurs in 1% to 2% of cases, and is a devastating complication for the patient and the surgeon. Reoperation to salvage the flap occurs in 5% of the cases (45).

Perforator Transverse Rectus Abdominis Myocutaneous Flaps

The harvesting of the free TRAM flap has been taken another step by dissecting the flap as the deep inferior epigastric perforator (DIEP) flap (50). The advantage of this technique is the decrease in donor site morbidity, hernias, and bulging due to the rectus muscle harvesting (51). However, the somewhat tedious dissection of the perforators adds 1 to 5 hours to the operative time, depending on the abilities of the surgeon. Flap necrosis and partial flap loss is increased due to the decrease in the perforators to the skin paddle.

Flap loss can be improved if the DIEP flap reconstruction is limited to patients with a a palpable perforator pulse and a perforator vein greater than 1 mm (52,53).

Other Free Flaps

Other autologous flaps include the superior gluteal free flap, which provides adequate amounts of skin and subcutaneous fat in selected patients. The inferior gluteal free flap is also available and provides a substantial amount of tissue and longer pedicle than the superior gluteal flap. However, vein grafts are frequently needed. Perforator versions of these flaps are also possible, which can improve donor site defects. The lateral transverse thigh flap and the Rubens peri-iliac free flap are also available if the TRAM flap is not possible due to previous surgeries or insufficient tissue. These flaps leave more obvious door site defects, and the Rubens flap violates the lateral abdominal wall and may result in a hernia.

OUR PREFERRED APPROACH

After gaining experience in a variety of reconstructive techniques, we now prefer autogenous tissue using the free TRAM. Any time local excision or re-excision of a breast tumor will significantly affect the final shape and size of the breast, some type of reconstruction should be considered. Of course, radiotherapy effects on the breast need also be taken into consideration. For women with ample breast tissue, particularly if they have had symptoms of neck and back discomfort, incorporation of the local excision into a pattern for reduction mammaplasty with reduction of the opposite breast concurrently, can be an excellent way of treating early breast cancer or premalignant conditions such as DCIS. Small-breasted patients may be left with defects not unlike a mastectomy if a large excision is necessary. These patients may prefer to complete the excision of the remainder of the gland in order to avoid radiation therapy and their concern for lifetime monitoring. Alternatively, a local flap such as the latissimus dorsi can be used to fill out an anticipated hollow in the final shape.

Clearly, patients in whom negative margins cannot be achieved, or where re-excisions are likely to produce significant deformity, conversion to mastectomy and reconstruction might be considered.

PLANNING AND LOGISTICS

Mastectomy and immediate reconstruction require that the oncologic surgeon and the plastic surgeon communicate and work well together. Considerations include the type of breast pathology, the preferred method of reconstruction, and the necessary alterations of the opposite breast. The best incision is then determined so that an adequate and safe mastectomy can be combined with the best possible reconstruction.

If autogenous reconstruction is selected as the method of choice, the TRAM flap is our preferred technique. When transferred as a free flap, advantages include better and more reliable blood supply, less sacrifice of abdominal musculature (rectus abdominis), ease of shaping, and lack of a "bulge" in the upper abdomen from the tunneled muscle (as often seen in the conventional pedicled TRAM). Better blood supply translates into less partial necrosis and fat necrosis.

However, the free TRAM is a serious undertaking for both patient and surgical team and, therefore, planning needs to include prophylaxis for deep vein thrombosis, the possibility of blood transfusion, and a 4 to 5 day hospitalization. Scheduling of mastectomy and immediate reconstruction also requires that the office staffs of both the oncologic surgeon and the plastic surgeon communicate and coordinate scheduling so that the procedure can be performed in a timely fashion.

PREFERRED TECHNIQUE

The present state-of-the-art procedure for immediate reconstruction is skin-sparing mastectomy and free TRAM flap. The plastic surgeon needs to preoperatively mark the patient with the patient preferably in the in the standing position. Immediately after the patient is under general anesthesia, the previously marked inframammary fold needs to be established. We use 2/0 silk sutures that traverse the deep tissue planes so that during the oncologic procedure the inframammary fold can easily be identified. Minimizing the use of a high-temperature bovie to perform the dissection under the skin flaps may also aid in skin flap survival. With a little planning and cooperation, both the mastectomy and the flap preparation can be carried out by the two teams working simultaneously. Instrument sets and operative fields are kept separate. In our experience, the donor flap is ready for transfer about the same time that the mastectomy is completed. The mastectomy may be more technically difficult because of the longer skin flaps. The mastectomy specimen and the TRAM flap are weighed intraoperatively to estimate the quantity of TRAM tissue required for the breast reconstruction. Circulation to the skin must be carefully assessed after the mastectomy. Any area where the perfusion is in question should be excised and replaced with skin from the abdominal flap.

The free TRAM flap is based on the deep inferior epigastric artery and its accompanying veins. The flap is elevated and only a small island of rectus muscle is harvested with the perforating vessels. Recipient vessels are usually a branch of the subscapular system in the axilla. The thoracodorsal artery and vein just proximal to the serratus arterial branch is usually ideal. These vessels can be anastomosed using loupes or the operating microscope. Once circulation is restored, the flap is molded into the shape of the opposite side. If the opposite side is to be corrected, this is best done first and the flap should then match the corrected and anticipated shape of the opposite breast.

When insetting the flap, it is essential to restore the axillary soft tissues and lateral breast skin to their original position to avoid ptosis of the reconstructed breast and bothersome axillary fullness. All buried portions of the flap are de-epithelialized, and a small skin island is left exteriorized at the future position of the nipple areolar complex to aid in monitoring of the circulation of the flap.

POSTOPERATIVE CARE AND SECONDARY SURGERY

The primary reason for postoperative hospitalization is to recover from the abdominal portion of the procedure and to monitor the flap. Patients are encouraged to be up and around the first postoperative morning. Monitoring of the flap is by conventional doppler and laser doppler as well as simple direct observation. Most are ready for discharge on the fourth or fifth postoperative day.

The reconstruction can usually be completed in one additional outpatient procedure in which the nipple is reconstructed and any corrections of the breast mound, opposite breast, or abdomen are performed.

RESULTS

From 1988 to 1999, we performed breast reconstructions on 314 patients with an average age of 47.3 years. The free TRAM was used in 233 cases (74.7%), pedicled TRAM in 46 cases (15.7%), latissimus dorsi flap in 9 cases (2.9%), and other techniques in 22 cases (6.9%). The histology of the primary breast lesion was DCIS in 85 cases (27.2%). The incidence of minor mammary skin necrosis was 18.3%, but all healed spontaneously. The incidence of major breast skin flap necrosis was 1.3%. All patients were eventually successfully reconstructed (Fig. 51.3).

CONCLUSION

Our experience has demonstrated the safety of the skin-sparing technique when coupled with immediate reconstruction. We are particularly pleased with the long-term stability and aesthetic results of the free TRAM. With experience, this method is predictable and has a low rate of serious complications. We believe that this treatment should be given serious consideration for at least some patients who require surgical treatment of DCIS.

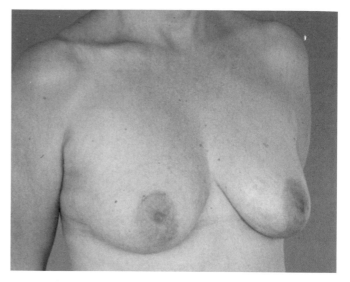
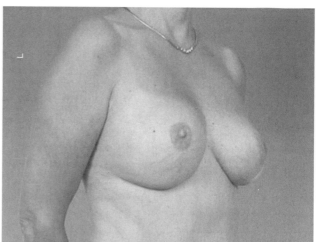

FIGURE 51.3. Pre- and postoperative photographs of a 53-year-old patient with extensive DCIS with components of comedo, solid, cribriform, and papillary subtypes of intermediate nuclear grade. She underwent skin-sparing mastectomy with immediate free transverse rectus abdominis myocutaneous reconstruction and a left mastopexy.

REFERENCES

1. Fisher B. From Halsted to Prevention and Beyond: Advances in the Management of Breast Cancer during the Twentieth Century. *Eur J Cancer* 1999;35(14):1963–1973.
2. Pusic A, Thompson TA, Kerrigan CL. Surgical Options for Early-Stage Breast Cancer: Factors Associated with Patient Choice and Postoperative Quality of Life. *Plast Reconstr Surg* 1999;104(5):1325–1333.
3. Lopez MJ, Proter KA. The Current Role of Prophylactic Mastectomy. *Surg Clin North Am* 1996;76(2):231–242.
4. Wilkins EG, Cederna PS, Lowery JC. Prospective Analysis of Psychosocial Outcomes in Breast Reconstruction: One-year Postoperative Results from the Michigan Breast Reconstruction Outcome Study. *Plast Reconstr Surg* 2000;106(5):1014–1025.
5. Bland KI, Menck HR, Scott-Conner CE, et al. The National Cancer Database 10-year survey of breast carcinoma treatment at hospitals in the United States. *Cancer* 1998;83:1262–1273.

6. Hughes KS, Lee AK, Rolfs A. Controversies in the Treatment of Ductal Carcinoma In Situ. *Surg Clin North Am* 1996;76(2): 243–265.

7. Ernst VL, Barclay J. Increases in ductal carcinoma in situ (DCIS) of the breast in relation to mammography: a dilemma. *J Natl Cancer Inst Monogr* 1997;22:151–156.

8. Silverstein MJ, Lagios MD, Martino S, et al. Margin width: A critical determinant of local control in patients with ductal carcinoma in situ of the breast. *Proc Am Soc Clin Oncol* 1998;17:120a.

9. Silverstein MJ, Lagios MD, Craig PH, et al. A prognostic index for ductal carcinoma in situ of the breast. *Cancer* 1996;77: 2267–2274.

10. Hughes KS, Lee AK, Rolfs A. Controversies in the Treatment of Ductal Carcinoma In Situ. *Surg Clin North Am* 1996;76(2): 243–246.

11. Hwang ES, Eserman LJ. Management of Ductal Carcinoma In Situ. *Surg Clin North Am* 1999;79(5):1007–1029.

12. Anderson LG, Smeds S, Fagerberg G, et al. Follow-up of two treatment modalities for ductal cancer in situ of the breast. *Br J Surg* 1989;76:762–765.

13. Malata CM, McIntosh SA, Purushotham AD. Immediate Breast Reconstruction After Mastectomy for Cancer. *Br J Surg* 2000;87: 1455–1472.

14. Tzaferta K, Ahmed O, Bahia H. Evaluation of the Factors Related to Postmastectomy Breast Reconstruction. *Plast Reconstr Surg* 2001;107(7):1694–1701.

15. Chang DW, Wang B, Robb GL. Effect of Obesity on Flap and Donor-site Complications in Free Transverse Rectus Abdominis Myocutaneous Flap Breast Reconstruction. *Plast Reconstr Surg* 2000;105(5):1640–1648.

16. Chang DW, Reece GP, Wang B. Effect of Smoking on Complications in Patients Undergoing Free TRAM Flap Breast Reconstruction. *Plast Reconstr Surg* 2000;105(7):2374–2380.

17. Lin KY, Patterson JW, Simmons J. Effects of External Beam Irradiation on the TRAM Flap: An Experimental Model. *Plast Reconstr Surg* 2001;107(5):1190–1200.

18. Laronga C, Kemp B, Johnston D. The Incidence of Occult Nipple-Areola Complex Involvement in Breast Cancer Patients Receiving a Skin Sparing Mastectomy. *Ann Surg Oncol* 1999;6(6): 609–613.

19. Rubio IT, Mirza N, Sahin AA, et al. Role of specimen radiography in patients treated with skin-sparing mastectomy for ductal carcinoma in situ of the breast. *Ann Surg Oncol* 2000;7(7): 544–548.

20. Carlson GW, Losken A, Moore B. Results of Immediate Breast Reconstruction After Skin Sparing Mastectomy. *Ann Surg* 2001; 46(3):222–228.

21. Carlson GW, Moore B, Thornton JF. Breast Cancer after Augmentation Mammaplasty: Treatment by Skin Sparing Mastectomy and Immediate Reconstruction. *Plast Reconstr Surg* 2001; 107(3):687–692.

22. Hwang TG, Wilkins EG, Lowery JC. Implementation and Evaluation of a Clinical Pathway for TRAM Breast Reconstruction. *Plast Reconstr Surg* 2000;105(2):541–548.

23. Kroll SS, Baldwin B. A Comparison of Outcomes Using Three Different Methods of Breast Reconstruction. *Plast Reconstr Surg* 1992;90(3):455–462.

24. Carlson GW, Bostwick J, Styblo TM. Skin-Sparing Mastectomy Oncologic and Reconstructive Considerations. *Ann Surg* 1997; 225(5):570–577.

25. Rubio IT, Mirza N, Sahin AA. Role of Specimen Radiography in Patients Treated with Skin-Sparing Mastectomy for Ductal Carcinoma In Situ of the Breast. *Ann Surg Oncol* 2000;7(7): 554–548.

26. Buehler PK. Patient Selection for Prophylactic Mastectomy: Who Is At High Risk? *Plast Reconstr Surg* 1983;72(3):324–330.

27. Clough KB, O'Donoghue JM, Fitoussi AD. Prospective Evaluation of Late Cosmetic Results Following Breast Reconstruction: I. Implant Reconstruction. *Plast Reconstr Surg* 2001;107(7): 1702–1709.

28. Vandeweyer E, Hertens D, Nogaret J-M. Immediate Breast Reconstruction with Saline-filled Implants: No Interference with the Oncologic Outcome. *Plast Reconstr Surg* 2001;107(6): 1409–1412.

29. Spear SL, Spittler CJ. Breast Reconstruction with Implants and Expanders. *Plast Reconstr Surg* 2001;107(1):177–187.

30. Burden WR. Skin-Sparing Mastectomy with Staged Tissue Expander Reconstruction Using a Silicone Gel Prosthesis and Contralateral Endoscopic Breast Augmentation. *Ann Plas Surg* 2001; 46(3):234–237.

31. Spear SL, Slack C, Howard MA. Postmastectomy Reconstruction of the Previously Augmented Breast: Diagnosis, Staging, Methodology, and Outcome. *Plast Reconstr Surg* 2001;107(5): 1167–1176.

32. Kroll SS, Evans GRD, Reece GP. Comparison of Resource Costs Between Implant-Based and TRAM Flap Breast Reconstruction. *Plast Reconstr Surg* 1996;97(2):364–372.

33. De La Torre JI, Fix RJ, Gardner PM. Reconstruction with the Latissimus Dorsi Flap After Skin Sparing Mastectomy. *Ann Plas Surg* 2001;46(3):229–233.

34. Grotting JC, Urist MM, Maddox WA. Conventional TRAM Flap versus Free Microsurgical TRAM Flap for Immediate Breast Reconstruction. *Plast Reconstr Surg* 1989;83(5):828–844.

35. Clough KB, O'Donoghue JM, Fitoussi AD. Prospective Evaluation of Late Cosmetic Results Following Breast Reconstruction. II. TRAM Flap Reconstruction. *Plast Reconstr Surg* 2001;107(7): 1710–1716.

36. Charanek AM, Carramaschi FR, Curado JH. Refinements in Transverse Rectus Abdominis Myocutaneous Flap Breast Reconstruction: Projection and Contour Improvements. *Plast Reconstr Surg* 2000;106(6):1262–1275.

37. Hartrampf CR, Scheflan M, Black PW. Breast Reconstruction with a Transverse Abdominal Island Flap. *Plast Reconstr Surg* 1982;69(2):216–225.

38. Kroll SS, Evans GRD, Reece GP. Comparison of Resource Costs of Free and Conventional TRAM Flap Breast Reconstruction. *Plast Reconstr Surg* 1996;98(1):74–77.

39. Schusterman MA, Kroll SS, Weldon ME. Immediate Breast Reconstruction: Why the Free TRAM over the Conventional TRAM Flap? *Plast Reconstr Surg* 1992;90(2):255–261.

40. Paige KT, Bostwick J, Bried JT. A Comparison of Morbidity from Bilateral, Unipedicle and Unilateral, Unpedicled TRAM Flap Breast Reconstructions. *Plast Reconstr Surg* 1998;101(7): 1819–1827.

41. Clugston PA, Gingrass MK, Azurin D. Ipsilateral Pedicled TRAM Flaps: The Safer Alternative? *Plast Reconstr Surg* 2000; 105(1):77–82.

42. Gherardini G, Arnander C, Gylbert L. Pedicled Compared with Free Transverse Rectus Abdominis Myocutaneous Flaps in Breast Reconstruction. *Scand J Plast Reconstr Hand Surg* 1994;28: 69–73.

43. Larson DL, Yousif NJ, Sinha RK. A Comparison of Pedicled and Free TRAM Flaps for Breast Reconstruction in a Single Institution. *Plast Reconstr Surg* 1999;104(3):674–680.

44. Tran NV, Evans GRD, Kroll SS. Postoperative Adjuvant Irradiation: Effects on Transverse Rectus Abdominis Muscle Flap Breast Reconstruction. *Plast Reconstr Surg* 2000;106(2): 313–320.

45. Kroll SS, Gherardini G, Martin JE. Fat Necrosis in Free and Pedicled TRAM Flaps. *Plast Reconstr Surg* 1998;102(5): 1502–1507.

46. Esander-Nord A, Jurell G, Wickman M. Donor-site Morbidity

after Pedicle or Free TRAM Flap Surgery: A Prospective and Objective Study. *Plast Reconstr Surg* 1998;102(5):1508–1516.

47. Codner MA, Bostwick J, Nahai F. TRAM Flap Vascular Delay for High-Risk Breast Reconstruction. *Plast Reconstr Surg* 1995; 96(7):1615–1622.

48. Edsander-Nord A, Wickman M, Hansson P. Somatosensory Status after Pedicled or Free TRAM Flap Surgery: A Retrospective Study. *Plast Reconstr Surg* 1999;104(6):1642–1648.

49. Baldwin BJ, Schusterman MA, Miller MJ. Bilateral Breast Reconstruction: Conventional versus Free TRAM. *Plast Reconstr Surg* 1994;93(7):1410–1417.

50. Allen RJ, Treece P. Deep Inferior Epigastric Perforator Flap for Breast Reconstruction. *Ann Plas Surg* 1994;32(1):32–38.

51. Blondeel PN, Vanderstraeten GG, Monstrey SJ. The Donor Site Morbidity of Free DIEP Flaps and Free TRAM Flaps for Breast Reconstruction. *Br J Plast Surg* 1997;50:322–330.

52. Kroll S, Reece GP, Miller MJ. Comparison of Cost for DIEP and Free TRAM Flap Breast Reconstruction. *Plast Reconstr Surg* 2001;107(6):1413–1418.

53. Kroll SS. Fat Necrosis in Free Transverse Rectus Abdominis Myocutaneous and Deep Inferior Epigastric Perforator Flaps. *Plast Reconstr Surg* 2000;106(3):576–583.

52

DUCTAL CARCINOMA IN SITU WITH MICROINVASION

MELVIN J. SILVERSTEIN
MICHAEL D. LAGIOS

Things have changed since we last looked at ductal carcinoma in situ with microinvasion (DCIS-Mi). In 1997, we published a chapter on DCIS-Mi in the first edition of this textbook. At that time, we suggested that DCIS-Mi should be recognized as a separate pathologic entity, distinct from DCIS without microinvasion, and that this should be reflected in the TNM staging system. In the next version of the staging system, that happened (1).

Within the section on primary tumors (T category), a fourth category has been added to T1 and it is named T1mic. T1mic is defined as invasion 1 mm or less in greatest diameter and, hence, microinvasion. Previously, the category of T1a contained all invasive lesions 5 mm or smaller. This has now been subdivided. The staging system does not limit the number of T1mic foci; as with larger invasive lesions, multiple foci should not be added together. Noninvasive tumors are classified as Tis (tumor in situ), N0, M0, and are stage 0. Their size is recorded as the greatest dimension of the entire DCIS lesion. If a focus of invasion 1 mm or less is found, the lesion is classified as T1mic. Its size is recorded as the greatest diameter of the invasive component, regardless of the size of the accompanying DCIS. If axillary lymph nodes are negative, the lesion is stage 1.

Although it is theoretically possible for a 1 mm invasive tumor to exist without DCIS (or other noninvasive component), we have never seen it in our experience. Virtually all T1mic lesions are an area of DCIS with one or more tiny 1 mm or less foci of invasive breast cancer. In essence, they are minute invasive ductal carcinomas with an extensive intraductal component. T1mic may also be an invasive lobular carcinoma within an area of lobular carcinoma in situ (LCIS). Microinvasive breast cancer arises from a preexisting area of noninvasive breast cancer.

T1mic or DCIS-Mi (in this chapter we will use the terms interchangeably) is a true invasive breast carcinoma whose treatment should be based on a number of variables, including

number of invasive foci,
margin status of the noninvasive and invasive components,

breast size,
extent of the noninvasive component,
nuclear grade and presence of necrosis,
age of the patient,
ability to follow the patient mammographically, and
patient's desires.

In other words, all of the prognostic and predictive factors discussed throughout this book.

T1mic is a relatively new lesion having only been formally defined in 1997 (1). However, all of the problems and issues concerning DCIS are generally applicable to DCIS-Mi. There is controversy regarding the classification, biology, pathologic criteria for, and treatment of DCIS when tiny foci of invasive carcinoma are found within it. Can experienced pathologists reliably, reproducibly, and routinely discriminate between DCIS and T1mic? Should it be treated less aggressively, like DCIS without microinvasion, or more aggressively, like invasive cancer, with decisions being made on nuclear grade, tumor margins, immunochemical prognostic factors, nodal status, etc.? Is some form of axillary lymph node dissection necessary for DCIS-Mi? This chapter will address these concerns and attempt to resolve them.

PATIENTS AND DEFINITIONS

We will look at some of the issues raised above by comparing two patient populations. The DCIS patient population of the University of Southern California/Van Nuys series (USC/Van Nuys, discussed in numerous chapters throughout this book) and all of the additional patients seen during the same time period who meet the new criteria for T1mic (DCIS-Mi). Through December 2000, there were 909 patients with DCIS without microinvasion: 326 treated with mastectomy, 237 treated with excision plus radiation therapy, and 346 treated with excision alone.

The DCIS-Mi population is quite small, with only 24 patients meeting the new strict 1 mm or less criteria. In an earlier report (2), our group employed a broader definition of microinvasion and reported 47 patients with DCIS-Mi. However, central pathology review of all 47 cases revealed that some of the smaller foci of questionable invasion were not unequivocal and, as suggested by Lagios, were better classified as DCIS without microinvasion. In addition, when the ocular micrometer was used to measure all unequivocal foci of invasion, many measured between 1 to 2 mm and were then reclassified as T1a invasive lesions, rather than DCIS-Mi.

RESULTS

Through December 2000, our DCIS series was comprised of 909 patients with pure DCIS. These patients are compared with 24 patients with DCIS-Mi in Table 52.1. Some prognostic markers (ER, PR, ploidy, HER2/neu, p53 and s-phase) were available in limited numbers of patients, and are noted in Table 52.1. In general, because prognostic markers are expensive and of no proven benefit for patients with DCIS, they were seldom obtained. Because the DCIS-Mi group is so small, p values are not provided.

Patients with DCIS-Mi trended toward having palpable lesions and involved margins after their initial markers, a reflection of the fact that DCIS-Mi lesions were larger than pure DCIS without microinvasion.

Local recurrence–free survival was greater for patients with DCIS (80% at 12 years) when compared with DCIS-Mi (73% at 12 years) (Fig. 51.1) but the difference was not

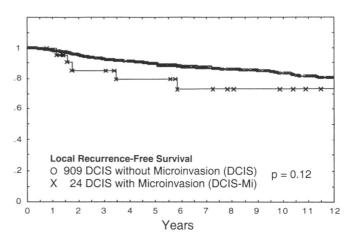

FIGURE 52.1. Local recurrence–free survival for 909 patients with DCIS and 24 patients with DCIS-Mi.

significant. It is important to note that 14 DCIS-Mi patients were treated with mastectomy, two of whom recurred locally (Table 52.2). Because DCIS-Mi lesions were larger and more difficult to excise with clear margins, they were more likely to be treated with mastectomy (58% of 24 patients), whereas only 36% (326 of 909) of patients with pure DCIS received mastectomy. Six patients with DCIS-Mi were treated with excision plus radiation therapy, none of whom recurred. Four patients were treated with excision only and three recurred (Table 52.2). Table 52.3 analyzes the local and distant recurrences among 24 patients with DCIS-Mi by size, with the DCIS components being

TABLE 52.1. COMPARISON OF CLINICAL FACTORS FOR PATIENTS WITH DUCTAL CARCINOMA IN SITU WITH MICROINVASION OR DUCTAL CARCINOMA IN SITU WITHOUT MICROINVASION

Factor	DCIS-Mi	DCIS
Number of patients	24	909
Average age (years)	50	53
Median follow-up (months)	91	83
Palpable	7 (29%)	126 (14%)
Calcifications	20 (83%)	723/868 (83%)
Size DCIS (mm)	38	26
ER positive	5/8 (63%)	98/149 (66%)
PR positive	5/8 (63%)	90/144 (63%)
Average nuclear grade	2.22	2.25
Necrosis	18 (75%)	623 (67%)
Aneuploid	4/5 (80%)	36/74 (47%)
HER2/neu positive	5/9 (56%)	73/204 (36%)
p53 positive	2/8 (25%)	22/153 (14%)
S-phase >6	3/4 (75%)	25/66 (38%)
Initial excision margins <1 mm	18 (75%)	517 (57%)
Recurrences	5 (21%)	111 (12%)
Invasive recurrences	5 (100%)	49 (44%)
Positive nodes by H&E	0/20 (0%)	2/427 (0.5%)
Positive nodes by IHC	0/1 (0%)	6/71 (8%)
Distant mets	2 (8%)	8 (0.8%)
BC deaths	1 (4%)	5 (0.6%)

DCIS-Mi, ductal carcinoma in situ with microinvasion; DCIS, ductal carcinoma in situ without microinvasion.

TABLE 52.2. TREATMENT FOR PATIENTS WITH DUCTAL CARCINOMA IN SITU WITH MICROINVASION OR DUCTAL CARCINOMA IN SITU WITHOUT MICROINVASION

Treatment	DCIS-Mi No. of Patients (Recurrences)	DCIS No. of Patients (Recurrences)
Mastectomy	14 (2)	326 (2)
Excision plus radiation therapy	6 (0)	237 (48)
Excision only	4 (3)	346 (61)
Total	24 (5)	909 (111)

DCIS-Mi, ductal carcinoma in situ with microinvasion; DCIS, ductal carcinoma in situ without microinvasion.

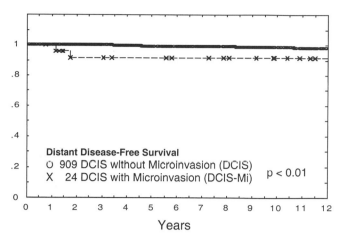

FIGURE 52.2. Distant recurrence–free survival for 909 patients with DCIS and 24 patients with DCIS-Mi.

grouped by those less than 45 mm versus those 45 mm or greater. The two distant recurrences in patients with DCIS-Mi occurred in patients with larger DCIS components.

A total of 427 node dissections or samplings were done in patients with DCIS, two of which were positive (0.05%) by hematoxylin and eosin (H&E) staining. Twenty node dissections were done in patients with DCIS-Mi, none of which contained metastases by H&E.

Since 1995, we have done 76 sentinel node biopsies for patients with DCIS who were being treated with mastectomy. All were negative by H&E but six (8%) contained cytokeratin-positive cells by immunohistochemistry (IHC). As a general rule, we have made it a policy not to upstage these patients to stage 2 disease based on IHC results and, therefore, not to treat these patients with chemotherapy. Only one patient with DCIS-Mi underwent sentinel node biopsy during the last 6 years. That node was negative by H&E and IHC.

Eight of 909 patients (0.9%) with DCIS developed local invasive recurrences followed by distant metastatic disease; whereas two of 24 patients (8%) with DCIS-Mi developed metastatic disease (Fig. 51.2) ($p < 0.01$). The two patients with DCIS-Mi who developed distant disease should be commented on. One patient had a 10 cm area of microcalcifications. A generous biopsy revealed high-grade DCIS spanning the entire biopsy specimen. Multiple areas of true microinvasion (1 mm or less) were noted and mastectomy

TABLE 52.3. PATIENTS WITH MICROINVASION DIVIDED BY THE SIZE OF THEIR DUCTAL CARCINOMA IN SITU LESION

Characteristic	Less Than 45 mm	Equal or Greater Than 45 mm
No. of patients	18	6
Average age (years)	53	43
Necrosis present	14 (78%)	5 (83%)
Local recurrence	3 (17%)	1 (17%)
Distant recurrence	0 (0%)	2 (33%)

was strongly advised. Unfortunately, the patient refused all further conventional therapy at that time, opting for various forms of alternative medicine. She returned two years later with inflammatory breast cancer and soon developed metastatic breast cancer. Had the appropriate treatment (a mastectomy) been originally performed, it is possible that larger areas of invasion might have been found. Transecting a large DCIS-Mi and following that with no further treatment doomed that patient to recurrence.

The second patient had a 45 mm high-grade DCIS, again, with multiple tiny foci of invasion. She was treated with a mastectomy and immediate reconstruction. Twenty lymph nodes were negative by H&E. She developed distant metastases two years later without a local recurrence and died 1 year after that.

Both of these patients have outcomes not readily predicted by the existing TMN staging system. They were both stage 1 at the time of diagnosis (T1mic, N0, M0), (although the first patient was incompletely evaluated because multiple margins were positive and no nodes were analyzed; perhaps she should not be included in this series). In any event, the T category that we assigned both patients (T1mic) did not truly reflect the significance of their disease. It has long been appreciated that a large area of high-grade DCIS with multiple small foci of invasion is a lesion with a poorer prognosis than a small area of DCIS with a single microinvasive focus (3), yet both are staged identically. The T category of the staging system currently does not permit for differentiation between these two lesions.

Lagios et al. (4,5) reported a subset of DCIS patients who were treated with standard modified radical mastectomy for a diagnosis of DCIS established by open surgical biopsy. This subset was characterized by the large extent of disease pathologically ($\geq$ 50 mm) and generally extensive linear branching microcalcifications occupying a quadrant or more of the breast. Nearly half of these patients exhibited identifiable invasion at mastectomy when the entire breast was extensively sampled histopathologically using the serial subgross technique. Three of 25 (12%) such patients developed subsequent distant or loco-regional recurrences within 24 months of mastectomy. Although one of these patients had multifocal invasive disease of substantial size (the largest focus was 12 mm), the remaining two exhibited only microinvasion. All three patients were H&E node negative with a standard level I to II axillary dissection.

More recently, Tabar et al. (3) identified a similar low stage but prognostically poor subset of patients. Among 343 patients with carcinomas less than or equal to 14 mm in size, the subset was identified on the basis of casting-type microcalcifications noted in the preoperative mammograms. Although the majority of the T1aN0/T1bN0 patients in this database had a very high cause-specific survival (97%) at 16 years, those with casting-type microcalcifications fared poorly (3,6). Eight of 19 (42%) patients with invasive carcinomas that were less than or equal to 9 mm in size and had cast-type microcalcifications died of breast cancer after 20 years of follow-up.

Our experience and that of Tabar (3,6) suggest that patients with extensive DCIS and multiple foci of minimal invasion, in spite of node negative status, may not be as prognostically favorable a subgroup as previously thought, even when treated with mastectomy.

DISCUSSION

Using the current definition of T1mic (DCIS-Mi), an area of DCIS with one or more foci of invasion, each measuring 1 mm or less, it is a rare lesion. We have reported 24 cases that meet this strict definition within our database of more than 3,800 patients with breast cancer. This is a rate of 6.3 cases of DCIS-Mi per 1,000 breast cancer patients (0.6%).

Twenty years ago, DCIS-Mi essentially did not exist. Today, with the dramatic increase in the number of cases of DCIS, microscopic foci of invasive carcinoma are more readily recognized, and the problem of defining the significance of such areas has become a clinical issue.

Many cases of high-grade DCIS and DCIS with comedo-type necrosis show marked intralobular and periductal stromal fibroplasia, lymphoid infiltration, and may exhibit cancerization of lobules, which can make it difficult to distinguish microinvasion from distortion of ductile structures with cancerization.

DCIS may also occur in foci of sclerosing adenosis, a frequent and often difficult pitfall in the microscopic identification of microinvasive disease. However, more recent use of immunochemistry for type IV collagen or smooth muscle actin have put this differential on a more certain foundation.

For the practicing pathologist, the presence of stromal microinvasion is occasionally difficult to assess. This is illustrated in Fisher and colleague's (7) analysis of the pathologic findings of the National Surgical Adjuvant Breast Project

Protocol (NSABP) B-06. In their review of the biopsy material from 2,072 patients who had been diagnosed with invasive breast cancer, 80 (4%) were found to have noninvasive lesions: 77 were DCIS, two were LCIS, and one patient had both. Similar results were note by Bijker et al. (8), who identified numerous cases of invasive disease included within the European Organization for Research and Treatment of Cancer (EORTC) DCIS trial (protocol 10853) via central review.

How many slides per centimeter of DCIS must be evaluated before we are convinced that no microinvasion or margin involvement exists? There is no uniform agreement here. Our group routinely sections all nonpalpable lesions at 2 to 3 mm intervals, submitting all tissue. We have found that we cannot reliably exclude microinvasion unless all tissue is serially sectioned and sequentially submitted. No matter how many slides are examined, the evaluation of a DCIS lesion is limited by the sampling process and pathologists can never be absolutely certain that microinvasion or margin involvement is absent. However, the likelihood of missing a focus of microinvasion or margin involvement decreases as the number of slides evaluated increases. We continue to recommend complete tissue processing as the best method to characterize the disease that is present and we cannot overemphasize the importance of this.

The in situ component of a microinvasive lesion is often large, averaging 38 mm in this series. In the series of Lagios et al. (4), the average in situ component of a microinvasive lesion was greater than 50 mm in diameter. Complete tissue processing for these large lesions is more time consuming. Yet, even in a nonacademic setting and despite the realities of today's clinical/financial world, most community pathologists are willing to serially section these lesions at 2 to 3 mm intervals to perform a thorough evaluation and look for foci of invasion. In spite of this, we must accept the fact that with larger lesions, true areas of invasive cancer may be missed.

Lagios (4) showed that as DCIS lesions get larger, invasion is more likely. The series reported here supports that conclusion. Because DCIS-Mi lesions were larger than DCIS, they were extremely difficult to completely excise with clear margins. Even though most of these lesions were excised using a multiple-wire bracketing technique (9) (Chapter 15), the initial excision margins were involved in DCIS-Mi patients 75% of the time compared with 57% for DCIS without microinvasion (Table 52.1). By choosing a subgroup of DCIS lesions with the same average size as the DCIS-Mi lesions, we found that margins were involved as frequently, which suggests that it is not the microinvasive component that makes complete excision of these lesions difficult; rather, it is the size of the DCIS component and the fact that the entire DCIS or DCIS-Mi is not always marked by microcalcifications.

There was no statistical difference in the local recurrence–free survival at 12 years between DCIS (80%) and

DCIS-Mi (73%) (p = not significant) (Fig. 52.1). In reality, there were too few patients in the DCIS-Mi group (n = 24) to feel comfortable with the level of accuracy of the actuarial analysis of their local recurrence–free survival. Nonetheless, distant metastases only occurred in our small subset of DCIS-Mi patients in those with disease greater than or equal to 45 mm (two of six). Although there was a statistical difference when distant disease–free survival was analyzed (Fig. 52.2), there are simply too few DCIS-Mi patients for us to draw any firm conclusion. More patients and longer follow-up are required for the DCIS-Mi group. It is worth noting, however, that there were no local recurrences in six patients with DCIS-Mi treated with excision and postoperative radiation therapy, whereas, there were three local recurrences out of four patients with DCIS-Mi treated with excision alone. This suggests that DCIS-Mi is more likely to contain additional foci of invasion and should be treated with postoperative radiation therapy if the patient elects breast conservation.

DCIS-Mi evolves from DCIS but it is qualitatively distinct and should not be grouped with DCIS as we ill advisedly did in a previous paper published in 1990 (10). The DCIS component of DCIS-Mi is generally larger, has a higher DNA index, is more often aneuploid, and overexpresses HER2/neu more frequently. It is a more advanced lesion that has achieved the molecular genetics necessary to develop invasive growth. DCIS-Mi is no longer a potential or borderline cancer; it is a real cancer, regardless of the small size of its invasive component. Microinvasion, however, is not synonymous with the ability to metastasize. Large DCIS lesions with multiple tiny foci of microinvasion, although they are stage 1 at this time, should be treated with great caution.

Axillary Node Dissection for Ductal Carcinoma in Situ-Mi

Because of the large number of negative node dissections or samplings in patients with pure DCIS (425 of 427), our group abandoned this procedure in the late 1980s as a routine part of the treatment for patients with DCIS (11,12). DCIS-Mi, however, is an invasive lesion and a decision regarding node dissection for these patients lagged behind. In 1993, we suggested that node dissection be abandoned as a routine procedure for patients with DCIS-Mi (2). This became a moot point in 1995 with the introduction of sentinel node biopsy. At this point, we recommend sentinel node biopsy for all patients with DCIS-Mi, even though the vast majority are likely to be node negative.

With early invasion, there is clearly a potential for metastasis to axillary nodes. But how much is the risk, and does it justify axillary node dissection? In 1995, we published the results of an analysis comparing palpable and nonpalpable invasive breast carcinomas by T category. The rate of axillary node metastases in patients with nonpalpable T1a lesions was 4%; with palpable T1a lesions, it was 6% (13). Extrapolating from these results, the rate of axillary node positivity for DCIS-Mi should be no more than 5% and is probably less. If this is true, it hardly seems worth recommending axillary dissection on a routine basis. However, in light of our current thinking regarding the tumor biology of breast cancer and the possible therapeutic role of node dissection (14), we would like to re-examine whether axillary node dissection has any role for patients with DCIS-Mi.

Wong and associates (15) reviewed the records of the University of California Los Angeles Medical Center from 1965 to 1988 and found 41 patients who met their definition of DCIS with microinvasion: "breast cancer cells confined to the duct system with only a microscopic focus of malignant cells invading beyond the basement membrane." They give no maximum size of the invasive focus for inclusion in the DCIS-Mi category. Thirty-three patients underwent axillary node dissection; all were negative. There have been no local or distant recurrences and no deaths with a median follow-up of 47 months. Like us, they suggested that axillary node dissection be abandoned for DCIS-Mi.

Taking the opposite approach, Rosner et al. (16) and Solin et al. (17) suggested that axillary node dissection be continued as an integral part of the staging and treatment for patients with DCIS-Mi. Rosner and associates (16) reported a single positive node dissection out of 37 performed for patients with DCIS-Mi. Their definition of DCIS-Mi was broader ("DCIS with limited microscopic stromal invasion below the basement membrane in one or several ducts but not invading more than 10% of the surface of the histologic sections examined"). In spite of this liberal definition, only 3% of their node dissections were positive. Never the less, they concluded that node dissection was indicated for DCIS-Mi.

Solin and associates (17), using no more than 2 mm of invasion or less than 10% invasive cancer as their definition for DCIS-Mi, found two positive node dissections out of 37 (5%) and recommended that axillary staging remain an integral part of the treatment of DCIS-Mi.

As a prognostic or staging modality, complete axillary node dissection is neither cost effective nor in the DCIS-Mi patient's best interest. It should be abandoned if prognosis is the only reason for its performance. If one performs 100 node dissections for DCIS-Mi patients, 2% to 5% would likely be positive, depending on the definition of DCIS-Mi used. One hundred node dissections cannot be justified in an attempt to find no more than five node-positive patients to treat with chemotherapy because, at most, only one or two will be helped (18).

Alternatively, axillary lymph node dissection for microinvasive lesions could be justified if it can be proven to be a therapeutic procedure rather than just a prognostic one. Harris and Osteen (19) believe that approximately 5% to 10% of patients with invasive carcinomas are cured by axillary dissection. In other words, they believe that the procedure is therapeutic in some patients. They believe that NS-ABP protocol B-04 (20), which showed no statistical difference in survival whether or not the axilla was treated, was flawed because one-third of the patients randomized to receive no treatment to the axilla had 1 to 10 nodes removed during their initial surgery (21). Ultimately, this yielded a smaller group of patients without the statistical power to rule out a small therapeutic benefit from axillary dissection. Fifteen-year follow-up data from NSABP protocol B-04 continue to reveal a 4% to 5% (statistically insignificant) survival benefit in favor of patients whose axillary nodes were treated with either surgical removal or radiation therapy.

In the Karnofsky Lecture at the 1994 Annual Meeting of the American Society of Clinical Oncology, Hellman (14) stated that both the Halstedian Hypothesis and Fisher's Systemic Hypothesis (22) were too restrictive. He said, "The hypothesis most consistent with the data is that breast cancer is a spectrum of disease with increasing proclivity for metastasis as a function of tumor size. Although lymph node involvement can be a marker of increased risk of distant disease, it may be the only site of metastasis in many patients, especially those with small tumors." If axillary node dissection is therapeutic in some cases, then patients with the smallest lesions are the ones mostly likely to benefit; for example, patients with DCIS-Mi, T1a or T1b lesions. It is entirely possible that many patients with DCIS-Mi, T1a, or T1b lesions who were treated years ago with radical or modified radical mastectomy were cured because this surgery removed lymph nodes with micrometastases that were not identified on routine, single section, hematoxylin and eosin stained lymph node examination.

Axillary node dissection may be therapeutic in a very small percentage of breast cancers and early lesions are the ones most likely to benefit. A large DCIS-Mi is a different lesion when compared with a small unifocal invasive carcinoma without an extensive intraductal component. We fear that larger lesions, like DCIS-Mi, may not be completely sampled during routine microscopic evaluation (thereby missing foci of invasion) or that permanent sections may indeed show foci of true invasion that were not appreciated during mastectomy. Taking all of this into account, we recommend that a sentinel lymph node biopsy be performed on all patients with DCIS-Mi.

For patients with pure DCIS lesions that are large enough to require a mastectomy, we recommend sentinel node biopsy at the time of mastectomy. Because the lower axilla is exposed during a total mastectomy, sentinel node biopsy can be done without added morbidity. If a small focus of true invasive cancer is found on permanent sections, there will be no need to redissect the axilla if the sentinel node is negative. For patients with smaller pure DCIS lesions and clear margins that are being treated conservatively, we do not routinely recommend sentinel node biopsy.

Treatment of the Breast in Patients with Ductal Carcinoma in Situ-Mi

Treatment of the breast for patients with DCIS-Mi has never been well defined. Because the majority of DCIS-Mi lesions are large (the DCIS component), many of these patients will, by necessity, undergo mastectomy. Immediate reconstruction should be the routinely available, if desired. The mastectomy should be skin-sparing and, for most patients, autologous tissue will often yield an aesthetically superior reconstruction.

When the patient is appropriate for breast preservation, there may be some debate regarding whether radiation therapy should be added to every case. We generally believe that it should be, because DCIS-Mi is an invasive breast cancer. There are no studies randomizing conservatively treated patients with DCIS-Mi to excision only versus excision plus radiation therapy. The prospective study that most closely approximates this scenario was done by Schnitt et al (23). They treated small (2 cm or less), histologically favorable invasive tumors (low-grade, well-differentiated, tubular, etc.) with widely clear margins (1 cm or more). Patients treated with excision alone recurred at a statistically higher rate than those treated with excision plus radiation therapy in a historical comparison group. The recommendation was made that all patients with invasive breast cancer, no matter how histologically favorable, be treated with postoperative radiation therapy if the breast was to be preserved.

CONCLUSION

We believe that the treatment of the breast for both DCIS and DCIS-Mi should be similar and should be based on the size of the DCIS component relative to breast size, margin status, the ability to follow the patient mammographically, and patient preferences. All conservatively treated patients with DCIS-Mi should receive postoperative radiation therapy. A sentinel node biopsy should be performed at the time of mastectomy for patients treated with mastectomy. Sentinel node biopsy should also be routinely performed for breast preservation patients. With time and longer follow-up, we believe that patients with DCIS-Mi will not do quite as well as patients with DCIS without microinvasion, and that other prognostic markers such as HER2/neu, ER, PR, p53, etc. may play a more predictive role.

REFERENCES

1. Sobin LH, Wittekind CH, eds. *Breast Tumors in TNM Classification of Malignant Tumors*, 5th ed. New York: Wiley-Liss, 1997:123–130.
2. Silverstein MJ, Waisman JR, Colburn WJ, et al. Intraductal breast carcinoma (DCIS) with and without microinvasion (Mi): Is there a difference in outcome? *Proc Am Soc Clin Oncol* 1993;12:56(abst).

3. Tabar L, Chen HH, Duffy S, et al. A novel method for prediction of long-term outcome of women with T1a, T1b, and 10–14 mm invasive breast cancers: a prospective study. *Lancet* 2000;355: 429–433.

4. Lagios MD, Westdahl PR, Margolin FR, et al. Duct carcinoma in situ: Relationship of extent of noninvasive disease to the frequency of occult invasion, multicentricity, lymph node metastases and short-term treatment failures. *Cancer* 1982;50: 1309–1314.

5. Lagios MD, Margolin FR, Westdahl PR, et al. Mammographically detected duct carcinoma in situ. Frequency of local recurrence following tylectomy and prognostic effect of nuclear grade on local recurrence. *Cancer* 1989;63:618–624.

6. Tabar L, Duffy SW, Vitak B, et al. The natural history of breast carcinoma: What have we learned from screening? *Cancer* 1999; 86:449–462.

7. Fisher ER, Sass R, Fisher B, et al. Pathologic findings from the National Surgical Adjuvant Breast Project (Protocol 6) I. Intraductal carcinoma (DCIS). *Cancer* 1986;57:197–208.

8. Bijker N, Peterse JL, Duchateau L, et al. Risk factors for recurrence and metastasis after breast conserving therapy for ductal carcinoma in situ: Analysis of European Organization for Research and Treatment of Cancer Trial 10853. *J Clin Oncol* 2001; 19:2263–2271.

9. Silverstein MJ, Gamagami P, Colburn WJ, et al. Nonpalpable breast lesions: Diagnosis with slightly overpenetrated screen-film mammography and hook wire–directed breast biopsy in 1,014 cases. *Radiology* 1989;171:633–638.

10. Silverstein MJ, Waisman JR, Rosser RJ, et al. Intraductal carcinoma of the breast (208 cases): Clinical factors influencing treatment choices. *Cancer* 1990;66:102–108.

11. Silverstein MJ, Rosser RJ, Gierson ED, et al. Axillary Lymph node dissection for intraductal carcinoma—is it indicated? *Proc Am Soc Clin Oncol* 1986;5:265(abst).

12. Silverstein MJ, Rosser RJ, Gierson ED, et al. Axillary Lymph node dissection for intraductal carcinoma—is it indicated? *Cancer* 1987;59:1819–1824.

13. Silverstein MJ, Gierson ED, Waisman JR, et al. Predicting axillary node positivity in patients with invasive carcinoma of the breast by using a combination of T category and palpability. *J Am Coll Surg* 1995;180:700–704.

14. Hellman S. The Natural History of Small Breast Cancers. *J Clin Oncol* 1994;12:2229–2234.

15. Wong JH, Kopald KH, Morton DL. The impact of microinvasion on axillary node metastases and survival in patients with intraductal breast cancer. *Arch Surg* 1990;125:1298–1302.

16. Rosner D, Lane WW, Penetrante R. Duct carcinoma in situ with microinvasion: A curable entity using surgery alone without need for adjuvant therapy. *Cancer* 1991;67:1498–1503.

17. Solin LJ, Fowble BL, I-Tien Y, et al. Microinvasive ductal carcinoma of the breast treated with breast conserving surgery and definitive irradiation. *Int J Radiat Oncol Biol Phys* 1992;23: 961–968.

18. Cady B. The need to reexamine axillary lymph node dissection in invasive breast cancer. *Cancer* 1994;73:505–508.

19. Harris JR, Osteen RT. Patients with early breast cancer benefit from effective axillary treatment. *Breast Cancer Res Treat* 1985; 5:17–21.

20. Fisher B, Redmond C, Fisher ER, et al. Ten-year results of a randomized clinical trial comparing radical mastectomy and total mastectomy with or without radiation. *N Engl J Med* 1985;312: 674–681.

21. Fisher B, Montague E, Redmond C, et al. Comparison of radical mastectomy with alternative treatments for primary breast cancer. *Cancer* 1977;39:2827–2839.

22. Fisher B. The surgical dilemma in the primary therapy of invasive breast cancer: A critical appraisal. *Curr Probl Surg* Oct 1970: 1–53.

23. Schnitt SJ, Hayman J, Gelman B, et al. A prospective study of conservative surgery alone in the treatment of selected patients with stage 1 breast cancer. *Cancer* 1996;77:1094–1100.

53

MANAGEMENT OF THE CONTRALATERAL BREAST

SONJA EVA SINGLETARY

Deciding how to manage the contralateral breast when a patient is diagnosed with unilateral breast cancer is an emotional and intellectual challenge for both the patient and the physician. It is difficult to estimate a woman's risk of developing a contralateral breast cancer. The clinician must take into account not only the woman's personal risk factors for breast cancer but also the probability of relapse and death from the initial breast cancer and the possibility of other causes of death. Furthermore, the value of any risk estimate is somewhat limited because of the controversy surrounding which risk factors are significant and how they interact. The dilemma is heightened for women with ductal carcinoma in situ (DCIS) because the prognosis is excellent but the amount of time women are exposed to the risk of a second cancer is increased. This chapter will address the incidence and impact on survival of contralateral breast cancer in patients with DCIS and the clinical decision-making process used to determine which patients are candidates for chemoprevention or prophylactic mastectomy.

INCIDENCE OF METACHRONOUS CONTRALATERAL BREAST CANCER

Predictors of metachronous contralateral primary breast cancer in patients with DCIS have not been examined to date. In general, most clinicians have assumed that the annual risk of developing cancer in the second breast is similar for women with DCIS and women with invasive cancer, about 0.5% to 0.7% per year from the date of diagnosis of the first breast cancer [1].

The effect of risk factors such as family history on the risk of contralateral breast cancer is unclear. In Anderson and Badzioch's study [2] of 556 patients at The University of Texas M. D. Anderson Cancer Center with a diagnosis of unilateral breast cancer (any type) and a history of breast cancer in the mother, a sister, or a second-degree relative, the risk of contralateral disease became relatively constant over time after an initial high risk in the immediate postoperative period. After 14 years, the risk eventually reached a

plateau. However, this may have been due to the small number of patients remaining at risk. In contrast, Harris et al. [3] described the risk of contralateral disease in women with familial breast cancer as elevated in the first 5 years and then peaking again at 14 years.

Anderson and Badzioch [2,4] also reported a three to four times greater risk for developing bilateral cancer when a relative had bilateral breast cancer, was diagnosed with breast cancer before menopause, or both. Others have found the risk of bilateral breast cancer to be associated more with young age itself than with family history, particularly in the case of metachronous breast cancer [5–7], invasive lobular carcinoma or lobular carcinoma in situ [8,9], tubular carcinoma [9–11], or multicentricity [5,7,12,13].

To determine if there is a subset of unilateral breast cancer patients who face a particularly high risk for developing contralateral disease, Newman et al. [14] studied 70 patients with a history of bilateral breast cancer who were treated at M. D. Anderson Cancer Center between 1983 and 1994 and 70 age-matched control patients with unilateral breast cancer who had a survival duration equal to at least the interval between cancers in the bilateral cases. Patients with bilateral breast cancer were significantly more likely to have multicentric disease and to have a positive family history for breast cancer compared with the unilateral breast cancer group. There were no significant differences regarding history of exogenous hormone exposure, lobular histology, hormone receptor status, or HER2/neu expression. The 5-year disease-free survival rate was 94% for the unilateral breast cancer patients and 91% for the bilateral breast cancer patients ($p = 0.16$).

Patients with DCIS are usually diagnosed in the fifth decade of life [15]. Whether a younger age at diagnosis or a family history of breast cancer increases the risk of contralateral breast cancer has not been specifically addressed in most series of DCIS cases. Even in large trials such as the National Surgical Adjuvant Breast and Bowel Project (NSABP) B-17 trial, the overall cumulative incidence of contralateral breast cancer as a first event through almost 8 years of follow-up of the 814 treated patients was only 4.5%, and

TABLE 53.1. OVERALL INCIDENCE OF CONTRALATERAL BREAST CANCER IN PATIENTS WITH DUCTAL CARCINOMA IN SITU

Series (Year, Reference)	No. of Patients	Follow-Up (Months)	Contralateral Breast Cancer			
			Synchronous		Metachronous	
			IS	IC	IS	IC
Farrow (1970, 17)	200	48+	2	6	2	6
Webber et al. (1981, 18)	113	108	2	1	0	1
Sunshine et al. (1985, 19)	70	120	7	0	0	1
Silverstein et al. (1990, 20)	203	45	4	9	3	6
Baird et al. (1990, 21)	38	39	0	0	0	0
Ward et al. (1992, 22)	220	120	3	0	12	39
Fisher et al. (1991, 23) (NSABP B-06)	76	83	0	0	4	1
Solin et al. (1993, 24)	172	84	0	0	1	6
Archer et al. (1994, 15)	68	134	0	0	2	0
Fisher et al. (1998, 16) (NSABP B-17)	814	90	0	0	10	22
Fisher et al. (1999, 25) (NSABP B-24 placebo)	902	74	0	0	13	23
Total	2,880	86	18[a]	16	47[b]	105
Percentage			(0.6%)	(0.6%)	(1.6%)	(3.6%)

IC, invasive carcinoma; IS, all in situ carcinomas, including lobular carcinoma in situ (LCIS).
[a] 5 LCIS.
[b] 4 LCIS.

the incidence of invasive contralateral cancer was only 3% (16). Table 53.1 shows the incidence of contralateral breast cancer in patients with DCIS in 11 series. According to these data, the likelihood of developing an invasive contralateral breast cancer is only 4% in women who have had DCIS, and that of developing a noninvasive lesion (including lobular carcinoma in situ) is only 2%.

IMPACT OF CONTRALATERAL BREAST CANCER ON SURVIVAL

The impact of contralateral breast cancer on survival has usually been examined in patients with invasive breast cancer. Many studies of invasive breast cancer that were conducted before adjuvant therapy was routinely used showed similar survival rates for patients with bilateral breast cancer and those with unilateral breast cancer (1,9,26–30). In a review of 1,036 patients with operable breast cancer treated postoperatively with doxorubicin-containing combination chemotherapy at M. D. Anderson Cancer Center, the prognosis of patients with bilateral breast cancer (44 with synchronous cancers and 17 with metachronous cancers) was similar to that of patients with unilateral breast cancer (31). The minimal effect on survival of the second breast cancer may explain why the use of contralateral breast biopsies at the time of initial diagnosis to detect occult disease has not been clearly shown to improve survival rates (9,28,32,33).

Is this same survival pattern true for patients with DCIS and contralateral disease? Although most studies have not

specifically addressed the issue of survival after contralateral breast cancer in patients with an initial diagnosis of DCIS, this patient population usually has an excellent breast cancer-specific survival outcome. In series reporting treatment failure after mastectomy for DCIS (19,34–39), approximately 3% of patients had a recurrence, and only 2% died of breast cancer. Similarly, in series describing recurrence and survival after excision plus radiotherapy for DCIS (16,37,40–42), 6% to 11% of patients had a recurrence, but the survival rate was 99%.

Another survival consideration is the possibility of primary cancers at other sites. Rosen et al. (30) reported that patients with breast cancer are just as likely to develop a second primary tumor that is not in the breast as they are to develop a contralateral breast cancer. A non-breast primary tumor is more likely than a second breast cancer to be life-threatening (43). Of the 1,324 consecutive breast cancer patients who underwent breast-conservation therapy between 1970 and 1994 at M. D. Anderson, 130 patients (10%) had a second primary malignancy; 44% of these had a second primary malignancy prior to their breast cancer diagnosis and 56% after treatment of the breast cancer (45). The sites of second primary tumors were gastrointestinal in 22%, gynecologic in 19%, lung in 18%, hematologic in 8%, thyroid in 7%, and other sites in 26%. Contralateral breast cancer occurred in only 9%.

Thus, given the low risk of clinically significant contralateral breast cancer, the similar prognoses of patients with unilateral and those with bilateral breast cancer, and the potential of death from other causes (including cancers not associated with the breast), careful surveillance of the opposite breast by physical examination and yearly mammography appears to be a reasonable option in women with DCIS. Alternatively, patients may be counseled regarding the benefits versus risks of chemoprevention with tamoxifen and the role, if any, of prophylactic mastectomy.

CHEMOPREVENTION

Recent studies have confirmed the efficacy of tamoxifen for the chemoprevention of breast cancer. In the NSABP P-1 study, Fisher et al. (44) prospectively randomized more than 13,000 women to receive either tamoxifen or a placebo for 5 years. All study participants were determined to be at high risk for breast cancer based on age greater than 60 years, a history of lobular carcinoma in situ, or a 5-year risk for breast cancer of at least 1.66% based on Gail model calculations (45). After a median follow-up of only 4.5 years, the study was unblinded because of the magnitude of the difference in breast cancer incidence between the two arms of the study. Tamoxifen use resulted in a 49% decrease in the incidence of breast cancer in this study. However, tamoxifen was effective in decreasing the incidence of estrogen receptor–positive tumors only; there was no impact on the incidence of estrogen receptor–negative tumors. Unfortunately, tamoxifen use in high-risk postmenopausal women is associated with an increase in the risk of endometrial cancer and thromboembolic events such as deep vein thrombosis and pulmonary embolism.

Data from the NSABP B-24 study of 1,804 patients randomized to receive tamoxifen or placebo after lumpectomy and irradiation for DCIS support the use of tamoxifen to lower the incidence of ipsilateral tumor recurrence and contralateral breast cancer (25). With a median follow-up of 74 months, 36 contralateral breast cancers (23 invasive and 13 noninvasive) occurred as first events in the placebo group, as compared with only 18 contralateral breast cancers (15 invasive and 3 noninvasive) in the tamoxifen group. Although there was an increase in the rate of endometrial cancer in patients who received tamoxifen (1.53 versus 0.45 per 1,000 patients per year in the placebo group), no deaths from endometrial cancer occurred in the tamoxifen group.

Raloxifene, a newer selective estrogen receptor modulator, has been investigated as a therapy for postmenopausal osteoporosis. Preliminary data indicate that raloxifene may be at least as effective as tamoxifen in reducing the incidence of estrogen receptor–positive breast cancers (46), possibly without the increased risk of endometrial cancer seen with tamoxifen. However, patients should be discouraged from taking raloxifene as a breast cancer chemopreventative agent until more data are available from clinical trials. The NSABP Study of Tamoxifen and Raloxifene (STAR) trial is rapidly accruing high-risk postmenopausal women to compare the breast cancer risk reduction with raloxifene versus tamoxifen.

Genetic testing is now available to detect mutated genes that substantially increase the risk of breast cancer (e.g., BRCA1, BRCA2, p53, and ataxia-telangiectasia), but the role of chemopreventative agents in women with documented mutations is unknown. Participants in the Royal Marsden Hospital study of breast cancer chemoprevention were selected on the basis of high risk as determined by a family history of breast cancer (47). The study showed no benefit from tamoxifen, and the negative results were speculated to be related to an excessive rate of inclusion of patients who had BRCA1 mutations and, thus, a higher likelihood of estrogen receptor–negative breast cancer. However, the low rate of incident cancers in the study population does not support this theory. In contrast, the NSABP P-1 study demonstrated that tamoxifen reduces risk in women at high risk for breast cancer based on family history or overall Gail model risk calculations (45). A subset of the NSABP P-1 participants is currently being evaluated for the incidence of BRCA1 mutations, with the results unpublished at this time.

Another chemopreventative strategy in patients at risk for hereditary breast cancer is prophylactic oophorectomy. Rebbeck et al. (48) reported a case-control series of 43 BRCA1 mutation carriers who underwent bilateral prophylactic oophorectomy and 79 control patients who were also BRCA1 mutation carriers but had not undergone prophylactic surgery. With a median follow-up of more than 8 years, prophylactic oophorectomy resulted in a 50% lower incidence of breast cancer regardless of whether hormone replacement therapy was used.

PROPHYLACTIC MASTECTOMY

Unfortunately, prophylactic mastectomy does not guarantee freedom from breast cancer. Experimental studies of prophylactic mastectomies in rats given chemical carcinogens have shown that tumors still occur in residual breast tissue despite total mastectomy (49). Even in mice not exposed to mammary carcinogens, prophylactic mastectomy does not prevent spontaneous breast malignancies from developing in residual breast tissue (50). In humans, Temple et al. (51) found that careful pathologic examination of the chest wall and axilla in women undergoing mastectomy for breast cancer demonstrated extension of breast tissue into the axilla and pectoralis fascia. Thus, although a total mastectomy is defined as the complete removal of breast tissue, some breast tissue may in fact remain after mastectomy. In women who undergo less extensive subcutaneous mastectomies, which leave more residual breast tissue, subsequent invasive carcinomas have been reported in up to 1% of cases (52–54).

Hartmann et al. (55) reported an update of the Mayo Clinic database of prophylactic mastectomies. Of the 1,065 women who underwent bilateral prophylactic mastectomies (90% of which were subcutaneous mastectomies) between 1960 and 1993, 639 women had a family history of breast cancer. These 639 women were then stratified into two risk groups based on the extent of breast and ovarian cancer in the patient's family pedigree. The incidence of subsequent breast cancer in the 214 patients in the high-risk group who had prophylactic mastectomies was compared with that in 403 female siblings who did not have prophylactic surgery. The 425 women in the moderate-risk group who had prophylactic mastectomies were evaluated by determining the number of breast cancers that would have been expected based on the Gail model for risk calculations (45). At a median follow-up of 14 years, only seven cancers had developed in women who had undergone prophylactic mastectomies: three (1.4%) in the high-risk group and four (0.9%) in the moderate-risk group. In contrast, 156 cancers developed in the female siblings of patients in the high-risk group, and 37.4 cancers would have been expected in the moderate-risk group; this represents an approximately 90% reduction in breast cancer risk for both prophylactic surgery groups. Recently, Hartmann et al. (56) performed testing for BRCA1 and BRCA2 mutations in a subset of 110 high-risk families within their database. With a median follow-up of 16.1 years, breast cancer has not developed in any of the BRCA mutation carriers who underwent prophylactic mastectomy.

A review of the M. D. Anderson Cancer Center experience with prophylactic mastectomy included 155 patients with operable unilateral primary breast cancer who elected to have a contralateral mastectomy despite negative physical and mammographic findings in the contralateral breast (57). The patients ranged in age from 25 to 69 years (median, 46 years). All of the women underwent bilateral mastectomy and immediate breast reconstruction. The review identified specific factors that may have influenced a woman's decision to undergo prophylactic contralateral mastectomy (Table 53.2). Fifty-four percent of patients had a family history of breast cancer, although only 30% had a first-degree relative with a history of breast cancer. Approximately one-fourth of patients had one or more histologic features of the primary tumor that were associated with an increased risk of developing breast cancer. In 48% of the patients, a significant factor in the decision-making process was the anticipated difficulty in subsequent breast surveillance. The histologic findings in the prophylactic contralateral breast specimens were also reviewed; findings included DCIS in 3% of contralateral breasts, invasive cancer in 1%, atypical hyperplasia in 12%, and lobular carcinoma in situ in 7%.

Even though the likelihood of finding a significant occult cancer in the opposite breast is low, the patient is often concerned about whether reconstruction after mastectomy for a

TABLE 53.2. FACTORS AFFECTING DECISION OF WOMEN WITH UNILATERAL BREAST CANCER TO ALSO UNDERGO PROPHYLACTIC CONTRALATERAL MASTECTOMY

Factor	% of Patients
Family history of breast cancer	
First-degree relative	30
Any family history	54
Histopathology of index cancer	
Multicentric primary cancer	28
Associated lobular carcinoma in situ	23
Associated atypical hyperplasia	22
Other	
Anticipated difficulty of breast surveillance[a]	48
Age less than 40 years	21
Surgery needed on contralateral breast to achieve symmetry in reconstruction	14

[a] Includes severe fibrocystic disease; extremely dense, nodular breasts; diffuse microcalcifications; and multiple prior breast biopsies.

second cancer will be feasible, especially if the first reconstruction employed a transverse rectus abdominis myocutaneous (TRAM) flap. An M. D. Anderson review of 469 patients who had a mastectomy with unilateral breast reconstruction between 1988 and 1994 with at least 5 years of follow-up from the initial breast cancer revealed that only 18 (4%) of the patients developed contralateral breast cancer (58). The median age of the patients was 43 years for the initial breast cancer and 48 years for the second breast cancer. The reconstructive management after the initial mastectomy in the 18 patients who developed second breast cancers included 16 TRAM flaps (seven free and nine pedicled), one latissimus dorsi (LD) flap with an implant, and one superior gluteal free flap. Surgical management of the second breast cancers included breast conservation in two patients, mastectomy without reconstruction in four, and mastectomy with reconstruction in 12 (one free TRAM flap, three extended LD flaps, two LD flaps with implants, three implants, two Ruben's flaps, and one superior gluteal free flap). No major complications were detected after the reconstruction of the second breast. The best symmetry was obtained when similar methods and tissues were used on both sides. Patients should be reassured that if they do not elect to have prophylactic mastectomy for unilateral cancer and a contralateral breast cancer does occur and mastectomy is chosen or needed, breast-conservation therapy or reconstruction is feasible.

Although prophylactic mastectomy does not completely eliminate the risk of breast cancer, the procedure may be appropriate for selected women who are known to be at very high risk for breast cancer, who are extremely anxious about breast surveillance alone as follow-up, or who are not candidates for chemoprevention with tamoxifen (59). In helping

TABLE 53.3. QUESTIONS TO HELP CLINICIAN DETERMINE WHETHER PROPHYLACTIC CONTRALATERAL MASTECTOMY IS AN APPLICABLE TREATMENT OPTION

Is mastectomy the treatment choice for the ipsilateral breast?

Is the patient planning to undergo immediate reconstruction that will necessitate surgical reshaping of the contralateral breast?

Does the patient fully understand her risk of contralateral breast cancer?

Is the patient aware of risk reduction with tamoxifen?

Is the patient certain that prophylactic mastectomy is the best choice for her?

a patient decide whether prophylactic mastectomy is in her best interest, the clinician may find it useful to use a series of questions (Table 53.3) as a guide. First, is the choice of cancer therapy for the ipsilateral breast total mastectomy? The next question is whether the patient is interested in immediate reconstruction and, if so, the type of reconstruction and anticipated cosmetic outcome. If the plastic surgeon will need to surgically alter the opposite breast to achieve symmetry with the reconstructed breast mound, then bilateral mastectomy may be a reasonable option because the contralateral breast will have to be operated on anyway.

Another question to be addressed is whether the patient understands her true risk for contralateral breast cancer. Most patients overestimate their risk or fail to put their relative risk in proper perspective with other potential health problems. The patient also needs to understand that removal of both breasts will not guarantee freedom from breast cancer.

In addition, the patient should be aware of possible out-of-pocket expenses when a prophylactic procedure is considered. Many insurance carriers will refuse to pay or individualize the approval required to cover the costs of prophylactic surgery. Kuerer et al. (60) surveyed 150 different third-party payer agencies and found that private insurance plans were more likely to have a policy allowing coverage for prophylactic mastectomy than were governmental plans (Medicare and Medicaid); however, approximately half of all plans had no explicit policy at all, with coverage determined on a case-by-case basis.

Finally, as a compassionate listener, the physician has the important role of aiding the patient in sorting out her emotional needs (61). If the patient has any doubt about proceeding with prophylactic mastectomy, she is not a candidate for this procedure.

CONCLUSION

In the current information age, patients spend hours educating themselves with books and electronic media. When they seek medical advice, they expect the clinician to be their personal advocate and to assist them in sorting through information that is sometimes confusing. A thoughtful and careful evaluation of the risks of contralateral breast cancer usually reassures the patient with a newly diagnosed breast cancer and allows her to appropriately focus on the management of the known cancer. For patients who are extremely anxious concerning the potential risk of cancer in the opposite breast, an unhurried discussion of the available information to date on chemoprevention strategies and the role, if any, of prophylactic mastectomy should be provided by a clinician with expertise in this field.

REFERENCES

1. Singletary SE, Taylor SH, Guinee VF, et al. Occurrence and prognosis of contralateral breast cancer. *J Am Coll Surg* 1994; 178:390–396.
2. Anderson DE, Badzioch MD. Bilaterality in familial breast cancer patients. *Cancer* 1985;56:2092–2098.
3. Harris RE, Lynch HT, Guirgis HA. Familial breast cancer: risk to the contralateral breast. *J Natl Cancer Inst* 1978;60:955–960.
4. Anderson DE. Some characteristics of familial breast cancer. *Cancer* 1971;28:1500–1504.
5. Robbins GF, Berg JW. Bilateral primary breast cancers: prospective clinicopathologic study. *Cancer* 1964;17:1501–1527.
6. Slack N, Bross KOJ, Nemoto T, et al. Experiences with bilateral primary carcinoma of the breast. *Surg Gynecol Obstet* 1973;136:433–440.
7. Leis HP. Managing the remaining breast. *Cancer* 1980;46:1026–1030.
8. Singletary SE. Lobular carcinoma in situ of the breast: a 31-year experience at The University of Texas M. D. Anderson Cancer Center. *Breast Disease* 1994;7:157–163.
9. Fisher ER, Fisher B, Sass R, et al. Pathologic findings from the National Surgical Adjuvant Breast Project (protocol No. 4). XI. Bilateral breast cancer. *Cancer* 1984;54:3002–3011.
10. Lagios MD, Rose MR, Margolin FR. Tubular carcinoma of the breast: Association with multicentricity, bilaterality, and family history of mammary carcinoma. *Am J Pathol* 1980;73:25–30.
11. Winchester DJ, Sahin AA, Tucker SL, et al. Tubular carcinoma of the breast: Predicting axillary nodal metastases and recurrence. *Ann Surg* 1996;223:342–347.
12. Lesser ML, Rosen PP, Kinne DW. Multicentricity and bilaterality in invasive breast carcinoma. *Surgery* 1982;91:234–240.
13. Vlastos G, Rubio I, Mirza N, et al. The impact of multicentricity on clinical outcome in patients with T1-2, N0-1, M0 breast cancer. *Ann Surg Oncol* 2000;7:581–587.
14. Newman LA, Sahin AA, Bondy M, et al. A case-control study of unilateral and bilateral breast cancer patients. *Cancer* 2001;91:1845–1853.
15. Archer SG, Kemp BL, Gadd M, et al. Ductal carcinoma in situ of the breast: comedo versus noncomedo subtype nonpredictive of recurrence or contralateral new breast primary. *Breast Disease* 1994;7:353–360.
16. Fisher B, Dignam J, Wolmark N, et al. Lumpectomy and radiation therapy for the treatment of intraductal breast cancer: findings from National Surgical Adjuvant Breast and Bowel Project B-17. *J Clin Oncol* 1998;16:441–452.
17. Farrow JH. Current concepts in the detection and treatment of the earliest of the early breast cancers. *Cancer* 1970;25:468–477.

18. Webber BL, Heise H, Neifeld JP, et al. Risk of subsequent contralateral breast carcinoma in a population of patients with in-situ breast carcinoma. *Cancer* 1981;47:2928–2932.

19. Sunshine JA, Moseley HS, Fletcher WS, et al. Breast carcinoma in situ. A retrospective review of 112 cases with a minimum 10 year follow-up. *Am J Surg* 1985;150:44–51.

20. Silverstein MJ, Waisman JR, Gamagami P, et al. Intraductal carcinoma of the breast (208 cases). Clinical factors influencing treatment choice. *Cancer* 1990;66:102–108.

21. Baird RM, Worth A, Hislop G. Recurrence after lumpectomy for comedo-type intraductal carcinoma of the breast. *Am J Surg* 1990;159:479–481.

22. Ward BA, McKhann CF, Ravikumar TS. Ten-year follow-up of breast carcinoma in situ in Connecticut. *Arch Surg* 1992;127:1392–1395.

23. Fisher ER, Leeming R, Anderson S, et al. Conservative management of intraductal carcinoma (DCIS) of the breast. *J Surg Oncol* 1991;47:139–147.

24. Solin LJ, Yeh I-T, Kurtz J, et al. Ductal carcinoma in situ (intraductal carcinoma) of the breast treated with breast-conserving surgery and definitive irradiation. Correlation of pathologic parameters with outcome of treatment. *Cancer* 1993;71:2532–2542.

25. Fisher B, Dignam J, Wolmark N, et al. Tamoxifen in treatment of intraductal breast cancer: National Surgical Adjuvant Breast and Bowel Project B-24 randomised controlled trial. *Lancet* 1999;253:1993–2000.

26. Adair F, Berg J, Joubert L, et al. Long-term follow-up of breast cancer patients: the 30-year report. *Cancer* 1974;33:1145–1150.

27. Robinson E, Rennert G, Rennert HS, et al. Survival of first and second primary breast cancer. *Cancer* 1993;73:172–176.

28. McCredie JA, Inch WR, Alderson M. Consecutive primary carcinoma of the breast. *Cancer* 1975;35:1472–1477.

29. Mueller CB, Ames F. Bilateral carcinoma of the breast: frequency and mortality. *Can J Surg* 1978;21:459–465.

30. Rosen PP, Groshen S, Kinne DW, et al. Contralateral breast carcinoma: an assessment of risk and prognosis in stage I (T1N0M0) and stage II (T1N1M0) patients with 20-year follow-up. *Surgery* 1989;106:904–910.

31. Berte E, Buzdar AU, Mith TL, et al. Bilateral primary breast cancer in patients treated with adjuvant therapy. *Am J Clin Oncol* 1988;11:114–118.

32. Al-Jurf AS, Jochimsen PR, Urdanetta LF, et al. Factors influencing survival in bilateral breast cancer. *J Surg Oncol* 1981;16:343–348.

33. King RE, Terz JJ, Lawrence WJR. Experience with opposite breast biopsy in patients with operable breast cancer. *Cancer* 1976;37:43–45.

34. Ashikari R, Hajdu SI, Robbins GF. Intraductal carcinoma of the breast (1960–1969). *Cancer* 1971;28:1182–1187.

35. Brown PW, Silverman J, Owens E, et al. Intraductal "noninfiltrating" carcinoma of the breast. *Arch Surg* 1976;111:1063–1067.

36. Carter D, Smith RL. Carcinoma in situ of the breast. *Cancer* 1977;40:1189–1193.

37. Fisher ER, Sass R, Fisher B, et al. Pathologic findings from the National Surgical Adjuvant Breast Project (protocol B-06). I. Intraductal carcinoma (DCIS). *Cancer* 1986;57:197–208.

38. Lagios MD, Westdahl PR, Margolin FR, et al. Duct carcinoma in situ: relationship of extent of noninvasive disease to the frequency of occult invasion, multicentricity, lymph node metastases and short-term treatment failure. *Cancer* 1982;50:1309–1314.

39. Von Rueden DG, Wilson RE. Intraductal carcinoma of the breast. *Surg Gynecol Obstet* 1984;158:105–111.

40. Montague ED. Conservative surgery and radiation therapy in the treatment of operable breast cancer. *Cancer* 1984;53:700–704.

41. Recht A, Danoff BS, Solin LJ, et al. Intraductal carcinoma of the breast: results of treatment with excisional biopsy and radiation. *J Clin Oncol* 1985;3:1339–1343.

42. Zafrani B, Fourquet A, Vilcoq JR, et al. Conservative management of intraductal breast carcinoma with tumorectomy and radiation therapy. *Cancer* 1986;57:1299–1301.

43. Mirza NQ, Vlastos G, Meric F, et al. Incidence and survival impact of non-breast second primary malignancies following breast conserving therapy. San Antonio Breast Symposium December 2000.

44. Fisher B, Costantino JP, Wickerham DL, et al. Tamoxifen for prevention of breast cancer: report of the National Surgical Adjuvant Breast and Bowel Project P-1 study. *J Natl Cancer Inst* 1999;90:1371–1388.

45. Gail MH, Brinton LA, Byer DP, et al. Projecting individualized probabilities of developing breast cancer for white females who are being examined annually. *J Natl Cancer Inst* 1989;1: 1879–1886.

46. Cummings SR, Eckert S, Krueger KA, et al. The effect of raloxifene on risk of breast cancer in postmenopausal women: results from the MORE randomized trial. *JAMA* 1999;281:2189–2197.

47. Powles T, Eeles R, Ashley S, et al. Interim analysis of the incidence of breast cancer in the Royal Marsden Hospital tamoxifen randomized chemoprevention trial. *Lancet* 1998;352:98–101.

48. Rebbeck TR, Levin AM, Eisen A, et al. Breast cancer risk after bilateral prophylactic oophorectomy in BRCA 1 mutation carriers. *J Natl Cancer Inst* 1999;91:1475–1479.

49. Wong JH, Jackson CF, Swanson JS, et al. Analysis of the risk reduction of prophylactic partial mastectomy in Sprague-Dawley rats with 7,12-dimethylbenzanthracene–induced breast cancer. *Surgery* 1986;99:67–71.

50. Nelson H, Miller SH, Buck D, et al. Effectiveness of prophylactic mastectomy in the prevention of breast tumors in C3H mice. *Plast Reconstr Surg* 1989;83:662–669.

51. Temple WJ, Lindsay RL, Magi E, et al. Technical considerations for prophylactic mastectomy in patients at high risk for breast cancer. *Am J Surg* 1991;161:413–415.

52. Goodnight JE Jr, Quagliania JM, Morton DL. Failure of subcutaneous mastectomy to prevent the development of breast cancer. *J Surg Oncol* 1984;26:198–201.

53. Pennisi VR, Capozzi A. Subcutaneous mastectomy data: a final statistical analysis of 1,500 patients. *Aesthetic Plast Surg* 189;13:2115–2122.

54. Ziegler LD, Kroll SS. Primary breast cancer after prophylactic mastectomy. *Am J Clin Oncol* 1991;14:451–454.

55. Hartmann LC, Schaid DJ, Woods JE, et al. Efficacy of bilateral prophylactic mastectomy in women with a family history of breast cancer. *N Engl J Med* 1999;340:77–84.

56. Hartmann LC, Schaid D, Sellers T, et al. Bilateral prophylactic mastectomy in BRCA 1/2 mutation carriers abstract. *Proc Am Assoc Cancer Res* 2000;41:222–223.

57. Gershenwald JE, Hunt KK, Kroll SS, et al. Synchronous elective contralateral mastectomy and immediate bilateral breast reconstruction in women with early-stage breast cancer. *Ann Surg Oncol* 1998;5:529–538.

58. Chang DW, Kroll SS, Dackiw A, et al. Reconstructive management of contralateral breast cancer in patients who previously underwent unilateral breast reconstruction. *Plast Reconstr Surg* 2001;108:352–360.

59. Kroll SS, Miller MJ, Schusterman MA, et al. Rationale for elective contralateral mastectomy with immediate bilateral reconstruction. *Ann Surg Oncol* 1994;1:457–461.

60. Kuerer HM, Hwang ES, Anthony JP, et al. Current national health insurance coverage policies for breast and ovarian cancer prophylactic surgery. *Ann Surg Oncol* 2000;7:325–332.

61. Newman LA, Kuerer HM, Hunt KK, et al. Prophylactic mastectomy. *J Am Coll Surg* 2000;191:322–330.

54

EXTENSIVE INTRADUCTAL COMPONENT IN ASSOCIATION WITH INVASIVE BREAST CANCERS

STUART J. SCHNITT

The term "extensive intraductal component" (EIC) was first used in the mid 1980s to describe a distinctive pattern of ductal carcinoma in situ (DCIS) that is seen in association with a subset of invasive breast cancers (1). Since that time, studies from a number of institutions in the United States and Europe have evaluated the relationship between the presence of an EIC and the risk of local recurrence in the treated breast in women with invasive breast cancer treated with conservative surgery (CS) and radiation therapy (RT). These studies differ with regard to the precise definition of EIC, patient selection criteria, extent of surgery, details of radiation therapy, and length of follow-up. Despite these differences, these studies have generally shown that invasive tumors that have an EIC are associated with a significantly higher risk of local recurrence than tumors that lack an EIC, at least when information regarding the status of the microscopic margins is not available (2–10) (Table 54.1).

At our institution, tumors with an EIC (EIC-positive tumors) are defined as invasive carcinomas that show the simultaneous presence of prominent ductal carcinoma in situ (DCIS) within the tumor (usually comprising 25% or more of the area of the tumor) and DCIS beyond the edges of the invasive tumor. Tumors that lack one or both of these features are categorized as EIC-negative. Also included among the EIC-positive cases are tumors that are predominantly DCIS with one or more foci of microinvasion. Of note, approximately two-thirds of EIC-positive tumors can be suspected on mammography, and this may serve as a useful guide to the surgeon in planning the extent of the excision (11).

A number of studies have attempted to determine the reason for an association between EIC-positive tumors and an increased risk of local recurrence after CS and RT. In a study of patients who underwent a re-excision of the primary site after an initial gross excision in which there were positive or close margins, investigators at the Joint Center for Radiation Therapy in Boston (JCRT) found that the likelihood of residual cancer was significantly higher in EIC-

positive than in EIC-negative cases (88% versus 48%, p = 0.002). Moreover, for patients in the EIC-positive group, this residual tumor was composed primarily of DCIS and was often widespread. Prominent residual DCIS was seen in the re-excision specimen in 44% of EIC-positive cases compared with only 2% of patients in the EIC-negative group ($p < 0.0001$). In contrast, the residual tumor found in the EIC-negative patients typically consisted of only scattered microscopic foci of infiltrating cancer and/or DCIS (12). In a subsequent study, Holland et al. (13) related the presence or absence of an EIC in the primary tumor to the type and extent of residual tumor in the remainder of the breast in mastectomy specimens using a correlated radiologic-pathologic mapping technique. In that study, patients with EIC-positive tumors were significantly more likely than those with EIC-negative lesions to have residual DCIS in the breast. Furthermore, in about 30% of patients with EIC-positive tumors, this residual DCIS was prominent and extended at least 2 cm beyond the edge of the primary tumor. In contrast, such extensive residual intraductal disease was seen in only 2% of patients with EIC-negative tumors ($p < 0.0001$) (13). The results of these two studies indicate that EIC-positive tumors are lesions in which the associated intraductal involvement is often more extensive than can be appreciated clinically or at the time of surgery. Therefore, EIC-positive patients who undergo a limited resection of the clinically evident tumor frequently have considerable residual DCIS in the vicinity of the tumor site. The most likely explanation for the high risk of local recurrence observed in EIC-positive patients is that the residual tumor burden in such patients is too large to be eradicated by cosmetically acceptable doses of irradiation. It is also possible that this residual DCIS contains a hypoxic compartment that renders it relatively radioresistant (14).

Several studies have not found an association between the presence of an EIC and increased risk of local recurrence. In particular, investigators from the NSABP B-06 trial failed to find an adverse effect of an EIC on the rate of local recur-

TABLE 54.1. RELATIONSHIP BETWEEN THE PRESENCE OF AN EXTENSIVE INTRADUCTAL COMPONENT AND THE RISK OF LOCAL RECURRENCE IN PATIENTS WITH INVASIVE BREAST CANCER TREATED WITH CONSERVATIVE SURGERY AND RADIATION THERAPY

Study (Reference)	No. of Patients	Follow-Up (mo)	Local Recurrence	
			EIC-Positive (%)	EIC-Negative (%)
Paterson (3)	236	44 (mean)	11	3
Jacquemier (4)	496	60 (act)	18	8
Voogd (10)	879	120 (act)	21	9
Yeh (8)	275	60 (act)	22	4
Lindley (6)	293	24 (min)	22	10
Fourquet (7)	434	120 (act)	23	5
Boyages (2)	584	60 (act)	24	6
Veronesi (TART) (9)	345	84 (act)	28	10
Locker (5)	263	60 (act)	50	25

TART, tumorectomy, axillary dissection and radiation therapy; act, actuarial; min, minimum; EIC, extensive intraductal component.

rence (15). However, in that trial patients with positive microscopic margins of excision were excluded from the breast-conserving arms of the study. Because EIC-positive patients frequently have positive microscopic margins after a local excision (16), it is likely that many EIC-positive patients were excluded from the conservative treatment arms in that trial.

The results of more recent studies (16–19) have indicated that the presence of an EIC is not an independent predictor of local recurrence when the microscopic margin status is also taken into consideration. Therefore, in current practice where microscopic margin assessment has become routine, EIC has evolved into more of a patient selection factor than a prognostic factor for local recurrence. In particular, identification of an EIC in association with an invasive breast cancer is one of the major factors taken into consideration in evaluating the suitability of a patient for treatment with CS and RT and in helping to determine the extent of the surgical excision prior to RT.

It should be evident from the foregoing discussion that there are a number of important similarities between invasive cancers with an EIC and cases of pure DCIS with regard to patient evaluation and management. In both instances, intraductal involvement by neoplastic cells may be more extensive than is appreciated clinically or at the time of surgery. Therefore, careful mammographic and pathologic evaluation are essential to help define the extent of the lesion and to determine the adequacy of excision (20–22). Mammographic evaluation includes preoperative mammography, specimen radiography (if the indication for biopsy was a mammographically detected, nonpalpable lesion), and, in many instances, post-biopsy mammography to determine if the full extent of the mammographic abnormalities have been completely excised. In all of these situations, the use of magnification views is of great value in defining the extent of the radiographic lesion. Pathologic evaluation must in-

clude inking of the specimen margins and microscopic assessment of the status of the inked margins, because this provides important information with regard to the likelihood of residual disease and the risk of local recurrence following breast-conserving treatment (17,23–28).

REFERENCES

1. Recht A, Connolly JL, Schnitt SJ, et al. Conservative surgery and radiation therapy of early breast cancer: Results, controversies and unsolved problems. *Semin Oncol* 1986;13:434–449.
2. Boyages J, Recht A, Connolly JL, et al. Early breast cancer: predictors of breast recurrence for patients treated with conservative surgery and radiation therapy. *Radiother Oncol* 1990;19:29–41.
3. Paterson DA, Anderson TJ, Lack WJL, et al. Pathological features predictive of local recurrence after management by conservation of invasive breast cancer: importance of non-invasive carcinoma. *Radiother Oncol* 1992;25:176–180.
4. Jacquemier J, Kurtz JM, Amalric R, et al. An assessment of extensive intraductal component as a risk factor for local recurrence after breast-conserving therapy. *Br J Cancer* 1990;61:873–876.
5. Locker AP, Ellis IO, Morgan DAL, et al. Factors influencing local recurrence after excision and radiotherapy for primary breast cancer. *Br J Surg* 1989;76:890–894.
6. Lindley R, Bulman A, Parsons P, et al. Histologic features predictive of an increased risk of early local recurrence after treatment of breast cancer by local tumor excision and radical radiotherapy. *Surgery* 1989;105:13–20.
7. Fourquet A, Campana F, Zafrani B, et al. Prognostic factors of breast recurrence in the conservative management of early breast cancer: a 25-year follow-up. *Int J Radiat Oncol Biol Phys* 1989; 17:719–725.
8. Yeh I, Fowble B, Viglione MJ, et al. Pathologic assessment and pathologic prognostic factors in operable breast cancer. In Fowble B, Goodman RL, Glick JH, Rosato EF, eds. *Breast Cancer Treatment. A Comprehensive Guide to Management*. St. Louis: Mosby–Year Book, 1991:167–208.
9. Veronesi U, Luini A, Galimberti V, et al. Conservation approaches for the management of stage I/II carcinoma of the breast: Milan cancer institute trials. *World J Surg* 1994;18:70–75.

10. Voogd AC, Nielsen M, Peterse JL, et al. Differences in risk factors for local and distant recurrence after breast-conserving therapy or mastectomy for stage I and II breast cancer: Pooled results of two large European randomized trials. *J Clin Oncol* 2001; 19:1688–1697.
11. Healey EA, Osteen RT, Schnitt SJ, et al. Can the clinical and mammographic findings at presentation predict the presence of an extensive intraductal component in early stage breast cancer? *Int J Radiat Oncol Biol Phys* 1989;17:1217–1221.
12. Schnitt SJ, Connolly JL, Khettry U, et al. Pathologic findings on re-excision of the primary site in breast cancer patients considered for treatment by primary radiation therapy. *Cancer* 1987;59: 675–681.
13. Holland R, Connolly JL, Gelman R, et al. The presence of an extensive intraductal component following a limited excision correlates with prominent residual disease in the remainder of the breast. *J Clin Oncol* 1990;8:113–118.
14. Mayr NA, Staples JJ, Robinson RA, et al. Morphometric studies in intraductal breast carcinoma using computerized image analysis. *Cancer* 1991;67:2805–2812.
15. Fisher ER, Sass R, Fisher B, et al. Pathologic findings from the National Surgical Adjuvant Breast Project (Protocol 6). II. Relation of local breast recurrence to multicentricity. *Cancer* 1986;57:1717–1724.
16. Schnitt SJ, Abner A, Gelman R, et al. The relationship between microscopic margins of resection and the risk of local recurrence in patients with breast cancer treated with breast-conserving surgery and radiation therapy. *Cancer* 1994;74:1746–1751.
17. Park CC, Mistumori M, Nixon A, et al. Outcome at 8 years after breast-conserving surgery and radiation therapy for invasive breast cancer: influence of margin status and systemic therapy on local recurrence. *J Clin Oncol* 2000;18:1668–1675.
18. Gage I, Schnitt SJ, Nixon A, et al. Pathologic margin involvement and the risk of local recurrence in patients treated with breast-conserving therapy. *Cancer* 1996;78:1821–1928.
19. Smitt MC, Nowels KW, Zdeblick MJ, et al. The importance of lumpectomy surgical margin status in long term results of breast conservation. *Cancer* 1995;76:259–267.
20. Schnitt SJ, Connolly JL. Processing and evaluation of breast excision specimens. A clinically-oriented approach. *Am J Clin Pathol* 1992;98:125–137.
21. Schnitt SJ, Silen W, Sadowsky NL, et al. Ductal carcinoma in situ (intraductal carcinoma) of the breast. *N Engl J Med* 1988;318: 898–903.
22. Pierce SM, Schnitt SJ, Harris JR. What to do about mammographically detected ductal carcinoma in situ? *Cancer* 1992;70: 2576–2578.
23. Solin LJ, Fowble BL, Schultz DJ, et al. The significance of the pathology margins of the tumor excision on the outcome of patients treated with definitive irradiation for early stage breast cancer. *Int J Radiat Oncol Biol Phys* 1991;21:279–287.
24. Borger J, Kemperman H, Hart A, et al. Risk factors in breast conservation therapy. *J Clin Oncol* 1994;12:653–660.
25. Kurtz JM, Jacquemier J, Amalric R, et al. Risk factors for breast recurrence in premenopausal and postmenopausal patients with ductal cancers treated by conservation therapy. *Cancer* 1990;65: 1867–1878.
26. Anscher MS, Jones P, Prosnitz LR, et al. Local failure and margin status in early-stage breast carcinoma treated with conservation surgery and radiation therapy. *Ann Surg* 1993;218:22–28.
27. Spivack B, Khanna MM, Tafra L, et al. Margin status and local recurrence after breast-conserving surgery. *Arch Surg* 1994;129: 952–957.
28. Heimann R, Powers C, Halpern HJ, et al. Breast preservation in stage I and II carcinoma of the breast. The University of Chicago experience. *Cancer* 1996;78:1722–1730.

55

SALVAGE OF LOCAL-REGIONAL FAILURE

ABRAM RECHT

The major goal of surveillance after treatment of patients with ductal carcinoma in situ (DCIS) is to detect and treat ipsilateral local-regional recurrences (and new ipsilateral or contralateral primary tumors) as soon as possible. A secondary goal is to allow the use of a second breast-conserving approach, at least for selected individuals with a low risk of subsequent local recurrence. Even with effective surveillance schemes and local salvage therapy, some patients with a local recurrence might be at sufficient risk of distant failure to warrant systemic treatment also.

This chapter will review

the characteristics of local recurrences after breast-conserving therapy (BCT);

the presentation, differential diagnosis, and evaluation of suspected local recurrences after BCT;

the results of salvage mastectomy and further BCT for such recurrences;

the characteristics and prognosis of local recurrences after mastectomy; and

axillary node recurrence.

CHARACTERISTICS OF LOCAL RECURRENCE AFTER BREAST-CONSERVING THERAPY

Most local failures after BCT for DCIS are in the same quadrant as the initial tumor (i.e., usually at or near the original biopsy site), whether or not radiotherapy is given (1–11). Recurrences are found over the entire period of observation in these series, with little evidence for a "plateau" occurring until more than 10 years after initial therapy. For example, in an international collaborative study of patients treated with lumpectomy and radiotherapy with a median follow-up time of 124 months, the 5-, 10-, and 15-year actuarial local failure rates were 7%, 16%, and 19%, respectively (4,12). The median time to failure was 62 months (range, 17 to 202 months). Prolonged time to recurrence has also been found in series of patients treated without radiotherapy (13,14).

It is important to realize that lesions labeled as local "recurrences" after BCT might actually represent new primary ipsilateral cancers rather than regrowth of residual tumor cells from the index lesion. One observation supporting this hypothesis is that an increasing proportion of recurrences are seen in other quadrants of the breast with increasing time for patients treated initially for invasive cancers (15,16). For example, in a series of 1,628 patients treated for invasive cancer at the Joint Center for Radiation Therapy (JCRT), the annual hazard rate for developing a recurrence at or near the lumpectomy site was very low in the first year after completion of radiotherapy but was between 1.3% to 1.8% per year for years two through seven and then decreased slowly until year 10, from which point on it remained stable at approximately 0.4% per year (17). In contrast, the risk of failure elsewhere in the breast rose slowly to reach a rate of approximately 0.7% per year at 8 years and then remained stable.

This issue is less well understood for patients with DCIS because of the shorter follow-up time and smaller numbers of patients in the available studies. However, it seems likely that a similar pattern will eventually emerge. These different mechanisms of local failure might have different implications for patient management and outcome, but at present there are few data comparing the histology and subsequent outcome for these two groups.

About one-half the recurrences are invasive in nearly all series of patients treated initially with BCT, whether treated with or without radiotherapy [with rare exceptions (2,18)]. The risk of developing an invasive recurrence may be related to the initial histology of the lesion. In a study from the Southern Health Care region of Sweden, there were 24 recurrences at a median of 3 years follow-up (four, four, and 16 in each group, respectively) (19). The original tumor was comedo DCIS with high nuclear grade in 16 patients, nine of which recurred as invasive cancers. Only two recurrences were invasive among the eight patients who originally had a noncomedo lesion with moderate nuclear grade. The location of the local failure (which as noted above may help distinguish between truly "recurrent" disease and the development of new ipsilateral tumors) may also impact this risk, but very few data are available on this subject. In a series from William Beaumont Hospital near Detroit, six of nine recurrences at or near the original tumor after treatment with lumpectomy and radiotherapy were invasive; in contrast, all four "recurrences" in other portions of the breast were invasive (11).

The risk of axillary lymph node involvement in patients with recurrence after initial BCT is uncertain. In the international collaborative series, one of 25 patients undergoing axillary dissection at the time of salvage mastectomy had a single positive node (3). In another series, none of nine patients undergoing dissection had positive nodes (11). However, the risk has been higher in some studies. In a series from Sweden, six of 11 patients with invasive disease had positive axillary nodes (19), and four of five patients had positive nodes in another study (20). However, the selection factors leading to the decision to perform axillary dissection in these series were not reported.

PRESENTATION, DIFFERENTIAL DIAGNOSIS, AND EVALUATION OF SUSPECTED LOCAL RECURRENCE

The majority of local failures after BCT are detected by mammography with no physical signs of disease present. However, some patients have presented with a palpable mass as the first sign of recurrence (3,20). Rarely, patients may present with an inflammatory-type recurrence (21) or even concurrent local and distant metastases (3,20). The chance of a lesion being palpable may depend on its histology but does not seem to be strongly influenced by whether radiotherapy was used or not. For example, in the Van Nuys series, when patients had a noninvasive recurrence, 6% of patients treated initially with excision alone had a palpable lesion, compared with 12% of patients treated initially with excision plus radiotherapy (20). However, when the recurrent lesion was invasive, it was palpable in 25% of patients treated with excision alone and 35% of those treated with excision plus radiotherapy.

The differential diagnosis of new findings on physical examination or mammography includes both treatment-related and benign breast diseases. The most common of these is probably fat necrosis. This may create a palpable mass (22–24) or mimic carcinoma on mammography (24) or magnetic resonance imaging (25). Occasionally, breast abscesses or cellulitis may mimic an inflammatory-type recurrence (26,27). The presence of pain, possible systemic symptoms of infection, and the time-course of development usually make the diagnosis clear, but biopsy is sometimes required to distinguish between infection and recurrence. Rarely, patients may develop patches of white or yellowish, well-circumscribed sclerosis and induration after radiotherapy. These may be surrounded by a more highly pigmented,

bruise-like area, and sometimes may be preceded by the development of erythema. This phenomenon has been termed "post-irradiation morphea" or "circumscribed scleroderma." Such lesions may appear weeks (28) to years (29) after treatment. Again, biopsy is required to confirm the clinical impression.

Radiation-related sarcomas are the most dangerous treatment-related diagnoses to be distinguished from local failure. These tend to occur 8 to 10 years or longer after treatment, but the shortest reported interval is 16 months (30). At the Marseilles Cancer Institute, two of 2,850 patients developed soft-tissue sarcomas at 5 and 5.5 years after BCT for invasive cancers, which is 9 cases per 100,000 patient-years of observation (31). In a series from the Institut Gustav-Roussy near Paris, nine of 7,620 patients developed a sarcoma, which is an estimated excess of 9.9 per 100,000 patient-years of observation (32). The actuarial incidence was 0.2% at 10 years, 0.43% at 20 years, and 0.78% at 30 years.

In recent years, angiosarcomas appear to be reported more frequently than other types of radiation-related sarcomas are. On average, these tend to occur earlier than other sarcomas. The best data allowing for an estimate of their incidence come from a collaborative study in France (33). A total of nine angiosarcomas of the breast were found among 18,115 patients treated between 1963 and 1996, with a median latency of 74 months (range, 57 to 108 months). The prevalence was, therefore, five cases per 10,000. However, no attempt was made to adjust this figure for the actual length of follow-up of patients prior to a censoring event (such as the development of metastases or death due to intercurrent illness). A survey of cancer centers in the Netherlands found 21 cases of angiosarcomas arising in patients irradiated from 1987 to 1995 (34). These studies estimated that approximately 16,500 patients were treated during this time, for a prevalence of 12.7 per 10,000 patients. However, the actual number treated was unknown.

Mammography and physical examination are by no means always conclusive as to the nature of new lesions found in follow-up. In one series of patients with DCIS treated with lumpectomy and radiotherapy, 28% of patients who had suspicious, palpable, masses that were also seen on mammography had no evidence of recurrence on biopsy (35). Other technologies (such as ultrasound, magnetic resonance imaging, and scintimammography) have been used with varying degrees of success to further evaluate patients (predominantly treated initially for invasive cancers) with abnormal findings on physical examination or mammography (36). It is debatable whether these modalities should be used routinely in the evaluation of patients with suspected recurrence, however, given the ease, high accuracy, and relatively low cost of core biopsy.

Mammogram- or ultrasound-directed core-needle biopsy is an increasingly popular tool for evaluating patients with worrisome radiologic findings (37). However, when used in the initial evaluation of suspicious findings in previously-untreated patients, core biopsies may show only atypical ductal hyperplasia in patients who are found at open biopsy to have DCIS, and only DCIS may be found in patients who truly have invasive cancer. The exact incidence of such understaging in patients previously treated for DCIS is not known. In addition, it is also sometimes difficult to distinguish between radiation-induced cellular atypia and recurrent malignancy after BCT—even on larger, open-biopsy specimens (38–41). Hence, considerable care needs to be taken in making treatment decisions based on core biopsies.

RESULTS OF SALVAGE MASTECTOMY

Most patients suffering local failure after initial BCT have been treated with mastectomy. Although the great majority of patients do not suffer further local-regional or distant recurrences, the correlates of subsequent outcome have not been well studied. However, the major factor appears to be the histology of the recurrent lesion. In a large collaborative study of patients treated with conservative surgery and radiotherapy from 1967 through 1985 with a median follow-up after recurrence of 56 months, the 3-year actuarial distant failure rate was 20% among 23 patients with an invasive recurrence (3). In contrast, none of 19 patients with noninvasive recurrences recurred after mastectomy.

Similar results have been reported in the Van Nuys series, in which patients were treated with or without radiotherapy (20). None of 39 patients with noninvasive recurrences developed metastatic disease. However, the 35 patients with invasive recurrences fared much worse. Only 51% of them presented with clinical stage I disease; 11% had stage IIIB disease, and one presented with simultaneous metastases. With a median follow-up of 69 months after recurrence, seven of 35 patients had developed metastatic disease. The actuarial 8-year risks of distant failure and breast-cancer–specific mortality were 27% and 14%, respectively.

There are few data on whether the initial use of radiotherapy affects outcome after salvage mastectomy. In the Van Nuys series, patients initially treated with excision and radiotherapy did worse than those treated with excision alone, but the invasive recurrences were much larger in the former group than the latter (median sizes, 30 mm and 12 mm, respectively) (20). This difference may reflect differences in surveillance of patients (i.e., more careful follow-up in patients treated with excision alone), but it may also reflect difficulty in detecting recurrences early in patients treated with an interstitial radiation implant in the earlier part of their series. No difference in salvage results were seen between the two arms in the NSABP B-17 trial, where such potential biasing forces were not present (10).

There are no data on how the time to development of an ipsilateral breast recurrence or its location in relation to the original lesion affects outcome, when histology is controlled for.

Many patients treated with mastectomy for local failure after BCT desire breast reconstruction. The risk of complications is slightly greater than for patients who have not had prior radiotherapy, and overall cosmetic results are not as favorable (42). However, the results are still likely to be acceptable to most patients. Complication rates in one series were higher when latissimus flaps were used (47%) than when rectus abdominis flaps were employed (25%) (42), but many of these were minor. Complete flap loss has not been reported (42,43). Submuscular tissue expanders have been poorly tolerated by previously irradiated patients (44,45). Other types of subpectoral prostheses appear less subject to complications, at least in carefully selected individuals (46–48).

RESULTS OF SALVAGE BREAST-CONSERVING THERAPY

It is not clear how often salvage BCT might be employed for patients with local failure, nor how successful such treatment is likely to be when compared with salvage mastectomy. The largest experience in this regard is from the NSABP B-17 trial. Fifty-two percent of patients (54 of 104) initially treated with surgery alone underwent salvage BCT (10). The risk of developing a second breast failure was 6% (3 of 54). (Fourteen of these 54 patients also received radiotherapy, but results were not divided according to its use.) All three failures occurred among the 26 patients with only DCIS present at recurrence; one of these three patients subsequently developed distant metastases. In comparison, one of 25 patients with noninvasive recurrence treated by mastectomy suffered a further local-regional failure, and two of the 25 patients with invasive recurrence treated with mastectomy developed subsequent failures (one local-regional, one distant).

Thirty-six percent of patients (18 of 47) in the B-17 trial initially treated with lumpectomy and radiotherapy who failed locally underwent salvage lumpectomy. There were four further ipsilateral local failures (and one distant failure) among 15 patients with noninvasive recurrences in this group. None of three patients with invasive recurrences so treated had a further recurrence. There was one distant failure among 15 patients with noninvasive recurrences and two distant failures among 14 patients with invasive recurrences after salvage mastectomy in this arm of the trial.

Unfortunately, no information was given in this study about the correlates of success or failure of secondary BCT (e.g., tumor size, margin width, etc.). Such information, however, is difficult to acquire in such retrospective analyses, particularly in a multi-institutional cooperative group study. Compared with other studies, the relatively high rates of local-regional and distant failure after the treatment of supposedly noninvasive recurrences raise questions about the pathologic assessment of these specimens, which were not centrally reviewed.

Some patients with recurrences after initial BCT including radiotherapy for invasive primary cancers have been re-treated with wide excision followed by interstitial implantation or external-beam irradiation to a small part of the breast. In the largest such series, 25 patients in Marseille were treated with re-excision and brachytherapy between 1974 and 1992; six patients were treated with brachytherapy alone (49). With a mean follow-up of 4 years, seven patients (23%) suffered further local failure (four in the same quadrant as the recurrence and three in another quadrant). One patient developed necrosis in the tumor bed. Cosmetic results were considered "fair" in 24 of the 25 cases. At the University of Pittsburgh, 16 patients were treated with repeat lumpectomy and reirradiation of the operative site (50). However, only eight patients had a minimum potential follow-up of 5 years; two of these patients recurred locally within that time and another at 62 months after re-treatment. There are no comparable studies of this approach for patients initially treated for DCIS, however.

LOCAL FAILURE AFTER INITIAL MASTECTOMY

Chest-wall failure rarely occurs after initial treatment of DCIS with mastectomy. For example, in one series, three of 103 patients suffered local recurrence at 50 to 62 months after surgery (13). This rate may be much higher after subcutaneous mastectomy if the nipple-areola complex is preserved. One group reported a 9% incidence of local recurrence (three of 34 cases) within 3 years of treatment of DCIS, and one of these recurrences was invasive (51). Noninvasive chest-wall recurrences have been described (52), but the majority are invasive.

As for patients treated with BCT, some "recurrences" (especially after prolonged intervals) may actually be new primary tumors, because mastectomy does not remove all breast tissue from the chest wall (53–55). For example, in one report, DCIS was found on the chest wall of a patient 11 years after mastectomy for papillary DCIS, but whether the new lesion was histologically similar to the initial one was not stated (56). In another case report, one patient developed a chest-wall lesion 27 years after mastectomy (57).

The largest series investigating salvage therapy for chest-wall recurrences after treatment of initially noninvasive cancers was reported by investigators at the Fox Chase Cancer Center (58). The median time to recurrence for these six patients was 5 years (range, 2.8 to 9.3 years). All recurrences were invasive. None had metastatic disease at presentation. They were treated with wide excision plus chest-wall irradiation (with concurrent regional nodal irradiation in four patients). All except one also received chemotherapy and/or tamoxifen. Four of the six patients were alive without further recurrence at 1.4 to 10.7 years after salvage treatment. One patient developed a further chest wall recurrence 7 years later and then metastases 4.8 years after this event. Another patient developed distant metastases at 3.3 years. The 5- and 10-year disease-free survival rates were 83% and 63%, respectively; overall survival rates were 80% at both time points.

AXILLARY NODAL RECURRENCE

Axillary recurrence in the absence of concurrent breast recurrence appears to be quite rare, despite reports suggesting a 6% to 12% incidence of initial axillary nodal involvement for patients undergoing sentinel node biopsy whose specimens were analyzed by immunohistochemical techniques (59,60). In the EORTC randomized trial, one patient treated with excision without radiotherapy developed an isolated axillary recurrence and subsequently developed distant failure (61). One of 87 patients treated with excision and radiotherapy at the M.D. Anderson Cancer Center developed an axillary recurrence 5 years after treatment; she developed a contralateral invasive breast cancer 1 year later, and then metastases (62). Details of treatment of these patients were not reported, however.

MANAGEMENT SUMMARY

The great majority of patients with local recurrence after BCT can be cured by mastectomy. A level I/II axillary dissection should be performed routinely for patients with an invasive recurrence and for selected individuals with large noninvasive recurrences, particularly if it is high-grade. To my knowledge, there is no experience using sentinel node biopsy in this situation. I recommend that prostheses should not be used in reconstructions when patients have previously been irradiated. Systemic therapy should be considered for patients with invasive recurrences, using the same policies employed for patients with *de novo* cancers. It may be possible to treat selected individuals who have had a local failure with further BCT, with or without radiation therapy. However, the long-term success rates of such treatment are uncertain. This approach seems reasonable for previously irradiated patients only when the recurrence is small, purely noninvasive, and can be excised with widely negative margins. Patients with invasive chest-wall recurrence after initial mastectomy or regional nodal recurrence after BCT or mastectomy should probably be staged and managed similarly to patients treated initially for an invasive cancer (36).

REFERENCES

1. Lagios MD. Duct carcinoma in situ: biological implications for clinical practice. *Semin Oncol* 1996;23(suppl 2):6–11.
2. Schwartz GF. Sub-clinical ductal carcinoma in situ of the breast: selection by local excision and surveillance alone. *Breast J* 1996;2:41–44.
3. Solin L, Fourquet A, McCormick B, et al. Salvage treatment for local recurrence after breast-conserving surgery and definitive irradiation for ductal carcinoma *in situ* (intraductal carcinoma) of the breast. *Int J Radiat Oncol Biol Phys* 1994;30:3–9.
4. Solin L, McCormick B, Recht A, et al. Mammographically detected, clinically occult ductal carcinoma in situ (intraductal carcinoma) treated with breast-conserving surgery and definitive breast irradiation. *Cancer J* 1996;2:158–165.
5. Silverstein MJ, Lagios MD, Groshen S, et al. The influence of margin width on local control of ductal carcinoma in situ. *N Engl J Med* 1999;340:1455–1461.
6. White J, Levine A, Gustafson G, et al. Outcome and prognostic factors for local recurrence in mammographically detected ductal carcinoma *in situ* of the breast treated with conservative surgery and radiation therapy. *Int J Radiat Oncol Biol Phys* 1995;31:791–797.
7. Kuske RR, Bean JM, Garcia DM, et al. Breast conservation therapy for intraductal carcinoma of the breast. *Int J Radiat Oncol Biol Phys* 1993;26:391–396.
8. Hiramatsu H, Bornstein B, Recht A, et al. Local recurrence after conservative surgery and radiation therapy for ductal carcinoma-in-situ: the possible importance of family history. *Cancer J* 1995;1:55–61.
9. Hetelekidas S, Collins L, Silver B, et al. Predictors of local recurrence following excision alone for ductal carcinoma in situ. *Cancer* 1999;85:427–431.
10. Fisher B, Dignam J, Wolmark N, et al. Lumpectomy and radiation therapy for the treatment of intraductal breast cancer: findings from the National Surgical Adjuvant Breast and Bowel Project B-17. *J Clin Oncol* 1998;16:441–452.
11. Kestin LL, Goldstein NS, Lacerna MD, et al. Factors associated with local recurrence of mammographically detected ductal carcinoma in situ in patients given breast-conserving surgery. *Cancer* 2000;88:596–607.
12. Solin L, Kurtz J, Fourquet A, et al. Fifteen-year results of breast-conserving surgery and definitive breast irradiation for the treatment of ductal carcinoma in situ of the breast. *J Clin Oncol* 1996;14:754–763.
13. Cataliotti L, Disante V, Ciatto S, et al. Intraductal breast cancer: review of 183 consecutive cases. *Eur J Cancer* 1992;28A:917–920.
14. Gallagher WJ, Koerner FC, Wood WC. Treatment of intraductal carcinoma with limited surgery: long-term follow-up. *J Clin Oncol* 1989;7:376–380.
15. Recht A. Breast carcinoma: in situ and early-stage invasive cancers. In: Gunderson LL, Tepper JE, eds. *Clinical Radiation Oncology*. New York: Churchill Livingstone, 2000:968–998.
16. Morrow M, Harris JR. Local management of invasive breast cancer. In: Harris JR, Lippman ME, Morrow M, et al., eds. *Diseases of the Breast,* 2nd ed. Philadelphia: Lippincott Williams & Wilkins, 2000:515–560.
17. Gage I, Recht A, Gelman R, et al. Long-term outcome following breast-conserving surgery and radiation therapy. *Int J Radiat Oncol Biol Phys* 1995;33:245–251.
18. Fowble B, Hanlon AL, Fein DA, et al. Results of conservative surgery and radiation for mammographically detected ductal carcinoma *in situ* (DCIS). *Int J Radiat Oncol Biol Phys* 1997;38:949–957.
19. Ringberg A, Idvall I, Anagnostaki L, et al. Morphological and clinical characteristics in patients with ipsilateral recurrence after DCIS. *Eur J Cancer* 1994;30A(suppl 2):S74(abst).
20. Silverstein MJ, Lagios MD, Martino S, et al. Outcome after invasive local recurrence in patients with ductal carcinoma in situ of the breast. *J Clin Oncol* 1998;16:1367–1373.
21. Chan KC, Knox WF, Sinha G, et al. Extent of excision margin width required in breast conserving surgery for ductal carcinoma in situ. *Cancer* 2001;91:9–16.
22. Stefanik DF, Brereton HD, Lee TC, et al. Fat necrosis following breast irradiation for carcinoma: clinical presentation and diagnosis. *Breast* 1982;8(4):4–7.
23. Rostom AY, El-Sayed ME. Fat necrosis of the breast: an unusual complication of lumpectomy and radiotherapy in breast cancer. *Clin Radiol* 1987;38:31.
24. Boyages J, Bilous M, Barraclough B, et al. Fat necrosis of the breast following lumpectomy and radiation therapy for early breast cancer. *Radiother Oncol* 1988;13:69–74.
25. Solomon B, Orel S, Reynolds C, et al. Delayed development of enhancement in fat necrosis after breast conservation therapy: a potential pitfall of MR imaging of the breast. *AJR Am J Roentgenol* 1998;170:966–968.
26. Keidan RD, Hoffman JP, Weese JL, et al. Delayed breast abscesses after lumpectomy and radiation therapy. *Ann Surg* 1990;56:440–444.
27. Staren E, Klepek S, Hartsell B, et al. The dilemma of breast cellulitis after conservation surgery and radiation therapy. *Breast Cancer Res Treat* 1993;27:188(abst).
28. Trattner A, Figer A, David M, et al. Circumscribed scleroderma induced by postlumpectomy radiation therapy. *Cancer* 1991;68:2131–2133.
29. Colver GB, Rodger A, Mortimer PS, et al. Post-irradiation morphoea. *Br J Derm* 1989;120:831–835.
30. Shapiro LL, Recht A. Side effects of adjuvant therapy for breast cancer. *N Engl J Med* 2001;244:1997–2008.
31. Kurtz JM, Amalric R, Brandone H, et al. Contralateral breast cancer and other second malignancies in patients treated by breast-conserving therapy with radiation. *Int J Radiat Oncol Biol Phys* 1988;15:277–284.
32. Taghian A, de Vathaire F, Terrier P, et al. Long-term risk of sarcoma following radiation treatment for breast cancer. *Int J Radiat Oncol Biol Phys* 1991;21:361–367.
33. Marchal C, Weber B, de Lafontan B, et al. Nine breast angiosarcomas after conservative treatment for breast carcinoma: a survey from French comprehensive cancer centers. *Int J Radiat Oncol Biol Phys* 1999;44:113–119.
34. Strobbe LJA, Peterse HL, van Tinteren H, et al. Angiosarcoma of the breast after conservation therapy for invasive cancer, the incidence and outcome. An unforeseen sequela. *Breast Cancer Res Treat* 1998;47:101–109.
35. Solin LJ, Fowble BL, Schultz DJ, et al. The detection of local recurrence after definitive irradiation for early stage carcinoma of the breast: an analysis of the results of breast biopsies performed in previously irradiated breasts. *Cancer* 1990;65:2497–2502.
36. Recht A, Come SE, Troyan S, et al. Local-regional recurrence after mastectomy or breast-conserving therapy. In: Harris JR, Lippman ME, Morrow M, et al., eds. *Diseases of the Breast,* 2nd ed. Philadelphia: Lippincott Williams & Wilkins, 2000:731–748.
37. Venta LA. Image-guided biopsy of nonpalpable breast lesions. In: Harris JR, Lippman ME, Morrow M, et al., eds. *Diseases of the Breast,* 2nd ed. Philadelphia: Lippincott Williams & Wilkins, 2000:149–164.
38. Schnitt SJ, Connolly JL, Harris JR, et al. Radiation-induced changes in the breast. *Hum Pathol* 1984;15:545–550.

39. Schnitt SJ, Connolly JL, Recht A, et al. Breast relapse following primary radiation therapy for early breast cancer. II. Detection, pathologic features and prognostic significance. *Int J Radiat Oncol Biol Phys* 1985;11:1277–1284.

40. Connolly JL, Schnitt SJ. Evaluation of breast biopsy specimens in patients considered for treatment by conservative surgery and radiation therapy for early breast cancer. *Pathol Annu* 1988;23(1): 1–23.

41. Peterse JL, Van Heerde P. Fine needle cytology of breast lesions after breast conserving treatment: cytology of radiation induced changes in normal breast epithelium. Fourth EORTC Breast Cancer Working Conference. London, 1987.

42. Kroll SS, Schusterman MA, Reece GP, et al. Breast reconstruction with myocutaneous flaps in previously irradiated patients. *Plast Reconstr Surg* 1994;93:460–469.

43. Howrigan P, Slavin SA. Salvage mastectomy and chest wall reconstruction using myocutaneous flaps. *Breast Dis* 1991;4: 39(abst).

44. Dickson MG, Sharpe DT. The complications of tissue expansion in breast reconstruction: a review of 75 cases. *Br J Plast Surg* 1987;40:629–635.

45. Olenius M, Jurell G. Breast reconstruction using tissue expansion. *Scand J Plast Reconstr Hand Surg* 1992;26:83–90.

46. Fowble B, Solin L, Schultz D, et al. Breast recurrence following conservative surgery and radiation: patterns of failure, prognosis, and pathologic findings from mastectomy specimens with implications for treatment. *Int J Radiat Oncol Biol Phys* 1990;19: 833–842.

47. Barreau-Pouhaer L, Lê MG, Rietjens M, et al. Risk factors for failure of immediate breast reconstruction with prosthesis after total mastectomy for breast cancer. *Cancer* 1992;70:1145–1151.

48. LaRossa D. Reconstructive surgery. In: Fowble B, Goodman RL, Glick JH, et al., eds. *Breast Cancer Treatment: A Comprehensive Guide to Management.* St. Louis: Mosby–Year Book, 1991: 311–324.

49. Cowen D, Altschuler C, Blanc B, et al. Second conservative surgery and brachytherapy for isolated breast carcinoma recurrence. Abstract presented at the European Society of Mastology meeting, 1994, in Venice, Italy.

50. Mullen EE, Deutsch M, Bloomer WD. Salvage radiotherapy for local failures of lumpectomy and breast irradiation. *Radiother Oncol* 1997;42:25–29.

51. Abbès M, Caruso F, Bourgeon Y. Subcutaneous mastectomy: a review of 130 cases. *Int Surg* 1988;73:107–111.

52. Fisher DE, Schnitt SJ, Christian R, et al. Chest wall recurrence of ductal carcinoma in situ of the breast after mastectomy. *Cancer* 1993;71:3025–3028.

53. Hicken NF. Mastectomy: a clinical pathologic study demonstrating why most mastectomies result in incomplete removal of the mammary gland. *Arch Surg* 1940;40:6–14.

54. Goldman LD, Goldwyn RM. Some anatomical considerations of subcutaneous mastectomy. *Plast Reconstr Surg* 1973;51: 501–505.

55. Barton FE, English JM, Kingsley WB, et al. Glandular excision in total glandular mastectomy and modified radical mastectomy: a comparison. *Plast Reconstr Surg* 1991;88:389–392.

56. Graham MD, Lakhani S, Gazet JC. Breast conserving surgery in the management of in situ breast carcinoma. *Eur J Surg Oncol* 1991;17:258–264.

57. De Jong E, Peterse JL, van Dongen JA. Recurrence after breast ablation for ductal carcinoma *in situ*. *Eur J Surg Oncol* 1992;18: 64–66.

58. Montgomery RC, Fowble BL, Goldstein LJ, et al. Local recurrence after mastectomy for ductal carcinoma in situ. *Breast J* 1998;4:430–436.

59. Pendas S, Dauway E, Giuliano R, et al. Sentinel node biopsy in ductal carcinoma in situ patients. *Ann Surg Oncol* 2000;7:15–20.

60. Klauber-DeMore N, Tan LK, Liberman L, et al. Sentinel lymph node biopsy: is it indicated in patients with high-risk ductal carcinoma-in-situ and ductal carcinoma-in-situ with microinvasion? *Ann Surg Oncol* 2000;7:636–642.

61. Julien J-P, Bijker N, Fentiman IS, et al. Radiotherapy in breast-conserving treatment for ductal carcinoma in situ: first results of the EORTC randomised phase III trial 10853. *Lancet* 2000;355: 528–533.

62. Mirza NQ, Vlastos G, Meric F, et al. Ductal carcinoma-in-situ: long-term results of breast-conserving therapy. *Ann Surg Oncol* 2000;7:656–664.

OUTCOME AFTER INVASIVE LOCAL RECURRENCE IN PATIENTS WITH DUCTAL CARCINOMA IN SITU OF THE BREAST

MELVIN J. SILVERSTEIN
JAMES R. WAISMAN

As stated numerous times throughout this text, ductal carcinoma in situ (DCIS) has become a more common diagnosis because of the increasing use of mammography (1). Until the early to mid-1980s, most cases of DCIS were treated with mastectomy, and local recurrence rates were low, generally around 1% to 2% (2–4). Most of the earlier lesions were large and many were palpable. With the small, nonpalpable lesions that are commonly found today, local recurrence rates after mastectomy should be less than 1%.

With the acceptance of breast-conservation therapy for invasive breast cancer (5–7), an increasing number of DCIS cases have been treated with breast conservation with or without radiation therapy. For most patients, breast conservation yields a better cosmetic result when compared with mastectomy (even when state-of-the-art skin-sparing mastectomy and autologous tissue reconstruction are used). But, in order to achieve the generally superior cosmetic result of breast preservation, patients must be willing to accept a higher risk of local recurrence with rates ranging from 5% to 40%, depending on a variety of factors (3,4,8–21). These include but are not limited to: tumor size, nuclear grade, the presence or absence of necrosis, margin width, and age of the patient.

Local recurrence after breast-conservation treatment for DCIS is demoralizing and, if invasive (as approximately 40% to 50% are) (3,4,8–10,14,15,22–24), is also a potential threat to life. None of the retrospective or observational studies reported to date have shown a significant difference in breast cancer–specific survival for patients with DCIS, regardless of treatment. The same is true for the prospective randomized trials. Among the prospective randomized trials that have been published by the National Surgical Adjuvant Breast Project (NSABP) (25–30), the European Organization for Research and Treatment of Cancer (EORTC) (31,32), and the United Kingdom Coordinating Committee on Cancer Research (UKCCCR) (commonly referred to as the U.K. Trial) (33) (Chapter 44), none show any difference in breast cancer—specific or overall survival, regardless of treatment.

For properly selected patients with invasive breast cancer, numerous prospective randomized studies have concluded that there is no difference in survival, regardless of whether a patient is treated with mastectomy or breast conservation. Furthermore, the NSABP has suggested that a local invasive recurrence that occurs in a patient previously treated for invasive breast cancer is a marker of poor prognosis but not an instigator of distant disease (34). This concept, which is not unequivocally accepted for invasive breast cancer, certainly cannot be extended to patients with DCIS. An invasive recurrence in a patient previously treated for DCIS upstages that patient from stage 0 disease to at least stage I breast cancer. Stage 0 disease has a breast cancer fatality rate of less than 1%. Stage I disease has a breast cancer fatality rate of approximately 15% to 20%. An invasive recurrence in a patient who previously had noninvasive disease has profound implications. This chapter will focus on the stage of presentation and outcome for 49 patients with local invasive recurrence after initial treatment for DCIS, as measured by the probability of distant disease and breast cancer fatality.

PATIENTS AND METHODS

A total of 909 patients with DCIS were accrued from 1971 through December 2000. The treatment selection process was not randomized; it evolved over time, and it has been described in numerous prior publications (4,5,8,15,16) and in Chapter 17 by Poller and Silverstein. The average follow-up time for all patients was 83 months.

In this series, patients with lesions 40 mm or smaller and with all margins clear by at least 1 mm were generally advised to undergo breast preservation. Patients with lesions larger that 40 mm or with persistently positive surgical margins after re-excision were generally advised to accept mastectomy, usually with immediate reconstruction. These guidelines were not absolute and some patients who could have been treated with breast preservation elected mastectomy and vice versa.

Radiation therapy was routinely added to most breast-preservation patients' treatment regimen until 1989; thereafter most breast-preservation patients were treated with excision alone. Whole-breast external beam irradiation (40 to 50 Gy) was performed on a 4 or 6 Mv linear accelerator with a boost of 10 to 20 Gy to the tumor bed by iridium 192 implant or external beam. Ninety-three of 237 patients treated with radiation therapy received a boost by interstitial iridium 192; 107 patients were boosted with photons or electrons but the nature of the boost is unknown in 20; and 17 patients received no boost. Ninety-three patients were treated 4 days per week while 144 were treated 5 days per week (see radiation therapy detain in Chapter 37). Disease-free survival and breast cancer–specific survival probabilities were determined by the Kaplan-Meier method and all results are estimates at 5 and 10 years.

RESULTS

There were 111 local recurrences: two after mastectomy and 109 after breast conservation (48 after excision plus radiation therapy and 61 after excision alone). Of the 111 total local recurrences, 62 were noninvasive (DCIS) and 49 were invasive. Table 56.1 details the number of patients, the type and rate of local and distant recurrence, the size of the original lesion and the size of the recurrence, follow-up time, and fatality, by initial treatment method and by treatment groups. In addition, Table 56.1 reports these parameters by analyzing all patients with local recurrences and invasive local recurrences as separate subgroups. Table 56.1 has a great deal of information and is worth careful review.

For the entire cohort of 909 patients, at 10 years, the probability of local recurrence (both invasive and noninvasive) was 16%, the probability of local invasive recurrence was 8%, the breast cancer–specific fatality was 1%, and the overall fatality rate (death from any cause) was 10%.

For 326 patients treated with mastectomy, the 10-year probability of a local invasive recurrence was 1% and the probability of a breast cancer–specific fatality was zero. For the cohort of patients treated with breast conservation (n = 583) (346 received excision alone and 237 were treated with excision plus radiation therapy), the 10-year probability of a

TABLE 56.1. PATIENT DATA BY SPECIFIC TREATMENT, TREATMENT GROUPS, AND RECURRENCES

Data Point	All Patients	Mastectomy	All BCT	Excision + Radiation	Excision Only	All Recurrences	Invasive Recurrences
Number of patients	909	326	583	237	346	111	49
Total recurrences	111	2	109	48	61	111	49
Noninvasive (DCIS) recurrences	62	0	62	26	36	62	0
Invasive recurrences	49	2	47	22	25	NA	49
Local only	41	1	40	16	24	NA	41
Local + distant	8	1	7	6	1	NA	8
Breast cancer—specific deaths	5	0	5	4	1	NA	5
Average (median) size original DCIS (mm)	26 (15)	42 (33)	16 (12)	18 (15)	15 (10)	23 (18)	24 (18)
Average (median) size original DCIS (mm) in patients who recurred	23 (18)	73 (73)	22 (18)	22 (19)	23 (17)	23 (18)	24 (180)
Average (median) size of recurrence (mm)	26 (17)	21 (21)	26 (17)	28 (20)	25 (18)	—	—
Average follow-up (months)	83	81	84	106	70	109 (101)	127 (123)
5/10-yr local recurrence probability (invasive + DCIS)	10%/16%	0.4%/1%	15%/23%	12%/20%	19%/28%	65%/84%	NA
5/10-yr local invasive recurrence probability	4%/8%	0.4%/1%	6%/11%	4%/9%	7%/14%	NA	48%/74%
5/10-yr distant recurrence probability	0.6%/1.1%	0.4%/0.4%	0.8%/1.4%	1%/2.2%	0.6%/0.6%	4%/7%	8%/16%
5/10-yr breast cancer—specific fatality probability	0.2%/1%	0%/0%	0.3%/1.5%	0.5%/2.3%	0%/0.7%	1%/6%	2%/11%
5/10-yr overall fatality probability	3%/10%	1%/10%	4%/9%	2%/9%	5%/9%	1%/8%	2%/11%

All probabilities are Kaplan-Meier estimates at 10 years.
BCT, breast—conservation therapy; NA, not applicable; DCIS, ductal carcinoma in situ.

local invasive recurrence was 11% and the probability of a breast cancer–specific fatality was 1.4%.

The probability of local invasive recurrence was higher for patients treated with excision alone than for patients treated with excision plus radiation therapy (14% versus 9%) but the difference was not significant ($p = 0.19$). Paradoxically, the probability of distant disease was higher for patients treated with excision plus radiation therapy than for patients treated with excision alone (2.2% versus 0.6%, $p = $ not significant). In addition, the breast cancer–specific fatality was higher for patients treated with excision plus radiation therapy than for patients treated with excision alone (2.3% versus 0.7%, $p = $ not significant) (Table 56.1). This might be explained by the fact that mammography is somewhat more difficult to interpret after radiation therapy, if there is any degree of radiation fibrosis. This, in turn, may cause a delay in the diagnosis of an invasive recurrence, allowing more time for the development of metastatic disease.

For the cohort of 111 patients who recurred locally, the probability of developing distant disease at 10 years was 7% and breast cancer–specific fatality was 6%. Because no patient with a noninvasive recurrence (DCIS) developed distant disease or died of breast cancer, it may be more appropriate to analyze these data considering only the 49 invasive recurrences as events. When this is done, the 10-year probability of developing distant disease for a patient with a local invasive recurrence was 16% and the breast cancer–specific fatality was 11%. This is a surprisingly good prognosis.

Patients originally treated for DCIS who then develop a local invasive recurrence have a much better prognosis when compared with patients who were originally treated for invasive breast cancer and later develop a local invasive recurrence. In other words, all invasive recurrences are not equal. Figures 56.1 through 56.4 detail this comparison. Figure

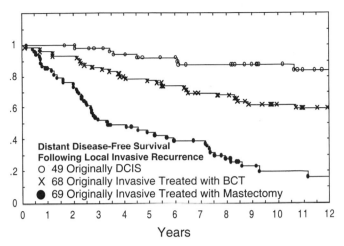

FIGURE 56.2. The patients in Figure 56.1 who originally had invasive breast cancer subdivided by treatment: 68 breast-conservation patients (excision plus radiation therapy) versus 69 patients who initially underwent mastectomy. It is clear that those patients treated with mastectomy who then recur locally have a poorer prognosis than those originally treated with breast preservation.

56.1 compares distant disease-free survival for all 49 patients with DCIS who developed a local invasive recurrence with a group of 137 invasive breast cancer patients who subsequently developed a local invasive recurrence. All original treatment modalities are included. Figure 56.2 subdivides the patients who originally had invasive breast cancer by treatment, 68 breast-conservation patients (excision plus radiation therapy) versus 69 patients who initially underwent mastectomy. It is clear that those patients treated with mastectomy who then recur locally have a poorer prognosis than those originally treated with breast preservation. Figures 56.3 and 56.4 use breast cancer–specific survival as the end point for the same groups of patients.

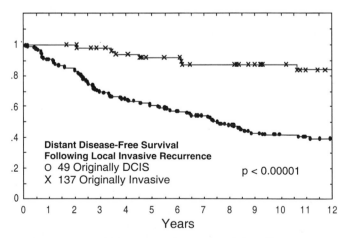

FIGURE 56.1. Distant disease-free survival for all 49 patients with ductal carcinoma in situ who developed a local invasive recurrence compared with a group of 137 patients with invasive breast cancer who subsequently developed a local invasive recurrence. All original treatment modalities are included.

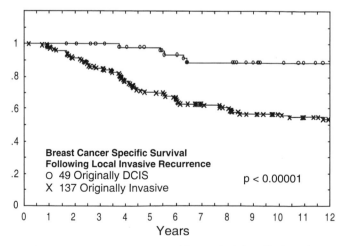

FIGURE 56.3. Breast cancer–specific survival for all 49 patients with ductal carcinoma it situ who developed a local invasive recurrence compared with a group of 137 patients with invasive breast cancer who subsequently developed a local invasive recurrence. All original treatment modalities are included.

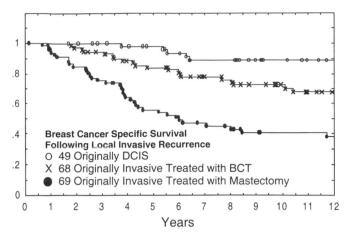

FIGURE 56.4. The patients in Figure 56.3 who originally had invasive breast cancer subdivided by treatment: 68 breast-conservation patients (excision plus radiation therapy) versus 69 patients who initially underwent mastectomy. It is clear that those patients treated with mastectomy who then recur locally have a poorer prognosis than those originally treated with breast preservation.

Figure 56.5 shows the time from original diagnosis (x-axis) for all local recurrences (both invasive and noninvasive) by treatment (excision alone versus excision plus radiation therapy). The median time to local recurrence after excision alone was 25 months; after excision plus radiation therapy, it was 57 months ($p < 0.01$).

Figure 56.6 shows the time from original diagnosis to local recurrence by the type of local recurrence (noninvasive versus invasive). The median time to a noninvasive local recurrence was 27 months; for an invasive local recurrence, it was 57 months ($p < 0.01$).

Table 56.2 shows the median time to local recurrence, the median size of the local recurrence, and the percent of

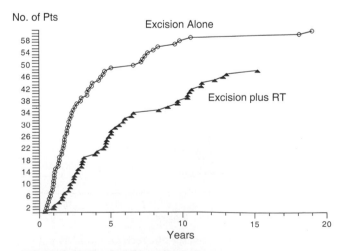

FIGURE 56.5. The number of recurrences (both invasive and noninvasive) by treatment (excision alone versus excision plus radiation therapy) are plotted over time. The median time to local recurrence after excision alone was 23 months; after excision and radiation therapy, it was 56 months.

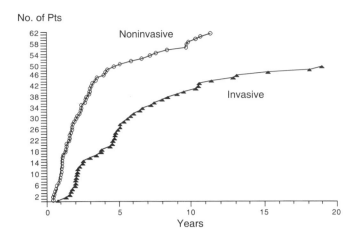

FIGURE 56.6. The number of recurrences by type of recurrence (invasive versus noninvasive) are plotted over time. The median time to a noninvasive recurrence was 22 months; for an invasive recurrence, it was 58 months.

local recurrences that were palpable analyzed by both treatment (radiation therapy versus excision alone) and type of recurrence (invasive versus noninvasive). Invasive recurrences in patients undergoing radiation therapy had the longest median time from initial treatment until the diagnosis of recurrence. Invasive recurrences were almost twice as large as noninvasive recurrences (median size 23 mm versus 12 mm, respectively) (p < 0.01), and the largest recurrences were invasive recurrences in patients undergoing radiation therapy (median 26 mm). One should also remember that the size of the invasive recurrence is the size of the invasive component. The noninvasive component is disregardes if the recurrence has any invasive breast cancer.

TABLE 56.2. MEDIAN TIME TO RECURRENCE, MEDIAN SIZE AND PERCENT PALPABLE FOR ALL RECURRENCES BY BOTH TREATMENT (RADIATION VERSUS EXCISION ONLY) AND TYPE OF RECURRENCE (INVASIVE VERSUS DUCTAL CARCINOMA IN SITU)

Factor	Excision Only	Radiation
Median time to recur by type of recurrence and treatment		
Invasive (months)	45	66
DCIS (months)	19	37
Median size of recurrence by treatment		
Invasive (mm)	21	26
DCIS (mm)	15	10
Percent palpable by type of recurrence and treatment		
Invasive (%)	44	45
DCIS (%)	6	8

DCIS, ductal carcinoma in situ.

Twenty-one of 47 (45%) invasive recurrences in breast conservation patients were palpable at the time of diagnosis compared with only four of 62 (6%) noninvasive recurrences (*p* < 0.0001).

The ability to predict which patients are likely to develop an invasive local recurrence is important. Unfortunately, at the current time, known risk factors such as nuclear grade, necrosis, size, etc., are unable to predict which patients are likely to develop an invasive local recurrence rather then a noninvasive local recurrence after treatment for DCIS (35) (Chapter 21 Sposto, Epstein and Silverstein). The only factor that appears to predict the type of local recurrence is the disease-free interval (time) from initial treatment to local recurrence (35). The association between the disease-free interval and invasion is most likely attributable to delay in diagnosis, reflecting a failure to diagnose the recurrence during the noninvasive stage, or conversely, the earlier diagnosis of persistent or recurrent in situ disease.

Fourteen of 22 patients who had invasive recurrences and were treated with radiation therapy during the 1980s received a 2,000 cGy boost to the tumor bed using a minimum two-plane interstitial iridium 192 implant. Of the six patients who received radiation therapy but developed distant disease, five were boosted in this manner.

None of 62 patients with noninvasive recurrences developed metastatic disease or died of breast cancer. Of the 49 patients who had invasive recurrences, eight developed metastatic disease: one patient originally treated with mastectomy, one patient originally treated with excision alone, and six patients originally treated with excision plus radiation therapy. Five of eight patients with metastatic disease died of breast cancer: one patient originally treated with excision alone and four patients originally treated with excision plus radiation therapy (three of the four were treated with an interstitial boost during the 1980s).

Figure 56.7 shows the stage of disease at the time of diagnosis of recurrence for all 49 patients who developed invasive recurrences. Slightly less than half (24 of 49) (49%)

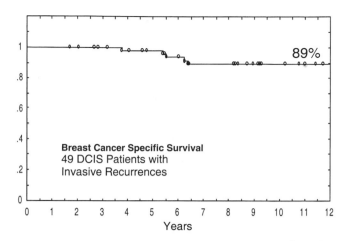

FIGURE 56.8. Breast cancer–specific survival is shown from the time of initial ductal carcinoma in situ diagnosis for 49 patients with invasive recurrences. The probability of a breast cancer–specific fatality at 12 years of follow-up is 11%.

were diagnosed with stage I disease; the remainder had more advanced disease at the time of diagnosis. Nine patients presented with stage IIA disease, ten with stage IIB, five with stage IIIB, and one with stage IV disease. No patient presented with stage IIIA disease.

When stage was assessed by whether or not radiation therapy was given, a higher percentage of patients who did not receive radiation therapy presented with stage I disease. The average patient who received radiation therapy with an invasive recurrence presented with a slightly higher stage of disease. Fifty-two percent (13 of 25) of excision-only patients presented with stage I disease at the time of recurrence, whereas only 44% (10 of 22) of those previously receiving radiation therapy presented with stage I disease (*p* = not significant). The median follow-up for the 49 patients with invasive recurrence from the time of the initial DCIS diagnosis was 127 months (57 months from initial diagnosis to invasive recurrence and 70 additional follow-up months after recurrence). The breast cancer–specific fatality rate for the subgroup of DCIS patents with invasive recurrences was 11% at 10 years (Fig. 56.8), and the distant recurrence rate for this subgroup was 16% at 10 years (Fig. 56.9).

DISCUSSION

Invasive local recurrence after breast-preservation treatment for patients with DCIS is a serious event, converting patients with previous stage 0 disease to patients with disease ranging from stage I to stage IV. The results of staging, however, may be somewhat misleading. Many patients in this series were treated in the 1980s when it was common to perform a standard axillary lymph node dissection for patients with DCIS. The axillary nodes, therefore, had already been removed in most patients and were not available for staging purposes at the time of local invasive recurrence. There were

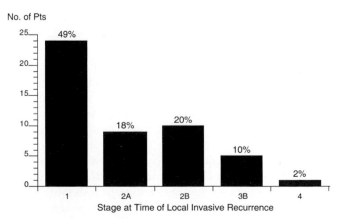

FIGURE 56.7. The percentage of patients with each stage of disease at the time of diagnosis of invasive recurrence is shown.

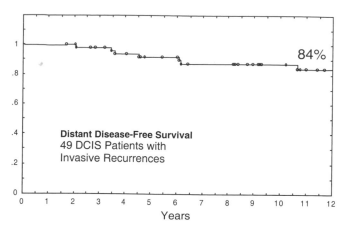

FIGURE 56.9. Distant disease-free survival is shown from the time of initial ductal carcinoma in situ diagnosis for 49 patients with invasive recurrences. The probability of developing distant metastatic disease at 12 years of follow-up is 16%.

only 13 of 49 patients with invasive recurrences in this series in whom axillary nodes were available at the time of local invasive recurrence; in 5 of those (38%), one or more nodes contained metastatic cancer. The staging for the remaining 36 patients was based on recurrence size, skin involvement, and metastatic workup without benefit of current axillary node status. It is probable that some of those 36 patients would have had positive nodes if axillary nodes had been available for evaluation. This would be particularly important for the 24 patients evaluated as stage I at the time of invasive recurrence. In all likelihood, this group of 36 patients is probably understaged because of the lack of axillary nodal data at the time of local invasive recurrence. In spite of this, their prognosis has been remarkably good, somewhat better than patients with untreated invasive cancer and similar staging.

In our experience, the diagnosis of recurrent breast cancer after conservative treatment for DCIS has been more difficult following radiation therapy than in patients treated with excision alone, particularly in those patients who received an interstitial boost to the tumor bed. Radiation therapy causes some degree (from very mild to severe) of radiation fibrosis and scarring that may obscure the earliest mammographic signs of local recurrence in some patients. In this series, recurrences in the irradiated breast were larger (Tables 56.1 and 56.2), more commonly palpable, slightly higher stage, and their diagnosis possibly delayed (longer median time from initial treatment until diagnosis of recurrence) (Fig. 56.5). The inability to detect the earliest possible signs of recurrence in patients who received radiation therapy may be due to the radiation techniques of the 1980s, which often included higher daily doses than currently employed today and more importantly, interstitial boosts.

In the results section, we noted that 14 of 22 of those patients who received radiation therapy and reported invasive recurrences were boosted with a 2000 cGy iridium 192 in-

terstitial implant to the tumor bed. Most of these patients (12 of 14, 86%) received 200 cGy per day 4 days per week (rather than 5 days per week) to a total dose of 5,000 cGy. We raise this issue to emphasize that this treatment technique, which was common in the 1980s, often yielded more internal fibrosis and external skin changes than current radiation therapy techniques (for example, 180 cGy/day, 5 days per week to a total of 4,500 to 5,000 cGy followed by a 1,000 cGy to 1,600 cGy electron boost).

When local recurrence-free survival is analyzed by whether or not patients are treated 4 or 5 days per week, there is no difference in outcome (36) (Chapter 37 by Lewinsky, Streeter and Silverstein). In other words, both treatment methods are equally effective at reducing cancer recurrences. Our concern is not the number of days per week of treatment but rather the fact that patients who received a boost by interstitial implant are more likely to develop radiation fibrosis; should they develop a local recurrence, its diagnosis could be delayed. Of 93 patients in this series who were treated with interstitial implants (median follow-up of 149 months), five developed metastatic disease, three of whom presented with inflammatory (dermal lymphatic carcinomatosis) type recurrences. Only one of 144 patients who received photon or electron boosts, an unknown boost, or no boost at all developed metastatic disease (median follow-up of 76 months). To some extent, this difference may be explained by the longer median follow-up of radiation therapy patients treated with interstitial implants.

Current radiation therapy methods yield a better external cosmetic result with less internal scarring (fibrosis), which therefore results in a patient who is easier to follow clinically and mammographically, making an earlier diagnosis of recurrence more likely. In support of this, it should be noted that in this series, the median time from initial treatment until diagnosis of local recurrence was 74 months for 22 patients who received radiation therapy and were treated with interstitial implants, and 35 months for the remaining 26 patients who received radiation therapy but did receive interstitial implants.

It has always been our policy to follow conservatively treated patients with DCIS (both irradiated and nonirradiated) with mammography every six months on the ipsilateral breast and yearly on the contralateral breast. However, the mobile population of California and changes in the health care delivery system have often made that difficult. Two of our patients who presented at the time of local recurrence with stage IIIB disease were followed for more than 5 years at other facilities with a diagnosis of progressive radiation fibrosis.

We caution all physicians who follow conservatively treated patients with DCIS to carefully evaluate any patient who presents with increasing radiation fibrosis more than 2 to 3 years after initial treatment. This may represent the development of an invasive recurrence, and biopsy is probably indicated. Recurrent breast cancer after conservative treatment for DCIS may present mammographically as microcalcifications, a mass, an architectural distortion, or any combination of the three (37). In some patients, there may be a palpable mass with false-negative mammography. An occasional patient with recurrent breast cancer may present with progressive breast shrinkage (37). Any suspicious or progressive change must be biopsied.

We suggest that surgeons who perform conservative procedures for patients with DCIS mark the biopsy cavity with metallic clips. This will focus the radiologist's attention on the exact area of the original DCIS and make long-term mammographic follow-up easier.

The absence of radiation fibrosis permits better mammographic follow-up of the excision-alone patients and may be one explanation why the median time to local recurrence for excision-alone patients is 27 months compared with 57 months for a patient treated with excision plus radiation therapy. Another explanation is that radiation therapy delays local recurrence. Both explanations are likely to play a role here.

The probability of local recurrence and local invasive recurrence is higher for excision-only patients when compared with excision plus radiation therapy patients (Table 56.1). Paradoxically, the probability of distant disease and breast cancer–specific fatality is higher for excision plus radiation therapy patients than for patients treated with excision alone. The differences in distant disease probability and breast cancer–specific fatality in favor of excision-alone patients when compared with excision plus radiation therapy patients, although statistically insignificant, requires discussion. The radiation therapy patients in this series had larger initial lesions (median 15 mm versus 10 mm) and have been followed for a longer period of time (106 versus 70 months). Hence, a higher recurrence rate might be expected. On the other hand, this is balanced to some extent by the fact that the median time to recurrence after excision alone is 27 months compared with 57 months for patients treated with excision plus radiation therapy (Fig. 56.5). As follow-up of the excision-only patients lengthens, there may be a small increase in the distant disease rate and breast cancer–specific fatality. Although radiation therapy decreases the local recurrence rate for both invasive and noninvasive disease, if patients do recur with invasive breast cancer, the recurrence may carry a worse prognosis because of a delay in the diagnosis and/or because a DCIS that survives radiation therapy and becomes an invasive cancer may be biologically more aggressive.

If the breast-conservation patients were evenly matched by tumor size, margin width, and nuclear grade and prospectively randomized, excision-alone patients would be expected to experience a significantly higher rate of local failure than excision plus radiation therapy patients (27,31,33). It is interesting to note that a similar percentage of each group presented with stage IIA disease or more. Twelve of 22 (55%) radiation therapy patients who recurred

with invasive disease presented with stage IIA or more disease at the time of recurrence and 12 of 25 (48%) excision-only patients presented with stage IIA or more recurrences (*p* = not significant).

Overall, after 83 months of median follow-up, the probability of breast cancer fatality for 326 patients with DCIS in this series treated with mastectomy was zero. With longer follow-up, the fatality rate is not likely to rise beyond 0.5%. This confirms other long-term studies that report an extremely low fatality rate after mastectomy for DCIS (2–4). However, this figure is low because it excludes those patients with a biopsy diagnosis of DCIS in whom an invasive focus was found at the time of mastectomy. These patients were then reclassified as having invasive carcinoma and were no longer included in this DCIS series. Patients treated with breast preservation do not benefit from this exclusion (unless invasion is found at re-excision and then, of course, they too are excluded) and therefore, some breast-preservation patients, albeit a very small percentage, likely harbor occult undocumented foci of invasion. This contention is supported by the fact that the prospective randomized trials have a small percentage of patients (2% to 3%) who present with distant disease without ever having had a local invasive recurrence (27,31).

The 10-year probability of breast cancer fatality for all 583 patients treated conservatively was 1.5%. With increased follow-up, we expect this rate to rise slightly, perhaps to as high as 3%. This occurs because any ipsilateral breast cancer event, regardless of which quadrant, is scored as a local recurrence despite the fact that it may be a new cancer distant from the index lesion. Any ipsilateral invasive event in a patient with previous DCIS may lead to metastatic cancer and death.

The 10-year probability of breast cancer fatality for the subgroup of 237 patients treated with excision plus radiation therapy was 2.3%, a result similar to that reported by Solin et al (23) (Chapter 33). This multi-institutional group reported a 15-year breast cancer—specific survival rate of 4% for 268 women with DCIS treated with excision and radiation therapy with a median follow-up of 10.3 years. In 2001, they reported on 418 women with mammographically detected DCIS. The 15-year breast cancer–specific survival rate was 98% with 6% of patients having developed metastatic disease (38). There is no doubt that radiation therapy decreases the local recurrence rate (27,31,33). But when patients recur despite radiation therapy, it is possible that their recurrences will be more difficult to diagnose and, therefore, larger in size; the lesion may also be more aggressive and more difficult to manage, so prognosis may suffer.

Breast preservation for patients with DCIS is not without a theoretical fatality risk. Mastectomy eliminates almost all of the breast tissue and almost all chance of recurrence, but for many patients it is overtreatment. Breast preservation preserves significant residual tissue, much of it at risk for local recurrence or a new breast cancer in another quadrant.

Patients committed to breast preservation must also be committed to careful, close clinical follow-up, and should be examined physically and mammographically twice a year for at least 10 years.

The results of this series indicate that most patients with local recurrence can be salvaged. Overall, the 10-year breast cancer–specific fatality probability for all 111 patients who recurred locally (both invasive and noninvasive) was 6%, an outcome similar or slightly better than patients with T1a or T1b breast carcinoma (39,40). For the small subgroup of 49 patients who recurred with invasive breast cancer, there was an 11% risk of death from metastatic disease within 10 years of initial treatment, a fatality rate similar or slightly better than a patient with stage T1c node negative breast cancer (39,40).

CONCLUSION

DCIS is an extremely favorable disease. Regardless of treatment choice, the overall fatality rates are low. Fatality rates are likely to be a few percentage points higher for breast preservation than for mastectomy, but cosmetic results will be superior. Patients who develop significant or progressive radiation fibrosis after radiation therapy should be followed extremely closely, as local recurrence may be obscured. Patients should be informed of these data and allowed to participate in the treatment selection process. Invasive local recurrence after breast-preservation treatment for patients with DCIS is a serious event, converting patients with previous stage 0 disease to patients with disease ranging from stage 1 to stage 4. These results, however, indicate that most patients with DCIS with local invasive recurrence can be salvaged and do far better than patients who were originally treated for invasive breast cancer and who then recur locally with invasive breast cancer.

REFERENCES

1. Greenlee RT, Hill-Harmon MB, Murray T, et al. Cancer Statistics, 2001. *CA Cancer J Clin* 2001;51:15–36.
2. Sunshine JA, Moseley HS, Fletcher WS, et al. Breast Carcinoma in situ. A retrospective review of 112 cases with a minimum 10 year follow-up. *Am J Surg* 1986;150:44–51.
3. Morrow M. Surgical overview in the treatment of ductal carcinoma in situ. In: Silverstein MJ, ed. *Ductal Carcinoma In Situ of the Breast.* Baltimore: Williams and Wilkins, 1997:469–478.
4. Silverstein MJ, Barth A, Poller DN, et al. Ten-year results comparing mastectomy to excision and radiation therapy for ductal carcinoma in situ of the breast. *Eur J Cancer* 1995;31:1425–1427.
5. Veronesi U, Saccozzi R, Del Vecchio M, et al. Comparing radical mastectomy with quadrantectomy, axillary dissection, and radiation therapy in patients with small cancers of the breast. *N Engl J Med* 1981;305:6–11.
6. Fisher B, Redmond C, Fisher E, et al. Ten-year results of a randomized clinical trial comparing radical mastectomy and total mastectomy with or without radiation. *N Engl J Med* 1985;312: 674–681.
7. Fisher B, Anderson S, Redmond C, et al. Reanalysis and results after 12 years of follow-up in a randomized clinical trial comparing total mastectomy and lumpectomy with or without irradiation in the treatment of breast cancer. *N Engl J Med* 1995;333: 1456–1461.
8. Silverstein MJ, Lagios MD, Craig PH, et al. A prognostic index for ductal carcinoma in situ of the breast. *Cancer* 1996;77: 2267–2274.
9. Lagios NM, Margolin FR, Westdahl PR, et al. Mammographically detected duct carcinoma in situ. Frequency of local recurrence following tylectomy and prognostic effect of nuclear grade on local recurrence. *Cancer* 1989;63:619–624.
10. Solin LJ, Yet I-T, Kurtz J, et al. Ductal carcinoma in situ (intraductal carcinoma) of the breast treated with breast-conserving surgery and definitive irradiation. Correlation of pathologic parameters with outcome of treatment. *Cancer* 1993;71:2532–2542.
11. Bellamy COC, McDonald C, Salter DM, et al. Noninvasive ductal carcinoma of the breast. The relevance of histologic categorization. *Hum Pathol* 1993;24:16–23.
12. Fisher ER, Constantino J, Fisher B, et al. Pathologic findings from the National Surgical Adjuvant Breast Project (NSABP) Protocol B-17. *Cancer* 1995;75:1310–1319.
13. Silverstein MJ. Prognostic Factors that Predict Recurrence of DCIS. In: Silverstein MJ, ed. *Ductal Carcinoma In Situ of the Breast.* Baltimore: Williams and Wilkins, 1997:271–284.
14. Silverstein MJ. Prognostic factors and local recurrence in patients with ductal carcinoma of the breast. *Breast J* 1998;4:349–362.
15. Silverstein MJ, Poller DN, Waisman JR, et al. Prognostic Classification of breast duct carcinoma in situ. *Lancet* 1995;345:1154–1157.
16. Silverstein MJ, Lagios MD, Groshen, S, et al. The influence of margin width on local control in patients with ductal carcinoma in situ (DCIS) of the breast. *N Engl J Med* 1999;340:1455–1461.
17. Vicini FA, Kestin LL, Goldstein NS, et al. Impact of young age on outcome in patients with ductal carcinoma in situ treated with breast-conserving therapy. *J Clin Oncol* 2000;18:296–306.
18. Szelei-Stevens KA, Kuske R, Yantos VA, et al. The influence of young age and positive family history of breast cancer on the prognosis of ductal carcinoma in situ treated by excision with or without radiation therapy or mastectomy. *Int J Radiat Oncol Biol Phys* 2000;48:943–949.
19. Goldstein NS, Vicini FA, Kestin LL, et al. Differences in the pathologic features of ductal carcinoma in situ of the breast based on patient age. *Cancer* 2000;88:2552–2560.
20. Kestin LL, Goldstein NS, Lacerna MD, et al. Factors associated with local recurrence of mammographically detected ductal carcinoma in situ in patients given breast conserving therapy. *Cancer* 2000;88:596–607.
21. Van Zee K, Borgen PI. Memorial Sloan Kettering Cancer Center Experience. In: Silverstein MJ, ed. *Ductal Carcinoma In Situ of the Breast.* Baltimore: Williams and Wilkins, 1997:455–462.
22. Solin LJ, Fourquet A, McCormick B, et al. Salvage treatment for local recurrence following breast conserving surgery and definitive irradiation for ductal carcinoma in situ (intraductal carcinoma) of the breast. *Int J Radiat Oncol Biol Phys* 1994;30:3–9.
23. Solin LJ, Kurtz J, Fourquet A, et al. Fifteen-year results of breast conserving surgery and definitive breast irradiation for the treatment of ductal carcinoma in situ of the breast. *J Clin Oncol* 1996; 14:754–763.
24. Silverstein MJ, Lagios MD, Martino S, et al. Outcome After Invasive Local Recurrence in Patients with Ductal Carcinoma in Situ of the Breast. *J Clin Oncol* 1998;16(4):1367–1373.
25. Fisher B, Costantino J, Redmond C, et al. Lumpectomy compared with lumpectomy and radiation therapy for the treatment of intraductal breast cancer. *N Engl J Med* 1993;328:1581–1586.

26. Fisher B, Dignam J, Wolmark N, et al. Lumpectomy and radiation therapy for the treatment of intraductal breast cancer: Findings from National Surgical Adjuvant Breast and Bowel Project B-17. *J Clin Oncol* 1998;16:441–452.

27. Fisher B, Land S, Mamounas E, et al. Prevention of invasive breast cancer in women with ductal carcinoma in situ: An update of the National Surgical Adjuvant Breast and Bowel Project Experience. *Semin Oncol* 2001;28:400–418.

28. Fisher ER. Pathobiological considerations relating to the treatment of intraductal carcinoma (ductal carcinoma in situ) of the breast. *CA Cancer J Clin* 1997;47:52–64.

29. Fisher ER, Dignam J, Tan-Chiu E, et al. Pathologic findings from the National Surgical Adjuvant Breast Project (NSABP) eight-year update of Protocol B-17: Intraductal Carcinoma. *Cancer* 1999;86:429–448.

30. Fisher B, Dignam J, Wolmark N. Tamoxifen in treatment of intraductal breast cancer: National Surgical Adjuvant Breast and Bowel Project B-24 randomised controlled trial. *Lancet* 1999; 353:1993–2000.

31. Julien JP, Bijker N, Fentiman I, et al. Radiotherapy in breast conserving treatment for ductal carcinoma in situ: First results of EORTC randomized phase III trial 10853. *Lancet* 2000;355: 528–533.

32. Bijker N, Peterse JL, Duchateau L, et al. Risk factors for recurrence and metastasis after breast conserving therapy for ductal carcinoma in situ: Analysis of European Organization for Research and Treatment of Cancer Trial 10853. *J Clin Oncol* 2001;19:2263–2271.

33. George WD, Houghton J, Cuzick J, et al. Radiotherapy and tamoxifen following complete local excision (CLE) in the management of ductal carcinoma in situ (DCIS): preliminary results from the U.K. DCIS trial. *Proc Am Soc Clin Oncol* 2000;19: 70a(abst).

34. Fisher B, Anderson S, Fisher E, et al. Significance of ipsilateral breast tumour recurrence after lumpectomy. *Lancet* 1991;338: 327–331.

35. Skinner KA, Sposto R, Silberman H, et al. Risk of invasive local recurrence following therapy for DCIS is a function primarily of time. *Breast Cancer Res Treat* 2001;59.

36. Beron P, Lewinsky BS, Silverstein MJ. Van Nuys experience with excision plus radiation therapy. In: Silverstein MJ, ed. *Ductal Carcinoma In Situ of the Breast*. Baltimore: Williams and Wilkins, 1997:405–412.

37. Gamagami P. Follow-up mammography after treatment of breast cancer. In: Gamagami P, ed. *Atlas of Mammography: New early signs in breast cancer*. Cambridge, MA: Blackwell Science, 1996.

38. Solin LJ, Fourquet A, Vicini FA, et al. Mammographically detected ductal carcinoma in situ of the breast treated with breast conserving surgery and definitive breast irradiation: Long-term outcome and prognostic significance of patient age and margin status. *Int J Radiat Oncol Biol Phys* 2001;50:991–1002.

39. Rosen PP, Groshen S, Saigo PE, et al. A long-term follow-up study of survival in stage I (T1N0M0) and Stage II (T1N1M0) breast carcinoma. *J Clin Oncol* 1989;7:355–366.

40. Rosen PP, Groshen S, Kinne DW, et al. Factors influencing prognosis in node-negative breast carcinoma: Analysis of 767 T1N0M0/T2N0M0 patients with long-term follow-up. *J Clin Oncol* 1993;11:2090–2100.

57

AXILLARY DISSECTION FOR DUCTAL CARCINOMA IN SITU

NORA M. HANSEN
ARMANDO E. GIULIANO

Ductal carcinoma in situ (DCIS) has increased dramatically over the last 20 years due largely to the increased use of screening mammography. Although the mainstay of treatment for breast cancer is still surgical resection, the type and extent of resection have changed. The radical resections that were popular in the 1950s and 1960s have been replaced by a more conservative surgical approach that reflects better understanding of the systemic nature of breast cancer.

For most of this century, axillary lymph node dissection (ALND) was thought to be both prognostic and therapeutic; however, in the 1970s Fisher (1) suggested that breast cancer was a systemic disease at presentation. If small tumors were an early manifestation of metastatic disease, then nodal involvement becomes not an orderly contiguous extension as described by Halsted but rather a marker of distant disease. Thus, the presence or absence of lymph node metastasis is the most important prognostic factor in patients with potentially curable invasive carcinomas of the breast, and the development of effective adjuvant systemic therapies has made recognition of axillary metastases critical to patient management (2–4).

The prognostic importance of axillary lymph node metastases has been examined almost exclusively in invasive rather than noninvasive breast cancers. Thus, there is no consensus on optimal management of the regional lymphatics in patients with DCIS who are treated with surgical intervention ranging from biopsy to mastectomy. This chapter addresses the question of axillary lymph node dissection and axillary staging in patients with DCIS.

EVOLUTION OF SURGERY FOR BREAST CARCINOMA

The first reported case of breast cancer is in the Edwin Smith papyrus, written around 1500 B.C. The operative treatment of breast cancer was not reported until the first century A.D., when Leonides described repeated applications of cautery to the breast. He did not mention the axillary lymph nodes. In fact, axillary lymph node metastasis was not identified until the 1500s, when Ambrose Pare observed that breast cancer often caused swelling of the axillary glands (5). Servetus believed that these glands and the underlying muscle should be removed (6). Pieter Camper first described the drainage to the internal mammary nodes while Pable Mascgni described pectoral lymphatic drainage. Henri Le Dran contradicted Lagen's humoral theory when he concluded that spread to lymph nodes signaled a worse prognosis. Jean Louis Petit, first director of the French Academy of Surgery, recommended removal of the breast, underlying pectoral muscle, and axillary lymph nodes—the earliest radical mastectomy (7).

The 19th century brought two major advances in surgery of the breast (8). In 1846, William Morton introduced anesthesia; in 1867 Joseph Lister, an English surgeon, developed the principle of antisepsis. Joseph Lister advocated division of the origins of both pectoral muscles to gain better exposure of the axilla for nodal dissection. In 1877, Mitchell Banks recommended removal of axillary nodes in all breast operations (9).

In 1844, Joseph Pancoast described the first *en bloc* removal of the breast with its axillary lymphatic contents. Samuel Gross, in the mid-1800s, removed the axillary lymph nodes only if grossly involved; however, his son in 1887 advocated the removal of axillary glands regardless of their gross appearance (5). In 1908, Lord Moynihan stated that surgery of malignant disease is not the surgery of organs; it is the anatomy of the lymphatic system. William Halsted believed in this concept and revolutionized the treatment of breast cancer with the radical mastectomy (10). Cushman Haagensen classified breast cancers according to size, clinical findings, and nodal status; he remained a strong proponent of the radical mastectomy. Patey and Dyson popularized the modified radical mastectomy (11).

Since the 1970s, the approach to breast cancer has favored limited surgical resection plus nonsurgical adjuvant therapy. Fisher et al. (12), who demonstrated no significant difference in disease-free or overall survival after modified radical mastectomy versus segmental mastectomy and axillary lymph node dissection, popularized the concept of breast conservation. Adjuvant radiation therapy decreased the incidence of local recurrence after conservative surgery. All of these advances in surgical management have been applied to DCIS.

AXILLARY DISSECTION IN BREAST CANCER

Axillary dissection in breast cancer has three main goals.

First, it should act as a guide to staging and prognosis.
Second, it should provide a rational basis for adjuvant chemotherapy, irradiation, or hormonal therapy.
Third, it should provide a basis for control of disease in the axilla.

The effect of axillary lymph node dissection on survival remains controversial; it may contribute to long-term survival in a small subset of patients.

The axilla is bordered superiorly by the axillary vein, laterally by the latissimus dorsi muscle, and medially by the serratus anterior muscle; its inferior extent is not well defined. Anatomically, the lymph nodes of the axilla are divided into six different groups. The external mammary nodes run along the medial side of the axilla following the course of the long thoracic nerve. The scapular nodes are found along the subscapular vessels and their thoracodorsal branches, while the central nodes are embedded in the fat of the central axilla. The interpectoral nodes, otherwise known as Rotter's nodes, lie between the pectoralis major and minor muscles. The axillary vein nodes lie along the lateral portion of the axillary vein. The subclavian nodes, the highest nodes in the axilla, are medial to the origin of the thoracoacromial vein and extend to the apex of the axilla; the tendon of the subclavius muscle known as Halsted's ligament (13).

In 1955, Berg (14) subdivided the axilla into three functional levels based on their relationship to the pectoralis minor muscle. Level I nodes are lateral and inferior to the pectoralis minor muscle, level II nodes are directly beneath the pectoralis minor muscle, and level III nodes are medial and superior to the pectoralis minor muscle. Total axillary lymph node dissection removes Berg levels I, II, and III; partial axillary lymph node dissection removes Berg levels I and II; and low axillary lymph node dissection removes only Berg level I (6). Removal of Berg levels I and II has been the standard practice of most surgeons performing axillary lymph node dissection for early invasive breast cancer and was recommended by the 1991 NIH Consensus Conference (15).

STAGING THE AXILLA

Definitive diagnosis of axillary metastases requires histologic examination of an axillary specimen. Noninvasive staging techniques are not satisfactory; the detection of axillary involvement by physical exam has a high error rate. Fisher et al. (16) demonstrated that up to 35% of lymph nodes judged normal on physical exam proved to contain metastases on histologic exam, and 25% of patients with clinical evidence of lymph node metastases did not have histologic evidence of tumor in the nodes. Haagensen (13) reported a false-positive rate of 26% and a false-negative rate of 27% for breast cancer detected by physical exam.

Other noninvasive methods of evaluating the axilla such as mammography, computed tomography (CT), and magnetic resonance imaging (MRI) have not been successful in differentiating between benign and malignant nodes. Positron emission tomography (PET) with intravenous 18-fluoro-2-deoxy-glucose may identify abnormal nodes, but only when they are larger than 1 cm (17). Also, PET scanning is very expensive and its low sensitivity and specificity make it a poor diagnostic choice at this time.

The incidence of axillary nodal involvement is related to tumor size. Studies have reported a 12% to 37% incidence of nodal metastases associated with tumors measuring 1 cm or less in diameter. Silverstein et al. (18) documented nodal metastasis in 3% of 96 patients with tumors less than 0.5 cm; however, some of those patients had DCIS with microinvasion. The reported incidence of axillary nodal involvement is also related to the method of tumor detection. The incidence of metastases was 24% for palpable lesions and 7% for mammographically detected lesions (19).

COMPLICATIONS OF AXILLARY LYMPH NODE DISSECTION

The wide range of complications associated with axillary lymph node dissection has received little attention because this procedure has been considered a necessary component of breast cancer therapy. Major complications, such as injury to the motor nerves of the axilla or injury or thrombosis to the axillary vein, are rare. Much more common are seroma formation, shoulder dysfunction, numbness of the inner aspect of the upper arm, and edema of the arm and breast. Lymphedema affects approximately 15% to 20% of women after breast cancer treatment and is the most widely recognized complication of axillary lymph node dissection (20). It causes substantial psychological and functional morbidity and predisposes patients to cellulitis. The most traditional method of evaluating lymphedema involves using a tape to measure arm circumference 10 cm above and below either the olecranon or the lateral epicondyle of the forearm; lymphedema is generally defined as a 2-cm difference. A body mass index greater than 27.3 kg/m^2 and age over 60 years may be the most significant risk factors for arm edema (21,22). In addition, the risk is twice as high after total, compared with partial, axillary lymph node dissection (23).

Many studies have examined the incidence of lymphedema. Werner et al. (22) reported a 5-year actuarial rate of 16% in 282 patients treated at Memorial Sloan-Kettering Cancer Center; most of whom underwent breast conservation. Ivens et al. (24) reported an 18% incidence in 126 patients who were all treated with breast conservation. These rates are similar to a study reporting a 17% rate of postoperative lymphedema in 57 patients undergoing modified radical mastectomy (25). This study also concluded that chest wall irradiation increased the incidence of lymphedema.

Seroma formation is a common complication of axillary lymph node dissection and results in an abnormal collection of fluid in the axillary space. Siegel et al. (26) reported a 4.2% incidence of seroma formation in patients undergoing breast conservation without a postoperative drain. Somers et al. (27) conducted a study of 227 postoperative patients randomized to receive an axillary drain for 24 hours or to be followed expectantly. Patients who received an axillary drain had a quicker resolution of seroma, fewer aspirations, and a smaller aspirate.

In a study of 106 patients who underwent axillary lymph node dissection, 70% complained of numbness, 30% complained of pain, and 25% described weakness (24). Of these patients, 15% reported that their symptoms interfered with daily living. Lin et al. (20) reported similar results: 78% of 122 patients had numbness, 22% had numbness and pain, and 17% had some restriction of shoulder motion. The most common complication related to injury or division of the intercostobrachial nerve is numbness, but the most troublesome complication is intercostobrachial nerve syndrome. This syndrome is characterized by paresthesias and pain in the upper arm, shoulder, axilla, and, occasionally, the anterior portion of the chest wall (28).

In addition to the potential complications, another factor of axillary lymph node dissection to consider is its cost. A lumpectomy can be performed in an outpatient setting with local anesthesia and i.v. sedation, but the addition of axillary lymph node dissection requires general anesthesia and usually an overnight stay—a significant expense. Morrow's survey of costs related to axillary lymph node dissection predicted a savings of 160 million dollars annually if this procedure were used selectively (29). Thus, axillary lymph node dissection is not a benign procedure; it should be undertaken only when the benefit outweighs its possible complications.

PROGNOSTIC IMPACT OF AXILLARY METASTASIS

The tumor status of the axillary lymph nodes remains the most important prognostic factor in patients with potentially curable breast cancers. Axillary metastasis is a major determinant for adjuvant therapy and represents important staging information. In a study from Memorial Sloan-Kettering Cancer Center, multivariate analysis of breast cancer patients followed for 30 years after mastectomy revealed that survival was most closely related to axillary nodal status (30). The rate of long-term survival was 75% for patients with tumor-negative axillary nodes compared with 40% for patients with tumor-involved nodes.

Prognosis has been correlated to the extent of lymph node involvement and, more directly, to the total number of tumor-involved nodes (14,31). Numerous trials have shown that increasing numbers of tumor-involved lymph nodes are associated with a progressively greater incidence of treatment failure. Most oncologists base postoperative chemotherapy on the presence and extent of axillary lymph node metastasis.

DUCTAL CARCINOMA IN SITU

The concept of an in situ or preinvasive breast cancer did not emerge until this century. One of the earliest reports of DCIS described a pure comedo tumor that showed no evidence of axillary node metastasis (32). Prior to screening mammography, DCIS was believed to be relatively uncommon: a 1970 survey conducted by the American College of Surgeons found that only 2% of 10,000 new breast cancer cases were DCIS (33). The most common presenting symptom in these cases was a palpable mass or nipple discharge. Since then, the use of screening mammography has dramatically increased the detection of DCIS; between 1979 and 1986 the incidence of DCIS in women over the age of 50 increased 235%; whereas the incidence of localized breast cancer increased 50% (34). Now, most cases of DCIS are usually identified by microcalcifications on a screening mammogram.

Axillary Metastasis in Ductal Carcinoma in Situ

Initially, the incidence of axillary lymph node metastasis in DCIS was thought to be high, and these patients were treated with radical mastectomy. Some of the problems in determining the incidence of axillary metastases in DCIS were due to the definition of DCIS and whether there was evidence of microinvasion. Haagensen and Bodian (35) considered all patients with DCIS to have microinvasion, and all patients were treated with a radical mastectomy. Their definition allowed up to 50% of such lesions to be invasive. It is not surprising that up to 25% of patients in that study had positive axillary nodes and that survival after radical mastectomy was about 75%.

Many studies have documented axillary node status in DCIS. In the American College of Surgeons study, the incidence of axillary involvement associated with in situ cancers was 1% to 4% (33). Silverstein et al. (18) reported no tumor-positive axillary nodes in 189 patients undergoing axillary lymph node dissection as treatment for DCIS. He has updated his axillary node data for this text. Silverstein performed a total of 427 node dissections or samplings for patients with DCIS, two of which were positive (0.05%) by hematoxylin and eosin (H&E) staining. Since 1995, he has done 76 sentinel node biopsies for patients with DCIS who were being treated with mastectomy. All were negative by H&E but six (8%) contained cytokeratin-positive cells by immunohistochemistry (IHC). Silverstein and colleagues effectively argued against routine axillary lymph node dissection for cases of DCIS.

Gump et al. (36) divided 70 patients with DCIS into those with gross disease and those with microscopic disease. Most patients were treated with mastectomy and limited axillary lymph node dissection. Residual disease was common in both groups but slightly more prevalent in patients with gross disease. One patient with gross disease had a tumor-positive axillary lymph node dissection specimen and microscopic invasion in the mastectomy specimen. Lagios et al. (37) reported two cases of axillary micrometastasis in 87 patients; both patients had large (68 and 160 mm) in situ cancers and very extensive high-grade lesions with demonstrable areas of microinvasion in the mastectomy specimen. Ashikari et al. (38) reported only one tumor-positive specimen in 109 patients undergoing axillary lymph node dissection for DCIS; even so, these investigators advocated mastectomy and axillary lymph node dissection because the breast might harbor occult invasive carcinoma. In the National Surgical Adjuvant Breast and Bowel Project (NSABP) trial (39), none of the 78 patients undergoing axillary lymph node dissection for DCIS had tumor-positive axillary specimens. Rosen (40) described eight patients undergoing mastectomy and axillary lymph node dissection for axillary lymph node metastasis without an obvious primary lesion in the breast. Three patients had DCIS, four had lobular cancer in situ, and one patient had both entities. There was no evidence of invasion in the mastectomy specimen. The high incidence of axillary metastasis in this group may be due to sampling error and the inability to detect invasion in the mastectomy specimen. There is evidence that invasion through the basement membrane may take place before it is detectable by light microscopy. Ozello and Sampitak (41) identified carcinoma cells outside the basement membrane in electron micrographs of histologically noninvasive breast cancers. Carter and Smith (42) reported that four of 29 patients undergoing axillary lymph node dissection had axillary metastasis, but three of these also had invasive disease in the mastectomy specimen.

Table 57.1 summarizes studies examining the incidence of axillary lymph node metastasis in DCIS (19,33,36–39, 42–48). Among 1,235 patients who underwent axillary lymph node dissection, 20 (1.6%) axillary specimens revealed metastatic disease. Only four of 20 tumor-positive axillary specimens were associated with invasion in the mastectomy specimen. However, in several studies, the method of detection was not well characterized and the incidence of invasion may be underestimated secondary to sampling techniques. Data from the National Cancer Database in 1991 indicated that 58.5% of patients with DCIS underwent axillary lymph node dissection despite a nodal positivity rate of 2% or less. Obviously, an overwhelming number of axillary dissections are performed for a very limited benefit.

Because axillary metastasis without demonstrable invasion in the primary tumor is rare in DCIS, we cannot recommend routine axillary lymph node dissection for patients with DCIS. The Consensus Conference on the Treatment of DCIS stated that an axillary dissection is not required in patients with DCIS (49). However, some type of nodal staging might be beneficial in a subset of patients who are more

TABLE 57.1. INCIDENCE OF AXILLARY METASTASIS IN PATIENTS WITH DUCTAL CARCINOMA IN SITU

Author (Reference)	No. Patients	No. Axillary Dissections	No. Positive Nodes
Ashikari et al. (38)	112	113	1
Brown et al. (43)	40	21	1
Carter and Smith (42)	38	26	1
Fisher et al. (39)	78	78	0
Gump et al. (36)	70	64	1
Lagios et al. (37)	87	87	2
Patchefsky (53)	51	51	3
Recht et al. (45)	40	13	0
Rosner et al. (33)	210	210	8
Schuh et al. (46)	52	52	1
Silverstein et al. (Chap. 17,52)	427	427	2
Sunshine et al. (47)	70	61	0
Von Rueden et al. (48)	53	32	0
Total	1,328	1,235	20

From Swain SM, Lippman ME. In: Lippman ME, Lichter AS, Danforth DN Jr, eds. *Diagnosis and management of breast cancer.* Philadelphia: WB Saunders, 1988:296–325.

likely to develop lymph node metastasis because they harbor a focus of invasive disease. It would be beneficial to determine which subset of patients with DCIS is at an increased risk for occult invasion because this group has an increased risk of axillary metastases. In theory, DCIS lacks the ability to metastasize and, therefore, only DCIS with a microinvasive component can spread to the axillary lymph nodes.

Ductal Carcinoma in Situ and Occult Invasion

Traditional DCIS classification is based primarily on the architectural pattern of the lesion: comedo, cribriform, micropapillary, papillary, and solid. More recently, there has been a trend toward categorizing DCIS into comedo and noncomedo types and by nuclear grade and necrosis. In situ comedocarcinoma carries a greater long-term risk for infiltrating cancer and is more likely to become invasive. Lagios et al. (50) correlated high tumor grade and aneuploidy with comedocarcinoma, tumor necrosis, and increased risk of local recurrence. In their series of 79 patients who underwent lumpectomy without axillary lymph node dissection or postoperative radiotherapy for mammographically detected foci of DCIS of less than 25 mm, the incidence of recurrence was correlated with high-grade, nuclear morphology and comedo-type necrosis. Lagios and colleague's recurrence data are updated in Chapter 35.

The incidence of occult invasion near the primary tumor or in other parts of the breast has been examined in mastectomy series and reportedly ranges from 0% to 26% (51), which would account for the small number of patients with DCIS with positive lymph nodes. The likelihood of occult invasion appears to be related to the size of the index lesion. In a series of 53 breast specimens analyzed using the Egan serial subgross technique, lesions greater than 25 mm were more likely to have occult invasion (50). The Egan method can detect smaller lesions by correlating directed sampling with radiographic examination (52). The breast is sectioned into 20 to 30 segments approximately 5 mm in thickness and radiographs are taken of each section. The radiologist and pathologist together examine each area of interest. This technique is associated with a three-fold increase in the probability of finding occult invasion when compared with directed sampling of randomly selected quadrants (52). Using this technique, Lagios et al. (50) demonstrated a 21% incidence of occult invasion and a 32% incidence of multicentricity. The incidence of invasion was significantly related to tumor size: occult invasion was found in 11 of 24 lesions greater than 25 mm, but in none of the 29 lesions less than 25 mm. Most (82%) of the occult invasion was found in lesions greater than 50 mm; the one patient with axillary lymph node metastasis had a lesion of 160 mm. Increasing size also increased the incidence of multicentricity; multicentricity was found in 13 of 24 lesions greater than 25 mm, but in only four of 29 lesions less than 25 mm.

The incidence of occult invasion appears to be much more common in comedo lesions. Patchefsky et al. (53) found evidence of microinvasion in 63% of comedo-DCIS lesions but only 11% of noncomedo lesions. The amount of DCIS was measured by counting the number of duct structures with tumor. Even small comedocarcinomas showed a significant propensity toward microinvasion. Comedo-type DCIS cytologically appears more malignant; it is more often associated with microinvasion and more often exhibits biologic markers indicative of high-grade malignant lesions. Comedo lesions are more likely to lack estrogen receptors (54), demonstrate a high proliferative rate (55), exhibit aneuploidy (56), and overexpress HER-2/neu as well as mutations of p53 (57).

Occult invasion also seems to be related to the method of initial detection. Gump et al. (36) found evidence of invasive cancer in 11% of patients with DCIS who had a palpable mass, nipple discharge, or Paget's disease on physical exam but in only one of 16 patients whose nonpalpable tumors were mammographically detected. These findings indicate that patients with tumors larger than 2.5 cm with comedo-type histopathology have a higher risk of invasive diseases, which may increase the rate of axillary metastasis. However, even in this subset of patients with DCIS, the incidence of axillary metastasis is too small to justify routine axillary lymph node dissection. Axillary sampling might be quite useful if it could be performed with minimal morbidity, low expense, and high accuracy. But even axillary sampling should only be applied to very specific clinical situations.

SELECTIVE SENTINEL LYMPHADENECTOMY USING VITAL BLUE DYE

Morton et al. (58) demonstrated the accuracy of intraoperative lymphatic mapping and selective sentinel lymph node dissection (lymphadenectomy) (SLND) to identify lymph node metastases in patients with primary cutaneous melanoma; they reported a false-negative rate less than 1% in over 500 cases. The sentinel node is the initial lymph node on the path of lymph draining a primary tumor, and its tumor status therefore indicates whether regional lymphatic metastasis has occurred. Giuliano et al. (59) adapted SLND to stage the axilla of patients with breast cancer. In his initial study, 172 patients with 174 potentially curable breast cancers underwent SLND during modified radical mastectomy or breast conservation procedures. All patients then underwent axillary lymph node dissection that removed level I, II, and part of level III lymph nodes.

In this study of 174 breast cancers, a 1% isosulfan blue dye was used to identify the sentinel node. The sentinel node (SN) was identified in 66% of patients overall, but the identification rate improved as the investigator developed the technique and indications. The 59% rate of SN detection in the first 87 cases increased to 72% in the remaining 87 cases, and the detection rate reached 78% by the last 50 cases in this series. The technique was modeled after the melanoma model (a cutaneous tumor identification system), but had to be adapted to breast cancer (a parenchymal tumor system), which led to significant changes in the technique. Although the initial identification rate using the blue dye technique was only 66%, this was at first interpreted as the "learning curve." Although experience is needed before mastering this technique, much of this learning curve was due to the improvements in the technique itself, along with better patient selection. The volume of dye injected, the site of injection, the timing of the axillary incision, the histopathologic workup of the sentinel node, and the addition of massage to the injection site all aided in improving the probability of identifying the sentinel node. Using this mature technique, the SN was identified in 93% of patients and was 100% predictive of nodal status (60). Based on the results of this study, in 1995 we abandoned complete axillary lymph node dissection in patients whose sentinel nodes were tumor free.

SELECTIVE SENTINEL LYMPHADENECTOMY USING RADIOACTIVE COLLOID

Krag et al. (61) published the first pilot study of sentinel lymphadenectomy in patients with invasive breast cancer. In this study of 22 patients, an unfiltered radioactive colloid (technetium sulfur colloid) injected 1 to 9 hours prior to surgery was used to map the lymphatic tract and identify the SN. The SN was identified in 82% of patients using a hand-held Geiger counter and was 100% predictive of the axillary status—implying that if the SN was negative, the remainder of the axillary nodes were also negative. Krag updated his results in 248 cases (62). The SN was identified in 95.5% of patients with a true false-negative rate of 6.5%. This led to the initiation of a multicenter trial to evaluate the success of intraoperative lymphatic mapping and sentinel lymph node biopsy (SLNB) using a radioactive colloid. The multicenter validation study reported a 90% identification rate; however, marked variability in the success and accuracy of sentinel node identification was found (63). Among 11 experienced breast surgeons, the false-negative rate varied from 0% to 30%. This emphasizes the point that there needs to be a learning process before abandoning axillary lymph node dissection in patients with invasive breast cancer.

SELECTIVE SENTINEL LYMPHADENECTOMY USING A COMBINATION OF VITAL BLUE DYE AND RADIOACTIVE COLLOID

Albertini and co-workers (64) combined both techniques in an effort to improve the detection rate and reduce the learn-

ing curve. This technique combined a filtered radioactive colloid with a 1% isosulfan blue dye. In a study of 62 patients, the sentinel node was identified in 92% of patients and the sentinel node was 100% predictive of the axillary status. Cox updated their experience and reported the results in 466 consecutive patients (65). The SN was successfully identified in 94.4% of patients with only one false-negative case.

Other investigators have reported their success with SLND. Veronesi et al. (66) reported their probe-directed mapping with a subdermal injection of Tc-99m–labeled human serum albumin colloid in 163 consecutive breast cancer patients who underwent SLND followed by ALND (66). The SN was identified in 98.2% of the patients; however, there was a 2.5% false-negative rate. In a large California-based health maintenance organization (HMO), Guenther et al. (67) had a 71% identification rate using blue dye alone in a cohort of 145 patients. Although this identification rate is low, when the SN was identified, it was 97% accurate. Similarly, Dale (68) published his results using blue dye alone in 21 patients where the SN was identified in only 66% of cases but was 100% predictive of the axillary status. Pijpers et al. (69) reported the use of a peritumoral injection of Tc-99m–labeled colloidal albumin in 37 patients. They reported a 92% success rate and the SN was 100% predictive of the axillary status. Borgstein et al. (70) used Tc-99m–labeled colloidal albumin in patients with a T1 or T2 tumor. There was a 94% identification rate and a 1.7% false-negative rate. Miner et al. (71) applied the use of ultrasound to aid in the peritumoral injection of unfiltered Tc-99m sulfur colloid. The SN was identified in 98% of patients and was 98% accurate. Offodile et al. (72) used Tc-99m–labeled dextran as the radioactive tracer in 41 patients with an identification rate of 98% and an accuracy rate of 100%. Crossin et al. (73) used a peritumoral injection of Tc-99m sulfur colloid to identify the SN. The SN was successfully identified in 84% of cases and was 98% accurate. Barnwell et al. (74) reported a 90% identification rate and 100% accuracy rate using the combined technique. The group at Memorial Sloan-Kettering Cancer Center (75) was successful at identifying the SN in 93% of cases, but the SN was only 95% accurate in predicting the status of the axilla. Koller et al. (76) recently reported their results using either a methylene blue or patent blue dye. A SN was successfully identified in 98% of patients and was 97% accurate in predicting the status of the axilla.

From these studies using a variety of techniques, it is clear that the success rate of identifying the SN is generally greater than 90%. More importantly, the accuracy of the SN in predicting the nodal status of the axilla is consistently over 95%. The average number of SNs excised in all of these studies ranged from 1 to 2.9 and was similar whether dye or a radioactive colloid was used alone or in combination. SLND can be successfully performed in a variety of centers, and in an academic or private setting.

HISTOPATHOLOGIC EXAMINATION

Although SLND can accurately identify the axillary lymph nodes most likely to contain tumor cells, the detection of tumor-positive nodes ultimately depends on the sensitivity of the pathologic examination (which depends not only on the extent of dissection, but also on the choice of staining technique). Lymph nodes determined to be tumor-negative by routine H&E staining may become positive when examined by IHC antibodies for specific breast epithelial cell products such as cytokeratin, mucin, or milk fat globulin (77,78). Although IHC is impractical for routine examination of the axillary lymph node dissection specimen, it is feasible for focused histopathologic examination of much smaller SLND specimens.

We examined the potential of focused histopathologic examination by comparing the rate of axillary node metastases detected in patients undergoing axillary lymph node dissection and patients undergoing SLND followed by axillary lymph node dissection (79). SLND specimens were examined initially by frozen section to confirm nodal tissue, and then processed for permanent sections. Each node was blocked to create two section levels per paraffin block. A cytokeratin stain was performed with an antibody cocktail to low and intermediate molecular weight cytokeratin, with approximately six to eight histologic levels for each sentinel node staining negative with H&E. Axillary lymph node dissection specimens were dissected fresh per routine surgical pathology techniques for isolation of lymph nodes. Multiple nodes were embedded per block and one or two levels examined per node using H&E.

The two patient groups were similar with respect to age, size of primary tumor, and total number of axillary nodes examined. Axillary metastases were identified in 39 (29%) of the axillary lymph node dissection group and 68 (42%) of the SLND group, a significant difference ($p < 0.03$). In 26 of the 68 tumor-involved sentinel nodes, metastases were less than 2 mm; 11 of these micrometastatic foci were missed by H&E and detected only by subsequent IHC staining.

Dowlatshahi et al. (80) reported that 52% of H&E node-negative T1a and T1b tumors were positive when the sentinel node was serially sectioned and examined by IHC. In an update to the Ludwig trial, Cote et al. (81) demonstrated the increase of nodal metastases with the addition of IHC stains to the lymph nodes (in this case, not sentinel nodes); however, these "occult" metastases were not significant for disease-free or overall survival in the premenopausal patient but were found to be significant in the postmenopausal patient.

Turner et al. (82) applied IHC to all non–sentinel nodes in a cohort of patients who had undergone a SLND followed by a completion ALND. The purpose of this study was to determine if the enhanced detection of metastatic tumor reflected a more intensive histopathologic workup of the SN rather than the presumed biologic significance of the SN. A total of 1,087 non–sentinel nodes were examined at two levels using IHC, and only one non–sentinel node was found to have a micrometastasis. Therefore, if the SN is negative on H&E and IHC, the probability of a non–sentinel node metastasis is less than 0.1%. The addition of IHC to the entire axillary specimen is impractical due to both time and financial constraints; however, the addition of IHC to the sentinel node alone may improve the detection of micrometastases and the natural history of micrometastases may eventually be elucidated.

The conclusion of this study was that the detection of axillary metastases might be significantly enhanced by the focused histopathologic examination of the SLND specimen with a combination of H&E and IHC evaluation. It is clear that the addition of IHC stains does increase the incidence of detecting sentinel node metastases, but the significance of these metastases remains unknown and often leads to overtreatment of the patient with adjuvant chemotherapy. This is particularly evident in the group of patients with DCIS who are found to have a positive sentinel node with IHC. The significance of axillary metastases (particularly IHC-detected metastases) in this group is unknown and is inconsistent with the natural history of DCIS. The presence of metastases in the sentinel node often leads to confusion and overtreatment. The role of IHC stains has become controversial and is now the focus of a multi-institutional randomized study through the American College of Surgeons Oncology Group.

SENTINEL LYMPH NODE DISSECTION AS AN INTRAOPERATIVE STAGING TOOL

SLND has been validated by many groups throughout the United States and abroad and has become a recognized staging procedure for patients with early breast cancer. It is currently being tested in several national and international trials and will likely become the standard of care for evaluating the axilla of patients with breast cancer.

SLND is particularly useful in patients with early breast cancers. We studied 250 patients with T1 tumors and reported the incidence of axillary metastases was 29% with T1c tumors, 13% with T1b tumors, and 10% with T1a tumors, based on histologic examination of the sentinel node alone with H&E staining. These rates increased to 33% in T1c, 15% in T1b, and 15% in T1a using IHC stains (83).

The disadvantage of sentinel lymph node biopsy is that, even in experienced hands, the lymphatic channel or sentinel lymph node cannot always be found. If the breast cancer drains to internal mammary nodes rather than axillary nodes, then the surgeon must decide what to do with the axillary lymph nodes and whether or not to biopsy the internal mammary nodes. At our center, we perform preoperative lymphoscintigraphy in patients with medially placed breast cancers to identify the drainage pattern of that particular cancer. In selected cases, we do biopsy the internal mammary lymph node if it is the primary drainage site of the cancer.

When used properly, SLND is a simple, low-cost procedure that has minimal morbidity and is extremely accurate. It can be performed as an outpatient procedure under local anesthesia with intravenous sedation and is an ideal alternative to standard axillary lymph node dissection in patients with invasive cancer; the question is should it be used to evaluate the axilla in patients with DCIS?

SENTINEL LYMPH NODE DISSECTION IN PATIENTS WITH DUCTAL CARCINOMA IN SITU

Most of the published literature on SLND focuses on invasive disease, and the role of SLND in patients with invasive cancer is clear. The role of SLND in patients with DCIS is unclear.

The natural history of DCIS, a disease with a breast cancer–specific mortality rate of only 1% after mastectomy, suggests that DCIS has little or no metastatic potential while in the in situ phase. A small subset of patients with DCIS is found to have metastatic disease. Data derived from the time when a level I and II axillary dissection was routinely performed for patients with DCIS show a nodal positivity rate of less than 1% (84). Although an invasive component was not identified in the mastectomy specimens of this group, rather than this component not being present, it was thought that it simply was not identifiable. Proponents of SLND in DCIS argue that, due to a smaller specimen size, a pathologist has an easier time identifying a metastatic deposit in a sentinel node than a segmental mastectomy or mastectomy specimen. However, Lagios et al. (50) argue that invasive foci are more commonly detected with a thorough, standard H&E examination. At mastectomy, as many as 48% of patients with DCIS of an extent greater than 5.5 cm may exhibit identifiable microinvasion. The majority of such occult microinvasive foci will range from T1mic to T1b size groups, and almost all are node-negative by conventional H&E staining. The question should not be which is easier; it should be whether or not it is indicated!

Several reports have examined the incidence of sentinel node metastases in patients with DCIS. Pendas et al. (85) reported on 87 patients undergoing SLND for DCIS. Of the 177 sentinel nodes evaluated with both H&E and IHC stains, five of 87 patients (6%) were found to have metastatic disease in the sentinel node. Sixty percent of metastases were identified only with IHC, and 40% were both H&E- and IHC-positive. An IHC-positive node was defined as cohesive clusters of immunoreactive cells present within the lymph node. The primary tumor was reevaluated in these five patients, and one patient was found to have a

focus of microinvasive disease with additional sections and staining with basement membrane stains. Eighty percent of patients had at least one focus of high-grade solid or comedocarcinoma associated with DCIS, and one patient had a 9.5 cm low-grade cribriform and micropapillary type of DCIS. All five patients underwent a completion axillary lymph node dissection, and the sentinel node was the only positive node in all cases. It was not stated whether the non–sentinel nodes were examined by H&E stains and IHC or just H&E stains alone. This group recommended using SLND in patients with DCIS and selectively treating high-risk patients with DCIS (those with a positive sentinel node) with a completion axillary lymph node dissection and adjuvant therapy.

Klauber-DeMore et al. (86) report a 12% incidence of sentinel node metastases in 76 patients with DCIS using H&E and IHC stains. A micrometastasis defined as less than 2 mm and only identified with IHC was found in seven of nine (78%) patients. Of the nine patients with a positive sentinel node, six underwent a completion axillary lymph node dissection and one patient was found to have a non–sentinel node macrometastasis. On re-evaluation of the primary tumor, one patient was found to have a focus of microinvasion (< 1 mm) that was not previously identified. Another patient was found to have a contralateral invasive breast cancer with a single positive sentinel node. Two patients had non–high-grade DCIS with evidence of lymphovascular invasion, and the remaining five patients had high-grade DCIS.

Cox et al. (87) report a 13% incidence of nodal metastases in 195 patients with DCIS. Fifty percent were detected with H&E stains while 50% were detected only with IHC. The risk of lymph node metastases in these patients did not correlate with grade, presence of comedonecrosis, or predominant histologic pattern.

Our group has recently analyzed the incidence of sentinel node metastases in our patients with DCIS. Of 170 patients analyzed, 6% were found to have lymph node metastases, the majority of which (80%) were identified only with IHC stains. Due to the sentinel node findings, all patients were offered adjuvant therapy and 60% of patients accepted treatment. The problem with this approach is that we are assuming that IHC-detected metastases are significant, which is clearly unknown at this time; we are also assuming that adjuvant therapy is appropriate and beneficial for such patients. The natural history of DCIS does not support this assumption.

SENTINEL LYMPH NODE DISSECTION IN PATIENTS WITH DUCTAL CARCINOMA IN SITU WITH MICROINVASION

Ductal carcinoma in situ with microinvasion (DCIS-Mi) is defined as proliferating malignant ductal cells limited to the ductal units with occasional cancerization of the lobular units with evidence of invasion outside the myoepithelial layer of mammary ducts or lobules in foci 1 mm in size or smaller. Although DCIS-Mi is clearly defined, a DCIS-Mi diagnosis is subject to interpretive error because true macroinvasion into tangentially sectioned ducts may appear to only represent microinvasion. With the breach of the basement membrane, lymph node metastases are possible. However, it is unclear if the risk is high enough to warrant surgical staging of the axilla. Some believe that axillary lymph node dissection is not necessary for DCIS-Mi because it is generally not associated with lymph node metastases and has a favorable natural history (88,89). Other groups report rates of lymph node metastases ranging from 2.7% to 20% and advocate axillary lymph node dissection (90–92).

Several groups have used SLND in patients with DCIS-Mi and have found a positive SN in 10% to 20% of patients (86,87,93). Of the 60 patients from these three series, seven (11.6%) were found to have a positive sentinel node. Fifty-seven percent of patients had a metastases detected with IHC alone. The significance of these findings with regard to disease-free survival and overall survival is unknown.

SHOULD SENTINEL LYMPH NODE DISSECTION BE PERFORMED IN PATIENTS WITH DUCTAL CARCINOMA IN SITU?

The significance of axillary metastases, particularly IHC-detected metastases, in DCIS is unknown and is inconsistent with the natural history of DCIS. The presence of sentinel node metastases often leads to confusion and overtreatment. Although the National Surgical Adjuvant Breast and Bowel Project B-17 trial (94), a prospective randomized trial of treatment for DCIS, reported that 1.5% of patients died of metastatic disease at an 8-year follow-up, it cannot be extrapolated to this group of sentinel node–positive patients. Most patients with DCIS who develop metastatic disease often first develop a local recurrence. Solin et al. (95) recently presented an update of the collaborative trial in which only one of 270 patients exhibited a distant first event at 15 years of follow-up. Silverstein et al. (96) reported that none of almost 900 patients in the University of Southern California/Van Nuys database developed a distant event first, although a small fraction developed metastatic disease after local invasive recurrence.

Although SLND is less invasive and less morbid than an axillary dissection, the ease of this technique should not be an excuse for its use. Our group has abandoned the routine use of SLND in the majority of patients with DCIS. Indications for SLND in our patients with DCIS include those patients who have elected to proceed with a mastectomy as the treatment of choice. If an invasive component was found in the mastectomy specimen, the only options for that pa-

tient would be an axillary dissection or observation of the axilla. By offering the patient a SLND with frozen section analysis of the sentinel node at the time of mastectomy, the morbidity of an axillary lymph node dissection could be avoided in a majority of patients and the evaluation of the axilla accomplished. The use of IHC staining in this group of patients should be avoided until the significance of these metastases is understood. The American College of Surgeons Oncology Group Z0010 study is evaluating the significance of IHC-detected metastases in patients with early invasive breast cancer by blinding the results of the IHC stains and treating the patient based on the primary tumor characteristics. By blinding the results of the IHC stains, the true significance of these metastases will be identified. If these IHC-detected metastases are significant in invasive disease, perhaps this could be applied to patients with DCIS. However, until such data are available, SLND should be discouraged for patients with DCIS. Our group does offer patients with any degree of invasion an SLND. A majority of our patients enroll in the American College of Surgeons Oncology Group Z0010 study and, therefore, the IHC results are blinded. For those patients who do not participate in this study, the decision to use IHC stains is left to the pathologist. The surgeons in our group discourage its use.

REFERENCES

1. Fisher B. The surgical dilemma in the primary therapy of invasive breast cancer: a critical appraisal. *Curr Probl Surg* 1970;Oct:1–53.
2. Fisher B, Carbone P, Economou SG, et al. l-Phenylalanine mustard (l-Pam) in the management of primary breast cancer. A report of early findings. *N Engl J Med* 1975;292:117–122.
3. Bonadonna G, Brusamolino E, Valagussa P, et al. Combination chemotherapy as an adjuvant treatment in operable breast cancer. *N Engl J Med* 1976;294:405–410.
4. Controlled trial of tamoxifen as single adjuvant agent in management of early breast cancer. Analysis of six years by Nolvadex Adjuvant Trial Organization. *Lancet* 1985;1(8433):836–840.
5. Robinson JO. Treatment of breast cancer through the ages. *Am J Surg* 1986;151:317–333.
6. Lewison EF. The surgical treatment of breast cancer: a historical and collective review. *Surgery* 1953;34:904–913.
7. Cooper WA. The history of radical mastectomy. *Ann Med History* 1941;3:36–54.
8. DeMoulin D. *A Short History of Breast Cancer*. Boston: Martinus Nijhoff, 1983.
9. Banks WM. A plea for the more free removal of cancerous growths. *Liverpool Manchester Surg Rep* 1878;192–206.
10. Haagensen CD. The history of the surgical treatment of breast carcinoma from 1863–1921. In: Haagensen CD, ed. *Diseases of the breast*, 3rd ed. Philadelphia: WB Saunders, 1986:864–872.
11. Robbins GF, ed. *Silvergirl's surgery; the breast*. Austin, TX: Silvergirl, Inc., 1984.
12. Fisher B, Bauer M, Margolese R, et al. Five-year results of a randomized clinical trial comparing total mastectomy and segmental mastectomy with or without radiation in the treatment of breast cancer. *N Engl J Med* 1985;312:666–673.
13. Haagensen CD. Lymphatics of the breast. In: Haagensen CD, ed.

Diseases of the breast, 3rd ed. Philadelphia: WB Saunders, 1986:300–321.

14. Kinne DW. Controversies in primary breast cancer management. *Am J Surg* 1993;166:502–508.
15. National Institutes of Health Consensus Conference. Treatment of early stage breast cancer. *JAMA* 1991;265:391–395.
16. Fisher B, Wolmark N, Bauer M, et al. The accuracy of clinical nodal staging and of limited axillary dissection as a determinant of histologic nodal status in carcinoma of the breast. *Surg Gynecol Obstet* 1981;152:765–771.
17. Nieweg O, Kim E, Wong W, et al. Positron emission with fluorine 18-deoxyglucose in the detection and staging of breast cancer. *Cancer* 1993;71:3920–3925.
18. Silverstein MJ, Gierson ED, Waisman JR, et al. Axillary lymph node dissection for T1a breast carcinoma: is it indicated? *Cancer* 1994;73:664–667.
19. Silverstein M, Gierson E, Waisman J, et al. Predicting axillary node positivity in patients with invasive carcinoma of the breast by using a combination of category and palpability. *J Am Coll Surg* 1995;180:700–704.
20. Lin PP, Allison DC, Wainstock J, et al. Impact of axillary lymph node dissection on the therapy of breast cancer patients. *J Clin Oncol* 1993;11:1536–1544.
21. Pezner R, Patterson M, Hill L. Arm edema in patients treated conservatively for breast cancer. Relationship to patient age and axillary node dissection technique. *Int J Radiat Oncol Biol Phys* 1986;12:2079–2083.
22. Werner R, McCormick B, Petrek J, et al. Arm edema in conservatively managed breast cancer. Obesity is a major predictive factor. *Radiology* 1991;180:177–184.
23. Aitken D, Minton J. Complications associated with mastectomy. *Surg Clin North Am* 1983;63:1331–1352.
24. Ivens D, Hoe AL, Podd CR, et al. Assessment of morbidity from complete axillary dissection. *Br J Cancer* 1992;66:136–138.
25. Ryttov N, Holm NV, Qvist N, et al. Influence of adjuvant irradiation on the development of late arm lymphedema and impaired shoulder mobility after mastectomy for carcinoma of the breast. *Acta Oncol* 1988;27(6A):667–670.
26. Siegel BM, Mayzel KA, Love SM. Level I and level II axillary dissection in the treatment of early-stage breast cancer: An analysis of 259 consecutive patients. *Arch Surg* 1990;125:1144–1147.
27. Somers RG, Jablon LK, Kaplan MJ, et al. The use of closed suction drainage catheter after lumpectomy and axillary node dissection for breast cancer. A prospective randomized trial. *Ann Surg* 1992;215:146–149.
28. Wood KM. Intercostobrachial nerve entrapment syndrome. *South Med J* 1978;71:662–663.
29. Morrow M. Axillary node dissection: what role in managing breast cancer? *Contemp Oncol* 1994;8:16–28.
30. Adair F, Berg J, Joubert L, et al. Long-term follow-up of breast cancer patients: The 30-year report. *Cancer* 1974;33:1145–1150.
31. Fisher B, Ravdin RG, Ausman RK, et al. Surgical adjuvant chemotherapy in cancer of the breast: results of a decade of cooperative investigation. *Ann Surg* 1968;168:337–356.
32. Bloodgood JC. Comedo carcinoma of the female breast. *Am J Cancer* 1943;22:842–853.
33. Rosner D, Bedwani RN, Vana J, et al. Noninvasive breast carcinoma: results of a national survey by the American College of Surgeons. *Ann Surg* 1980;192:139–147.
34. Kessler CG, Feur EJ, Brown ML. Projections of the breast cancer burden to US women 1990–2000. *Prev Med* 1991;20:170.
35. Haagensen CD, Bodian C. A personal experience with Halsted's radical mastectomy. *Ann Surg* 1984;199:143–150.
36. Gump FE, Jicha DL, Ozello L. Ductal carcinoma in situ (DCIS): a revised concept. *Surgery* 1987;102:790–795.

37. Lagios MD, Margolin FR, Westdahl PR, et al. Mammographically detected duct carcinoma in situ. *Cancer* 1989;63:618–624.
38. Ashikari R, Hajdu SI, Robbins GF. Intraductal carcinoma of the breast (1960–1969). *Cancer* 1971;28:1182–1187.
39. Fisher ER, Sass R, Fisher B, et al. Pathologic findings from the National Surgical Adjuvant Breast Project (protocol 6). I. Intraductal carcinoma (DCIS). *Cancer* 1986;57:197–208.
40. Rosen PP. Axillary lymph node metastasis in patients with occult noninvasive breast carcinoma. *Cancer* 1980;46:1298–1306.
41. Ozello L, Sampitak P. The epithelial stromal junction of intraductal carcinoma of the breast. *Cancer* 1970;26:1186–1198.
42. Carter D, Smith RL. Carcinoma in situ of the breast. *Cancer* 1977;40:1189–1193.
43. Brown PW, Silverman J, Owens E, et al. Intraductal noninfiltrating carcinoma of the breast. *Arch Surg* 1976;111:1063–1067.
44. Rosen P, Senic R, Schottenfeld D, et al. Noninvasive breast carcinoma: frequency of unsuspected invasion and implications for treatment. *Ann Surg* 1979;189:377–382.
45. Recht A, Danoff BS, Solin LJ, et al. Intraductal carcinoma of the breast: results of treatment with excisional biopsy and irradiation. *J Clin Oncol* 1985;3:1339–1343.
46. Schuh ME, Nemoto T, Penetrante RB, et al. Intraductal carcinoma. Analyzing presentation, pathologic findings and outcome of disease. *Arch Surg* 1986;121:1303–1307.
47. Sunshine JA, Moseley HS, Fletcher WS, et al. Breast carcinoma in situ: a retrospective review of 112 cases with a minimum of 10-year follow-up. *Am J Surg* 1985;150:44–51.
48. Von Rueden DG, Wilson RE. Intraductal carcinoma of the breast. *Surg Gynecol Obstet* 1984;158:105–111.
49. Schwartz GF, Colin LJ, Olivotto IA, et al. The Consensus Conference on the treatment of in situ ductal carcinoma of the breast. April 22–25, 1999. *Semin Breast Disease* 2000;3:209–219.
50. Lagios MD, Westdahl PR, Margolin FR, et al. Duct carcinoma in situ: relationship of extent of noninvasive disease to the frequency of occult invasion, multicentricity, lymph node metastases and short-term treatment failures. *Cancer* 1982;50:1309–1314.
51. Fowble B. In situ breast cancer. In: Fowble B, Goodman R, Glick J, Rosato E, eds. *Breast cancer treatment. A comprehensive guide to management.* St. Louis: Mosby Year Book, 1991:325–344.
52. Egan RL, Ellis JR, Powell RW. Team approach to the study of disease of the breast. *Cancer* 1969;23:847–854.
53. Patchefsky AS, Schwartz GF, Finkelstein SD, et al. Heterogeneity of intraductal carcinoma of the breast. *Cancer* 1989;63:731–741.
54. Bur ME, Zimarowski MJ, Schnitt SJ, et al. Estrogen receptor immunohistochemistry in carcinoma in situ of the breast. *Cancer* 1992;69:1174–1181.
55. Meyer JS. Cell kinetics of histologic variants of in situ breast carcinoma. *Breast Cancer Res Treat* 1986;7:171–180.
56. Killeen JL, Namiki H. DNA analysis of ductal carcinoma in situ of the breast. A comparison with histologic features. *Cancer* 1991;68:2602–2607.
57. Bartkova J, Barnes DM, Miller RR, et al. Immunohistochemical demonstration of c-erbB-2 protein in mammary ductal carcinoma in situ. *Hum Pathol* 1990;21:1164–1167.
58. Morton D, Wen D-R, Wong J, et al. Technical details of intraoperative lymphatic mapping for early stage melanoma. *Arch Surg* 1992;127:392–399.
59. Giuliano AE, Kirgan DM, Guenther JM, et al. Lymphatic mapping and sentinel lymphadenectomy for breast cancer. *Ann Surg* 1994;220:391–401.
60. Giuliano AE, Jones RC, Brennan M, et al. Sentinel lymphadenectomy in breast cancer. *J Clin Oncol* 1997;15:2345–2350.
61. Krag DN, Weaver DL, Alex JC, et al. Surgical resection and radiolocalization of the sentinel lymph node in breast cancer using a gamma probe. *Surg Oncol* 1993;2:335–339.

62. Krag D, Harlow S, Weaver D, et al. Technique of sentinel node resection in melanoma and breast cancer: probe-guided surgery and lymphatic mapping. *Eur J Surg Oncol* 1998 24(2):89–93.

63. Krag D, Weaver D, Askikaga T, et al. The sentinel node in breast cancer: A multicenter validation trial. *N Engl J Med* 1998;339: 941–945.

64. Albertini JJ, Lyman GH, Cox C, et al. Lymphatic mapping and sentinel node biopsy and lymphatic mapping of patients with breast cancer. *Ann Surg* 1998;227:645–653.

65. Cox CE, Pendas S, Cox JM, et al. Guidelines for sentinel node biopsy and lymphatic mapping of patients with breast cancer. *Ann Surg* 1998;227:645–653.

66. Veronesi U, Paganelli G, Galimberti V, et al. Sentinel-node biopsy to avoid axillary dissection in breast cancer with clinically negative lymph-nodes. *Lancet* 1997;349:1864–1867.

67. Guenther JM, Krishnamoorthy M, Tan LR. Sentinel lymphadenectomy for breast cancer in a community managed care setting. *Cancer J* 1997;3:336–340.

68. Dale PS, Williams JT, IV. Axillary staging utilizing selective sentinel lymphadenectomy for patients with invasive breast carcinoma. *Am Surg* 1998;64:28–32.

69. Pijpers R, Meijer S, Koekstra OS, et al. Impact of lymphoscintigraphy on sentinel node identification with Technetium-99m—colloidal albumin in breast cancer. *J Nucl Med* 1997;38:366–368.

70. Borgstein PJ, Pijpers R, Comans EF, et al. Sentinel lymph node biopsy in breast cancer: guidelines and pitfalls of lymphoscintigraphy and gamma probe detection. *J Am Coll Surg* 1998;186: 275–283.

71. Miner TJ, Shriver CD, Jaques DP, et al. Ultrasonographically guided injection improves localization of the radiolabeled sentinel lymph node in breast cancer. *Ann Surg Oncol* 1998;5:315–321.

72. Offodile R, Hoh C, Barsky SH, et al. Minimally invasive breast carcinoma staging using lymphatic mapping with radiolabeled dextran. *Cancer* 1998;82:1704–1708.

73. Crossin JA, Hohnson AC, Stewart PB, et al. Gamma-probe–guided resection of the sentinel lymph node in breast cancer. *Am Surg* 1998;64:666–669.

74. Barnwell JM, Arredondo MA, Kollmorgen D, et al. Sentinel node biopsy in breast cancer. *Ann Surg Oncol* 1998;5:126–130.

75. O'Hea BJ, Hill ADK, El Shinrbiny AM, et al. Sentinel lymph node biopsy in breast cancer: Initial experience at Memorial Sloan-Kettering Cancer Center. *J Am Coll Surg* 1998;186:423–427.

76. Koller M, Barsuk D, Zippel D, et al. Sentinel lymph node involvement—a predictor for axillary node status with breast cancer—has the time come? *Eur J Surg Oncol* 1998;24:166–168.

77. Fisher ER, Swanidoss S, Lee CH, et al. Detection and significance of occult axillary node metastases in patients with invasive breast cancer. *Cancer* 1978;42:2025–2031.

78. Hainsworth PJ, Tjandra JJ, Stillwell RG, et al. Detection and significance of occult metastases in node-negative breast cancer. *Br J Surg* 1993;80:459–463.

79. Giuliano AE, Dale PS, Turner RR, et al. Improved axillary staging of breast cancer with sentinel lymphadenectomy. *Ann Surg* 1995;222:394–401.

80. Dowlatshahi K, Fan M, Bloom KJ, et al. Occult metastases in sentinel lymph nodes of patients with early stage breast carcinoma: A Preliminary Study. *Cancer* 1999;86:990–996.

81. Cote RJ, Peterson HF, Chaiwun B, et al. Role of immunohistochemical detection of lymph-node metastases in management of breast cancer. *Lancet* 1999;354:896–900.

82. Turner RR, Ollila DW, Krasne DL, et al. Histopathological validation of the sentinel lymph node hypothesis for breast carcinoma. *Ann Surg* 1997;226:271–278.

83. Ollila DW, Brennan MB, Giuliano AE. Therapeutic effect of sentinel lymphadenectomy in T1 breast cancer. *Arch Surg* 1998;133(6):647–651.

84. Silverstein MJ, Rosser RJ, Gierson ED, et al. Axillary lymph node dissection for intraductal breast carcinoma—is it indicated? *Cancer* 1987;59:1819–1824.

85. Pendas S, Dunway E, Giuliano R, et al. Sentinel node biopsy in ductal carcinoma in situ patients. *Ann Surg Oncol* 2000;7:15–20.

86. Klauber-DeMore N, Tan LK, Liberman L, et al. Sentinel lymph node biopsy. Is it indicated in patients with high-risk DCIS and DCIS with microinvasion? *Ann Surg Oncol* 2000;7:636–642.

87. Cox CE, Keoni N, Gray R, et al. Importance of lymphatic mapping in ductal carcinoma in situ (DCIS): Why map DCIS? *Am Surg* 2001;67:513–521.

88. Wong JH, Kopald KH, Morton DL. The impact of microinvasion on axillary node metastases and survival in patients with intraductal breast cancer. *Arch Surg* 1990;25:1298–1302.

89. Silver SA, Tavassoli FA. Microinvasive carcinoma of the breast: is axillary lymph node dissection indicated? *Mod Pathol* 1997;10: 25A(abst).

90. Rosner D, Lane WW, Pentrant R. Ductal carcinoma in situ with microinvasion: a curable entity using surgery alone without the need for adjuvant therapy. *Cancer* 1991;67:1498–1503.

91. Shuch ME, Nemoto T, Penetrante RB, et al. Intraductal carcinoma: Analysis of presentation, pathologic findings, and outcome of disease. *Arch Surg* 1986;121:1303–1307.

92. Penault-Liorca F, Le Bouedec G, Pomel C, et al. Microinvasive carcinoma of the breast: is axillary lymph node dissection indicated? *Mod Pathol* 1998:11:25A(abst).

93. Zavotsky J, Hansen N, Brennan MB, et al. Lymph node metastasis from ductal carcinoma in situ with microinvasion. *Cancer* 1999;85:2439–2443.

94. Fisher B, Digman J, Wolmark N, et al. Lumpectomy and radiation therapy for the treatment of intraductal breast cancer: findings from National Surgical Adjuvant Breast and Bowel Project B-17. *J Clin Oncol* 1998;16:441–452.

95. Solin LJ, Recht A, Fourquet A, et al. Ten-year results of breast-conserving surgery and definite irradiation for intraductal carcinoma (ductal carcinoma in situ) of the breast. *Cancer* 1991;68: 2337–2344.

96. Silverstein MJ, Lagios MD, Martino S, et al. Outcome after invasive local recurrence in patients with ductal carcinoma in situ of the breast. *J Clin Oncol* 1998;16:1367–1373.

58

THE ROLE OF SENTINEL LYMPH NODE BIOPSY IN DUCTAL CARCINOMA IN SITU: THE MEMORIAL SLOAN-KETTERING OPINION

HIRAM S. CODY III
PATRICK I. BORGEN
KIMBERLY J. VAN ZEE

Sentinel lymph node (SLN) biopsy is a new standard of care for axillary node staging in the patient with invasive breast cancer. The large majority of breast cancer patients have clinical stage T1–2N0 disease, and numerous validation studies worldwide confirm the potential of SLN biopsy to replace routine axillary lymph node dissection (ALND) in this setting (1). The role of SLN biopsy in patients with ductal carcinoma in situ (DCIS), a group currently comprising 20% to 25% of new breast cancer diagnoses in the United States, is more controversial. Current treatment guidelines (2), standard texts (3), and a recent consensus statement (4) find no indication for axillary staging in patients with DCIS. Some even argue that SLN biopsy for DCIS is a "dangerous and unwarranted direction" (5).

Only three publications to date, two from the Moffitt Cancer Center (6,7) and one from Memorial Sloan-Kettering Cancer Center (8), report the results of SLN biopsy for DCIS (Table 58.1). This chapter will

  i) review the rationale for SLN biopsy in DCIS,
 ii) summarize the results of the above preliminary studies,
iii) suggest guidelines for the use of SLN biopsy for DCIS, and
 iv) outline directions for future study.

DOES DUCTAL CARCINOMA IN SITU EVER REQUIRE AXILLARY NODE STAGING?

The simplest answer to this question is "no." By definition, in situ cancer cannot metastasize, and local treatment [surgical excision with or without radiotherapy (RT)] should be curative in virtually all cases. Three major randomized clinical trials [National Surgical Adjuvant Breast and Bowel Project (NSABP) B-17 (9), NSABP B-24 (10), and the Eu-

ropean Organization for the Research and Treatment of Cancer (EORTC) 10853 (11)], none of which included axillary staging, largely support this concept. The addition of RT or RT plus tamoxifen reduces local recurrence but has not (at 4 to 8 years of follow-up) improved survival over that obtained by surgical excision alone: 98% to 99%. Large retrospective series support the same conclusion. Silverstein et al. (12) found axillary nodal metastases in fewer than 1% of their carefully studied patients with DCIS; their only patients with DCIS who died of breast cancer first developed an *invasive* local recurrence (13). Kestin et al. (14) recently cite a 10-year disease-specific survival of 99% to 100% for their patients with DCIS treated with breast conservation without axillary staging.

A more nuanced answer to this question is "yes, selectively," and this is our preferred position. The hallmark of breast cancer is heterogeneity, and DCIS is a morphologically and biologically heterogeneous mix of lesions with varying malignant and/or metastatic potential. There are many reasons for the skeptical clinician to question a diagnosis of DCIS. The strongest justification for SLN biopsy in DCIS is the inability of conventional pathologic techniques to reliably rule out invasive cancer.

IS IT REALLY DUCTAL CARCINOMA IN SITU?

Even in the smallest invasive cancers (15), axillary node metastases are present in about 10% of cases, and no diagnostic test can completely exclude the presence of invasion in a patient with DCIS.

  i) A fine-needle aspiration (FNA) diagnosis of DCIS is automatically suspect: FNA simply cannot distinguish between DCIS and invasive cancer (16).

TABLE 58.1. STUDIES OF SENTINEL LYMPH NODE BIOPSY IN DUCTAL CARCINOMA IN SITU

Study	Case Selection	SLN + (%)	H&E + (%)	IHC + (%)[a]	Completion ALND + (%)
Moffitt I (6) (n = 87)	Consecutive cases	5 (6%)	2 (2%)	3 (4%)	0 (0%)
MSKCC (8) (n = 76)	"High risk" cases[b] (21% of DCIS)	9 (12%)	2 (3%)	7 (9%)	1 (17%)
Moffitt II (7) (n = 95)	All recent cases[c] (70% of DCIS)	26 (13%)	13 (7%)	13 (7%)	Not stated

Percentages rounded to nearest percent.
[a] SLN-positive only on IHC.
[b] DCIS patients felt to be at increased risk for having invasive cancer.
[c] SLN biopsy recommended for all recent patients, but not done in 30% of DCIS cases overall.
SLN, sentinel lymph node; H&E, hematoxyin-eosin; IHC, immunohistochemical; ALND, axillary lymph node dissection.

ii) A core-needle biopsy showing DCIS is subject to histologic underestimates: depending on technique, 0% to 35% of patients with DCIS diagnosed by core biopsy will prove to have invasive cancer on surgical excision (17).

iii) A surgical biopsy diagnosis of DCIS is fallible as well: pathologic review detects missed invasive foci in 2% to 3% of surgical excision specimens initially read as DCIS (18,19). In one series (7), invasive cancer was found in 13% of patients having definitive surgery for a diagnosis of DCIS based on a prior surgical biopsy.

iv) Invasion must be suspected in any patient with DCIS presenting as a palpable or mammographic mass, or as Paget's disease.

v) Invasion is especially likely in patients with DCIS that is extensive enough to require mastectomy because sampling error increases proportionate to specimen size. Following mastectomy for a diagnosis of DCIS, Morrow et al. (20) needed to perform reoperative ALND in 12% of patients when unexpected invasion was found in the breast specimen. In contrast, by performing SLN biopsy, Cox et al. (7) were able to avoid reoperative ALND in the 18% of "DCIS" patients who were found on mastectomy to have invasion.

vi) Occasionally, patients with DCIS will have lymphovascular invasion (LVI) within the breast, yet no other evidence of invasive disease (8).

vii) The mechanical displacement of ductal epithelium into the breast stroma by FNA or core needle biopsy may artifactually simulate invasion (21).

viii) In the most difficult borderline cases, expert pathologists may be unable to agree whether a given lesion is atypical hyperplasia, DCIS, or invasive cancer (22).

In summary, every decision regarding axillary nodal staging in the DCIS patient must take into account the diagnostic uncertainty of conventional pathologic techniques.

CAN DUCTAL CARCINOMA IN SITU METASTASIZE?

By definition, in situ cancer cannot metastasize, yet patients diagnosed as having DCIS can indeed die of metastatic breast cancer. Most historic series of DCIS treatment by mastectomy report a breast cancer–specific mortality of 1% to 2% (23), as do more recent studies from the era of breast conservation (14). In the series of Silverstein et al. (13), all deaths from metastatic disease occurred in patients with DCIS who had developed *invasive* breast recurrence prior to the appearance of distant disease, and one might reasonably argue that the invasive recurrence was the source of metastasis. However, in both the NSABP B-17 (9) and EORTC trials (11), nine of 13 and four of 24 patients, respectively, who died of disease developed distant metastasis *as a first event* or after a *locoregional non-breast recurrence*. Considering the methodological limitations of conventional pathologic assessment, it is reasonable to suspect that this subgroup of patients with "DCIS" really had occult invasive cancers from the outset and to hypothesize that SLN biopsy might have disclosed this metastatic potential.

ARE MICROMETASTASES CLINICALLY SIGNIFICANT?

Enhanced pathologic analysis of lymph nodes with serial sectioning and immunohistochemical (IHC) stains for cytokeratins is logistically prohibitive for routine ALND specimens but has become feasible with SLN biopsy and substantially increases the yield of positive nodes for invasive tumors of comparable size (24). The prognostic significance of micrometastases detected only by IHC remains a matter of controversy.

Both Rosser (25) and Carter (26) suggest that IHC-detected "micrometastases" may not represent biologic metastasis at all, but rather the passive transport to the SLN of tumor cells and debris from the trauma of a core-needle or surgical biopsy. In contrast, two lines of data (retrospective studies of "negative" axillary nodes and prospective studies of bone marrow aspirates taken at the time of surgery) suggest that IHC-detected micrometastatic disease is indeed significant. Retrospective enhanced pathologic analysis by serial sections and/or IHC staining of "negative" axillary nodes detects micrometastases in 10% to 20% of cases and suggests a 10% to 15% worse survival rate for these patients (27–29). Two elegant prospective trials (30,31) demonstrate that occult IHC-detected bone marrow micrometastases detected at the time of initial surgery have an *independent* prognostic impact exceeding that of conventional criteria. Two prospective trials of SLN biopsy by the American College of Surgeons Oncology Group (ACSOG) (32) and the NSABP (33) are now in progress; both studies include *blinded* IHC staining of both the SLN and the bone marrow and promise a definitive answer to this question.

None of the above studies address the patient with DCIS. One might reasonably ask whether the finding of SLN micrometastases in 6% to 13% of patients with DCIS (Table 58.1) could possibly have prognostic relevance in a disease with 99% long-term survival. In fact, these figures are quite consistent with the natural history of DCIS. If one assumes that

i) SLN-negative patients with DCIS have no systemic risk,

ii) ten percent of patients with DCIS are SLN-positive, and

iii) ten percent of these SLN-positive patients with DCIS might be expected to die of distant disease,

then projected disease-specific mortality for DCIS overall would be 1% (10% of 10%), quite consistent with historic data (23). It is important to emphasize that only a fraction of SLN-positive patients with DCIS (10% at most) will ever die of their disease. Nevertheless, by identifying a subset of patients with DCIS whose risk of systemic disease is perhaps 10% instead of 1%, SLN biopsy has the potential to alter treatment: 10% is the risk threshold at which current guidelines (2) dictate the use of systemic adjuvant therapy.

STUDIES OF SENTINEL LYMPH NODE BIOPSY IN DUCTAL CARCINOMA IN SITU

The First Moffitt Cancer Center Study

Pendas et al. (6) were the first to report on SLN biopsy for DCIS, in a presentation given to the Society of Surgical Oncology in March of 1999. Among 87 *consecutive* patients with pure DCIS, they observed positive SLN in 6% (five of 87). In two patients, the SLN were positive on both H&E and immunohistochemical (IHC) stains for cytokeratin, and in three patients they were positive on IHC only. On completion ALND, none had residual axillary nodal disease.

Four of five SLN-positive patients had a high-grade comedo subtype, and the remaining patient had a very large (9.5 cm) tumor of low-grade cribriform/papillary type. The authors concluded that

i) SLN biopsy should not be considered routine for all patients with DCIS, but may be suitable for selected patients with large and/or poorly differentiated tumors, and

ii) SLN biopsy may be the most efficient way to screen the breast for occult invasive disease.

The Memorial Sloan-Kettering Cancer Center Study

In March of 2000, Klauber-DeMore et al. (8) reported the results of SLN biopsy in a series of 76 selected patients with "high-risk" DCIS. These patients comprised 21% of all patients seen with DCIS during the same period. They were selected for SLN biopsy based not on a diagnosis of DCIS *per se*, but *on the suspicion of invasive disease*. All had one or more of the following: a palpable or mammographic mass, pathology suggesting but not diagnostic of invasion, high-grade histology and/or necrosis, or extensive disease requiring a mastectomy. Positive SLN were present in 12% (nine of 76). Two were positive on H&E and seven only on IHC. Of six patients who had completion ALND, one (with a SLN micrometastasis) had an H&E-positive non–sentinel node. Seven of nine SLN-positive patients had high-grade histology, two of nine had LVI, and one of nine proved to have microinvasion on pathologic review. Among patients with DCIS with microinvasion (DCIS-Mi), 10% (three of 31) had a positive SLN. The authors conclude that SLN biopsy is reasonable in the subset of patients with DCIS at increased risk for having occult invasive disease.

The Second Moffitt Cancer Center Study

Cox et al. (7) recently updated their early experience. Among 341 consecutive patients with DCIS or DCIS-Mi, 240 (70%) had SLN biopsy. Within this group, the study addresses the issues of

i) tumor upstaging,

ii) SLN metastasis, and

iii) cost effectiveness.

Among patients with a preoperative diagnosis of DCIS, 10% were upstaged to invasive cancer and an additional 3% were upstaged to DCIS-Mi by the subsequent definitive surgical excision. Upstaging from DCIS to invasive cancer was equally frequent whether the initial diagnosis had been by core-needle biopsy or surgical excision. These 13% of patients would have required a reoperative ALND had the SLN biopsy not been done concurrently.

The SLN proved positive in 13% of patients with a final diagnosis of DCIS (26 of 195). Half of these were positive only on IHC, and half were positive on H&E. Neither DCIS type nor histologic grade was significantly related to the frequency of SLN metastasis. By comparison, the SLN were positive in 20% of patients with DCIS-Mi (three of 15, two of these on H&E), and 27% of patients with invasive cancer (eight of 30, all of these on H&E). That is, of 240 patients initially thought to have either DCIS or DCIS-Mi, 23 (10%) became candidates for systemic adjuvant therapy through the detection of H&E-positive metastases in their SLN.

The authors estimate an additional cost of $384 per patient from routine SLN biopsy for DCIS/DCIS-Mi, or of $134 per patient in the subgroup having mastectomy. Balanced against this small added cost is the benefit of identifying H&E-positive nodal metastasis in about 10% of cases and the avoidance of reoperative ALND in mastectomy patients unexpectedly found to have invasive cancer.

The study concluded that SLN biopsy is justified in *all* patients with DCIS, based on

i) the high incidence of unsuspected invasive cancers in patients with DCIS and DCIS-Mi,
ii) the inability of histologic type or grade to reliably predict SLN metastasis, and
iii) the avoidance of reoperative ALND in patients with DCIS found at mastectomy to have invasion.

THE TECHNIQUE OF SENTINEL LYMPH NODE BIOPSY IN DUCTAL CARCINOMA IN SITU

The technique of SLN biopsy in DCIS is identical to that used for invasive cancer. The basic elements of our own approach, summarized in detail elsewhere (34), are based on an experience to date of more than 4,000 procedures and include:

i) the use of both blue dye and isotope in combination to map the SLN (35),
ii) preoperative lymphoscintigraphy in all patients (36, 37),
iii) the intradermal injection (38–40) of unfiltered Tc-99m sulfur colloid in a volume of 0.05 cc of saline at a single site directly over the tumor (or just cephalad from the biopsy scar), with a dose of 0.1 mCi (3.7 MBq) on the morning of surgery or 0.5 mCi (18.5 MBq) the afternoon before (36,37),
iv) the intraparenchymal injection around the tumor or biopsy site of 4 to 5 cc of isosulfan blue dye at the start of surgery (41),
v) the removal at surgery of all blue and of all focally "hot" SLN (using a hand-held gamma probe) (42),

vi) the removal of any clinically suspicious nodes palpated at surgery (43), and
vii) pathologic examination to include serial sectioning of all SLN, with both routine H&E and IHC stains for cytokeratins (CAM 5.2 and AE1:AE3) (34).

Many patients with DCIS have nonpalpable lesions requiring preoperative needle localization. In this setting, a localizing wire is placed on the morning of surgery, and the subsequent isotope injection is guided by the position of the wire. Our success in identifying the SLN has been identical for nonpalpable and palpable lesions (35,44,45).

Some authors have considered tumor multicentricity to be a contraindication to SLN biopsy (46), although it appears increasingly clear that the entire breast and its overlying skin drain to the same few SLNs in most patients (40,47–51). Accordingly, when DCIS is sufficiently extensive to require mastectomy, we simply inject the isotope and dye over the approximate center of the lesion or just cephalad to the recent biopsy scar.

For patients with invasive cancer, we normally perform intraoperative frozen section (FS) of the SLN, allowing the immediate performance of a completion ALND when the SLN is positive (52). The yield of intraoperative FS diminishes with tumor size: only 4% of our patients with T1a invasive cancers and none with "high-risk" DCIS have had a positive FS. Accordingly, FS is not done for DCIS, and the entire SLN is submitted for enhanced pathologic analysis. For those patients with DCIS in whom the SLN proves positive and a completion ALND is done, the non–SLNs are examined routinely with a single H&E-stained section per node.

CONCLUSIONS AND RECOMMENDATIONS

SLN biopsy is indicated in *any DCIS patient suspected of having an underlying invasive cancer.* Suitable patients with DCIS include:

i) those presenting with a palpable or mammographic mass,
ii) those in whom the pathologist cannot rule out invasion,
iii) those with LVI,
iv) those with extensive and/or high-grade tumors, and
v) *all of those having mastectomy.* In the latter group, SLN biopsy (if negative) allows the avoidance of a reoperative ALND if invasion is found in the breast specimen.

FUTURE DIRECTIONS

The role of SLN biopsy in DCIS is incompletely defined and requires further study with larger numbers of patients. A number of unanswered questions remain.

i) Regarding case selection, it remains unclear whether SLN biopsy should be done in all patients with DCIS or limited to certain "high-risk" subsets.

ii) The exact definition of "high-risk" is itself a matter for further study; the factors that predict SLN metastasis are not necessarily the same as those that predict local relapse after breast conservation.

iii) Regarding surgical treatment of the positive SLN in DCIS, too few data exist to make a confident recommendation either for or against routine completion ALND.

iv) Regarding systemic treatment for positive SLN, the few patients with DCIS found to have H&E-positive SLN should be considered conventionally node-positive and are candidates for systemic adjuvant therapy. Of note, the 6.5% frequency of H&E-positive SLN in the second Moffitt series (7) is surprisingly high, and this discordance with the two other studies [and with the DCIS literature in general (23)] requires confirmation.

v) The prognostic significance SLN micrometastases found only by IHC is unknown. Pending the results of studies in progress, these patients should not be treated as conventionally node-positive.

REFERENCES

1. Cody HS. Clinical aspects of sentinel node biopsy. *Breast Cancer Res Treat* 2001;3:104–108.
2. Carlson RW, Anderson BO, Bensinger W, et al. Update: NCCN practice guidelines for the treatment of breast cancer. *Oncology* 1999;13:187–212.
3. In: Silverstein MJ, ed. *Ductal Carcinoma In Situ of the Breast.* Baltimore: Williams and Wilkins, 1997.
4. Schwartz GF, Solin LJ, Olivotto IA, et al. The consensus conference on the treatment of in situ ductal carcinoma of the breast, April 22–25, 1999. *Breast J* 2000;6:4–13.
5. Lagios MD, Silverstein MJ. Sentinel node biopsy for patients with DCIS: a dangerous and unwarranted direction. *Ann Surg Oncol* 2001;8:275–277.
6. Pendas S, Dauway E, Giuliano AE, et al. Sentinel node biopsy in duct carcinoma in situ patients. *Ann Surg Oncol* 2000;7:15–20.
7. Cox CE, Nguyen K, Gray RJ, et al. Importance of lymphatic mapping in ductal carcinoma in situ (DCIS): Why map DCIS? *Am J Surg* 2001;67:513–519.
8. Klauber-DeMore N, Tan LK, Liberman L, et al. Sentinel lymph node biopsy: is it indicated in patients with high-risk ductal carcinoma-in-situ and ductal carcinoma-in-situ with microinvasion? *Ann Surg Oncol* 2000;7:636–642.
9. Fisher B, Dignam J, Wolmark N, et al. Lumpectomy and radiation therapy for the treatment of intraductal breast cancer: Findings from the National Surgical Adjuvant Breast and Bowel Project B-17. *J Clin Oncol* 1998;16:441–452.
10. Fisher B, Dignam J, Wolmark N, et al. Tamoxifen in the treatment of intraductal breast cancer: National Surgical Adjuvant Breast and Bowel Project B-24 randomised controlled trial. *Lancet* 1999;353:1993–2000.
11. Julien J-P, Bijker N, Fentiman IS, et al. Radiotherapy in breast-conserving treatment for ductal carcinoma in situ: first results of the EORTC randomised phase III trial 10853. *Lancet* 2000; 355:528–533.
12. Silverstein MJ, Gierson ED, Colburn WJ, et al. Axillary lymphadenectomy for intraductal carcinoma of the breast. *Surg Gynecol Obstet* 1991;172:211–214.
13. Silverstein MJ, Lagios MD, Martino S, et al. Outcome after invasive local recurrence in patients with ductal carcinoma in situ of the breast. *J Clin Oncol* 1998;16:1367–1373.
14. Kestin LL, Goldstein NS, Martinez AA, et al. Mammographically detected ductal carcinoma in situ treated with conservative surgery with or without radiation therapy: Patterns of failure and 10-year results. *Ann Surg* 2000;231:235–245.
15. Rush-Port E, Tan LK, Borgen PI, et al. Incidence of axillary lymph node metastases in T1a and T1b breast carcinoma. *Ann Surg Oncol* 1998;5:23–27.
16. Chieng DC, Fernandez G, Cangiarella JF, et al. Invasive carcinoma in clinically suspicious breast masses diagnosed as adenocarcinoma by fine-needle aspiration. *Cancer* 2000;90: 96–101.
17. Liberman L. Centennial dissertation. Percutaneous imaging-guided core breast biopsy: State of the art at the millennium. *AJR Am J Roentgenol* 2000;174:1191–1199.
18. Fisher ER, Costantino J, Fisher B, et al. Pathologic findings from the National Surgical Adjuvant Breast Project (NSABP) Protocol B-17. Intraductal carcinoma (ductal carcinoma in situ). The National Surgical Adjuvant Breast and Bowel Project Collaborating Investigators. *Cancer* 1995;75:1310–1319.
19. Bijker N, Peterse JL, Duchateau L, et al. Risk factors for recurrence and metastasis after breast-conserving therapy for ductal carcinoma-in-situ: Analysis of European Organization for Research and Treatment of Cancer Trial 10853. *J Clin Oncol* 2001; 19:2263–2271.
20. Morrow M, Venta L, Stinson T, et al. Prospective comparison of stereotactic core biopsy and surgical excision as diagnostic procedures for breast cancer patients. *Ann Surg* 2001;233: 537–541.
21. Liberman L, Vuolo M, Dershaw DD, et al. Epithelial displacement after stereotactic 11-gauge directional, vacuum-assisted breast biopsy. *AJR Am J Roentgenol* 1999;172:677–681.
22. Rosai J. Borderline epithelial lesions of the breast. *Am J Surg Pathol* 1991;15:209–221.
23. Swallow CJ, Van Zee KJ, Sacchini V, et al. Ductal carcinoma in situ of the breast: Progress and controversy. *Curr Probl Surg* 1996;33:556–600.
24. Giuliano AE, Dale PS, Turner RR, et al. Improved staging of breast cancer with sentinel lymphadenectomy. *Ann Surg* 1995;3: 394–401.
25. Rosser RJ. A Point of View: Trauma is the Cause of Occult Micrometastatic Breast Cancer in Sentinel Axillary Lymph Nodes. *Breast J* 2000;6:209–212.
26. Carter BA, Jensen RA, Simpson JF, et al. Benign transport of breast epithelium into axillary lymph nodes after biopsy. *Am J Clin Pathol* 2000;113:259–265.
27. Dowlatshahi K, Fan M, Snider HC, et al. Lymph node micrometastases from breast carcinoma: Reviewing the dilemma. *Cancer* 1997;80:1188–1197.
28. International (Ludwig) Breast Cancer Study Group. Prognostic importance of occult axillary lymph node micrometastases from breast cancers. *Lancet* 1990;335:1565–1568.
29. Cote RJ, Peterson HF, Chaiwun B, et al. Role of immunohistochemical detection of lymph-node metastases in management of breast cancer. International Breast Cancer Study Group [see comments]. *Lancet* 1999;354:896–900.
30. Diel IJ, Kaufmann M, Costa SD, et al. Micrometastatic breast cancer cells in bone marrow at primary surgery: prognostic value

in comparison with nodal status. *J Natl Cancer Inst* 1996;88:1652–1664.

31. Braun S, Pantel K, Muller P, et al. Cytokeratin-positive cells in the bone marrow and survival of patients with stage I, II, or III breast cancer. *N Engl J Med* 2000;342:525–533.

32. Grube BJ, Giuliano AE. Observation of the breast cancer patient with a tumor-positive sentinel node: Implications of the ACOSOG Z0011 trial. *Semin Surg Oncol* 2001;20:230–237.

33. Krag DN, Harlow S, Weaver D, et al. Radiolabeled sentinel node biopsy: collaborative trial with the national cancer institute. *World J Surg* 2001;25:823–828.

34. Cody HS, Borgen PI. State-of-the-art approaches to sentinel node biopsy for breast cancer: Study design, patient selection, technique, and quality control at Memorial Sloan-Kettering Cancer Center. *Surg Oncol* 1999;8:85–91.

35. Cody HS, Fey J, Akhurst T, et al. Complementarity of blue dye and isotope in sentinel node localization for breast cancer: univariate and multivariate analysis of 966 procedures. *Ann Surg Oncol* 2001;8:13–19.

36. Yeung HWD, Cody HS, Turlakow A, et al. Lymphoscintigraphy and sentinel node localization in breast cancer patients: a comparison between one-day and two-day protocols. *J Nucl Med* 2001;42:420–423.

37. McCarter MD, Yeung H, Yeh SDJ, et al. Localization of the sentinel node in breast cancer: identical results with same-day and day-before isotope injection. *Ann Surg Oncol* 2001;8:682–686.

38. Linehan DC, Hill ADK, Akhurst T, et al. Intradermal radiocolloid and intraparenchymal blue dye injection optimize sentinel node identification in breast cancer patients. *Ann Surg Oncol* 1999;6:450–454.

39. Boolbol SK, Fey J, Borgen PI, et al. Intradermal isotope injection: a highly accurate method of lymphatic mapping in breast carcinoma. *Ann Surg Oncol* 2001;8:20–24.

40. Martin RCG, Derossis A, Fey J, et al. Intradermal isotope injection is superior to intramammary in sentinel node biopsy for breast cancer. *Surgery* 2001;130:432–438.

41. O'Hea BJ, Hill ADK, El-Shirbiny A, et al. Sentinel lymph node biopsy in breast cancer: initial experience at Memorial Sloan-Kettering Cancer Center. *J Am Coll Surg* 1998;186:423–427.

42. Martin RCG, Fey J, Yeung H, et al. Highest isotope count does not predict sentinel node positivity in all breast cancer patients. *Ann Surg Oncol* 2001;8:592–597.

43. Hill ADK, Tran KN, Akhurst T, et al. Lessons learned from 500 cases of lymphatic mapping for breast cancer. *Ann Surg* 1999;229:528–535.

44. Liberman L, Cody HS, Hill ADK, et al. Sentinel lymph node biopsy after percutaneous diagnosis of nonpalpable breast cancer. *Radiology* 1999;211:835–844.

45. Liberman L, Cody HS, III. Percutaneous biopsy and sentinel lymphadenectomy: minimally invasive diagnosis and treatment of nonpalpable breast cancer. *AJR Am J Roentgenol* 2001;177:887–891.

46. Veronesi U, Paganelli G, Galimberti V, et al. Sentinel node biopsy to avoid axillary dissection in breast cancer with clinically negative lymph-nodes. *Lancet* 1997;349:1864–1867.

47. Borgstein P, Meijer S. Historical perspective of lymphatic tumour spread and the emergence of the sentinel node concept. *Eur J Surg Oncol* 1998;24:85–89.

48. Borgstein PJ, Meijer S, Pijpers R, et al. Functional lymphatic anatomy for sentinel node biopsy in breast cancer; echoes from the past and the periareolar blue dye method. *Ann Surg* 2000;232:81–89.

49. McMasters KM, Wong SL, Martin RCG, et al. Dermal injection of radioactive colloid is superior to peritumoral injection for breast cancer sentinel lymph node biopsy: results of a multi-institutional study. *Ann Surg* 2001;233:676–687.

50. Kern KA. Sentinel lymph node mapping in breast cancer using subareolar injection of blue dye. *J Am Coll Surg* 1999;189:539–545.

51. Klimberg VS, Rubio IT, Henry R, et al. Subareolar versus peritumoral injection for location of the sentinel lymph node. *Ann Surg* 1999;229:860–865.

52. Weiser MR, Montgomery LL, Susnik B, et al. Is routine intraoperative frozen section of sentinel lymph nodes in breast cancer patients worthwhile? *Ann Surg Oncol* 2000;7:651–655.

59

EXPLAINING DUCTAL CARCINOMA IN SITU TO PATIENTS: THE ROLE OF SPECIFIC INFORMATION AND ABSOLUTE RISKS

PATRICIA T. KELLY

"If patients do not understand their prognoses accurately, then their decisions about trade-offs between treatment choices may not reflect their true values" (1).

Providing information about ductal carcinoma in situ (DCIS) to a newly diagnosed patient can be a daunting and time-consuming process. Even after lengthy discussion with physicians, many women say they remain confused about treatment choices and uncertain about recurrence risks. Others continue to wonder, even years later, if their "cancer" has or will soon metastasize. As one said some months after her diagnosis, "Now that I've had breast cancer—and I am so lucky that my DCIS was a small one—there is an uncertainty that lingers uncomfortably and that I will probably have for the rest of my life."

To understand enough to make decisions about treatment and follow-up care and to regain their sense of peace and security, women with a DCIS diagnosis need specific, clear information, time in which to reflect and internalize new information, and help in making decisions that best reflect their comfort level and values. This chapter reviews five topics that are essential in helping women to achieve these ends, and emphasizes the value of presenting information:

- In specific terms, including methodological problems that compromise study results, and
- As absolute risks instead of as relative risks or comparison risks.

DISTINCTION BETWEEN INVASIVE AND IN SITU DISEASE

Many women report that from the time they heard their diagnosis they were unable to focus or think critically. As one remembered, "After the doctor said that word 'carcinoma,' I didn't hear anything else." Another recalls ". . . it became a terrifying issue that put my life on hold" (2). To these women, the term "carcinoma" in DCIS meant that they had a life threatening illness. Many believed that metastatic disease was present or that it might be found any day. As soon as possible, therefore, it is important for patients to learn that DCIS cells lack the biologic capacity to metastasize. Many patients appear to be unaware that although these cells can develop a metastatic capacity in the future if they become invasive, in their present state they cannot metastasize.

When women are told that their DCIS "has not spread beyond the breast ducts," many wonder how the doctor can be so sure. They relate instances in which friends or relatives with a cancer diagnosis were told "we got it all," only to learn they had widespread disease a few years later. Here again, it is important to distinguish between the capacity of in situ and invasive cells. Generalizations are often more confusing than specifics, even when the specifics are complex or involve sophisticated concepts. According to one woman with a diagnosis of DCIS, "I was routinely told, often in the same appointment, that I have cancer and that I do not have cancer" (2). Specific information is not only more useful, it also helps to reduce anxiety. For example, women generally find it useful and reassuring to learn of a study of 319 women with DCIS in which only two were found to have lymph node metastases (3). These metastases were probably due to occult invasive cancer in the breast, not to the DCIS.

Patients tend to be confused by the term "precancer," which is commonly used to describe DCIS. To many, this term suggests that they will certainly have invasive disease, probably quite soon, if not already. In fact, some question how, if they have a "precancer," the doctor can be so certain that "it hasn't turned to cancer already." Because the term "precancer" could be used to describe almost any cell in the body, it is not useful in helping women to appreciate the difference between normal, in situ, and invasive cells. Women with DCIS benefit by learning about the genetic changes that transform a normal cell to an in situ cell and an in situ cell to one that is invasive (4). Information of this type helps to remove the mystique that often surrounds DCIS (and invasive disease), and also helps to re-enforce the difference between DCIS and invasive cancer.

LIKELIHOOD THAT INVASION IS PRESENT IN OTHER PARTS OF THE BREAST

Many women worry that once they are found to have DCIS in one part of the breast, areas of invasive disease are likely to be present elsewhere in it. Fortunately, specific information is available to help women determine this probability. Small amounts of DCIS are associated with little or no risk of invasive disease elsewhere in that breast. In one very careful study, for example, only one woman whose DCIS measured less than 56 mm in size had invasive disease elsewhere in the breast (5). However, when DCIS was 56 mm or greater in extent, invasive disease was present nearly half the time. Therefore, when DCIS measures less than 56 mm, when adequate margins have been obtained (see below), and when the mammogram shows no other area of abnormality, there is little chance that either more DCIS or invasive cancer is present in other areas of the breast.

RECURRENCE RATES IN WOMEN CHOOSING BREAST CONSERVATION

In discussing treatments for DCIS, care must be taken to ensure that patients realize the term "recurrence" refers to future disease *in that breast only*, not to metastatic disease. Women with DCIS benefit by clearly understanding that survival rates are the same for those treated with mastectomy and those treated with breast conservation (with or without radiation therapy) (6,7). In fact, one study found that in the 10 years after their diagnosis, women with DCIS had a *lower* overall death rate than women in the general population (8).

Risk Over Time

Most patients are unaware that risk information without a time frame is meaningless. If, for example, a woman does not know whether a 10% risk applies to today, to this year, or to the next 10 years, she has no way to evaluate the significance of that risk to her. To be clinically meaningful, recurrence risks need to be presented as risk over time, such as "8% to 8 years, with a risk of 1% per year." As a woman goes through each year without a recurrence, she leaves the risk associated with that year behind her just as she leaves behind the risk of accident on a road already traveled (4). So, using

the 8% risk just given, at the end of 2 years, her risk is no longer 8% to 8 years, but 8% minus 2%, or 6%.

Risks in Perspective

In thinking about recurrence risks after a DCIS diagnosis, patients generally find that information about invasive breast cancer risks associated with other breast lesions can help to provide perspective. For example, women with a diagnosis of atypical hyperplasia have a subsequent invasive breast cancer risk of 0.5% to at most 1% per year (9,10). For lobular carcinoma in situ (LCIS), the subsequent invasive breast cancer risk is about 1% per year (11,12). Careful follow-up alone is generally recommended for these lesions.

Information about prognosis after an invasive breast cancer diagnosis is also relevant, because most women with DCIS are concerned that in the future they might develop an invasive recurrence that metastasizes. The results of recent studies suggest that when breast cancers are found at a small size, the prognosis is excellent. For example, with node-negative breast cancers less than 1 cm, the survival to 20 years is over 90% in several studies (13,14). Therefore, important components in making decisions about treatment and follow-up include ease of detection and the latest data on the excellent prognosis associated with small invasive breast cancers.

Clear Margins

Regardless of grade or size, DCIS is less likely to recur when adequate margins are obtained (15–21). When DCIS does recur, it tends to do so near the site of the original lesion (22). Optimal margin size has yet to be determined; however, when margins are 1 cm or greater, 8-year recurrences are few, with or without radiation therapy (23). In one study, with results shown in Table 59.1, margins of 10 mm and greater were associated with recurrences of less than 0.5% per year, and were about equal for those who did and did not receive radiation therapy. These results suggest that

TABLE 59.1. MARGIN SIZE AND EIGHT-YEAR RECURRENCE[a] AFTER DUCTAL CARCINOMA IN SITU

Margin Size	Lumpectomy	Lumpectomy and Radiation Therapy
10 mm +	3%	4%
1–10 mm[b]	20%	12%
Less than 1 mm[c]	58%	30%

[a] Includes both ductal carcinoma in situ and invasive breast cancer.
[b] Difference is not statistically significant, so the difference is more likely to be due to other factors, not the treatment.
[c] Difference is statistically significant, and so is more likely to be due to the treatment.
From ref.23, with permission.

when margins are adequate, radiation therapy does *not* further decrease recurrence rates; that is, removal of all DCIS and exclusion of occult invasion are essential and sufficient for local control. In a number of studies, radiation therapy does not appreciably reduce recurrence rates when margins are clear (18,21,23). More studies will be needed to determine optimal margin size and to learn whether this size differs for DCIS of different grades.

With margins of 1 to 10 mm, also shown in Table 59.1, the recurrence rates were 2.5% per year with lumpectomy and 1.5% per year with lumpectomy and radiation therapy. The 1% difference per year is not statistically significant, so factors other than treatment may well be responsible for differences found between the two study groups (24). When margins are 1 mm or less, rates of recurrence are high: 58% for lumpectomy and 30% with both lumpectomy and radiation therapy. These results suggest that radiation therapy does not compensate for inadequate margin size.

An 8-year national study [National Surgical Adjuvant Breast Project (NSABP) study B-17] reported a reduction in local recurrence rates when women with DCIS who were treated with lumpectomy also received radiation therapy (19). These 8-year results are shown in Table 59.2. An approximately 13% invasive recurrence rate without radiation therapy and a 4% recurrence with its use was found, which is a difference of approximately 1% per year over the course of the study. For noninvasive disease (both DCIS and LCIS appear to be included), there was a 13% invasive recurrence without radiation therapy and an 8% recurrence with it, which is a difference of about 0.6% per year.

Unfortunately, this study had a number of methodological problems that make it difficult to use its results to assess the role of radiation therapy in reducing local recurrence rates after a diagnosis of DCIS. A major problem is that more than one-fourth of the surgical specimens were not reviewed at all, with the remainder receiving only partial review. Because the tissue was not completely examined, the presence of occult invasive disease could not be ruled out. A significant number of subjects appear to have entered the study with invasive disease, because fourteen deaths due to breast cancer occurred within the 8 years of the study (10 in the group that received both lumpectomy and radiation

TABLE 59.2. EIGHT-YEAR RECURRENCE FOLLOWING DUCTAL CARCINOMA IN SITU TREATED WITH LUMPECTOMY ONLY OR LUMPECTOMY AND RADIATION THERAPY

Type of Recurrence in Breast	Lumpectomy	Lumpectomy and Radiation Therapy
Invasive	13%	4%
Non-invasive	13%	8%
Total	26%	12%

From ref. 19, with permission.

therapy). This is a far higher mortality rate than would be expected and that has been found in other studies of women with DCIS.

A 15-year study from multiple institutions in the United States and Europe reported a 19% local failure rate in women with DCIS treated with excision and radiation therapy (25). About half the recurrences were invasive. At 10 years, the local failure rate was 16%, close to the 20% 8-year recurrence rate shown in Table 59.1 with lumpectomy alone when margins were adequate (1 to 10 mm). Margin status was unknown in 47% of the specimens from the multiple institution study, which probably accounts for the high local failure rate. The results of this study further support the importance of clear margins in reducing recurrence rates and suggest that radiation therapy does not control residual disease.

To provide information about recurrence rates when DCIS is treated with lumpectomy with and without radiation therapy, a number of investigators have called for large-scale studies using a methodology that includes:

- complete investigation of entire lumpectomy samples
- measurement of the extent of DCIS
- clear margins around DCIS
- measurement of margin size
- classification of DCIS by type

In making treatment decisions, women need to be aware of the limitations of study results when these methodologies were not used.

RECURRENCE RATES AFTER TAMOXIFEN USE

Tamoxifen is sometimes suggested as a way to reduce ipsilateral and contralateral recurrence after a diagnosis of DCIS. A large national study, NSABP B-24, compared 5-year breast cancer recurrence in women with DCIS who did and did not receive tamoxifen after their diagnosis (26). All were treated with lumpectomy followed by radiation therapy. Unfortunately, the methodology in this study did not require specimen margins to be clear. Invasive cancer was apparently present in a number of study subjects at the onset, because 10 women developed regional or distant metastases in only 5 years of follow-up.

Recurrence risks for those who did and did not take tamoxifen are shown in Table 59.3. For ipsilateral invasive disease, there was a 2% difference between the tamoxifen and placebo group spread over 5 years, which is less than half a percent a year. For ipsilateral in situ disease (both DCIS and LCIS appear to be included), there was a 1% difference between the two groups over the 5 years of the study, which is a benefit of about 0.2% per year. Contralateral invasive risks were small for both groups. Due to this study's short follow-up and methodological problems, which in-

TABLE 59.3. TAMOXIFEN AND FIVE-YEAR RECURRENCE RISKS AFTER LUMPECTOMY AND RADIOTHERAPY FOR DUCTAL CARCINOMA IN SITU

Recurrence	No Tamoxifen	Tamoxifen
Ipsilateral invasive	4%	2%
Ipsilateral in situ[a]	5%	4%
Contralateral invasive	2%	2%
Contralateral in situ[a]	1%	0.2%
Non-breast	3%	4%
Regional/distant metastasis	n = 7	n = 3

[a] Ductal carcinoma in situ and lobular carcinoma in situ.
From ref. 26, with permission.

clude a failure to exclude women with invasive disease, it does not provide clinically useful information regarding the effectiveness of tamoxifen in reducing recurrence rates in women with DCIS.

Some have used the results of another study, NSABP P-1, in advocating the use of tamoxifen in treating women with DCIS. This study, reported a 49% reduction in invasive breast cancer risk to "high-risk" women, including some with a diagnosis of atypical hyperplasia and LCIS (27). When applying study results such as these, physicians need to be aware that risks framed in comparison terms (such as a percent reduction, a percent increase, or a relative risk) are less useful in a clinical setting than absolute risks are and can be misleading to patients and physicians alike (4,28). Generally, the clinical relevance of a risk is more readily apparent when it is presented in absolute terms. As Laupacis et al. (29) note ". . . absolute risk reduction is superior to the relative risk reduction because it incorporates both the baseline risk and the magnitude of the risk reduction." For example, "A 25% relative risk reduction, after all, can be reported whether the absolute rates in the two arms are 40% and 30% or 4% and 3%" (30).

As shown in Table 59.4, the 49% reduction in breast cancer risk to high-risk women who took tamoxifen means in absolute (actual) terms that in nearly 6 years only 1.8 fewer invasive breast cancers would be found in 100 women who took tamoxifen compared with nonusers. Many

TABLE 59.4. TAMOXIFEN USE IN WOMEN WITHOUT A BREAST CANCER DIAGNOSIS AND BREAST CANCER RATES AT 5.75 YEARS

No./Rate	No Tamoxifen	Tamoxifen
No. of women	6,599	6,576
No. of breast cancers	175	89
Average annual rate per 100 women	0.6	0.3
Cumulative rate per 100 women	3.8	2.0

From ref. 27, with permission.

women (and their physicians), who are enthused about tamoxifen as a preventive agent reported to reduce breast cancer risk by 49%, are understandably less impressed when they realize this is a difference of fewer than two breast cancers in 100 women followed nearly 6 years. Therefore, the 49% reduction means that 333 women would need to be treated with tamoxifen for 1 year to avoid one case of breast cancer. The term "avoid" is more precise than "prevent" in this instance, because this study followed women for less than 6 years. Most breast cancers are detected only after 7 to 10 years, so all or most of the cancers diagnosed during the course of this study were undoubtedly present but subclinical at the time the women entered the study. At nearly 6 years, tamoxifen users and non-users rates of in situ disease (LCIS or DCIS) differed by less than one breast cancer in 100 women.

RECURRENCE RATES AFTER HORMONE REPLACEMENT THERAPY

Hormone replacement therapy (HRT) frequently becomes an emotional topic after DCIS diagnosis, because some physicians are comfortable about its use and others strongly advise against it. Few studies of breast cancer risk to HRT users with DCIS are available. In one, no significant increase in invasive breast cancer or DCIS was found among women who used HRT for up to 10 years before their DCIS diagnosis or who used hormones after their diagnosis (31).

Many studies with pertinent information about the association of hormone use and the development of invasive breast cancer are available and either find no increase in invasive breast cancer risk or find a risk that is quite small. In several women with various types of benign breast disease, including atypical hyperplasia, do not have a further increase in breast cancer risk if they take HRT (32–34). Another compelling group of studies suggests that HRT use does not cause hormone users' invasive breast cancers to grow more rapidly than those of nonusers. In these studies, women who were taking HRT at the time of their invasive breast cancer diagnosis had tumors that were no larger and of no higher grade than those of nonusers (35–39). These results are congruent with those in which breast cancer mortality rates in HRT users were no higher than those of nonusers (40–42).

Many studies find no significant increase in invasive breast cancer risk with hormone use of 15 or more years (43–45). One frequently cited study did find a statistically significant 1.5-fold increase in risk with 5 or more years of use (46). However, these study results were presented as a relative risk of 1.5 or an increase of 50%. For this reason, it is important to investigate the meaning of this relative risk in clinical and in absolute terms.

When the results of epidemiologic studies are used in a clinical setting, relative risks less than three should be viewed with caution, because even when differences are statistically significant, the difference may well be due to the way in which the study groups were selected, not to the agent being studied (such as hormones) (4,24). The 1.5-fold increase in risk found in this study may therefore be due to other differences between the study and control groups, and not to hormone use, because 1.5 is far less than a three-fold increase.

Here, also, it is important to learn what the 1.5-fold increase in risk actually means. Even if the 1.5 increase in breast cancer risk in this study was due to hormone use, in absolute terms the increase means that less than one additional breast cancer would occur in 100 women who used estrogen for 10 years (47)! The point is that unless clinicians have access to absolute risk information, they are unable to fully evaluate the clinical implications of risks to an individual patient.

More recently, as the number of studies finding either no increase or no clinically important increase in invasive breast cancer risk to estrogen users has accumulated, questions are being raised about breast cancer risks associated with progesterone use. In one study an 8% increase in breast cancer risk per year was reported for women who used estrogen and progestin (48). Thin women who used progestin had a 12% per year increase. When presented in this manner, the risks seem large. However, in actual (absolute) numbers, the risk is surprisingly small. In absolute terms, the 8% increase per year, for example, means that 2,000 women would need to take estrogen and progestin for a year to result in the detection of even one additional breast cancer. In this study, risks were reported to only 4 years, so all of the cancers detected were probably present before hormone use began.

As a group, then, the many studies find either exceedingly small increases or no increase in invasive breast cancer risk to HRT users compared with nonusers. No significant increase in risk has been found to women with a diagnosis of DCIS or with other types of benign breast disease. Women who were taking hormones at the time of their breast cancer diagnosis do not have larger or more aggressive tumors. These studies suggest that either hormone replacement therapy does not increase breast cancer risk, or does so to an extent that is so small it is difficult to measure.

CONCLUSION

In making decisions about treatments and follow-up regimens, women with a DCIS diagnosis benefit by having access to information that helps them to clearly understand:

- the inability of DCIS to metastasize
- the likelihood that invasive disease or more DCIS is present in the affected breast
- the importance of clear margins in reducing recurrence, whether or not radiation therapy is used
- recurrence risks in percentages over time

- similar mortality rates in women with DCIS whether they are treated with mastectomy or breast conservation with or without radiation therapy
- absolute recurrence rates per year after lumpectomy and lumpectomy followed by radiation therapy
- recurrence rates after treatment with radiation therapy and/or tamoxifen in absolute terms not as relative or comparison risks
- methodological problems in several large studies that compromise findings about recurrence rates after radiation therapy and tamoxifen treatments
- recurrence rates in groups using HRT in absolute terms, not as relative risks

Women who receive this information and who are helped to understand their risks in absolute terms are generally less anxious and better prepared to participate in meaningful discussions about treatment options than are those who lack this information. And, with greater understanding, their confidence in treatment is likely to increase and their anxiety to decrease.

REFERENCES

1. Fogarty LA, Curbow BA, Wingard JR, et al. Can 40 seconds of compassion reduce patient anxiety? *J Clin Oncol* 1999;17:371–379.
2. Godby CJ. A formerly clueless patient responds [Letter]. *BMJ* 2000;321:1409.
3. Silverstein MJ. Ductal carcinoma in situ with microinvasion. In: Silverstein MJ, ed. *Ductal Carcinoma In Situ of the Breast*. Baltimore: Williams & Wilkins, 1997:557–562.
4. Kelly PT. *Assess Your True Risk of Breast Cancer*. NY: Henry Holt and Company, 2000.
5. Lagios MD, Margolin FR, Westdahl PR, et al. Mammographically detected duct carcinoma in situ. *Cancer* 1989;63:618–624.
6. Silverstein MJ, Lagios MD. Benefits of irradiation for DCIS: a Pyrrhic victory. *Lancet* 2000;355:510–511.
7. Schwartz LM, Wolosin S, Sox HC, et al. US women's attitudes to false positive mammography results and detection of ductal carcinoma in situ: cross sectional survey. *BMJ* 2000;320:1635–1640.
8. Ernster VL. Mortality among women with ductal carcinoma in situ of the breast in the population-based Surveillance, Epidemiology and End Results Program. *Arch Intern Med* 2000;160:953–958.
9. Bodian CA, Perzin KH, Lattes R, et al. Prognostic significance of benign proliferative breast disease. *Cancer*1993;71:3896–3907.
10. Page DL, Dupont WD, Rogers LW, et al. Atypical hyperplastic lesions of the female breast. *Cancer* 1985;55:2698–2708.
11. Haagensen CD, Lane N, Lattes R, et al. Lobular neoplasia (so-called lobular carcinoma in situ) of the breast. *Cancer* 1978;42:737–769.
12. Abner AL, Connolly JL, Recht A, et al. The relation between the presence and extent of lobular carcinoma in situ and the risk of local recurrence for patients with infiltrating carcinoma of the breast treated with conservative surgery and radiation therapy. *Cancer* 2000;88:1072–1077.
13. Tabar L, Vitak B, Chen H-H, et al. The Swedish Two-County Trial twenty years later. *Radiol Clin North Am* 2000;38:625–665.

14. Joensuu H, Pylkkanen L, Toikkanen S. Late mortality from pT1N0M0 breast carcinoma. *Cancer* 1999;85:2183–2189.

15. Silverstein MJ. Predicting local recurrences in patients with ductal carcinoma in situ. In: Silverstein MJ, ed. *Ductal Carcinoma in Situ of the Breast*. Baltimore: Williams & Wilkins, 1997:271–283.

16. Weng EY, Juillard GJF, Parker RG, et al. Outcomes and factors impacting local recurrence of ductal carcinoma in situ. *Cancer* 2000;88:1643–1649.

17. Page DL, Simpson JF. Ductal carcinoma in situ—the focus for prevention, screening, and breast conservation in breast cancer. *N Engl J Med* 1999;340:1499–1500.

18. Vicini FA, Kestin LL, Goldstein NS, et al. Impact of young age on outcome in patients with ductal carcinoma-in-situ treated with breast-conserving therapy. *J Clin Oncol* 2000;18:296–306.

19. Fisher B, Dignam J, Wolmark N, et al. Lumpectomy and radiation therapy for the treatment of intraductal breast cancer: Findings from National Surgical Adjuvant Breast and Bowel Project B-17. *J Clin Oncol* 1998;16:441–452.

20. Fisher B, Dignam J, Tan-Chiu, et al. Pathologic findings from the National Surgical Adjuvant Breast Project (NSABP) eight-year update of Protocol B-17. *Cancer* 1999;86:429–438.

21. Chan KC, Knox WF, Sinha G, et al. Extent of excision margin width required in breast conserving surgery for ductal carcinoma in situ. *Cancer* 2001;91:9–16.

22. Silverstein MJ, Poller DN, Waisman JR, et al. Prognostic classification of breast ductal carcinoma-in-situ. *Lancet* 1995;345:1154–1157.

23. Silverstein MJ, Lagios MD, Groshen S, et al. The influence of margin width on local control of ductal carcinoma in situ of the breast. *N Engl J Med* 1999;340:1455–1461.

24. Taubes G. Epidemiology faces its limits. *Science* 1995;269:164–169.

25. Solin LJ, Kurtz J, Fourquet A, et al. Fifteen-year results of breast-conserving surgery and definitive breast irradiation for the treatment of ductal carcinoma in situ of the breast. *J Clin Oncol* 1996;14:754–763.

26. Fisher B, Dignam J, Wolmark N, et al. Tamoxifen in treatment of intraductal breast cancer: National Surgical Adjuvant Breast and Bowel Project B-24 randomised controlled trial. *Lancet* 1999;353:1993–2000.

27. Fisher B, Costantino JP, Wickerham DL, et al. Tamoxifen for prevention of breast cancer: Report of the National Surgical Adjuvant Breast and Bowel Project P-1 Study. *J Natl Cancer Inst* 1998;90:1371–1388.

28. Hoffrage E, Lindsey S, Hertwig R, et al. Communicating statistical information. *Science* 2000;290:2261–2262.

29. Laupacis A, Sackett DL, Roberts RS. An assessment of clinically useful measures of the consequences of treatment. *N Engl J Med* 1988;318:1728–1733.

30. Naylor CD, Chen E, Strauss B. Measured enthusiasm: Does the method of reporting trial results alter perceptions of therapeutic effectiveness? *Ann Intern Med* 1992;117:916–921.

31. Habel LA, Daling JR, Newcomb PA, et al. Risk of recurrence after ductal carcinoma *in situ* of the breast. *Cancer Epidemiol Biomarkers Prev* 1998;7:689–696.

32. Byrne C, Connolly JL, Colditz GA, et al. Biopsy confirmed benign breast disease, postmenopausal use of exogenous female hormones, and breast carcinoma risk. *Cancer* 2000;89:2046–2052.

33. Dupont WD, Page DL, Rogers LW, et al. Influence of exogenous estrogens, proliferative breast disease, and other variables on breast cancer risk. *Cancer* 1989;63:948–957.

34. Dupont WD, Page DL, Pari FF. Estrogen replacement therapy in women with a history of proliferative breast disease. *Cancer* 1999;85:1277–1283.

35. Bonnier P, Romain S, Giacalone PL, et al. Clinical and biologic prognostic factors in breast cancer diagnosed during postmenopausal hormone replacement therapy. *Obstet Gynecol* 1995;85:11–17.

36. Strickland DM, Gambrell RD, Butzin CA, et al. The relationship between breast cancer survival and prior postmenopausal estrogen use. *Obstet Gynecol* 1992;80:400–404.

37. Fowble B, Hanlon A, Freedman G, et al. Postmenopausal hormone replacement therapy: Effect on diagnosis and outcome in early-stage invasive breast cancer treated with conservative surgery and radiation. *J Clin Oncol* 1999;17:1680–1688.

38. Harding C, Knox WF, Faragher EB, et al. Hormone replacement therapy and tumour grade in breast cancer: prospective study in screening unit. *BMJ* 1996;312:1646–1647.

39. Jernstrom H, Frenander J, Ferno M, et al. Hormone replacement therapy before breast cancer diagnosis significantly reduces the overall death rate compared with never-use among 984 breast cancer patients. *Br J Cancer* 1999;80:1453–1458.

40. Grodstein F, Stampfer MJ, Colditz GA, et al. Postmenopausal hormone therapy and mortality. *N Engl J Med* 1997;336:1769–1775.

41. Willis DB, Calle EE, Miracel-McMahill L, et al. Estrogen replacement therapy and risk of fatal breast cancer in a prospective cohort of postmenopausal women in the United States. *Cancer Causes Control* 1996;7:449–457.

42. Sellers TA, Mink PJ, Cerhan JR, et al. The role of hormone replacement therapy in the risk for breast cancer and total mortality in women with a family history of breast cancer. *Ann Intern Med* 1997;127:973–980.

43. Brinton LA, Hoover R, Fraumeni JF. Menopausal oestrogens and breast cancer risk: An expanded case-control study. *Br J Cancer* 1986;54:825–832.

44. Kaufman DW, Palmer JR, de Mouzon J, et al. Estrogen replacement therapy and the risk of breast cancer: Results from the case-control surveillance study. *Am J Epidemiol* 1991;134:1375–1385.

45. Palmer JR, Rosenberg L, Miller DR, et al. Breast cancer risk after estrogen replacement therapy: Results from the Toronto breast cancer study. *Am J Epidemiol* 1991;134:1386–1395.

46. Colditz GA, Hankinson SE, Hunter DJ, et al. The use of estrogens and progestins and the risk of breast cancer in postmenopausal women. *N Engl J Med* 1995;332:1589–1593.

47. Collaborative Group on Hormonal Factors in Breast Cancer. Breast cancer and hormone replacement therapy: Collaborative reanalysis of data from 51 epidemiological studies of 52,705 women with breast cancer and 108,411 women without breast cancer. *Lancet* 1997;350:1047–1059.

48. Schairer C, Gail M, Byrne C, et al. Estrogen replacement therapy and breast cancer survival in a large screening study. *J Natl Cancer Inst* 1999;91:264–270.

60

DUCTAL CARCINOMA IN SITU OF THE MALE BREAST

BRUNO CUTULI

Male breast cancer (MBC) is a rare disease, accounting for approximately 0.5% of all cases of breast carcinoma in Western countries (1,2). In other populations, such as in Africa, the incidence of MBC appears to be higher. An increased incidence of MBC has also been reported in American blacks and Jews, compared with whites (3). Risk factors for the development of MBC have not yet been clearly identified (3a). No consistent endocrine abnormalities have been identified in MBC patients, although testicular failure and increased estrogen production have been thought by some to be associated with an increased risk of MBC. Other hypothesized risk factors include radiation exposure, estrogen administration (i.e., for treatment of prostate carcinoma), Klinefelter syndrome, and some hepatic diseases (i.e., cirrhosis) that produce relative hyperestrogenism. Whether there is a causal relationship between gynecomastia and MBC remains uncertain. An increased risk of MBC has also been reported in families who carry a mutation in the BRCA2 gene.

Although there is extensive literature on invasive MBC (1–7), few data are available on DCIS in the male breast. To date, 290 cases of pure DCIS have been reported in series dealing with MBC (Table 60.1) (7–34). The proportion of MBC that was DCIS varied from 0% to 17%, with an average of 7%. The proportion of DCIS may be increasing with time. For example, the proportion increased from 3% in 1953 through 1984 to 8% in 1985 through 1995 among patients with MBC in a study in Milwaukee, Wisconsin (7).

This chapter will review what is known about the clinical and pathologic features of DCIS in males and the outcome when treated with either mastectomy or breast-conserving therapy.

CLINICAL FEATURES

The clinical features of DCIS in males have been described in detail in only a few series. The two largest are those of 31 patients seen at French cancer centers from 1970 to 1992 (18), and a series of 84 patients collected by the United States Armed Forces Institute of Pathology (AFIP) from 1957 to 1995 (34). However, case ascertainment methods were very different between these two studies. The French series formed a portion of a much larger study of 621 patients with MBC. The AFIP series was selected from 280 cases of DCIS registered by the AFIP, but the selection criteria for why only 30% of this entire population was analyzed were not specified. Four patients with DCIS treated at the Lahey Clinic near Boston were also reported in detail (33,35). These series are summarized in Table 60.2.

In the French and Lahey Clinic series, the median ages at diagnosis of men with pure DCIS were 58 and 56 years, respectively, compared with 63 and 64 years for patients with invasive cancers. In the AFIP series, the median age of patients with DCIS was 65 years, but no comparison group with invasive cancers was analyzed. Six patients (19%) in the French series were younger than age 40, a much higher proportion than among females with DCIS.

Patients in these series commonly presented with either a subareolar mass, serosanguineous nipple discharge, or both (Table 60.2).

The incidence of unilateral or bilateral gynecomastia among patients in these series varied substantially. However, gynecomastia is defined in extremely different ways by different authors. Its incidence may also depend on other factors, such as long-term use of certain drugs (36). True gynecomastia (i.e., breast enlargement due to hypertrophy of the glandular tissue of the breast) also must be differentiated from pseudogynecomastia (breast enlargement due to excess subcutaneous fat in obese patients). In the French series, true gynecomastia was histologically confirmed in seven of 11 patients with a clinical diagnosis.

The median duration from onset of the symptoms to the first physician visit was shorter in the two largest series (3 and 2 months, respectively) than in the Lahey Clinic series (9 months), and these are also shorter than is usually the case with invasive MBC. However, this interval was unknown for a number of patients in these series.

Three cases in each of these series had a family history of breast cancer in first and/or second-degree relatives. However, this incidence may be underestimated due to missing data for patients accrued in the earlier years of these studies.

TABLE 60.1. FREQUENCY OF DUCTAL CARCINOMA IN SITU IN PUBLISHED SERIES OF MALE BREAST CANCER

Author (Reference)	n (Total)	# DCIS	%
Visfeldt (8)	187	0	0
Erlichmann (9)	89	1	1
Ramantanis (10)	138	2 [2]	1
Ribeiro (11)	385	8 [8]	2
Salvadori (12)	170	4	2
Scheicke (13)	176	5	3
Guinee (14)	346	11[a]	3
Goss (15)	229	10 [6]	4
Stierer (16)	169	8	5
Treves (17)	146	7	5
Cutuli (18)	621	31	5
Holleb (19)	198	12	6
Vanderbilt (20)	52	3	6
Donegan (7)	152	10	7
Norris (21)	113	8	7
Gadenne (22)	73	5	7
Langlands (23)	88	6	7
Vercoutere (24)	45	3	7
Heller (25)	97	8	8
Stranzl (26)	31	3	10
Izquierdo (27)	50	5 [4]	10
Wang (28)	33	4	12
Tan (29)	22	3	14
Hill (30)	142	21	15
Borgen (31)	104	16 [8]	15
Ouriel (32)	50	8	16
Camus (33)	23	4[b]	17
Hittmair (34)	NA	84	NA

NA, not assessed; DCIS, ductal carcinoma in situ; numbers in square brackets, cases presenting with Paget's disease.
[a] Cases not described in detail.
[b] These four cases were also reported in a later work by Joshi et al. in 1996 (35), but with a larger denominator (46 patients).

HISTOLOGIC FEATURES

The predominant histologic subtypes of DCIS in patients of these three series are described in Table 60.3. In accordance with other studies (18,33), papillary and/or cribriform subtypes were the most common. Papillary architecture predominated in the larger ducts, whereas other subtypes were observed more frequently in smaller, more peripheral ducts.

The most detailed analysis of the histologic features of DCIS in the male breast is the report from the AFIP (34). One-fourth of the cases showed histologically mixed patterns. Fifty-seven percent were classified as grade 1 and 43% as grade 2; no grade 3 lesions were found. Intraductal tumor necrosis and microcalcifications were present in 26% and 38% of the cases, respectively. Atypical intraductal hyperplasia was present in adjacent mammary tissue in 36%. Pagetoid tumor cell infiltration within the epidermis was observed in one case.

In the French series, the size of the lesions was specified in 12 of 31 cases, ranging from 3 to 45 mm. However, in many cases, only few foci of DCIS were noted (18).

Estrogen and/or progesterone receptors in breast tumors are positive in about 85% and 75% of invasive MBC, respectively (a higher proportion than among women). However, no data on their expression are available in male DCIS. Similarly, no data are available on the incidence of overexpression of the C-erbB-2 oncoprotein and nuclear p53 protein accumulation in male DCIS.

No positive lymph nodes were found among the 19 patients in the French series who underwent axillary dissection (with an average of 12 recovered nodes) (18). Dissections were also negative for the three patients undergoing them in the Lahey Clinic series (33). In contrast, one case of axillary involvement among four patients undergoing dissection was found in the AFIP series (34).

TABLE 60.2. CLINICAL FEATURES OF MALE DUCTAL CARCINOMA IN SITU IN SELECTED SERIES

Characteristic	French Cancer Centers (18)	AFIP (34)	Lahey Clinic (33,35)
No. of cases	31	84	4
Median age (range) (years)	58 (26–74)	65 (25–94)	56 (53–69)
No. of patients younger than 40	6 (19%)	NA	0
First symptom			
Nipple discharge	12 (39%)	29 (35%)	1 (25%)
Mass	11 (35%)	49 (58%)	3 (75%)
Both nipple discharge and mass	4 (13%)	NA	0
Not specified	4 (13%)	NA	0
Gynecomastia	11 (35%)	16 (19%)	0
Median duration of symptoms (months)	3	2	9
Family history of breast cancer	3 (10%)	3 (4%)	NA

AFIP, Armed Forces Institute of Pathology; NA, not assessed.

TABLE 60.3. PREDOMINANT HISTOLOGY OF MALE DUCTAL CARCINOMA IN SITU IN SELECTED SERIES

Characteristic	French Cancer Centers (18)	AFIP (34)	Lahey Clinic (33,35)
Total no. of cases	31	84	4
Papillary	7 (23%)	40 (48%)	4 (100%)[a]
Cribriform	3 (10%)	16 (19%)	0
Papillary + cribriform	5 (16%)	23 (27%)	0
Apocrine	1 (3%)	0	0
Solid	0	5 (6%)	0
Comedo	3 (10%)	0	0
Not otherwise specified	12 (39%)	0	0

AFIP, Armed Forces Institute of Pathology.
[a] One papillary and three intracystic papillary.

PAGET'S DISEASE

Paget's disease results from the spread of intraductal carcinoma cells into the skin of the nipple and areola. Its estimated incidence varies from 3% to 5% of all breast cancer (37). Cytologically, a Paget's cell is a large pleomorphic cell with few intranuclear bridges containing a large, hyperchromatic nucleus and pale cytoplasm. The actual origin of Paget's cells is still debated. Some authors believe the cells are of pure intraepidermal origin, but the majority thinks that they originate from an intraductal cancer and spread to the nipple by migration.

Paget's disease of the male breast is extremely rare. Paget's disease was reported in eight cases among 385 patients (2%) with MBC in one series, but no details were given as to whether invasive cancer was present or not (11). In three other studies of MBC, Paget's disease represented approximately half of the cases of DCIS (15,25,31).

In a recent literature review, only five of 33 cases (15%) of Paget's disease were associated with pure DCIS rather than an underlying invasive cancer (38). The average age of these five patients was 63.6 years. Their first symptoms included nipple bleeding, irritation, ulceration, or erythema of the nipple. The duration of symptoms before diagnosis was highly variable. All five underwent mastectomy, with or without axillary dissection. Three were alive at 1, 3, and 5 years after surgery, respectively, but two patients were lost to follow-up.

RESULTS OF TREATMENT

Few data are published on the outcome of different therapies for male DCIS (Table 60.4) (18,25,33,39). Only one of 35 patients (3%) treated with simple, radical, or modified radical mastectomy suffered a local recurrence. In contrast, six of nine patients (67%) treated with lumpectomy or partial mastectomy without irradiation developed a local recurrence from 12 to 108 months after surgery. However, no details of margin status, histology, or other features were reported. Three recurrences were noninvasive (intracystic papillary in two cases), and three were already invasive. Two of these latter three patients also had extensive axillary nodal involvement found on dissection and subsequently developed metastases.

RISK OF CONTRALATERAL BREAST CANCER

To our knowledge, only two cases of metachronous contralateral DCIS of the male breast have been reported. In the French series (18), a 43-year-old patient presented with nipple discharge from the right breast 6 months after undergoing modified radical mastectomy for a left-sided papillary intracystic DCIS. Modified radical mastectomy was again performed. Histology showed a cribriform DCIS. He was still alive without disease 8 years after the second operation.

TABLE 60.4. LOCAL RECURRENCE AFTER TREATMENT OF MALE DUCTAL CARCINOMA IN SITU

Author/reference	Mastectomy	Lumpectomy	Lumpectomy + RT
Cutuli (18)	4% (1/25)[a]	60% (3/5)	0 (0/1)
Heller (25)	0 (0/8)	—	—
Camus (33)	0 (0/2)	100% (2/2)	—
Cole (39)	—	50% (1/2)	—

[a] Five patients underwent chest wall irradiation after mastectomy.
RT, radiation therapy.

CONCLUSIONS

DCIS in men is a very rare disease. As a result, there is little information about it. Because men do not undergo routine screening mammography, patients present with a palpable mass, nipple discharge, or both. Other clinical and histologic features of DCIS in men appear roughly similar to those of DCIS in women. Breast-conserving therapy has been increasingly used over the past years for women with DCIS, but for men the cosmetic aspects of treatment are of minor importance. Therefore, the optimal treatment for DCIS in men is simple mastectomy. Axillary dissection or sentinel node biopsy should not be performed, except perhaps for patients with lesions larger than 2.5 cm, because the risk of occult microinvasion increases with tumor size (40,41,42).

To date, 290 cases of pure DCIS have been reported in series dealing with MBC (Table 60.1) (7–34). The proportion of all cases of MBC that were DCIS varied from 0% to 17%, with an average of 7%. As observed in women, DCIS occurs in men earlier than invasive carcinoma (6 to 10 years earlier); similarly, DCIS is frequently associated with an infiltrating ductal carcinoma in both sexes. These facts suggest that DCIS represents the first step in the breast cancer process in both sexes. Therefore, a definitive treatment at this stage offers an excellent prognosis. Early diagnosis is important, and breast mass and/or bloody discharge in men require a thorough assessment.

REFERENCES

1. Axelsson J, Andersson A. Cancer of the male breast. *World J Surg* 1983;7:281–287.
2. Ravandi-Kashani F, Hayes TG. Male breast cancer: a review of the literature. *Eur J Cancer* 1998;34:1341–1347.
3. Gateley CA. Male breast disease. *The Breast* 1998;7:121–127.
3a. Lenfant-Pejovic MH, Cabanne NM, Bouchardy C, et al. Risk factors for male breast cancer: a Franco-Swiss case-control study. *Int J Cancer* 1990;45:661–665.
4. Spence R, Mackenzie G, Anderson JR, et al. Long term survival following cancer of the male breast in Northern Ireland. A report of 81 cases. *Cancer* 1985;55:648–651.
5. Cutuli BF, Lacroze M, Dilhuydy JM, et al. Male breast cancer. Results of the treatments and prognostic factors in 397 cases. *Eur J Cancer* 1995;31A:1960–1964.
6. Crichlow RW, Galt SW. Male breast cancer. *Surg Clin North Am* 1990;70:1165–1177.
7. Donegan WL, Redlich PN. Breast cancer in men. *Surg Clin North Am* 1996;76:343–363.
8. Visfeldt J, Scheike O. Male breast cancer. I. Histologic typing and grading of 187 Danish cases. *Cancer* 1973;22:985–990.
9. Erlichman C, Murphy KC, Elhakim T. Male breast cancer: a 13 year review of 89 patients. *J Clin Oncol* 1984;2:903–909.
10. Ramantanis G, Besbeas S, Garas JG. Breast cancer in the male: a report of 138 cases. *World J Surg* 1980;4:621–624.
11. Ribeiro GG, Swindell R, Harris M, et al. A review of the management of the male breast carcinoma based on an analysis of 420 treated cases. *The Breast* 1996;5:141–146.
12. Salvadori B, Saccozzi R, Manzari A, et al. Prognosis of breast cancer in males: an analysis of 170 cases. *Eur J Cancer* 1994;30A:930–935.
13. Scheike O. Male breast cancer. 5. Clinical manifestations in 257 cases in Denmark. *Br J Cancer* 1973;28:552–561.
14. Guinee VF, Olsson H, Moller T, et al. The prognosis of breast cancer in males. A report of 335 cases. *Cancer* 1993;71:154–161.
15. Goss PE, Reid C, Pintilie M, et al. Male breast carcinoma. A review of 229 patients who presented to the Princess Margaret Hospital during 40 years: 1955–1996. *Cancer* 1999;85:629–639.
16. Stierer M, Rosen H, Weitensfelder W, et al. Male breast cancer: Austrian experience. *World J Surg* 1995;19:687–693.
17. Treves N, Holleb A. Cancer of the male breast. A report of 146 cases. *Cancer* 1955;8:1239–1250.
18. Cutuli BF, Dilhuydy JM, De Lafontan B, et al. Ductal carcinoma in situ of the male breast: analysis of 31 cases. *Eur J Cancer* 1997;33:35–38.
19. Holleb AI, Freeman HP, Farrow JH. Cancer of the male breast I. *N Y State J Med* 1968;68:544–553.
20. Vanderbilt P, Warren SE. Forty year experience with carcinoma of the male breast. *Surg Gynecol Obstet* 1973;133:629–633.
21. Norris HJ, Taylor HB. Carcinoma of the male breast. *Cancer* 1969;23:1428–1435.
22. Gadenne C, Contesso G, Travagli JP, et al. Tumeurs du sein chez l'homme. Etude anatomo-clinique. 73 observations. *Nouv Presse Méd* 1982;11:2331–2334.
23. Langlands AO, Maclean N, Kerr GR. Carcinoma of the male breast: Report of a series of 88 cases. *Clin Radiol* 1976;27:21–25.
24. Vercoutere AL, O'Connell TX. Carcinoma of the male breast. An update. *Arch Surg* 1984;119:1301–1304.
25. Heller KS, Rosen PP, Schottenfeld D, et al. Male breast cancer: a clinicopathologic study of 97 cases. *Ann Surg* 1978;188:60–65.
26. Stranzl H, Mayer R, Quehenberger F, et al. Adjuvant radiotherapy in male breast cancer *Radiother Oncol* 1999;53:29–35.
27. Izquierdo MA, Alonso C, De Andres L, et al. Male breast cancer. Report of a series of 50 cases. *Acta Oncol* 1994;33:767–771.
28. Wang Y, Abreau M, Hoda S. Mammary duct carcinoma in situ in males: pathological findings and clinical considerations. *Mod Pathol* 1997;10:27A.
29. Tan PH, Sng IT. Male breast cancer: a retrospective study with immunohistochemical analysis of hormone receptor expression. *Pathology* 1997;29:2–6.
30. Hill A, Yagmour Y, Tran KN, et al. Localized male breast carcinoma and family history. An analysis of 142 patients. *Cancer* 1999;86:821–825.
31. Borgen PI, Wong GY, Vlamis V, et al. Current management of male breast cancer. A review of 104 cases. *Ann Surg* 1992;215:451–459.
32. Ouriel K, Lotze MT, Hinshaw JR. Prognostic factors of carcinoma of the male breast. *Surg Gynecol Obstet* 1984;159:373–376.
33. Camus MF, Joshi MG, Mackarem G, et al. Ductal Carcinoma in situ of the male breast. *Cancer* 1994;74:1289–1293.
34. Hittmair AP, Lininger RA, Tavassoli FA. Ductal carcinoma in situ (DCIS) in the male breast. A morphologic study of 84 cases of pure DCIS and 30 cases of DCIS associated with invasive carcinoma. A preliminary report. *Cancer* 1998;83:2139–2149.
35. Joshi MG, Lee AKC, Loda M, et al. Male breast carcinoma: an evaluation of prognosis factors contributing to a poorer outcome. *Cancer* 1996;77:490–498.
36. Bland RI, Page DL. Gynecomastia. In: Bland KI, Copeland EM, eds. *The Breast. Comprehensive Management of Benign and Malignant Diseases.* Philadelphia: WB Saunders, 1991:135–168.
37. Banerjee SN, Estabrook A, Schnabel FR. Surgical treatment of Paget's disease. In: Silverstein MJ, ed. *Ductal Carcinoma In Situ of the Breast.* Baltimore: Williams & Wilkins, 1997:551–554.
38. Desai DC, Brennan EJ, Carp NZ. Paget's disease of the male breast. *Am Surg* 1996;62:1068–1072.
39. Cole FM, Qizilbash AH. Carcinoma in situ of the male breast. *J Clin Pathol* 1979;32:1128–1134.

INTERSTITIAL THERAPY OF DUCTAL CARCINOMA IN SITU: WHERE DOES IT STAND?

DAVID S. ROBINSON

During the last decade, a six-fold increase in the number of women seeking screening mammography coupled with advances in imaging technology have yielded both a decreased average size of primary infiltrating carcinoma and a growing number of patients diagnosed with ductal carcinoma in situ (DCIS). Over this same time, progressive improvements in stereotactic biopsy technology have sparked an interest in image-guided, minimally invasive interstitial therapy (ITT). In the same way that automobiles of 100 years ago competed with one another in a protean array, ITT in its technological adolescence has taken several forms, including laser interstitial therapy (LITT) (1), radiofrequency (RF) ablation (2), cryotherapy (3), and the use of focused, directed external energy sources such as ultrasound. Where all of this will settle out remains to be seen.

Although attention has been directed thus far to treating small, primary infiltrating breast cancers, here we give consideration to interstitial therapy for ductal carcinoma in situ. Why not transpose the same ITT technology used to treat invasive cancer to the treatment of ductal carcinoma in situ? This would seem an obvious choice for those lesions of minimal volume that are currently being surgically excised. We will explore the existing technology, its biopsy and imaging requirements, and expectation of outcome with consideration of treating DCIS.

BIOLOGY OF INTERSTITIAL THERAPY

If a cancer is to be treated without being removed, then the means used to destroy it must be complete and thorough. The two approaches to this problem have both dealt with thermal change—heating (4) or cooling (5) the tumor. Laser interstitial therapy, radiofrequency, and external focused energy sources are designed to increase the temperature far above the physiologic norm to bring about perturbation of viable cellular metabolism, which leads to apoptosis and cell death of all tissue within the treatment field. This differs from the hyperthermic therapy of a quarter century ago. Previously, the goal was to destroy only the tumor cells, leaving normal tissues and architecture intact; the current goal is to bring the tissues to even higher temperatures in order to destroy not only the tumor cells but also their surrounding, supportive stroma (6). Cryotherapy involves a mechanical approach in which serial freezing and thawing disrupts the cancer cell's membranes, leading to death.

In LITT, near-infrared laser light is delivered by an optical fiber to the tissues, where laser radiation is absorbed and scattered by the tissue (7). Absorption of these photons and heat diffusion to the surrounding tissue creates a controlled heating zone with higher temperatures closer to the optical fiber. Cell death begins when the tissue temperature reaches 43°C and increases beyond that with protein denaturation and coagulation at temperatures between 50°C and 60°C. The volume of this denaturation and subsequent necrosis is a function of the thermal properties of the tissue, its vascular perfusion, the dispersion characteristics of the energy employed, the nature of the energy-tissue transition, the amount of power and duration of the administration, and the shape, size, and emission pattern of the optical probe itself.

The same basic tenants apply to hyperthermia delivered through a metal RF probe when the energy source is electrons rather than photons. For the treatment of complex tissues, the heat distribution through more and less dense tissues made up of different components such as fat, fibrous tissue, and blood vessels is a far more complicated determination than the evaluation of the cancer cells as a single component. Clearly, presence of a circulating blood volume alone will syphon away heat to some extent (8). For that reason and to achieve the goal of complete destruction of the tumor and its surrounding stroma, adaptation of a hyperthermic approach to interstitial therapy would be best applied by taking the temperature to a level above the point of known cell kill of both neoplastic and normal tissues. This should not be taken to the boiling point in the tissues because production of bubbles would change the direction of laser light or to an even higher level in which charring could lead to changes in the distribution of electrical and light energy. The desired goal is a zone of total tissue destruction around the cancer encompassing complete destruction of the cells and tissues within the field for a determined distance with a definitive, finite, sharp border that leaves tissues beyond the narrow zone undamaged (4). The present commercially available sources of RF, either through a single antenna or multiple antennae, and of LITT through a single laser fiberoptic probe with a defusing tip all aspire to achieve this end point. Bringing the tissue to between 50°C and 60°C would be appropriate for such a zone of necrosis.

Cryotherapy to bring about a rapid decrease in temperature by passing liquid nitrogen through a metal probe inserted into the tumor has adapted hardware using a larger probe (designed to treat liver metastases of colon cancer) to a smaller probe (for image guidance in the treatment of both benign breast lesions and primary breast cancer). Early reports indicate that a diminution of probe size and the ice sphere's volume would be necessary if this is to become a clinically useful approach.

THE CANCER

Clearly, when taking the initial steps into a new paradigm such as ITT, the optimal course would be to select a cancer that could be completely treated with a high probability of cure. Information in the literature suggests that smaller cancers would be preferable. Infiltrating duct cancers of 10 mm or less (T1a and T1b) treated with modified radical mastectomy alone in patients with no lymph node involvement have shown a 91% survivorship at 10 years (9). Low to intermediate-grade DCIS of a 10 mm diameter or smaller treated with wide excision also has a remarkable chance of cure (10). Thus, for both infiltrating and in situ carcinoma, if we were to select the tumor that would give us the best chance of demonstrating early ITT success, we would elect to treat tumors of 10 mm or less in the greatest diameter. Arguably, this poses a problem in patient accrual for early studies; using today's demographic analyses, approximately 60,000 women will have infiltrating cancers of an appropriate size for ITT in the United States each year. What fraction of the 35,000 diagnosed cases of DCIS would be small enough remains a guess. An inclusion of larger tumors accelerates accrual, but risks early failure in this developing technology. Although certainly not good for patients, clinical failures may also be critically viewed with alarm that

could lead to abandonment of this promising approach. It would be better to succeed early with smaller tumors and have a goal of expanding the trial to those eligible for treatment as the technology demonstrates its efficacy.

FIELD SIZE

Using the same clinical descriptions of optimal tumor size and depth of margin, the optimal field size appears to be a 10 mm radius of disease-free tissue circumferentially around the tumor. This is true for both infiltrating ductal carcinoma treated with lumpectomy and standard radiation therapy (11) and for ductal carcinoma in situ (10). Therefore, the optimal field size would encompass a tumor of 10 mm or less in diameter and an additional 10 mm completely around the tumor leading to a total diameter of approximately 3 cm. This depth may be decreased as efficacy is demonstrated with the "optimal" field of treatment. Thus, to be successful, the tumor must be at least 2 cm below the surface of the skin and have ample noninvolved tissue surrounding it that could be treated. Clearly, this becomes more difficult in both the thin patient with a smaller breast and in the older woman with very ptotic breasts.

PREVIOUS BIOPSY TECHNIQUE

Although the interstitial treatment of a small, primary breast cancer should offer the same level of cure as conventional excision, it probably will not decrease local recurrence or improve the rate of survival. Consequently, the only advantage is the enhanced cosmetic outcome that eliminates the skin incision and tissue removal and replaces it with a 2 to 3 mm incision site (for placement of the interstitial probe). This becomes important when considering which biopsy technique to employ in diagnosing the cancer. A standard excisional biopsy would leave a longer scar that could no longer merit the use of interstitial therapy. Therefore, in order for ITT to be a valuable treatment approach, patients must have had a stereotactically guided biopsy through a small incision (12); anything larger would be self defeating.

DETERMINATION OF THE VOLUME AND TEMPERATURE OF THE TREATMENT FIELD

If cryotherapy is used, the size of the treatment field is currently determined by ultrasonographic imaging (3,5). The treatment temperature is below the point of freezing, which gives rise to an ice ball that can be visualized. The actual temperature is not appreciable without introduction of a thermocouple, but that is not necessary in this setting because the formation of ice at 0°C is the goal. With LITT or RF, the size and temperature of the treatment field become significant to recognize the volume of heat distribution sphere around the cancer and to determine the temperatures within the field to bring about cell kill. A single thermal measurement probe at a known distance from the treatment probe can be placed to provide a quantitative and qualitative determination at that point (13). An assumption is made that the dispersion of heat is uniform and symmetrical through the heterogeneous tissues, creating a treatment sphere that is uniform in shape. A fiber optic probe has been used in LITT—not to determine temperature as much as to demonstrate a change of light distribution through tissue on denaturation. Metallic temperature probes, such as copper-constantan thermocouples, have been used to measure heat experimentally at different distances from the central treatment probe. Both fiberoptic and metallic probes can be attached to a computer for chart recording. In developing studies, the thermal field has been determined by a decrease in tissue density measured by digital mammography of tissue immobilized during the treatment period (14). The images of the tissue taken during and after the heat treatment are digitally subtracted from the pre-treatment image. With image enhancement, changes in density can demonstrate the heated area in a two-dimensional (2-D) field. Further modification of this technology will bring it to a point where it can be clinically tested in the near future.

IMAGING THE TUMOR

The disease itself or the biopsy site to be treated must be clearly seen, and the treatment probe must be placed to this site using image guidance. Where cryotherapy has employed ultrasound for cryoprobe placement, the stereotactic approach uses 2-D digital mammography images at two known angles to compute the coordinates within the breast for three-dimensional placement of either the laser fiberoptic cable or the radiofrequency probe. At the time of a stereotactic biopsy, it is important to leave a marker to later locate the lesion for treatment. This should allow highly accurate placement of the probe using digital mammographic guidance through a stereotactic technique. When a magnetic resonance imaging (MRI) nonmetallic biopsy instrument can be brought to clinical use, we may be able to place a treatment probe such as a laser fiberoptic cable with a proper diffusing tip for treatment (15). A metallic probe similar to those currently use for RF ablation would not be possible using MRI.

The same microcalcifications used to locate DCIS for biopsy may present a limitation in defining the field size for interstitial therapy of ductal carcinoma in situ. The small cluster of microcalcifications lying within the central domain of ductal carcinoma in situ often is left in the wake of the advancing phalanx of disease within a duct (16). Consequently, the leading edge of its progressive growth along ducts cannot be seen. For that reason, the true size of the lesion cannot necessarily be determined mammographically.

The placement of a treatment probe central to the site is certainly possible, but of major concern is the edge of the site of disease. How could we be certain that the entire area of DCIS was completely encompassed within the treatment sphere? One possible solution would be peripheral stereotactic core sampling taken at compass points at the edge of a treatment field to validate the absence of ductal carcinoma beyond the edge of the sphere.

An area of advancing technology that could provide an answer to this problem may be MRI. At present, this evolving technology appears very promising in the demonstration of ductal carcinoma in situ, but a detailed demonstration of true-positives and false-negatives has not yet been determined. When this technology becomes mature, it may well be appropriate for the placement of a fiberoptic laser cable, but it is less likely a metallic radiofrequency probe will be employed because of the interference of metal with the MRI signal (17).

SUMMARY

To date, infiltrating ductal carcinoma has been treated using a stereotactic approach with laser interstitial therapy through a fiberoptic cable, by a radio frequency beacon, and by cryotherapy placed intraoperatively using an ultrasound-guided approach. Preliminary feasibility studies are under way, but clinical prospective trials have not yet come to maturity. From reports available at present, several beams of externally focused ultrasound and other energy sources directed within the breast tissue have not produced a high enough temperature in a short time to induce total cell kill. Whether interstitial therapy can encompass the field of ductal carcinoma in situ, in which the edges cannot currently be well determined, remains to be seen. In the future, perhaps light-activated therapy of materials such as protoporphyrin injected along ducts may be useful, but that technology, too, has not reached a level of maturity where it would be appropriate for a clinical trial at this time.

Interstitial therapy for ductal carcinoma in situ has not yet been employed in clinical studies, but the available technology would be applicable for this disease if the volume of cancer can be imaged accurately enough to determine the appropriate treatment volume.

REFERENCES

1. Robinson DS, Parel JM, Denham DS, et al. Interstitial laser hyperthermia model development for minimally invasive therapy of breast carcinoma. *J Am Coll Surg* 1998;186:284–292.
2. Jeffrey SS, Birdwell RL, Ihedu DM, et al. Radiofrequency ablation of breast cancer: a first report of an emerging technology. *Arch Surg* 1999;134:1064–1068.
3. Staren ED, Sabel MS, Gianakakis LM, et al. Cryosurgery of breast cancer. *Arch Surg* 1997;132:28–32.
4. Schoben R, Bettag M, Sabel M, et al. Fine structure of zonal

changes in experimental ND:YAG laser-induced interstitial hyperthermia. *Lasers Surg Med* 1993;13:234–241.

5. Ravikumar TS, Kane R, Cady B, et al. A 5-year study of cryosurgery in the treatment of liver tumors. *Arch Surg* 1991;126:1520–1523.

6. Fajardo LF, Egbert B, Marmor J, et al. Effects of hyperthermia in a malignant tumor. *Cancer* 1980;45:613–623.

7. Milne PJ, Parel JM, Manns F, et al. Development of stereotactically guided laser interstitial thermotherapy of breast cancer: In situ measurement and analysis of the temperature field in ex vivo and in vivo adipose tissue. *Lasers Surg Med* 2000;26:67–75.

8. Lyng H, Monge OR, Bohler PJ, et al. The relevance of tumor and surrounding normal tissue vascular density in clinical hyperthermia of locally advanced breast carcinoma. *Int J Radiat Biol Phys* 1991;60:189–193.

9. Rosen PP, Groshen S, Kinne DW, et al. Factors influencing prognosis in node negative breast carcinoma: analysis of 767 $T_1N_0M_0/T_2N_0M_0$ patients with long term follow-up. *J Clin Oncol* 1993;11:2090–2100.

10. Silverstein MJ. Current management of noninvasive (in situ) breast cancer. *Adv Surg* 2000;34:17–41.

11. Barterlink H, Borger JH, vanDongen JA, et al. The impact of tumor size and histology on local control after breast-conserving therapy. *Radiother Oncol* 1988;11:297–303.

12. Burak WE Jr, Owens KE, Tighe MB, et al. Vacuum assisted stereotactic breast biopsy; histologic underestimation of malignant lesions. *Arch Surg* 2000;135:700–703.

13. Dowlatshahi K, Fan M, Sherkaloo M, et al. Stereotaxic interstitial laser therapy of early-stage breast cancer. *Breast J* 1996;2:304–311.

14. Minhaj AM, Manns F, Milne PJ, et al. X-ray monitoring of laser interstitial therapy (LITT) in ex vivo porcine tissue. SPIE Optical Engineering, Bellingham, Washington. Proceedings SPIE vol. 4244, p. 500–507, *Lasers in Surgery* 2001.

15. Harms SE. MR-guided minimally invasive procedures. *Magn Reson Imaging Clin N Am* 2001(May);9:381–392.

16. Ohtake T, Abe R, Kimijima I, et al. Intraductal extension of primary invasive breast carcinoma treated by breast conserving surgery; computer graphic three dimensional reconstruction of the mammary duct lobular systems. *Cancer* 1995;76:32–45.

17. Hall-Craggs MA. Interventional MRI of the breast: minimally invasive therapy. *Eur Radiol* 2000;10:59–62.

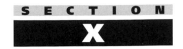

THE DUCTAL CARCINOMA IN SITU CONSENSUS CONFERENCES

THE EUROPEAN ORGANIZATION FOR RESEARCH AND TREATMENT OF CANCER DUCTAL CARCINOMA IN SITU CONSENSUS MEETINGS

EMIEL J. T. RUTGERS
ABRAM RECHT
NINA BIJKER

In the 'old days,' ductal carcinoma in situ (DCIS) was clinically detected with physical findings or symptoms (e.g., a mass or nipple discharge). It was treated in the same way as invasive cancer; that is, with mastectomy and axillary clearance. However, the increasing incidence of clinically occult DCIS during the last several decades, due to the widespread use of screening mammography, has triggered great interest in this particular form of breast cancer and has led investigators to conduct a multitude of trials.

These trials were designed predominantly to investigate aspects of breast-conserving therapy (BCT), for which little information was available. For example, in 1986, the European Organization for Research and Treatment of Cancer (EORTC) breast cancer group started a randomized trial (trial 10853) assessing the value of radiotherapy in patients with DCIS treated with complete local excision (see Chapter 43). However, many other questions also arose. What is the long-term outcome of BCT, i.e., is there any risk of death due to breast cancer? Will every lesion evolve to an invasive breast cancer, i.e., do subtypes with different clinical behavior exist that can be distinguished from one another? Do the randomized trials have sufficient statistical power to accurately assess outcomes for these subtypes? Can trials be grouped together into meta-analysis, or are the methodological differences between them so large that such an exercise is meaningless?

These questions prompted the EORTC breast cancer group, under the leadership of Joop van Dongen, to organize consensus meetings on DCIS. The aims of these meetings were three-fold:

to bring together a group of experts to try to answer the questions raised above;
to reach consensus on guidelines for managing DCIS; and

to bring together researchers working in the field of DCIS (both basic scientists and clinicians) to exchange experiences, look for new ways to answer unresolved questions, and help resolve problems in ongoing research activities.

This chapter describes the main foci and conclusions of the four EORTC DCIS consensus meetings. In an attempt to judge what impact these meetings had in the management of patients with DCIS, we analyzed the diagnostic and therapeutic procedures in patients entered in the EORTC DCIS trial and the treatment policies and outcome in five large centers during the period in which this trial was open. These results are also reported here. Because these consensus meetings were held during an 11-year period (1988 to 1998), they collectively provide a unique historical overview into the evolution of our concepts about DCIS and into how current clinical practice evolved.

THE 1988 MEETING

The main focus of this meeting, held in November 1988 near Amsterdam, was to inventory what were considered "established" facts about the biology and treatment of DCIS, and to review the retrospective clinical series and, more importantly, prospective trials on this subject (1). Consensus was achieved as to the following points:

i) DCIS constitutes 10% to 15% of all screen-detected cancers and 2% to 3% of all clinically detected cancers (data from hospital-based series).
ii) Mastectomy results in nearly 100% local control and cure rates.
iii) Local relapse rates of 5% to 30% are seen after BCT in series with relatively short follow-up.

iv) Nodal involvement is seen in 2% of cases. Therefore, a "watch policy" for the axilla is considered to be safe.

v) DCIS has a wide range of morphologic subtypes, which were felt to have different biologic behavior. The need for adopting a uniform classification system was stressed.

vi) Given the high percentage of DCIS found in contralateral "mirror" biopsies and in necropsy series, it is likely that not all DCIS evolves into clinically significant cancers.

vii) Over 50% of DCIS (both in clinically and screen-detected series available at the time) are over 5 cm in size and not suitable for treatment by BCT.

viii) The value of radiotherapy in BCT (in addition to wide local excision) is unknown. The indications for using radiotherapy cannot be determined from the available retrospective studies.

ix) The annual risk of developing an ipsilateral invasive breast cancer after biopsy showing lobular carcinoma in situ is 0.9%, comparable to that of developing a new contralateral primary cancer after treatment of an invasive ductal cancer. Ablative surgery (mastectomy) is considered excessive treatment for the majority of patients with LCIS, and "watchful waiting" is advised.

Part of the meeting was devoted to determining the meaning of an extensive intraductal component (EIC) in relation to the risk of recurrence after BCT for invasive cancers. It was concluded that EIC was not a risk factor for recurrence if complete excision was performed (i.e., uninvolved histologic margins).

THE 1991 MEETING

This meeting, held in Leuven, Belgium in September 1991, was largely devoted to discussing

the clinical, pathologic, and biologic factors pertinent to managing DCIS,

the assessment of lesion size and margin involvement, and

the methodological aspects of ongoing prospective trials (2).

Correlations were shown between the mammographic appearance, architectural growth patterns, and biologic characteristics of DCIS, but the relationships were by no means uniform or constant. The available evidence from retrospective studies was considered insufficient to use any of these characteristics (other than tumor size and the completeness of excision) to decide between the treatment options of wide local excision alone, excision plus radiotherapy, or mastectomy.

It was agreed that accurately measuring tumor size is extremely difficult for DCIS.

Traditional clinical and pathologic measurements of size (i.e., the largest diameter of a palpable lesion or gross mass in the excised specimen) are not applicable to screen-detected lesions. The mammographic extent of microcalcifications (particularly small, rounded ones, usually associated with well-differentiated DCIS) often markedly underestimates the pathologic spread of the lesion. Thus, mammography in itself is not sufficient to accurately measure the size of DCIS. However, pathologic estimation of size was also considered to present difficult problems, particularly because of the lack of a standardized approach to this task. Therefore, the group felt strongly that having a standardized protocol for pathologic evaluation of DCIS is mandatory, including inking of the margins, slicing of a properly-oriented specimen at fixed intervals, and obtaining specimen radiography to guide the cutting of slides for histologic review. There was strong consensus that a number of histologic features should be documented routinely by the pathologist to allow eventual analysis of their impact on treatment outcome (Table 62.1). Assessment of specimen margins is critical, and the distance of tumor from the inked specimen edges should be quantitatively recorded. However, there were insufficient clinical data to define what constitutes a truly "free" or "negative" margin (i.e., one where there is a minimum risk of DCIS left after local excision).

At the time of the meeting, eight randomized trials for patients with DCIS were open. Seven trials randomized patients to observation or radiation therapy after excision with negative margins. Two trials randomized between taking tamoxifen or a placebo in addition to BCT; one of these also randomized patients between observation and radiotherapy, using a 2 × 2 design. However, many of these trials were accruing patients very slowly. The main reasons for this were

TABLE 62.1. CONSENSUS ON HISTOLOGIC FEATURES TO BE EVALUATED

Should be described routinely
  Tumor size
  Margin involvement
  Nuclear grade
  Size
  Pleomorphism
  Mitoses
  Necrosis
  Architecture

Description optional
  Nuclear features: chromatin pattern; nucleoli
  Microcalcifications
  Host reaction (cellular or stromal)

Additional studies of interest
  Oncogenes (especially c-erbB-2)
  Hormone receptors
  Ploidy
  Morphometric analysis

felt to be that 40% to 60% of the DCIS were considered too large for BCT, the varying availability of mammographic screening, and the increasing reluctance of physicians and patients to enter trials.

In any event, results from these prospective trials were not yet available, and hence could not be used to devise evidence-based treatment guidelines. It was also felt that treatment guidelines could not be derived from the existing retrospective studies, due to

the heterogeneity of the patients included in them,

the changing biology of DCIS during the periods of patient accrual (due to the advent of screening),

the shifting indications for different treatments over time, and

insufficient length of follow-up.

In particular, treatment recommendation could not be given for particular subtypes of DCIS.

THE 1994 MEETING

A major topic of this meeting, held in Venice in February 1994, was the subclassification of DCIS (3). Was it possible to classify DCIS in a reproducible and objective manner that would predict treatment outcome? Due to the lack of consistent outcome data for any of the proposed classifications, no consensus on this point could be reached. Again, it was stressed that the histologic evaluation should be standardized, adequate margin assessment should be performed, and that all the features of DCIS listed in Table 62.1 should be described in the pathology report.

Ongoing biologic studies were described at this meeting. These incited intense interest but were not felt to give sufficient clues as to the clinical behavior of DCIS to be useful yet in patient management.

The National Surgical Adjuvant Breast and Bowel Project (NSABP) B-17 trial, which was the first trial to be published, was extensively discussed. An updated report of this trial with an average follow-up time of 57 months was given. This trial clearly showed the value of adjuvant radiotherapy in reducing the risk of ipsilateral invasive breast recurrences (see Chapter 42). Despite this positive result, it was felt that the indications for using radiotherapy in BCT for patients with DCIS were far from being settled given the relatively short follow-up and the lack of adequate subgroup analysis to distinguish subgroups that may hardly benefit from radiotherapy.

Progress reports were also given on nonrandomized retrospective studies and the other randomized trials still underway. These were felt, again, to be very interesting but still not sufficient (for the same reasons noted above) to allow specific treatment recommendations. Substantial differences in outcome were seen not only between studies from different institutions, but also for earlier and later studies from the same institutions!

THE 1998 MEETING

There were two main questions at this meeting, held near Amsterdam in January 1998 (4).

First, can we identify subtypes of DCIS that have a low risk of local recurrence when patients are treated with breast-conserving surgery without radiotherapy, or, should initial BCT fail, for which the likelihood of developing a potentially life-threatening invasive cancer are small?

Second, how can we optimally treat patients with BCT so as to minimize their risks of recurrence while still attempting to maximize the quality of their lives?

By this meeting, a lot more information was available from the retrospective studies, but no data were yet available from randomized trials, except for the NSABP B-17 trial. Agreement could be reached by the participants on a large number of points. The most important are summarized as follows:

i) There is a high chance (approximately 50%, averaged over all subtypes) that DCIS that has not been completely eradicated will be associated with an invasive breast cancer by the time of clinical recurrence.

ii) Indirect evidence suggests that when DCIS recurs with an invasive component, the grade of the latter is likely to reflect the grade of the initial DCIS. Consequently, a local recurrence resulting from initial breast-conserving therapy of a low-grade DCIS probably has less lethal potential than that after treatment of a high-grade DCIS. However, further prospective and retrospective studies were felt needed to confirm this contention.

iii) The pathologic reporting of DCIS according to the criteria outlined at the Philadelphia Consensus Conference in April 1997 was endorsed (5). However, neither the Philadelphia conference nor this gathering committed themselves to a preferred classification scheme for general use.

iv) The risk of patients dying of breast cancer appeared to be numerically similar for atypical ductal hyperplasia, atypical lobular hyperplasia, lobular carcinoma in situ, and low-grade DCIS.

v) Core-needle biopsy reduces the need for open surgical biopsy when the histologic findings are unequivocally benign and correspond to the clinical and radiologic features of the case. However, core biopsies that show only ADH may be markers of an underlying DCIS or invasive cancer and should lead to open biopsy. Similarly, invasive cancer may be present when core-needle biopsy shows only DCIS.

vi) Approximately 20% of patients will have involved microscopic resection margins on the initial attempt at excision, even when performed by experienced surgeons. Improved radiologic, surgical, and pathologic techniques that decrease this proportion should be sought and, when found, widely adopted.

vii) The use of electrocautery in BCT was condemned, because it makes adequate pathologic evaluation of specimen margins much more difficult.

viii) The risk of relapse after BCT depends predominantly on microscopic margin width, histologic features, and probably tumor size, particularly when radiotherapy is not used. No consensus existed as to precisely which groups of patients can be treated with surgery alone.

ix) Patients with extensive high-grade DCIS should undergo mastectomy. However, there is interest as to whether BCT can be used for patients with extensive low-grade lesions without facing excessive risk of ultimately developing a fatal invasive breast cancer.

x) Adjuvant therapies may allow patients to be successfully treated with BCT who cannot be treated with breast-conserving surgery alone without the use of such wide excision that the cosmetic results would be unacceptable. However, the value of adjuvant therapies depends not only on the magnitude of the residual tumor burden after surgery but on the evolutionary potential of the lesion and its responsiveness to such therapy.

xi) With regard to patient management outside a trial or protocol, it was generally felt that patients with "small" lesions (less than 2 to 3 cm) with "low-grade" DCIS that is "widely excised" will be likely to do well after surgery alone; therefore, offering such patients a "wait and see" option is reasonable, provided that careful follow-up is performed. However, there was no consensus as to precisely how to define these terms and on which subgroups of patients can be adequately treated with surgery alone. Radiotherapy should probably play a more important role in the management of patients with intermediate or high-grade DCIS, although some of these patients may also be adequately treated with surgery alone. Regardless of grade or the planned use of radiotherapy, when cosmetically acceptable, re-excision should be performed when margins are incompletely excised. Otherwise, simple mastectomy (with or without immediate reconstruction) may be superior.

VARIATIONS IN DIAGNOSTIC AND THERAPEUTIC PROCEDURES: RESULTS FROM A QUALITY CONTROL PROJECT OF THE EUROPEAN ORGANIZATION FOR RESEARCH AND TREATMENT OF CANCER TRIAL 10853

From October 1995 until March 1996, thirty of the forty-six institutes participating in the EORTC trial 10853 on DCIS underwent a site visit from at least one of the members of the EORTC DCIS task force (6). The aim of these

visits was to perform a quality check on all data collected and sent to the central data center. The medical records of 842 patients were reviewed. Patients were entered from 1986 to 1995. Detailed data regarding clinical presentation, mammographic findings, surgical procedures, pathologic findings, and the delivery of radiotherapy were retrieved and analyzed.

DCIS was detected by clinical symptoms in 28% of patients (20% with palpable lesions, 8% with nipple discharge) and in 72% by mammography (one-third from patients participating in screening projects). Only 10% of the patients with mammographic microcalcifications underwent additional magnification views, and only 49% of the mammogram reports estimated the size of the abnormality. In 90% of patients with mammographically detected lesions, a specimen x-ray was performed to document the excision of the mammographic abnormality.

Table 62.2 lists the surgical procedures performed. In 29% of the cases, the surgeon performed cavity shavings, random biopsies, or re-excisions immediately during surgery to check for completeness of excision. Two-thirds of patients had more than one excised specimen. Twenty percent (166 patients) had axillary lymph node sampling or clearance. Interestingly, whether an axillary procedure was performed was related to whether frozen section was employed. When frozen section was performed and showed "malignancy," 18 of 20 such patients had an axillary node dissection. If frozen section showed DCIS, 33% of patients had dissection. Only 6% of patients for whom frozen section was not performed (54% of the cases) underwent dissection. These results clearly showed that frozen section should not be performed for lesions considered to be DCIS.

Pathologic procedures varied substantially (Table 62.3). In particular, inking of the margins and performing mammography of sections of lesions were performed only in a minority of patients. Gross microscopic size was mentioned in 28% of the pathology reports, and the microscopic size of the lesion was reported in only 11%. Margin status was not noted in 14% of cases.

TABLE 62.2. SURGICAL PROCEDURES PERFORMED IN REVIEWED CASES IN THE EORTC DCIS TRIAL

Procedure	No. of Patients (%)
Breast surgery	
Single simple excision	299 (36)
Shaving of biopsy cavity	239 (29)
Two-step procedure	279 (34)
More than two steps	7 (1)
Axillary dissection	166 (20)
Sampling	105 (63)
Complete	52 (31)
Unknown	9 (5)

TABLE 62.3. HISTOLOGIC PROCESSING AND EVALUATION PERFORMED IN REVIEWED CASES IN THE EORTC DCIS TRIAL

Processing and Evaluation	No. of Patients (%)
Histological measurement	
Macroscopic size	228 (28)
Microscopic size	138 (17)
Conclusive size	94 (11)
Microscopic or conclusive size[a]	187 (23)
Any size reported	368 (45)
Inking of specimen	
No	594 (72)
Yes	206 (25)
Unknown	24 (3)
Use of specimen radiography for selecting sections for histology (mammographically detected lesions only)	
No	495 (84)
Yes	78 (13)
Unknown	18 (3)
Margin status	
"Free"	213 (26)
Exact distance reported	38 (5)
Re-excision showed no residual tumor	179 (22)
"Surrounded by normal breast tissue"	7 (1)
Shaving of biopsy cavity	208 (25)
"Near/doubtful/not sure/not evaluable"	37 (4)
Involved	4 (0.5)
Not reported	116 (14)
Unknown	22 (3)

[a] Microscopic and/or conclusive (size as concluded by the pathologist) size given in report.

This study shows that substantial variations in diagnostic and therapeutic procedures existed in the EORTC trial. This trial was designed in 1984 when there was relatively limited knowledge of the biology of DCIS and the risk factors for recurrence after BCT. Since then, more insight has been gained into the optimal diagnostic and therapeutic approach. With 46 participating institutes, numerous participating radiologists, surgeons, pathologists, radiation oncologists, and patient entry over a span of 10 years, it is not surprising that it was difficult to maintain protocol compliance. As a result, it is likely that the results of the trial reflect this heterogeneity. These variations will *not* influence the main goal of the trial, i.e., the evaluation of the effect of radiotherapy in BCT for DCIS, as it may be assumed that these variations will be balanced between the two randomization arms. However, the risk of local recurrence may be directly related to the quality of the initial evaluation and surgery. Complete excision of a nonpalpable lesion is a technically difficult procedure and requires expertise. The present study shows large variations in surgical procedures.

This supports the need for clearly defined guidelines for BCT for DCIS, with special emphasis on the surgical procedure and the pathologic workup. If the quality of the surgical procedure is an important prognostic factor for the outcome of treatment, quality assurance is of the utmost importance.

TREATMENT OF DUCTAL CARCINOMA IN SITU IN FIVE LARGE EUROPEAN ORGANIZATION FOR RESEARCH AND TREATMENT OF CANCER CENTERS: ARE THE OUTCOMES DIFFERENT BETWEEN PATIENTS TREATED IN OR OUTSIDE OF THE TRIAL?

The consensus meetings repeatedly emphasized the importance of treating patients with DCIS within prospective randomized trials. It was also stressed that there was no evidence that treatment decisions could be made on the basis of subtype. Therefore, we decided to investigate what proportion of eligible patients were actually entered the EORTC DCIS trial, and why patients were not entered (7). Further, we were anxious to know whether there was any difference in outcome between patients treated with BCT within or outside the trial. For this purpose, we needed to analyze an unselected, prospectively-registrated cohort of patients with DCIS. Five centers participating in the EORTC 10853 DCIS trial routinely recorded the incidence, treatment, and outcome of all cancer cases. These five institutes (the Centre Henry Becquerel in Rouen, the Policlinico di Careggi in Florence, Guy's Hospital in London, the Institut Bergonié in Bordeaux, and the Netherlands Cancer Institute in Amsterdam) entered 27% of all patients on the trial.

During the period of participation in the trial, 910 patients were diagnosed with DCIS and treated in the five institutes (Table 62.4), constituting, on average, 7% of all breast cancer cases. Of those 910 patients, 477 (52%) were ineligible for the study. The ineligibility rate ranged from 44% to 66% between the institutions. The main reasons for ineligibility were the size of the lesion, margin involvement, patient age (older than 70 years), or a history of an earlier or simultaneous contralateral breast cancer. Of the eligible patients, 64% entered the trial (range, 41% to 100%). Patient refusal and physician preference were the most important reasons why patients did not enter. One center preferred to treat patients with comedo-type DCIS with mastectomy or excision plus radiotherapy. Consequently, 78% of randomized patients from this institute had well-differentiated DCIS, although in other institutes the proportion of the three subtypes was more equal. Two other institutes preferred to treat well-differentiated DCIS without radiotherapy: Fifty-two of the 54 eligible but nonparticipating patients with well-differentiated DCIS had local excision alone.

TABLE 62.4. ELIGIBILITY AND ENTRY THE EORTC DCIS TRIAL FOR FIVE STUDY INSTITUTIONS

	Institute					Total	p Value
	A	B	C	D	E		
Years of participation	86–96	92–95	86–96	90–95	86–96	86–96	—
No. DCIS/year	22	10	25	58	10	125	—
No. operable breast cancer/year	320	200	465	595	155	1735	—
% DCIS	7%	5%	5%	10%	7%	7%	< 0.001
Total patients with DCIS	224	40	252	292	102	910	—
% entered of eligible	41%	100%	76%	61%	66%	64%	< 0.001
Not entered due to patient refusal (% of eligible)	27 (36)	0 (0)	3 (2)	5 (3)	6 (14)	41 (9)	— < 0.001
Not entered due to doctor preference (% of eligible)	18 (24)	0 (0)	28 (22)	59 (36)	9 (20)	114 (26)	— < 0.001

Values in parentheses are percentages.
DCIS, ductal carcinoma in situ.

Of the 910 patients, 60% were treated with BCT. The proportion of patients who were treated conservatively outside the trial was similar in four institutes (30% to 36%), although in one institute this rate was 60%. The median follow-up for the trial patients was 51 months; it was 39 months for non-trial patients. Follow-up was complete for 96% of all patients.

Treatment results are given in Table 62.5. After mastectomy (usually performed for extensive lesions), the 4-year

TABLE 62.5. ACTUARIAL 4-YEAR RATES OF FREEDOM FROM LOCAL RECURRENCE IN PATIENTS ENTERED IN THE EORTC DCIS TRIAL, THOSE ELIGIBLE BUT NOT PARTICIPATING, AND THOSE INELIGIBLE IN THE FIVE STUDY INSTITUTIONS

	Treatment		
	M	LE	LE + RT
Entered in EORTC DCIS trial			
No. of patients	—	135	133
No. of events	—	19	12
4-year FFLR (%)	—	89	98
Eligible but not participating			
No. of patients	33	93	29
No. of events	0	6	4
4-year FFLR (%)	100	93	74
Ineligible			
No. of patients	329	83	65
No. of events	5	11	6
4-year FFLR (%)	98	85	86

FFLR, freedom from local recurrence; LE, local excision; LE + RT, local excision plus radiotherapy; M, mastectomy.

actuarial rate of freedom from local recurrence was 98%. For patients treated with local excision alone, this rate did not vary significantly between ineligible patients (85%), patients eligible for but not participating in the trial (93%), or patients treated in the trial (89%). When nonparticipating patients treated with local excision alone (whether eligible or ineligible) were grouped together, the rates were the same as the patients who were treated in the trial (both 89%). Larger differences were seen when patients were treated with local excision plus radiotherapy; rates of freedom from local failure were 86%, 74%, and 98% in the three groups, respectively. When nonparticipating patients treated with local excision and radiotherapy (whether eligible or ineligible) were grouped together, their local control rate was substantially lower than those patients entered in the trial and randomized to local excision plus radiotherapy (83% versus 98%, *p* = 0.031).

This study showed that only approximately 70% of patients with DCIS seen during this period could be offered BCT. Only two-thirds of eligible patients were entered in the trial, with the reasons for nonparticipation varying substantially between the centers. The observed selection with respect to histologic subtype was especially disconcerting. Randomized patients treated with local excision plus radiotherapy had better local control rates than patients treated outside the trial. This indicates that the quantitative overall result of this trial (i.e., the reduction of the 4-year local recurrence rate by 38% by the addition of radiotherapy to local excision) might not be generalized to all patients with DCIS eligible for BCT. Therefore, our findings indicate the importance of prospective registration and follow-up of nonrandomized patients for evaluating the applicability of the trial results to the general population with the disease.

CONCLUSIONS

This chapter shows that much has been learned about DCIS over the last 13 years, but there are still many unresolved questions. The most important lesson is that if DCIS is to be treated with BCT, the risk of local relapse is predominantly related to the completeness of the resection as measured by margin status, and that this risk can be substantially reduced by the addition of radiotherapy to local excision. However, performing a 'complete' resection is the most difficult part of the overall treatment program. It is still not clear how to optimally interpret the results of breast imaging results, how technically to perform a complete resection, how to assess the margin status, and what the optimal definition of a complete resection should be. Over half of the patients with DCIS still are treated with mastectomy.

The risk of recurrence does not appear to be strongly related to the subtype of DCIS. However, the majority of patients who eventually develop metastatic disease after BCT for DCIS had an ipsilateral invasive breast cancer that developed from a poorly differentiated DCIS. In this regard, it is disturbing to see that, even in experienced centers, patients treated with BCT and RT outside a trial ('the real world') have an 11% breast relapse rate at four years. Half of them will have an invasive cancer. It is still unknown to what extent performing BCT in patients with DCIS will result in an excess of breast-cancer related deaths, as compared with initial treatment with mastectomy.

Substantial insight into the biology of DCIS has been gained during this period. Morphologic features have been found to correlate (although by no means perfectly) with molecular characteristics and genetic changes. But there is still too little known about these matters to translate this knowledge into better strategies for managing patients with DCIS.

At present, the main conclusion from these consensus meetings is that patients with DCIS should be treated by a multidisciplinary team. Optimizing the outcome of patients depends on the experience and cooperation of all members of this team:

the radiologist (optimal imaging for preoperative diagnosis and characterization of the lesion, as well as aid in excising nonpalpable lesions);

the surgeon (experience and skill in translating knowledge of the growth pattern of DCIS into an "anatomical" segmental or sector resection, which achieves adequate margins while preserving good cosmesis);

the pathologist (optimal histologic workup that provides all relevant information);

the radiation oncologist (information about the pros and cons of radiation therapy); and

the medical oncologist (information about the pros and cons of adjuvant tamoxifen).

Every woman with DCIS may ask for, and deserves, such a team.

REFERENCES

1. Van Dongen JA, Fentiman IS, Harris JR, et al. In-situ breast cancer: the EORTC consensus meeting. *Lancet* 1989;2:25–27.
2. Van Dongen JA, Holland R, Peterse JL, et al. Ductal carcinoma in-situ of the breast: second EORTC consensus meeting. *Eur J Cancer* 1992;28A:626–629.
3. Recht A, van Dongen JA, Fentiman IS, et al. Third meeting of the DCIS Working party of the EORTC (Fondazione Cini, Isola S. Giorgo, Venezia, 28 February 1994)-conference report. *Eur J Cancer* 1994;30A:1895–1901.
4. Recht A, Rutgers EJ, Fentiman IS, et al. The fourth EORTC DCIS consensus meeting (Château Marquette, Heemskerk, The Netherlands, 23–24 January 1998)-conference report. *Eur J Cancer* 1998;34:1664–1669.
5. Consensus Conference Committee. Consensus conference on the classification of ductal carcinoma in situ. *Cancer* 1997;80:1798–1802.
6. Bijker N, Rutgers EJ, Peterse JL, et al. Variations in diagnostic and therapeutic procedures in a multicenter randomized clinical trial (EORTC 10853) investigating breast conserving treatment for DCIS. *Eur J Surg Oncol* 2001;27:135–140.
7. Bijker N, Peterse JL, Fentiman IS, et al. "Effects of patient selection on the applicability of results from a randomized clinical trial (EORTC 10853). Investigating breast conserving treatment for DCIS." In: Bijker N, thesis, University of Amsterdam, 2000:61.

63

THE CLASSIFICATION AND TREATMENT OF DUCTAL CARCINOMA IN SITU OF THE BREAST: SUMMARY OF THE 1997 AND 1999 CONSENSUS CONFERENCES

GORDON FRANCIS SCHWARTZ

Ductal carcinoma in situ (DCIS) constitutes a spectrum of noninvasive but malignant epithelial lesions confined within the basement membrane of the ducts of the breast. As screening mammograms have become commonplace, this diagnosis has emerged from relative obscurity a generation ago to represent currently up to one-fourth of breast cancer diagnoses in some institutions. Although lacking the ability to metastasize *sui generis*, it has been considered an initial step in a process that may potentially progress to invasive cancer if not treated. For this reason, until the late 1970s, mastectomy was standard treatment.

As greater knowledge about the behavior of DCIS has become available and in keeping pace with treatment changes for invasive cancer, the goal of treatment for DCIS evolved so that most women with DCIS are currently treated with breast conservation with or without radiation therapy. Mastectomy is reserved for selected cases of DCIS or if the patient demands it. Adding tamoxifen to whichever treatment option is chosen has also emerged within the last several years, hopefully to reduce the risk of recurrence in the ipsilateral breast and to reduce the risk of a new primary lesion in the contralateral breast. Differences in treatment recommendations abound because physicians have been unable to determine precisely which patients with DCIS fit best into each of these treatment categories, and if any women are well served by a recommendation for treatment that does not include the whole breast. Additionally, pathologists do not agree on the features that define DCIS or those histologic or other characteristics that might predict risk of recurrence of further DCIS or invasive cancer. It is not, therefore, surprising that optimal treatment has become equally controversial.

To try to establish reasonable guidelines to help physicians who encounter these patients to sift through the myriad of information available, two DCIS consensus conferences were convened in Philadelphia; the first occurred in April 1997 to focus on the classification of DCIS, and the second was in April 1999 to discuss treatment. Both of these conferences were sponsored by the Breast Health Institute and the Fashion Group International—Philadelphia, and brought together recognized "experts" in DCIS, representing the disciplines of surgical oncology, radiation oncology, medical oncology, breast imaging (radiology), pathology, epidemiology, and biostatistics. Consensus was achieved at both of these meetings, and the proceedings of the conferences were subsequently published concurrently in three peer-reviewed journals (1,2).

These two conferences limited their discussions to DCIS only, recognizing the occasional difficulties in separating DCIS from atypical ductal hyperplasia (ADH) on one end of the spectrum, and DCIS from microinvasive ductal carcinoma (pT1mic) on the other. Treatment of these two conditions was not part of the conference discussions, nor was lobular carcinoma in situ (LCIS) except as it might occur as an incidental finding in a biopsy that disclosed DCIS. (With respect to the latter, the finding of LCIS should not influence the treatment of DCIS.) The following information is a condensed summary of these two consensus conferences, with additional editorial comments.

THE MICROSCOPIC CLASSIFICATION OF DUCTAL CARCINOMA IN SITU

The traditional classification of DCIS had formerly been on the basis of architecture, but newer systems to stratify DCIS are based primarily on nuclear grade and secondarily on the presence and amount of necrosis and cell polarization. Any classification of DCIS should reflect the biologic potential for local recurrence and/or progression to invasive carcinoma. Pathology reports should document the following:

  i) Nuclear grade.
  ii) Necrosis.

iii) Polarization.
iv) Architectural pattern(s).

The following additional information should also be documented in pathology reports:

v) Margins (distance from any margin to the nearest focus of DCIS, and focal or diffuse involvement of margins.
vi) Size (extent and size of DCIS).
vii) Microcalcifications associated with DCIS and those outside the area of DCIS.
viii) Correlation of tissue specimens with specimen x-ray and mammographic findings.

Nuclear grade is considered the most important single characteristic of DCIS to predict outcome, so stratifying DCIS by nuclear grade leads to the following definitions:

I. Low-grade nuclei (NG1).
   A. Appearance: Monotonous, monomorphic.
   B. Size: 1.5 to 2.0 normal red blood cell (RBC) or duct epithelial nucleus dimensions.
   C. Features: Diffuse, finely dispersed chromatin, occasional nucleoli and mitotic figures; (Caveat: The presence of pleomorphic nuclei precludes a low-grade classification even if of similar size).
II. High-grade nuclei (NG3).
   A. Appearance: Markedly pleomorphic.
   B. Size: Nuclei usually more than 2.5 RBC or duct epithelial cell nuclear diameters.
   C. Features: Usually vesicular and exhibit irregular chromatin distribution and prominent, often multiple, nucleoli. Mitoses may be conspicuous.
III. Intermediate-grade nuclei (NG2). Nuclei that do not fit into either NG1 or NG3.

Necrosis probably increases the risk associated with nuclear grade. True necrosis, however, should be distinguished from secretory material by the presence of ghost cells and karyorrhectic debris. Necrosis should be quantified as comedonecrosis (any central zone necrosis within a duct, usually exhibiting a linear pattern if sectioned longitudinally) or as punctate necrosis (nonzonal foci of necrosis that do not exhibit this linear pattern when sectioned longitudinally).

Cell polarization reflects the radial orientation of the apical portion of tumor cells toward intercellular spaces. The presence of this feature is characteristic of lower grade DCIS.

These features, i.e., nuclear grade, necrosis, and cell polarization, may not apply to a small proportion of DCIS cases. For these, stratification has not yet been established.

Although architecture alone does not satisfactorily stratify DCIS with regard to outcome, the traditional terms that have been used should also be cited in the pathology report, in the order of decreasing amounts, because several patterns may coexist in the same specimen. These include comedo, cribriform, papillary, micropapillary, and solid. Necrosis

may occur in any of these patterns. The term "comedo" refers specifically to solid intraepithelial growth within the basement membrane with central (zonal) necrosis. Such lesions are often but not invariable of high nuclear grade. This is a major departure from prior classification systems that used "comedo" to indicate both central necrosis and high nuclear grade. Nuclear grade and architecture should be separately documented.

DCIS may exhibit heterogeneity of nuclear grade, and it is not certain how the relative proportions of each nuclear grade may affect outcome. Therefore, any report should note the nuclear grades present and the proportions of each when possible.

SIZE (EXTENT, DISTRIBUTION) AND MARGINS

Several methods exist to assess size of the area of DCIS and the adequacy of the margins around the area. Previously, the traditional surgical procedure has been a needle-guided (also known as wire-directed) localization and excision of an area of calcifications. A specimen radiograph confirms the successful excision of the suspicious area. In the last few years, less invasive procedures have become more popular as the initial biopsy step, but irrespective of the mode of detection and diagnosis, if breast conservation is chosen, the definitive surgical step is the local excision of the area of calcifications.

Whenever possible, the specimen must be oriented by the surgeon for the pathologist, correlating the specimen radiography with the preoperative films. A metallic clip placed in the specimen at or near the site of calcifications may help. If the surgical margins are not submitted as individual specimens, the surfaces of the specimen should be inked in some reproducible manner to permit orientation of the specimen. If margins are not separately submitted, the surfaces of the specimen should be inked to permit orientation of the specimen, whether by one color or several. The principle is the identification of the margins to measure distance from the surgical margins to any focus of DCIS.

The specimen can be processed in several ways but, when feasible, the entire specimen should be processed in sequence in separate cassettes after being "breadloafed" into 2 to 3 mm sections. Another technique is to section the specimen and x-ray the slices; only those exhibiting the radiographic abnormality and adjacent ones are further processed. Remaining tissue is then examined only when DCIS is identified in the initial sections. Using this technique, the margins of the specimen are determined by measuring the distance between the DCIS and the closest inked resection margin.

An alternative technique is to shave the margins of the biopsy cavity as arcs of tissue following the contour of the cavity, as if peeling an onion from the inside out. The separate marginal biopsies are labeled, submitted, and processed separately. Any involvement within the tissue submitted is considered a positive margin. Using this technique, if a single margin is positive, it may be addressed at a subsequent procedure if breast conservation is employed, because the exact location of the positive margin is unequivocal. This is our personal preference for margin assessment, because trying to paint India ink or other colored inks onto the surface(s) of a specimen is like trying to paint the surface of an English muffin! Moreover, when the specimen is excised from the breast, its edges always retract toward the center, and the margins may appear narrower than they were *in vivo*. Moreover, the surgeon is concerned about what is left behind, not by what has been removed. The additional shaving of margins offers this information without equivocation.

TREATMENT CONSIDERATIONS

The first consensus conference concluded with the above classification of DCIS being accepted, along with the techniques of measuring size and determining margin status. Once consensus had been reached on these fundamental issues, attention could then be directed to diagnosis and therapy. DCIS is usually detected by mammography as a screening examination in an asymptomatic woman or for another unrelated reason. The diagnosis of DCIS as a palpable mass or as nipple discharge was not discussed, except in the context of a mammographic finding. Although other imaging techniques are currently used for the detection of breast abnormalities, such as ultrasound, digital mammography, and magnetic resonance imaging (MRI), none is a current substitute for a high-quality, film-screen mammogram. Digital mammography and MRI are potentially the most helpful, and both are being actively studied.

From the 1997 consensus conference to the 1999 conference (and through the present time) greater experience has been gained with the minimally invasive technique of stereotactic core biopsy using a large-gauge, usually vacuum-assisted, needle. This conference (and a subsequent consensus conference on image-detected breast biopsy) endorsed the minimally invasive biopsy as the preferred procedure when feasible, prior to a recommendation for definitive treatment (3). Needle-guided (also known as wire-directed) surgical excision of the area of calcifications (or mass with calcifications) using preoperative needle localization with specimen radiography to confirm the successful excision of the suspicious areas remains the traditional biopsy technique. Also, there may be suspicious areas on a mammogram that cannot be sampled adequately by a stereotactic core biopsy for several reasons, such as the scattered distribution of the calcifications, their location in the breast, or the size of breast. In these circumstances, surgical, needle-guided localization is required. Whether a core biopsy or an open biopsy is performed, concordance between the biopsy findings and the mammograms must be assured.

When used as the first diagnostic step, open surgical, needle-guided biopsy may be performed as a wide excision (with the intent of achieving microscopically clear margins) or as a more limited procedure (to make the diagnosis only). With a wide primary excision, if the findings are benign, a larger volume of tissue may be removed than is necessary. If the first procedure is a limited excision and the diagnosis is malignant, a second procedure is required to achieve wider margins. If feasible, a single, open procedure is preferred. This can be facilitated by preoperative diagnosis by core biopsy. Specimen radiography is mandated regardless of the manner in which the biopsy is performed.

When a patient requires surgical excision after core biopsy or re-excision of an area of DCIS after an initial needle-guided biopsy, a post-biopsy mammogram is essential. Because the treatment of DCIS is not an emergency, enough time should elapse between the initial procedure and the post-biopsy mammogram to optimize the visualization of possible residual calcifications. This may take as long as 2 to 3 months in some patients. When core biopsy is performed, a specimen radiograph and a radiograph of the breast immediately following the biopsy should be performed to insure removal of the most significant calcifications. A radioopaque clip should be placed at the site of calcifications so that this area can be localized again if (when) further surgery is performed. Not infrequently, core biopsy may remove most or even all of the calcifications. Without the clip, the area cannot be accurately identified if the calcifications have all been removed by the initial procedure.

TREATMENT OF THE BREAST

The goal of treatment for DCIS is breast conservation, with optimal cosmesis and a minimum risk of subsequent invasive or in situ recurrence. There are some women for whom mastectomy remains the optimal treatment, but most women with DCIS are candidates for breast conservation. Each patient should be apprised of her own situation and each option should be discussed with her in detail, including local excision and radiation therapy, local excision alone, or mastectomy.

Mastectomy

The factors that influence the recommendation for any treatment of the breast are the size of the area of DCIS, its biology, and margin status. Although there are no randomized clinical trials that compare total mastectomy with breast conservation, total ("simple") mastectomy is the "gold standard" against which any other treatment must be compared. Ample data from retrospective studies of the treatment of DCIS and the treatment of invasive cancers permit this extrapolation. Because, by definition, DCIS lacks the ability to metastasize, systemic failure after mastectomy implies the presence of undiagnosed (clinically occult) invasive carcinoma. Local failure could also be related to undetected DCIS or invasive carcinoma in the removed breast, or to DCIS or invasive cancer that remains or develops anew in residual breast tissue. Local failure after mastectomy, however, is rarely encountered.

Regardless of the goal of breast conservation, mastectomy is an acceptable treatment option for patients with DCIS, irrespective of their eligibility for breast conservation. This statement should not be misconstrued as a recommendation that all, or even most, patients with DCIS should undergo mastectomy. A minority of patients with DCIS require mastectomy, probably less than 25%, but mastectomy could be performed if it were the patient's preference.

Mastectomy is recommended, however, for patients with DCIS presenting as follows:

i) Patients with large areas of DCIS where the size of the lesion prevents an oncologically acceptable excision (see discussion of margins following) while conserving a cosmetically acceptable breast.
ii) Patients with multiple areas of DCIS in the same breast that cannot be encompassed through a single incision. (There may be a subgroup of these patients who might be treated with excision alone without radiation therapy, but as of this time, radiation oncologists are uncomfortable treating patients with more than one site of DCIS in the breast).
iii) Patients who cannot undergo radiation therapy because of prior therapeutic irradiation to the chest for another illness, for other medical problems, e.g., collagen vascular diseases, or for patients in whom treatment by excision alone is not appropriate.

Reconstruction should be offered to each patient who chooses mastectomy. The patient should discuss the timing and technique with her oncologist and reconstructive surgeon. Women with DCIS who undergo mastectomy are ideal candidates for reconstruction, and there are few, if any, contraindications to an immediate reconstruction if the patient desires one.

With respect to the technique of mastectomy employed, "skin-sparing" mastectomy for DCIS is appropriate, because this technique still removes all of the breast tissue, including the nipple and areola. When the biopsy site can reasonably be included within the skin sacrificed, it should be removed with the nipple/areola and adjacent skin; when the biopsy site is at some distance from the central portion of the breast, separate excision of the biopsy site should be considered if skin-sparing mastectomy is performed. This caveat should not apply for the site of a needle/core biopsy in DCIS. Skin-sparing mastectomy is not recommended if the patient does not undergo an immediate reconstruction, because the wound closure would result in too much redundant skin, and leaving this redundant skin is not usually appropriate.

There are situations where the location or the extent of the DCIS within the breast brings it close to the posterior margin of the mastectomy specimen. The proximity of DCIS to this particular margin is not considered similar to the other margins within the breast itself. There is no glandular breast tissue, i.e., ducts or lobules, deep to the deep layer of the superficial fascia of the breast. Moreover, the deep layer of superficial fascia of the breast that invests the back of the breast and the fascia of the pectoralis major muscle deep to the breast itself are effective barriers to the posterior penetration of malignant cells. DCIS cells cannot penetrate these fascial planes. Proximity to them is irrelevant in the treatment of DCIS. A so-called close posterior margin after mastectomy does not imply the need for adjuvant radiation therapy as it might for an invasive cancer.

A formal dissection of the axilla is not part of the procedure for DCIS (see treatment of the axilla section below). However, it is virtually impossible to perform a total mastectomy without some lymph nodes in the axillary tail of the breast being part of the breast dissection. These are variable in number and location, and the pathologist will often find several nodes in this portion of the breast as he dissects the specimen.

Breast Conservation

The majority of women with DCIS are candidates for breast conservation. This implies wide local excision of the disease within the breast. All patients for whom breast conservation is anticipated should undergo a post-excision mammogram to insure that all of the suspicious calcifications have been removed. This step may be avoided only if the specimen radiograph performed at the time of initial biopsy shows all of the suspicious calcifications to be well within the excised tissue, and the margins are widely clear (> 10 mm) microscopically. Even then, there is no harm done nor is it redundant if a post-biopsy mammogram is performed prior to a final recommendation about treatment. The timing of the post-biopsy mammogram is flexible. Because any residual calcifications must be imaged, the mammogram should not be performed until the patient is comfortable enough to undergo the compression that is necessary to achieve a technically optimal mammogram. Magnification films of the biopsy site are also advisable. In some patients, this post-biopsy mammogram may not be feasible for 2 or 3 months after the initial biopsy. Patients and physicians should not feel intimidated by any delay necessary to complete this important step, because the treatment of DCIS is not an emergency. In fact, contraction of the surgical biopsy site is an advantage if re-excision is planned; the volume of tissue removed at the second operation is usually less if the procedure is performed later rather than sooner after the initial procedure.

Whether radiation therapy, surveillance alone, or either of these plus tamoxifen, is optimal treatment when breast conservation is employed remains controversial. There are groups of patients with DCIS who fall into each of these categories, but no one has yet defined the selection criteria for each of them precisely enough to make dogmatic recommendations. Clinical trials have shown that local excision and radiation therapy in patients with negative margins provide excellent rates of local control. Patients treated with excision alone have a greater chance of local recurrence. There is evidence that recurrence is decreased with wider surgical margins around the area of DCIS. The available data indicate that the likelihood of developing invasive cancer of the breast after treatment with breast conservation with or without radiation therapy is about 1% or less per year after the initial diagnosis and treatment.

Although adding radiation therapy to wide local excision benefits all groups of patients with DCIS who are candidates for breast conservation, the magnitude of that benefit may be small enough in some patient subgroups that the radiation therapy can be omitted. However, patients who may avoid radiation therapy have not been reproducibly and reliably identified by any clinical trials. There are institutional and individual reports of large series of such patients treated with wide excision alone who achieve a risk of invasive recurrence of 1% or less per year.

To consider treatment of DCIS with wide excision alone without radiation therapy, patients should meet at least the following criteria:

i)   The area of DCIS, whether measured by the pathologist or on the mammogram, should be small, preferably less than 2 to 3 cm in diameter. Occasionally, larger areas of calcifications may be encountered that can be well excised because the breast is large enough to accommodate the loss of a greater volume of tissue without significant deformity.

ii) Margins around any site of DCIS should be 10 mm or greater (see discussion of margins below).

iii) The nuclear grade of the DCIS should usually be low or intermediate grade (as defined above), although patients with high nuclear grade DCIS also may be candidates for local excision alone, if wider margins than 10 mm can be achieved.

iv) The aesthetic appearance of the breast after local excision should be appropriate. A well-performed mastectomy may be preferable to local excision that is so large with respect to the volume of the breast that the patient is unhappy with her appearance.

Candidates for breast conservation who do not fit these guidelines are best treated with the addition of radiation therapy after wide local excision. Radiation oncologists usually prefer that the size of the area of DCIS is less than 5 cm in its greatest dimension. This is for technical reasons and due to the difficulty in achieving a wide local excision with negative margins and an acceptable cosmetic result when the area is larger. Any grade or subtype of DCIS is appropriate

for radiation therapy. Margins preferably should be clear (as described below).

Margins

Clear surgical margins are a major criterion for treatment of DCIS with breast conservation; it is generally accepted that the wider the margin, the lower the rate of local recurrence. Margin status is of crucial importance because it is the one variable that the physician can control. The biologic character, i.e., nuclear grade and architecture, and the size of the area of DCIS cannot be influenced by treatment, but the margins can. A 10 mm margin is the best compromise between removal of so much tissue that the cosmetic result would be less than desirable and the likelihood of local recurrence. When treatment with local excision alone without radiation therapy is considered, a clear margin of at least 10 mm is essential. Re-excision to achieve clear margins is appropriate if an initial attempt is unsuccessful. How many attempts at re-excision are acceptable before admitting that clear margins cannot be achieved? The answer is uncertain, but in theory, whatever might be necessary to clear the margins is acceptable as long as it is consistent with the patient's desire for breast conservation and the final aesthetic result. However, a well-performed mastectomy and reconstruction are often better than multiple attempts at re-excision that destroy the contour and size of the breast.

When breast conservation includes radiation therapy, the initial target volume is the whole ipsilateral breast. The whole-breast irradiation is delivered with tangential fields. Treatment is given using daily (Monday through Friday) fractions. Daily fraction sizes typically range from 1.8 to 2.0 Gy, and whole-breast doses typically range from 45 to 50 Gy delivered over 4.5 to 5 weeks. Megavoltage photon irradiation is used. Some radiation oncologists use a boost to the primary tumor site in all patients. The boost dose is 10 to 20 Gy delivered over 1 to 2 weeks, most commonly with electrons, although other boost methods, including implants, have been described. A boost is mandatory when the margins of resection are not confirmed as histologically negative. A boost is required when the whole-breast dosage is less than 50 Gy.

Irradiation of regional lymph nodes (axillary and supraclavicular) is contraindicated in patients with DCIS. Although incidental (generally partial) nodal volumes are sometimes included in standard tangential volumes because of anatomical considerations, specific techniques to include nodal volumes should be avoided.

TREATMENT OF THE AXILLA

An axillary dissection is not required in patients with DCIS. The incidence of occult invasive carcinoma that might have spread to axillary nodes is so infrequent that this possibility should not provoke a therapeutic recommendation to dissect the axilla. For patients undergoing mastectomy, some lymph nodes situated in the axillary tail of the breast may be incidentally removed, but an intentional dissection of the axilla is not warranted.

As sentinel node biopsy has become a popular treatment plan for the axilla in addressing invasive cancers; however, the role of sentinel node biopsy in DCIS has emerged as another point of controversy. Although sentinel node biopsy using either radioactive isotope or blue dye to locate the node(s) is less invasive and less morbid than the customary axillary dissection performed for invasive cancer, the ease of sentinel node biopsy should not be an excuse for its use. If, by definition, DCIS does not spread to lymph nodes, a procedure to prove lymph node status should not be necessary, however free from complications it might be.

ADJUVANT THERAPY

There is no indication for adjuvant cytotoxic chemotherapy in patients with DCIS. In patients undergoing mastectomy, the patient should be treated as for any other stage I carcinoma (of the same size) in the breast in the unlikely event that a focus of invasive carcinoma is found in the specimen.

A randomized clinical trial has demonstrated that the addition of tamoxifen, 20 mg daily for 5 years, to the treatment of DCIS by local excision and radiation therapy decreased the incidence of invasive cancer recurrence. This benefit was seen independent of margin status or the presence of comedo-type necrosis. However, no overall survival benefit was observed during the course of the study.

Whether these observations are justification for the routine use of tamoxifen in all patients with DCIS remains unclear, because the subgroups of patients who would benefit the most have not been defined. It is likely that many women with DCIS have been given prescriptions for tamoxifen on the assumption that all of them will benefit. Because the use of tamoxifen is not without complications and the likelihood of developing invasive cancer in the ipsilateral breast after treatment for DCIS is already small, whether treated with radiation therapy or with surveillance alone, the incremental benefit from tamoxifen may not be great enough to warrant its use in all women who undergo breast conservation. Also, although the measurement of steroid hormone receptors is recommended for DCIS as it is for invasive cancers, no data indicate whether it is only the women with estrogen receptor–positive DCIS who might benefit from the use of tamoxifen. Although the role of tamoxifen in patients undergoing breast conservation for DCIS is promising, these data must be considered immature. Other agents, such as selective estrogen receptor modulators (SERMs), e.g., raloxifene, are currently considered investigational.

TREATMENT OF RECURRENCE AFTER BREAST CONSERVATION

Recurrence as invasive cancer is an end point that affects disease-specific survival. Evidence suggests that this event does increase the patient's risk of death from breast cancer, however "early" the diagnosis is made. It also affects treatment recommendations, because attention to the axilla is usually mandated in invasive cancer. Although a "censoring event" in the statistical analysis of the data, recurrence as DCIS alone may not be of this same significance.

If invasive cancer is the recurrence, its treatment should be as for any other invasive cancer of the same stage. The prognosis should be excellent, because most of these are detected as new areas of calcifications on follow-up mammograms and are often microinvasive in character (T1mic). However, a small number of these women are destined for metastasis, and this possibility is truly the crux of the treatment dilemma in breast conservation.

When DCIS is the recurrence, a different question exists. When DCIS only (i.e., without invasive cancer) occurs after treatment by local excision alone, the usual treatment is radiation therapy or mastectomy, based on the same selection criteria as for DCIS treatment when it occurs for the first time. However, no data extant address the likelihood of further recurrence (for either DCIS or invasive cancer) if this second event is treated with local excision alone. The choice between radiation therapy and mastectomy would be based on the same criteria as noted at the time of initial diagnosis. We have several patients who have been treated three and even four times with re-excision only for recurrent DCIS, without the development of invasive cancer (to date). Therefore, for the women who underwent local excision alone, the choices include re-excision, re-excision and radiation therapy, or mastectomy. Highly motivated women may choose additional attempt(s) at local excision alone presuming that the recurrence is entirely DCIS and recognizing the lack of information about their long-term outcome. Because radiation therapy to the same area cannot be safely undertaken, the recommendation for the treatment of recurrence in patients who underwent radiation therapy at the time of the initial diagnosis is usually mastectomy. There may be selected occasions when local excision alone may be employed; but these infrequently encountered occasions do not vitiate the opinion that mastectomy is the recommended treatment for recurrence of DCIS after initial treatment by radiation therapy.

BIOLOGIC MARKERS

The use of prognostic markers as predictors of local recurrence after breast conservation for DCIS remains investigational. Among these are estrogen and progesterone hormone receptors, apoptosis inhibitor bcl-2, nuclear proliferation marker Ki-67, tumor suppressor gene and apoptosis mediator p53, membranous growth factor c-erbB2 (Her2/neu), and p21waf/cip. In our own institutional experience thus far, hormone receptor information, as well as bcl-2, have not predicted recurrence. Ki-67 and p53 displayed potential predictive value for tumor recurrence, but the *p* values for both were greater than 0.05. The combination of high Ki-67 and high p53 seemed to predict recurrence better than either alone.

Two markers did demonstrate statistical significance for recurrence: c-erbB2 and p21waf/cip. For c-erbB2, the difference between none or marginal expression and any greater expression was significant, and a similar stratification between high and low risk for recurrence was seen when p21 was greater than 15% positive.

These data should not yet influence physicians to use them to determine treatment for DCIS. They are, however, an inducement to further study prognostic markers as potential selection criteria to choose, for example, between treatment by local excision and radiation therapy and local excision alone. As data continue to accumulate about the importance of these markers and others, and because virtually all markers can be determined from paraffin blocks of formalin fixed tissue, the paraffin blocks should never be discarded.

FOLLOW-UP

All patients undergoing treatment for DCIS, particularly breast conservation, require lifetime follow-up. Early detection of local recurrence after breast conservation is especially important because of the high salvage rate for these patients and the need to detect contralateral carcinoma. The lengthy time course for both ipsilateral and contralateral events also implies the need for lifetime surveillance. When possible, the same team should follow these patients because of the changes in physical examination and mammography that the treatment produced and the difficulties differentiating benign changes from recurrence. Unfortunately, insurance considerations, especially in the United States, might affect these recommendations. Insurance carriers may insist that follow-up be conducted by the patient's primary care physician and may dictate the venue for mammography. Additionally, patients who traveled far from home to undergo their treatment may prefer that their follow-up be carried out locally.

Bilateral mammography should be performed annually for the patient undergoing breast conservation, with the first post-treatment mammogram performed about 6 months after completion of treatment. Our own protocol advises 6 month interval mammograms of the involved breast for the first 3 years after initial diagnosis and treatment. Clinical examination of both breasts is recommended at 6-month intervals for the first 3 years after treatment, then annually. The argument for physical examination is less well supported from the literature, particularly because the majority of recurrences are detected by mammography. No role has been established for imaging modalities other than mam-

mography. Other surveillance studies, such as serum chemistries or chest x-ray, are not indicated.

REPORTING END POINTS

Uniform reporting is required to compare various reports of treatment, both for randomized trials and retrospective studies. These include a careful description of the patient population, because selection bias affects the apparent efficacy of different treatments. For example, it is likely that patients chosen for breast conservation with radiation therapy are different from those women selected for local excision alone without radiation therapy. Reportable demographic characteristics include, but are not restricted to, family history, age, parity, hormone use, and menopausal status. Tumor factors to be reported include size, nuclear grade, architecture, and margin status (including width). Treatment factors include type of surgery, radiation therapy data (if used), and adjuvant systemic treatment (if used).

The following end points should be reported:

overall survival,
deaths from breast cancer,
local failure (DCIS/invasive cancer),
metastatic rate,
contralateral breast cancer,
extent of disease at recurrence (loco-regional or systemic), and
treatment for recurrence.

Breast conservation rates and cosmetic outcome reporting were encouraged. Definitions of the method of calculation of events and definitions of censoring methods should be defined.

The treatment of DCIS is constantly being refined, and the observations and recommendations made at this time may be influenced by new data reported contemporaneously as well as in the future. Because this report is based on opinions and experience as of the date written, these opinions must not be construed as dogmatic guidelines for treatment. Management of individual patients should be based on each patient's unique clinical circumstances. Recommendations for treatment must be made by the responsible physician(s) with the participation of the patient.

REFERENCES

1. The Consensus Conference Committee. Consensus Conference on the Classification of Ductal Carcinoma in Situ, April 25–28, 1997. *Cancer* 1997;80:1798–1802.
2. Schwartz GF, Solin LJ, Olivotto IA, et al. Consensus Conference on the Treatment of In Situ Ductal Carcinoma of the Breast. *Cancer* 2000;88:946–954.
3. International Breast Consensus Conference Committee. Image-Detected Breast Cancer: State of the Art Diagnosis and Treatment. *J Am Coll Surg* 2001;193:297–302.

OTHER NONINVASIVE BREAST CANCERS AND PRENEOPLASTIC DISEASES

64

BREAST-CONSERVING TREATMENT OF PAGET'S DISEASE OF THE BREAST WITH RADIOTHERAPY

ALAIN FOURQUET
BRIGITTE SIGAL-ZAFRANI
FRANÇOIS CAMPANA
KRISHNA B. CLOUGH

In principle, it would seem that breast-conservation therapy should be a good alternative to mastectomy for patients with isolated Paget's disease of the nipple, as it is for patients with other forms of early-stage breast cancer. However, because this disease is rare, few publications have addressed the issue of breast-conserving treatment for these patients (1–8). In 1987, we published the results of a series of 20 patients treated with breast-conservation therapy using radiotherapy, with a median of 7.5 years (9). We concluded that radiotherapy could be an alternative to radical surgery in patients with disease limited to the nipple but that further studies were needed to confirm these results.

The current study updates the original series, includes more patients, and extends the follow-up of the initial series.

MATERIAL AND METHODS

Between November 1962 and December 1997, 121 patients with Paget's disease of the nipple without an associated breast tumor were accrued in the Institut Curie database. They represent 0.5% of all patients with nonmetastatic breast cancer treated during this period. The median age at diagnosis was 63 years (range, 33 to 87 years). The first sign of disease was an eczematous rash (76 patients, 63%), nipple discharge (15 patients, 12%), or ulceration (30 patients, 25%). Retroareolar microcalcifications were present in 52 patients (43%).

Seventy-one patients (59%) underwent modified radical mastectomy. Intraductal carcinoma within the lactiferous ducts was found in all patients, with microinvasive foci also found in 16 patients (23%). No involved axillary nodes were found. There were no recurrences in these patients at a median follow-up of 7 years.

One patient was treated with excision of the nipple and areola complex (NAC) without irradiation. Histologic analysis showed intraductal carcinoma with microinvasion. She had an invasive breast recurrence 50 months after treatment and then underwent mastectomy. She died of intercurrent disease 28 months after recurrence.

The present study focuses on the remaining 49 patients (40% of the entire population) who underwent breast-conserving treatment with irradiation, with or without complete gross excision of the NAC. The median age at diagnosis of this group was 56 years (range, 33 to 78 years). Twenty-eight patients (57%) were postmenopausal. An eczematous rash of the NAC was the first sign of disease in 31 patients (63%). Diagnosis of Paget's disease was established by a nipple and/or areolar biopsy in all 49 patients. Grading was done in ten cases, all of which were poorly differentiated intraductal carcinoma with high nuclear grade (10). Twelve patients (24%) underwent wide surgical excision of the NAC that included part of the underlying tissue. Ductal carcinoma in situ in the underlying breast parenchyma was found in nine of the 12 patients (75%); microinvasive cancer was associated with intraductal disease in three patients. Thirty-seven patients (76%) had no further surgery after incisional biopsy and were treated with radiation therapy alone.

All 49 patients underwent radiation therapy to the breast using cobalt 60. The median dose was 54 Gy (range, 30 to 67 Gy). Additional irradiation to the tumor site (a boost) was given to 46 patients (94%), using cobalt 60 for 17 patients, electrons (usually 9 MeV) for 27 patients, and 200-kV x-rays for two patients. Electron boosts were delivered through a single field directed at the NAC, using a bolus in 19 of the 27 treated patients (70%). The cobalt 60 and 200-kV boosts were given using two small opposed lateral fields, using a bolus in six of the 17 patients (35%) who had a cobalt 60 boost. Three of the 12 patients who had excision of the NAC were not given a radiation boost. The median dose to the tumor site was 74 Gy (range, 52 to 83 Gy). Median tumor doses for the 37 patients treated with irradiation

TABLE 64.1. PATIENTS AND TUMOR CHARACTERISTICS

	All Patients	1962–1984	1984–1997
No. of patients	49	20	29
Age (yr)			
Median	56	52	57
Range	33–78	33–72	40–78
Menopausal status			
Premenopausal	21	12	9
Postmenopausal	28	8	20
First sign of disease			
Eczematous rash	31	10	21
Ulceration	10	6	4
Nipple discharge	8	4	4
Retroareolar microcalcifications			
Yes	18	7	12
No	26	13	17

alone and the 12 patients treated with excision and irradiation were 75 Gy (range, 57 to 83 Gy) and 64.5 Gy (range, 52 to 80 Gy), respectively. Twenty-six patients (53%) received internal mammary and axillary lymph node irradiation.

Because the patients in the study were treated over a long period (30 years), they were divided into two cohorts. The first cohort included 20 patients treated between November 1962 and February 1984 (the results for whom were originally published in 1987). The second cohort comprised 29 patients treated between 1984 and 1997. The two cohorts represented 39% and 43 % of all patients with Paget's disease treated at the Institut Curie during each period, respectively. Patients in the second cohort were older than patients in the first cohort. Regional nodal irradiation was rarely performed after 1984, whereas it was given to all patients treated before 1984. Other characteristics were similar between the groups (Tables 64.1 and 64.2).

Recurrence rates were determined by using Kaplan-Meier estimates. Patients were censored at the time of death or last follow-up.

RESULTS

The median follow-up for surviving patients was 11 years (range, 1 to 34 years). Six patients (12%) died of intercurrent disease; no patient died of breast cancer. One patient developed an isolated bone metastasis 28 months after diagnosis, without ipsilateral or contralateral recurrence. She was alive without disease 108 months after diagnosis. Nine patients had a breast recurrence, one patient had an axillary lymph node recurrence, and seven patients developed a contralateral breast cancer. The 10-year rates of breast recurrence and contralateral breast cancer were 18% and 16%, respectively. Because all breast recurrences were treated with

TABLE 64.2. TREATMENT

	All Patients	1962–1984	1984–1997
No. of patients	49	20	20
Surgery			
Nipple/areola biopsy	37	17	20
Nipple-areolar complex excision	12	3	9
Radiotherapy			
Breast alone	23	0	23
Breast + nodes	26	20	6
Median dose (range) (Gy)			
Whole breast	54 (30–67)	57 (50–65)	54 (30–67)
Tumor site	74 (52–83)	73.5 (52–83)	75 (52–80)
Follow-up (yr)			
Median	10	20	8
Range	1–34	4–34	1–15

TABLE 64.3. BREAST RECURRENCES AFTER TREATMENT WITH RADIATION THERAPY WITHOUT TUMOR EXCISION

Age at Diagnosis (yr)	Retroareolar Microcalcifications	Tumor Dose (Gy)	Type of Boost	Time to Recurrence (mo)	Recurrence Histology	Follow-Up After Recurrence (mo)
43	Present	78	Electrons	17	Paget' disease	124
60	Present	83	Electrons	23	Paget' disease	201
60	Absent	75	Electrons	27	Paget' disease	138
50	Present	66	Electrons	34	Paget' disease + microinvasive	148
58	Absent	74	Cobalt	49	Paget' disease	199
40	Present	64	Electrons	50	Paget' disease + microinvasive	90
61	Absent	71	Electrons	58	Paget' disease	125
42	Present	75	Electrons	63	Invasive	19
57	Present	81	Electrons	400	Invasive	11

mastectomy, the 10-year ipsilateral breast preservation rate for all 49 patients was 82%.

The median follow-up for the 12 patients treated with NAC excision followed by breast irradiation was 6 years (range, 2.5 to 30 years). None experienced a breast recurrence. One developed an isolated ipsilateral axillary node recurrence 24 months after initial treatment, which included nodal irradiation. Microinvasive cancer was present in the initial excision. After this recurrence, she was treated with axillary dissection and chemotherapy and was in remission 92 months later.

The median follow-up for the 37 patients who were treated by radiation therapy alone was 12 years (range, 1 to 34 years). There were nine breast recurrences (24%). Characteristics of these patients and their recurrences are listed in Table 64.3. The 5- and 10-year cumulative risks of breast recurrence were 21% ($\pm$ 14%). The median time to breast recurrence was 43 months (range, 17 to 400 months). Only one patient had a recurrence more than 5 years after treatment (at 33 years). Five of the nine recurrences were Paget's disease only, two were Paget's disease associated with microinvasive cancer, and two were invasive cancer (at 63 and 400 months).

The recurrence rate was not influenced by age at diagnosis, period of treatment, or the breast or total tumor dose.

TABLE 64.4. BREAST RECURRENCE RATES IN RELATION TO TREATMENT

Treatment Group	Follow-Up (yr)		Recurrence
	Median	Range	
NAC excision + WBRT[a]	6	2.5–30	0% (0/12)
WBRT + photon boost	11	4.5–20	8% (1/12)
WBRT + electron boost	14	1–34	32% (8/25)

[a] One patient developed axillary recurrence without breast recurrence.
NAC, nipple-areolar complex; WBRT, whole-breast radiation therapy.

Patients without retroareolar microcalcifications had fewer recurrences than those with microcalcifications on diagnostic mammography, but the difference was not significant. The rate of local recurrence varied according to treatment combinations (Table 64.4). Eight of the nine recurrences developed in the 25 patients treated with radiotherapy without NAC excision who received an electron boost (which included the use of bolus in 18 patients or 72%); only one recurrence occurred in the 12 patients treated with a boost using opposed tangential photons fields.

All patients who had a recurrence were treated with mastectomy. The median follow-up after breast recurrence was 10 years (range, 1 to 17 years). No patients developed further recurrences within this period.

DISCUSSION

This study analyzed the patterns of recurrence in a series of 49 patients with isolated Paget's disease treated with breast-conserving treatment using radiotherapy with or without resection of the NAC in a single institution over a 30-year period. These results confirm that breast-conserving treatment in patients with Paget's disease of the nipple without an associated breast mass did not impair survival, as was found in an earlier analysis of this series (9) and as has been shown by others (1,2,5–8).

Two of the nine breast recurrences were invasive cancer without evidence of recurrent Paget's disease. They occurred at 5 and 33 years after treatment, thus probably representing new ipsilateral primary breast cancers. All other recurrences were of Paget's disease, either alone or associated with microinvasive cancer. This is a different pattern from that observed in patients treated for ductal carcinoma in situ (11). All breast recurrences developed in the 37 patients treated with radiotherapy alone who underwent only a diagnostic (incisional) biopsy. The results of this study also underline the importance of the radiotherapy technique:

eight of the nine recurrences were observed in the 25 patients who received a boost using a single electron field encompassing the NAC. Low energy (e.g., 9 MeV) was used, and in 72% of patients, a bolus was applied, increasing the dose at the surface but decreasing the dose in depth. Of the 12 patients who received a boost dose through opposed tangential fields, only one had a recurrence. This was similar to what was observed with shorter follow-up in the 12 patients treated with excision of the NAC and radiotherapy (i.e., no breast recurrences and one regional recurrence).

Although this study has a long follow-up, the number of patients is too small to have sufficient statistical power to reliably determine which factors are associated with local recurrence. Whether breast irradiation can be omitted for patients treated with NAC excision with free margins, as it often is for patients with pure ductal carcinoma in situ, remains to be determined. There is too little information available in the literature to resolve this issue. Low recurrence rates were observed in several published series of patients treated with excision alone (3,12,13), but the numbers of patients treated were very small and follow-up in these series was short. The need for whole-breast irradiation in Paget's disease is supported by the fact that the underlying ductal carcinoma in situ is poorly differentiated in most cases and that microinvasive cancer was present in 23% of the cases treated with mastectomy in our series. Additionally, Paget's cells, like poorly differentiated high-grade ductal carcinoma in situ, overexpress c-erbB-2/HER2-neu in most cases (14,15). These features suggest that a high recurrence rate can be expected if patients with Paget's disease are treated with wide excision without radiotherapy.

CONCLUSIONS

Experience in breast-conserving treatment of isolated Paget's disease of the nipple is limited because this is a rare presentation of breast cancer. The current Institut Curie policy is to make breast-conserving treatment available to all patients who desire it. Our results suggest that excision of the nipple and areola with free margins, followed by breast irradiation, will give the highest probability of a cure. However, this results in the cosmetic and functional loss of the nipple and areola. Plastic surgery (reconstruction of the nipple and tattooing of the areola) can be performed after completion of irradiation. Treatment with irradiation without surgery should be considered as an alternative to resection of the NAC, provided that an effective boost technique is used (i.e., one adequately encompassing the NAC and underlying breast tissue, which contains ductal carcinoma in situ in most patients). This requires accurate pretreatment evalua-

tion of the extent of disease, best performed using magnification mammography (16) and magnetic resonance imaging (17). Studies comparing the results of both treatment strategies and their cosmetic consequences should be initiated.

REFERENCES

1. Bulens P, Vanuytsel L, Rijnders A, et al. Breast conserving treatment of Paget's disease. *Radiother Oncol* 1990;17:305–309.
2. El-Sharkawi A, Waters JS. The place for conservative treatment in the management of Paget's disease of the nipple. *Eur J Surg Oncol* 1992;18:301.
3. Lagios MD, Westdahl PR, Rose MR, et al. Paget's disease of the nipple: alternative management in cases without or with minimal extent of underlying breast carcinoma. *Cancer* 1984;54:545–551.
4. Rissanen PM, Holsti P. Paget's disease of the breast. *Oncology* 1969;23:209–216.
5. Stockdale AD, White WF, Brierley JD, et al. Radiotherapy for Paget's disease of the nipple: a conservative alternative. *Lancet* 1989;2:664–666.
6. Pierce LJ, Haffty BG, Solin LJ, et al. The conservative management of Paget's disease of the breast with radiotherapy. *Cancer* 1997;80:1065–1072.
7. Fu W, Mittel VK, Young SC. Paget disease of the breast. Analysis of 41 patients. *Am J Clin Oncol* 2001;24:397–400
8. Bijker N, Rutgers EJT, Duchateau L, et al. Breast-conserving therapy for Paget disease of the nipple. A prospective European Organization for Research and Treatment of cancer study of 61 patients. *Cancer* 2001;91:474–477.
9. Fourquet A, Campana F, Vielh P, et al. Paget's disease of the nipple without detectable breast tumor: conservative management with radiation therapy. *Int J Radiat Oncol Biol Phys* 1987;14:1463–1465.
10. Holland R, Peterse JL, Millis RR, et al. Ductal carcinoma in situ: a proposal for a new classification. *Semin Diagn Pathol* 1994;11:167–180.
11. Fourquet A, Zafrani B, Campana F, et al. Breast-conserving treatment of ductal carcinoma in situ. *Semin Radiat Oncol* 1992;2:116–124.
12. Paone J, Baker RR. Pathogenesis and treatment of Paget's disease of the breast. *Cancer* 1981;48:825–829.
13. Dixon AR, Galea MH, Ellis IO, et al. Paget's disease of the nipple. *Br J Surg* 1991;78:722–723
14. Vielh P, Validire P, Kheirallah S, et al. Paget's disease of the nipple without clinically and radiologically detectable breast tumor. *Pathol Res Pract* 1993;189:150–155.
15. Zafrani B, Leroyer A, Fourquet A, et al. Mammographically detected ductal in situ carcinoma of the breast analyzed with a new classification. A study of 127 cases: correlation with estrogen and progesterone receptors, p53 and c-erbB-2 proteins, and proliferative activity. *Semin Diagn Pathol* 1994;11:208–214.
16. Holland R, Hendriks JHCL. Microcalcifications associated with ductal carcinoma in situ: mammographic-pathologic correlations. *Semin Diagn Pathol* 1994;11:181–192.
17. Gilles R, Zafrani B, Guinebretiere JM, et al. Ductal carcinoma in situ: MR imaging-histopathologic correlation. *Radiology* 1995;196:415–419.

65

PAGET'S DISEASE

MARK R. WICK
SUZIE M. DINTZIS

Paget's disease is an unusual adenocarcinoma of the breast that is typified by epidermal involvement and usually accompanied by an underlying breast carcinoma. The disease is not uncommon, constituting 0.7% to 4.3% of all breast carcinomas (1–7). Paget's disease has been well described morphologically, but its fundamental tumorigenesis remains unclear. This review describes the histopathology of Paget's disease of the breast and discusses in detail the progress that has been made in understanding its molecular pathogenesis. Prognosis and treatment of Paget's disease of the breast are discussed in Chapter 64.

CLINICAL FEATURES OF MAMMARY PAGET'S DISEASE

The epidemiology of mammary Paget's disease does not appear to differ from that of other breast carcinomas. The age distribution of the disease is similar to that of other patients with mammary cancers. Although only small numbers of cases of mammary Paget's disease in men have been reported, the mean age and clinical behavior appear to be similar to those reported in women (8–11). No unique predisposing clinical or epidemiologic factors have been identified. Clinically, the lesion of mammary Paget's disease appears first on the nipple and may extend secondarily to involve the areola and, rarely, the surrounding skin of the breast. The clinical appearance varies from that of erythema of the nipple and areola to the development of overt eczematoid change with eventual nipple distortion, erosion, or ulceration (Fig. 65.1). Paget's disease should not be confused with involvement of dermal lymphatics by invasive carcinoma, commonly called inflammatory carcinoma of the breast. Unlike Paget's disease, inflammatory carcinoma presents characteristically with diffuse breast tenderness and enlargement as well as epidermal edema, erythema, and thickening.

In approximately 95% of cases, mammary Paget's disease is accompanied by an underlying malignancy, either an intraductal or invasive ductal carcinoma (1,3,12–14). Invasive carcinomas are preponderant among the 50% to 60% of patients who present with a palpable mass in a breast that also exhibits Paget's disease. The overwhelming majority of such invasive neoplasms are ductal in origin (Figs. 65.2 and 65.3). In the absence of a clinically apparent tumor, in situ ductal lesions are seen in most instances. It is a peculiarity of mammary Paget's disease that lobular mammary neoplasia is not often encountered as an underlying disorder.

HISTOLOGIC FINDINGS IN MAMMARY PAGET'S DISEASE

Microscopically, Paget's disease is characterized by the presence of foreign epithelioid tumor cells within the keratinizing epithelium of the nipple epidermis (Figs. 65.4 and 65.5). The adjacent skin may show hyperkeratosis and acanthosis. The cells tend to occur as small clusters in the basal epidermal layers. Isolated pagetoid cells may also be found singly in the basalis or superficial surface epithelium where they can be distinguished from surrounding squamous keratinocytes by the absence of intercellular bridges. Typically, tumor cells in mammary Paget's disease are round to ovoid and contain abundant pale, amphophilic cytoplasm that can be vacuolated. The nuclei vary in character, but most contain evenly distributed or vesicular chromatin, often with a discernible, but not prominent, nucleolus. Nuclei also can be hyperchromatic with irregular nuclear outlines. Mitotic figures are infrequent. An anaplastic variant of Paget's disease has also been described (15). This subtype features marked variation in the size, shape, and density of tumor cell nuclei as well as variable configurations of the cells themselves. Such findings may be problematic in reference to histologic differential diagnosis with other intraepidermal malignancies, but they do not appear to have an adverse effect on the biologic behavior of mammary Paget's disease.

Another microscopic peculiarity of Paget's disease relates to its potentially confluent growth in the basal epidermis. Because the neoplastic elements in mammary Paget's disease have relatively poor intercellular cohesion, they may undergo

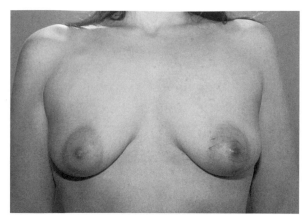

FIGURE 65.1. Mammary Paget's disease of the left nipple. The left nipple epithelium is smooth, reddened, and thickened.

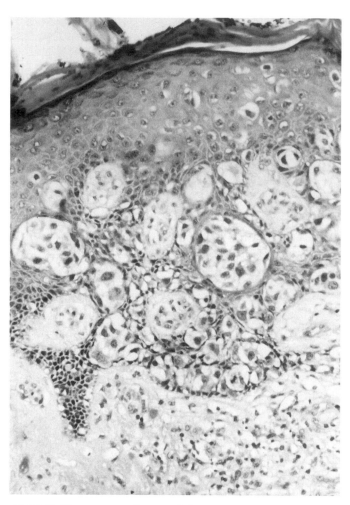

FIGURE 65.4. Paget's disease of the nipple shows basically located groups and scattered single tumor cells within the epidermis.

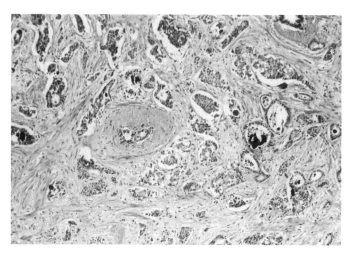

FIGURE 65.2. Invasive ductal carcinoma is seen in only a minority of breast cancers that are associated with mammary Paget's disease.

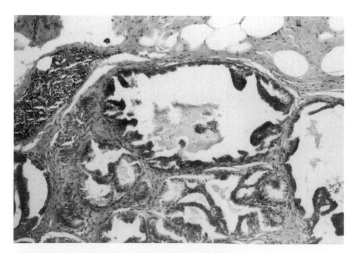

FIGURE 65.3. Ductal carcinoma in situ is most often found in breast tissue subjacent to mammary Paget's disease.

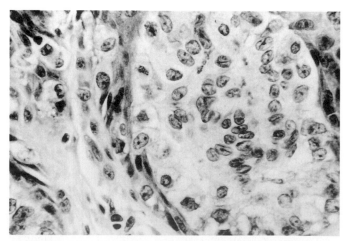

FIGURE 65.5. The tumor cells in mammary Paget's disease are characterized by abundant pale cytoplasm and evenly distributed nuclear chromatin, often with a nucleolus.

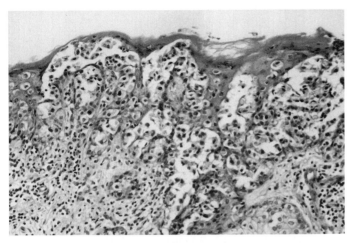

FIGURE 65.6. Some examples of mammary Paget's disease have confluent growth in the basal epidermis. Lack of cohesion between tumor cells produces pseudobullae that may result in confusion with non-neoplastic entities such as pemphigus vulgaris.

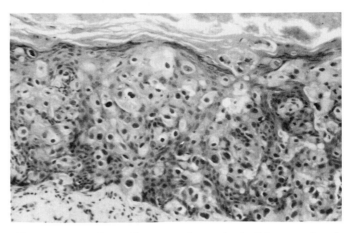

FIGURE 65.8. The malignant melanocytes in this example of amelanotic superficial spreading malignant melanoma closely resemble the tumor cells of mammary Paget's disease.

detachment from one another with even modest distortion of the tissue that is introduced during biopsy or processing. This phenomenon produces pseudobullae that may, to the uninitiated, simulate the acantholysis that typifies variants of pemphigus. Indeed, the authors have encountered several cases of mammary Paget's disease in which this diagnostic error had been made (Fig. 65.6). Attention to the foreign cytologic attributes of more superficially located Paget's cells in such instances should prevent interpretative mishaps. Paget's cell cytoplasm contains neutral and acid mucopolysaccharides that may confer positivity with the periodic acid–Schiff-diastase, mucicarmine, aldehyde fuchsin, and Alcian blue methods. Fifty percent to 60% of mammary Paget's cells will demonstrate staining for mucin (Fig. 65.7).

DIFFERENTIAL DIAGNOSIS OF MAMMARY PAGET'S DISEASE

Potential diagnostic difficulties arise especially when fixation or tissue preparation is suboptimal or when tumor cells are rare. The differential diagnosis principally includes superficial spreading amelanotic melanoma and bowenoid forms of intraepidermal squamous carcinoma (Figs. 65.8 and 65.9). In particular, Paget's cells may contain granules of melanin, which are produced by neighboring melanocytes and secondarily engulfed by the tumor cells. The presence of melanin pigment within the cells obviously may lead to diagnostic confusion with malignant melanoma (15a). Conventional histochemistry can be helpful in determining the glandular nature of Paget's disease because neither melanoma nor squamous carcinoma produces epithelial mucin; however, only a

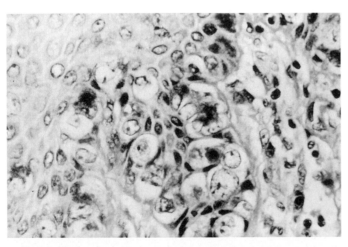

FIGURE 65.7. Neutral mucin present within the cytoplasm of Paget's cells stains with the periodic acid–Schiff method.

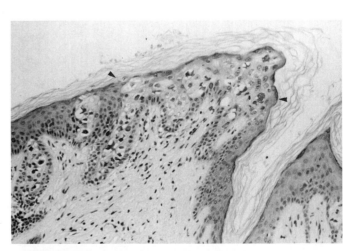

FIGURE 65.9. In intraepidermal squamous cell carcinoma (pagetoid Bowen's disease) (*arrows*), the pale tumor cells may be confused with those of mammary Paget's disease.

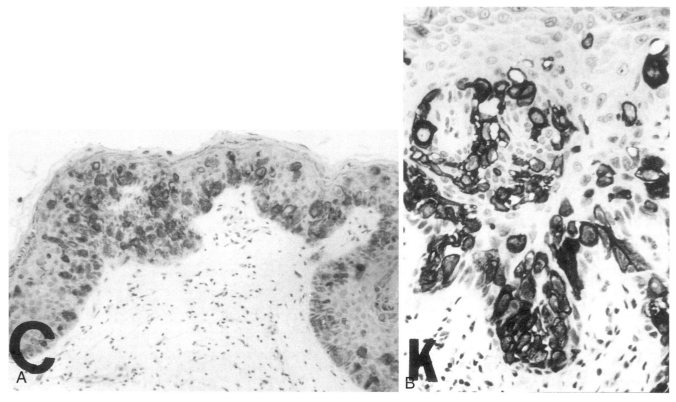

FIGURE 65.10. Immunoreactivity for carcinoembryonic antigen (C) **(A)** or cytokeratin type 7 (K) **(B)** is expected in mammary Paget's disease and excludes the diagnosis of superficial spreading malignant melanoma or squamous cell carcinoma.

proportion of Paget's cells may contain mucin in any given case and mucin-negative cases are also well recognized.

Immunostains may be exploited diagnostically if mucin stains are unrevealing. Various antibodies directed against the structural cellular components and secretions of apocrine and eccrine glands have been applied to the study of mammary Paget's disease. Immunoreactivity of Paget's cells

for carcinoembryonic antigen or cytokeratin type 7 confirm the diagnosis in the cited context (Fig. 65.10). However, as discussed later, labeling with these and other antibodies in Paget's disease has not been universal, and they also may decorate normal elements of the nipple-areolar complex known as Toker cells (15b). S100 protein has also been used to distinguish malignant melanoma, which shows nuclear and cytoplasmic positivity from Paget's disease, which is negative (16) or demonstrates cytoplasmic staining. The HMB-45, MART-1, and tyrosinase antigens are likewise restricted to melanoma in this narrow context.

Amplified expression of e-*erb*B-2 oncoprotein has been shown to be present in a high proportion of Paget's cells. One study combining antibodies against low-molecular weight keratin and the c-*erb*B-2 protein reported absolute sensitivity and specificity in a small number of mammary Paget's disease cases (Fig. 65.11) (17), in comparison with other histologically similar proliferations.

HISTOGENESIS OF MAMMARY PAGET'S DISEASE

Because most cases of mammary Paget's disease are associated with an intraductal or infiltrating carcinoma, conventional teaching holds that Paget's disease is a manifestation

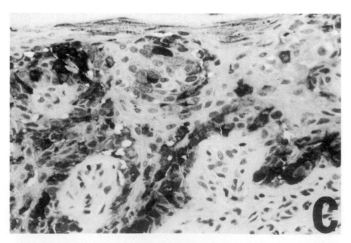

FIGURE 65.11. Immunopositivity for the c-erbB-2 oncoprotein (C) correlates with gene overexpression and is present in most Paget's disease cases.

of the migration of ductal breast cancer into the epidermis. However, this concept remains a largely untested and unproven hypothesis.

In support of the migration hypothesis, several groups have performed immunohistochemical studies on both Paget's cells and accompanying ductal carcinomas to demonstrate the presence of common antigens. Paget's disease and associated ductal carcinomas have been found, in selected studies, to coexpress specific low-molecular weight keratin subclasses, epithelial membrane antigen, carcinoembryonic antigen, κ-casein, α-lactalbumin, carcinoma-associated antigens such as TAG-72, gross cystic disease fluid protein-15, lysozyme, S100 protein, and the c-*erb*B-2 oncoprotein (5,18–28). Many authors contend that concordant immunostaining results suggest that the tumor cells of Paget's disease and breast cancer originate from the same neoplastic population. However, similar staining profiles are not definitive evidence of clonality. Antigens may be shared by virtually all derivatives of the embryonic epidermis and may be aberrantly expressed on neoplastic transformation of the Paget's cells. The alternative possibility of concomitant but independent malignant transformation of ductal epithelium and intraepidermal cells has certainly not been excluded by data from immunohistochemical studies. Indeed, discordance between the carcinoembryonic antigen and gross cystic disease fluid protein-15 profiles of Paget's cells and ductal adenocarcinomas has been demonstrated in some cases and cited as evidence that Paget's cells probably emanate from the epidermis itself (28).

Ultrastructural studies provide another approach to establishing whether Paget's disease originates in underlying carcinomas or in the epidermis. Electron micrographic studies performed on Paget's cells have yielded variable results and interpretations. Most evaluations describe a variable degree of plasma membrane specialization, with the presence of desmosomes and microvilli (5,29–31). The presence of large junctional complexes between Paget's cells and adjacent keratinocytes suggests that Paget's cells do not migrate into intact epithelium but are instead transformed from native epidermal constituents (30–31a). Others have compared the ultrastructural features of Paget's cells with those of ductal breast carcinomas (5) or normal mammary secretory cells (32), and these assessments have found instead putative similarities supportive of the epidermotropic hypothesis. In corroboration of a ductal origin for Paget's cells, selected dissimilarities have been noted between keratinocytes and Paget's cells such as the relative scarcity of elaborate cell junctions, tonofilaments, and keratohyaline granules in mammary Paget's disease. General markers of glandular derivation such as prominent endoplasmic reticulum, numerous mitochondria, secretory vacuoles, and lipid droplets also have been used to argue for a ductal origin of Paget's cells. Nevertheless, no distinctive ultrastructural features uniquely determine their nature.

In support of the in situ evolution of mammary Paget's disease in the epidermis, Toker (29) reported the presence of glandular epithelial heterotopias within the normal nipple skin in 12% of 109 autopsy cases in both sexes. This finding suggests that nonneoplastic glandular populations of cells may provide the substrate for the development of a primary intraepidermal adenocarcinoma. The existence of mammary Paget's disease in the epidermis in the absence of an underlying breast carcinoma (1,26,31,33–36) and the occurrence of mammary Paget's disease with no evidence of a direct connection to underlying carcinomas (3) also would strongly support an origin of Paget's cells within the epidermis.

In considering the histogenesis of mammary Paget's disease, it is tempting to consider its similarity to extramammary Paget's disease. Extramammary Paget's disease is a rare adenocarcinoma, which is most often observed in the vulva, scrotum, and perianal skin. These sites are included in the "milk line" and overlie apocrine gland–bearing tissue. Extramammary Paget's disease is morphologically identical to the mammary variety, but, unlike mammary Paget's disease, it is almost exclusively confined to the epidermis. In our experience, less than 1% of extramammary Paget's disease cases demonstrate invasive involvement of the dermis or an association with a regional visceral carcinoma.

Although it has been posited that extramammary Paget's disease is caused by the spread of an underlying sweat gland carcinoma into the epidermis, most cases of extramammary Paget's disease feature tumor cells that are confined to the surface epithelium (37). When concomitant carcinomas are discovered in association with vulvar extramammary Paget's disease, adenocarcinoma of the vulvar apocrine glands is most common. Interestingly, carcinoma of the breast, either synchronous or metachronous, is next most frequently associated with vulvar Paget's disease (38). Paget's disease of the genitoperineal skin has rarely been reported in association with regional visceral malignancies such as cancers of the urinary bladder, rectum, periurethral glands, Bartholin's glands, or endocervix (39–42). Hence, the frequency of underlying malignancy represents the main difference between mammary Paget's disease and extramammary Paget's disease.

There is a lack of consensus in the literature on the issue of synonymity of mammary and extramammary Paget's disease. The main body of evidence from immunohistochemistry and enzyme histochemistry tends to support predominantly apocrine differentiation in both mammary and extramammary Paget's disease (43,44). Both disorders appear to differentiate toward glandular epithelium and may express restricted keratin subclasses, epithelial membrane antigen, human milk fat globule proteins, carcinoembryonic antigen, tumor-associated glycoprotein-72, and gross cystic disease fluid protein-15 (19,20,24,44–49).

If Paget's disease is a unified histopathologic entity regardless of its mammary or extramammary location, as we believe it is, the lack of associated underlying malignancies in some cases of each form constitutes the strongest evidence for an intraepidermal pathogenesis. Both mammary Paget's disease and extramammary Paget's disease probably represent local epidermal proliferations, which serve as markers for an increased susceptibility to a variety of regional, but independent, neoplastic processes (49a). In the breast, this marker function of mammary Paget's disease is great; in other sites, it is much more limited. The concept that certain cutaneous diseases are indicators of risk for noncutaneous malignancies is not a new one. Over the years, dermatologists have learned that certain forms of acanthosis nigricans, eruptive seborrheic keratosis, basal cell carcinomas, sebaceous proliferations, and other dermal adnexal neoplasms may be attended by carcinomas of visceral organs.

MOLECULAR OBSERVATIONS ON PAGET'S DISEASE

Because neither immunohistochemical nor ultrastructural analyses have definitively accounted for the morphogenesis and unique pathologic features of Paget's disease, investigators have recently turned to molecular genetic studies. The epidermotropic hypothesis for mammary Paget's disease requires the presence of an underlying breast carcinoma in which the cells of the latter tumor have migrated into the surface epithelium. Solid tumors are commonly known to spread by directly invasive growth or embolic metastasis. However, the extension of such neoplasms by migration into an otherwise intact adjacent tissue is largely speculative and the molecular mechanisms whereby it would occur are unclear. Several groups have evaluated the expression of the c-*erb*B-2 (HER-2) oncoprotein by Paget's disease, as well as HER-3 and HER-4 (49b). It has been suggested that these moieties may function to promote the intraepithelial spread of adenocarcinoma cells. The proteins in question are transmembrane glycoproteins with mitogenic activities; in particular, the HER polypeptides show a close homology to the epidermal growth factor receptor. In support of the migration theory for Paget's disease, Schelfhout et al. (49a) have proposed a mechanism wherein HER gene products on Paget's cells serve as receptors for Heregulin-alpha, a motility factor produced by epidermal keratinocytes (in the skin of the breast and elsewhere). Amplification of the gene encoding the c-*erb*B-2 oncoprotein has been demonstrated in 30% of primary breast carcinomas (50–54). Gene amplification results in elevated intracellular levels of both c-*erb*B-2 RNA and translated protein. Immunohistochemical studies, in which positive staining correlates with gene overexpression, have revealed a higher incidence of positivity in ductal carcinoma in situ (DCIS) than in invasive carcinoma of the breast (55–57). Intraductal carcinomas (DCIS) with high-grade comedo-type morphology demonstrate c-*erb*B-2 immunopositivity in 80% to 100% of cases.

Investigators evaluating the expression of c-*erb*B-2 protein in Paget's disease have likewise reported immunolabeling in 79% to 100% of cases (25–27).

Many evaluations have reported that the extent of intraductal breast cancer is greatest and the incidence of postexcisional recurrence more frequent in the comedo-type of DCIS (58,59). The linkage between c-*erb*B-2 overexpression in comedo DCIS with extensive intraductal spread and Paget's disease with its intraepithelial growth is intriguing but unproven. Indeed, in the final analysis, it may represent an epiphenomenon rather than a basic pathogenic mechanism.

The role that HER oncoproteins play, if any, in the motility of tumor cells is similarly unclear. De Potter et al. (60) attempted to address this question using tissue cultures derived from human breast carcinomas. These authors reported that incubation of tumor cells that overexpress the c-*erb*B-2 protein with medium that had been conditioned by epidermal keratinocytes induced motility of the cells and may therefore have acted as a chemotactic factor that could attract Paget's cells into the nipple epidermis. However, it should be stated forthrightly that this experimental milieu is quite unlike the anatomic context of clinical mammary and extramammary Paget's disease.

SUMMARY AND FUTURE DIRECTIONS

Evidence exists to support either of two antithetical hypotheses to explain the histogenesis of mammary Paget's disease. The migration hypothesis proposes that Paget's cells are derived from underlying breast carcinomas that have spread through migration into the epidermis. The in situ hypothesis suggests an origin for mammary Paget's disease from stem cells that differ from those of associated, underlying breast carcinomas. The migration model, therefore, necessarily implies a monoclonal derivation of Paget's cells, whereas the in situ hypothesis would allow multiclonal derivation of Paget's cells and those of possibly associated breast carcinomas. Molecular genetics provides a number of methods to investigate these issues further. Conventionally, tumor tissues have been analyzed by the Southern blot method to detect gene rearrangements, restriction fragment length polymorphisms, or oncogene insertions. In specific reference to mammary Paget's disease, however, this technique has limited value because it requires large numbers of tumor cells and is an insensitive measure of clonality in tissues that contain large numbers of non-neoplastic cells.

Strategies have evolved for the determination of clonality using small numbers of tumor cells in either fresh or paraffin-embedded tissues (61–64). Such procedures rely on the differential methylation that occurs in females with X chromosome inactivation. By targeting polymorphic loci and using the polymerase chain reaction, it is possible to determine which of the two X chromosomes have been inactivated in a tumor cell population. One could obviously employ this technique in the study of Paget's disease. Given a suitably large statistical sample, demonstration of identical allele inactivation in Paget's cells and those of underlying breast carcinomas would establish a monoclonal derivation. Conversely, variable X chromosome allele activation between the cells of mammary Paget's disease and those of DCIS of the breast would argue strongly for the in situ tumorigenesis model.

The recent identification of susceptibility loci for familial breast cancer, namely, BRCA-1 and BRCA-2 (65–68), may also provide tools for investigating the pathogenesis of mammary Paget's disease. It remains to be demonstrated whether mutant alleles of these genes predispose carriers to the development of Paget's disease as they do for other forms of breast cancer. Again, molecular techniques that utilize the polymerase chain reaction would permit a retrospective analysis of mutations in the *BRCA* genes in Paget's disease and associated ductal mammary carcinomas. This, among other eventualities, represents an exciting prospect for future research on this enigmatic disorder.

REFERENCES

1. Ashikari R, Park K, Huvos AG, et al. Paget's disease of the breast. *Cancer* 1970;26:680–686.
2. Nance FC, DeLoach DH, Welsh RA, et al. Paget's disease of the breast. *Ann Surg* 1970;171:864–874.
3. Paone JF, Baker RR. Pathogenesis and treatment of Paget's disease of the breast. *Cancer* 1981;48:825–829.
4. Chaudary NM, Millis RR, Lane EB, et al. Paget's disease of the nipple: a ten-year review including clinical, pathological, and immunohistochemical findings. *Breast Cancer Res Treat* 1986; 8:139–146.
5. Ordonez NG, Awalt H, Mackay B. Mammary and extramammary Paget's disease; an immunohistochemical and ultrastructural study. *Cancer* 1987;59:1173–1183.
6. Bulens P, Vanuytsel L Rijnders A, et al. Breast conserving treatment of Paget's disease. *Radiother Oncol* 1991;17:305–309.
7. Berg JW, Hutter RV. Breast cancer. *Cancer* 1995;75:257–269.
8. Satiani B, Powell RW, Mathews WE. Paget disease of the male breast. *Arch Surg* 1977;112:587–592.
9. Lancer HA, Moschella SL. Paget's disease of the male breast. *J Am Acad Dermatol* 1982;7:398–396.
10. Muretto P, Polizzi V, Staccioli MP. Paget's disease in gynecomastia: immunohistochemical study of a case. *Tumori* 1988;74:183–190.
11. Sano Y, Inoue T, Aso M, et al. Paget's disease of the male breast-report of a case and histopathologic study. *J Dermatol* 1989; 16:237–241.
12. Kister SJ, Haagensen CD. Paget's disease of the breast. *Am J Surg* 1970;119:606–609.
13. Salvadori B, Fariselli G, Saccozzi R. Analysis of 100 cases of Paget's disease of the breast. *Tumori* 1976;62:529–535.
14. Du Tait RS, Van Rensburg PS, Goedhals L. Paget's disease of the breast. *SAMJ* 1988;73:95–97.
15. Rayne SC, Santa Cruz DJ. Anaplastic Paget's disease. *Am J Surg Pathol* 1992;16:1085–1091.
15a. Nakamura S, Ishida-Yamamoto A, Takahashi H, et al. Pigmented Paget's disease of the male breast: a case report. *Dermatology* 2001; 202:134–137.
15b. Zeng Z, Melamed J, Symmans PJ, et al. Benign proliferative nipple duct lesions frequently contain CAM5.2 and anti-cytokeratin 7 immunoreactive cells in the overlying epidermis. *Am J Surg Pathol* 1999; 23:1349–1355.
16. Glasgow BJ, Wen DR, Al-Jitawi S, et al. Antibody to S100 protein aids the separation of pagetoid melanoma from mammary and extramammary Paget's disease. *J Cutan Pathol* 1987;14: 223–226.
17. Hitchcock A, Tophain S, Bell J, et al. Routine diagnosis of mammary Paget's disease. *Am J Surg Pathol* 1992;16:58–61.
18. Bussolati G, Pich A. Mammary and extramammary Paget's disease. *Am J Pathol* 1975;80:117–124.
19. Nadji M, Morales AR, Girtanner RE, et al. Paget's disease of the skin: a unifying concept of histogenesis. *Cancer* 1982;50:2203–2206.
20. Kariniemi AL, Forsman L, Wahlstrom T, et al. Expression of differentiation antigens in mammary and extramammary Paget's disease. *Br J Dermatol* 1984;110:203–210.
21. Kariniemi AL, Ramaekers F, Lehto VP, et al. Paget cells express cytokeratins typical of glandular epithelia. *Br J Dermatol* 1985; 112:179–183.
22. Kirkham N, Berry N, Jones DE, et al. Paget's disease of the nipple: immunohistochemical localization of milk fat globule membrane antigens. *Cancer* 1985;55:1510–1512.
23. Lee AX, DeLellis RA, Rosen PP, et al. Alpha-lactalbumin as an immunochemical marker for metastatic breast carcinomas. *Am J Surg Pathol* 1984;8:93–100.
24. Guamer J, Cohen C, DeRose PB. Histogenesis of extramammary and mammary Paget cells: an immunohistochemical study. *Am J Dermatopathol* 1989;11:313–318.
25. Lammie GA, Barnes DM, Millis RR, et al. An immunohistochemical study of the presence of c-*erb*B-2 protein in Paget's disease of the nipple. *Histopathology* 1989;15:505–514.
26. Meissner K, Riviere A, Haupt G, et al. Study of neu-protein expression in mammary Paget's disease with and without underlying breast carcinoma and in extramammary Paget's disease. *Am J Pathol* 1990;137:1305–1309.
27. Wolber RA, Dupuis EA, Wick MR. Expression of c-*erb*B-2 oncoprotein in mammary and extramammary Paget's disease. *Am J Clin Pathol* 1991;96:243–247.
28. Cohen C, Guarner J, DeRose PE. Mammary Paget's disease and associated carcinoma: an immunohistochemical study. *Arch Pathol Lab Med* 1993;117:291–294.
29. Toker C. Clear cells of the nipple epidermis. *Cancer* 1970;25: 601–610.
30. Sagebiel RW. Ultrastructural observations on epidermal cells in Paget's disease of the breast. *Am J Pathol* 1969;57:49–65.
31. Lagios MD, Westdahl PR, Rose MR, et al. Paget's disease of the nipple: alternative management in cases without or with minimal extent of underlying breast carcinoma. *Cancer* 1984;54: 545–551.
31a. Mai KT. Morphological evidence for field effect as a mechanism for tumour spread in mammary Paget's disease. *Histopathology* 1999;35:567–576.
32. Jahn H, Osther PJ, Nielsen EH, et al. An electron microscopic study of clinical Paget's disease of the nipple. *APMIS* 1995; 103:628–634.
33. Muir R. The pathogenesis of Paget's disease of the nipple and associated lesions. *Br J Surg* 1935;22:728–737.
34. Jones RE. Mammary Paget's disease without underlying carcinoma. *Am J Dermatopathol* 1985;7:361–365.
35. Mori O, Hachisuka H, Nakano S, et al. A case of mammary Paget's disease without an underlying carcinoma: microscopic analysis of the DNA content in Paget cells. *J Dermatol* 1994; 21:160–165.
36. Vielh P, Validire P, Kheirallah S, et al. Paget's disease of the nip-

ple without clinically and radiologically detectable breast tumor. Histochemical and immunohistochemical study of 44 cases. *Res Pract* 1993;189:150–155.

37. Jones RE, Ackerman AB. Extramammary Paget's disease: a critical reappraisal. *Am J Dermatopathol* 1979;1:101–132.

38. Friedrich EG, Wilkinson EJ, Steingraeber PH, et al. Paget's disease of the vulva and carcinoma of the breast. *Obstet Gynecol* 1975;46:130–134.

39. Takeshita K, Izumoi S, Ebuchi M, et al. A case of rectal carcinoma concomitant with pagetoid lesion in the perianal region. *Gastroenterol Jpn* 1978;13:85–95.

40. McKee PH, Hertogs KT. Endocervical adenocarcinoma and vulvar Paget's disease: a significant association. *Br J Dermatol* 1980;103:443–448.

41. Degefu S, O'Quinn AG, Dhurandhar HN. Paget's disease of the vulva and urogenital malignancies. *Gynecol Oncol* 1986;25:347–354.

42. Ojeda VJ, Heenen PJ, Watson SH. Paget's disease of the groin associated with adenocarcinoma of the urinary bladder. *J Cutan Pathol* 1987;14:227–231.

43. Wick MR, Lillemoe TJ, Copland GT, et al. Gross cystic disease fluid protein-15 as a marker for breast cancer. *Hum Pathol* 1989;20:281–287.

44. Mazoujian G, Pinkus GS, Haagensen DE. Extramammary Paget's disease: evidence for an apocrine origin. *Am J Surg Pathol* 1984;8:43–50.

45. Vanstapel MJ, Gatter KC, De Wolf-Peeters C, et al. Immunohistochemical study of mammary and extra-mammary Paget's disease. *Histopathology* 1984;8:1013–1023.

46. Nagle RE, Lucas DO, McDaniel KM, et al. New evidence linking mammary Paget cells to a common cell phenotype. *Am J Clin Pathol* 1985;83:431–438.

47. Mariani-Constantini R, Andreola S, Rilke F. Tumour-associated antigens in mammary and extramammary Paget's disease. *Virchows Arch* 1985;405:333–340.

48. Tazawa T, Ito M, Fujiwara H, et al. Immunologic characteristics of keratins in extramammary Paget's disease. *Arch Dermatol* 1988;124:1063–1068.

49. Imam A, Yoshida SO, Taylor CR. Distinguishing tumour cells of mammary from extramammary Paget's disease using antibodies to two different glycoproteins from human milk-fat-globule membrane. *Br J Cancer* 1988;58:373–378.

49a. Lloyd J, Flanagan AM. Mammary & extramammary Paget's disease. *J Clin Pathol* 2000;53:742–749.

49b. Schelfhout VR, Coene ED, Delaey B, et al. Pathogenesis of Paget's disease: epidermal Heregulin-alpha, motility factor, and the HER receptor family. *J Natl Cancer Inst* 2000;92:622–628.

50. Van de Vijver MJ, van de Bersselaar R, Devilee P, et al. Amplification of the neu (c-*erb*B-2) oncogene in human mammary tumors is relatively frequent and is often accompanied by amplification of the linked c-*erb*A oncogene. *Mol Cell Biol* 1987;7:2019–2023.

51. Varley JM, Swallow JE, Brammar WJ, et al. Alterations to either the c-*erb*B-2(neu) or c-*myc* protooncogenes in breast carcinomas correlate with poor short-term prognosis. *Oncogene* 1987;1:423–430.

52. Berger MS, Locher GW, Saurer S, et al. Correlation of c-*erb*B2 gene amplification and protein expression in human breast carcinoma with nodal status and nuclear grading. *Cancer Res* 1988;47:1238–1243.

53. Barnes DM, Lammie GA, Millis RR, et al. An immunohistochemical evaluation of c-*erb*B-2 expression in human breast carcinoma. *Br J Cancer* 1988;58:448–453.

54. Slamon DJ, Godolphin W, Jones LA, et al. Studies of the HER-2/*neu* proto-oncoprotein in human breast and ovarian cancer. *Science* 1989;244:707–712.

55. Van de Vijver MJ, Petersen JL, Mooi WJ, et al. Neu-protein overexpression in breast cancer: association with comedo-type ductal carcinoma in situ and limited prognostic value in stage 11 breast cancer. *N Engl J Med* 1988;319:1239–1245.

56. Gusterson BA, Machin LG, Gullick WJ, et al. Immunohistochemical distribution of c-*erb*B-2 in infiltrating and in situ breast cancer. *Int J Cancer* 1988;42:842–846.

57. Allred DC, Clark GM, Molina R, et al. Immunohistochemical analysis of Her-2/*neu* oncogene expression in *in situ* and invasive breast carcinomas: evaluation of pathological characteristics and biological significance. *Lab Invest* 1990;62:3A.

58. Bellamy CO, McDonald C, Salter DM, et al. Noninvasive ductal carcinoma of the breast: the relevance of histologic categorization. *Hum Pathol* 1993;24:16–23.

59. Lagios MD, Margolin FR, Westdahl PR, et al. Mammographically detected duct carcinoma in situ: frequency of local recurrence following tylectomy and prognostic effect of nuclear grade on local recurrence. *Cancer* 1989;63:618–624.

60. De Potter CR, Eeckhout L, Schelfhout AM, et al. Keratinocyte induced chemotaxis in the pathogenesis of Paget's disease of the breast. *Histopathology* 1994;24:349–356.

61. Thompson L, Chang B, Barsky SH. Monoclonal origins of malignant mixed tumors (carcinosarcomas). Evidence for a divergent histogenesis. *Am J Surg Pathol* 1996;20:277–285.

62. Busque L, Zhu J, DeHart D, et al. An expression based clonality assay at the human androgen receptor locus (HUMARA) on chromosome X. *Nucleic Acids Res* 1994;22:697–698.

63. Gilliland DG, Blanchard KL, Levy J, et al. Clonality in myeloproliferative disorders: analysis by means of the polymerase chain reaction. *Proc Natl Acad Sci U S A* 1991;88: 6846–6852.

64. Willman C, Busqne L, Griffith BB, et al. Langerhans'-cell histiocytosis (histiocytosis X)—a clonal proliferative disease. *N Engl J Med* 1994;331:191–193.

65. Cannon-Albright LA, Skolnick MH. The genetics of familial breast cancer. *Semin Oncol* 1996;23:1–5.

66. Radford DM, Zehnbauer BA. Inherited breast cancer. *Surg Clin North Am* 1996;76:205–220.

67. Tavtigian SV, Simard J, Rommers J, et al. The complete BRCA2 gene and mutations in chromosome 13q-linked kindreds. *Nat Genet* 1996;12:222–227.

68. Szabo CL, King MC. Inherited breast and ovarian cancer. *Hum Mol Genet* 1995;4:1811–1817.

LOBULAR CARCINOMA IN SITU

BENJAMIN O. ANDERSON   **KRISTINE RINN**   **DIANNE GEORGIAN-SMITH**
THOMAS LAWTON   **CHRISTOPHER I. LI**   **ROGER E. MOE**

Although it is commonly accepted that ductal carcinoma in situ (DCIS) represents a spectrum of pathologic entities that range in aggressiveness, the general view has been that lobular carcinoma in situ (LCIS) is a monotonously indolent lesion lacking significant invasive potential. LCIS has come to be viewed as a nonsurgical disease, an ambiguous marker of risk for future breast cancer in either breast. This view may underestimate the biologic variability of LCIS and its potential for disease progression in selected cases. In his preface to the first edition of this textbook (1), Silverstein observes that, "Our current approaches to DCIS are based on morphology rather than etiology, on phenotype rather than genotype." This observation applies equally well to LCIS. Recent compelling molecular genetic and immunohistochemical evidence suggests that LCIS may include more aggressive lesions having homologies to both invasive lobular carcinoma (ILC) and low-grade DCIS. As our knowledge of the underlying genetic makeup of LCIS, DCIS, and invasive cancer increases, we may find that highly selected cases of LCIS warrant surgical treatment, just as low-grade DCIS does. The challenge will be to understand and predict the biology of this disorder well enough so correct patient selection can occur.

LCIS is confounding to categorize. The unique borderline behavior of LCIS challenges our definitions of "breast cancer risk factor" versus "premalignant lesion" versus "preinvasive cancer." Our driving desire to fit LCIS into one discrete category is powered by the requirement that we make specific clinical treatment recommendations to our patients with LCIS. However, LCIS repeatedly illustrates the inadequacy of "black-and-white" descriptors for a pathologic entity that manifests a spectrum of biologic activity. The thesis of this chapter is that although LCIS is clearly a risk factor for future development of separate and distinct invasive breast cancers, it also has features of a premalignant lesion and even a preinvasive cancer, albeit in unusual circumstances. Ultimately, clinical recommendations for patients diagnosed with LCIS probably must be provided in the absence of a neat definition for LCIS as cancer or noncancer.

The goals of this chapter are to

1. review the early historical concepts of LCIS, before and after the term lobular neoplasia came into vogue,
2. present new data regarding the rising incidence of LCIS, which is associated with a concomitant rising incidence of ILC,
3. describe the spectrum of histopathology that characterizes LCIS compared with the microscopic features of low-grade DCIS,
4. examine the clinical presentations associated with LCIS and describe the subtle radiographic features of LCIS, which differ from the stereotypic belief that LCIS is devoid of mammographic findings,
5. discuss the parallels between LCIS and low-grade intraductal carcinoma in terms of risk of future breast cancer,
6. explore the kinetic and genetic relationships between LCIS and low-grade DCIS and the molecular genetic relationship between LCIS and ILC,
7. suggest principles of LCIS clinical management regarding biopsy, diagnosis, and chemoprevention treatment with particular attention directed toward the evaluation and management of pleomorphic LCIS.

HISTORICAL BACKGROUND AND LOBULAR CARCINOMA IN SITU CLASSIFICATION

Why Did Early Pathologists Describe Lobular Carcinoma in Situ as a Cancer?

Rosen's (2) outstanding historical review of carcinoma in situ (CIS) and precancerous lesions of the breast illustrates work by various authors dating back to 1865, when Cornil (3) described intraepithelial breast carcinoma in lobules. In 1919, Ewing (4) published photomicrographs of atypical proliferation of acinar cells, photographs that show the lesion that we today call LCIS. Early reports on lobular carcinomas (acinar carcinomas) primarily dealt with invasive carcinomas coexisting with intraepithelial carcinoma cells, not just intraepithelial lobular carcinomas. For example, Cheatle and Cutler (5) published an extensively illustrated book on tumors of the breast in 1931. Challenging the concept that malignant-appearing cells confined to the lobules and ducts were merely precancerous, they argued that these cells look cytologically identical to those from invasive cancers: "In the earliest carcinomata of the breast there is always present an epithelial neoplasia that is still confined within normal boundaries. The morphological characteristics of the epithelial cells within the normal boundaries are identical with those that have invaded, and there can be no doubt that they form the primary tumour from which these invading cells originated. In these instances, there is no doubt that these epithelial cells inside the normal boundaries are as biologically malignant as those that have transgressed them and are trespassing in the surrounding tissues" (5).

Indeed, the cytologically malignant appearance of LCIS provides the basis for arguing that LCIS is itself a preinvasive cancer. LCIS cells look cancerous to the point that a diagnosis of malignancy is sometimes made when LCIS is sampled by fine needle aspiration. Furthermore, no lobular cells other than LCIS cells have even been identified as possible precursors of ILC.

The term LCIS was first coined by Foote and Stewart (6) in 1941, who wrote about this uncommon form of in situ neoplasia affecting the lobules and most distal microscopic ducts of the breast. Foote and Stewart noted that, "Examples of entirely noninfiltrative lesions of a definitely cancerous cytology have been accumulated for almost every mucosa-lined structure." Accordingly, they reviewed 300 mastectomy specimens collected over a year at New York's Memorial Hospital (known today as Memorial Sloan-Kettering Cancer Center). Among the 300, they identified two cases of strict intraepithelial carcinoma in lobules, which they labeled LCIS. They observed a proliferation of small, uniform, discohesive cells filling and often distending the acinar units within a lobule. Foote and Stewart described a "graded progressive increase in cell size so gradual that demarcation is impossible." In that same year, Muir (7) published a report on the evolution of carcinoma of the mamma, including intra-acinous carcinoma as well as other types of breast cancer. Muir stated that the epithelial cells of the acini became larger, often more columnar, with increasing dedifferentiation. Both articles describe patterns of LCIS combined with ILC, similar to earlier descriptions by Ewing and Cheatle.

By the 1940s, the concept was becoming well established that CIS can exist within the duct or lobule and progressively infiltrate the native glandular structure to form an invasive malignancy (8). Foote and Stewart's landmark publication thereby set the stage for performing mastectomies as treatment for LCIS. A surgeon at that time who read their article would have learned that "a breast in which this process occurs in the slightest degree constitutes an extreme hazard." The authors warned that it would be a tragic mistake to miss the diagnosis of LCIS. They reported: "In our first case, local excision revealed this process, and we were

unfortunately not aware of its significance. Within a few months, that patient had infiltrating cancer with axillary metastases, and bone metastases not long after that" (7).

Today, we recognize that the patient of Foote and Stewart almost certainly had coexisting but clinically occult invasive cancer in the breast. Her underlying invasive and metastatic disease was missed by the excisional biopsy. Surgeons from the 1940s and 1950s were unaware of the frequency with which clinically occult cancer exists in the breast because they lacked the breast imaging technology that we have today. They dealt almost exclusively with palpable breast cancers. We now realize that breast cancer progression is much more gradual than Foote and Stewart believed to have occurred in their patient with LCIS.

It becomes easy to see how subsequent surgeons in the mid-twentieth century became primed to perform mastectomies for LCIS. In 1952, Godwin (9) published a case report in which he formally suggested that LCIS evolves into ILC, cementing the idea developed by Foote and Stewart that LCIS is itself a preinvasive malignancy that demands clinical intervention. Godwin's theory dominated clinical thinking for the next three decades. Mastectomy seemed like a reasonable, logical approach to the management of what they thought must be a life-threatening disorder.

Why was Lobular Carcinoma in Situ Redefined as Lobular Neoplasia?

After the original description by Foote and Stewart's of LCIS as a preinvasive cancer, investigators increasingly questioned the histopathologic distinction between LCIS and atypical lobular hyperplasia (ALH) and the associated prognostic significance of each. In particular, Haagensen debated the premalignant potential of the LCIS, believing LCIS, like ALH, to be a fundamentally benign process. In 1978, Haagensen and colleagues (10) reported a long-term follow-up study of 211 patients with ALH and LCIS, collectively grouped together under the term lobular neoplasia. Diagnosis was based on surgical breast biopsies only, mastectomy having not been routinely performed in these women. Over a 15-year period, only a small percentage of these patients developed subsequent breast cancers. Among the 211 patients, 10% were later diagnosed with another cancer in the same breast, and 9% were diagnosed with a cancer in the opposite breast. Haagensen et al. omitted the term cancer from the nomenclature to dissuade surgeons from performing routine mastectomies for LCIS. He reasoned that this restriction was appropriate because of the low incidence of subsequent breast cancer and the nearly equal hazard of contralateral breast cancer, which would be left unaddressed by a unilateral mastectomy.

Also in 1978, Rosen et al. (11) reported a series of 84 cases of LCIS in which only a surgical breast biopsy was performed. Unlike the study of Haagensen et al., this report did not include patients who had only ALH on biopsy. With a follow-up period averaging 24 years after biopsy, 38% of these patients developed a breast cancer other than the initial LCIS, with 14% of these in the same breast as the LCIS, 14% in the opposite breast, and 8% with bilateral cancers. Thus, the study of Rosen et al. reported a higher incidence of subsequent breast cancer development than did the study of Haagensen et al. but described the same bilateral cancer risk. In 1993, Bodian and colleagues (12) published a follow-up study based on the original patients of Haagensen et al. Among the 211 patients with lobular neoplasia (including both ALH and LCIS), there were 99 on whom adequate data were available for 21 years of follow-up. Of these 99 patients, 24% developed another cancer, demonstrating that the potential incidence of subsequent cancers was higher than suggested in Haagensen's original report (10).

Gradually, the medical community increasingly accepted Haagensen's conceptual model of lobular neoplasia, concomitantly recognizing that surgical treatment for the disorder is generally not required or indicated. By the 1990s, the dominant thinking had become the same position taken by Haagensen that LCIS (or lobular neoplasia) is fundamentally not a cancer but rather is simply a risk factor for the development of cancer.

Why is the Term Lobular Carcinoma in Situ Regaining Significance?

Several investigators use the term lobular neoplasia but not necessarily with the same implications intended by Haagensen. Cheatle and Cutler (5) had earlier used the term epithelial neoplasia. Primary epithelial neoplasia pertained to noninfiltrating carcinoma in lobules and ducts, but these authors clearly were not using this term to avoid the cancer designation. Rather, they were trying to define in situ neoplasia in a broad collective sense as precursors of invasive cancer.

Currently, Tavassoli (13) at the Armed Forces Institute of Pathology uses the term lobular neoplasia to represent the entire spectrum of preinvasive lobular pathology. The term can help one avoid the sticky issue of defining absolute criteria by which ALH and LCIS are differentiated. Tavassoli also uses a related term, ductal intraepithelial neoplasia, to describe preinvasive ductal pathology. She defines several substratifying grades within both lobular neoplasia and ductal intraepithelial neoplasia, pointing out the similarities between ductal and lobular preinvasive disease. Although Tavassoli's grading system is well devised, we do not know of other pathologists who currently use this grading system for lobular neoplasia nor are we aware of data about how her data might compare with those from other institutions.

By contrast to Haagensen's perspective, Rosen (14) presents a cogent argument against the ongoing use of the term lobular neoplasia. He points out that present-day treatment of breast cancer commonly involves breast conservation, so the need for a term other than carcinoma no longer exists to

prevent unnecessary mastectomies. Rosen points out that the spectrum of lesions encompassed by lobular neoplasia is so broad as to render it a misleading and useless diagnostic term: "In clinical practice, the use of this term creates a situation in which a single diagnosis does not discriminate between the patient with a minimal proliferative lesion that might be only mildly atypical hyperplasia and fully developed LCIS. ... The term lobular neoplasia disguises our limitations and creates a false sense of specificity for the patient and clinician. The range of morphological changes covered by lobular neoplasia is very broad, making this one of the least specific diagnoses in breast pathology and one that is not recommended " (14).

The risk of invasive cancers developing among women with LCIS is greater than the risk among women with atypical hyperplasia (whether lobular or ductal). As a result, several professional groups continue to use the term LCIS to be distinguished from ALH rather than allowing the all-encompassing term lobular neoplasia in their categorization systems. The National Surgical Adjuvant Breast and Bowel Project (NSABP) P-01 study is a clinical trial using tamoxifen for the prevention of breast cancer (15). This trial revealed a 100% increase in the average annual rate of invasive cancer among women in the placebo group who had a history of LCIS but only a 57% increase in this rate among women with a history of ALH or atypical ductal hyperplasia (ADH). Distinction between the different gradations of lobular neoplasia appears to have prognostic significance and the NSABP continues to collect data in this fashion.

Like the NSABP, the population-based cancer registries that make up the Surveillance, Epidemiologic, and End Results Program continue to categorize LCIS as a specific histopathology entity. Similarly, the National Comprehensive Cancer Network has continued to discuss LCIS in the context of their breast cancer treatment algorithms, although observation remains the preferred "treatment" for the disease (16). Finally, the American Joint Committee on Cancer continues to list LCIS among stage 0 breast diseases, just like DCIS. Even in the most recent staging reclassification, LCIS staging has not been changed, acknowledging the complexity of its biologic behavior. The comment of the American Joint Committee on Cancer committee is that "LCIS is increasingly defined as a risk factor for subsequent breast cancer, although there is some evidence that it may occasionally be a precursor of ILC" (17).

More recently, pathologists have begun to discuss the concept of more aggressive variants of LCIS such as pleomorphic LCIS. Pleomorphic LCIS has higher grade features than does classic LCIS and may have a biologic behavior more typical of DCIS. Recent molecular genetic data support the concept that LCIS is a direct precursor of ILC in some cases. Although it is premature to make specific treatment suggestions for pleomorphic LCIS, future groups could begin to recommend local treatment for selected cases of this disorder, just as we already do for low-grade DCIS.

INCIDENCE

Estimating the incidence of LCIS among the general population is challenging because it generally is diagnosed as an incidental finding on breast biopsies. This makes it unclear what proportion of women who have not undergone breast tissue sampling has undiagnosed LCIS. Nonetheless, different approaches have been used to evaluate the incidence of LCIS including autopsy series, biopsy series from individual institutions, and population-based studies. Each of these study methods introduces a different set of problems and limitations in trying to identify the true incidence of the disease.

Autopsy Series

Autopsy series suggest that LCIS is a rare lesion, occurring in less than 1% of the general population. In 1951, Frantz and colleagues (18) found no cases of LCIS among 225 autopsies of women whose median age was 45 years at death. A limitation of this study was that relatively few slides were prepared from each patient because an average of only two microscopic slides per breast was evaluated. More recently, Kramer and Rush (19) reported an autopsy study of women 70 years of age or older. The investigators looked at an average of 40 slides per breast but also found no cases of LCIS among 70 women from this postmenopausal population. A subsequent Danish autopsy series (20) that extensively evaluated breast tissue from 88 autopsy subjects (57 to 166 blocks per breast) found three cases of LCIS alone and three cases of LCIS with DCIS. However, this study did not specify the ages of the subjects with LCIS and has been criticized for using an overly broad definition of LCIS. A later study (21), with tissue analyses equally rigorous as those in the Danish study, found no cases of LCIS among 101 randomly selected subjects.

The strength of autopsy series is that they avoid the selection bias seen among series of patients who have already been selected to undergo breast biopsy. However, the problem with them is that they are performed on subjects who have come to the end of life. As such, these populations may have characteristics or findings that may not be representative of those of younger women. This would be particularly problematic if LCIS, like normal lobules, tends to regress after menopause in the absence of hormonal stimulation.

Individual Institution Series

Surgical biopsy series from individual institutions suggest that the incidence rates of LCIS among women undergoing biopsy for benign breast lesions range from 0.5% to 3.6% and are higher than the rates for women in the general population. Haagensen and colleagues (10) reported the highest rate among breast biopsy patients (3.6%), identifying 211 lobular neoplasia cases among 5,560 benign epithelial breast lesions diagnosed at Columbia-Presbyterian Medical Center

between 1930 and 1972. Other institutional series, using more restrictive pathologic criteria for inclusion, have reported lower rates ranging from 0.5% to 1.5% (22–24). The lowest incidence (0.5%) was reported by Page and colleagues (24) who identified 48 cases of LCIS among 10,542 benign breast biopsy specimens obtained between 1950 to 1968. The primary reason that they found fewer cases of LCIS is that they demanded strict diagnostic criteria for diagnosing LCIS in contrast to the generous inclusion criteria of Haagensen et al. for lobular neoplasia that encompassed both LCIS and ALH.

Population-Based Studies

Few population-based studies have assessed the incidence rate of LCIS. A Swiss study of nearly 300,000 women reported that the LCIS incidence rate increased from 1.0 per 100,000 person-years in 1977 to 1979 to 2.3 per 100,000 person-years in 1992 to 1994 (25). Similarly, a study in the Detroit metropolitan area showed that the LCIS incidence rates increased between 1975 and 1988 from 1.0 to 2.8 per 100,000 person-years in whites and from 0.8 to 1.9 per 100,000 person-years in blacks (26). Also, a study from Connecticut found that from 1973 to 1992, LCIS incidence rates increased from approximately 1.0 to 2.0 per 100,000 person-years in both whites and blacks (27). The major limitation of population-based studies is that they require outside reporting of LCIS on biopsy specimens. Because many pathologists and clinicians consider LCIS to be a benign disorder, it can be underreported in these registry-based series.

To further study the incidence of LCIS, we examined all cases identified collectively by nine population-based cancer registries in the United States that participate in the Surveillance, Epidemiologic, and End Results program (Fig. 66.1A). Three patterns in LCIS incidence are apparent.

1. Among all ages, the incidence of LCIS is increasing, having more than doubled over the past quarter century from 1.2 per 100,000 women in 1977 to 1980 to 2.8 per 100,000 in 1993 to 1995.
2. The highest incidence of LCIS occurs in middle-aged women around the age of menopause. Like invasive cancer, the incidence of LCIS is low among very young women, but, unlike invasive cancer rates, the incidence of LCIS does not continue to rise. Instead, as women move into the seventh, eighth, and ninth decades of life, LCIS incidence steeply declines.
3. The peak age at diagnosis of LCIS has gradually been shifting upward over the past three decades. In the mid-1970s, the peak incidence of LCIS occurred among women in their 40s at a rate of 4.1 per 100,000. By the end of the 1990s, the peak incidence of LCIS incidence shifted to women in their 50s and rose to 10.2 per 100,000.

These findings are consistent with the hypothesis that LCIS tends to regress over time among postmenopausal

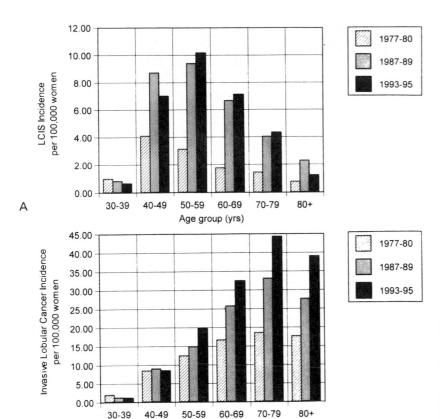

A

B

FIGURE 66.1. Age-adjusted incidence rates of **(A)** LCIS and **(B)** invasive lobular carcinoma comparing three time periods and distributed by decade of life among women from nine Surveillance, Epidemiologic, and End Results (SEER) registry regions. Data from nine SEER registries in Connecticut, Hawaii, Iowa, New Mexico, and Utah and the urban areas surrounding Atlanta, Detroit, San Francisco–Oakland, and Seattle–Puget Sound were analyzed by methods previously described (102).

women. The upward shift in peak age could be related to the increased use of hormone replacement therapy (HRT) during this period (28–31). Hypothetically, HRT could inhibit the natural regression of LCIS that would occur in the absence of hormonal stimulation. Another factor that could contribute to the increased incidence of LCIS in recent years is the increased use of mammographic screening (32–34). Although LCIS is generally not seen on mammograms, screening mammograms often reveal findings that precipitate tissue biopsy. As a result, the number of breast biopsies performed has increased, and concomitantly the number of LCIS cases diagnosed has increased (35).

Increasing Incidence of Both Lobular Carcinoma in Situ and Invasive Lobular Carcinoma

We recently published population-based data demonstrating an increasing incidence in ILC among postmenopausal women from the 1970s to 1990s (31). Comparing these figures with those for LCIS (Fig. 66.1B), similarities and differences can be observed:

1. Like LCIS, the overall incidence of ILC has been increasing from the 1970s to the 1990s.
2. Unlike LCIS, the incidence of ILC does not drop off immediately after menopause. Instead, ILC incidence rates peak in the eighth decade of life before beginning to de-

cline. Thus, the peak age at ILC diagnosis occurs approximately 20 years later in life than does the peak age at diagnosis of LCIS.

During the past 20 years, progestin-containing HRT regimens were increasingly used, specifically to protect women who have not undergone hysterectomy against endometrial cancer. However, progesterone also stimulates lobular development in the breast during the second and third trimesters of pregnancy in preparation for lactation. It would be reasonable to postulate that the increased incidence of LCIS among postmenopausal women may be partly owing to the increased use of progestins.

We have shown that the increased usage of progestin-containing HRT during the 1980s and 1990s directly corresponds to the increased incidence of ILC (36). We hypothesize that the mechanism by which progesterone-containing HRT would do so is through some supportive or stimulatory effect on LCIS. We speculate that progestin-containing HRT may cause LCIS to persist in the breast and that it might facilitate the progression of LCIS into ILC in selected cases.

PATHOLOGY

Anatomy and Physiology of Lobules

A normal duct has branching segments with tiny arborizing acini of lobules on the perimeter of each segment (Fig. 66.2).

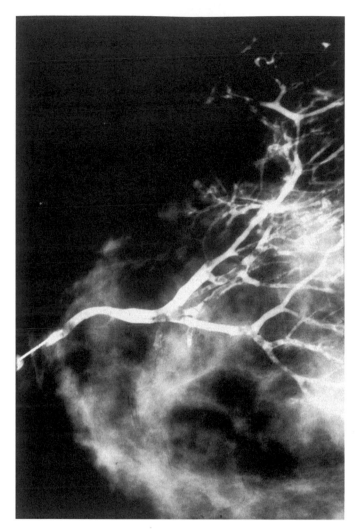

FIGURE 66.2. Ductogram of a normal ductal segment shows radio-opaque dye injected into the central sinuses via the nipple.

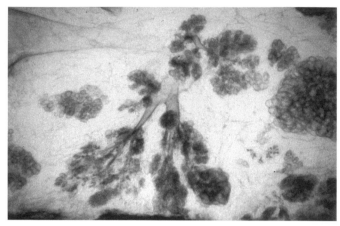

FIGURE 66.3. Thick section of normal human breast tissue observed at low magnification (subgross anatomy), with the epithelium stained with hematoxylin to stand out against the background stroma. (Specimen provided by Dr. Hanna Jensen, Davis, CA.)

veloping mammary carcinoma. They suggest that these persistent atypical mammary lobules could be precancerous in humans.

Histopathologic Features of Classic Lobular Carcinoma in Situ

In their original 1941 description of LCIS, Foote and Stewart (6) described a proliferation of small, uniform, discohesive cells filling and often distending the acinar units within a lobule. The cells of classic LCIS are small, relatively uniform in size, with round to oval nuclei with scanty cytoplasm lacking prominent nucleoli (Fig. 66.5A). The cells frequently contain intracytoplasmic lumina. These classic

Lobules do not appear on the sides of the larger ducts. Branching ducts terminate in lobules, much like stems terminating in tiny grape-like clusters (Fig. 66.3). The functional unit of lactation, called the terminal ductal–lobular unit, contains blind-end ductules that merge into lobules and bulge with acini (Fig. 66.4). Using a three-dimensional technique of subgross histopathology preparation, Wellings et al. (37) analyzed 119 whole human breasts. They reported that, with the exception of intraductal papillomata that occur in larger ducts, most breast lesions begin in the terminal ductal–lobular units or in the lobules themselves. These peripherally developing lesions include most benign masses, DCIS, and LCIS.

In general, lobules become atrophic and disappear after menopause unless the patient is taking HRT. Conversely, Wellings et al. (38) reported that some human mammary lobules persist after menopause, and some atypical lobules are morphologically similar to preneoplastic alveolar nodules that occur in strains of mice with a propensity for de-

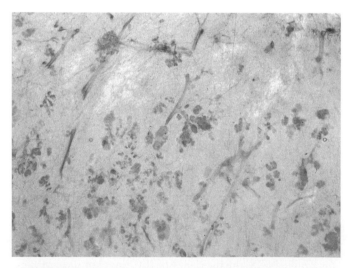

FIGURE 66.4. Subgross specimen showd terminal ductal-lobular units at higher magnification. (Specimen provided by Dr. Peggy Porter, Seattle, WA.)

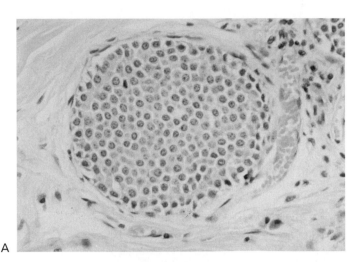
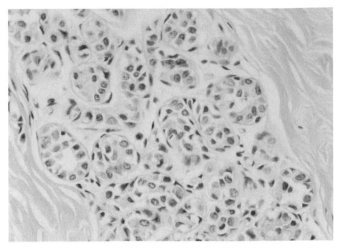

A   B

FIGURE 66.5. Photomicrograph of classic lobular carcinoma in situ (LCIS) **(A)** and atypical lobular hyperplasia (ALH) **(B)** stained by standard hematoxylin and eosin. Classic LCIS cells are small, relatively uniform in size, with round to oval nuclei without prominent nucleoli and scanty cytoplasm. LCIS is distinguished from ALH by having at least half of the acinar units within the lobule filled with neoplastic cells. LCIS lobules are typically distended with cells, although this is not required for a LCIS diagnosis to be made.

cytologic features have been referred to as type A cells (10). Type A cells of classic LCIS are contrasted with type B cells, which are also seen in the lobules of some LCIS cases but are larger and more pleomorphic. Type B cells are cytologically reminiscent of DCIS, suggesting a more aggressive cellular biology that define pleomorphic LCIS as discussed below. Cytologic alterations in some cases of LCIS include intracellular mucin, signet ring cell formation, clear cell change, and apocrine differentiation (39–44).

Histologically, one of the defining features of LCIS is the characteristic discohesiveness of the cells as they fill individual acinar units (6,10). Although the discohesiveness of the cells and intracytoplasmic vacuoles can give the false impression of secondary lumina, cribriform growth and true lumen formation are not seen in classic LCIS (10). In some instances, the cells grow in a mosaic pattern within the acini, resulting in more distinct cell borders (44).

Foote and Stewart (6) did not define quantitative criteria for the fraction of involved acinar units or lobules necessary for diagnosing LCIS in their original description. Since that publication, several authors have attempted to develop quantitative criteria for LCIS to distinguish it from ALH (Fig. 66.5B). Most authors now believe that the diagnosis can be made with as little as one lobule containing neoplastic cells (10,11,45). However, within a lobular unit, there is still disagreement as to how many acinar units need to be involved and how extensive that involvement must be to make a diagnosis of LCIS versus ALH. Some authors believe that at least half of the acinar units in a lobule need to be filled and distended by neoplastic cells (46,47). Others believe that three-fourths of the acini should be involved (48), but that distention of acinar units is not a requirement for the diagnosis of LCIS (10,44).

Although the neoplastic cells begin within the lobule, they can extend up into the most peripheral microscopic ducts, splitting the ductal epithelial layer off from the surrounding myoepithelial layer (Fig. 66.6). This extension process, called pagetoid spread, can sometimes be challenging to distinguish from some forms of DCIS, particularly when the DCIS extends in an analogous manner up into the lobules,

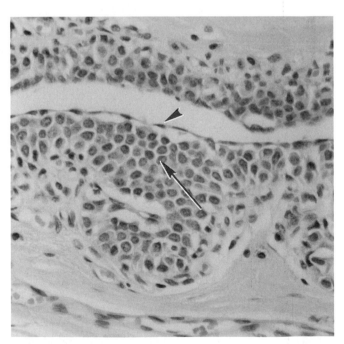

FIGURE 66.6. Photomicrograph of lobular carcinoma in situ demonstrates pagetoid spread from a lobule into the adjacent duct. Lobular neoplastic cells (*arrow*) extend up into the most peripheral microscopic ducts by splitting the ductal epithelial layer (*arrowhead*) off the surrounding myoepithelial layer.

so-called cancerization of the lobules. The clinical significance of LCIS pagetoid spread, whether it represents a more aggressive biologic variant of LCIS, is unknown at this time.

Pleomorphic Lobular Carcinoma in Situ

Since the 1941 description by Foote and Stewart (6) of classic LCIS, there have been multiple descriptions of CIS with the classic lobular pattern of growth but with more pleomorphic cytology (10,13,44,49–57). These lesions have been variably called type B LCIS, pleomorphic LCIS, and mixed ductal-lobular CIS to name a few. In almost all these descriptions, the cells in question grow in the pattern of classic LCIS with acinar distention, discohesiveness, and pagetoid extension along terminal ducts. However, the cytology is more pleomorphic, the cells contain more cytoplasm, nucleoli can be prominent, and central necrosis is often identified (Fig. 66.7). Although relatively rare in classic LCIS, Tavassoli (13) notes that necrosis itself does not rule out a diagnosis of LCIS. This histopathologic pattern is visually reminiscent of DCIS, but the loss of E-cadherin staining confirms that the lesion is lobular rather than ductal in origin as discussed below (Fig. 66.8).

We prefer the term pleomorphic LCIS to the other descriptions of nonclassic LCIS because the lesion tends to be associated with ILC and, in particular, the pleomorphic form of ILC (49,50,54,55). Many of the cytologic features of pleomorphic LCIS bear more similarity to those of classic DCIS and are vastly different from the small, uniform,

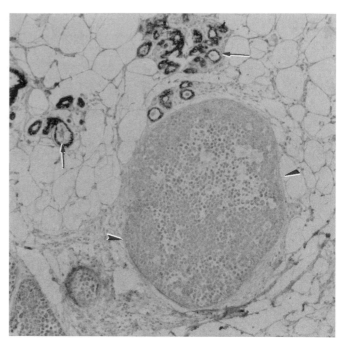

FIGURE 66.8. E-cadherin immunostaining distinguishes pleomorphic lobular carcinoma in situ (LCIS) from ductal carcinoma in situ. E-cadherin is a transmembrane glycoprotein responsible for cell-cell adhesion (103). Membranous staining of cells in benign lobules (*arrows*) is absent in cells within the LCIS lobule (*arrowheads*). E-cadherin expression is lost in lobular but not ductal carcinomas. E-cadherin immunostaining image (100×). (From Georgian-Smith D, Lawton TJ. Calcifications of lobular carcinoma in situ of the breast: radiologic-pathologic correlation. *AJR Am J Roentgenol* 2001;176:1255–1259, with permission.)

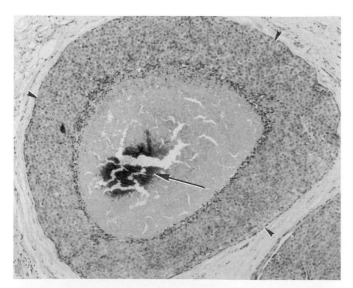

FIGURE 66.7. Photomicrograph of pleomorphic lobular carcinoma in situ (LCIS) demonstrates central necrosis and calcifications (*arrow*) within LCIS-containing lobule (*arrowheads*). These calcifications are associated with the pleomorphic LCIS and to a much lesser degree with the surrounding benign tissue. Hematoxylin and eosin image (400×). (From Georgian-Smith D, Lawton TJ. Calcifications of lobular carcinoma in situ of the breast: radiologic-pathologic correlation. *AJR Am J Roentgenol* 2001;176:1255–1259, with permission.)

round cells of classic LCIS. Because the therapy for classic LCIS and DCIS differs so drastically, it is important to better determine whether this large-cell type of LCIS is more similar to classic LCIS or to DCIS in terms of prognosis. Long-term follow-up data on this histologic subset of LCIS are not yet available, partly because pathologists from the 1940s and 1950s were only beginning to understand and diagnose lobular pathology.

Microcalcifications and Lobular Carcinoma in Situ

Calcifications sometimes occur in conjunction with LCIS. Prior investigators suggested that calcifications always represent a coincident, serendipitous finding unrelated to the development of malignancy (56). Supporting this view, classic LCIS tends to develop microcalcifications that appear similarly within both the LCIS and the adjacent tissues with benign proliferative change (Fig. 66.9). Pleomorphic LCIS, conversely, may promote microcalcification deposition within the lobules that are specific to LCIS (Fig. 66.7). In some settings of pleomorphic LCIS, microcalcifications are seen within the lobular changes but are not seen in surrounding benign tissues, as our group recently reported (58).

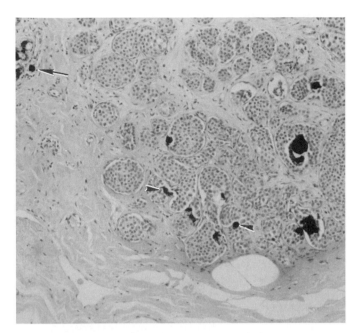

FIGURE 66.9. Photomicrograph of classic lobular carcinoma in situ (LCIS) shows microcalcifications. The calcifications within the LCIS (*arrowheads*) appear similar to those in the adjacent area of benign adenosis (*arrow*). Hematoxylin and eosin image (100×). (From Georgian-Smith D, Lawton TJ. Calcifications of lobular carcinoma in situ of the breast: radiologic-pathologic correlation. *AJR Am J Roentgenol* 2001;176:1255–1259, with permission.)

Immunohistologic Features of Lobular Carcinoma in Situ

Several studies were recently published that looked at E-cadherin in an attempt to better classify the large-cell type of pleomorphic LCIS. E-cadherin is a transmembrane glycoprotein involved in calcium dependent cell-cell adhesion whose expression has been shown to be lost in ILC of the breast (49,54,59–63). Although E-cadherin expression is similarly lost in LCIS (Fig. 66.8), it is not altered in DCIS or invasive ductal carcinoma (IDC) (49,53,54,60,62,64,65). Thus, several studies were performed that looked at the usefulness of E-cadherin immunostaining for distinguishing LCIS from DCIS, with particular reference to the pleomorphic LCIS. E-cadherin membrane staining is absent in classic LCIS and in those CIS with typical lobular growth pattern. Similarly, E-cadherin membrane staining is lost in cases of pleomorphic LCIS, despite the appearance of larger, more cytologically atypical cells akin to those seen in DCIS (49,53,57,59,63). These data suggest that pleomorphic LCIS lesions are more immunophenotypically related to classic LCIS than to DCIS.

Differential Diagnosis

LCIS in some circumstances can be difficult to distinguish from low-grade, solid-type DCIS extending into lobules. Ductal extension of LCIS can be seen in which the cells appear to extend from the acinar units within the lobule to grow along terminal ducts. They grow in a pagetoid pattern, undermining the overlying ductal epithelium and often resulting in a cloverleaf pattern (Fig. 66.6) (10,44,66,67). The discohesiveness of the cells, uniform small cell cytology, and lack of secondary lumina can help in this distinction. In addition, E-cadherin immunostaining can assist in this differential, because it will be negative in LCIS.

Benign Disease Associated with Lobular Carcinoma in Situ

The most common benign breast disorders associated with LCIS have changed over time, probably because LCIS is generally diagnosed incidentally on surgical biopsies. The indications for surgical diagnosis in the breast have been changing with our technology. Before screening mammography became established, most cases of LCIS were diagnosed in conjunction with gross cystic disease of the breast. In Haagensen's (68) series of 297 patients, 199 (67%) had associated gross cysts. In Rosen's (11) 1978 series of 99 patients, the most common indications for biopsy were cysts, mastitis, and fibroadenomas, all of which were appreciated on clinical breast examination (CBE). The association between cysts and LCIS was not observed in later studies, presumably because cysts were increasingly being found by fine needle aspiration and high-resolution ultrasonography without going to surgery.

As screening mammography became established in the 1980s, the indication for LCIS-yielding biopsy more commonly became an abnormal mammogram, although this remains the indication for biopsy in only approximately one-third of patients (69,70). Other findings associated with an LCIS diagnosis have included papilloma, dense fibrous changes in the breast, phyllodes tumor, ductal ectasia, subareolar abscess, and fat necrosis. It is believed that there is no etiologic link between any of these disorders and LCIS. Generally, LCIS remains an incidental finding on breast biopsies performed for some other clinical indication.

Published series from the radiology literature have noted that LCIS is found adjacent to or even within a fibroadenoma in 7% to 8% of cases (Table 66.1). In each of these cases, the fibroadenoma itself is the primary radiographic indication for the tissue biopsy. Again, LCIS appears to be an incidental finding in relationship to the benign mass rather

TABLE 66.1. RADIOGRAPHY SERIES ASSOCIATING LOBULAR CARCINOMA IN SITU WITH FIBROADENOMAS

Study	Total No. of LCIS Cases	No. of LCIS Cases with Fibroadenomas
Pope et al., 1988 (83)	26	2 (8%)
Sonnenfeld et al., 1991 (84)	41	3 (7%)
Buete et al., 1991 (80)	73	5 (7%)

than being connected by some common etiologic mechanism. LCIS can occur within a fibroadenoma and does so more commonly than does invasive carcinoma or DCIS (71). Because it is a relatively rare occurrence, it is difficult to know whether LCIS occurring within a fibroadenoma has the same implication for increased breast cancer risk as LCIS occurring within common breast parenchyma.

Malignant Disease Associated with Lobular Carcinoma in Situ

Between 2.9% and 8.4% of invasive breast cancers are reported to have LCIS coexisting within the same tumor (72–74). Some authors believe that LCIS is an incidental finding in these cases of invasive cancer. If this supposition were true, then one might anticipate that the invasive cancers associated with LCIS would be typical invasive cancers with average histopathologic features. To the contrary, Haagensen and colleagues (75) observed that most invasive cancers found coexisting with lobular neoplasia are well-differentiated lesions. The associated invasive cancers tend to be small cell, intraductal, and/or tubular carcinomas with a more favorable prognosis than typical invasive breast cancers. The combined lesions tend to occur in women older than those diagnosed with lobular neoplasia alone. The findings of Haagensen et al. suggest that well-differentiated invasive cancers and LCIS have some common etiology and/or cellular mechanisms. Haagensen et al. also noted that some microscopic features were considerably more frequent in the lobular neoplasia coexisting with invasive carcinoma compared with lobular neoplasia without invasive cancer: (i) loss of cohesion of the cells filling up the lobules, (ii) macroacini, and (iii) a maximal amount of lobular neoplasia. These findings would suggest that more extensive or extreme cases of LCIS are more likely to be associated with or progress to invasive cancer.

The observations of Haagensen et al. challenge the concept that LCIS found adjacent to invasive carcinoma is truly coincidental, particularly when the associated disease is ILC. Wheeler and colleagues (22) noted that among 57 patients with coexisting LCIS and invasive cancer, 13 of them had associated ILC and eight had associated combined invasive lobular and IDC. This incidence of 21 of 57 cases (37%) of ILC is 18 times higher than the expected frequency for the disease. These findings led these investigators to conclude that LCIS is a preinvasive form of cancer because the association of LCIS was so much more frequent than would be expected. These data provide the greatest support for the concept that, in selected circumstances, LCIS can progress to ILC and that it is not simply a risk factor for breast cancer.

CLINICAL PRESENTATION AND DIAGNOSIS
Clinical Features of Lobular Carcinoma in Situ

Generally, LCIS is asymptomatic and clinically occult. Unlike invasive breast cancer, LCIS rarely (if ever) forms palpable masses. This is the primary reason that LCIS is most commonly diagnosed as an incidental finding among women undergoing breast biopsy for some other reason, such as a benign palpable mass or an indeterminate mammographic finding. It seems self-evident that a significant number of women has LCIS who have never been diagnosed because there has been no indication for performing a breast biopsy on them.

Multifocality, Multicentricity, and Bilaterality

A major clinical theme for LCIS is its propensity for being multifocal, multicentric, and bilateral. Multifocality and multicentricity are often confused but conceptually distinct terms, each implying diffuse distribution in the breast, albeit in different ways. *Multifocality* is a microscopic finding in which disease is sprinkled in a discontinuous fashion throughout a given region of the breast. *Multicentricity,* conversely, refers to how disease is grossly distributed in the breast, implying that distinct regions or quadrants of the breast are involved. LCIS exhibits both of these features and bilaterality as well, although these features are not necessarily all present in every case.

The concept of multifocal, multicentric distribution of LCIS if often attributed to original publications by Foote and Stewart (6) and Muir (7). Both articles emphasized that LCIS occurs in multiple foci and multiple lobules of the breast. Foote and Stewart did not use the terms multicentric and multifocal. Nonetheless, they observed that when patients underwent mastectomy after surgical biopsy showing LCIS, the mastectomy specimen commonly had residual disease in areas outside the biopsy cavity. Muir used the terms "multiplicity of independent foci" and "the multicentric origin of cancer." Although he provided no data of his own on the topic, Muir referenced Cheatle and Cutler (5) for the information on which his conclusions were based.

LCIS is clearly multifocal in many cases, tending to demonstrate a speckled, microscopic distribution in multiple lobules throughout large regions of the breast. By contrast, multicentricity with LCIS is more difficult to prove. Although Foote and Stewart noted the propensity for residual cancer to be present in mastectomy specimens after surgical biopsy, this does not necessarily illustrate multicentricity of the disease. Holland and Faverly (76) have shown that cancers can have a multifocal but unicentric distribution over large areas of the breast, as much as 10 cm in diameter. Rosen et al. (77) analyzed 50 mastectomy specimens from patients who underwent surgical biopsy showing LCIS, providing one of the most definitive studies regarding multicentricity. They observed that LCIS was present in quadrants other than the one in which the initial surgical biopsy was performed in 24 of 50 cases (48%). One recent summary (78) states that "LCIS is characterized by a diffuse involvement throughout all breast tissue, and it should be assumed as present throughout both breasts whenever it is found in a biopsy specimen." To the contrary, we can find no direct data to support such a concept that LCIS involves all breast tissue in a diffuse distribution in all cases as suggested here.

Regarding the bilaterality of LCIS, Swain's (79) review of 15 studies reveals bilaterality rates varying from 9% to 69%. Rosen (14) comments that there is compelling evidence that both breasts are frequently affected by LCIS, but it has not been shown that all women with LCIS always have bilateral disease. In 1991, Beute and colleagues (80) reviewed mammographic-pathologic features of 104 cases of LCIS identified from biopsies and mastectomy specimens. Cases of LCIS associated with invasive carcinoma were excluded. Among the 104 patients, 82 had both breasts sampled either by mirror-image biopsy or contralateral mastectomy. LCIS was found to be bilateral in half of these patients (41 of 82).

RADIOGRAPHIC FEATURES OF LOBULAR CARCINOMA IN SITU

The general belief accepted today that LCIS lacks distinctive mammographic features has not always been accepted. The hypothesis is currently being revisited in the literature. It remains a possibility that LCIS may have some radiographic correlates in selected circumstances.

Lobular Carcinoma in Situ and Mammographic Breast Density

Pope and colleagues (83) observed an association of LCIS with mammographically dense breast tissue. Among the 26 women who underwent mammographic imaging followed by biopsy showing LCIS, 22 were noted to have dense breast tissue. Similarly, Beute and colleagues (80) noted a distinct association between LCIS and increased mammographic breast density. Compared with age-matched controls and postmenopausal women, LCIS was seldom found in a fatty breast (1% versus 29%) or in a breast with less than 25% of its parenchymal area occupied by fibroglandular density (3% versus 33%). Compared with the control group, breasts with LCIS had more than 50% fibroglandular density (85% versus 45%).

Mammographic Calcifications and Lobular Carcinoma in Situ

Historically, it has been debated whether LCIS has distinctive mammographic patterns of microcalcifications that distinguish LCIS from other lesions. In 1966, Snyder (81) proposed that there was a particular set of calcifications, "minute punctuate or linear flecks, grouped, fading in distinctness" that was strongly indicative of LCIS. However, the same group refuted their own findings 3 years later in a

follow-up publication that included the same set of patients plus an additional 34 patients in whom the mammographic features did not appear to be consistently observed (82).

Subsequent studies in the 1980s and early 1990s performed to correlate the mammographic and pathologic features of LCIS corroborated the latter publication's findings of the lack of imaging correlation (80,83,84). In 1988, Pope and colleagues (83) reviewed mammographic findings among 26 cases of LCIS. The authors found that, although calcifications were the most common mammographic indication for biopsy, the calcium that was seen microscopically was present in the benign tissue adjacent to the LCIS rather than within the LCIS itself. Less commonly, they noted microcalcifications present within the LCIS itself but in general observed no distinctive mammographic features of LCIS. Three years later, Sonnenfeld and colleagues (84) reviewed 41 cases of LCIS in whom preoperative mammograms had been obtained. Like the study of Pope et al., these authors found that most of the calcifications were present in benign tissue adjacent to the LCIS. For the patients in whom the microcalcifications and LCIS did coincide, the authors speculated that the calcifications had originated in "pre-existing benign changes and were subsequently engulfed" as the LCIS progressed through the tissues (84).

It still may be that there is a subset of cases in which LCIS forms mammographically concordant microcalcifications, particularly as related to the more aggressive pleomorphic form of LCIS. Liberman and colleagues (85) reviewed the Memorial Sloan-Kettering experience of 1,315 consecutive stereotactic biopsies and identified 14 core needle biopsies (1.2%) in patients who underwent subsequent surgical excision. Seventy-nine percent (11 of 14) of the LCIS cases were confirmed incidental cases, but in three cases, the mammographically detected microcalcifications actually were concordant and colocalized with the LCIS. Two cases had calcifications within the LCIS and the third had abundant calcification immediately surrounding the benign breast tissue. Sapino and colleagues (57) presented two cases of mammographically detected calcifications in which LCIS was directly associated with the mammographic findings. The radiographic features of the calcifications were described as "coarse, granular, arranged in round or oval clusters." There were some areas of "casting and powdery calcifications suggestive of a ductal distribution." Notably, the calcifications were secondary to necrosis in the LCIS lobules. These studies suggest that if there is a subset of patients for whom microcalcifications seen on mammogram actually do represent LCIS itself, it is a relatively small subgroup of the population of women with LCIS.

Our group reviewed the mammographic-histologic correlation among seven cases of LCIS presenting with microcalcifications (58). Two patterns of microcalcifications were observed. The classic form of LCIS microcalcifications with small, uniform cells, similar to the description by Snyder (81), was seen in two cases (Fig. 66.10). These calcifications

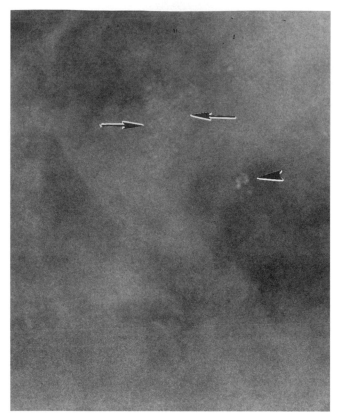

FIGURE 66.10. Mammographic findings associated with classic lobular carcinoma in situ (LCIS). The clustered punctate calcifications in the LCIS (*between arrows*) appear similar to those in adjacent benign tissues (*arrowhead*). Mammographic image (spot magnification, 1.7×). (From Georgian-Smith D, Lawton TJ. Calcifications of lobular carcinoma in situ of the breast: radiologic-pathologic correlation. *AJR Am J Roentgenol* 2001;176:1255–1259, with permission.)

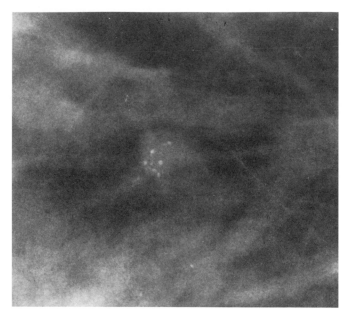

FIGURE 66.11. Mammographic findings associated with pleomorphic lobular carcinoma in situ (LCIS). Cluster of punctate calcifications 0.5 mm or smaller confined to the area of pleomorphic LCIS. Mammographic image (spot magnification, 1.7×). (From Georgian-Smith D, Lawton TJ. Calcifications of lobular carcinoma in situ of the breast: radiologic-pathologic correlation. *AJR Am J Roentgenol* 2001;176:1255–1259, with permission.)

were observed both in the LCIS and in the surrounding benign breast tissue. A second pattern of calcifications was seen in five LCIS cases that were of the pleomorphic form characterized by larger cells that were more pleomorphic in appearance. With pleomorphic LCIS, the calcifications were associated with central necrosis within the pleomorphic LCIS lobules (Fig. 66.11). These calcifications were larger and varied from oval to nearly linear in shape with slight angular margins. In particular, there were no amorphous or indistinct calcifications with the pleomorphic LCIS. These necrotic calcifications were intimately associated with LCIS and were not found in the surrounding tissues. In two of the five cases, a small focus of ILC was found adjacent to the pleomorphic LCIS. The clinical significance of each type of LCIS is unknown at this time because the distinction between classic and pleomorphic LCIS is only recently becoming fully recognized. However, the finding is of concern in that two of five pleomorphic LCIS cases had associated ILC, suggesting that it could represent a more virulent form of LCIS with an increased propensity for progression and invasion (58).

NATURAL HISTORY AND BIOLOGIC SIGNIFICANCE OF LOBULAR CARCINOMA IN SITU

Risk of Subsequent Invasive Carcinoma

Women who have been diagnosed with LCIS are at increased risk of developing breast cancer in both the ipsilateral and contralateral breasts. Page and colleagues (24) reported the absolute risk of ipsilateral breast cancer after LCIS to be 17% at 15 years, which translates to a relative risk of 8.0 in the first 15 years of follow-up compared with the general population. Mathematical modeling suggested that during the first 15 years after biopsy, women with LCIS had 10.8 times the risk of breast cancer compared with women of comparable age who underwent biopsy and who lacked proliferative disease.

Women who have developed an invasive cancer in one breast are at increased risk for developing a contralateral breast cancer. The contralateral risk appears to be increased if their ipsilateral breast cancer was associated with LCIS. Haagensen and colleagues (75) observed that invasive carcinoma developed in the contralateral breast three times more frequently in patients with lobular neoplasia preceding or coexisting with unilateral carcinoma than it did in patients without lobular neoplasia.

Multiple studies examined the long-term relative incidence of invasive breast cancer in the ipsilateral and contralateral breasts of women diagnosed with LCIS by surgical

TABLE 66.2. SELECTED LONG-TERM FOLLOW-UP STUDIES OF PATIENTS WITH LOBULAR CARCINOMA IN SITU

Study	Mean Follow-Up (yr)	Cancer in Ipsilateral Breast	Cancer in Contralateral Breast
Haagensen, 1986 (68)	14.7	27/257 (11%)	27/258 (10%)
Anderson, 1974 (104)	15	9/46 (20%)	9/52 (17%)
Wheeler et al., 1974 (22)	15.7	1/25 (4%)	5/34 (15%)
Page et al., 1991 (24)	19	6/39 (15%)	4/39 (10%)
Rosen et al., 1978 (11)	24	18/83 (22%)	17/83 (20%)

biopsy (Table 66.2). The major clinical issue with LCIS is the repeated demonstration that the risk of developing subsequent invasive breast cancer is approximately equal in the two breasts. Long-term studies with 15- to 25-year follow-up show equally in both breasts chances of breast cancer developing of 10% to 22%.

The implication of these studies is that if one were to embark on surgical therapy for LCIS, the only logical operation would be a bilateral mastectomy. These studies concomitantly show that if one were to perform such an operation, it would have been unnecessary approximately 80% of the time. So whether one views LCIS as a risk factor for subsequent invasive cancer or as a well-differentiated premalignant lesion with low potential for progression to invasion, the conclusion remains the same. In general, bilateral mastectomy is an overly aggressive treatment for a lesion with this low likelihood of promoting life-threatening disease.

The new question, then, is whether the subset of patients with pleomorphic LCIS has a particularly heightened risk of the development of invasive disease. If so, this may identify a subset of LCIS patients who actually do warrant surgical intervention, just as is now done for low-grade DCIS.

Parallels Between Lobular Carcinoma and Low-Grade Ductal Carcinoma in Situ

Most investigators describe DCIS and LCIS as fundamentally different lesions. They imply that DCIS warrants treatment as a cancer whereas LCIS warrants management as a high-risk breast cancer marker. Clearly, most cases of LCIS carry different clinical implications from those of high-grade DCIS (Table 66.3), but LCIS may not be so different from low-grade DCIS, which also tends to have a particularly indolent course. Silverstein (1) points out that some DCIS lesions, if untreated, may progress to invasive breast cancer whereas others, if untreated, may change very little over 5 to 50 years. Page and colleagues (86) studied a group of 28 women with small, noncomedo DCIS who were treated with biopsy alone and then followed for an average of 30 years. They concluded that it might take more than two decades for small, noncomedo DCIS to evolve into invasive breast cancer in the ipsilateral breast in the same area in which DCIS had been biopsied. It is possible that LCIS, particularly of the more aggressive pleomorphic variant, might have a similar time course for evolution into invasive malignancy.

The common assumption that LCIS and DCIS are very different in terms of contralateral breast cancer risk has also been challenged. Our group reviewed the experience in western Washington State of women who were diagnosed between 1974 and 1993 with either DCIS (1,929 women) or LCIS (282 women) and then were followed for contralateral breast cancer, as recorded in the local Surveillance, Epidemiologic, and End Results registry (87). Adjusting for age and year of diagnosis, we found that the risk of contralateral invasive breast cancer was elevated for at least 5 years after a diagnosis for both DCIS and LCIS compared with the rate of first primary breast cancers developing in the same population. The rate of contralateral invasive disease was increased approximately twofold for women with DCIS and threefold for women with LCIS. This difference between LCIS and DCIS narrowed when contralateral invasive and noninvasive breast cancers were considered conjointly.

There are morphologic parallels between LCIS and low-grade DCIS as well. The cytology of these two histologic categories can look identical in some instances. Fechner (88), an authoritative breast cancer pathologist, described a personal experience of sorting out DCIS from LCIS: "During the late 1960's I became interested in LCIS because of a few papers (in the surgical literature and in *Cancer*) regard-

TABLE 66.3. COMPARATIVE FEATURES OF DUCTAL CARCINOMA IN SITU AND LOBULAR CARCINOMA IN SITU

High-Grade DCIS	LCIS
Propagates within ducts	Propagates within lobules
Tends to be localized and unilateral	Tends to be diffuse and bilateral
Increases risk of subsequent IDC	Risk of subsequent ILC or IDC
DCIS microcalcifications seen on mammogram	Few characteristic mammographic changes (with exception of pleomorphic LCIS)
Preinvasive cancer	Risk factor or preinvasive cancer?

DCIS, ductal carcinoma in situ; LCIS, lobular carcinoma in situ; IDC, invasive ductal carcinoma; ILC, invasive lobular carcinoma.

ing microscopic diagnosis and follow-up of untreated cases. The emphasis on detecting LCIS led me to search for lesions in ducts that might be a clue for LCIS located elsewhere in the unsampled breast. In 1972, I published a paper illustrating 'epithelial proliferations' in the ducts of patients who had LCIS when additional blocks were submitted. I accurately noted that the ducts were populated by cells 'cytologically identical' to the characteristic cells of LCIS. The proper categorization of these proliferations as either low-grade cribriform or micropapillary DCIS went unrecognized, and the diagnosis of DCIS was also missed by the reviewer or reviewers of the manuscript as well."

A St. Louis group of investigators concur that low-grade solid carcinoma of the breast can be difficult to classify (54). Using E-cadherin expression to distinguish ductal from lobular lesions, they evaluated 12 cases of CIS with equivocal features and correlated the results with the histologic features of associated invasive breast cancers. Conventional histologic criteria used to distinguish low-grade, solid DCIS from LCIS (sharply defined cell membranes, necrosis, or presence of microacini) could not reliably separate low-grade DCIS from LCIS, as subsequently proven by E-cadherin expression.

A Boston group used E-cadherin expression to demonstrate that CIS with indeterminate features (CIS-IF) can represent LCIS, DCIS, or a combination of the two (53). Based on standard histologic criteria, Jacobs and colleagues (53) divided CIS-IF cases into three groups: group 1 cases looked like LCIS but had comedonecrosis; group 2 cases had CIS comprised of small, uniform neoplastic cells either growing in a solid pattern with focal microacinar-like structures but with cellular discohesiveness or were growing in a cohesive mosaic pattern but with occasional intracytoplasmic vacuoles; group 3 cases showed marked cellular pleomorphism and nuclear atypia but had the discohesive pattern characteristic of LCIS (pleomorphic LCIS). All CIS-IF cases in groups 1 and 3 were negative for E-cadherin expression, consistent with lobular histologic origin. The group 2 cases were heterogeneous for E-cadherin expression (n = 17). Six cases were E-cadherin negative like LCIS, five cases were E-cadherin positive like DCIS, and six cases had both E-cadherin–positive and E-cadherin–negative cells.

In both studies, necrosis was seen in E-cadherin–negative cells (LCIS). In the second paper, the CIS-IF group with the marked cellular pleomorphism and nuclear atypia were E-cadherin negative, like LCIS. In common practice, such pleomorphic cells are often categorized incorrectly as DCIS. It is evident that one cannot draw a clean histologic line between LCIS and low-grade DCIS based on histologic criteria alone.

Molecular Genetics Comparing Ductal Carcinoma in Situ and Lobular Carcinoma in Situ

In addition to the morphologic and immunohistochemical data showing homology between LCIS and DCIS, there is also molecular genetic and cellular kinetic information suggesting that LCIS and DCIS are biologically related lesions. Buerger and colleagues (89) studied LCIS, DCIS, and associated invasive carcinoma of the breast using comparative genomic hybridization after microdissection and E-cadherin staining. They noted a high degree of genetic homology between LCIS and well-differentiated DCIS. Interestingly, genetic alterations seen in invasive carcinoma were not necessarily seen in the adjacent precursor lesions. They hypothesized that LCIS and a subgroup of DCIS are different phenotypic forms of a common genotype. Meyer (90) reported a thymidine-labeling study of cell kinetics in 61 CIS cases. He found that the thymidine-labeling index was significantly lower in cribriform or papillary DCIS cases (mean, 1.83%) and LCIS (mean, 0.63%) than in comedo (high-grade) DCIS (mean, 5.15%). Meyer concluded that cribriform-papillary intraductal carcinoma is "relatively bland" biologically, similar to LCIS. The striking genetic similarities seen in this study led him to hypothesize that LCIS and a subgroup of DCIS are actually different phenotypic forms of a common genotype.

Is Lobular Carcinoma in Situ a Marker for Breast Cancer Risk or is it a Precursor of Invasive Lobular Carcinoma?

Lishman and Lakhani (46) studied loss of heterozygosity among cases of LCIS with associated adjacent invasive carcinoma. Loss of heterozygosity at chromosomal arms exhibiting imbalance at high frequency in invasive carcinoma can also be found with LCIS associated with invasive carcinoma and with pure LCIS. The investigators interpreted these data to confirm the neoplastic nature of LCIS. Suspecting that LCIS is likely a direct precursor of ILC, Vos and colleagues (63) studied E-cadherin gene mutations in ILC, IDC, DCIS, and in LCIS associated with ILC. Using mutation analysis, they demonstrated the same truncating mutations and loss of heterozygosity of the wild-type E-cadherin in the LCIS component as in the adjacent ILC. These data indicate that these LCIS cells are not just markers of some sort for increased risk for breast cancer. To the contrary, these data appear to be direct confirmation that these LCIS cells are direct precursors of ILC in some cases.

Pleomorphic Lobular Carcinoma in Situ May Represent Biologically Aggressive Disease

Pleomorphic LCIS and pleomorphic ILC have received little attention in the past. This diagnosis is seldom made, in part because some of these cases are diagnosed as DCIS by virtue of the pleomorphic cytology. In 1991, Page and co-workers (24) wrote about cancer risk implications among different patterns of the LCIS spectrum. Thirty-nine patients with a diagnosis of isolated LCIS underwent surgical biopsy but not mastectomy and were followed for an average of 19 years. The absolute risk of invasive cancer was 17% at 15 years. The histologic pattern of ten invasive carcinomas developing in nine patients was predominantly of the lobular type, with three pure and four variant types representing 70% of the developed carcinomas. Three of those women with invasive breast cancer died at an average interval of 5.3 years. All three had a histologic pattern of pleomorphic ILC. They pointed out that this represents a much stronger association with the tubular and lobular types of invasive cancer than reported by Haagensen or by Rosen. "The reason for this may be our selection of more completely developed examples of lobular neoplasia" (24).

Pleomorphic ILC coexisting with LCIS is associated with poor outcome. In a 1992 report from Italy, the authors described 10 cases of pleomorphic ILC, six cases of which included LCIS (91). Six of ten patients died within 42 months of diagnosis. Three other patients developed recurrence or distant metastases at short intervals. The authors concluded that pleomorphic ILC is a highly lethal variant of invasive carcinoma. In 1994, Weidner and Semple (92) at the University of California compared the clinical course of 25 cases of classic invasive lobular carcinoma and a group of 16 cases of pleomorphic ILC. Survival until recurrence was significantly worse in the patients with pleomorphic ILC. Patients with positive nodes and pleomorphic histology were 30 times more likely to experience breast cancer recurrence than were patients with classic ILC histology. A more recent article by Bentz et al. (50) from the University of Utah evaluated 12 patients with pleomorphic ILC, 11 of whom had long-term clinical follow-up. Of the 12 cases, seven had coexisting pleomorphic LCIS. Among the 11 cases with follow-up, nine developed fatal metastatic disease with a median survival of 2.1 years.

These findings suggest that pleomorphic ILC is as aggressive as most forms of IDC and that pleomorphic LCIS could be a warning for that aggressive underlying biology. This part of the spectrum of LCIS may warrant different management than classic LCIS. Just what such management should be remains to be determined. Our policy at the University of Washington, in the absence of more definitive data, has been to recommend treating these unusual cases of pleomorphic LCIS like DCIS with surgical resection for clear margins and radiation if the breast is conserved.

CLINICAL MANAGEMENT

Surgical Excision Biopsy Specimens Showing Lobular Carcinoma in Situ

Because classic LCIS generally does not itself require surgical treatment, surgical biopsy showing LCIS should not itself demand further intervention. The implication is that surgical margins for LCIS, as with ADH, are not clinically relevant. Unlike surgical treatment for DCIS or invasive cancer, it is not necessary to remove more breast tissue surgically simply because the tissue that was excised had LCIS at the edge of the excision specimen. A possible exception to this is patients with pleomorphic LCIS, although no long-term follow-up data are yet available to make definitive recommendations. Although future study could reveal that subgroups of patients with LCIS warrant surgical treatment, no such subgroup has yet been identified based on prospective analysis.

Should Core Needle Samples Showing Lobular Carcinoma in Situ be Surgically Excised?

At more debatable question is whether LCIS on core needle sampling warrants a subsequent wire-localization surgical biopsy for definitive diagnosis. When ADH is seen on core needle biopsy, a subsequent excisional procedure is performed because a percentage of these needle-diagnosed cases will ultimately prove to contain DCIS or even invasive cancer. The question is whether the same principle might apply to the management of LCIS.

O'Driscoll and colleagues (93) noted that the finding of isolated LCIS is relatively uncommon. In the Cambridge and Huntingdon breast screening programs, 47,975 women underwent mammographic screening, 749 (1.6%) underwent core needle biopsy, but only seven were found to have isolated LCIS on that needle sampling. All seven patients subsequently underwent surgical excision, which revealed one case of LCIS with ILC, two cases of LCIS with DCIS, and one case with a probable focus of IDC. LCIS was the only abnormality on both core needle and surgical biopsy in only three of the seven cases. These authors concluded that, in general, LCIS seen on core needle biopsy should undergo surgical excision for definitive diagnosis.

Other investigators have taken a more selective approach to management. As discussed above, Liberman and colleagues (85) retrospectively reviewed the Memorial Sloan-Kettering experience of 1,315 consecutive stereotactic biopsies of which 16 were found to have LCIS on percutaneous core needle biopsies (1.2%). Of these, 14 lesions from 13 women underwent subsequent surgical excision. Five of the 14 stereotactic biopsies showed LCIS together with a high-risk lesion (radial scar in three and ADH in two). Of these five, one (20%) was found to have DCIS on subsequent surgical excision. In four of the 14 lesions, the LCIS in the percutaneous biopsy had histologic features overlapping those of DCIS. Of these four, one had DCIS and one had infiltrating lobular carcinoma on subsequent surgical excision. Based on these findings, Liberman et al. identified three scenarios in which the finding of LCIS on core biopsy should be considered for further surgical excision: (i) the histologic finding of LCIS is discordant with the imaging findings suggesting other forms of breast pathology, (ii) when there may be confusion or overlap in the histologic features of LCIS and DCIS on the core needle sample, and (iii) when LCIS is present with other high-risk lesions such as radial scar or ADH, which are themselves indications for wire-localization biopsy.

Breast Conservation in Patients who Have Lobular Carcinoma in Situ Coincident with Invasive Cancer

It has been debated whether patients with extensive LCIS combined with invasive carcinoma are still reasonable candidates for breast-conserving surgery. The concern would be that a patient who developed invasive carcinoma among a field of LCIS might be at heightened risk for local recurrence, i.e., that they had a particularly bad form of LCIS.

Some studies have not shown an increased risk of ipsilateral breast cancer recurrence after breast conservation for invasive breast cancer coincident with LCIS (73,74). Abner and colleagues (74) from Harvard's Joint Center for Radiation Therapy retrospectively reviewed their experience with this issue. They found that the 8-year local recurrence rate was 13% among the 119 patients with associated LCIS adjacent to the tumor compared with 12% for the 1,062 patients without associated LCIS ($p =$ NS). The extent of LCIS did not appear to affect the risk of recurrence. Furthermore, the risks of contralateral disease and distant failure were similarly not affected by the presence or extent of LCIS within the ipsilateral breast. The authors concluded that breast-conserving therapy with lumpectomy and radiation therapy remains an appropriate method for treating patients with invasive breast carcinoma with or without associated LCIS. Analogous studies of invasive breast cancers associated with atypical hyperplasia have also suggested that ALH and ADH are not contraindications to breast-conserving therapy (94).

However, a more recent study from the Fox Chase Cancer Center had different results, suggesting that there may be subsets of patients with invasive breast cancer and coincident LCIS who may be at markedly increased risk of ipsilateral breast tumor recurrence (IBTR) (95). Sasson and colleagues (95) retrospectively reviewed 1,274 patients with stage I or II treated with lumpectomy and radiation between 1979 and 1995, identifying 65 women (5%) who had LCIS in the lumpectomy specimens. The 10-year cumulative incidence rate of IBTR was 6% in women without LCIS versus 29% in women with LCIS ($p = 0.0003$). Risk factors for IBTR included age older than 50, small invasive tumor (<2 cm), negative lymph node status, and the absence of any adjuvant systemic treatment ($p < 0.001$).

Although Sasson and colleagues were able to identify patient risk factors for IBTR after breast conservation for invasive breast cancer with coexistent LCIS, they stopped short of recommending mastectomy for these. They noted that women who had LCIS in their lumpectomy specimens and who also received tamoxifen was markedly lower at only 8%. They suggest that tamoxifen should be considered in these women for decreasing IBTR risk when they choose breast conservation.

Chemoprevention of Invasive Cancer with Tamoxifen

Because LCIS marks an increased risk of ipsilateral and contralateral breast cancer development, it makes biologic sense to consider systemic chemoprevention strategies in this patient population. Literature from randomized trials directly addressing breast cancer risk reduction among patients with LCIS remains limited. At the time of this writing, the only chemoprevention agent with published randomized data is tamoxifen.

Tamoxifen is a selective estrogen receptor (ER) modulator with both agonist and antagonist properties. Initially approved by the U.S. Food and Drug Administration in 1978 for the treatment of metastatic breast cancer, tamoxifen has been widely studied in clinical trials involving nearly 35,000 women. The safety and efficacy of tamoxifen are well established. In addition to treating known hormone-receptor–positive invasive breast cancers in the adjuvant and metastatic setting, tamoxifen has also been shown to decrease the risk of contralateral breast cancer (96). For this reason, tamoxifen was initially chosen for breast cancer prevention trials. Of the three worldwide tamoxifen prevention trials published to date, only the NSABP P-01 trial specifically evaluates the subset of participants with LCIS (15,97,98). The NSABP study is also the only study to date showing a statistically significant benefit from tamoxifen in the prevention setting, although the trials have considerable differences in the patient populations enrolled.

The NSABP P-01 trial is a randomized, double-blinded trial initiated in 1992 that enrolled 13,388 women at increased risk of breast cancer by virtue of an elevated Gail model score (5-year risk of 1.66% of developing breast cancer), age older than 60 years, or a history of biopsy-proven LCIS or ADH. Participants in this trial were randomized to tamoxifen, 20 mg daily, or to a placebo for a planned duration of 5 years. At the time of randomization, there were 411 women with a history of LCIS on the placebo arm and 415 on the tamoxifen arm. Among these women, there were 18 cases of invasive breast cancer on the placebo arm and eight on the tamoxifen arm. Although the absolute numbers are small, this translates to a notable increase in the average annual rate of invasive breast cancer for patients with LCIS compared with the subgroup of women without a history of LCIS (12.99 cases per 1,000 women versus 5.69 cases per 1,000 women).

The P-01 trial reports a 56% relative reduction in the risk of breast cancer among patients with LCIS from the use of tamoxifen (95% confidence interval, 0.16 to 1.06). Although this is based on a limited number of events, it represents the only available literature specifically addressing LCIS as a breast cancer risk factor. These data compare with a 49% risk reduction between the two arms for all women enrolled in the trial and an 86% reduction for patients with ADH. Overall benefit was seen regardless of patient age or eligibility subgroup. The absolute reduction in invasive breast cancer at 5 years for all participants was 1.3%. All breast cancer risk reduction was seen in the occurrence of ER-positive tumors, with no difference in ER-negative tumors comparing the tamoxifen and placebo groups (15). No difference in survival was observed or expected between the two arms, particularly with short-term follow-up. Based on these results, the trial was terminated early at the recommendation of an independent monitoring committee. The Food and Drug Administration has now approved tamoxifen for breast cancer prevention (99).

Ongoing and Future Chemoprevention Trials

Confirmatory prevention trials using tamoxifen as well as studies involving other agents are currently underway. A randomized, double-blinded, placebo-controlled trial is ongoing in the United Kingdom and Europe (United Kingdom Co-ordinating Committee on Cancer Research-IBIS, EU94041) also evaluating tamoxifen as a chemoprevention agent. Women with a history of LCIS are eligible for this trial. U.S. studies enrolling participants with LCIS include the NSABP P-2 STAR trial (study of tamoxifen and raloxifene) in postmenopausal women and a phase II study of raloxifene as a chemoprevention agent for premenopausal women at high risk of developing invasive breast cancer (NCI-98-C-0123, MB-402) (100). As more selective ER modulators, antiestrogens, retinoids, and other chemoprevention agents are developed, more clinical trials for patients with a history of LCIS may be anticipated.

Is There a Defined Role for Surgical Prophylaxis with Lobular Carcinoma in Situ?

In general, LCIS is not a pathologic entity that warrants surgery. The risk of developing invasive breast cancer with LCIS is significantly heightened above the general population, but most women with this diagnosis will not develop invasive breast cancer. Of those women who do get breast cancer, the relative risk appears to be similar in both breasts. Thus, if one were to perform surgery for LCIS, the only logical operation would be a bilateral total mastectomy. Such a procedure seems excessively morbid for the moderate risk associated with LCIS.

Conversely, there may be circumstances with LCIS in which surgery is a reasonable consideration. Bilateral prophylactic mastectomy (with or without reconstruction) confers an approximate 90% risk reduction for the development of subsequent cancer (101). A diagnosis of LCIS might contribute to one's decision regarding the use of this procedure. If a patient is otherwise a reasonable candidate for prophylactic surgery, such as a woman from a high-risk family in which genetic testing is noninformative and if that

same woman is then found to have LCIS, she might have heightened consideration for such a procedure. Any use of prophylactic surgery for breast cancer must be highly individualized and selected, given the paucity of data on this topic, and the huge personal impact that such a procedure is going to have on a woman's life. It becomes virtually impossible to make generalized recommendations about how this procedure should be applied in women with LCIS. Any prophylactic intervention warrants considerable introspection. Counseling for both medical and psychological issues is mandatory as well as ample time (measured in months) to make an appropriate personal decision.

Probably the most unclear area today is the proper treatment of higher grade pleomorphic LCIS. This lesion has many cytologic characteristics resembling DCIS but expresses the immunocytologic profile of LCIS as measured by E-cadherin immunostaining. Is this lesion best treated by observation, as in classic LCIS, or should there be heightened consideration for surgical intervention, just as is done for DCIS? Pleomorphic ILC represents biologically aggressive high-grade disease (91). If pleomorphic LCIS specifically predisposes toward the development of pleomorphic ILC, then the risk increases of leaving untreated pleomorphic LCIS in the breast. Tamoxifen with or without surgery could also be particularly protective for women diagnosed with pleomorphic LCIS. Unfortunately, there are no current long-term follow-up data on pleomorphic LCIS because the reported numbers of cases are relatively few. Only recently has this form of LCIS received significant attention in the literature. Further study and subset analyses are mandatory.

FUTURE DIRECTIONS

The dilemma of LCIS relates to its biologic heterogeneity combined with its diffuse localization within the breast. The debate about whether LCIS is a risk factor for or a precursor of invasive breast cancer may not have a definitive answer. Thus, it remains unclear how LCIS can best be categorized—as a breast cancer risk factor, a premalignant lesion, or an indolent preinvasive malignancy. In fact, LCIS may be both.

The future for LCIS management, then, may be hidden within biologic investigation. The study of immunohistochemical markers such as E-cadherin may be the first of a series of analyses that may help to distinguish between LCIS of lower or higher propensities for malignant degeneration and transformation into invasive disease. Haagensen was the first to fully acknowledge that LCIS may not warrant surgical treatment because of its diffuse anatomic nature combined with its generally indolent course. However, the lumping together of ALH, classic LCIS, and pleomorphic LCIS as lobular neoplasia may cause us to underestimate the diversity of the malignant biology that this family of disorders may express. We may find that future scientific investigation, as it uncovers the underlying cellular and genetic mechanisms by which LCIS develops, will take us in the opposite direction. We may start to differentially respond to a LCIS diagnosis in a given patient-based approach by using cytogenetic subtyping and molecular analysis that permit us to better predict that patient's outcome in the absence of intervention.

REFERENCES

1. Silverstein MJ. Preface. In: Silverstein MJ, ed. *Ductal carcinoma in situ of the breast.* Baltimore: Williams & Wilkins, 1997:vii.
2. Rosen P. In situ (intra-epithelial) carcinoma and precancerous lesions: historical perspective. In: Rosen P, ed. *Breast pathology.* Philadelphia: Lippincott–Raven, 1997:209–217.
3. Cornil A-V. Contributions a l'histoire du developpement histologique des tumeurs epitheliales (sqirrhe, encephaloide, etc.). *J Anat Physiol* 1865;2:266–276.
4. Ewing J. *Neoplastic diseases.* Philadelphia: WB Saunders, 1919.
5. Cheatle GL, Cutler M. *Tumours of the breast.* London: Edward Arnold, 1931.
6. Foote FJ, Stewart F. Lobular carcinoma in situ: a rare form of mammary carcinoma. *Am J Pathol* 1941;17:491–496.
7. Muir J. The evolution of carcinoma of the mamma. *J Pathol Bacteriol* 1941;52:155–172.
8. Broders AC. Carcinoma in situ contrasted with benign penetrating epithelium. *JAMA* 1932;99:1670–1674.
9. Godwin JT. Chronology of lobular carcinoma of the breast: report of a case. *Cancer* 1952;5:259–266.
10. Haagensen CD, Lane N, Lattes R, et al. Lobular neoplasia (so-called lobular carcinoma in situ) of the breast. *Cancer* 1978;42:737–769.
11. Rosen PP, Lieberman PH, Braun DWJ, et al. Lobular carcinoma in situ of the breast. Detailed analysis of 99 patients with average follow-up of 24 years. *Am J Surg Pathol* 1978;2:225–251.
12. Bodian CA, Perzin KH, Lattes R, et al. Prognostic significance of benign proliferative breast disease. *Cancer* 1993;71:3896–3907.
13. Tavassoli F. Lobular neoplasia. In: Tavassoli F, ed. *Pathology of the breast,* 2nd ed. Stamford, CT: Appleton & Lange, 1999:373–400.
14. Rosen PP. Lobular carcinoma in situ versus lobular neoplasia. In: Rosen PP, ed. *Breast pathology.* Philadelphia: Lippincott–Raven, 1997:536–537.
15. Fisher B, Costantino JP, Wickerham DL, et al. Tamoxifen for prevention of breast cancer: report of the National Surgical Adjuvant Breast and Bowel Project P-1 Study. *J Natl Cancer Inst* 1998;90:1371–1388.
16. Carlson RW, Anderson BO, Benzinger W, et al. Update: NCCN practice guidelines for the treatment of breast cancer. *Oncology* 1999;13:187–212.
17. Eva Singletary, MD, personal communication.
18. Frantz VK, Pickren JW, Melcher GW, et al. Incidence of chronic disease in so-called "normal breasts." *Cancer* 1951;4:762–783.
19. Kramer WM, Rush BF. Mammary duct proliferation in the elderly: a histopathologic study. *Cancer* 1973;31:130–137.
20. Nielsen M, Jensen J, Andersen J. Precancerous and cancerous breast lesions during lifetime and at autopsy: a study of 83 women. *Cancer* 1984;54:612–615.

21. Alpers CE, Wellings SR. The prevalence of carcinoma in situ in normal and cancer-associated breasts. *Hum Pathol* 1985;16:796–807.
22. Wheeler JE, Enterline HT, Roseman JM, et al. Lobular carcinoma in situ of the breast: long-term followup. *Cancer* 1974;34:554–563.
23. Andersen JA. Lobular carcinoma in situ of the breast: an approach to rational treatment. *Cancer* 1977;39:2597–2602.
24. Page DL, Kidd TE Jr, Dupont WD, et al. Lobular neoplasia of the breast: higher risk for subsequent invasive cancer predicted by more extensive disease. *Hum Pathol* 1991;22:1232–1239.
25. Levi F, Te VC, Randimbison L, et al. Trends of in situ carcinoma of the breast in Vaud, Switzerland. *Eur J Cancer* 1997;33:903–906.
26. Simon MS, Lemanne D, Schwartz AG, et al. Recent trends in the incidence of in situ and invasive breast cancer in the Detroit metropolitan area (1975–1988). *Cancer* 1993;71:769–774.
27. Zheng T, Holford TR, Chen Y, et al. Time trend of female breast carcinoma in situ by race and histology in Connecticut, USA. *Eur J Cancer* 1997;33:96–100.
28. Kennedy DL, Baum C, Forbes MB. Noncontraceptive estrogens and progestins: use patterns over time. *Obstet Gynecol* 1985;65:441–446.
29. Hemminki E, Kennedy DL, Baum C, et al. Prescribing of noncontraceptive estrogens and progestins in the United States. *Am J Public Health* 1988;78:1478–1481.
30. Wysowski DK, Golden L, Burke L. Use of menopausal estrogens and medroxyprogesterone in the United States, 1982–1992. *Obstet Gynecol* 1995;85:6–10.
31. Li CI, Anderson BO, Porter P, et al. Changing incidence rate of invasive lobular breast carcinoma among older women. *Cancer* 2000;88:2561–2569.
32. Lantz PM, Remington PL, Newcomb PA. Mammography screening and increased incidence of breast cancer in Wisconsin. *J Natl Cancer Inst* 1991;83:1540–1546.
33. Feuer EJ, Wun LM. How much of the recent rise in breast cancer incidence can be explained by increases in mammography utilization? A dynamic population model approach. *Am J Epidemiol* 1992;136:1423–1436.
34. Miller BA, Feuer EJ, Hankey BF. The increasing incidence of breast cancer since 1982: relevance of early detection. *Cancer Causes Control* 1991;2:67–74.
35. Simon MS, Lemanne D, Schwartz AG, et al. Recent trends in the incidence of in situ and invasive breast cancer in the Detroit metropolitan area (1975–1988). *Cancer* 1993;71:769–774.
36. Li CI, Weiss NS, Stanford JL, et al. Hormone replacement therapy in relation to risk of lobular and ductal breast carcinoma in middle-aged women. *Cancer* 2000;88:2570–2577.
37. Wellings SR, Jensen HM, Marcum RG. An atlas of subgross pathology of the human breast with special reference to possible precancerous lesions. *J Natl Cancer Inst* 1975;55:231–273.
38. Wellings SR, Jensen HM, DeVault MR. Persistent and atypical lobules in the human breast may be precancerous. *Experimentia* 1976;32:1463–1465.
39. Andersen J, Vendelboe M. Cytoplasmic mucous globules in lobular carcinoma in situ. Diagnosis and prognosis. *Am J Surg Pathol* 1981;5:251–255.
40. Barwick K, Kashgarian M, Rosen P. "Clear cell" change within duct and lobular epithelium of the human breast. *Pathol Annu* 1982;17:319–328.
41. Breslow A, Brancaccio M. Intracellular mucin production by lobular breast carcinoma cells. *Arch Pathol Lab Med* 1976;100:620–621.
42. Eusebi V, Betts C, Haagensen D, et al. Apocrine differentiation in lobular carcinoma of the breast: a morphologic, immunologic and ultrastructural study. *Hum Pathol* 1984;15:134–140.

43. Gad A, Azzopardi J. Lobular carcinoma of the breast: a special variant of mucin-secreting carcinoma. *J Clin Pathol* 1975; 28:711–716.
44. Rosen P. Lobular carcinoma and hyperplasia. In: Rosen P, ed. *Breast pathology*. Philadelphia: Lippincott–Raven, 1997:507–544.
45. Hutter R. The management of patients with lobular carcinoma in situ of the breast. *Cancer* 1984;53:798–802.
46. Lishman S, Lakhani S. Atypical lobular hyperplasia and lobular carcinoma in situ: surgical and molecular pathology. *Histopathology* 1999;35:195–200.
47. Page D, Anderson T, Rogers L. Carcinoma in situ (CIS). In: Page D, Anderson T, eds. *Diagnostic histopathology of the breast*. New York: Churchill-Livingstone, 1987:174–184.
48. Rosen P. Lobular carcinoma in situ and intraductal carcinoma of the breast. In: McDivitt R, Oberman H, Ozzello L, et al., eds. *The breast*. Baltimore: Williams & Wilkins, 1984:59–105.
49. Acs G, Lawton T, Rebbeck T, et al. Differential expression of E-cadherin in lobular and ductal neoplasms of the breast and its biologic and diagnostic implications. *Am J Clin Pathol* 2001; 115:85–98.
50. Bentz J, Yassa N, Clayton F. Pleomorphic lobular carcinoma of the breast: clinicopathologic features of 12 cases. *Mod Pathol* 1998;11:814–822.
51. Fisher E, Constantino J, Fisher B, et al. Pathologic findings from the National Surgical Adjuvant Breast Project (NSABP) Protocol B-17: five year observations concerning lobular carcinoma in situ. *Cancer* 1996;78:1403–1416.
52. Frost A, Tsangaris T, Silverberg S. Pleomorphic lobular carcinoma in situ. *Pathol Case Rev* 1996;1:27.
53. Jacobs T, Pliss N, Kouria G, et al. Carcinomas in situ of the breast with indeterminate features: role of E-cadherin staining in categorization. *Am J Surg Pathol* 2001;25:229–236.
54. Maluf H, Swanson P, Koerner F. Solid low-grade in situ carcinoma of the breast: role of associated lesions and E-cadherin in differential diagnosis. *Am J Surg Pathol* 2001;25:237–244.
55. Middleton L, Palacios D, Bryant B, et al. Pleomorphic lobular carcinoma: morphology, immunohistochemistry, and molecular analysis. *Am J Surg Pathol* 2000;24:1650–1656.
56. Schnitt S, Morrow M. Lobular carcinoma in situ: current concepts and controversies. *Semin Diagn Pathol* 1999;16:209–223.
57. Sapino A, Frigerio A, Peterse J, et al. Mammographically detected in situ lobular carcinoma of the breast. *Virchows Arch* 2000;436:421–430.
58. Georgian-Smith D, Lawton TJ. Calcifications of lobular carcinoma in situ of the breast: radiologic-pathologic correlation. *AJR Am J Roentgenol* 2001;176:1255–1259.
59. De Leeuw W, Berx G, Vos C, et al. Simultaneous loss of E-cadherin and catenins in invasive lobular breast cancer and lobular carcinoma in situ. *J Pathol* 1997;183:404–411.
60. Gamallo C, Palacios J, Suarez A, et al. Correlation of E-cadherin expression with differentiation grade and histological type in breast carcinoma. *Am J Pathol* 1993;142:987–993.
61. Kanai Y, Oda T, Tsuda H, et al. Point mutation of the E-cadherin gene in invasive lobular carcinoma of the breast. *Jpn J Cancer Res* 1994;85:1035–1039.
62. Moll R, Mitze M, Frixen U, et al. Differential loss of E-cadherin expression in infiltrating ductal and lobular breast carcinomas. *Am J Pathol* 1993;143:1731–1742.
63. Vos C, Cleton-Jansen A, Berx G, et al. E-cadherin inactivation in lobular carcinoma in situ of the breast: an early event in tumorigenesis. *Br J Cancer* 1997;76:1131–1133.
64. Gupta S, Douglas-Jones A, Jasani B, et al. E-cadherin (E-cad) expression in duct carcinoma in situ (DCIS) of the breast. *Virchows Arch* 1997;430:23–28.
65. Kashiwaba M, Tamura G, Suzuki Y, et al. Epithelial-cadherin gene is not mutated in ductal carcinomas of the breast. *Jpn J Cancer Res* 1995;86:1054–1059.
66. Andersen J. Lobular carcinoma in situ of the breast with ductal involvement. Frequency and possible influence on prognosis. *Acta Pathol Microbiol Scand* 1974;82A:655–662.
67. Fechner R. Epithelial alterations in extralobular ducts of breasts with lobular carcinoma. *Arch Pathol* 1972;93:164–171.
68. Haagensen CD. Lobular neoplasia (lobular carcinoma in situ). In: Haagensen CD, ed. *Diseases of the breast*. Philadelphia: WB Saunders, 1986:192–241.
69. Singletary SE. Lobular carcinoma in situ of the breast; a 31-year experience at the University of Texas M.D. Anderson Cancer Center. *Breast Dis* 1994;7:157–163.
70. Carson W, Sanchez-Forgach E, Stomper P, et al. Lobular carcinoma in situ: observation without surgery as an appropriate therapy. *Ann Surg Oncol* 1994;1:141–146.
71. Pick PW, Iossifides IA. Occurrence of breast carcinoma within a fibroadenoma. A review. *Arch Pathol Lab Med* 1984;108: 590–594.
72. Davis N, Baird RM. Breast cancer in association with lobular carcinoma in situ. Clinicopathologic review and treatment recommendation. *Am J Surg* 1984;147:641–645.
73. Moran M, Haffty BG. Lobular carcinoma in situ as a component of breast cancer: the long-term outcome in patients treated with breast-conservation therapy. *Int J Radiat Oncol Biol Phys* 1998;40:353–358.
74. Abner AL, Connolly JL, Recht A, et al. The relation between the presence and extent of lobular carcinoma in situ and the risk of local recurrence for patients with infiltrating carcinoma of the breast treated with conservative surgery and radiation therapy. *Cancer* 2000;88:1072–1077.
75. Haagensen CD, Lane N, Bodian C. Coexisting lobular neoplasia and carcinoma of the breast. *Cancer* 1983;51:1468–1482.
76. Holland R, Faverly DRG. Whole-organ studies. In: Silverstein MJ, ed. *Ductal carcinoma in situ of the breast*. Baltimore: Williams & Wilkins, 1997:233–240.
77. Rosen PP, Senie R, Schottenfeld D, et al. Noninvasive breast carcinoma: frequency of unsuspected invasion and implications for treatment. *Ann Surg* 1979;189:377–382.
78. Frykberg ER. Lobular carcinoma of the breast. *Breast J* 1999;5:296–302.
79. Swain SM. Overview and treatment of lobular carcinoma in situ. In: Silverstein MJ, ed. *Ductal carcinoma in situ of the breast*. Baltimore: Williams & Wilkins, 1997:595–609.
80. Beute BJ, Kalisher L, Hutter RVP. Lobular carcinoma in situ of the breast: clinical, pathologic and mammographic features. *AJR Am J Roentgenol* 1991;157:257–265.
81. Snyder RE. Mammography and lobular carcinoma in situ. *Surg Gynecol Obstet* 1966;122:255–260.
82. Hutter RVP, Snyder RE, Lucas JC, et al. Clinical and pathologic correlation with mammographic findings in lobular carcinoma in situ. *Cancer* 1969;23:826–839.
83. Pope TL, Fechner RE, Wilhelm MC, et al. Lobular carcinoma in situ of the breast: mammographic features. *Radiology* 1988;168:63–66.
84. Sonnenfeld MR, Frenna TH, Weidner N, et al. Lobular carcinoma in situ: mammographic-pathologic correlation of results of needle-directed biopsy. *Radiology* 1991;181:363–367.
85. Liberman L, Sama M, Susnik B, et al. Lobular carcinoma in situ at percutaneous breast biopsy: surgical biopsy findings. *AJR Am J Roentgenol* 1999;173:291–299.
86. Page DL, Dupont WD, Rogers LW, et al. Continued local recurrence of carcinoma 15–25 years after a diagnosis of low grade ductal carcinoma in situ of the breast treated only by biopsy. *Cancer* 1995;76:1197–200.
87. Habel LA, Moe RE, Daling JR, et al. Risk of contralateral breast cancer among women with carcinoma in situ of the breast. *Ann Surg* 1997;225:69–75.

88. Fechner RE. History of ductal carcinoma in situ. In: Silverstein MJ, ed. *Ductal carcinoma in situ of the breast.* Baltimore: Williams & Wilkins, 1997:18–19.

89. Buerger H, Simon R, Schafer KL, et al. Genetic relation of lobular carcinoma in situ, ductal carcinoma in situ, and associated invasive carcinoma of the breast. *Mol Pathol* 2000;53:118–121.

90. Meyer JS. Cell kinetics of histologic variants of in situ breast carcinoma. *Breast Cancer Res Treat* 1986;7:171–180.

91. Eusebi V, Magalhaes F, Azzopardi JG. Pleomorphic lobular carcinoma of the breast: an aggressive tumor showing apocrine differentiation. *Hum Pathol* 1992;23:655–662.

92. Weidner N, Semple JP. Pleomorphic variant of invasive lobular carcinoma of the breast. *Hum Pathol* 1992;23:1167–1171.

93. O'Driscoll D, Britton P, Bobrow L, et al. Lobular carcinoma in situ on core biopsy—what is the clinical significance? *Clin Radiol* 2001;56:216–220.

94. Fowble B, Hanlon AL, Patchefsky A, et al. The presence of proliferative breast disease with atypia does not significantly influence outcome in early-stage invasive breast cancer treated with conservative surgery and radiation. *Int J Radiat Oncol Biol Phys* 1998;42:105–115.

95. Sasson AR, Fowble B, Hanlon AL, et al. Lobular carcinoma in situ increases the risk of local recurrence in selected patients with stages I and II breast carcinoma treated with conservative surgery and radiation. *Cancer* 2001;91:1862–1869.

96. Early Breast Cancer Trialists' Collaborative Group. Tamoxifen for early breast cancer: an overview of the randomised trials. *Lancet* 1998;351:1451–1467.

97. Powles T, Eeles R, Ashley S, et al. Interim analysis of the incidence of breast cancer in the Royal Marsden Hospital tamoxifen randomised chemoprevention trial. *Lancet* 1998;352:98–101.

98. Veronesi U, Maisonneuve P, Costa A, et al. Prevention of breast cancer with tamoxifen: preliminary findings from the Italian randomised trial among hysterectomised women. Italian Tamoxifen Prevention Study. *Lancet* 1998;352:93–97.

99. Chlebowski RT, Collyar DE, Somerfield M, et al. American Society of Clinical Oncology technology assessment on breast cancer risk reduction strategies: tamoxifen and raloxifene. *J Clin Oncol* 1999;17:1939–1955.

100. NCI CancerNet Clinical Trial Database. 2001;vol 2001.

101. Hartmann LC, Schaid DJ, Woods JE, et al. Efficacy of bilateral prophylactic mastectomy in women with a family history of breast cancer. *N Engl J Med* 1999;340:77–84.

102. Surveillance, epidemiology, and end results: incidence and mortality data, 1973–77. *Natl Cancer Inst Monogr* 1981:1–1082.

103. Grumbiner BM. Cell adhesion: the molecular basis of tissue architecture and morphogenesis. *Cell* 1996;84:345–357.

104. Anderson JA. Multicentric and bilateral appearance of lobular carcinoma in situ of the breast. *Acta Pathol Microbiol Scand* 1974;82A:730–734.

67

PATHOLOGY OF DUCTAL CARCINOMA IN SITU: PROLIFERATIVE AND NONPROLIFERATIVE BENIGN BREAST DISEASE

JAMES L. CONNOLLY

This book deals with in situ carcinoma, specifically with ductal carcinoma in situ (DCIS). Proliferative lesions that histologically approach but do not fulfill the criteria for the diagnosis of in situ carcinoma are classified as atypical hyperplasias. At one end of the spectrum of benign breast changes, the proliferation may be so mild as to be considered a normal variant, whereas at the other end of the spectrum, it may be difficult to differentiate from small in situ carcinomas.

Pathologists have long recognized that benign breast tissue in women with carcinoma often shows more proliferation and atypicality than breast tissue in women without cancer (1). Several retrospective studies verify that atypicality in benign breast biopsies signifies an increased subsequent cancer risk (2–5). These studies used various definitions for proliferation and atypicality, and the patient populations were small. The first large study of benign breast disease and subsequent risk of breast cancer was published in 1985 by Dupont and Page (6). In this retrospective cohort study, pathologists evaluated biopsy specimens from more than 3,000 women in the Nashville, TN, area. All these women had a benign breast biopsy specimen, and a minority ultimately developed breast cancer. Using women with nonproliferative changes as a control group, the study found that women had a slightly increased risk for the subsequent development of breast cancer if their biopsy specimens revealed proliferative changes without atypicality and a substantially increased risk if the specimens revealed atypical hyperplasia. Based on the size of the patient population involved in this study and the relatively well-defined categories of benign breast disease, there was optimism that the findings of this study could be useful in counseling women with benign breast disease on the risk of subsequent breast cancer. Questions remained of the usefulness and reproducibility of the Dupont and Page study; therefore, the National Cancer Institute of the United States funded a number of studies to determine whether the results of Dupont

and Page could be duplicated in other patient populations by independent pathologists. At this time, two of these studies have been published (7,8). They were both population-based, retrospective cohort studies. The two groups that have published to date using standardized criteria and independent pathologists are the Nurses' Health Study (NHS) (7) and the Breast Cancer Detection Demonstration Project (BCDDP) (8). This type of study requires a large study population to identify a relatively small number of women who had evaluable benign breast biopsy specimens and who subsequently developed breast cancer. These patient populations are illustrated in Table 67.1.

In all three studies, the pathologists were unaware of patient outcome while performing the histologic evaluations. In the NHS and BCDDP studies, the pathologists agreed to use the criteria of Page and Rogers (9) and standardized their criteria with Dr. Page before the onset of the study. The benign biopsies were classified into three categories: (i) nonproliferative changes, which included normal breast tissue, apocrine metaplasia, cysts, and mild ductal hyperplasia of the usual type; (ii) proliferative changes without atypia, which included fibroadenomas, sclerosing adenosis, intraductal papillomas, and moderate or florid ductal hyperplasia of the usual type; and (iii) atypical hyperplasias, which could be of either the ductal or lobular type. The atypical hyperplasias were defined as epithelial proliferative lesions with intermediate features between ordinary hyperplasia and carcinoma in situ.

Atypical ductal hyperplasia is a lesion with some of the architectural and cytologic features of a low-grade or noncomedo DCIS. These features include nuclear monomorphism, regular cell placement, and round regular spaces. These changes are usually limited to one space or, commonly, to one part of a space. A more detailed description of the histologic and cytologic criteria for the diagnosis of atypical hyperplasia is outlined by Page and Rogers (9).

TABLE 67.1. NUMBER OF WOMEN WITH EVALUABLE BENIGN BIOPSIES WHO SUBSEQUENTLY DEVELOPED BREAST CANCER (CASES), CONTROLS, AND NUMBER OF ELIGIBLE WOMEN FROM THE THREE SERIES

Series	Cases	Controls	Total Population
Nashville	134	—	3,303
NHS	401	1702	240,000
BCDDP	95	190	>280,000

Nashville, study by Dupont and Page (6); NHS, Nurses' Health Study (7); BCDDP, Breast Cancer Detection Demonstration Project (8).

TABLE 67.3. EFFECT OF INTERACTION OF FAMILY HISTORY [+ FAMILY HISTORY IN A FIRST-DEGREE RELATIVE (MOTHER, SISTER, DAUGHTER)] AND HISTOLOGIC SUBTYPE OF BENIGN BIOPSY ON RELATIVE RISK OF BREAST CANCER

	Nashville	NHS	BCDDP
Nonproliferative	1	1	1
PWA (+ FH)	2.7	4.5	2.6
AH (+ FH)	8.9	7.3	22.0

Nashville, study by Dupont and Page; NHS, Nurses' Health Study (7); BCDDP, Breast Cancer Detection Demonstration Project (8); PWA, proliferation without atypia; AH, atypical hyperplasia (ductal or lobular).

As illustrated in Table 67.2, the results of these three studies are remarkably similar. Using the nonproliferative group as the reference group, patients with proliferation without atypia had a slightly elevated relative risk for the subsequent development of cancer (1.6- to 1.9-fold), whereas patients with atypical hyperplasia had a substantially elevated relative risk for the subsequent development of breast cancer (3.7- to 5.3-fold).

Women who had a positive family history of breast cancer in a first-degree relative (mother, sister, or daughter) had a substantially elevated risk for developing breast cancer compared with women without a positive family history in all three studies. This increase in risk was seen in women with proliferation without atypia but was especially prominent in the group with atypical hyperplasia and a positive family history. In patients with atypical hyperplasia and a positive family history, the risk approaches that of patients with DCIS or lobular carcinoma in situ (Table 67.3).

The NHS and the BCDDP were able to evaluate the effect of menopausal status as a risk factor. Both studies found it an important modulator of risk. The relative risk for premenopausal patients with atypical hyperplasia was 5.9 in the NHS and 12.0 in the BCDDP. However, if these patients reached menopause without developing breast cancer, the risk was substantially reduced (Table 67.4). Studies such as this have led to proposals of placing women at high risk on chemoprevention such as the estrogen blocker tamoxifen.

Epidemiologic studies have shown that women taking hormone replacement therapy are at an elevated risk for de-

veloping breast cancer (10). This raises the question of the influence of hormone replacement therapy on the risk of breast cancer in women with documented types of benign breast disease. Surprisingly, the use of hormone replacement therapy did not increase the risk in women with proliferative breast disease with or without atypical hyperplasia in both the Dupont and Page study (11) and the NHS (12). In the NHS, the relative risk in patients with atypical hyperplasia was 3.4 for those who had not used hormone replacement therapy, 3.0 for past users, and 2.5 for current users (12). This would lead one to conclude, based on the available data, that the use of hormone replacement therapy is not contraindicated in women with atypical hyperplasia.

In addition to the three broad categories of benign breast disease, there are numerous specific proliferative lesions in the breast. Two of these lesions have been assessed for risk of breast cancer within the confines of these large clinical studies. The first was sclerosing adenosis, which was found to have a similar risk as other components of proliferative breast disease without atypia (relative risk, 1.7) (13). Another lesion that mammographically and clinically may mimic invasive breast cancer is a radial scar or complex sclerosing lesion. The presence of a radial scar in a benign breast biopsy specimen increased the relative risk threefold compared with patients with nonproliferative disease (14). In patients who had radial scars plus atypical hyperplasia, the relative risk increased to 5.8-fold compared with 3.8-fold for patients with atypical hyperplasia without a radial scar (14). In addition, the risk increased with increasing size of the radial scar and increasing numbers of radial scars.

TABLE 67.2. RELATIVE RISK OF BREAST CANCER ASSOCIATED WITH HISTOLOGIC SUBTYPE OF BENIGN BREAST BIOPSY

	Nashville	NHS	BCDDP
Nonproliferative	1	1	1
PWA	1.9	1.6	1.6
AH	5.3	3.7	4.3

Nashville, study by Dupont and Page (6); NHS, Nurses' Health Study (7); BCDDP, Breast Cancer Detection Demonstration Project (8); PWA, proliferation without atypia; AH, atypical hyperplasia (ductal or lobular).

TABLE 67.4. EFFECT OF MENOPAUSAL STATUS ON RELATIVE RISK OF BREAST CANCER IN PATIENTS WITH ATYPICAL HYPERPLASIA

Status	NHS	BCDDP
Premenopausal	5.9	12.0
Postmenopausal	2.3	3.3

NHS, Nurses' Health Study (7); BCDDP, Breast Cancer Detection Demonstration Project (8).

Although some controversy remains, classic papers on lobular carcinoma in situ indicate that it is associated with a bilaterally increased risk for the subsequent development of breast cancer (15,16). In contrast, low-grade or noncomedo DCIS has been shown to be associated primarily with an ipsilaterally increased risk (17–19). One would predict, therefore, that atypical lobular hyperplasia, like its more well-developed counterpart lobular carcinoma in situ, would be associated with a bilateral risk. One would predict that atypical ductal hyperplasia, which has features similar to but not as fully developed as low-grade (noncomedo) DCIS would therefore be a predictor of an ipsilaterally increased risk of breast cancer. Surprisingly, the risk of subsequent breast cancer in patients with both atypical lobular and atypical ductal hyperplasia has been shown to be approximately equal in both breasts (20–22). The fact that atypical ductal hyperplasia is associated with a bilateral risk for the subsequent development of carcinoma indicates that at least some of these lesions are biologically different from diagnostic low-grade DCIS. What this biologic difference is remains to be determined.

There is a good correlation between the differentiation or grade of DCIS and associated infiltrating ductal carcinomas (23). In particular, low-grade DCIS is usually associated with low-grade infiltrating carcinoma. Given that atypical hyperplasias of the breast are lesions with some features of low-grade in situ carcinomas, it has been speculated that the carcinomas that develop in these patients would tend to be low-grade carcinomas. A recent study of women in the NHS has examined these issues (24). Breast cancers from women with a previous benign biopsy specimen showing nonproliferative changes, proliferative lesions without atypia or atypical hyperplasias were compared. The carcinomas were categorized by histologic grade, histologic type, tumor size, nodal status, lymphatic–small vessel invasion, extensive intraductal component, and hormone receptor status. The cancers that developed in the women with the three types of benign breast disease did not differ with respect to any of these variables. Of particular interest was that the breast cancers that arose in patients with atypical hyperplasias were not primarily low-grade cancers. Given that and the fact that the carcinomas that arose in women with the different categories of benign breast disease were as likely to be contralateral as ipsilateral indicates that the atypical hyperplasias, at least in most instances, are not direct precursors of invasive carcinoma.

At least one study has attempted to use size as a major criterion for the diagnosis of atypical ductal hyperplasia versus low-grade (or noncomedo) DCIS. This study included cases of low-grade DCIS (≤2 mm) as atypical intraductal hyperplasia as well as lesions that would have been classified as atypical ductal hyperplasia in the studies outlined here (25). In this study, approximately 75% of the recurrences were ipsilateral. Therefore, many cases in this study have behaved biologically as small cases of DCIS and recurred ipsilaterally.

Therefore, I do not believe that a size criterion is the best determinant of what is low-grade DCIS versus atypical ductal hyperplasia. If a lesion is otherwise diagnostic of low-grade DCIS but is smaller than 2 mm, it should, I believe, be considered a small example of DCIS and treated accordingly.

The diagnosis of atypical ductal proliferative lesions remains a highly controversial and difficult area in breast pathology (21,26). It is clear that the definitions of atypical hyperplasia used in the three major studies, as elaborated here, carry clinically significant and relevant information. If pathologists use definitions for atypical hyperplasia that are different from those used in these studies, it is unclear what the clinical significance would be (27). When a standardized set of criteria is not used, there will be little if any interobserver concordance between the diagnosis of atypical hyperplasia and proliferation without atypia, at one end of the spectrum, and low-grade DCIS at the other end. This was graphically illustrated in a study by Rosai (28) in 1991. In contrast, Schnitt et al. (29) demonstrated that, by using standardized criteria and pathologists, this interobserver variability can be substantially reduced. The diagnosis of atypical hyperplasia versus low-grade DCIS is becoming an increasingly common problem. Before extensive use of mammography, atypical hyperplasia was found in approximately 4% of biopsies done for a palpable abnormality (6). The incidence of finding atypical hyperplasia has increased to 15% to 20% of mammographically directed biopsies for microcalcifications (30,31).

Given the difficulty in separating atypical ductal hyperplasia from low-grade DCIS, investigators have sought to define molecular and genetic characteristics that may help to differentiate the two. Unfortunately, atypical ductal hyperplasia and low-grade DCIS have been shown to be very similar in most studies. Both lesions are usually estrogen receptor positive (32), do not show overexpression of HER-2/neu (33,34), do not show increases in p53 protein (34–37), and do show Bcl-2 protein expression (38). Cyclin D1 overexpression was initially thought to be seen much more frequently in low-grade DCIS than in atypical ductal hyperplasia (39), but in a more recent study, atypical ductal hyperplasia and low-grade DCIS showed essentially no difference in overexpression of cyclin D1 protein. A promising area of investigation involves the use of differential cytokeratin staining for distinguishing among proliferative breast lesions (41,42). Although currently there is no reliable molecular or genetic study that can differentiate between benign and malignant in situ proliferations, it is an important area for further investigation.

In conclusion, one can assess the risk of subsequent development of cancer in patients with benign breast biopsies depending on the pathologic changes found in those biopsies. Women whose biopsies reveal nonproliferative changes are not, based on their biopsy, at an elevated risk for the subsequent development of breast cancer. Women whose biopsies reveal proliferative changes without atypicality are at a slightly elevated risk for breast cancer. Women whose biopsies reveal either atypical ductal or atypical lobular hyperplasia are at a substantially increased risk for the subsequent development of breast cancer. Women with a family history of breast cancer in a first-degree relative are at elevated risk if their biopsy reveals proliferation without atypicality, and these women are at a substantially elevated risk if the biopsy reveals atypical hyperplasia. Atypical hyperplasia is especially significant for patients who are premenopausal. Patients with atypical hyperplasia who reach menopause without developing breast cancer show a decrease in relative risk for developing cancer, although their absolute risk is still substantially greater than patients without atypical hyperplasia. The increased risk associated with atypical hyperplasia is a bilateral increase in risk in contrast to that seen with DCIS, which is primarily an ipsilateral increase in risk.

ACKNOWLEDGMENT

This work was supported by research grant CA-46475.

REFERENCES

1. Foote FW, Stewart FW. Comparative studies of cancerous versus noncancerous breasts. *Ann Surg* 1945;121:197–222.
2. Black MM, Barclay THC, Cutler SJ, et al. Association of atypical characteristics of benign breast lesions with subsequent risk of breast cancer. *Cancer* 1972;29:338–343.
3. Kodlin D, Winger EE, Morgenstern NL, et al. Chronic mastopathy and breast cancer: a follow-up study. *Cancer* 1977;9:2603–2607.
4. Donnelly PK, Baker KW, Carney JA, et al. Benign breast lesions and subsequent breast carcinoma in Rochester, Minnesota. *Mayo Clin Proc* 1975;50:650–656.
5. Hutchinson WB, Thomas DB, Hamlin WB, et al. Risk of breast cancer in women with benign breast disease. *J Natl Cancer Inst* 1980;65:13–20.
6. Dupont WD, Page DL. Risk factors for breast cancer in women with proliferative breast disease. *N Engl J Med* 1985;312:146–151.
7. London SJ, Connolly JL, Schnitt SJ, et al. A prospective study of benign breast disease and the risk of breast cancer. *JAMA* 1992;267:941–944.
8. Dupont WD, Parl FF, Hartmann WH, et al. Breast cancer associated with proliferative breast disease and atypical hyperplasia. *Cancer* 1993;71:1258–1265.
9. Page DL, Rogers LW. Combined histologic and cytologic criteria for the diagnosis of mammary atypical ductal hyperplasia. *Hum Pathol* 1992;23:1095–1097.
10. Collaborative Group on Hormonal Factors in Breast Cancer. Breast cancer and hormone replacement therapy: collaborative re-analysis of data from 51 epidemiological studies of 52,705 women with breast cancer and 10,8411 women without breast cancer. *Lancet* 1997;350:1047–1059.
11. Dupont WD, Page DL, Rogers LW, et al. Influence of exogenous estrogens, proliferative breast disease, and other variables on breast cancer risk. *Cancer* 1989;63:948—957.
12. Byrne C, Connolly JL, Colditz GA, et al. Biopsy confirmed benign breast disease, postmenopausal use of exogenous female hormone, and breast carcinoma risk. *Cancer* 2000;89:2046–2052.
13. Jensen RA, Page DL, Dupont WD, et al. Invasive breast cancer risk in women with sclerosing adenosis. *Cancer* 1989;64:1977–1983.
14. Jacobs TW, Byrne C, Colditz G, et al. Radial scars and breast cancer risk: A case control study. *N Engl J Med* 1999;340:430–436.
15. Rosen PP, Kosloff C, Lieberman PH, et al. Lobular carcinoma in situ of the breast: detailed analysis of 99 patients with average follow-up of 24 years. *Am J Surg Pathol* 1978;2:225–251.
16. Haagensen CD, Lane N, Lattes R, et al. Lobular neoplasia (so-called lobular carcinoma in situ) of the breast. *Cancer* 1978;42:737–769.
17. Rosen PP, Braun DW, Kinne DW. The clinical significance of preinvasive breast carcinoma. *Cancer* 1980;46:919–925.
18. Page DL, Dupont WD, Rogers LW, et al. Intraductal carcinoma of the breast: follow-up after biopsy only. *Cancer* 1982;49:751–758.
19. Eusebi V, Foschini MP, Cook MG, et al. Long-term follow-up of in situ carcinoma of the breast with special emphasis on clinging carcinoma. *Semin Diagn Pathol* 1989;6:165–173.
20. Connolly J, Schnitt S, London S, et al. Both atypical lobular hyperplasia (ALH) and atypical ductal hyperplasia (ADH) predict for bilateral breast cancer risk. *Lab Invest* 1992;66:13(abst).
21. Connolly JL, Schnitt SJ. Benign breast disease: resolved and unresolved issues. *Cancer* 1993;71:1187–1189.
22. Connolly JL, Schnitt SJ. Clinical and histologic aspects of proliferative and nonproliferative benign breast disease. *J Cell Biochem* 1993;17G:45–48.
23. Lampejo OT, Barnes DM, Smith P, et al. Evaluation of infiltrating ductal carcinomas with a DCIS component: correlation of the histologic type of the in situ component with grade of the infiltrating component. *Semin Diagn Pathol* 1994;11:215–222.
24. Jacobs TW, Byrne C, Colditz G, et al. Pathologic features of breast cancers in women with prior benign breast disease. *Am J Clin Pathol* 2001;115:362–369.
25. Tavassoli FA, Norris HJ. A comparison of the result of long-term follow-up for atypical intraductal hyperplasia and intra-ductal hyperplasia of the breast. *Cancer* 1990;65:518–529.
26. Rosen PP. Proliferative breast "disease": an unresolved diagnostic dilemma. *Cancer* 1993;71:3798–3807.
27. Bodian CA, Perzin KH, Lattes R, et al. Prognostic significance of benign proliferative breast disease. *Cancer* 1993;71:3896–3907.
28. Rosai J. Borderline epithelial lesions of the breast. *Am J Surg Pathol* 1991;15:209–221.
29. Schnitt SJ, Connolly JL, Tavassoli FA, et al. Interobserver reproducibility in the diagnosis of ductal proliferative lesions using standardized criteria. *Am J Surg Pathol* 1992;16:1133–1143.
30. Rubin E, Visscher DW, Alexander RW, et al. Proliferative disease and atypia in biopsies performed for nonpalpable lesions detected mammographically. *Cancer* 1988;61:2077–2082.
31. Owings DW, Hann L, Schnitt SJ. How thoroughly should needle localization breast biopsies be sampled for microscopic examination? A prospective mammographic-pathologic correlative study. *Am J Surg Pathol* 1990;14:578–583.
32. Gillett CE, Lee AH, Millis RR, et al. Cyclin D1 and associated proteins in mammary ductal carcinoma in situ and atypical ductal hyperplasia. *J Pathol* 1998;184:396–400.
33. Lodato RF, Maguire HC, Greene MI, et al. Immunohistochemical evaluation of c-erbB-2 oncogene expression in ductal carcinoma in situ and atypical ductal hyperplasia of the breast. *Mod Pathol* 1990;3:449–454.
34. Millikan R, Hulka B, Thor A, et al. P53 mutations in benign breast tissue. *J Clin Oncol* 1995;13:2293–2300.
35. Humphrey PA, Franquemont DW, Geary WA, et al. Immunodetection of p53 protein in noninvasive epithelial proliferative breast disease. *Appl Immunohistochem* 1994;2:22.

36. Eriksson ET, Schimmelpenning H, Aspenblad U, et al. Immunohistochemical expression of the mutant p53 protein and nuclear DNA content during the transition from benign to malignant breast disease. *Hum Pathol* 1994;25:1228–1233.

37. Younes M, Lebovitz RM, Bommer KE, et al. P53 accumulation in benign breast biopsy specimens. *Hum Pathol* 1995;26: 155–158.

38. Siziopikou KP, Prioleau JE, Harris JR, et al. Bcl-2 expression in the spectrum of preinvasive breast lesions. *Cancer* 1996;77: 499–506.

39. Weinstat-Saslow D, Merino MJ, Manrow RE, et al. Overexpression of cyclin D1 mRNA distinguishes invasive and in situ breast carcinomas from non-malignant lesions. *Nat Med* 1995;1: 1257–1260.

40. Alle KM, Henshall SM, Field AS, et al. Cyclin D1 protein is overexpressed in hyperplasia and intraductal carcinoma of the breast. *Clin Cancer Res* 1998;4:847–854.

41. Jarasch E-D, Nagle RB, Kaufmann M, et al. Differential diagnosis of benign epithelial proliferations and carcinomas of the breast using antibodies to cytokeratins. *Hum Pathol* 1988;19:276–289.

42. Moinfar F, Man YG, Lininger RA, et al. Use of keratin 34betaE12 as an adjunct in the diagnosis of mammary intraepithelial neoplasia-ductal type—benign and malignant intraductal proliferations. *Am J Surg Pathol* 1999;23:1048–1058.

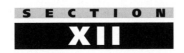

SECTION
XII

CONCLUSION

68

EDITORS' CONSENSUS

MELVIN J. SILVERSTEIN
ABRAM RECHT
MICHAEL D. LAGIOS

In October 2001, the three editors began working on a consensus statement to be inserted as the last chapter. As in the first edition of this text, we decided to write a number of independent final statements from the point of view of our specialties and to integrate them into a single chapter.

GENERAL COMMENTS

Throughout this text, we have read that ductal carcinoma in situ (DCIS) is an architecturally and biologically heterogeneous group of lesions with varying malignant potential. Although there continues to be no internationally accepted classification system and a variety of classifications exist based on histologic architecture, nuclear grade, necrosis, or cytonuclear differentiation, some progress was made in 1997 when an international consensus conference on the pathology of DCIS was held in Philadelphia (1) (Chapter 63).

Therapeutic approaches continue to range from excision only to all types of wider excisions, including segmental resection and quadrant resection, all of which may or may not be followed by radiation therapy. The 1997 Surveillance, Epidemiologic, and End Results program data show that treatment in the United States is evenly divided with approximately one-third of patients with DCIS being treated with mastectomy, one-third with excision plus radiation therapy, and one-third with excision alone. Since the last edition of this text, there has been greater emphasis on an oncoplastic approach to wide segmental resection (Chapter 15). For patients treated with mastectomy, the skin-sparing approach with immediate reconstruction has become common.

Because DCIS is a heterogeneous group of lesions, no single approach, based on current knowledge, will be appropriate for all forms of the disease, and methods must be developed to determine the most appropriate treatment for each individual patient. In the future, as we understand more about the etiologic factors of DCIS, treatments that interfere with malignant transformation or progression from DCIS to invasive cancer are indeed a possibility.

Today, the most innocuous-appearing forms of DCIS (e.g., low nuclear grade, small cells without necrosis, estrogen and progesterone receptor positive, HER 2/neu [c-erbB2] negative), if untreated, may never become an invasive lesion or cause clinical problems, leading us to wonder whether these lesions should have been labeled as cancer in the first place. Conversely, the most aggressive phenotypic forms, if left untreated, may develop into invasive carcinomas in relatively short periods of time.

The immediate questions, then, are quite simple. Which lesions, if left untreated, are going to become invasive and how long will this take? For those who require treatment, what treatment is most appropriate? Which lesions, if treated conservatively, demonstrate such high recurrence rates that mastectomy is preferable? In those patients in whom mastectomy is not required, which patients can be treated with excision alone and which ones require radiation therapy? The questions are simple, the answers are not, and they are the focus of worldwide study and debate.

THE RADIATION ONCOLOGIST'S POINT OF VIEW: ABRAM RECHT

There remain several major controversies regarding the management of patients with DCIS as mentioned previously. I give my views on the selection of patients for breast-conserving therapy (BCT) rather than mastectomy; the definition of patient subgroups that have a low risk of recurrence after BCT without radiotherapy; the use of tamoxifen; and the optimal follow-up schedule.

Breast-Conserving Therapy Versus Mastectomy

Patients with positive lumpectomy margins have had a substantial risk of local failure despite radiation therapy in some series (2), but other groups have not found higher risks of failure among patients with positive margins than among those with negative margins (3–5). Even for patients with negative margins, the risk of recurrence (including the development of new primary cancers in the ipsilateral breast) is higher for patients treated with BCT than for those treated with mastectomy. On average, 50% of local failures after BCT are invasive. Salvage treatment does not always prevent further local/regional or distant relapse in this setting.

Therefore, there may be long-term differences of 1% to 2% in survival rates in patients treated with mastectomy and BCT, even for patients who are candidates for the latter approach (6). In my experience, most patients are willing to accept this risk to preserve their breast. Indeed, some patients will even forego substantial long-term advantages in survival time (which, however, would not be enjoyed until some point in the distant future) to avoid permanent (and immediate) reductions in their quality of life (7,8). Other patients are not willing to make such bargains.

Breast-Conserving Therapy: When can Radiotherapy be Omitted?

One can never be absolutely certain that there is no residual disease left after breast-conserving surgery. Therefore, the routine use of radiotherapy will reduce the risk of local failure in all patient subgroups, as was seen in the National Surgical Adjuvant Breast Project (NSABP) B-17 and European Organization for Research and Treatment of Cancer (EORTC) trials. However, some patient subgroups treated with wide excision after meticulous radiologic and pathologic evaluation appear to have very low ipsilateral failure rates even when not irradiated (5% to 10% at 10 years). For them, the absolute reduction in recurrence obtained by adding radiotherapy may be very small (a few percent). However, there is no agreement on exactly how to define these subgroups, nor is it clear how many institutions can offer the broad array of skills needed to yield such results without the aid of radiotherapy.

I believe that margin status is probably the most critical variable in selecting between the options of wide excision with or without radiotherapy. As discussed in my chapter on the randomized trials (Chapter 40), the minimum width of the tumor-free margin needed to achieve excellent results is not clear. Margins less than 1 mm are inadequate, but patients in some series with margin widths more than 1 mm or more than 5 mm had very similar results to those in series with margin widths of 10 mm or more. Histologic features, particularly nuclear grade and perhaps necrosis, also appear important in predicting the results of wide excision alone. The role of other histologic and biologic factors is uncertain. No consensus has been reached on whether combinations of features have superior prognostic significance than a single pathologic factor (1), nor is there agreement on how such features interact with margin status.

From the individual patient's point of view, decreased failure rates must be weighed against the short- and long-term toxicities of radiotherapy (9). The excess risk of death

owing to radiation-related heart disease, sarcomas, leukemia, and lung cancer will likely be less than 1% among patients irradiated using current techniques. Radiation-related breast cancer is of concern for patients age 45 or younger at diagnosis, but the absolute increase in the risk of developing breast cancer (perhaps 3% to 5% at 25 years) is small compared with the background risk (e.g., 15% to 25%). Because few patients in this age group (or their physicians) seem to consider prophylactic contralateral mastectomy to be of value, it would appear unlikely that this small additional risk will deter many from undergoing irradiation.

There are no studies specifically addressing what patients consider to be a sufficiently low risk of recurrence that they would be willing to forego radiotherapy after lumpectomy (or, conversely, at what point patients are more likely to elect mastectomy rather than BCT). However, in a study conducted in Hamilton, Ontario, 78 of 82 patients (95%) with early-stage invasive cancers treated with breast-conserving surgery chose to be irradiated rather than observed (10). Their reasons for doing so included equally their beliefs that this would improve survival, reduce the risk of local recurrence, and prevent the need for further breast surgery. In a study conducted in Toronto, patients with breast cancer were generally willing to forego irradiation only when the absolute reduction in the risk of any recurrence was less than 1% (11). Similar results were found in a study of patients who had undergone conservative surgery and radiotherapy at the Joint Center for Radiation Therapy (12).

It is important to point out that conflict may easily arise between patients, their families, and their health care providers regarding the minimum benefit needed to justify a particular treatment option. Healthy individuals clearly have very different ideas about what they would want to do in a hypothetical health care situation than do patients faced with real decisions (13–15). Perhaps the most important lesson to be learned from these studies is how variable individual patient's opinions are. Age, education, income, and other demographic factors correlate roughly or not at all with an individual's responses. Doctors usually recommend oncologic treatments only when they believe [often erroneously (16)] that the rates of return are much greater than what many patients are willing to settle for. Such differing views seem especially likely to occur when the absolute survival benefits of treatment are small or nil and the cost is high (as with radiotherapy in the management of DCIS).

Tamoxifen

The NSABP B-24 trial showed that tamoxifen reduced the risk of both ipsilateral recurrence and contralateral breast cancers (17). This was not surprising, given what was previously known about tamoxifen. The more interesting aspects of this study are to be found in their subgroup analysis. As discussed earlier (Chapter 40), the absolute benefits of tamoxifen were greatest for patients with positive margins or those younger than age 50 at diagnosis. Unfortunately, a 2 × 2 analysis of the impact of age and margin status together was not performed.

The early results of the United Kingdom-Australia-New Zealand trial (18) suggest that tamoxifen is not an adequate substitute for radiotherapy in patients treated with excision alone. Similarly, tamoxifen does not appear to substitute for adequate margin width. In a nonrandomized study conducted in Manchester, England, with a median follow-up of 47 months, the risk of local failure for patients treated with excision alone or excision plus tamoxifen were 40% (17 of 43 patients) and 33% (five of 15), respectively, for patients with tumor-free margin widths 1 mm or less (19). [For patients with margin widths greater than 1 mm, the respective local failure rates were 8% (seven of 86) and 0% (none of 12).]

Tamoxifen may cause life-threatening side effects, the incidence of which increase with increasing patient age. In the NSABP B-24 trial, deep vein thromboses and pulmonary emboli occurred in 0.3% and 1.2% of patients on the placebo and tamoxifen arms, respectively (17). In addition, one patient in the placebo arm and five in the tamoxifen arm had strokes (20). The rate of endometrial cancer was 0.45 cases per 100 patient-years in the placebo arm and 1.53 cases per 100 patient-years in the tamoxifen arm (17). No deaths from these events have occurred in either arm yet. However, to date, tamoxifen has not improved the overall or breast cancer–specific survival rate, in either this trial or the NSABP P-1 trial (21).

Follow-Up

Many different follow-up schemes for patients with DCIS have been suggested. For example, both the National Comprehensive Cancer Network breast group and a joint panel of the American College of Radiology, the American College of Surgeons, the College of American Pathologists, and the Society of Surgical Oncology have suggested that physical examination be performed every 6 months for the first 5 years, then annually thereafter (22,23). Both groups also recommended yearly bilateral mammograms.

It is important to realize the arbitrary nature of these schemes, that is, they rest on expert opinion almost totally unsupported by comparative data specific to this setting. Further, these schemes often appear to be based on misunderstandings of the time course of recurrence and changes in the breast caused by BCT. As I discussed earlier (Chapter 55), the risk of recurrences at or near the ipsilateral primary tumor site probably does not decline sharply until 8 to 10 years after treatment. Fibrosis after radiotherapy may develop over the first 3 years after treatment but then remains stable (24). Similarly, the radiologic appearance may take 2 to 3 years after treatment to reach its final state. Hence, the 5-year break point chosen by these panels appears to have little justification. In addition, the risk of developing new ipsilateral or contralateral primary tumors is likely to be

fairly constant over time. This risk will also probably vary from patient to patient owing to factors such as BRCA1-2 status and age at presentation.

There are no data of which I am aware that compare the effectiveness of different intervals between routine histories and physical examinations for patients with DCIS (or invasive breast cancer, for that matter). There are limited data on this point for mammography. In a study of patients with invasive cancers treated at the Moffitt Cancer Center in Tampa, FL, only eight of 15 recurrences in the ipsilateral breast were detected first by mammography performed routinely at 6-month intervals; however, eight of ten new primaries occurring in the contralateral breast were detected first by annual mammography (25). Some studies of screening (in patients without a history of breast cancer) have shown annual mammography to be markedly more effective than biennial or triennial mammography (26,27), but in other studies, the differences in tumor size, stage, and so on between annual and less frequent mammography have been minimal or nil (28,29).

It is also unclear whether follow-up of patients with DCIS by a specialist yields better outcome than follow-up by general practitioners. A randomized trial performed in England that included patients with predominantly invasive tumors found no difference in time to diagnosis, survival rates, or quality of life (30), but no analysis was performed of the means of detection for different sites of failure. Further, the number of recurrences was small (26 of 296 patients), and the median follow-up was short (18 months). Because most failures in patients with invasive cancer (particularly at short follow-up) will be distant, the implications of this trial for patients with DCIS are limited at best.

Conclusions

Mastectomy is always considered to be acceptable treatment for patients with DCIS. In addition, patients with evidence of tumor spread diffusely through one or more quadrants of the breast on physical examination or mammography are not good candidates for BCT unless these areas are shown to be benign by biopsy. Patients with well-localized lesions 2 to 2.5 cm or smaller radiologically and pathologically, with low or moderate nuclear grade, in whom negative histologic margins more than 1 mm (and preferably more than 3 mm, as in the current Eastern Cooperative Oncology Group observational study) have been achieved may be considered for treatment with excision only. Patients with larger lesions, high nuclear grade, or narrower margins should receive radiotherapy routinely unless they are participating in a prospective study designed to test the need for such treatment. Having histologically uninvolved margins is probably not necessary in all cases to ensure successful results when radiotherapy is used, but there are no data on what degree of margin involvement is sufficient to result in a high risk of recurrence. Patients with high nuclear grade and/or comedonecrosis may be at high risk of failure despite radiotherapy when margins are involved, and I usually recommend mastectomy in this situation. The case for using tamoxifen for patients with positive margins or those younger than age 50 is more compelling than the case for its universal use for patients with DCIS treated with radiotherapy. Even so, rates of local recurrence in patients treated today will probably be lower than in the NSABP B-17 and B-24 trials, and hence the benefits of tamoxifen will be diminished accordingly. Patients must understand that the benefits and risks of tamoxifen in this setting are not yet fully understood before deciding whether to take it. Finally, there is no evidence at present that tamoxifen can be substituted for radiotherapy to achieve adequate local tumor control.

It seems likely that the majority of recurrences or new primaries in patients with prior DCIS will be detected by annual mammography at a highly curable stage. However, some lesions can only be detected by physical examination. My preference is that this be performed twice yearly for patients presenting with premenopausal breast cancer, partly because of the greater difficulty of screening mammography in finding lesions in this population and partly because they are probably at greater risk of developing new ipsilateral or contralateral primaries than older patients. (I try to have patients alternate these visits between the surgeon and myself, so each of us sees the patient once yearly.) For patients at lower risk, annual breast examinations and interval histories may be sufficient. Given the minimal changes resulting from properly performed modern radiotherapy and surgery and the time courses of ipsilateral recurrence and new primary development, it seems reasonable to space mammograms and physical examinations at equal intervals over the entire duration of follow-up rather than changing the schedule at 3, 5, or 10 years. I believe (although I cannot prove) that specialists experienced in treating and following patients with breast cancer [surgeons, radiation oncologists, medical oncologists, or specially trained nurse-practitioners or physician assistants (31)] are more likely than nonspecialists to pick up subtle, potentially important findings on interval physical examination or history. The impact of such expertise will probably be very difficult to appreciate in outcome statistics for the population as a whole. However, I believe that specialist care may result in substantial differences in results for individual patients. Such care will almost certainly be more costly than nonspecialist care, however (32). Like many other aspects of the treatment of patients with DCIS, how much society is willing to spend on such care is a political question, not a medical one.

THE PATHOLOGIST'S POINT OF VIEW: MICHAEL D. LAGIOS

For more than two millennia, therapeutic intervention for breast cancer had been a bootless enterprise, without impact on survival. In the United States, in particular, for most of the past century, treatment was limited to Halsted radical mastectomy. The use of radiation therapy and adjuvant therapies became common only after 1975.

Mammographic technology, as it was introduced to the medical community at large beginning in the early 1970s, was a transforming event. A radiologic screening technique as opposed to a therapy had a dramatic effect on stage, outcome, and, as has recently been confirmed in randomized trials, reducing breast cancer mortality. As a young pathologist interested in breast cancer, I lived through this transformation, which at present results in mean sizes of 11 mm for image-detected breast cancers, 95% of which are node negative and exhibit a similar expectation of disease-free survival.

A significant and continually growing part of that transformation was the large number of small, clinically occult DCIS being detected. For the first time, a preinvasive breast cancer, DCIS, a variable obligate precursor to invasive growth, could be detected and treated in substantial numbers. DCIS had been an infrequently if not rarely detected cancer before the introduction of mammography, as has been noted repeatedly in multiple separate experiences, and largely had been detected as palpable disease, Paget's disease, or nipple discharge, features that are now known to generally reflect extensive disease and a high likelihood of invasion.

Treatment of DCIS, particularly of the image-detected lesions of limited extent, presents numerous advantages over the treatment of even small invasive carcinomas. These advantages include the fact that no axillary dissection, not even the sentinel node technique, is necessary, nor is chemotherapy and/or adjuvant tamoxifen or similar selective estrogen receptor modulators. Although controversy persists regarding the routine use of irradiation for conservatively treated DCIS, it is clear that subsets of patients defined based on grade, size, and margin status can be identified with a fair degree of reproducibility by practicing community pathologists. These subsets receive no benefit from adjuvant irradiation. Today, half of conservatively treated patients with DCIS are spared radiation therapy, which is certainly not the standard of care for this disease. These advantages translate into less morbidity and a better quality of life for the patient, an expectation of a near 100% cause-specific survival rate, and, even factoring in the costs of local invasive recurrences in conservatively treated patients, a very large reduction in the costs of treatment.

Therapeutic intervention for image-detected DCIS is a very cost-effective stratagem and results in virtual complete local control, in many cases for the cost of an adequate surgical resection alone. Unlike some trial data, the University of Southern California (USC)/Van Nuys database reveals a stable level of local control after an adequate excision, not a decreasing slope over time.

DCIS provides an excellent opportunity to develop less invasive ablative therapies, perhaps permitting thermal or photonic energy to be targeted intraductally in cases of

DCIS or developing gene therapies that can arrest the several avenues of neoplastic progression that have been hypothesized for DCIS. The possibility of such interventions and their practical development will be left to those whose imaginations have not been blunted by the implacable walls of conventional wisdom and tradition.

Pathologic examination plays a critical role in determining treatment options for patients with DCIS. Management of patients with DCIS should not be attempted in centers where a pathologist is unable or unwilling to provide the grade, size, and margin status of the lesion and to correlate the pathologic findings with mammographic microcalcifications to estimate the extent of disease in the breast. This information can only be generated by inking margins, correlating with preoperative mammography and specimen radiography, and completely processing tissue sequentially. Sequential processing is critical in estimating the size of a DCIS, which may only in part be associated with microcalcifications, determining margin width, and excluding invasive foci. Such processing was advocated by the DCIS Consensus Conference (1) and recommended as the ideal by the International Image Detected Breast Cancer Consensus Conference (33).

Intraoperative frozen sections for margin assessment have no role in the pathologic diagnosis or management of DCIS, except in the most unusual circumstances. Intraoperative estimation of the adequacy of excision should be based on specimen radiography.

Radiation therapy probably provides no significant benefit for local control of low- or intermediate-grade DCIS as a whole. However, high-grade DCIS or intermediate-grade lesions either of large size or with suboptimal margins or both are benefited to a limited extent by irradiation. Silverstein (34) reported a 13% benefit of irradiation for local recurrence–free survival for patients with Van Nuys Prognostic Index scores of 5, 6, or 7 after 81 months of median follow-up. Some previous studies (35–37) of excision and radiation therapy for DCIS have documented an increasing local recurrence rate beyond 5 years with a minimum twofold increase in recurrence rate at 8 years of follow-up and would suggest that the benefit demonstrated for irradiation is likely to diminish with increasing time (34–36). A recent update of the NSABP protocol B-17 (38) revealed a comparable increase in local recurrence (15.8 % at 12 years) but after a longer interval. The relative benefit of irradiation for local control in B-17 at 5 years was threefold and at 12 years 1.9-fold greater compared with the nonirradiated control arm. This represents a 37% reduction of the relative benefit of irradiation beyond 8 years.

Mastectomy is necessary for local control in cases in which the disease is too extensive for segmental resection or margins remain unequivocally positive or uncertain after attempts at re-excision. Although mastectomy achieves the highest level of local control, some patients with extensive disease will remain at risk because of residual DCIS left in skin flaps and/or the axilla. Although postmastectomy recurrence rates for all DCIS patients are very low (1% to 2%), for those with disease extents greater than 50 mm in which microinvasive foci occur more frequently, postmastectomy recurrence rates may be somewhat higher (39).

THE SURGICAL ONCOLOGIST'S POINT OF VIEW: MELVIN J. SILVERSTEIN

When the first edition of this book was published in 1997, the only prospective randomized data that existed were those from the NSABP B-17 trial. B-17 was first published after 43 months of median follow-up (40,41). By 2002, when this edition was published, 12-year results were available for NSABP-B17 (38,42,43), 7-year results were available for B-24 (17,38), and 6-year results were available for EORTC trial 10853 (44,45) (Chapter 43). For the United Kingdom-Australia-New Zealand (UK/ANZ) trial, results after 53 months of median follow-up were available (18,46) (Chapter 44). All these published randomized trials have shown an approximate 50% reduction in local recurrence for all subgroups at any point in time for irradiated patients. None of them has shown any benefit in survival, regardless of treatment.

The B-24 trial showed a small but statistically significant local recurrence benefit for irradiated patients who received tamoxifen (17,38); the UK/ANZ trial did not (18,46) (Chapter 44). Both trials showed a similar small reduction in contralateral breast cancers in patients who received tamoxifen.

The USC/Van Nuys DCIS data come from a large series of nonrandomized patients with pathology parameters defined and collected prospectively. These data have been criticized because patient treatment was not randomized. In 2000, the *New England Journal of Medicine* published an article detailing the value of observational studies such as those reported by the USC/Van Nuys group (47). Observational nonrandomized studies were particularly useful at defining variables that should be studied prospectively in a randomized fashion. Moreover, the results of well done observational studies were often nearly identical with formal prospective randomized trials. So it is with the results of the USC/Van Nuys patients with DCIS. With an average follow-up of 7 years, the overall results are essentially identical when compared with the prospective randomized trials, that is, an approximate 50% reduction in local recurrence and no survival benefit for patients treated with radiation therapy compared with patients treated with excision alone (48).

The differences between the USC/Van Nuys patients with DCIS and the prospective randomized trials become apparent when we examine the subgroup analyses. The randomized trials did not pay meticulous attention to margin width (a measurement was present in less than 5% of the cases) or tumor size, and these parameters, for the most part, had to be collected retrospectively. Such retrospective review of pathology cannot accurately establish these features. The protocols varied among the trials, but most of the NSABP cases did not have inked margins. Inking was required for the EORTC trial, and it was advised but not mandatory for the UK/ANZ trial. The NSABP did not require specimen radiography. It was performed more than 80% of the time in both the EORTC and UK/ANZ trials. Complete tissue processing was not required in any of the trials, although some of the patients may have benefited from this. Conversely, the USC/Van Nuys series inked or dyed all margins and used complete tissue processing and mammographic/pathologic correlation, collecting all data in a prospective fashion.

The published randomized trials are of great value because treatment was prospectively randomized, but much of the key pathologic data had to be determined retrospectively by central slide review, and some of it, such as margin width or true size across multiple histologic blocks, could not be determined retrospectively, making some subset analyses impossible, e.g., those by tumor size or margin width.

Conversely, the USC/Van Nuys database is of great value because the pathologic variables were meticulously collected prospectively, but the USC/Van Nuys data are compromised because treatment was not prospectively randomized.

Essentially, all the prospective randomized trials and the USC/Van Nuys Series show exactly the same thing: radiation therapy works when local recurrence is the end point. Radiation therapy reduces local recurrence by 50%. When breast cancer–specific survival, however, is the end point, radiation therapy adds little because there is no difference in outcome regardless of treatment in any of the studies cited.

If there is a survival benefit from the addition of radiation therapy, it is speculative at this time, based on the premise that reducing invasive local recurrences can lead to a reduction in breast cancer mortality. No current data have shown such a benefit, and if it is subsequently demonstrated, the benefit will be small (49) (Chapter 56).

Why Not Irradiate Every Patient?

Radiation therapy is time-consuming and expensive. It results in radiation fibrosis in a small percentage of patents and skin changes in a larger percentage (50). It may make future mammographic interpretation more difficult. It precludes the later use of breast conservation with radiation therapy if the patient has a recurrence with invasive breast cancer. Finally, and perhaps most important, it may do harm.

A recent meta-analysis details the results of 40 prospective, randomized trials of radiation therapy for invasive breast cancer involving 19,582 patients (51). The trials were conducted between 1960 and 1990. There was a 3.7% breast cancer survival benefit for patients treated with radiation therapy, but there was a 2.5% increase in cardiovascu-

lar mortality associated with radiation therapy, leaving a net benefit of 1.2% (51,52). Current radiotherapy techniques probably have eliminated much of the excess cardiovascular mortality, but long-term data do not exist. Furthermore, two recent randomized trials have addressed the survival benefit from breast irradiation in favorable patients with invasive cancer. Both trials randomized patients to receive excision plus tamoxifen or excision plus tamoxifen plus radiation therapy. Hughes et al. (53) randomized 636 women 70 years of age and older with clinical stage 1 estrogen receptor–positive invasive breast cancer. There were more local recurrences in the excision plus tamoxifen group but no difference in survival between groups after 28 months of median follow-up. Similarly, Fyles et al. (54) randomized 769 women 50 years of age and older with T1N0 or T2N0. Once again there were more local recurrences in the excision plus tamoxifen group compared with the excision plus tamoxifen plus radiation therapy group, but there was no difference in survival between groups after 41 months of median follow-up.

No DCIS trials to date have shown any benefit in survival regardless of treatment. Now two trials for invasive breast cancer are yielding similar results: no benefit in survival regardless of treatment, albeit after relatively short follow-up. In light of this, I continue to be unwilling to recommend radiation therapy for all patients with DCIS who elect breast conservation. There is more to treatment than simply the control of local recurrence.

We have clearly shown throughout this book that there are subgroups of patients with DCIS who, after wide local excision, have a local recurrence rate so low that the addition of radiation therapy provides no significant benefit and is of no practical importance. The harm that it may cause clearly outweighs its potential benefit for these subsets. Why give a morbid treatment to all if there is no survival benefit overall and no local control benefit to identifiable subsets?

REFERENCES

1. Consensus Conference Committee. Consensus conference on the classification of ductal carcinoma in situ. *Cancer* 1997;80:1798–1802.
2. Solin L, Kurtz J, Fourquet A, et al. Fifteen-year results of breast-conserving surgery and definitive breast irradiation for the treatment of ductal carcinoma in situ of the breast. *J Clin Oncol* 1996;14:754–763.
3. Hiramatsu H, Bornstein B, Recht A, et al. Local recurrence after conservative surgery and radiation therapy for ductal carcinoma-in-situ: the possible importance of family history. *Cancer J Sci Am* 1995;1:55–61.
4. Fowble B, Hanlon AL, Fein DA, et al. Results of conservative surgery and radiation for mammographically detected ductal carcinoma *in situ* (DCIS). *Int J Radiat Oncol Biol Phys* 1997;38:949–957.
5. Vicini FA, Lacerna MD, Goldstein NS, et al. Ductal carcinoma in situ detected in the mammographic era: an analysis of clinical, pathologic, and treatment-related factors affecting outcome with

breast-conserving therapy. *Int J Radiat Oncol Biol Phys* 1997;39: 627–635.

6. Hillner BE, Desch CE, Carlson RW, et al. Trade-offs between survival and breast preservation for three initial treatments of ductal carcinoma-in-situ of the breast. *J Clin Oncol* 1996; 14:70–77.

7. Singer PA, Tasch ES, Stocking C, et al. Sex or survival: trade-offs between quality and quantity of life. *J Clin Oncol* 1991;9: 328–334.

8. McNeil BJ, Weichselbaum R, Pauker SG. Speech and survival: tradeoffs between quality and quantity of life in laryngeal cancer. *N Engl J Med* 1981;305:982–987.

9. Shapiro CL, Recht A. Side effects of adjuvant therapy for breast cancer. *N Engl J Med* 2001;344:1997–2008.

10. Whelan TJ, Levine MN, Gafni A, et al. Breast irradiation postlumpectomy: development and evaluation of a decision instrument. *J Clin Oncol* 1995;13:847–853.

11. Palda VA, Llewellyn-Thomas H, MacKenzie RG, et al. Breast cancer patients' willingness to wait for, and forgo, radiation therapy. *Breast Cancer Res Treat* 1994;32[Suppl]:45(abst).

12. Hayman JA, Fairclough DL, Harris JR, et al. Patient preferences concerning the trade-off between the risks and benefits of routine radiation therapy after conservative surgery for early-stage breast cancer. *J Clin Oncol* 1997;15:1252–1260.

13. Slevin ML, Stubbs L, Plant HJ, et al. Attitudes to chemotherapy: comparing views of patients with cancer with those of doctors, nurses, and general public. *BMJ* 1990;300:1458–1460.

14. McQuellon R, Muss H, Hoffman S, et al. The influence of toxicity on treatment preferences of women with breast cancer. *Proc Am Soc Clin Oncol* 1994;13:76(abst).

15. Bremnes RM, Andersen K, Wist EA. Cancer patients, doctors and nurses vary in their willingness to undertake cancer chemotherapy. *Eur J Cancer* 1995;31A:1955–1959.

16. Rajagopal S, Goodman PJ, Tannock IF. Adjuvant chemotherapy for breast cancer: discordance between physicians' perception of benefit and the results of clinical trials. *J Clin Oncol* 1994; 12:1296–1304.

17. Fisher B, Dignam J, Wolmark N, et al. Tamoxifen in treatment of intraductal breast cancer: National Surgical Adjuvant Breast and Bowel Project B-24 randomised controlled trial. *Lancet* 1999;353:1993–2000.

18. George WD, Houghton J, Cuzick J, et al. Radiotherapy and tamoxifen following complete local excision (CLE) in the management of ductal carcinoma in situ (DCIS): preliminary results from the UK DCIS trial. *Proc Am Soc Clin Oncol* 2000;19:70a(abst).

19. Chan KC, Knox WF, Sinha G, et al. Extent of excision margin width required in breast conserving surgery for ductal carcinoma in situ. *Cancer* 2001;91:9–16.

20. Dignam J, Fisher B. Occurrence of stroke with tamoxifen in NSABP B-24 [Letter]. *Lancet* 2000;355:848–849.

21. Fisher B, Constantino JP, Wickerham DL, et al. Tamoxifen for prevention of breast cancer: report of the National Surgical Adjuvant Breast and Bowel Project P-1 study. *J Natl Cancer Inst* 1998;90:1371–1378.

22. Winchester DP, Strom EA. Standards for diagnosis and management of ductal carcinoma in situ (DCIS) of the breast. *CA Cancer J Clin* 1998;48:108–128.

23. National Comprehensive Cancer Network. NCCN practice guidelines for breast cancer. *Oncology (Huntingt)* 2000;14 (11A):33–49.

24. Olivotto IA, Rose MA, Osteen RT, et al. Late cosmetic outcome after conservative surgery and radiotherapy: analysis of causes of cosmetic failure. *Int J Radiat Oncol Biol Phys* 1989;17:747–753.

25. Joseph E, Hyacinthe M, Lyman GH, et al. Evaluation of an intensive strategy for follow-up and surveillance of primary breast cancer. *Ann Surg Oncol* 1998;5:522–528.

26. Hunt KA, Rosen EL, Sickles EA. Outcome analysis for women undergoing annual versus biennial screening mammography: review of 24,211 examinations. *AJR Am J Roentgenol* 1999; 173:285–289.

27. Carlson KL, Helvie MA, Robidoux MA, et al. Relationship between mammographic screening intervals and size and histology of ductal carcinoma in situ. *AJR Am J Roentgenol* 1999;172: 313–317.

28. Kaas R, Hart AAM, Rutgers EJT, et al. Is annual mammography better to detect a contralateral breast cancer than mammography at a greater interval? *Eur J Cancer* 1998;34[Suppl 5]:S93(abst).

29. Blamey RW, Day N, Young R, et al. The UKCCCR trial of frequency of breast screening. *The Breast* 1999;8:215(abst).

30. Grunfeld E, Mant D, Yudkin P, et al. Routine follow up of breast cancer in primary care: randomized trial. *BMJ* 1996;313:665–669.

31. Earnshaw JJ, Stephenson Y. First two years of a follow-up breast clinic led by a nurse practitioner. *J R Soc Med* 1997;90:258–259.

32. Grunfeld E, Gray A, Mant D, et al. Follow-up of breast cancer in primary care vs specialist care: results of an economic evaluation. *Br J Cancer* 1999;79:1227–1233.

33. Consensus Committee. Image-detected breast cancer: State-of-the-art diagnosis and treatment. An international consensus conference. *J Am Coll Surg* 2001;193:297–302.

34. Silverstein MJ. Van Nuys Prognostic Index. In: Silverstein MJ, ed. *Ductal carcinoma in situ of the breast.* Baltimore: Williams & Wilkins, 1997:491–504.

35. Solin L, Recht A, Fourquet A, et al. Ten-year results of breast conserving surgery and definitive irradiation for intraductal carcinoma (ductal carcinoma in situ) of the breast. *Cancer* 1991; 68:2337–2344.

36. Bornstein BA, Recht A, Connolly JL, et al. Results of treating ductal carcinoma in situ of the breast with conservative surgery and radiation therapy. *Cancer* 1991;67:7–13.

37. Solin LJ, Yeh IT, Kurtz J, et al. Ductal carcinoma in situ (intraductal carcinoma) of the breast treated with breast-conserving surgery and definitive irradiation: correlation of pathologic parameters with outcome of treatment. *Cancer* 1993;71:1532–1542.

38. Fisher B, Land S, Mamounas E, et al. Prevention of invasive breast cancer in women with ductal carcinoma in situ: an update of the National Surgical Adjuvant Breast and Bowel Project Experience. *Semin Oncol* 2001;28:400–418.

39. Lagios MD, Margolin FR, Westdahl PR, et al. Mammographically detected duct carcinoma in situ. Frequency of local recurrences following tylectomy and prognostic effect of nuclear grade on local recurrence. *Cancer* 1989;63:619–624.

40. Fisher B, Constantino J, Redmond C, et al. Lumpectomy compared with lumpectomy and radiation therapy for the treatment of intraductal breast cancer. *N Engl J Med* 1993;328:1581–1586.

41. Fisher ER, Constantino J, Fisher B, et al. Pathologic finding from the National Surgical Adjuvant Breast Project (NSABP) protocol B-17: intraductal carcinoma (ductal carcinoma in situ). *Cancer* 1995;75:1310–1319.

42. Fisher B, Dignam J, Wolmark N, et al. Lumpectomy and radiation therapy for the treatment of intraductal breast cancer: findings from National Surgical Adjuvant Breast and Bowel Project B-17. *J Clin Oncol* 1998;16:441–452.

43. Fisher ER, Dignam J, Tan-Chiu E, et al. Pathologic findings from the National Surgical Adjuvant Breast Project (NSABP) eight-year update of protocol B-17: intraductal carcinoma. *Cancer* 1999;86:429–438.

44. Julien JP, Bijker N, Fentiman I, et al. Radiotherapy in breast conserving treatment for ductal carcinoma in situ: first results of EORTC randomized phase III trial 10853. *Lancet* 2000;355: 528–533.

45. Bijker N, Peterse JL, Duchateau L, et al. Risk factors for recurrence and metastasis after breast conserving therapy for ductal carcinoma in situ: analysis of European Organization for Research and Treatment of Cancer Trial 10853. *J Clin Oncol* 2001;19:2263–2271.
46. UKCCCR DCIS Working Party. The UK, Australian and New Zealand randomized trial comparing radiotherapy and tamoxifen in women with completely excised ductal carcinoma in situ of the breast (*submitted*).
47. Pocock SJ, Elbourne DR. Randomized trials or observational tabulations? *N Engl J Med* 2000;342:1907–1909.
48. Silverstein MJ, Lagios MD, Groshen S, et al. The influence of margin width on local control in patients with ductal carcinoma in situ (DCIS) of the breast. *N Engl J Med* 1999;340:1455.
49. Silverstein MJ, Lagios MD, Martino S, et al. Outcome after invasive local recurrence in patients with ductal carcinoma in situ of the breast. *J Clin Oncol* 1998;16:1367–1373

50. Recht A. Side effects of radiation therapy. In: Silverstein MJ, ed. *Ductal carcinoma in situ of the breast.* Baltimore: Williams & Wilkins, 1997:347–352.
51. Early Breast Cancer Trialists' Collaborative Group. Favorable and unfavorable effects on long-term survival of radiotherapy for early breast cancer. *Lancet* 2000;355:1757–1770.
52. Kurtz JM. Radiotherapy for early breast cancer: was a comprehensive overview of trials needed? *Lancet* 2000;355:1739–1740.
53. Hughes KS, Schnaper L, Berry D, et al. Comparison of lumpectomy plus tamoxifen with and without radiation therapy in women 70 rears of age and older who have clinical stage 1, estrogen receptor positive breast carcinoma. *Proc Am Soc Clin Oncol* 2001;20:24a(abst 93).
54. Fyles A, McCready D, Manchul L, et al. Preliminary results of a randomized study of tamoxifen plus or minus breast radiation in T1/2 N0 disease in women over 50 years of age. *Proc Am Soc Clin Oncol* 2001;20:24a(abst 92).

INDEX

Page numbers followed by "f" denote figures; those followed by "t" denote tables.

NSABP-17 experience, 436–437, 437t, 438f
NSABP-24 experience, 427, 428f, 438, 439t
survival impact of, 531–532
synchronous, incidence of, 531t
in tamoxifen trials, 505–506
benefit analysis, 509–510, 509t
in UK/ANZ trial, 453–455, 454t
Cooper's ligaments, intersection with mass, ultrasound evaluation of, 135–136, 136f–137f, 161f
Core needle biopsy
absolute sensitivity for, 323, 325, 327
calcification indications for, 114–115, 114f
consensus conferences (1997/1999) on, 596
for DCIS recurrence, 540–541
diagnostic limitations of, 566, 589
evolution of, 173, 174f
guidance modalities for, 174–178, 174f–177f
ultrasound as, 130–131, 137f, 152, 165, 179, 180f
of LCIS, as surgical excision indication, 629–630
pre-oncoplastic surgery, 187–189, 188f–189f
serial
Lagios experience, 303–304
from preexistent pathology, 14, 214–215
stereotactic. *See* Stereotactic core biopsy
tissue acquisition instruments for, 178–179, 180f–182f, 182–183
for treatment selection, 283
Coronary heart disease
hormone replacement therapy for, 503
risks of, 504
prevention strategies for, 497, 499, 501
Correlative studies
of contralateral breast tumors, 50, 365
French Regional Comprehensive Cancer Centers, 403–404, 404t
of ipsilateral breast tumors, 50, 589
special challenges in, 44, 49–50, 50t
Cosmetic outcomes, of surgery
clear tumor margins for, 470–471
example of poor, 189, 189f
partial-breast irradiation impact on, 407–408, 410–411
strategies for optimal. *See* Breast reconstruction; Oncoplastic surgery
Cost(s)
of adjuvant therapies, 208–209, 208t–209t
of axillary node dissection, 556, 558, 561, 568
of complete sequential tissue processing, 208, 208t
out-of-pocket, for prophylactic mastectomy, 534
Cost-benefit analysis
of complete sequential tissue processing, 208–209, 209t

of macrosection histology, 253–254
of radiation therapy, 461
with tamoxifen, 208–209, 208t–209t
Cotton bias wrap
post-biopsy, 188, 188f
post-segmentectomy, 196f
Counseling, for DCIS patients
of absolute risks
with breast-conservation therapy, 572–573, 572t–573t
with hormone replacement therapy, 574–575
with tamoxifen, 573–574, 574t
cautions with, 468
goals for, 571–572, 575
Cox model
of multivariate analysis
of local recurrence predictions, 256, 260, 261f, 363, 483f
in NSABP studies, 435
in Van Nuys Prognostic Index, 462, 463f
of recurrence based on margin width, 484
Cribriform DCIS
histologic appearance of, 17, 87, 89f
historical perspectives of, 5–6, 5f, 8–9
in male breasts, 578, 579t
mammographic appearances of, 106, 111f–112f
in Van Nuys classification, 222, 223f
Crushed stone-like calcifications, mammography findings of, 92, 94f–95f
in DCIS, 111, 113f
histologic correlations with, 88f, 102, 102f
Cryotherapy
for DCIS, 581–583
development of, 183
CST. *See* Complete sequential tissue processing (CST)
CTP. *See* Complete tissue processing (CTP)
Cuffing pattern, of angiogenesis, 236–238, 237f
Curvilinear lateral incision, for segmentectomy, 190–191, 194f–195f
Florence experience with, 351
Cyclin D1
as DCIS growth factor, 38
in DCIS vs. atypical hyperplasia, 637
Cyclin-dependent kinases, in DCIS proliferation, 38, 42
Cyclophosphamide, HER-2/*neu* gene overexpression response to, 55
Cyst(s)
carcinomatous, 5
fibrotic. *See* Fibrocystic disease
papillomatosis with, 149f, 152, 152f
Cytogenetic markers. *See* Chromosomes; Genetics
Cytokeratins
axillary node immunohistochemical staining for, 557, 560, 561–562, 568
prognostic significance of, 566–567
in Paget's disease diagnosis, 610, 610f

Cytokines, as DCIS growth factor, 43
Cytology
current applications of. *See* Histology
historical perspectives of, 3–5, 9–10

D

DCIS. *See* Ductal carcinoma in situ (DCIS)
DCIS-Mi. *See* Microinvasion in DCIS (DCIS-Mi)
Deep inferior epigastric perforator (DIEP) flap, for breast reconstruction, with mastectomy, 518–519
Deep venous thrombosis
from hormone replacement therapy, 504
from tamoxifen, 505
Depression, clinical, tamoxifen association with, 505
Desmoplakin, expression of, 42
Desmoplasia
microvessel density association with, 236
ultrasound evaluation of, 135–136, 136f
Desmosomes, 42
Detection and detection method. *See also* specific modality, e.g., Screening mammography
in EORTC 10853 trial, 448, 448t, 451t
recurrence correlation to
in international collaborative 15-year study, 362, 363t
Joint Center for Radiation experience, 375–376, 376t
as research focus, 12, 14
Diagnosis. *See also* Pathology; specific test, e.g., Biopsy(ies)
age at. *See* Age at diagnosis
controversial aspects of, 308–309, 320–321, 420–421, 421f, 474, 643
current trends in, 12–15, 13f, 308
EORTC consensus meetings on
1988 meeting, 587–588
1991 meeting, 588–589, 588t
1994 meeting, 589
1998 meeting, 589–590
exclusive nature of, 207
historical perspectives of, 3–4
standards for DCIS, 265–266, 295
Diagnostic mammography
DCIS features, 107–108, 107f–109f
exposure times for, 113
magnification importance with, 113–115, 114f
microfocus technique for, 97, 97f–99f, 101
in whole-organ studies, 244f, 245–246
Diagnostic reproducibility, of DCIS, 264–271
classification systems in, 70, 71f–72f, 264, 268
comparison of studies on, 269t–270t
conclusions about, 268, 270–271
EORTC consensus on, 589
pathology perspectives on, 264–271
problems with, 474–476, 478
statistical analysis of, 266–267, 267t
study limitations, 267–268
study methods, 264–266, 266t